Evidence-Based Practices in Behavioral Health

Series Editor

Nirbhay N. Singh, Medical College of Georgia, August University,
Augusta, ME, USA

This book series brings leading researchers and clinicians together to collaborate on books that present current research-based evidence for specific treatments across a broad range of subject areas. These books not only identify evidence-based practices, but also practice-based evidence. Furthermore, each book identifies the gaps in knowledge for future research. This series presents state-of-the-art knowledge in behavioral health, including but not limited to such disciplines as psychology, psychiatry, clinical social work, nursing, and rehabilitation therapies.

Gerald F. McKeegan

Behavior Change Interventions for Serious Mental Illness

Translating Research into Practice

Springer

Gerald F. McKeegan
Behavioryst Analytica
Conshohocken, PA, USA

ISSN 2366-6013 ISSN 2366-6021 (electronic)
Evidence-Based Practices in Behavioral Health
ISBN 978-3-032-18371-2 ISBN 978-3-032-18372-9 (eBook)
https://doi.org/10.1007/978-3-032-18372-9

This Springer imprint is published by the registered company Springer Nature Switzerland AG
The registered company address is: Gewerbestrasse 11, 6330 Cham, Switzerland

Preface

Serious mental illness has long held a contradictory position within human societies. Historically, the mentally ill have often been subjected to neglect, coercion, and abuse. From the asylums of the 16th through the 19th centuries to modern psychiatric institutions, individuals living with mental illness have often been placed in restrictive environments, subject to involuntary measures, and experienced reduced autonomy under practices justified as treatment or management. At various points in history, serious mental illness has been both feared and misunderstood, its origins often attributed to supernatural forces. Simultaneously, there has been recognition that individuals experiencing mental illness require help and support. Even within clinical settings, practices such as involuntary hospitalization, over-medication, and punitive interventions have raised ethical concerns. These abuses are not merely historical artifacts but reflect the enduring tensions between protection and paternalism, treatment and control. This duality is reflected in the way different cultures and eras have responded to those showing disturbances in thought, mood, or behavior.

Across cultures and throughout the centuries, responses to mental illness have ranged from reverence, where individuals were sometimes seen as possessing special insight or spiritual significance, to perceptions of vulnerability, leading to calls for compassionate assistance. However, these individuals have also been pathologized, subjected to institutionalization, victims of abuse, sterilized, and criminalized, depending on prevailing social attitudes and beliefs.

Presently, serious mental illness is acknowledged as a significant factor contributing to the global economic burden. Despite this recognition, stigma, marginalization, and systemic neglect remain persistent challenges for those affected by mental health conditions.

Consensus regarding the definition of mental illness continues to be elusive. For some, mental illness is primarily perceived as a societal label assigned to individuals exhibiting behaviors that differ from established social norms; this process of labeling may inadvertently exacerbate difficulties experienced by these individuals. Definitions of serious mental illness vary considerably across disciplines and conceptual frameworks. Typically, serious mental illness is characterized by disturbances in behavior, emotional regulation, or cognitive processes, and may also encompass impairments in interpersonal relationships and effective environmental interaction. Recurring patterns of maladaptive behavior are often interpreted as indicative of underlying psychological conditions. The etiology of such maladaptive presentations is explained through neurobiological or genetic paradigms, as well as models that consider conditioned or learned responses to environmental stressors. These diverse explanatory approaches augment traditional psychiatric classification and diagnostic systems, which have evolved since Kraepelin's foundational contributions.

The origins of mental illness are recognized as multifaceted and complex. Contemporary theoretical models emphasize the dynamic interaction among genetic predispositions, neurobiological dysregulation, developmental and environmental adversities, and psychosocial influences. Concepts such as the diathesis-stress model, advances in epigenetic research, and dimensional trait theories increasingly inform clinical understanding and guide intervention strategies. Historically, however, explanatory paradigms have been influenced not only by empirical research but also by prevailing ideological perspectives, including supernatural, moralistic, and reductionist biomedical viewpoints.

The impact of mental illness is profound and multidimensional. At the individual level, it can impair cognition, emotion regulation, interpersonal functioning, and occupational capacity. At the societal level, mental illness contributes to economic loss, strained healthcare systems, and social fragmentation. Perhaps most insidiously, it perpetuates cycles of exclusion, poverty, and discrimination, particularly for those with serious mental disorders such as schizophrenia, bipolar disorder, and severe personality pathology.

These differences in interpretation and viewpoints represent serious efforts to understand the patterns when problematic behaviors are perceived, resulting in distress for the individuals and others as well. How these problematic patterns of behavior, emotions, or thoughts are understood relate to the type of support and intervention offered to assist the person with attaining their goals and quality of life.

This book focuses on an analysis of these issues from the objective vantage point of behavior analysis and learning theory, emphasizing the impact of the environment on the ontogenesis and the amelioration of problematic behaviors that impede recovery. These constitute the understanding of both covert and overt behaviors as the outcome of past and present consequences and other environmental events. The problematic behaviors that are displayed by people living with serious mental illness are of diverse origins with the effects of environmental consequences as well as social and cultural influences upon diverse behaviors.

Central to contemporary efforts to address the challenges faced by individuals living with serious mental illness is the systematic assessment of the behaviors and symptoms that characterize the problematic behaviors linked to serious mental illness, including psychotic, mood, and severe personality disorders. Behavioral assessment provides a structured and objective lens through which clinicians and researchers can identify maladaptive patterns, functional impairments, and contextual triggers. When integrated with evidence-based behavioral principles, such as reinforcement, modeling, and skills training, these assessments inform targeted interventions that not only reduce problem behaviors but also promote adaptive functioning and psychosocial recovery.

The first five chapters present (1) an overview as to the definition of serious mental illness and the factors contributing to the definition; (2) the problematic behaviors and symptoms associated with serious mental illness; (3) the principles of applied behavior analysis and the application to problematic behaviors displayed by people living with serious mental illness; (4) discussions as to how to engage and collaborate with people living with serious mental illness in their recovery and the development of behavioral support strategies to alter challenging behaviors impeding their recovery; and (5) identifying ethical dilemmas that are common when supporting people with serious mental illness during their recovery. Examples of behavioral assessment tools are contained in the Appendices.

Chapters 6 through 18 present research findings and a dimensional analysis of problematic behaviors exhibited by individuals with serious mental illness. These chapters examine the typologies and contributing factors related to the development and persistence of such behaviors, explore their hypothesized origins, and review evidence-based behavioral support strategies for behavior modification. The final chapter addresses procedures for identifying and supporting individuals experiencing a mental health crisis and outlines relevant legal and regulatory considerations, including psychiatric hospitalization requirements, assent and consent to treatment, advanced psychiatric directives, and guardianship arrangements. This information is critical to ensuring comprehensive and successful service provision for individuals living with serious mental illness.

Conshohocken, PA, USA Gerald F. McKeegan

Acknowledgments

I want to acknowledge and thank the individuals living with serious mental illness who have shared their experiences, laughter, joy, and hope with me, especially rejoicing in the small but significant progress toward a more fulfilling life. They have been my most important teachers over the years, teaching me invaluable lessons during our conversations and life journey together. And for Debbie who has listened to my many meanderings and supported me while composing this text.

Competing Interests The author has no competing interests to declare that are relevant to the content of this manuscript.

Contents

Chapter 1
What Is Serious Mental Illness?

Introduction

Understanding serious mental illness (SMI) requires more than familiarity with diagnostic labels—it demands a nuanced grasp of the multidimensional nature of psychiatric symptoms, the limitations and evolution of classification systems, and the profound functional impairments that shape lived experience. While categorical frameworks such as the DSM-5-TR and ICD-11 offer structured criteria for identification and diagnosis of mental health problems, they often obscure the heterogeneity and complexity of individual presentations. A critical examination of the conceptual foundations and clinical realities of SMI is offered so as to move beyond static definitions to explore how symptom dimensions, insight deficits, trauma exposure, and substance use coalesce to influence prognosis, treatment engagement, and quality of life.

Historically rooted in Kraepelinian nosology, the classification of mental disorders has evolved toward increasingly behaviorally anchored systems. Yet, despite advances in reliability, categorical diagnoses frequently fail to capture the severity, chronicity, and functional impact that define SMI. Individuals with SMI often experience persistent impairments and challenges in adaptive functioning, social, occupational, self-care, and neurocognitive domains, compounded by anosognosia—a lack of awareness of illness—that undermines treatment adherence and recovery. Moreover, the intersection of SMI with trauma and substance use introduces additional layers of complexity, contributing to elevated rates of relapse, comorbidity, and involvement with the criminal justice system. These challenges underscore the need for dimensional, person-centered approaches that recognize variability in symptom expression and functional capacity.

Six interrelated domains central to the understanding of SMI are presented: (1) the dimensional nature of psychiatric symptoms, including positive, negative, and cognitive features; (2) the structure and limitations of contemporary classification

G. F. McKeegan, *Behavior Change Interventions for Serious Mental Illness*, Evidence-Based Practices in Behavioral Health,
https://doi.org/10.1007/978-3-032-18372-9_1

systems; (3) the scope and variability of functional impairments; (4) the clinical significance of insight deficits, particularly anosognosia; (5) the prevalence and impact of trauma across the lifespan; and (6) the role of substance use as both a co-occurring condition and a complicating factor in treatment. An in-depth analysis of the clinical, social, and systemic factors affecting individuals living with serious mental illness is presented and examines their significance for assessment, intervention strategies, and policy formulation.

Serious Mental Illness: History, Definitions, and Problematic Behaviors

At the end of the nineteenth century, Emil Kraepelin developed his classification system of mental health problems based on his observation of the individuals whom he was treating. The nosology that he developed divided the classification into exogenous and endogenous problems of mental health (Falkai et al., 2015). He differentiated exogenous conditions as caused by external factors such as lack of sleep, personal failures, and difficulties in relationships; in his view, the exogenous conditions responded to treatment and did not result in an insidious and life-long decline in the ability to function. Endogenous problems of mental health were the result of biological factors such as neurological insult, metabolic disorders, and/or genetics. Endogenous mental health problems often did not respond to treatment; the course of the condition was chronic and resulted in an individual not being able to function as an independent person in society. Kraepelin distinguished "manic depressive psychosis" as endogenous and dementia "dementia praecox" as endogenous; in the *Diagnostic and statistical manual of mental disorders* (DSM-V-TR) (American Psychiatric Association, 2022) these conditions presently are classified as bipolar and the schizophrenic spectrum mental health problems, respectively. According to Kraepelin, "dementia praecox" was characterized by a continuous and declining course in which the individual displayed behaviors that were not in touch with reality (such as delusions and hallucinations) but also worsening impairments in neurocognitions (i.e., attention, comprehension, abstract thinking, memory, executive functioning) and in adaptive functioning (i.e., interpersonal relationships, social skills, education, employment, self-care, and independent living skills).

With advances in mental health, practitioners and researchers realized that mental health problems are not unitary concepts but multidimensional (Helzer et al., 2008) although diagnostic systems are categorical. In the DSM-V-TR (American Psychiatric Association, 2022) and the *International Statistical Classification of Diseases and Related Health Problems*, 11th Edition (ICD-11) (World Health Organization, 2022), mental health conditions are defined by a set of observable behavioral criteria and specific rules regarding the number and patterns of criteria required to identify each condition. Individuals are assessed based on whether they meet the established criteria for a particular mental health condition (Keepers et al., 2020).

However, there are clinically significant individual differences among the persons living with a particular mental health condition (Halvorsen, 2016; Helzer et al., 2006, 2008). These differences may be in one category or across more than one. The difference may be in the ordinal number or frequency of a particular criterion or along a continuum of severity. Another dimension may be on a continuum on the person's ability to function in the various aspects of what is expected of an adult person who can function adaptively and independently. One person with the mental health problem of schizophrenia spectrum may hold a job, live independently, and have a social life; another person may live with her family, participate in a supportive work program, and attends a social clubhouse; and another may live in congregate housing with other persons with mental health conditions, rely on income from the government and does not want to participate in any social activities. In addition, responsiveness to rehabilitation interventions and rate of readmissions for inpatient mental health treatment differ as well among people with the same mental health problem.

Persons living with SMI differ in rates of relapses and readmissions to an inpatient psychiatric facility. Research has shown that relapses occur between 50% and 92% globally (Moges et al., 2021); factors associated with relapses are longer histories of living with SMI, poor premorbid adjustment, co-occurring substance use, stressful living conditions, and nonadherence to medications. During relapse, there is a rapid reemergence of psychotic symptoms to former intensity and magnitude; length of adherence to treatment does not affect the occurrence of relapse once the person discontinues treatment (Emsley et al., 2013; Machmutow et al., 2019; Moges et al., 2021; Porcelli et al., 2016).

Within the categories of mental health conditions, there have been attempts to develop subcategories (Jalensky, 2010). Crow (1980) proposed a subclassification of schizophrenia spectrum mental health problems based on the predominance of either positive or negative symptomatology. His classifications included two types. He characterized "Type 1" condition of schizophrenia spectrum by positive symptoms of psychosis such hallucinations, delusions, ideas of reference, paranoia and other first and second rank symptoms of a "formal thought disorder" (Suss & Parnas, 2017). Persons living with Type 1 responded well to available psychotropic medications, experienced fewer relapses, and had good premorbid functioning and fewer problems with adaptive functioning. People living with "Type 2" condition of schizophrenia spectrum displayed social withdrawal, loss of volition, affective flattening, poverty of speech, problems with being able to function independently, soft neurological signs, and neurocognitive impairments such as problems with memory and attention. People living with Type 2 also had minimal responsiveness to psychiatric medications and had more frequent and longer inpatient admissions. Research on the types of schizophrenia spectrum proposed was that none of the variables for the classifications have been definitively proven to possess the sensitivity and specificity expected of specific mental health problems. That is, people living with a schizophrenia spectrum condition display varied behaviors of differing severity, responsiveness to intervention and ability to function. In addition, mental health problems and symptoms are observed across many diagnostic categories; there is no symptom that is a necessary and sufficient condition to identify a particular mental health condition.

The most recent—and most utilized—attempt is the classification of severe or serious mental illness; the terms are interchangeable and depends on the organization using the label. However, "serious mental illness" is a broader term than "severe mental illness" and is usually defined by impairment, rather than by specific illnesses. The definition was first created by the Center for Mental Health Services in the 1990s for funding purposes to the states (Treatment Advocacy Center [TAC], n.d.).

While definitions may vary slightly by organization or locality, the National Institute of Mental Health (NIMH) defines serious mental illness as "a mental, behavioral, or emotional disorder resulting in serious functional impairment, which substantially interferes with or limits one or more major life activities" (TAC, n.d.). Therefore, serious mental illness is a broader term that includes a wider variety of psychiatric disorders but is commensurate with substantial impact on the lives of the individual living with SMI.

Serious mental illness also has been labeled as "serious and persistent mental illness" (SPMI); the term has been shortened to the word serious as having persistent symptoms for a longer duration and deficits in functioning would be redundant in that SMI has a significant impact on the individual living with SMI, their family, and society.

Presently, the definition of SMI refers to:

> ...a diagnosis of psychotic disorders, bipolar disorder, and either major depression with psychotic symptoms or treatment-resistant depression; SMI can also include anxiety disorders, eating disorders, and personality disorders, if the degree of functional impairment is severe. SMIs are long-term illnesses involving substantial functional impairment over multiple symptom domains. These impairments often lead to an inability to maintain gainful employment, poor social support, repeated psychiatric hospitalizations, homelessness, incarceration, and coexisting substance use disorders. (Evans et al., 2016, p. 7)

A person living with SMI must be identified as living with a DSM-V-TR mental health condition but, more importantly, has severe impairments in one or more socio-behavioral skills or expected social role performance (e.g., living independently, working, having friends, participating in leisure skills) that results in a disability. There is evidence that negative symptoms or functional behavioral and psychosocial deficits are correlated with higher rates of remission, poor real-life functioning, and lower quality of life indices. Studies have demonstrated that over 50% of people living with schizophrenia spectrum mental health problems have at least one negative symptom of moderate severity and 10–30% of individuals experienced two or more. Furthermore, between 50% and 90% of individuals determined to be living with a schizophrenic spectrum mental health problem show negative symptoms during their first hospital admission. Negative symptoms refer to a diminution or absence of normally expected behaviors related to motivation and interest (e.g., avolition, anhedonia, asociality) or expression (e.g., blunted affect, alogia) (Correll & Schooler, 2020).

An important and at times ignored aspect of SMI is that the duration of living with SMI is over two consecutive years (Ruggeri et al., 2000). People living with SMI account for the majority of people labeled as disabled (National Institute of Mental Health, n.d.; Ruggeri et al., 2000). A "disability" is defined as "a physical, mental, cognitive, or developmental condition that impairs, interferes with, or limits a person's ability to engage in certain tasks or actions or participate in typical daily activities and interactions" (Merriam-Webster On-line Dictionary, n.d.). By this definition a disability is a continuous impairment in the ability to function in daily life (Ustan & Kennedy, 2009); in the research in mental health, this concept has been labeled as "functional impairment," yet the description, frequency, and outcome of functional impairment is not well researched or defined (Mezzich & Ustun, 2002; Ustun, 2000). A person can display a deficit or failure in one area of social behavioral functioning to be classified as SMI and "disabled" if that deficit is severe and results in a chronic and limiting condition for that person. However, individuals living with SMI exhibit considerable variability in terms of disability; while some experience extensive deficits across multiple domains of social and behavioral functioning, others demonstrate minimal impairment.

Prevalence data show there were an estimated 14.1 million adults aged 18 or older in the United States living with SMI in 2021. People living with SMI account for over 5% of adults diagnosed with mental health problems in the United States (Terlizzi & Norris, 2021). The prevalence of SMI was higher among females (7%), young adults (aged 18–25 years) and among Native American adults (9.3%). From 2008 to 2019, there has been an increase in the percentage of adults who had been living with SMI, with increases from 3.7% (or 8.3 million people) to 5.2% (or 13.1 million people), with the largest increase being seen in young adults ages 18–25 years (Substance Abuse and Mental Health Services Administration [SAMHSA], 2020).

Besides impairments in social and daily functioning, people living with SMI have serious life consequences because of living with SMI. Research has shown that they have a lower life expectancy, greater incidents of substance use, physical and emotional trauma, being victims of violent crimes, and being arrested and incarcerated. Living with SMI decreases the person's life expectancy by 10–20 years. Although there is an increase in the cause of death because of suicide, it has been found that most of the years lost is attributable to physical health conditions which are similar in the general population. Individuals living with SMI have an increased likelihood of having a poor lifestyle, including lack of exercise, poor diet, and increased occurrence of smoking and obesity, resulting in increased rates of chronic somatic diseases leading to excess mortality rates. They seldom receive recommended medical treatment for their physical health conditions, which results in an increase in mortality. Efforts at providing lifestyle coaching to increase healthy living behaviors or coordination of care among providers has had a small impact on life expectancy among people living with SMI (de Mooij et al., 2019; Irurralde et al., 2021; Lomholt et al., 2019).

Adults living with SMI experience higher rates of trauma and the development of post-traumatic stress disorder (PTSD) than adults with either no or acute mental health problems (Mauritz et al., 2013). Rates of trauma experiences (e.g., experiencing or witnessing sexual or physical/verbal/emotional assaults, emotional and physical neglect) among individuals living with SMI range from 49% to 100% in some studies; trauma experiences include significant rates of both physical and sexual assault across the lifespan; childhood sexual abuse range from 13% to 64% and those who report childhood physical abuse range from 22% to 66%. In adulthood, individuals living with SMI report incidences of sexual assault ranging from 13% to 79% and 30% to 87% for physical assault. More than 25% of people living with SMI reported being a victim of violent crime in a 1-year period (Teplin et al., 2005). The annual rate of being a victim of a violent crime is four times the rate of the general population. Individuals living with SMI also suffer more repeated trauma experiences in a lifetime, including both trauma in adulthood and childhood.

Data also indicates that traumatic and harmful experiences, such as physical or sexual assaults, occur within inpatient psychiatric hospitals at an alarming rate. Trauma experiences in inpatient psychiatric settings include physical assault, sexual assault, and witnessing a trauma event (Teplin et al., 2005). Hospitalizations that include seclusion, restraint, administration of injectable medications, and police transport are frequently perceived as traumatic experiences. These events may result in reduced engagement with rehabilitation and recovery initiatives (Grubaugh et al., 2011).

Repeated exposure to traumatic events results in extreme stress that can lead to physical disorders (Monnat & Chandler, 2015) and exacerbations of the symptoms of SMI (Gibson et al., 2016). Results of studies have shown that psychosocial stressors such as exposure to trauma events and the resulting anxiety and other trauma-related symptoms (e.g., depression, thoughts of suicide, hypervigilance, flashbacks, and nightmares) can precipitate increases in symptoms or relapses in vulnerable individuals. There is recent evidence indicating that childhood abuse predicts severity of positive symptoms in adults, with greater overall number of types of trauma exposure increasing the probability of the development and severity of both positive and negative symptoms (Gibson et al., 2016; Loewy et al., 2019).

People with mental health problems are more likely to experience a substance use mental health problem than those not affected by a mental health problem (Flynn & Brown, 2008). Co-occurring conditions are defined as the coexistence of both a mental health problem and the determination of a substance use condition following the criteria in the DSM-5-TR (American Psychiatric Association, 2022). A co-occurring mental health condition includes the identification of a substance use problem and mental health condition. Criteria includes failed attempts to control the use of the substance, impairment in occupational and social functioning because of using the substance (e.g., family discord, decrease in leisure, and social activities), increased time thinking about obtaining and using the substance (i.e., craving), putting oneself at risk in obtaining and/or using the substance, increase in the use of the substance, and withdrawal symptoms if the person discontinues use of the substance (Hasin et al., 2013). Co-occurring problems involve the use of substances including benzodiazepines, sedative-hypnotics, opioids, stimulants, hallucinogens, nicotine, caffeine (if the person experiences withdrawal), cannabis, inhalants, and alcohol. The DSM-5-TR does not specifically identify any combination of mental health conditions and substance use issues as co-occurring mental health problems.

About 5.7% of individuals living with SMI have a co-occurring substance use problem. The largest group using substances are age 21–35, averaging about 11% of all individuals living with SMI in that age grouping (SAMHSA, 2021, 2024). Using either alcohol, drugs, or both range between a quarter to a third of samples in surveys conducted (RachBeisel et al., 1999; Virgio et al., 2001).

It is well established that the abuse of drugs and alcohol by people living with SMI is associated with many adverse impacts including increases in the severity of the symptoms associated with SMI, impairments in psychosocial functioning, decreases in adherence to treatment recommendations, the occurrence of disruptive behaviors, and higher rates of admissions to psychiatric facilities. People living with SMI and substance use are eight times more likely to discontinue treatment than a person living with SMI but not using substances. Living with SMI and co-occurring mental health problem led to increased health risks that are not only associated with use of substances (e.g., overdoses, anoxic events, head trauma, organ damage) but also the risk of sexually transmitted diseases. The presence of both SMI and a co-occurring mental health problem have been found to be associated with episodes of violence both in psychiatric wards and the community, increased hostility, negativity toward treatment and increased likelihood of contact with the legal system. The use of substances by a person living with SMI also puts the individual at greater risk for being traumatized by experiencing physical and sexual violence (RachBeisel et al., 1999).

Rates of substance dependency from national surveys show that rates were highly comparable across the surveys (Kessler & Zhao, 1999). Lifetime prevalence for alcohol use problem was 16.5% and 14.1% for the Epidemiological Catchment Area Program (ECA) and National Comorbidity Survey (NCS), respectively, with lifetime prevalence for drug use disorder being 6.1% for ECA and 7.5% NCS. Among individuals with drug use mental health condition (other than alcohol), rates of co-occurring mood and anxiety-related conditions were found to be 26% and 28%, respectively, while co-occurring psychotic thought disorders (i.e., schizophrenia spectrum mental health problems) was 7% and co-occurring antisocial personality problems was 18%. Regier et al. (1990) found that over half of individuals identified as having a drug use problem also presented with at least one additional mental health condition; however, the study did not differentiate between independent mental health disorders and those induced by substance use (Virgio et al., 2001).

Research has found that people living with SMI are overrepresented in the criminal justice system. Due to challenges in accurately assessing inmates' mental health and accounting for their environments, reliable estimates of how many people who live with SMI are incarcerated in jails or prisons remain uncertain. In addition, correctional settings do not have the resources or the inclination to participate in research studies. Results from studies have found that 6–31% of people in jails and 6–14% of people in prison are living with SMI (Prins, 2014). Results have shown that individuals living with SMI are re-incarcerated more quickly and frequently after their first encounter with the criminal justice system for reoffending, receiving minor charges, or not following through on demands after release such as meetings with probation officers, drug testing, and paying court costs (National Alliance on Mental Illness [NAMI], n.d.). Given the barriers that people living with SMI face including lifelong poverty, unemployment, victimization, family breakdown and discord, homelessness, substance use, general health problems, and stigma, contact with the criminal justice system can exacerbate social marginalization, disrupt treatment and linkages to service systems. Criminal behavioral activity is often linked to the untreated or worsening of symptoms of an individual living with SMI due to treatment nonadherence and/or discontinuation, use of substances, and the negative symptoms associated with neurocognitive disruptions, amotivation and lack of self-awareness in addition to the above-stated social factors (Wilson et al., 2020).

Failures in social-behavioral roles are seen by many as sine qua non for problems displayed by people living with SMI. For example, a person remaining in bed all day, not performing daily hygiene tasks, avoiding socializing with others and frequently smoking cigarettes and drinking coffee is viewed by others as "mentally ill" despite the absence of problematic behaviors or symptoms that are commonly associated with mental health problems such as hallucinations and delusions. Using the example above, the observed behaviors can be viewed not as abnormalities but as the absence of behaviors in the areas of leisure, social, self-control, and hygiene skills. Further assessment could be conducted with the goals of whether the absence of these behaviors is related to knowledge of the skills and when and where to perform the necessary behaviors. Spaulding et al. (2003) pointed out that using the word "deficit" does not connote an abnormality in which disruptions or disorganization in aspects of mental status prevent the person from performing in areas of psychosocial functioning; instead, such deficits are:

> predictable response to contingencies—a purposeful pursuit of a way of life, constrained by the environmental demands of institutions, cultural expectations, and stigma, and inability competed to perform key skills in support of alternative social roles. …. Behavioral failures can be understood as failures in people's repertoire of skills, and their ability to identify which skills are appropriate for which tasks, and the neurocognitive functions required to control performance of a particular scale or even in their ability to generate the degree of physiological arousal optimal for a particular task. (pp. 190–191)

The lack of certain behaviors displayed by people living with SMI can be a function of living and social environments where opportunities to engage in a variety of behaviors are limited by the impoverished conditions of many settings where people living with SMI reside (Chow & Priebe, 2013). Living in congregate living situations (e.g., hospitals, jails and prisons, group homes or adult care residences) limits the individuals' access to the outside world. In a study of psychiatric hospitals, Brown and Wing (1957) have found that the deficits noted in social and adaptive behaviors are associated with the social pressures from the institution, the length of time the person spends in these conditions, and the level of symptomatology displayed by the person living with SMI. Institutions are run on a strict routine schedule so that there are no disruptions in completing the daily tasks. Individuals are not given choices for basic daily activities such as what and when to eat, go to sleep, and what to wear. An individual may be dissuaded from acting independently or making requests to staff due to concerns about being reprimanded or labeled as a "demanding and problematic patient." For instance, some individuals living with SMI have reported that they began smoking while hospitalized because it provided the only opportunity to go outside for fresh air. They also observed that activities were limited; although the television was on throughout the day, it did not engage anyone, as programming was controlled by staff. A lack of independent behaviors, such as personal hygiene, dressing, toileting, and eating, in individuals experiencing SMI is frequently attributed to "amotivation," without further evaluation of the deficit. This approach often overlooks the environmental factors that may limit opportunities for these individuals to engage and be reinforced for manifesting independent activities and behaviors. In this setting, passivity is unintentionally encouraged, and individuals may find it in their best interest to refrain from exhibiting independence or self-motivation.

However, there is another view in the mental health literature that the absence of adaptive independent behavioral functioning is an aspect of SMI that is biologically determined. Behaviors observed in persons living with SMI have been categorized into two classes—"positive symptoms" and "negative symptoms." Positive symptoms are what behaviors are displayed by the person living with SMI—hallucinations, delusional speech, mood swings (or emotional dyscontrol), irritability, and aggression toward self and others. Negative symptoms are the absence of expected adaptive and independent behaviors—taking care of one's personal hygiene and physical health, pursuing leisure interests and activities, having friends, holding conversations, supporting oneself financially, and displaying emotions within expected norms (Correll & Schooler, 2020). Before the advent of the second-generation antipsychotic medications, it was hypothesized that the negative symptoms were the result of the side effects of the medications. Since the appearance and the wide use of the newer medications, the field of mental health has hypothesized that the deficits are biological as the negative symptoms are still problematic in people living with SMI. Studies have shown that 50–60% of people living with SMI have at least one negative symptom and between 10% and 30% have two or more negative symptoms. Negative symptoms have become an area on research and treatment because of the frequency of the occurrence in people living with SMI but also that there are strong relationships among low rates of remission (i.e., temporary improvement), poor life functioning, quality of life, and of perceptions of "burdensomeness" among caretakers, service providers and health care systems (Galderisi et al., 2021). The concept of a "deficit syndrome" has been introduced by Carpenter et al. (1988) to account for the wide range of negative symptoms. The deficit syndrome includes restricted affect, diminished emotional range, poverty of speech, curbing of interests, diminished sense of purpose, and diminished social drive. The deficits must be present during periods of clinical stability for a year and are not due to other mental health problems such as anxiety or depression. It was hypothesized that the deficit syndrome is a separate mental health entity and not just a more severe form of SMI and needs to be researched and treated separately. It was soon noted that the heterogeneity of the deficits compounded the difficulties of research and treatment (Galderisi et al., 2021).

Researchers suggested that the negative symptom of anosognosia is a significant factor in individuals living with SMI due to its persistent nature, severity, and influence on outcomes. As stated previously, negative symptoms are resistant to many efforts of treatment despite the advance in psychopharmacological and other biological interventions (Lutgens et al., 2017; Muyambi et al., 2023). A persistent and significant negative symptom observed in individuals living with SMIs is commonly described as a "lack of insight." This term denotes an individual's compromised capacity to recognize or comprehend their own condition. It is more than a denial of problems but a lack of self-awareness that the behaviors the person living with SMI is displaying—or not displaying—is problematic for themselves and others in their social environment. It is considered to be the most common reason for not seeking or maintaining treatment for people with SMI (Lutgens et al., 2017; Muyambi et al., 2023).

The lack of self-awareness is multidimensional—is the individual living with SMI lacking self-awareness in certain areas (e.g., need for treatment, acknowledging living with a SMI) or is the lack of self-awareness all encompassing? The degree of self-awareness can vary widely in terms of its severity. Impaired insight is observed not only among individuals living with SMI, but also among those without diagnosed mental health conditions (Markova & Berrios, 2011). For example, a person may live alone, seldom socialize, and states that he has many friends on social media sites but has never physically met the people. This same person may hold a job, have good relationships with co-workers and supervisors and go to an online college. The person in the example may have a deficit in his awareness of his social life but this aspect of his awareness is not burdensome to either himself or others. An example of a profound lack of self-awareness is a person living with SMI who denies that she is hearing voices as she is mumbling and responding to the auditory hallucinations.

Some researchers in mental health have compared the lack of insight or self-awareness as similar to a neurological symptom of "anosognosia." This lack of self-awareness is prevalent in in persons after suffering a confirmed neurological event or insult such as a traumatic or closed head injury, stroke, brain tumor, or a dementing condition such as Alzheimer's disease. Due to the parallels with impaired insight observed in individuals with SMI, it is postulated that diminished insight may result from anatomical brain damage, as demonstrated in cases of anosognosia (Acharya & Sánchez-Manso, 2023; TAC, n.d.). Neurological scans of individuals who are living with SMI and experiencing significant lack of awareness of the problem behaviors associated with living SMI do not reveal the distinct neurological abnormalities observed in confirmed cases of anosognosia following neurological injury (Acharya & Sánchez-Manso, 2023).

The presence of negative symptoms—or deficits in functioning—in people living with SMI results in poor outcomes and indicators of quality of life (QoL). In a review of available interventions for negative symptoms, Lutgens et al. (2017) concluded that most effects were "modest with high level of heterogeneity" (p. 324) and more research is needed for exploring interventions for ameliorating the impact of the behavioral deficits associated with negative symptoms.

As noted by others, there is a significant amount of heterogeneity in defining as to what constitutes impairments in adaptive functioning. Carpenter et al. (1988) defined deficit syndrome as compromising six domains including:

1. Restricted affect as shown by lack of facial expression, lack of verbal modulation, and gestures.
2. Diminished emotional range as shown by a reduction in the person's expressed range of emotional experiences.
3. Poverty of speech is observed by a reduced number of words used and information conveyed.
4. Curbing of interests as shown by the expressed interest shown by the person of the degree of what is occurring in the world and their environment.
5. Diminished sense of purpose as assessed by the person being able to make and pursue goals and participate in activities that are goal directed and not aimless or being inactive.
6. Diminished social drive is observed by the frequency to which the person seeks out or attempts social interactions.

   For the determination of "deficit syndrome," these symptoms—or lack of behaviors—must be present for at least 12 months (Carpenter et al., 1988).

However other researchers suggested other behavioral domains resulting in confusion as to definition of the targeted behaviors. NIMH published a review and census of the research on negative symptoms and proposed the following constructs be used when investigating and treating negative symptoms (Kirkpatrick et al., 2006). The consensus identified five main domains of negative symptoms:

1. Avolition refers to a reduction in the initiation and persistence of goal-directed activities due to a lack of motivation.
2. Anhedonia is defined as a reduction in participating in pleasurable activities. Subtypes include "consummatory anhedonia" that occurs during the activity and "anticipatory anhedonia" which is an inability to look forward to a pleasurable activity.
3. Asociality is a reduction of interacting with others due to a decrease in the drive to form and maintain relationships with others.
4. Blunted affect is a reduction of emotional expression verbally and nonverbally (also known as flat affect).
5. Alogia is a reduction in quantity of words spoken and the amount of spontaneous speech during an interaction.

For a person living with SMI to be identified as living with negative symptoms, it was recommended that the person had to exhibit at least three or more symptoms of "moderate severity" or two symptoms of being "moderately severe" as assessed on an objective measure such as the Positive and Negative Symptoms Scale (PANSS) (Kay et al., 1987) or other validated and reliable scales. In addition, the symptoms had to persist for at least 6 months and were not the result of a co-occurring depressive mental health problem or side-effects from prescribed medications.

There is a great deal of overlap in these areas both within and between the different domains. There also appears to be a lack of specificity as to the definition. It is unsure if blunted affect is not the result of a diminution in the pursuits of pleasurable activities. Is the negative symptom of diminished social interaction a function of not being motivated to engage in communication with others or is the targeted social avoidance aspects due to a lack of motivation or alogia (e.g., poverty of speech)? One can question if the negative symptoms are a function of the deficits that one finds in environments in which individuals living with SMI reside. As stated previously, negative symptoms may be a function of the impoverished environments in which the person living with SMI finds himself.

It is noticeable that the available scales for negative symptoms do not assess the presence or severity of anosognosia or lack of self-awareness (e.g., insight as to one's mental health). A web-based search of any valid and reliable instruments used for assessing deficits in self-awareness or anosognosia has shown that the scales being used were developed and being utilized in assessing individuals living with known neurological insults or disease such as Alzheimer's and other dementing conditions (de Ruijter et al., 2020). At present there is no objective scale to assess this problem in mental health conditions.

Spaulding et al. (2003) suggest a comprehensive view of impairments in adaptive functioning. They analyze each domain into components areas that can then be assessed by observable behaviors. Assessments in these areas need to be systematic and well defined as each domain may have multiple components; it is important to assess each of the components and the impact each component has on other areas of deficit. With assessment, interventions can be developed that target each component of the domain. There also is a need for a definition of the impairment being "clinically significant." Does clinical significance occur statistically when the change score is below a certain threshold or is there a range of change scores indicating clinical significance? What is the operational definition when a lack of a certain adaptive independent behavior becomes clinically significant?

Spaulding et al. (2003) also postulated that each problem area in functioning needs to be evaluated as to the impairment being a function of knowledge or performance. For example, an individual may know how to brush her teeth, but she seldom does the behavior. Both impairments in knowledge and performance have various aspects of intervention and target behaviors. Since the individual knows how to brush her teeth, her lack of performance is related to different variables and functions for not displaying the behavior, such as not having ready access to supplies or the bathroom, lack of privacy, and the time of day that she would like to brush her teeth. An example would be if an individual living with SMI was refusing to take a shower. After a very brief assessment, the results showed that he had always taken a bath in his younger years. He stated that he liked bathing instead of showering. An easy change in scheduling for him to take a bath resolved the "deficit."

Areas of Social Functioning

Spaulding et al. (2003) have specified skill deficits that are defined and each component behavior can be directly observed and assessed as to whether the impairment is a problem in knowing how to accomplish the assessed behavior, a problem in performing the component adequately, or a combination of both.

The impairments in skills that Spaulding et al. (2003) have recommended to be targeted for interventions are as follows:

1. Self-care impairments: Behaviors related to personal care, grooming, hygiene, nutrition, and health-related behaviors (e.g., refusing to bathe or shower and changing clothes).
2. Leisure recreational skills: Behaviors displayed by planning and participating in leisure time activities (e.g., watching TV all day and refusing to go for a walk).
3. Independent living skills: Behaviors displayed when keeping a routine for behaviors associated with adult living including housekeeping, laundry, cooking, shopping, budgeting finances to purchase what is needed or desired, and transportation (e.g., not using washer and dryer to wash clothes routinely).
4. Disorder management impairment: Behaviors displayed by the management of symptoms and problem behaviors of living with SMI including knowing and understanding the presence of symptoms, the warning signs of relapses, understanding the function of psychiatric medications, and the awareness and management of stress-related situations that can lead to relapse and worsening of symptoms (e.g., missing doses on medications, not being to differentiate episodes on energized and manic behavior).
5. Occupational skills impairments: Behaviors displayed in work-related activities such as getting to work timely, regulating boredom, pacing, following instructions, problem-solving, asking questions in novel situations, and developing and maintaining work relationships. These behaviors can be displayed in settings such volunteering or being a member of a clubhouse (e.g., using skills when bored with task instead of leaving work or hiding in bathroom).
6. Interpersonal skills impairments: Behaviors displayed during interpersonal interactions such as having conversations, expressing needs to others, making requests, identifying and resolving day-to-day conflicts, and establishing and maintaining mutually reinforcing relationships (e.g., friendships) (e.g., ability to hold a rational reciprocal conversation with another person).
7. Physiological dysregulations: Behaviors displayed during situations requiring self-control, the self-regulation of aversive emotional states and displaying adaptive alternative behavioral responses in stressful situations (e.g., skills related to stress management such as mindfulness, deep breathing, walking away).
8. Dysregulation of behavioral activation: Behaviors displayed during disruption in cycles of behavioral activity (i.e., rest or sleep difficulties) and adhering to a daily routine of necessary activities (e.g., sleeping too much or too little).

9. Dysregulation of mood: Behaviors displayed during episodes in alterations of mood and behavior (such as during episodes of dysthymia, major depression, hypomania, mania, and agitation due to paranoia) and when anger and hostility is persistent (e.g., staying away from others and not going to rehabilitation program when depressed).
10. Dysregulation of anger and aggression: Behaviors displayed during episodes of dysregulation associated with extreme explosive and or socially unacceptable anger and/or aggression (e.g., threatening or hitting others when frustrated, angry).
11. Dysregulation of fear and anxiety: Behaviors displayed during frequent episodes of intense psychophysiological and abnormal arousal resulting in behavioral avoidance of the anxiety producing situation (e.g., avoiding crowded social situations, sitting in corner with back to wall in social gatherings).
12. Dysregulation of appetitive behavior: Behaviors displayed that are associated with hunger and thirst that may be influenced by medication side effects, medical conditions, neurocognitive impairments, dysfunctional beliefs, deficient social problem-solving, and social-environmental situations. These behaviors may inlcude eating or drinking too much or too little or consuming excessive ammounts of caffeinated beverages.
13. Dysregulation of sexual behavior: Behaviors displayed in aspects of sexual functioning including an absence of appropriate sexual interests or hypersexuality (e.g., making sexualized statements to unfamiliar other persons; having sexual fetishes).
14. Rehabilitation adherence: Behaviors displayed in the participation of interventions and treatment for SMI as well as collaborating with service professionals in tailoring rehabilitation and recovery to the subjective experiences and/or expressed desires of the person living with SMI (e.g., participating in social clubhouse program, actively participating in group therapy).
15. Socialized psychiatric symptoms: Behaviors displayed as a function of social and/or tangible reinforcement to support the behaviors of the social role of an individual living with SMI (e.g., engaging in delusional speech during an evaluation for disability income).
16. Socially unacceptable behavior: Behaviors displayed that are not accepted and tolerated in normal social environments (e.g., taking coffee from convenience store and not paying, urinating in public).
17. Social environmental conflict: Behaviors displayed in situations of conflict between a person living with SMI and others in the individual's social environment (e.g., frequently asking others for cigarettes and coffee (may also be a problem in "socially unacceptable behaviors").
18. Restrictive legal status: Behaviors displayed as to the legal involvement of the person living with SMI such as probationary meetings, drug tests, restrictions from other people (such as family members).
19. Unstable living situations: Behaviors displayed during situations when the person living with SMI is removed from a residence, chooses to leave the residence, or is readmitted to a psychiatric facility and loses placement.

The above list of problems—impairments and dysregulations of behaviors—is extensive and can be seen that there is overlap among the categories. Each domain outlined represents a behavioral category of responses contributing to an identified impairment in adaptive functioning. Within each domain, multiple response classes are associated with behavioral impairments. For instance, challenges in personal hygiene encompass such response classes as bathing, showering, appropriate use of shampoo and soap during these activities, changing clothing, and correctly brushing teeth, among others.

Assessment of each behavioral problem or impairment can ascertain the behavioral response of a particular behavior. However, assessment of the behavior can determine if the behavior is a function or the result of another problematic area. For example, if an individual has few interactions with others, the assessment needs to determine if the lack of social interactions is due to social anxiety (i.e., is the individual worried about being evaluated by the other person when speaking, concerned about not having anything to talk about), problems with hearing, speaking clearly, or not understanding the language being spoken. The observed deficit in social interactions may be a function of avoiding others as the person living with SMI may be experiencing demeaning auditory hallucinations or paranoid beliefs that result in an increase in anger and aggression toward the other person with whom they are interacting. Spaulding et al. (2003) relate this to other problems in socio-cognitive functioning (i.e., positive symptoms of SMI) or neurocognitive impairments (i.e., problems with memory and attention).

Neurocognitive impairments and positive symptoms of SMI can contribute to any of the behavioral problems as outlined above. It is particularly important in the amelioration of the problem if the person has neurocognitive impairments or problems in the self-management of positive symptoms. If an individual living with SMI has difficulty in focusing, attending, and comprehending what is being told to her, then any implementation of a support plan or intervention will be impeded by the assessed neurocognitive impairments. If the person has delusions that she is being persecuted because she is the mother of a political figure, then attempts of that person complying with any intervention might be impaired given her belief that she is being persecuted. Neurocognitive impairments and problems in the self-management of positive symptoms of SMI should be addressed in any comprehensive plan of rehabilitation.

Given the above view of socio-behavioral challenges defining core aspects of SMI, these behaviors—or the absence of these behaviors—need to be addressed during rehabilitation and recovery efforts with the person living with SMI. Pharmacological interventions are, at most, moderately effective for treating negative symptoms and behavioral issues in SMI. In the clinical and scientific literature, "treatment resistant" usually means that the individual living with SMI does not have a maximal beneficial response to antipsychotic medications (Spaulding et al., 2008). The result is that the individual still experiences positive symptoms with no or slight change from baseline. In addition, people living with SMI frequently use substances that interfere with psychiatric medications; people living with SMI discontinue medications because of difficulties in socio-behavioral and neurocognitive behaviors (i.e., forgetting or refusing to take medications, lack of awareness of mental health problems, self-management of mental health problems). The result is that persons living with SMI chronically display many positive symptoms as well as complications in adaptive functioning, resulting in frequent hospitalizations, disruptions in care, interpersonal and family relationships, and unstable housing.

Despite the impediments of supporting a person living with SMI in their rehabilitation and recovery efforts, the behaviors associated with SMI—both positive symptoms and compromised socio-behavioral responses—can be managed using behavior analytic interventions. Effective interventions to improve social and adaptive functioning have been developed and implemented using behavioral principles of role modeling, prompting, shaping and reinforcement (Bellack, 2004; del Carmen Valiente, 1993; Liberman et al., 2001). Behavior analytic techniques have been used to effectively increase other adaptive behaviors in persons living with SMI (Bellus et al., 1999; Paul et al., 1997). Positive symptoms such as responding to hallucinations and talking about delusions were decreased using interventions based on behavior analytic principles (Layng & Andronis, 1984; Liberman et al., 1973). Social skills training is effective in reducing the observed problems in reacting to others. The use of contingency management interventions such as token economies and behavioral contracting has demonstrated improvement in area of adaptive functioning including self-management of symptoms.

The result is that the approach to treatment for people with mental health problems needs to be individualized and based on the needs and goals of the person living with a mental health problem (Spaulding et al., 2003). In assessing what changes in functioning are needed for each person living with SMI, interventions can be developed and implemented using the technology of behavior change. The person living with SMI can be empowered to become their own "agent of change" with support from other knowledgeable service providers. Each person can be assisted in developing a structure to support their efforts by using skills taught using instruction, modeling, prompting, and reinforcement. The goal is that when the adaptive behaviors are displayed the natural reinforcing contingencies will support the occurrence of the adaptive behavior and assist the person living with SMI in attaining their individual goals.

Summary

Researchers and practitioners in the identification and treatment of mental health problems have been aware that mental health problems are not unitary concepts and differ in certain dimensions. Kraepelin, the father of the classification system used in the identification of mental health conditions, was aware of the dimensions in his differentiation between conditions that he classified as exogenous or endogenous. The differentiation was based on dimensions as to the course of the condition, ability to adaptively function and responsiveness to treatment, including medications.

These dimensions were expanded to include the age when the behaviors of mental health problems appeared (i.e., age of onset), the functioning of the individual before the onset of the symptoms (i.e., premorbid) and assessed impairments in neurocognitive functioning. Individuals showing symptoms like hallucinations, delusions, mood swings, and poor adaptive functioning are considered to have severe and persistent mental illness (SPMI). These chronic positive and negative symptoms hinder independent adult functioning and generally do not improve with medication or current psychotherapy methods. Many of the people labeled as SPMI were diagnosed with some form of schizophrenia spectrum mental health and psychosis-related problems.

The label of SPMI has changed to either "serious mental illness" or "severe mental illness" (SMI). The mental health field realized that persons having nonpsychotic challenges such as depressive and anxiety-related problems, eating and personality-related mental health problems had chronic mental health conditions that did not respond to treatment; behavior and lack of behaviors displayed by individuals living with SMI interfered with basic abilities to function adaptively and at times, resulted in devastating consequences because of the inability to function, self-control, and self-manage.

Living with SMI has been shown to be associated with early mortality, frequent over-use of substances (including nicotine, caffeine, prescribed medications, and street drugs), reliance on disability income, legal involvement, unstable housing, and repeated trauma experiences, both as children and adults. The aspects of the problems in adaptive functioning differ according to the focus of the research. The amount and the labels given to the impairments vary; the identified challenges include the behavioral response classes of activities of daily living, social, employment, and leisure activity skills, being able to express and show emotions as expected by others, lack of enjoyment in reinforcing activities, and lack of motivation to change or engage in the expected behaviors, and problems with eating, sleeping, and sexual behaviors.

Hypotheses about the cause of the observed compromises in adaptive behaviors also differ. Biologically oriented service providers and researchers view the challenges as symptoms of a underlying neurological impairment with a genetic origin; socio-behavioral researchers view the behavioral difficulties as a function of the individual who is living with SMI having been deprived of necessary learning experiences, appropriate role modeling and social reinforcement, and living in impoverished and traumatic and punitive environments that result in the absence of expected behaviors.

A serious problem area is that the individual living with SMI often do not participate in treatment, rehabilitation, and recovery efforts; the challenges in participating in rehabilitation is cited as the reason for discontinuation of treatment by providers. The reason for this lack of involvement in treatment has been hypothesized as a function of the lack of awareness of the illness. The lack of self-awareness (or lack of insight) has been related to a neurological disorder, anosognosia, in which the individual is unaware of any problems or complication in their abilities after a traumatic neurological event. Others have hypothesized that the lack of insight may be related to social-environmental problems that the person has and is experiencing living with SMI.

The absence of considering the goals and desires of person living with SMI in the forefront of rehabilitation efforts, stigma, discrimination and marginalization, and lack of advocacy by others can result in the individual living with SMI to discontinue treatment to "escape" the daily reminders (e.g., going to appointments, social clubhouses, living in group homes, taking medications) of being a person living with SMI.

Lack of engagement in treatment may be related to the individual's concerns about treatment that is not considered by providers who have paternalistic attitudes and perceptions of the person living with SMI. Stigma of being labeled as SMI may result in the individual avoiding treatment to not be labeled and suffering the sociocultural consequences of the stigma of living with SMI.

Despite the negative perceptions supported by others, individuals living with SMI do recover and are able to function as in an adult role in society—being employed, attaining educational goals, living independently, and having friends. Research has demonstrated that evidence-based treatment can assist the person living with SMI manage the positive symptoms and acquire the skills in areas of challenges in social and adaptive functioning.

References

Acharya, A. B., & Sánchez-Manso, J. C. (2023). Anosognosia. In *StatPearls [Internet]*. StatPearls Publishing. https://www.ncbi.nlm.nih.gov/books/NBK513361/

American Psychiatric Association. (2022). *Diagnostic and statistical manual of mental disorders* (5th ed., text revision). https://doi.org/10.1176/appi.books.9780890425787

Bellack, A. S. (2004). Skills training for people with severe mental illness. *Psychiatric Rehabilitation Journal, 27*(4), 375–391. https://doi.org/10.2975/27.2004.375.391

Bellus, S. B., Vergo, J. G., Kost, P. P., Stewart, D., & Barkstrom, S. R. (1999). Behavioral rehabilitation and the reduction of aggressive and self-injurious behaviors with cognitively impaired, chronic psychiatric inpatients. *Psychiatric Quarterly, 70*(1), 27–37. https://doi.org/10.1023/A:1022075007384

Brown, G. W., & Wing, J. K. (1957). A comparative clinical and social survey of three mental hospitals. *The Sociological Review, 5*(1 Suppl), 145–171. https://doi.org/10.1111/j.1467-954X.1957.tb03571.x)

Buchanan, R. W. (2007). Persistent negative symptoms in schizophrenia: An overview. *Schizophrenia Bulletin, 33*(4), 1013–1022. https://doi.org/10.1093/schbul/sbl057

Carpenter, W. T., Heinrichs, D. W., & Wagman, A. M. (1988). Deficit and nondeficit forms of schizophrenia: The concept. *American Journal of Psychiatry, 145*(5), 578–583. https://doi.org/10.1176/ajp.145.5.578

Chow, W. S., & Priebe, S. (2013). Understanding psychiatric institutionalization: A conceptual review. *BMC Psychiatry, 13*(169), 1–14. https://doi.org/10.1186/1471-244X-13-169

Correll, C. U., & Schooler, N. R. (2020). Negative symptoms in schizophrenia: A review and clinical guide for recognition, assessment, and treatment. *Neuropsychiatric Disease and Treatment, 16*, 519–534. https://doi.org/10.2147/NDT.S225643

Crow, T. J. (1980). Molecular pathology of schizophrenia: More than one disease process? *British Medical Journal, 280*(6207), 66–68. https://doi.org/10.1136/bmj.280.6207.66

de Mooij, L. D., Kikkert, M., Theunissen, J., Beekman, A. T. F., de Haan, L., Duurkoop, P. W. R. A., van, H. L., & Dekker, J. J. M. (2019). Dying too soon: Excess mortality in severe mental illness. *Frontiers in Psychiatry, 10*, Article 855, 1–10. https://doi.org/10.3389/fpsyt.2019.00855

de Ruijter, N. S., Schoonbrood, M. G. A., van Twillert, B., & Hoff, E. I. (2020). Anosognosia in dementia: A review of current assessment instruments. *Alzheimer's & Dementia: Diagnosis, Assessment & Disease Monitoring, 12*, 1–5. https://doi.org/10.1002/dad2.12079

del Carmen Valiente, M. (1993). *Assessment of adherence of a social skills training intervention for serious mental illnesses*. (Doctoral dissertation, University of Arizona). University of Arizona Campus Repository. https://repository.arizona.edu/handle/10150/186141

Emsley, R., Chiliza, B., Asmal, L., & Harvey, B. H. (2013). The nature of relapse in schizophrenia. *BMC Psychiatry, 13*, Article 50. https://doi.org/10.1186/1471-244X-13-50

Emsley, R., Oosthuizen, P. P., Koen, L., Niehaus, D. J., & Martinez, G. (2012). Symptom recurrence following intermittent treatment in first-episode schizophrenia successfully treated for 2 years: A 3-year open-label clinical study. *Journal of Clinical Psychiatry, 73*(4), e541–e547. https://doi.org/10.4088/JCP.11m07061

Evans, T. S., Berkman, N., Brown, C., Gaynes, C. B., & Weber, R. P. (2016). *Disparities within serious mental illness* (Technical Briefs, No. 25.) Agency for Healthcare Research and Quality. https://www.ncbi.nlm.nih.gov/books/NBK368427/

Falkai, P., Rossner, M., Schulze, T., Hasan, A., Brzozka, M. M., Malchow, B., Honer, W. G., & Schmitt, A. (2015). Kraepelin revisited: Schizophrenia from degeneration to failed regeneration. *Molecular Psychiatry, 20*, 671–676. https://doi.org/10.1038/mp.2015.35

Flynn, P. M., & Brown, B. S. (2008). Co-occurring disorders in substance abuse treatment: Issues and prospects. *Journal of Substance Abuse Treatment, 34*(1), 36–47. https://doi.org/10.1016/j.jsat.2006.11.013

Galderisi, S., Mucci, A., Dollfus, S., Nordentoft, M., Falkai, P., Kaiser, S., Giordano, G. M., Vandevelde, A., Nielsen, M. Ø., Glenthøj, L. B., Sabé, M., Pezzella, P., Bitter, I., & Gaebel, W. (2021). EPA guidance on assessment of negative symptoms in schizophrenia. *European Psychiatry, 64*(1), Article e23. https://doi.org/10.1192/j.eurpsy.2021.11

Gibson, L. E., Alloy, L. B., & Ellman, L. M. (2016). Trauma and the psychosis spectrum: A review of symptom specificity and explanatory mechanisms. *Clinical Psychology Review, 49*, 92–105. https://doi.org/10.1016/j.cpr.2016.08.003

Grubaugh, A. L., Zinzow, H. M., Paul, L., Egede, L. E., & Frueh, B. C. (2011). Trauma exposure and posttraumatic stress disorder in adults with severe mental illness: A critical review. *Clinical Psychology Review, 31*(6), 883–899. https://doi.org/10.1016/j.cpr.2011.04.001

Halvorsen, J. O. (2016). Defining clinically significant change. *The British Journal of Psychiatry, 209*(1), 85. https://doi.org/10.1192/bjp.209.1.85

Hasin, D. S., O'Brien, C. P., Auriacombe, M., Borges, G., Bucholz, K., Budney, A., Compton, W. M., Crowley, T., Ling, W., Petry, N. M., Schuckit, M., & Grant, B. F. (2013). DSM-5 criteria for substance use disorders: Recommendations and rationale. *American Journal of Psychiatry, 170*(8), 834–851. https://doi.org/10.1176/appi.ajp.2013.12060782

Helzer, J. E., Kraemer, H. C., & Krueger, R. F. (2006). The feasibility and need for dimensional psychiatric diagnoses. *Psychological Medicine, 36*(12), 1671–1680. https://doi.org/10.1017/S003329170600821X

Helzer, J. E., Kraemer, H. C., Krueger, R. F., Wittchen, H.-U., Sirovatka, P. J., & Regier, D. A. (Eds.). (2008). *Dimensional approaches in diagnostic classification: Refining the research agenda for DSM-V*. American Psychiatric Association. https://doi.org/10.1176/appi.books.9780890428320

International Classification of Diseases, Eleventh Revision (ICD-11), World Health Organization (WHO) 2019/2021. https://icd.who.int/browse11

Iturralde, E., Slama, N., Kline-Simon, A. H., Young-Wolff, K. C., Don Mordecai, D., Stacy, A., & Sterling, S. A. (2021). Premature mortality associated with severe mental illness or substance use disorder in an integrated health care system. *General Hospital Psychiatry, 68*, 1–6. https://doi.org/10.1016/j.genhosppsych.2020.11.002

Jablensky, A. (2010). The diagnostic concept of schizophrenia: Its history, evolution, and prospects. *Dialogues in Clinical Neuroscience, 12*(3), 271–287. https://doi.org/10.31887/DCNS.2010.12.3/ajablensky

Kay, S. R., Fiszbein, A., & Opler, L. A. (1987). The positive and negative syndrome scale (PANSS) for schizophrenia. *Schizophrenia Bulletin, 13*(2), 261–276. https://doi.org/10.1093/schbul/13.2.261

Keepers, G. A., Fochtmann, L. J., Anzia, J. M., Benjamin, S., Lyness, J. L., Mojtabai, R., Servis, M., Walaszek, A., Buckley, P. F., Lenzenweger, M. F., Young, A. S., Degenhardt, A., & Hong, S. H. (2020). The American Psychiatric Association practice guideline for the treatment of patients with schizophrenia. *American Journal of Psychiatry, 177*(9), 868–872. https://doi.org/10.1176/appi.ajp.2020.177901

Kessler, R. C., & Zhao, S. (1999). The prevalence of mental illness. In A. V. Horwitz & T. L. Scheid (Eds.), *A handbook for the study of mental health: Social contexts, theories, and systems* (pp. 58–78). Cambridge University Press. https://psycnet.apa.org/record/1999-02431-003

Kirkpatrick, B., Fenton, W. S., Carpenter, W. T., Jr., & Marder, S. R. (2006). The NIMH-MATRICS consensus statement on negative symptoms. *Schizophrenia Bulletin, 32*(2), 214–219. https://doi.org/10.1093/schbul/sbj053

Layng, T. V. J., & Andronis, P. T. (1984). Toward a functional analysis of delusional speech and hallucinatory behavior. *The Behavior Analyst, 7*(2), 139–156. https://doi.org/10.1007/BF03391897

Liberman, R. P., Derisi, W. J., & Mueser, K. T. (2001). *Social skills training for psychiatric patients*. Allyn & Bacon. https://www.amazon.com/dp/0205144063

Liberman, R. P., Teigen, J., Patterson, R., & Baker, V. (1973). Reducing delusional speech in chronic, paranoid schizophrenics. *Journal of Applied Behavior Analysis, 6*(1), 57–64. https://doi.org/10.1901/jaba.1973.6-57

Loewy, R. L., Corey, S., Amirfathi, F., Dabit, S., Fulford, D., Pearson, R., & Vinogradov, S. (2019). Childhood trauma and clinical high risk for psychosis. *Schizophrenia Research, 205*, 10–14. https://doi.org/10.1016/j.schres.2018.05.003

Lomholt, L. H., Andersen, D. V., Sejrsgaard-Jacobsen, C., Øzdemir, C. M., Graff, C., Schjerning, O., Jensen, S. E., Straszek, S. P. V., Licht, R. W., Grøntved, S., & Nielsen, R. E. (2019). Mortality rate trends in patients diagnosed with schizophrenia or bipolar disorder: A nationwide study with 20 years of follow-up. *International Journal of Bipolar Disorders, 7*(1), Article 8. https://doi.org/10.1186/s40345-018-0140-x

Lutgens, D., Gariepy, G., & Malla, A. (2017). Psychological and psychosocial interventions for negative symptoms in psychosis: Systematic review and meta-analysis. *The British Journal of Psychiatry, 210*(5), 324–332. https://doi.org/10.1192/bjp.bp.116.197103

Machmutow, K., Meister, R., Jansen, A., Kriston, L., Watzke, B., Härter, M. C., & Liebherz, S. (2019). Comparative effectiveness of continuation and maintenance treatments for persistent depressive disorder in adults. *Cochrane Database of Systematic Reviews, 5*, Article CD012855. https://doi.org/10.1002/14651858.CD012855.pub2

Marková, I. S., & Berrios, G. E. (2011). Awareness and insight in psychopathology: An essential distinction? *Theory & Psychology, 21*(4), 421–437. https://doi.org/10.1177/0959354310375330

Mauritz, M. W., Goossens, P. J. J., Draijer, N., & van Achterberg, T. (2013). Prevalence of interpersonal trauma exposure and trauma-related disorders in severe mental illness. *European Journal of Psychotraumatology, 4*(1), Article 19985. https://doi.org/10.3402/ejpt.v4i0.19985

Merriam-Webster. (n.d.). Disability. In *Merriam-Webster.com dictionary*. Retrieved August 12, 2024, from https://www.merriam-webster.com/dictionary/disability

Mezzich, J. E., & Üstün, T. B. (Eds.). (2002). *International classification and diagnosis: Critical experience and future directions*. Karger Medical and Scientific Publishers. https://doi.org/10.1159/isbn.978-3-318-00655-0

Moges, S., Belete, T., Mekonen, T., & Menberu, M. (2021). Lifetime relapse and its associated factors among people with schizophrenia spectrum disorders who are on follow-up at Comprehensive Specialized Hospitals in Amhara region, Ethiopia: A cross-sectional study. *International Journal of Mental Health Systems, 15*(42). https://doi.org/10.1186/s13033-021-00464-0

Monnat, S. M., & Chandler, R. F. (2015). Long-term physical health consequences of adverse childhood experiences. *The Sociological Quarterly, 56*(4), 723–752. https://doi.org/10.1111/tsq.12107

Muyambi, K., Walsh, S., Bressington, D., Gray, R., Dennis, S., Brown, E., Chien, W. T., & Jones, M. (2023). Efficacy of behavioural activation in the treatment of negative symptoms in people with schizophrenia spectrum disorders: A systematic review. *International Journal of Nursing Studies Advances, 5*, Article 100132. https://doi.org/10.1016/j.ijnsa.2023.100132

National Alliance on Mental Illness (NAMI). (n.d.). *Mental health by the numbers*. https://www.nami.org/about-mental-illness/mental-health-by-the-numbers/

National Institute of Mental Health (NIMH). (n.d.). *Mental illness*. https://www.nimh.nih.gov/health/statistics/mental-illness

Paul, G. P., Stuve, P., & Cross, J. V. (1997). Real-world inpatient programs: Shedding some light—A critique. *Applied & Preventive Psychology, 6*(4), 193–204. https://doi.org/10.1016/S0962-1849(97)80008-X

Porcelli, S., Bianchini, O., de Girolamo, G., Aguglia, E., Crea, L., & Serretti, A. (2016). Clinical factors related to schizophrenia relapse. *International Journal of Psychiatry in Clinical Practice, 20*(2), 54–69. https://doi.org/10.3109/13651501.2016.1149195

Prins, S. J. (2014). Prevalence of mental illnesses in U.S. state prisons: A systematic review. *Psychiatric Services, 65*(7), 862–872. https://doi.org/10.1176/appi.ps.201300166

RachBeisel, J., Scott, J., & Dixon, L. (1999). Co-occurring severe mental illness and substance use disorders: A review of recent research. *Psychiatric Services, 50*(11), 1427–1434. https://doi.org/10.1176/ps.50.11.1427

Regier, D. A., Farmer, M. E., Rae, D. S., Locke, B. Z., Keith, S. J., Judd, L. L., & Goodwin, F. K. (1990). Comorbidity of mental disorders with alcohol and other drug abuse: Results from the Epidemiologic Catchment Area (ECA) study. *JAMA, 264*(19), 2511–2518. https://doi.org/10.1001/jama.1990.03450190043026

Ruggeri, M., Leese, M., Thornicroft, G., Bisoffi, G., & Tansella, M. (2000). Definition and prevalence of severe and persistent mental illness. *The British Journal of Psychiatry, 177*(2), 149–155. https://doi.org/10.1192/bjp.177.2.149

Sass, L., & Parnas, J. (2017). Thought disorder, subjectivity, and the self. *Schizophrenia Bulletin, 43*(3), 497–502. https://doi.org/10.1093/schbul/sbx032

Spaulding, W. D., Johnson, R. W., Nolting, J. R., & Collins, A. (2008). Treatment-resistant schizophrenia. In D. Castle, D. L. Copolov, T. Wykes, & K. T. Mueser (Eds.), *Pharmacological and psychosocial treatments in schizophrenia* (2nd ed., pp. 231–237). https://doi.org/10.3109/9780203091579

Spaulding, W. D., Sullivan, M. E., & Poland, J. S. (2003). *Treatment and rehabilitation of severe mental illness*. Guilford Press. https://psycnet.apa.org/record/2003-02546-000

Substance Abuse and Mental Health Services Administration (SAMHSA). (2020). *Key substance use and mental health indicators in the United States: Results from the 2019 National Survey on Drug Use and Health* (HHS Publication No. PEP20-07-01-001, NSDUH Series H-55). Center for Behavioral Health Statistics and Quality. https://www.samhsa.gov/data/

Substance Abuse and Mental Health Services Administration (SAMHSA). (2021). *Key substance use and mental health indicators in the United States: Results from the 2020 National Survey on Drug Use and Health* (HHS Publication No. PEP21-07-01-003, NSDUH Series H-56). Center for Behavioral Health Statistics and Quality. https://www.samhsa.gov/data/report/2020-nsduh-annual-national-report

Substance Abuse and Mental Health Services Administration (SAMHSA). (2024). *Co-occurring disorders and other health conditions: What are co-occurring disorders?* https://www.samhsa.gov/medications-substance-use-disorders/medications-counseling-related-conditions/co-occurring-disorders

Teplin, L. A., McClelland, G. M., Abram, K. M., & Weiner, D. A. (2005). Crime victimization in adults with severe mental illness: Comparison with the National Crime Victimization Survey. *Archives of General Psychiatry, 62*(8), 911–921. https://doi.org/10.1001/archpsyc.62.8.911

Terlizzi, E. P., & Norris, T. (2021). *Mental health treatment among adults: United States, 2020* (NCHS Data Brief No. 419). National Center for Health Statistics. https://www.cdc.gov/nchs/products/databriefs/db419.htm

Treatment Advocacy Center. (n.d.). *What is SMI?* https://www.treatmentadvocacycenter.org/what-is-smi/

Üstün, T. B. (2000). Unmet need for management of mental disorders in primary care. In G. Andrews & S. Henderson (Eds.), *Unmet need in psychiatry: Problems, resources, responses* (pp. 157–171). Cambridge University Press. https://www.cambridge.org/core/books/unmet-need-in-psychiatry/unmet-need-for-management-of-mental-disorders-in-primary-care/955DEE077C14A313EC8A19E6C5EE0845

Üstün, T. B., & Kennedy, C. (2009). What is "functional impairment"? Disentangling disability from clinical significance. *World Psychiatry, 8*, 82–85. https://doi.org/10.1002/j.2051-5545.2009.tb00222.x

Virgio, N., Bennetti, G., Higgins, D., Bennetti, L., & Thomas, P. (2001). The prevalence and characteristics of co-occurring serious mental illness (SMI) and substance abuse or dependence in the patients of Adult Mental Health and Addictions Services in eastern Dorset. *Journal of Mental Health, 10*(2), 175–188. https://doi.org/10.1080/09638230020023732

Wilson, A. B., Ishler, K. J., Morgan, R., Phillips, J., Draine, J., & Farkas, K. J. (2020). Examining criminogenic risk levels among people with mental illness incarcerated in US jails and prisons. *The Journal of Behavioral Health Services & Research*. Advance online publication. https://doi.org/10.1007/s11414-020-09737-x

World Health Organization (WHO). (2022). *ICD-11: International classification of diseases (11th revision)*. https://icd.who.int/

Chapter 2
Behaviors Associated with Serious Mental Illness

Introduction

Understanding serious mental illness (SMI) requires a nuanced appreciation of the behavioral, cognitive, and emotional phenomena that disrupt adaptive functioning and quality of life. While the term SMI encompasses a range of psychiatric conditions, most notably schizophrenia, schizoaffective disorder, and bipolar disorder with psychotic features, it is the behavioral manifestations of these disorders that most directly impact clinical care, social integration, and recovery. This chapter builds on the foundational overview of SMI by examining the core symptom domains and behavioral impairments that characterize its presentation, with particular attention to the multidimensional nature of these symptoms and their consequences.

Central to the clinical conceptualization of SMI is the distinction between positive and negative symptoms. Positive symptoms refer to the presence of atypical behaviors or experiences, such as hallucinations, delusions, disorganized speech, and affective lability, whereas negative symptoms reflect the absence or reduction of expected behaviors, including avolition, anhedonia, alogia, and deficits in social and self-care functioning. These symptoms vary not only in type but also in frequency, intensity, contextual appropriateness, and impact—dimensions that are critical for accurate assessment and intervention. Compounding these challenges is the frequent presence of impaired insight, which limits self-monitoring and adaptive behavior regulation, and contributes to treatment nonadherence and functional decline.

These domains are explored in depth, beginning with an overview of problem behaviors and the principles of dimensional assessment. Positive symptoms, including hallucinations and sensory deception, delusions, aggression, disorganized speech, and affective lability, followed by a discussion of negative symptoms and their implications for social and functional impairment will be examined. The

G. F. McKeegan, *Behavior Change Interventions for Serious Mental Illness*, Evidence-Based Practices in Behavioral Health,
https://doi.org/10.1007/978-3-032-18372-9_2

significance of utilizing individualized, multimodal assessment approaches and behavior analytic frameworks that address the heterogeneity and complexity of serious mental illness is underscored. Such strategies provide a comprehensive understanding of the interaction between symptom dimensions and behavioral deficits, which informs clinical presentation and supports recovery-oriented care planning.

Symptoms and Problematic Behaviors

The definition of serious mental illness (SMI) contains behaviors across multiple behavioral response classes and dimensions. Problem behaviors—or symptoms—displayed by individuals living with SMI differ along different dimensions. Problematic behaviors may manifest either through their occurrence—when they are displayed and observed (or self-reported)—or through their absence, resulting in the lack of expected behaviors such as showering, taking medications, or communicating effectively with others.

Problem behaviors can manifest in a range of contexts, such as when an individual is alone or with others, at home, or within a group home setting. These may include multiple behaviors classified under a "response class"—a term describing a group of behaviors that fulfill the same function or objective, regardless of their outward differences in appearance or presentation (i.e., topography) (Cooper et al., 2020).

Problem behaviors vary in the context in which the behavior is displayed. If a person is talking to himself in the privacy of their bedroom, it is not considered a problem. If talking to oneself occurs in crowded areas and loud enough for others to hear, it may result in the person living with SMI being avoided and stigmatized as "crazy." Many people yell at the television when watching a favorite sport team playing; others will label that behavior as "exuberant." If such "exuberance" occurs during a funeral service, the person doing that behavior would be asked to leave and more than likely be told not to return.

Behaviors differ depending on the dimension including the effects or consequences of the behavior that is or is not displayed. Behaviors that are or are not displayed have consequences that may benefit the individual or have harmful or negative results. The presence and absence of behaviors may be problematic because of the deleterious outcome that the person living with SMI could face, such as legal involvement, hospitalization or medical emergencies. An example would be refusing to attend court mandated treatment with the outcome being re-incarcerated for failure to attend. Another example may be forgetting to get a prescription for an anti-seizure medication, missing doses and experiencing "break-through" seizures.

Problem behaviors can vary in both the frequency with which they occur and do not occur; the rate at which these behaviors are exhibited may itself pose challenges. High-frequency behaviors, such as laughing or talking to oneself, expressing beliefs that are not based in reality, or engaging in repeated actions like smoking, can be disruptive to others, potentially resulting in social avoidance of the individual and contributing to stigmatizing labels. The problem behavior may differ in the severity, magnitude, or intensity of the behavior when it occurs. For instance, self-injurious behavior may be superficial and not require medical attention, such as repeated self-pinching. Alternatively, it could cause tissue injury that requires medical care, such as accidentally cutting oneself with a razor blade and experiencing heavy bleeding.

The absence of a behavior also may differ in magnitude or severity as well. An example may be in the response class of personal hygiene. The difference in severity of this particular "absence of behavior" (e.g., negative symptom) may differ from occasional body odor to the presence of abscess, skin lesions and infections due to lack of washing and using soap. Shortcomings (i.e., deficits) in the response class of dental hygiene behaviors may result in either halitosis, tooth decay, or gum disease. Aggressive behavior displayed by a person living with SMI may differ along the dimension of severity by yelling loudly and verbally threatening or hitting or physically assaulting another in some way; the harm caused by the aggression could be physical property damage (e.g., broken furniture or window) or result in physical damage to the assaulted person.

The behaviors associated with individuals living with SMI differ on the impact that certain behaviors have on other behaviors. The person may be living with a belief that they are being followed by aliens. The person can go about their daily life if it does not impact on other behaviors, such as self-control and intense personal distress that may result in maladaptive behaviors to reduce the distress by self-medicating with illegal or legal substances. A person may believe that aliens are watching him, but if he is able to function in other areas of daily life—personal hygiene, financial responsibilities, self-control, having friends, getting along with others, working—the impact of this false belief (a delusion) will be minimal. He may discuss this with others who accept this belief; to others what he says does not seem to be something about which to be concerned. However, if he begins to miss work, remains isolated for fear of the aliens, or frequently goes to the police to report this belief and ask the authorities to stop the aliens, then it becomes problematic for the person.

Behaviors that are determined as "problematic" in mental health are not problematic in general; the behaviors listed as symptoms by mental health service providers are displayed to some degree by everyone (e.g., talking to oneself when misplacing the cell phone or glasses, forgetting to take prescribed medications, drinking too much). The behavior being displayed is labeled as "symptomatic" if it results in an unfavorable outcome or consequence for the person emitting the behavior and on others as well. Many behaviors that are displayed by people living with SMI are not dangerous but make others feel uncomfortable, are annoying, or cause other individuals to be distressed. Behaviors can be labeled as abnormal if the behavior is displayed too often, too intensely or in the wrong settings. The behaviors that become problematic may not be under the control of setting events. The behaviors that are displayed in the wrong setting lack "stimulus control." Behavior is under stimulus control when the behavior appears more often in the context of the presence of a certain class of stimuli and not in the absence of that class of stimuli (Cooper et al., 2020). Behaviors lacking in stimulus control occur in settings or contexts in which the behaviors should not occur. People do not take off their clothes in public places if their clothes get wet after a rainstorm; they wait until they get home or change in private settings. The behavior of "taking off wet clothes" becomes abnormal when the behavior occurs in settings when it should not occur. Behavior lacking stimulus control is displayed in situations where behavior should not be displayed such as urinating in public or speaking or laughing loudly during a funeral.

The behavior of any person becomes abnormal when the behavior interferes with the display of other adaptive behaviors. Using the example above of the person believing that aliens are following him, the behavior of his false belief becomes abnormal if he also beliefs that the aliens can hear his thoughts through the shower heads. The belief becomes problematic if he refuses to take a shower and will only wash at public fire hydrants where he believes that the aliens cannot hear him.

The behavior becomes abnormal if the intensity or magnitude of the display of the behavior is high. Pinching oneself when in pain may not be a problem as some people pinch or rub in the part of the body where the pain is felt; the behavior is abnormal when the behavior is displayed with high intensity that it results in bruising, or the behavior occurs frequently. Research has shown that moods during the day fluctuate by time of day, physical status of the person, activities being performed and anticipation of events (Dysinger, 1938; Stone et al., 1996). Most persons have "good and bad days" depending on many factors that are often transient. "Bad days" or when mood is low becomes a problem if the low mood lasts too long, interferes with the ability to get out of bed, interact with others and function adaptively. A low mood becomes abnormal and problematic when the person remains isolated, does not take care of herself, has dysregulation of appetite, and sleep disturbances.

As stated previously, behaviors vary on different dimensions. If the "low mood" becomes so intense that the person keeps thinking that she is a burden to others, everyone would be better off if she was dead, has frequent and intense cognitions about committing suicide during periods of "low mood," and has difficulty decreasing the intensity and frequency of the suicidal thoughts, then her thoughts become abnormal and problematic.

Behaviors are multidimensional in terms of frequency, magnitude, settings, and effect. Behaviors also differ on how the behaviors can be assessed. Some behaviors are known as "private events" or "covert events" known only to the individual experiencing the behavior such as thoughts, feelings, perceptions, and sensations (Dougher, 2013). The private events can be accessed through self-reports from the individual. At times, assessing private events is unreliable and invalid—the person may be exaggerating or minimizing the pain they are experiencing and differentially reports the magnitude of the experienced pain as to the setting and the consequence. People are usually not aware of what they are thinking, especially if asking to recall what their thought was in the past. Additionally, language, cultural, and social differences can affect any verbal question and responses.

Another source of assessing private events is whether the behaviors have collateral sources of observation. Collateral sources can be reports from others about what the person is experiencing or behaviors that are associated with each other. For example, pain is a private and covert event. The person experiencing pain can inform others about where the pain is, how often it occurs, the intensity and what decreases the intensity and frequency. There are, however, other collateral behaviors that can be used to assess the pain. These may be facial expressions of discomfort, absence or slowness of physical movement, behavior changes observed by others familiar with a person experiencing pain (e.g., no longer performing leisure activities). There are assessments during which the person is asked to perform certain movements, called range of motion (ROM); the ease and fluidity of performing the movements can be used to assess how pain may be impacting the person's ability to function. The person experiencing the covert behavior is asked to communicate it to others but having collateral observable data aids in any assessment.

Positive and Negative Symptoms

As stated previously, a dimension of behavior that is a major focus for mental health practitioners is the presence or absence of certain behaviors. These are labeled positive and negative symptoms, respectively (Correll & Schooler, 2020). Positive symptoms are the symptoms of behaviors that are displayed by individuals living with SMI; examples of positive symptoms are the psychotic symptoms of delusions, hallucinations, disordered or disturbed thinking (which is displayed by certain aspects of verbal behavior). Negative symptoms are the absence of expected adaptive behaviors; examples include lack of interest and motivation to engage in expected behaviors (such as personal hygiene), poor social skills, social isolation, and a lack of awareness of problematic behaviors.

The positive and negative symptoms are conceptually both the present and the absence of behaviors. As stated previously, the positive symptoms are the behaviors that are displayed or occur. The negative symptoms are the behaviors that are not occurring but are expected from a person. However, the displays of positive symptoms also are the lack of a response class of self-monitoring and management; that is, the person living with SMI have may not have an awareness of the behavior that is being displayed and any adaptive alternative skills or behaviors associated with altering certain dimensions of the positive symptoms such as the frequency, intensity, stimulus control, and consequences.

An example that problem behaviors are both positive (i.e., being displayed) and negative (i.e., the absence of expected behavior) is with anger/frustration/fear and aggression (Sax et al., 1996). Aggressive behavior can be observed by perceiving the response class of aggressive behaviors (e.g., hitting. yelling, kicking, throwing items) or observing the product or outcome of the behavior such as physical damage to others or objects. The display of aggressive behaviors is also the absence or the lack of self-control and management behaviors when angry, fearful, frustrated and other associated emotional respondents. For every positive symptom there is a correlated impairment as well in self-awareness and management skills. Behavioral impairments vary on the same dimensions as positive symptoms in assessing the extent of the diminished abilities or capabilities. Individuals living with SMI display self-awareness and management behaviors but not at the rate, intensity, and/or in situations that result in the occurrence of self-control behaviors (Amador & Kronengold, 2004; Goldberg et al., 2001).

Positive Symptoms

There is a lack of agreement among researchers and practitioners in mental health as to the positive and negative symptoms displayed by people living with SMI. However, there is a consensus that the positive symptoms include the following:

1. Delusions are beliefs that are false, not agreed upon by others, have incorrect reference to reality and cannot be explained by religion or culture and are firmly sustained despite contrary evidence (Shahrokh & Hales, 2003). Delusional beliefs can be bizarre in that what the person is saying is implausible (American Psychiatric Association, 2022). An example would be if the person makes statements that he "eats buildings," has no legs (although the person is standing and walking), or has had his brain removed while asleep. Delusions differ on the dimension of the degree of conviction that the person expressing the belief has about the veracity of the belief (Bell et al., 2003). Individuals experiencing delusions can vary as to the firmness to which they hold onto the belief; studies have shown that grandiose and religious delusions are held more firmly by individuals experiencing the delusions than others delusional beliefs (Appelbaum et al., 1999). Delusions also vary as to the potential that the person experiencing a delusional belief act on the delusion. A person experiencing delusional religious beliefs will be more likely to act on the beliefs than other types of delusions (Appelbaum et al., 1999). An example would be a person firmly holding to the belief that she is the mother of the savior and kidnaps an infant believing that the infant is her child.

   Multiple forms of delusional beliefs are observed among individuals who live with SMI, each varying in prevalence (Bhuyan & Chaudhury, 2016; Paolini et al., 2016). Research indicates that persecutory delusions—defined as the conviction that one is being harassed, attacked, or conspired against—are the most common, followed by grandiose delusions, which involve an exaggerated sense of one's fame, importance, or abilities (Brucato et al., 2017).
2. Hallucinations are perceptual disturbances that occur with or without external stimulus (American Psychiatric Association, 2022). Hallucinations can occur in all sensory areas—visual, auditory, olfactory, tactile, gustatory (i.e., taste) and somatic (i.e., physical sensation on body such as snakes crawling under one's skin) (Shahrokh & Hales, 2003). A comprehensive definition of hallucinatory

experiences was reported by Slade and Bentall (1988); they defined hallucinations as a "perceptual-like" experience which:

(a) Occurs in the absence of an appropriate stimulus
(b) Has the same impact as a real perception in a particular sensory area
(c) Is not able to be voluntarily controlled by the person experiencing it

The definition accounts for some of the dimensional factors associated with hallucinations such as the misattribution of stimuli, the impact of the experience on the individual (e.g., distress, humor, guilt) and the subjective perception of control over the experience (Badcock et al., 2011).

Auditory hallucinations were by far the most common, followed by visual hallucinations, tactile, olfactory, and gustatory hallucinations; olfactory and gustatory hallucinations appear to be related as these two delusional beliefs frequently occur together (Mueser et al., 1990). Auditory hallucinations are frequently described as "hearing voices"; sometimes the individual experiencing an auditory hallucination can identify the voice. The content of what the person "hears" ranges from the humorous to derogatory; the auditory hallucination also is described as "white noise," one word or phrase repeated, or hearing a comment about what they are doing (Andrew, 2010).

A type of auditory hallucination is "command hallucination." The person experiencing an auditory hallucination is "commanded" by the hallucination to commit a certain act, sometimes of a dangerous nature, such as violence toward others or self (Andrew, 2010; Buccheri et al., 2007; Rogers et al., 1990). Command hallucinations are relatively common among individuals living with SMI with reported prevalence rates among adults ranging from 18% to 89% with a median of 53%. Prevalence rates for "dangerous or harmful" command hallucinations range from 7% to 70% with a median of 48% (Shawyer et al., 2003). Experiencing a command hallucination, the frequency and the intensity of the hallucination, and the emotional distress of experiencing the command hallucination has been found to be a risk factor for future dangerousness in persons living with SMI (Monahan et al., 2001). The studies have reported that the presence of command hallucinations often does not improve with treatment adherence (Andrew, 2010; Braham et al., 2004).

Visual hallucinations appear to be related to metabolic (e.g., withdrawal from alcohol, effects of some drugs) and neurogenerative disorders as well as seizures and other adverse neurologic events (Teeple et al., 2009). Typically, people see complex visual hallucinations, such as people, figures or faces. Less commonly, people experience simple visual hallucinations, such as lines, dots or flashes of light. Visual hallucinations occur in approximately 27% of people living with SMI (Aynsworth et al., 2017; Dudley et al., 2019; Janaki et al., 2017)

3. Disorganized speech and thinking—disordered thought patterns are evidenced by the person's speech being disorganized and incomprehensible, often characterized by rapid shifting from one unrelated topic to another (i.e., flight of ideas), juxtaposing unrelated topics (i.e., looseness of association), lacking a frame of reference to what is being discussed (i.e., incoherence) and incomplete sentences and made up words (i.e., neologisms) (Shahrokh & Hales, 2003). The

disorganization varies along dimensions of relatedness of topic and ideas that intrude in a person's speech, incoherence, and the degree of the lack of awareness by the person who is talking (Shahrokh & Hales, 2003). Disorganized speech can become incomprehensible to the listener when unrelatedness and juxtaposition of words and topics in a conversation becomes frequent and rapid.

4. Grossly disorganized or abnormal motor movements—impairment in motor movements can be displayed by a lack or deficit in motor responsiveness to external stimuli (e.g., not responding to questions or requests), bizarre posturing, or unpredictable excessive and not goal directed activity such as inability to sit down, pacing, and hand wringing (American Psychiatric Association, 2022; Shahrokh & Hales, 2003).
5. Inappropriate affect is "a display of emotion that is out of harmony with reality or with the verbal or intellectual content that it accompanies" (Shahrokh & Hales, 2003, p. 100). An example would be if the person displaying inappropriate affect laughed when discussing the death of his child, cried when talking about winning the lottery, or becoming angry and hitting others when told he had to wait in line for a piece of cake.

Brucato et al. (2017) found that the presence of delusions, bizarre thoughts and ideas, and disorganized speech predicted individuals who later would be identified as living with SMI. The presence of positive symptoms, however, are independent from the negative symptoms in people living with SMI and are not correlated; that is, positive symptoms do not predict the presence of negative symptoms and vice-versa. Practitioners and researchers report that positive symptoms respond to treatment, but negative symptoms often remain unchanged. About 20–30% of individuals living with SMI display negative symptoms that have a significant impact on functioning and do not improve with treatment (Buchanan, 2007).

Other Positive Symptoms There are other behaviors associated with living SMI that are not features of positive symptoms listed in the DSM-V-TR (American Psychiatric Association, 2022), yet are associated behaviors or symptoms of living with SMI. Following the definition of positive symptoms (behaviors that are present and observable during an assessment including review of records and history)—then aggressive behaviors, affective lability (i.e., mood swings), and substance use ought to be included. Like other positive behaviors, aggressive behaviors, affective lability, and substance use are multidimensional, varying on behavioral parameters as intensity/magnitude, frequency (e.g., rate), contexts (e.g., such as being displayed across multiple situations), motivational operations, consequences, and the presence of self-control skills.

Aggressive Behaviors Aggressive behaviors—defined as verbal or physical—is a serious behavior that is associated with people living with SMI. The aggressive behavior response class can be physical, verbal, or both; the behaviors can be directed toward a living organism or an inanimate object. Aggressive behaviors correlate with the respondent (i.e., emotion) of anger, annoyance, frustration, fear, and similar emotional respondents.

Aggressive behavior presents significant negative outcomes for individuals diagnosed with SMI and may further perpetuate societal stigma associated with such conditions. It is reasonable to consider aggressive behaviors as part of the positive symptomatology linked to SMI; accordingly, this text will address them as positive symptoms.

Aggressive behaviors have many topographies and can result in confusion as to what is an aggressive response class. Aggressive behaviors differ in behavioral dimensions and can vary within the response class of aggressive behaviors. For example, does the display occur more frequently or at a high intensity only with familiar people or with others as well? If an individual engages in hitting another person, does this behavior occur repeatedly—such as multiple instances of hitting directed toward one or more targets?

Describing and classifying aggressive behaviors can be difficult given the nuances of the behaviors involved. A summary of aggressive response classes includes the following:

1. Physical aggression includes hitting, kicking, punching, slapping, spitting, and other behaviors that may result in physical harm or injury to the person to whom the aggressive behavior is directed (Allen & Anderson, 2017; Gabbey, 2022). Physical aggression does not have to result in harming the intended "target." Spitting and a punch that misses the target does not result in physical harm to the victim but is still considered aggressive behavior. An item that is thrown against a wall or smashed under foot is aggressive behavior although the intent of the behavior is not to harm anyone.
2. Verbal aggression can include shouting, swearing, insults, and other comments that may cause emotional hurt and distress. It includes hostile threatening remarks that involve the statements of hurting someone or destroying something (Gabbey, 2022).
3. Passive aggression can include any indirect expression of anger or frustration toward another person. It can be both verbal and motoric. Sarcastic comments, forgetting to do what one promises to do, and blaming others are a few examples (Gabbey, 2022). Passive aggression can be "forgetting" to wash out your coffee cup and leaving it in the sink for your housemate or eating someone's snack that is in the office refrigerator. "Getting back" against a living organism or an organization is labeled as "revenge" as the revengeful person believes that they have been hurt or offended in some aspect.
4. Aggression and violence are often used interchangeably in the mental health literature. Violence (violent behavior) is defined as a severe form of an aggressive response class; the displayed behavior has the intention of causing physical, psychological, or emotional harm to the individual at whom the behavior is directed (i.e., victim). In forensic contexts, the term "violence" is often applied to describe behaviors within an aggressive response class. "Aggressive behavior" refers to actions and their observable consequences, whereas "violence" encompasses covert or internal events such as violent thoughts or intentions. Nevertheless, engaging in a violent act requires the individual to demonstrate

some form of aggressive behavior, thus the distinction between these terms is considered marginal (Allen & Anderson, 2017).

Aggressive behavior will be used to describe any behavior that results in an observable or potentially harmful, dangerous or destructive act. Intention to harm another person or destroy an item is a private event and only can be ascertained by asking the person and that person self-reporting the intent. Given the problems that are associated with living with SMI such as self-awareness, memory, attention, and verbal behaviors (e.g., disorganized speech and thought), one can conclude that self-reports can be unreliable especially coming from a person living with SMI and the behavioral impairments/symptoms that may be present.

Individuals living with mental health problems generally display less aggressive behaviors than other people living with no mental health problem. Research has shown that people living with SMI, however, have higher risk and incidences of violence than those with no mental or substance use conditions. Co-occurring mental health problems appear to increase the risk of a person living with SMI; irrespective of the presence of a co-occurring problem of substance use, individuals living with SMI do exhibit a higher incidence of violence and aggression (Junginger & McGuire, 2004; Van Dorn et al., 2011). Gopika et al. (2024) have postulated the factors associated with this higher incidence of aggressive behaviors are:

> …the presence of positive symptoms, history of aggression, involuntary admission, past or family history of substance abuse, and adverse environmental circumstance, including poor communication patterns, challenging living conditions, limited social support, overt criticality from caregivers, a longer period of hospitalization, provocative situations, and unemployment. (Gopika et al., 2024, p. 358)

Affective Lability ("Mood Swings") A person displays periods of intense anger and irritability, yelling and cursing others, making threats and accusing others of "cheating me" at work; within hours, the same person is laughing, is the "life of the party," making others laugh with his infectious humor. By the end of the day, the same person is crying, making derogatory statements about himself, and is threatening to kill himself saying, "I have nothing to live for!" This person is displaying affective lability, defined as fluctuations in a person's mood and affect over periods of time. The time of fluctuations can be in hours or days; the fluctuations may occur repeatedly. Marwaha et al. (2014) defines affective lability as:

> …frequent affective category shifts, disturbances in affect intensity, excessively rapid emotion rise-times and delayed return to baseline, excessive reactivity to psychosocial cues and overdramatic affective expression.... The term is used interchangeably with mood instability, affective instability, affective and emotional dysregulation and mood swings, by researchers and clinicians. (p. 3)

Affective lability is a problematic behavior across differing determinations of mental health problems and is associated with suicidality and higher rates of health care use. It has been shown that 13.9% of individuals living with SMI can be reliably identified as experiencing affective lability (Marwaha et al., 2013). It has been shown that individuals with a mental health problem have higher levels of affective lability and less control of their behavior than those people without a mental health problem (Marwaha et al., 2018). Interestingly, intensity of the affective stability was not found to be a determining variable in differentiating between individuals with and without a mental health problem (Marwaha et al., 2013).

Høegh et al. (2022) have found that affective instability is more prevalent with fluctuations between anxiety and depression, than between other affective states of anger and elation. Positive associations between affective lability, social functioning, and indicators of quality of life were also shown. Researchers have called for focusing on treating affective lability in people living with SMI to improve psychosocial functioning and rehabilitation efforts (Marwaha et al., 2018).

Substance Use Problematic substance use is the most common co-occurring condition among people living with a major mental health problem and is associated with poorer outcomes (Siegfried, 1998). Research on the use of substances with persons living with SMI have many inconclusive results given small size of samples, treatment drift and dropout, lack of an experimental design, short follow-up periods and inadequate assessment of use by the person (Siegfried, 1998). Using either drugs, alcohol or both range between a quarter to a third of samples in surveys conducted with people living with SMI (RachBeisel et al., 1999; Virgio et al., 2001).

It is well established that the use of drugs and alcohol by persons living with SMI is associated with adverse impacts including increases in the severity of the symptoms associated with SMI (i.e., increase in frequency, intensity, lowered self-control), psychosocial functioning, decreased adherence to treatment recommendations, disruptive and aggressive behaviors, and higher rates of admissions to psychiatric facilities. The use of substances by a person living with SMI puts the individual living with SMI at greater risk for being traumatized by experiencing physical and sexual violence (RachBeisel et al., 1999) as well as the associated physical health risks associated with use of drugs and/or alcohol. However, the "occasional" use of substances by individuals living with SMI—not meeting the criteria for a co-occurring mental health problem—has not been investigated thoroughly. The question remains if "occasional" use impacts the quality of life and recovery efforts. Given that most people living with SMI are prescribed medications, using alcohol and/or drugs can impact the body's metabolism of the prescribed medications and result in an increase in symptoms and side effects from the medications (Levin, n.d.).

Negative Symptoms

Negative symptoms are the absence or diminution of expected adaptive behaviors (Correll & Schooler, 2020); examples include lack of interest and motivation to engage in expected behaviors (such as personal hygiene), poor social skills, social isolation, and deficits in the awareness of problematic behaviors (Andreasen & Olsen, 1982; Andreasen et al., 1991). Negative symptoms are the lack of the occurrence of expected behaviors that are usually observed in functional adults. Although negative symptoms are a focus of research and treatment in the rehabilitation and recovery of people living with SMI, there is a lack of agreement as to the specificity of what are the negative symptoms. Studies have shown that 50–60% of people living with SMI have at least one negative symptom and between 10% and 30% have two or more negative symptoms (Galderisi et al., 2021). Negative symptoms include:

(a) Diminished emotional expression—include both verbal and nonverbal aspects of emotional expression such as facial expression, gestures, and verbal inflection and tone (i.e., prosody) (American Psychiatric Association, 2022, p. 88).
(b) Avolition—decrease or absence of self-initiated goal directed activity (American Psychiatric Association, 2022, p. 88).
(c) Alogia—deceased expressed verbal behavior (American Psychiatric Association, 2022, p. 88).
(d) Anhedonia—an inability to experience and express pleasure from an activity (American Psychiatric Association, 2022, p. 88).
(e) Asociality—lack of interest to engage in social interactions with others (American Psychiatric Association, 2022, p. 88).

The broad categories of negative symptoms listed in the DSM-V-TR (American Psychiatric Association, 2022) lack specificity as to the behavioral response classes in each category. As stated previously, behaviors vary along different measurable and defined behavioral dimensions; the categories presented above do not specify the dimensions of the response classes associated with each category. For example, avolition can include the total lack of self-initiated behaviors in one or several contexts. Is it still a problem in volition (i.e., self-initiation) if the frequency of a behavior in a response class occurs at a lower rate/frequency than what is expected or requested/prompted (e.g., taking a shower once a month or every other day)? Does this person then lack “self-initiation” in hygiene such as bathing? Is the problem in personal hygiene because the person is not changing dirty clothes? In a behavioral response class like personal hygiene, there are many possible responses along several dimensions that require assessment.

There may be an overlap as to the categories of negative symptomatology as well. “Asociality” can be an aspect of anhedonia or alogia. A person living with SMI may avoid social interaction because she does not have the skills to carry on a conversation or get negative feedback from others about her ability to talk and converse. The deficits are a part of a response class of social and conversational skills. Individuals living with difficulties in social skills would avoid a situation if the outcome or consequence was not positive and enjoyable. Behavior is displayed in situations that have a history of being reinforced. If the recent history of the individual living with SMI engaging in a specific behavior class has resulted in consequences that are punitive—or does not occasionally result in positive reinforcement—then the chances of the person engaging in that response class would decrease. The person living with SMI may not have opportunities to experience new situations or has “lost interest” in formerly reinforcing events because of not having the ability or resources to engage in those activities, such as recreational activities. The result would be an absence of behaviors in the context in which the behavior response class was not reinforced; the absence of the expected behaviors would be labeled as anhedonia, avolition, or asociality.

A possible interaction of positive and negative symptoms can impact the dimensions of either type of symptoms. A lack of awareness of positive symptoms being displayed in certain contexts can lead to problems in rehabilitation and recovery efforts; if an individual is not aware that she is talking and laughing loudly to herself while riding public transportation, other riders may become annoyed with her behavior and complain to authorities. If this happens in a social setting, there is a greater chance that others may avoid interacting with her; some may make punitive comments (e.g., "Why was she invited here? She is crazy and is scaring everyone."). Such a scenario also increases the stigmatization of the person.

Research has shown that certain dimensions of hallucinatory behaviors and delusional beliefs contribute to the chances of aggressive behavior being displayed (Appelbaum et al., 1999; Brucato et al., 2017). Use of substances also interact with the frequency and intensity of positive behaviors being displayed, including aggressive behaviors (RachBeisel et al., 1999). Command hallucinations can result in aggressive behaviors being displayed either toward self or others (Andrew, 2010). Delusional beliefs can have an impact on some of the dimensions of behavioral response classes of negative symptoms. For example, an individual may have paranoid beliefs that staff are attempting to hurt him. He may refuse to accept medications from certain staff members or interact with certain staff. The behavioral response class of daily hygiene may not be displayed as the person living with SMI may have the delusional belief that soap is harmful to his skin and hair. The interactions between positive and negative symptoms may make the treatment of the positive and negative symptoms more difficult. However, change can occur with collaboration among the service providers and the individual living with SMI in establishing person-centered support plans.

Other categories of negative symptoms cited in the literature include a lack of "ideational richness" and "deterioration in role functioning" (Piskulic et al., 2012). Research into negative symptoms in people living with SMI have included cognitive problems in attention and concentration. A lack of awareness of the deficits (i.e., anosognosia) has been identified as a negative symptom by some researchers (Mader & Galderisi, 2017). Brucato et al. (2017) reported that high ratings on social anhedonia, deficits in ideational richness, odd behavior or dress, and problems with attention and concentration significantly differentiated people living with SMI from others having mental health problems; the individuals experiencing the above-mentioned negative symptoms continue to experience problems in their recovery after discharge from a psychiatric admission.

The literature in negative symptoms have looked at the overlap between symptoms associated with depressive mental health problems and negative symptoms in mental health conditions, particularly psychotic-type mental health problems; the negative symptoms pertaining to psychomotor problems including avolition, disturbances in affective expressions, and poverty of speech or alogia are also problematic in persons living with a severe depressive conditions (Chaturvedi & Sarmukaddam, 1985; Pogue & Harrow, 1984). Negative symptoms are similar in severity and frequency in people living with either major depressive (MDD) or schizophrenia spectrum (SSD) mental health problems. The results have shown that negative symptoms are associated with the mood component in MDD. As the mood improves, the negative symptoms displayed in MDD improve. This is not the case with people living with SSD. There appears to be an enduring dimension of negative symptoms that is reported by the person as well as relatives; the negative symptoms are reported to be present 12 months prior to the first reported psychiatric admission whereas the negative symptoms associated with MDD do not intensify in severity until 3 months prior to a psychiatric admission (Bottlender et al., 2003); negative symptoms are similar on many behavioral dimensions during a mental health crisis for individuals living with MDD or SDD. Improvement occurs in the negative symptoms of MDD but the absence of behavior—negative symptoms—are persistent in people living with SDD. It appears that negative symptoms—deficits in adaptive functioning—continue to be a pervasive and persistent aspect of the mental health problem for individuals living with SDD.

An aspect of negative symptoms in individuals living with SMI are the problems in the areas of psychosocial functioning. Many areas of functioning are negatively affected by SMI, including activities of daily living (ADLs), vocational pursuits, academic role functioning, the ability to complete goals, managing finances, social and family relationships, leisure activities, taking care of one's possessions, and behaviors related to wellness and accessing health care (Brown & Velligan, 2016; Donat & McKeegan, 1990; Harvey & Strassnig, 2012). A study by Rubin and Panzano (2002) assessed a large catchment area in a mid-Western state using a rating scale completed by the case managers for over 3600 clients receiving mental health care. The results showed that the range of individuals living with SMI needing daily supervision in functional behaviors ranged from 15% to 29% of the sample. The assessment covered basic living skills, community resource use, medication management, and leisure or work activities. It was noted that those with the highest level of disability lived with family or in residential facilities.

The difficulties in functional capacities that are common in individuals living with SMI are persistent and not amenable to change with medications. Although positive symptoms may decrease along the behavioral dimensions cited above when the person living with SMI adheres to prescribed medications, the functional capacities of the individuals living with SMI remain unaltered (Harvey et al., 2011). Additionally, the functional issues presented have related contexts and outcomes in real-world situations. Individuals living with SMI have reduced opportunities to engage in mutually reinforcing social interactions. Meaningful academic and vocational opportunities are likewise diminished given the stigma associated with living with SMI. As an outcome of the lessened financial opportunities in job settings, many individuals living with SMI are dependent on disability payments; keeping those payments requires the person to continue to display functional impairments to qualify. Community resources also have limited availability to individuals living with SMI.

Assessing the problems in social functioning with people living with SMI confronts many challenges (Bellack et al., 2007; Harvey & Strassnig, 2012). A major limiting factor in the development of reliable and valid assessment instruments is the failure to develop a model of functional capacity and its primary mediators and moderators (Bellack et al., 2007). The development of reliable and valid measures of functioning is compounded by the multiple dimensions of the behavioral response classes in each of the functional capacities and the heterogeneity of functioning in individuals living with SMI.

It is difficult to capture "a snapshot" of the problems in daily functioning in an individual living with SMI given the dimensions of the various behavioral response classes involved. The domains of functional capacities in a person living with SMI are heterogeneous, complex, multidimensional, and multidirectional over the behavioral response classes that each functional impairment is constituted. The domains of diminished functional behavioral abilities and capacities are composed of several response classes that are made up of more than one behavior and vary on several behavioral dimensions.

Presently there are a plethora of instruments that are utilized. Bellack et al. (2007) concluded that every instrument has strengths and weaknesses and recommends that a multimodal and multimethod approach be used in assessing the functional problems of persons living with SMI; that is, a combination of self-reporting from the person living with SMI, surrogates and caretakers using multiple instruments and real-time observations of the functioning of the person. As the domains of functional capacities are heterogeneous and multidimensional, then the assessment needs to be individualized and based on the needs of the person living with SMI. Multimethod and multimodal individual assessment can ascertain the dimensions of the behaviors in each functional capacity on the amount of guidance and support needed for a person living with SMI to successfully initiate and complete the targeted task, the type and immediacy of reinforcement for the completion of the task to be maintained, and the need for shaping of the necessary behaviors.

The domain of psychosocial functional behaviors covers many behavioral response classes, some of which are interdependent and multidirectional; that is, improvement or impairment in one area may impact the person's ability in one or several additional areas. An example could be seen in a person's demonstrated challenge in recalling information that is verbally given to the person—someone telling her what needs to be done. The individual's problem in recalling what she has been instructed to do may interfere with her ability to function without reminders or follow-up requests in daily hygiene activities, getting to a vocational activity on time, and remembering tasks associated with the vocational activity. The assessment of a behavioral outcome being done "competently," "independently," and "completely" would be challenging unless the assessment measure was precise and the raters were reliable in understanding the criteria for each of the operationally defined concepts of competent, independent, and complete.

Items regarding functioning capacities may be general in the questions asked. For example, a question probing for the social skills may be phrased as "How do you or the person get along with others?" instead of more nuanced and detailed instances in the social skills domain. Less detailed assessment items may include phrases as "how often do you engage with others socially," "how well do you perform independent living skills," "how is the quality of your work," and "to what extent do you have problems with attention, memory, or planning that interfere with daily activities." One can substitute "you" with "the client" for the same obstacle in reports by surrogates/caretakers.

An assessment tool that includes more comprehensive questions regarding an individual's functional abilities will necessitate additional time for completion and should ensure respondents fully comprehend each item. For example, a more detailed question might include: "Do you maintain eye contact when conversing with others?" or "Do you wait until the other person has finished speaking before you respond?"

Assessing a specific behavioral response class by self-report from the person living with SMI may be unreliable given the challenges in intelligible and coherent speech as well as cognitive factors (e.g., memory) (Green, 2006; Harvey & Stassnig, 2012). Using surrogates/caretakers may be limited in the validity and reliability of the data given limitations in the opportunities to observe the person doing the targeted task or behavior across several contexts (Bellack et al., 2007).

Problems in the functional domains of neurocognition also must be considered for a complete picture of the individual's problems in psychosocial functioning. Studies have shown that individuals living with SMI demonstrate problems in composite scores on performance assessments of neurocognitive functioning. Long- and short-term memories, executive functioning and planning, vigilance, and psychomotor speed appear to be correlated with higher levels of functional capacities in certain domains (Green, 1996; Green et al., 2000; Heinrichs & Zakzanis, 1998). Executive functioning is composed of cognitive skills, such as task initiation, organization, flexibility, setting priorities, problem-solving, working memory, and control of impulsivity and emotions (Baggetta & Alexander, 2016).

However, these measures are not predictive of actual "real-life" functioning (Bowie et al., 2006; Harvey & Strassnig, 2012). Social functioning, such as interpersonal perception and interactions, have a better predictive value for adaptive functioning than scores on neuropsychological performance measures. Domains of social cognition include emotion recognition, in both visual and auditory modalities, inference of other's impressions of oneself, judgment of intentions, and other related domains appear to impact functional capacities in everyday life (Green, 1996; Harvey & Strassnig, 2012).

Self-monitoring and self-control skills are necessary skills to have and use in daily life. Both self-monitoring and self-control may be related to diminished self-awareness (e.g., "insight"); the lack of insight has similarities with the neurocognitive symptom of "anosognosia" that can be present in persons with neurogenerative disease and averse neurological events, such as CVAs (cerebrovascular accidents) and head trauma. If a person living with SMI is not aware of what they are doing, then the person is unable to monitor their behaviors; with a lack of self-monitoring, a person would have difficulty with refraining from doing a maladaptive problematic behavior and engaging in alternative adaptive behaviors. For example, when one gets angry, most individuals do not act maladaptively; they may walk away, sulk, yell, talk to others, and "basically cool off"; the context can be a "learning situation" in that the person will adjust what they will do when and if that situation repeats. When an individual is hungry, people with self-monitoring and control skills can determine when and how to reduce the impact of hunger and not act impulsively; poor self-control can result in maladaptive responses to reduce the aversive state of hunger (e.g., stealing food) and have worse aversive consequences for the individual (e.g., being arrested). Self-control skills are associated with better overall adjustment on a wide range of personal and interpersonal measures, including less alcohol use, binge eating, academic success, better emotional responses, and better interpersonal relationships (Tangney et al., 2018).

The problems with not having adequate self-control skills may be the result of an absence of certain skills. Most skills are learned from the environment; we learn what to do in situations by observing others (e.g., role-modeling), seeing what works and does not work for the role model, and engaging in the behaviors we have observed when similar situations occur. This includes cognitions (i.e., self-talk) that are associated with the behaviors as well. The behavioral responses that work are reinforced and will become part of the repertoire of skills; the behavioral responses that do not work will not be reinforced and will be extinguished…including the cognitions associated with the overt responses.

An individual living with SMI may not have had the opportunities to learn adaptive self-control skills. Many skills that are expected from functional adults are learned in mid-to-late adolescence. If the onset of living with SMI occurs during this period of adolescence, the person may not have chances to learn necessary skills. The young person living with SMI may have disruptions in their life due to being admitted to psychiatric facilities, entanglements with legal authorities, placements outside of the home and family, and problems with school attendance. The young person living with SMI may be experiencing the neurocognitive problems mentioned above such as in memory, attention, and planning; they will have fewer opportunities to engage in meaningful and practical skill acquisitions to improve quality of life. The results are the persistent and pervasive functional problems that are common across many contexts for the person living with SMI, including skills in self-control.

Summary

Individuals living with SMI display both behavioral excess and deficits across multiple domains of behaviors. The behaviors traditionally have been classified in the psychiatric literature as "positive symptoms" and "negative symptoms." Positive symptoms are behaviors that are displayed by the person living with SMI; negative symptoms are behaviors expected from functioning adults but the individual living with SMI does not engage in these behaviors at a rate, magnitude, or in the correct context. Positive and negative symptoms are transdiagnostic and heterogeneous;

that is, both types of symptoms and behaviors are an aspect of several diagnoses, including schizophrenic spectrum (SSD), affective, and personality mental health problems. Positive and negative symptoms differ in more than one dimension in persons living with SMI.

Positive symptoms include hallucinations; delusions; disorganized speech and thought processes; bizarre, abnormal, and disorganized motor behaviors; and disturbances of affective responses, including affective lability or "mood swings."

Hallucinations are perceptual experiences that occur in the absence of any external stimulus but are experienced as reality to the person. Hallucinations occur in all sensory modalities. Delusions are false beliefs that are firmly adhered to despite contrary evidence; delusions are not agreed upon by others, have incorrect reference to reality and cannot be explained by religion or culture. Delusions vary in dimensions of bizarreness, outlandishness and being unusual and eccentric. Some delusional beliefs do have elements of reality and although the beliefs may be possible, there is no supporting evidence to uphold or verify the beliefs. Hallucinations and delusions are heterogeneous on the frequency of the person acting on the hallucination or delusional belief. Lessened control occurs if the auditory hallucination is commanding or ordering the person to commit an act or if the content of the delusional belief is paranoid or of a religious nature. All positive symptoms can differ on dimensions of frequency, intensity, frequency of being reinforced in the environment and the contexts in which the symptoms are displayed.

Although not classified as "positive symptoms," both the occurrence of aggressive behaviors and substance use are problematic for individuals living with SMI. Displaying both aggressive behaviors and using substances occurs at a greater frequency and intensity in people living with SMI than for individuals not experiencing any mental health problems. Both the aggressive and substance use behavioral response classes result in deleterious outcomes for the individual living with SMI, contributing to the stigma that is experienced and interruptions in rehabilitation and recovery efforts with repeated psychiatric readmissions or even jail and prison. Aggressive and substance use behavioral response classes are heterogeneous in their display by individuals living with SMI and vary across multiple dimensions such as frequency, intensity/magnitude, and the extent of context dependency as other behavioral response classes in the positive system classifications.

Negative symptoms are persistent in individuals living with SMI and largely contribute to the stigma and disability associated with living with SMI. In the mental health literature, negative symptoms are listed in broad nonspecific categories; the negative symptoms include problems in expressing appropriate emotions; avolition; anhedonia; alogia; and asociality. Other areas may include a lack of "ideational richness" and a "deterioration in social role functioning." While psychiatric medications can improve positive symptoms in some people with SMI, negative symptoms often remain unaffected.

Negative symptoms also include the lack of functional adaptive behaviors being emitted by the person living with SMI. Negative symptoms are impairments in functional capacity to engage in adaptive behaviors expected from functioning adults in daily contexts. Negative symptoms are independent of the status of positive symptoms on multiple behavioral domains; that is, the positive symptoms that are displayed and evident have no effect on the dimensions of the negative symptoms. The absence and diminution of behavioral response classes in people living with SMI persist although the positive symptoms may improve (e.g., decrease in intensity and frequency) with treatment. The negative symptoms are composed of behavioral response classes that vary across multiple dimensions such as frequency, intensity/magnitude, extent of context dependency, need for supervision and prompting, levels of accuracy in completing the task.

The problems in functional capacity that is an aspect of negative symptoms are composed of several response classes including self-care behaviors, management of finances, academic and vocationally related behaviors, social and interpersonal skills, leisure skills, maintenance of one's own treatment and rehabilitation, lack of self-awareness (e.g., insight), self-control, and self-management. Individuals living with SMI score lower on assessments of neurocognitive abilities in attention, memory, motor speed, and executive functioning than people with no mental health problems and contribute to the treatment of the challenges in adaptive functional skills displayed by individuals living with SMI. The assessment of negative symptoms presents challenges given the complexity, multidimensionality, and heterogeneity of the behavioral response classes involved in the functional capacity domains.

Compounding the problem in the rehabilitation efforts with individuals living with SMI is the lack of opportunities to engage in adaptive learning situations in the contexts in which many people living with SMI resides. As pointed out, many individuals living with SMI resides in settings that are resource poor in leisure, academic, and vocational opportunities and impoverished in situations to engage in social interactions. An individual living with SMI may have had few opportunities to learn adaptive skills with disruptions in their life due to being admitted to psychiatric facilities, academic difficulties, entanglements with legal authorities, and problems within their families, especially when the onset of the SMI occurs during the developmental period of adolescence.

References

American Psychiatric Association. (2022). *Diagnostic and statistical manual of mental disorders* (5th ed., text rev.). https://doi.org/10.1176/appi.books.9780890425787

Allen, J. J., & Anderson, C. A. (2017). Aggression and violence: Definitions and distinctions. In P. Sturmey (Ed.), *The Wiley handbook of violence and aggression* (Vol. 1, pp. 1–14). Wiley-Blackwell. https://doi.org/10.1002/9781119057574.whbva001

Amador, X. F., & Kronengold, H. (2004). Understanding and assessing insight. In X. F. Amador & A. S. David (Eds.), *Insight and psychosis: Awareness of illness in schizophrenia and related disorders* (2nd ed., pp. 3–30). Oxford University Press. https://doi.org/10.1093/med/9780198525684.003.0001

Andreasen, N. C., & Olsen, S. (1982). Negative vs. positive schizophrenia: Definition and validation. *Archives of General Psychiatry, 39*(7), 789–794. https://doi.org/10.1001/archpsyc.1982.04290070025006

Andreasen, N. C., Flaum, M., Arndt, S., Alliger, R., & Swayze, V. W. (1991). Positive and negative symptoms: Assessment and validity. In A. Marneros, N. C. Andreasen, & M. T. Tsuang (Eds.), *Negative versus positive schizophrenia* (pp. 1–16). Springer. https://doi.org/10.1007/978-3-642-76841-5_3

Andrew, E. M. (2010). *Command hallucinations and the risks of violence and self-harm: What distinguishes compliers from non-compliers?* [Cardiff University]. ORCA. https://orca.cardiff.ac.uk/id/eprint/54381/

Appelbaum, P. S., Robbins, P. C., & Roth, L. H. (1999). Dimensional approach to delusions: Comparison across types and diagnoses. *American Journal of Psychiatry, 156*(12), 1938–1943. https://doi.org/10.1176/ajp.156.12.1938

Aynsworth, C., Collerton, D., & Dudley, R. (2017). Measures of visual hallucinations: Review and recommendations. *Clinical Psychology Review, 57*, 164–182. https://doi.org/10.1016/j.cpr.2017.05.001

Badcock, J. C., Paulik, G., & Maybery, M. T. (2011). The role of emotion regulation in auditory hallucinations. *Psychiatry Research, 185*(3), 303–308. https://doi.org/10.1016/j.psychres.2010.07.011

Baggetta, P., & Alexander, P. A. (2016). Conceptualization and operationalization of executive function. *Mind, Brain, and Education, 10*(1), 10–33. https://doi.org/10.1111/mbe.12100

Bell, V., Halligan, P., & Ellis, H. (2003). Beliefs about delusions. *The Psychologist, 16*(8), 418–423. https://www.bps.org.uk/psychologist/beliefs-about-delusions

Bellack, A. S., Green, M. F., Cook, J. A., Fenton, W., Harvey, P. D., Heaton, R. K., & Wykes, T. (2007). Assessment of community functioning in people with schizophrenia and other severe mental illnesses: A white paper based on an NIMH-sponsored workshop. *Schizophrenia Bulletin, 33*(3), 805–822. https://doi.org/10.1093/schbul/sbl035

Bhuyan, D., & Chaudhury, P. K. (2016). Nature and types of delusion in schizophrenia and mania–is there a difference. *IOSR Journal of Dental and Medical Sciences, 15*(5), 1–6. https://www.iosrjournals.org/iosr-jdms/papers/Vol15-Issue5/Version-2/A1505020106.pdf

Bottlender, R., Sato, T., Groll, C., Jager, M., Kunze, I., & Moller, H. J. (2003). Negative symptoms in depressed and schizophrenic patients: How do they differ? *Journal of Clinical Psychiatry, 64*(8), 954–958. https://www.psychiatrist.com/author/ronald-bottlender/

Bowie, C. R., Reichenberg, A., Patterson, T. L., Heaton, R. K., & Harvey, P. D. (2006). Determinants of real-world functional performance in schizophrenia subjects: Correlations with cognition, functional capacity, and symptoms. *American Journal of Psychiatry, 163*(3), 418–425. https://doi.org/10.1176/appi.ajp.163.3.418

Braham, L. G., Trower, P., & Birchwood, M. (2004). Acting on command hallucinations and dangerous behavior: A critique of the major findings in the last decade. *Clinical Psychology Review, 24*(5), 513–528. https://doi.org/10.1016/j.cpr.2004.04.002

Brown, M. A., & Velligan, D. I. (2016). Issues and developments related to assessing function in serious mental illness. *Dialogues in Clinical Neuroscience, 18*(2), 135–144. https://doi.org/10.31887/DCNS.2016.18.2/dvelligan

Brucato, G., Masucci, M. D., Arndt, L. Y., Ben-David, S., Colibazzi, T., Corcoran, C. M., Crumbley, A. H., Crump, F. M., Gill, K. E., Kimhy, D., Lister, A., Schobel, S. A., Yang, L. H., Lieberman, J. A., & Girgis, R. R. (2017). Baseline demographics, clinical features and predictors of conversion among 200 individuals in a longitudinal prospective psychosis-risk cohort. *Psychological Medicine, 47*(11), 1923–1935. https://doi.org/10.1017/S0033291717000319

Buccheri, R., Trygstad, L., & Dowling, G. (2007). Behavioral management of command hallucinations to harm in schizophrenia. *Journal of Psychosocial Nursing and Mental Health Services, 45*(9), 46–54. https://doi.org/10.3928/02793695-20070901-11

Buchanan, R. W. (2007). Persistent negative symptoms in schizophrenia: An overview. *Schizophrenia Bulletin, 33*(4), 1013–1022. https://doi.org/10.1093/schbul/sbl057

Chaturvedi, S. K., & Sarmukaddam, S. (1985). Negative symptoms in depression. *Indian Journal of Psychiatry, 27*(2), 139–144.

Cooper, J. O., Heron, T. E., & Heward, T. E. (2020). *Applied behavior analysis* (3rd ed.). Pearson. https://www.pearson.com/en-us/subject-catalog/p/applied-behavior-analysis/P200000000905/9780137477210

Correll, C. U., & Schooler, N. R. (2020). Negative symptoms in schizophrenia: A review and clinical guide for recognition, assessment, and treatment. *Neuropsychiatric Disease and Treatment, 16*, 519–534. https://doi.org/10.2147/NDT.S225643

Donat, D. C., & McKeegan, G. F. (1990). Brief report: Psychometric properties of the adaptive behavior scale with psychiatric inpatients. *Behavioral Interventions, 5*(1), 65–71. https://onlinelibrary.wiley.com/doi/10.1002/bin.2360050110

Dougher, M. J. (2013). Behaviorisms and private events. *Behavior Analysis, 36*(2), 223–227. https://doi.org/10.1007/BF03392308

Dudley, R., Aynsworth, C., Mosimann, U., Taylor, J. P., Smailes, D., Collerton, D., & Urwyler, P. (2019). A comparison of visual hallucinations across disorders. *Psychiatry Research, 272*, 86–92. https://doi.org/10.1016/j.psychres.2018.12.107

Dysinger, D. W. (1938). The fluctuations of mood. *Psychological Record, 2*, 115–123. https://doi.org/10.1007/BF03393214

Gabbey, A. E. (2022, March 3). *Aggressive behavior: Signs, causes, and treatment*. Healthline. https://www.healthline.com/health/aggressive-behavior

Galderisi, S., Mucci, A., Dollfus, S., Nordentoft, M., Falkai, P., Kaiser, S., Giordano, G. M., Vandevelde, A., Nielsen, M. Ø., Glenthøj, L. B., Sabé, M., Pezzella, P., Bitter, I., & Gaebel, W. (2021). EPA guidance on assessment of negative symptoms in schizophrenia. *European Psychiatry, 64*(1), Article e23. https://doi.org/10.1192/j.eurpsy.2021.11

Goldberg, R. W., Green-Paden, L. D., Lehman, A. F., & Gold, J. M. (2001). Correlates of insight in serious mental illness. *The Journal of Nervous and Mental Disease, 189*(3), 137–145. https://journals.lww.com/jonmd/Abstract/2001/03000/Correlates_of_Insight_in_Serious_Mental_Illness.1.aspx

Green, M. F. (1996). What are the functional consequences of neurocognitive deficits in schizophrenia? *The American Journal of Psychiatry, 153*(3), 321–330. https://doi.org/10.1176/ajp.153.3.321

Green, M. F. (2006). Cogntive impairment and fucntional outcome in schizophrenia and bipolar disorder. *Journal of Clinical Psychiatry, 67* (Suppl), 3–8

Green, M. F., Kern, R. S., Braff, D. L., & Mintz, J. (2000). Neurocognitive deficits and functional outcome in schizophrenia: Are we measuring the "right stuff"? *Schizophrenia Bulletin, 26*(1), 119–136. https://doi.org/10.1093/oxfordjournals.schbul.a033430

Gopika, G. G., Antony, S., Jayakumar, C., Moirangthem, S., Joseph, E., Gowda, G. S., & Reddi,V.S. K. (2024). Person-in-situation framework of aggression among persons with severe mental illness: A case series. *Indian Journal of Psychological Medicine, 46*(4), 358–362. https://doi.org/10.1177/02537176241251961

Harvey, P. D., & Strassnig, M. (2012). Predicting the severity of everyday functional disability in people with schizophrenia: Cognitive deficits, functional capacity, symptoms, and health status. *World Psychiatry, 11*(2), 73–79. https://doi.org/10.1016/j.wpsyc.2012.05.004

Harvey, P. D., Raykov, T., Twamley, E. W., Vella, L., Heaton, R. K., & Patterson, T. L. (2011). Validating the measurement of real-world functional outcomes: Phase I results of the VALERO study. *American Journal of Psychiatry, 168*(11), 1195–1201. https://doi.org/10.1176/appi.ajp.2011.10121723

Heinrichs, R. W., & Zakzanis, K. K. (1998). Neurocognitive deficit in schizophrenia: A quantitative review of the evidence. *Neuropsychology, 12*(3), 426–445. https://doi.org/10.1037/0894-4105.12.3.426

Høegh, M. C., Melle, I., Aminoff, S. R., Olsen, S. H., Lunding, S. H., Ueland, T., & Lagerberg, T. V. (2022). Affective lability and social functioning in severe mental disorders. *European Archives of Psychiatry and Clinical Neuroscience, 272*(5), 873–885. https://doi.org/10.1007/s00406-022-01380-1

Janaki, V., Suzaily, W., AR, A. H., Hazli, Z., & Azmawati, M. N. (2017). The dimensions of auditory hallucination in schizophrenia: Association with depressive symptoms and quality of life. *IIUM Medical Journal Malaysia, 16*(2). https://doi.org/10.31436/imjm.v16i2.325

Junginger, J., & McGuire, L. (2004). Psychotic motivation and the paradox of current research on serious mental illness and rates of violence. *Schizophrenia Bulletin, 30*(1), 21–30. https://doi.org/10.1093/oxfordjournals.schbul.a007064

Levin, H. (n.d.). *Can I drink alcohol while taking schizophrenia medications?* WebMD. https://www.webmd.com/schizophrenia/features/alcohol-schizophrenia-meds

Marder, S. R., & Galderisi, S. (2017). The current conceptualization of negative symptoms in schizophrenia. *World Psychiatry, 16*(1), 14–24. https://doi.org/10.1002/wps.20385

Marwaha, S., He, Z., Broome, M., Singh, S. P., Scott, J., Eyden, J., & Wolke, D. (2014). How is affective instability defined and measured? A systematic review. *Psychological Medicine, 44*(9), 1793–1808. https://doi.org/10.1017/S0033291713002407

Marwaha, S., Parsons, N., Flanagan, S., & Broome, M. (2013). The prevalence and clinical associations of mood instability in adults living in England: Results from the Adult Psychiatric Morbidity Survey 2007. *Psychiatry Research, 205*(3), 262–268. https://doi.org/10.1016/j.psychres.2012.09.036

Marwaha, S., Price, C., Scott, J., Weich, S., Cairns, A., Dale, J., Winsper, C., & Broome, M. R. (2018). Affective instability in those with and without mental disorders: A case control study. *Journal of Affective Disorders, 241*, 492–498. https://doi.org/10.1016/j.jad.2018.08.046

Monahan, J., Steadman, H. J., Silver, E., Appelbaum, P. S., Robbins, P. C., Mulvey, E. P., Roth, L. H., Grisso, T., Banks, S., & Simpson, J. (2001). *Rethinking risk assessment: The MacArthur study of mental disorder and violence*. Oxford University Press. https://global.oup.com/academic/product/rethinking-risk-assessment-9780195138825

Mueser, K. T., Bellack, A. S., & Brady, E. U. (1990). Hallucinations in schizophrenia. *Acta Psychiatrica Scandinavica, 82*(1), 26–29. https://doi.org/10.1111/j.1600-0447.1990.tb01350.x

Paolini, E., Moretti, P., & Compton, M. T. (2016). Delusions in first-episode psychosis: Principal component analysis of twelve types of delusions and demographic and clinical correlates of resulting domains. *Psychiatry Research, 243*, 5–13. https://doi.org/10.1016/j.psychres.2016.06.005

Piskulic, D., Addington, J., Cadenhead, K. S., Cannon, T. D., Cornblatt, B. A., Heinssen, R., & McGlashan, T. H. (2012). Negative symptoms in individuals at clinical high risk of psychosis. *Psychiatry Research, 196*(2–3), 220–224. https://doi.org/10.1016/j.psychres.2012.02.018

Pogue-Geile, M. F., & Harrow, M. (1984). Negative and positive symptoms in schizophrenia and depression: A follow-up. *Schizophrenia Bulletin, 10*(3), 371–387. https://doi.org/10.1093/schbul/10.3.371

RachBeisel, J., Scott, J., & Dixon, L. (1999). Co-occurring severe mental illness and substance use disorders: A review of recent research. *Psychiatric Services, 50*(11), 1427–1434. https://doi.org/10.1176/ps.50.11.1427

Rogers, R., Gillis, J. R., Turner, R. E., & Smith, T. (1990). The clinical presentation of command hallucinations. *American Journal of Psychiatry, 147*, 1304–1307. https://doi.org/10.1176/ajp.147.10.1304

Rubin, W. V., & Panzano, P. C. (2002). Identifying meaningful subgroups of adults with severe mental illness. *Psychiatric Services, 53*(4), 452–457. https://doi.org/10.1176/appi.ps.53.4.452

Sax, K. W., Strakowski, S. M., Keck, P. E., Upadhyaya, V. H., West, S. A., & McElroy, S. L. (1996). Relationships among negative, positive, and depressive symptoms in schizophrenia and psychotic depression. *The British Journal of Psychiatry, 168*(1), 68–71. https://doi.org/10.1192/bjp.168.1.68

Shahrokh, N. C., & Hales, R. E. (Eds.). (2003). *American psychiatric glossary* (8th ed.). American Psychiatric Publishing. https://www.appi.org/Products/Textbooks-and-References/Language-of-Mental-Health

Shawyer, F., Mackinnon, A., Farhall, J., Trauer, T., & Copolov, D. (2003). Command Hallucinations and Violence: Implications for Detention and Treatment. *Psychiatry, Psychology and Law, 10*(1), 97–107. https://doi.org/10.1375/pplt.2003.10.1.97

Siegfried, N. (1998). A review of comorbidity: Major mental illness and problematic substance use. *Australian and New Zealand Journal of Psychiatry, 32*(5), 707–717. https://doi.org/10.3109/00048679809113127

Slade, P. D., & Bentall, R. P. (1988). *Sensory deception: A scientific analysis of hallucination*. Johns Hopkins University Press. https://www.press.jhu.edu/books

Stone, A. A., Smyth, J. M., Pickering, T., & Schwartz, J. (1996). Daily mood variability: Form of diurnal patterns and determinants of diurnal patterns. *Journal of Applied Social Psychology, 26*(14), 1286–1305. https://doi.org/10.1111/j.1559-1816.1996.tb01781.x

Tangney, J. P., Boone, A. L., & Baumeister, R. F. (2018). High self-control predicts good adjustment, less pathology, better grades, and interpersonal success. In D. de Ridder, M. Adriaanse, & K. Fujita (Eds.), *Self-regulation and self-control* (pp. 173–212). Routledge. https://doi.org/10.4324/9781315175775-5

Teeple, R. C., Caplan, J. P., & Stern, T. A. (2009). Visual hallucinations: Differential diagnosis and treatment. *Primary Care Companion to the Journal of Clinical Psychiatry, 11*(1), 26–32. https://doi.org/10.4088/pcc.08r00673

Van Dorn, R., Volavka, J., & Johnson, N. (2011). Mental disorder and violence: Is there a relationship beyond substance use? *Social Psychiatry and Psychiatric Epidemiology, 47*, 487–503. https://doi.org/10.1007/s00127-011-0356-x

Virgo, G. B., Higgins, D., Bennett, L., & Thomas, P. (2001). The prevalence and characteristics of co-occurring serious mental illness (SMI) and substance abuse or dependence in the patients of Adult Mental Health and Addictions Services in eastern Dorset. *Journal of Mental Health, 10*(2), 175–188. https://doi.org/10.1080/09638230020023732

Chapter 3
Applied Behavior Analysis and Serious Mental Illness

Introduction

Serious mental illness (SMI) presents enduring challenges to adaptive functioning, social integration, and recovery. Individuals living with SMI often exhibit a complex interplay of behavioral excesses and deficits—ranging from psychotic symptoms and aggression to diminished motivation and impaired self-care—that interfere with daily living and quality of life. While pharmacological and psychotherapeutic interventions remain central to treatment, behavioral approaches offer a complementary and empirically grounded framework for understanding and modifying the environmental contingencies that sustain maladaptive behavior. Applied Behavior Analysis (ABA), rooted in the experimental analysis of behavior, provides a systematic methodology for assessing, interpreting, and intervening on the behaviors most relevant to clinical and rehabilitative outcomes in SMI.

The application of ABA in mental health settings is explored, emphasizing its utility in addressing both the overt and covert behaviors associated with SMI. Key concepts such as antecedent stimuli and conditions, motivating operations, discriminative stimuli, and reinforcement are introduced as foundational mechanisms through which behavior is shaped and maintained. The process of behavioral and functional assessments, which identify the environmental variables influencing behavior and guide the development of individualized support plans is outlined and explained. These plans aim to reduce maladaptive behaviors and promote skill acquisition, thereby enhancing autonomy, social participation, and overall well-being. The emphasis on observable, measurable behavior and data-driven decision-making distinguishes ABA as a pragmatic and person-centered approach to intervention.

Supplementary Information The online version contains supplementary material available at https://doi.org/10.1007/978-3-032-18372-9_3.

G. F. McKeegan, *Behavior Change Interventions for Serious Mental Illness*, Evidence-Based Practices in Behavioral Health,
https://doi.org/10.1007/978-3-032-18372-9_3

A comprehensive understanding of the application of behavior analytic principles is essential for effectively supporting individuals living with SMI in attaining significant and sustainable behavioral improvements. A four-part framework founded on the key principles of behavioral analysis is presented. The initial section provides a definition of ABA and places it within the wider field of behavioral science and psychiatric rehabilitation. The second part analyzes behavioral assessment methods, including operational definitions, antecedent analysis, and functional behavior assessments. The third section addresses intervention strategies, emphasizing reinforcement, skill development, and the creation of individualized support plans. The final segment reviews the implications of ABA for long-term recovery, interdisciplinary collaboration, and adherence to ethical standards in mental health practice.

Definition and Features of Applied Behavior Analysis

Applied Behavior Analysis (ABA) is an approach that deals with challenging maladaptive behaviors that are seen in many individuals with psychiatric, intellectual, and learning disorders. The objective of ABA is to decrease or extinguish challenging maladaptive behaviors and replace them with adaptive prosocial behaviors and skills that can be used to improve the quality of life of the individual living with SMI. The use of ABA principles decreases the need for more aversive, time-consuming or punishing interventions such as the use of additional medications, restriction of freedoms, being removed from programming, and other forms of coercive and restrictive techniques utilized in many settings, such as psychiatric hospitals, schools, and correctional facilities ABA focuses on what is happening or occurring around the individual (i.e., the situation or context) when the person does the challenging behavior. ABA asks the question "Why is this individual doing this specific behavior at this particular time and in this place or situation?" ABA seeks to address challenging behaviors by thoroughly examining all factors related to the individual, the circumstances preceding the behavior, and the outcomes achieved—whether these involve obtaining something desirable or avoiding an unwanted situation. This process is referred to as identifying the function of the behavior. ABA then aims to modify the environment or context in order to eliminate the necessity for challenging behavior to occur.

We do this all the time in our lives. We leave "post it" notes on our mirror in the morning because we know that is the first place we will look when we get up; we do this to make sure we do what is on the note but also to "improve our memory." If we are trying to lose weight, we may begin by keeping a "food diary" to see when, what, and how much we eat; we also may put down how we were feeling when we eat as we to become more aware that our emotions impacts our eating sometimes; we put food that is not on our diet on the upper shelves in cabinets so it takes more effort to access it to eat; if hungry, we replace high calorie food with food with less calories—and we "reinforce" ourselves with a movie or new shoes when we monitor our weight and see that we have lost a few pounds. By keeping this diary of our eating (i.e., self-monitoring), we become aware of those situations that precede our eating habits that may lead to eating high calorie foods and weight gain. We begin to change our eating habits and lose weight by changing what is occurring around us. We may do this by realizing that we tend to eat those potato chips when we are not busy and just sitting and watching television; we may become aware that when we eat the chips, we also tend to drink more soda. Since we like to watch television, we need to do something that changes what we are doing when we are eating; we may take up crocheting or play solitaire so that our hands are busy; we may place the chips on the other side of the house or out of easy access, so they are more difficult to get. We may also notice that we eat more when we are very tired and have not had a good night's sleep that day. We may take a short nap or do something relaxing before we watch television that night to make us more rested and less stressed (as not having a good sleep is an identified stressor for many). What we are doing is changing what is occurring around us to make the "maladaptive" eating behaviors less likely to occur.

In addition, ABA looks at the entire person and determines what strengths, hopes, and goals the individual brings with them to the situation that is happening around the person. ABA then uses all these factors to build new, more efficient, effective, and adaptive behaviors. ABA gives the person new skills and behaviors, so they do not have to rely on the maladaptive, challenging behaviors to either get what he wants or get her out of something that she does not want. ABA uses the strengths, hopes, and goals that the person wants to acquire; if adaptive behavior already occurs but at a low rate then the behavior needs to be reinforced or strengthened so that the more adaptive behaviors can replace the maladaptive challenging behavior that likely affects the quality of life that the person has. The use of ABA principles and technology can lead to both changes in a system (such as a ward, hospital, family, and group home) as well as changes with the individual (for example, Ayllon & Michael, 1959).

In the example of the person trying to lose weight, he notices that he eats more when he is stressed from work. He begins to realize that his job may be causing a lot of stress that is causing many unhealthy behaviors (including smoking and an occasional alcoholic drink with co-workers). The person decides that he will learn relaxation skills that he will use as soon as he gets home from work as he has become aware that he eats more on workdays and at home. Another behavior that may replace the targeted behavior of poor eating habits may be engaging in classes and learning a skill he wanted to try, such as tai chi that not only helps him to deal with the stress of his job but also may fulfill his goal of learning a martial art. He begins doing this instead of overeating. A more complicated behavior to learn may be to change jobs, go back to school and look for another career that does not cause so much stress. The key is that the person is learning a new behavior or skill to replace the maladaptive behavior of poor eating habits and overeating. His eating behaviors change without the use of extreme dieting and other punishing techniques (e.g., burning paper money when cheating occurs) or consequences, such as fasting and expensive and questionable supplements and medications that may have side effects.

What Does ABA Mean?

ABA is composed of three words that encompass what it is and what it does. The first word is "applied." The established principles of behavior change are "applied" in ABA to assist the individual in acquiring the adaptive behavior that takes the place of the maladaptive and challenging behavior. ABA uses these principles to make notable and significant changes in behaviors that impact the individual's quality of life and is acknowledged by others around the person. The interventions that come from ABA are individualized and based on an understanding of the person and their environment. The goal of ABA not only looks for the reduction and extinction of the maladaptive, challenging behavior but includes "quality of life" enhancements, such as improvements in social relationships, employment skills and opportunities, educational goals, living arrangements, spiritual needs, and other aspects of the whole person. These aspects of an individual are the positive reinforcers—or potential reinforcers—in the individual's life that can be used to change behaviors.

The second word is "behavior." ABA is based on the science and principles of the experimental analysis of behavioral or learning theory (Skinner, 1953). The principles of behavior and the application of the principles to everyday life have been studied in the field of science for well over half a century (Skinner, 1953). ABA focuses on what the person is doing and not looking for an underlying cause such as self-esteem or feelings towards one's mother. Problem behaviors have been shown to occur because it is followed by the "outcomes" or "consequences": the individual getting something positive (what he likes or wants) or escaping or avoiding something negative (what he does not like or want). By focusing on the antecedent situations and consequences of the behavior, it is possible to determine the functions of the behavior, understand what the problem behavior is likely getting the person that they want or do not want, and develop a more desired adaptive behavior able to meet the same needs of the person that the maladaptive behavior provides.

The principles of behavior have been proven repeatedly, and this technology has been used in schools, advertising, business and industry, the military, child rearing, and management. The principles of behavior are used in the training of animals both at home and for entertainment. The example used previously in losing weight is based on scientifically proven principles of behavior. ABA is the use of the principles of behavior, scientifically proven procedures, environmental/situational changes and an emphasis on outcomes that are important to the individual and society as well.

The last word in ABA is "analysis." ABA focuses on reliably demonstrating cause and effect relationships between behavior and the environment and the variables that interact with the individual in the environment. These may include other people, the physical setting, and the demands placed on the person. ABA always involves data-based decision-making, using functional behavioral assessments and ongoing monitoring of the intervention and the results. This often involves changing systems, altering environments or the situation and teaching new skills, as well as focusing on the problem behavior.

ABA looks at the whole person; ABA interventions usually consist of more than one strategy; and since it involves more than one strategy, it involves more than the provider of ABA services alone. ABA assists the service providers for the person living with SMI to work together with the individual in the center. One can view ABA plans as a circle with the individual in the center with all the stake holders—family, service providers, spiritual, occupational and academic advocates—supporting or helping individuals achieve their goals and highest quality of life whatever that may be. ABA is a collaborative effort among all individuals involved with commitment to the plan and its implementation. The ABA plan is dynamic; it is not "written in stone" and needs to change as the individual's situation and behaviors change as well, but always dictated by the individual living with SMI and observable data, and not just subjective impressions or "armchair" interventions (e.g., caregivers saying, "My parents raised me this way, and it was good enough for me."). Therefore, all service providers are seen as equal partners in implementing the ABA plan but also working collaboratively with all the other people in the individual's circle of support and change.

To summarize:

1. ABA is based on interventions in the acquisition of adaptive behaviors that take the place of the maladaptive behaviors; these behaviors are called replacement behaviors. The behaviors targeted for change need to be important to the quality of life of the individual. ABA is therefore based on person-centered values, treating the whole individual and respecting the dignity and goals of the person.
2. ABA is empirically derived and based on the principles of behavior. ABA is based on the principles of behavior, scientifically proven procedures, environmental change and an emphasis on outcomes important to the individual and society as well.
3. ABA interventions are focused on data. Interventions are based on assessments of targeted behaviors, involving when, where, and with whom the behaviors occur and what happens after the behavior occurs—the impact of the behavior on what occurs after the behavior is as well as when the targeted behavior is not exhibited. Therefore, ABA requires collaboration among all the service providers and the recovery team. ABA assessments and interventions include all those individuals who are involved with the individual and concerned about their recovery and problem behaviors and/or the absence of adaptive life enhancing behaviors that impede the recovery process.

Foundations of ABA

As stated previously, ABA is derived from the scientifically derived principles of behavior. From the study of behavior (i.e., the study of what living organisms do), it has been found that all behavior follows certain principles. One of the most important principles is that all behavior occurs as follows: there must be a situation (the antecedent) that sets up the conditions for the behavior to occur; this is then followed by the behavior, which in turn is followed by a result, a change, or a consequence in the environment that is around the person. Many individuals are familiar with the "A-B-Cs of behavior," which refers to the sequence of Antecedent (A), Behavior (B), and Consequence (C). All behaviors can be analyzed through this framework. Nevertheless, most behaviors are significantly more complex than a straightforward A-B-C pattern; they often consist of extended sequences of these events. Such intricate sequences are known as "behavioral chains."

The study of behavior is called the "experimental analysis of behavior." It studies components of complex behaviors. The study of human behavior and seeking to find ways to change behaviors is called "applied behavior assessment or analysis"—it assesses the components of the behavior that an individual is doing (that is the A-B-Cs) and assesses the relationship of each component within that particular environment for the individual; it then "analyzes" the relationship of each component to the behavior by methodically altering each component and then studying the impact of the alteration or change on the occurrence of the behavior (i.e., "behavior analysis"). It then "applies" this knowledge by changing one or more components that will have the most impact on changing the behavior of the individual in the environment or situation in which the behavior occurs. This is then "applied behavior analysis."

For example, eating a donut is seen as a simple behavior and taken for granted but it can be a behavior that is studied and changed using ABA. For a person to engage in this behavior, she must first see the donut, or it must be made available to her—that is it must be somewhere in her environment and to which she can have access. Having the stimulus of "donut" in her immediate environment—the smell of fresh donuts, seeing a box of donuts, seeing someone else with a donut or the donut in front of her, hearing the word "donut" spoken by someone—is called a "discriminative stimulus" (S^D); the absence of the stimulus "donut"—sight and smell—is the S_{delta} that is associated with the stimulus not being available (Cipani & Schock, 2010; Cooper et al., 2020).

Even before this, it is important to know the duration of time from when the person has eaten—simply put, is she hungry enough to eat a donut? The situations in the environment that impact the chances of this person eating a donut are called "motivating operations" (MOs). It assesses the value of some consequences, in this case having access to a donut. It is important to know how recently the person has eaten a donut, whether the person likes donuts (i.e., the history that the person has eating donuts; does she like donuts?) or whether the person can eat donuts due to health conditions (i.e., diabetes or swallowing difficulties) or wanting to lose weight.

MOs can increase the value of the outcome or consequence [i.e., "establishing operation" (EO)] or decrease the value [i.e., "abolishing operation" (AO)] (Cipani & Schock, 2010; Cooper et al., 2020; Whelan & Barnes-Holmes, 2010). The stimulus event in ABA is a change in the environment of the person; it can be different forms such as verbal, nonverbal, social, nonsocial, internal, and physiological. The stimuli event can act as a "signal" for a consequence, a behavior, or another signal.

These are some of the data that must be obtained during a behavior assessment. By using this data, ABA then can change each component one by one and see what effect it has on the behavior of the person eating a donut; that is, analyze what effect each change has on the occurrence of the behavior. The person can be presented with a donut after she has eaten a heavy meal; whether this has an impact on the person eating the donut can be observed. Hard and stale donuts can be made available to the individual or tell the individual that donuts are available to her, but she must go across a busy street and up five flights of stairs to get the donuts. This is changing the antecedent conditions, the MOs, and EOs. Another way is to berate, criticize, and "verbally punish" the person for "being a fat pig" after the person has eaten the donut and see whether the person will eat another donut that is given to her in the near future. This is changing the consequence. Each change in the "A" or the "C" of the "A-B-C" sequence and observing what impact the change has on whether the person engages in the behavior of donut eating (the "B") is part of behavior analysis. It becomes applied when the ABA practitioner then makes one of the changes so that the person will eat less or more donuts, whatever the goal of the change is. While donut consumption is not considered a significant challenging behavior, this example demonstrates how the principles of ABA can be effectively applied in everyday situations.

Using ABA to Intervene with Problem Behaviors Associated with SMI

SMI presents the mental health service provider with a myriad of challenges. The person living with SMI comes to the mental health service provider with severe and persistent problems; many have mental health problems that impact their ability to fulfill expected social roles. These individuals living with SMI are substantially impaired in their social, occupational, and general functioning. They are frequently admitted to inpatient psychiatry units and tend to have repeated admissions. An individual living with SMI may require a level of services in which they need to be involved with mental health centers where they receive case management and hands-on help in many areas of their lives such as taking medications, getting to appointments, or assisting with basic activities of daily living, such as showering, dressing, and cooking. To have the level of services needed, individuals living with SMI are more than likely to live in congregate living facilities with other individuals living with SMI or with family who provide the hands-on assistance the individual needs. People living with SMI usually are offered ongoing consultations for psychiatric medications and case management to assist with maneuvering through insurance, disability regulations, and applications. Outpatient individual and group therapies are sometimes offered to the person living with SMI, but availability can be a limitation (Torrey et al., 2001).

People living with SMI and their service providers face not only the social consequences of living with SMI and associated stigma but also the day-to-day challenges of living with the behavioral excesses and deficits of living with SMI. Caretakers, staff, family members, and various service providers frequently interact with people living with SMI who carry a range of mental health problems and who engage in challenging behaviors. The challenging behaviors include the positive symptoms of having SMIs such as hallucinations, delusions, disordered thinking and speaking, inappropriate affect, and disorganized or abnormal motor movements. Other problems behaviors that occur in people living with SMI include episodic aggressive behaviors, affective instability, and excessive or dangerous substance use. Rehabilitative efforts are confronted with behavioral response class deficits in activities of daily living (ADLs), vocational pursuits, academic role functioning, the ability to complete goals, managing finances, social and family relationships, leisure and social activities, taking care of one's possessions, treatment withdrawal and nonadherence, and behaviors related to wellness and accessing health care. An individual living with SMI may never have developed the necessary behavioral skills of self-awareness, self-monitoring, and self-control that would assist in rehabilitative efforts and allow the individual living with SMI to access resources in the community.

The prescribed treatment for each of these mental health problems can encompass a wide margin; consensus on the best course of action is not guaranteed. Individuals living with SMI who present symptoms of a major depressive condition will typically receive Cognitive-Behavioral Therapy (CBT) and antidepressant medications. Someone who displays symptoms of a schizophrenic spectrum mental health problems typically will receive medication as the primary (and sometimes only) intervention with supplemental case management. A person who is struggling with the co-occurring symptoms of substance "misuse" will typically receive therapy using different theoretical models and referred to a 12-step program. An individual living with an anxiety-based SMI may receive evidence-based therapy (EBT) for anxiety and an anti-anxiety medication. People living with an SMI that includes mental health problems related to personality may be provided with dialectical behavior therapy (DBT) and a cocktail of psychiatric medications including antipsychotic, antianxiety, antidepressant, and mood stabilizing medications.

ABA is a treatment approach which has its roots and is based on the principles of experimental analysis of behaviors as researched by B.F. Skinner (Skinner, 1953). ABA has been shown to be effective in ameliorating behavioral problems that are so persistent for a person living with SMI. The field of ABA was defined by a paper by Baer et al. (1968) in which the authors stated the following:

> Analytic behavioral application is the process of applying sometimes tentative principles of behavior to the improvement of specific behaviors and simultaneously evaluating whether any changes noted are indeed attributable to the process of application—and if so to what parts of that process. In short, analytic behavioral application is a self-examining, self-evaluating, discovery-oriented research procedure for studying behavior. (p. 91)

Cooper et al. (2020) defined ABA as:

> …the science in which tactics derived from the principles of behavior are applied systematically to improve socially significant behavior and experimentation is used to identify the variables responsible for the different for the behavior change. (p. 19)

The authors expounded on the definition and came up with six components that apply to the definition:

> First, applied behavior analysis is a science which means ABA practitioners are guided by the attitudes and methods of scientific inquiry. Second, all behavior change procedures are described and implemented in a systematic technological manner. Third, any means of changing behavior does not qualify as applied behavior analysis; the field circumscribes only those interventions that are conceptually derived from the basic principles of behavior. Fourth, the focus of applied behavior analysis is socially significant behavior. The fifth and sixth parts of the definition specify the twin goals of applied behavior analysis: improvement and understanding. Applied behavior analysis seeks to make meaningful improvement in important behavior and to achieve an analysis of the factors responsible for that improvement. (p. 19)

In its infancy, the scientific application of the principles of behavior expanded to include behaviors observed with individuals residing in state psychiatric facilities. Skinner applied the laboratory findings of operant conditioning at a state psychiatric facility beginning in 1953 (Rutherford, 2003). Psychotic behaviors were conceptualized and operationally defined following the principles of the experimental analysis of behavior. The application of the principles of behavior showed that the analyses and interventions were effective in reducing the occurrences of positive symptoms and increasing the occurrence of the functional behaviors that define the negative symptoms that are persistent in people living with SMI (Ayllon & Michael, 1959; Ayllon & Azrin, 1965; Bellus et al., 1999, 2003; Carey & Carey, 1999; Kazdin, 1982, 2017; Liberman, 1980; Öst et al., 1976). The principles of behavior have been utilized to alter delusional speech and hallucinatory behaviors (Layng & Andronis, 1984; Liberman et al., 1973), bizarre verbal behaviors (Wilder et al., 2001), major depressive disorder (Hopko et al., 2003), substance use (Preston et al., 2018), independent living skills (Wallace et al., 2000), polydipsia and psychotic behaviors (Pavalonis et al., 1992), negative symptoms of avolition, alogia, and functional daily living skills (Muyambi et al., 2023) and social skills (Liberman et al., 2001).

Implementation of ABA can alter the negative symptoms along the dimensions of the functional behavioral domains that are part of the clinical presentation of SMI. Given that ABA is scientifically based, what is targeted to be changed must first be clearly and concisely defined. The description of the targeted behavioral definition is a necessary step upon which all else is built. The behavior needs to be pinpointed and defined so that the picture that is painted of the targeted behavior can be observed and measured when it occurs and the intervention applied (Cipani & Schock, 2010). As the intervention is applied, the observation and measurement need to continue to ensure that the change in the targeted behavior is enduring and meaningful and if any modification in the intervention is needed as the behavior changes.

Defining Behaviors

ABA is an intervention based on scientifically based principles of behavior. An essential aspect of science is based on observable and descriptive data. Being based in science, ABA focuses on the observations of defined targeted behaviors so that it can then be determined when, where, and with whom the targeted behavior occurs (and does not occur) as well as measuring the dimensions of behavior, such as frequency, magnitude/intensity, and outcomes of behavior. Therefore, the first step is to define the targeted behavior in clear and unambiguous terms. The definition does not infer any private and internal states, events, emotions, or motivations. The behavior is "operationally defined," describing behaviors that can be objectively identified, avoiding vague or subjective terms and inferences about conditions that are not observable.

Many problematic behaviors or symptoms displayed by individuals living with SMI are multidimensional, heterogeneous, and transdiagnostic. Therefore, the operational definition needs to consider the various displays and dimensions of the targeted behaviors as well as the context in which the behaviors occur. For example, aggressive behavior is a response class that is composed of verbal and nonverbal behaviors; the aggressive behavior response class contains behaviors that may cause harm to a person, the intention to cause harm, or result in destruction of an object. However, intent is a private motivational state and should not be in any definition of a behavior; aggressive behavior may cause harm but that is an outcome of behavior and not a description of the behavior being defined. The operational definitions of aggressive behaviors in the response class are very different, yet they are all part of the behavioral response class of "aggression."

Below are some examples of the operational definition of some of the behavior that may occur in the response known as "aggression":

1. Hitting: Any occurrence of contacting any part of another person's body with an open or closed hand from a distance of 6 in. or more. An occurrence of hitting is scored as a single response unless 10 s have elapsed since the previous occurrence of hitting.
2. Kicking: Any occurrence of contacting any part of another person's body using a foot from a distance of 6 in. or more.
3. Throwing objects: Propelling objects at least 1 ft from their original location by movement of foot or leg in the direction of another person.
4. Spitting: Any occurrence of projecting matter or objects from the mouth, does not include drooling or saliva leaving the mouth during eating or speaking.

5. Throwing object: Any occurrence of propelling an object at least 1 ft from their original location by movement of hand or arm. Each object thrown is scored as another response of throwing.
6. Property destruction: Any occurrence of damaging personal or public property (e.g., breaking an object into two or more pieces, using an object to break other objects, ripping objects or parts of objects; throwing objects onto the walls, floors, or furniture and denting cars objects or walls). An episode of property destruction is scored as a single response unless at least 30 s have elapsed since the last break, tear, or dent.
7. Verbal aggression: Any occurrence of a verbal statement directed towards others that indicates any form of physical harm towards another person (e.g., "I'm going to hit you in the face!").

Positive symptoms can be similarly defined by what the observer will perceive with their senses—see, hear, smell, feel. The only way to assess a person experiencing a delusion is when the person is talking about it. Therefore, the operational definition would be "delusional speech." The following are examples of operational definitions of behaviors that are associated with positive symptoms of SMI:

- Delusional speech is any occurrence of verbal behavior that is intelligible but contextually inappropriate, events unrelated to the topic being discussed or talking about events that have not happened or are untrue as if they did happen or were true. Defining features include the fact that the belief is not one usually shared by others in one's culture nor is it credible when expressed as a value judgment, and that the person expressing the belief has difficulty in discussing the probability of the belief being true with objective facts.
- Hallucinatory behaviors can be defined behaviorally as any occurrence when a person informs another that they are experiencing a sensation when there is no external source of the sensation or behaving as if sensing something such as staring into space; gesturing, laughing or talking to oneself as if in a conversation; frequent occurrences of mumbling or smiling; rubbing body parts as if itching or something is on the skin; sniffing as if attempting to detect an odor when no odor is sensed by others; licking lips, sucking movements of the mouth or touching oral area as if tasting something.
  The definitions of hallucinatory behaviors can be refined by the type of hallucinations and the sensation the person is experiencing and reporting, whether auditory, visual, tactile, olfactory, somatic, and gustatory. An example would be an individual experiencing olfactory hallucinations, sniffing his arm and stating, "I smell rotting flesh from my arm."

Negative behaviors or the lack or absence of functional behaviors can by operationally defined according to each functional domain and the behavior in that domain. Hygiene skills entail many behaviors such taking a shower/bath; using soap and shampoo; changing dirty clothes into clean ones, brushing teeth, and grooming nails. Each of these behaviors can be operationally defined to consider the dimensions of the targeted behaviors as well as the contexts in which the behaviors do not occur but should occur. Taking a shower/bath can be operationally defined as follows:

> When asked to take a shower/bath, the person will have access to clean clothes, soap, shampoo, towel and washcloth. The person will turn on the water to adjust the temperature by placing their hand under the water and turning knob/handle to adjust temperature of water. The person will disrobe and place himself/herself into the shower area, stand under the shower water, get wet, and apply soap on the body areas by using rubbing motions of the soap, using the lather of the soap over the body. The person will use shampoo and apply it to hair and rub in the shampoo making a lather in hair. The person will rinse off the accumulated lather in hair and body areas. The person will then use a clean towel to dry off all body parts and hair with rubbing motions. The person will then put on clean clothes to which he/she has access.

Other problems in the domains of functional behaviors can be defined as well; the definitions would need to be individualized given the heterogeneity of problems in functional behaviors for individuals living with SMI. Given the example stated above, an individual may engage in the initial steps but then does not use soap or shampoo; the definition of the problems behavior needs to be modified to reflect what the individual is doing and not doing so that accurate observing and recording of the behavior can be accomplished.

Antecedents

Antecedents are defined as the stimuli that are present—or absent—in the environment of the person engaging in the behavior. As stated previously, antecedent stimuli can be anything occurring or not occurring around the person including the behavior or lack of behavior from others. Antecedents come before the targeted behavior and some "trigger" or set up the conditions for the behavior to occur. The antecedents are not a "casual factor" of the behavior but are stimuli that are present before the person engages in the behavior. For an occurrence of a behavior, there is an antecedent or a stimulus; this antecedent or stimulus may be observable; that is, it may be external. An antecedent may be a "private event" or only accessible by asking the individual (and then what the individual tells us may not be valid or true as people in general are not aware of many of their behaviors—but more about that later). For example, an individual walks to a water fountain to get a drink of water. The antecedent condition is that she has not had any fluids for a certain duration of time and is thirsty which is an internal sensation of "thirst." Not having any fluids is a motivating operation (MO) as this has increased the reinforcing properties of water. For the behavior of walking to the water fountain to occur, she must see the fountain and then engage in "self-talk" in which she tells herself that she is thirsty and that from her history she has had her thirst reduced by drinking from a water fountain. This may be one antecedent condition but there may be others. She may be on a diet and is drinking more water to help with losing weight; she may be on medication that requires her to take it at certain times with water; she may be bored (an internal condition) and she is getting a drink as her work is tedious. These are all antecedent conditions; for us to know the alternatives antecedent conditions, we must continuously observe the individual for long periods of time or ask the individual or others that are very familiar with her. These antecedent conditions of not having had any water for a while, being on a diet, needing to take a pill, or boredom are also MOs and EOs—motivating operations and establishing operations, respectively. MOs and EOs can alter the value of a stimulus such as water in the above example. The sight of a water fountain is a discriminative stimulus (S^D) for the person to engage in drinking water. MO, EO, and S^D are antecedent conditions that impact the chances of behavior occurring. If she gets a drink and is "reinforced" for her behavior of drinking from the fountain that she walked to, then the behavior occurring again has increased; if the fountain is broken and no water is available, then her using that fountain is not reinforced; her using that water fountain has decreased the next time she is experiencing thirst or one of the other MOs stated. If she uses that same broken water fountain again and again then that behavior is being extinguished for that particular water fountain. The sight of that water fountain is now an S^{delta} for not using that particular fountain to drink water.

Although behavior is sometimes confusing, hard to understand, and appears "to come out of the blue," it always has a purpose—that is, it has an impact on something that effects the condition of the individual by either getting what the individual wants (i.e., pleasurable) or getting rid of a condition that the individual does not want (i.e., aversive). This is the "function of a behavior."

Behavior occurs because it works for that individual in that situation. Because it works for the individual the behavior is more than likely to occur again. Some behavior may cause others grief, dismay, or consternation but it works for that individual in that moment. All behavior has a "consequence" or an effect on the condition of the individual doing the behavior. In the example above, the individual goes to the water fountain and drinks some water. The consequence may be that it decreases her thirst (an internal condition) or temporarily decreases her boredom with her work as she gets a "break" by going to the water fountain; another consequence is that she takes her medication and she tells herself that the medication will make her feel better; a consequence may be that this particular water fountain has very cold, good tasting water and she has had a drink from that fountain before and really likes the taste of the water. These are all possible consequences for the behavior and the different functions of the same behavior of getting a drink from that water fountain. In summary, one behavior can serve different functions in different situations by either getting the individual what they desire or like or getting rid of or decreasing what the individual does not like or desire. The function of a behavior depends on the consequences for that behavior for that individual in that context.

Consequences

All behavior affects the environment (what is occurring around us) through "consequences"; a consequence is what happens in the environment after a behavior occurs. Every behavior influences what is going on around us either externally or internally; that is,

(a) The effect is observed with our senses. We turn on a cold-water faucet and we can see the water coming out, hear it and feel it with our fingers.
(b) The effect alters an internal sensation, feeling, and thoughts (i.e., private events) that only can be accessed or known by asking the individual or by self-report (i.e., the individual telling us what is going on inside her). For example, we drink a glass of water, and we say to ourselves (or someone else) that it tastes good and cold and that it quenches our thirst.
(c) The effect may have collateral behaviors associated with the consequence that can be observed if the consequence impacts a "private event." Using the example above, the person drinks a glass of water; the person is asked if she wants another glass or has her thirst been satisfied. If she says that she is no longer thirsty (a change in the MO/EO), we can continue to observe her behavior to see if she returns in a short period to get more water, asks for more water, licks her lips, and other behaviors associated with thirst. By continued observation we can gather data about the reliability and validity of her self-report of thirst. Continued observation of her behavior that asking for water may be a way to get attention from the person or "escaping" from the request (i.e., demand) of doing a task that she is being prompted to do (such as eating the vegetables on her plate).

People learn several things when interacting with the environment around them. They learn that certain behaviors in certain situations lead to certain consequences (i.e., S^D). This occurs all the time, whether we are aware of it or not. We scratch an area on our body and the feeling of an itch decreases; we say something funny and others laugh; we put change into a soda machine, push a button and a cold bottle of soda comes out; we push a light switch and the light in the room comes on. These are all consequences of our actions or behaviors.

The consequences after an occurrence of a behavior make it more or less likely that the behavior will happen again in the future. If the consequences of an individual's behavior are appealing/pleasurable for that individual, the individual is more likely to behave that way in the future in a similar context. If the result "works" in some way for the individual, then the behavior is "reinforced." If the individual doesn't like the results of his behavior or the results do not work for him in some way, he is less likely to perform that behavior in the near future. If the results are not appealing to the individual and the behavior does not work for him, then the consequence is punitive or aversive for the individual and the chances of that behavior occurring again decrease. For example, a student realizes that if he does well on an assignment, then she will get a neat sticker that he likes. If the student does well on future assignments, then the sticker is a "reinforcement" as the chances of the student doing well on assignments has increased; the sticker is a "reinforcing consequence." Another student discovers that if she speaks out when the teacher is talking that she will receive reduced recess time that she really enjoys and looks forward to. If the student refrains from talking the next time the teacher is talking, then removing recess time is a "punishing consequence" as the consequence resulted in decreasing the chances of the student talking when the teacher is speaking. Removing recess time is labeled a punishment as it resulted in the decrease in the chance of the targeted behavior being emitted in the near future.

There are three kinds of consequences: reinforcing (or rewarding), punishing, and extinction (which is withholding a consequence after a targeted behavior occurs). Whether a consequence is reinforcing or punishing depends on the effect the consequence has on the probability of the behavior occurring in the near future. If the chances increase, then the consequence is "reinforcing"; the process is labeled "reinforcement" if the presentation of the consequential stimulus results in an increase of the behavior occurring again. If the probability decreases, then the application or the presentation of the consequential stimulus is an aversive stimulus; the application of an aversive stimulus resulting in a decrease in the chances of the targeted behavior occurring again in the near future is "punishment."

Any stimulus or event that increases the probability of the behavior occurring is called "reinforcement" and any stimulus or event that decreases the probability of the behavior occurring is called "punishment." If an event, item, or stimulus is presented or access is given to the individual after the response, it is called "positive" because something is added. If something is removed from the individual after the response, it is called "negative," that is something is subtracted. "Positive" and "negative" are often confused as being value labels meaning "good" and "bad"; the terms positive and negative when used in ABA and other behavioral interventions are *not* values like good and bad but are arithmetical terms.

Below is the summary describing the outcomes which typically occur after a consequential stimulus or event:

1. A consequence which presents a stimulus that results in an increase in behavior is labeled as reinforcement.
2. A consequence which presents a stimulus that results in a decrease in a behavior is labeled as punishment.
3. A consequence which does not allow any access to previously presented stimulus that results in either an increase or decrease in the targeted behavior is labeled as extinction. Extinction is the process of removing previously presented consequential stimulus after the targeted behavior occurs. Extinction is defined as "the removal of the functional reinforcer contingent upon the target behavior occurring" (Cipani & Schock, 2010).

Below is a summary for altering the chances of behavior occurring:

1. To increase the frequency, intensity, or probability of a behavior, administer a reinforcer following its occurrence.

2. To decrease the frequency, intensity, or likelihood of a behavior, apply a punishment when the behavior is exhibited.
3. If the objective is to eliminate a behavior entirely (i.e., to extinguish it), refrain from providing any positive consequence upon its occurrence, such as by withholding attention or reinforcement.

Table 3.1 presents the 4×4 contingency matrix for consequences that follows a behavioral analytic framework. Each square in the table gives the technical term, the effect on the behavior following the consequence, and an example. Each square gives one possibility of how the chances of a behavior occurring is either increased or decreased. For example, if an individual's rate of doing a behavior increases after a consequence is presented, we say that positive reinforcement has occurred; if it decreases then punishment has occurred. During extinction, there is initially a rapid rate of responding of the targeted behavior when the previous consequence is no longer available (i.e., extinction burst). The behavior will continue for a while but decrease as exposure to new contingency proceeds (Lattal et al., 2013).

We have used the behavior of going to the water fountain to get a drink of water to show that behaviors follow certain principles; that is something occurs or happens around the individual before the behavior (an antecedent) which is followed by a behavior which is then followed by an effect on the condition or the environment of the individual doing the behavior by either getting what the individual wants or likes or decreasing what the individual does not want or like (the function of the behavior). All behavior—simple or complex—follows the same principles. Because all behavior follows these principles, then all behavior can be changed by using the principles. If we become aware or knowledgeable about these aspects of targeted behavior, then manipulating the antecedents or the consequences can result in changing the occurrence of a behavior.

Using the example of the drinking from a water fountain, if that fountain sporadically works and delivers water and then does not, the person is being placed on a "intermittent schedule" of reinforcement and the behavior will continue. This

Table 3.1 A 4×4 contingency matrix for consequences

Stimulus	Give (+) or present	Take away (−) or remove
Consequence	Positive reinforcement	Negative reinforcement
Desired, pleasant, liked	The effect of the behavior is to increase the chances of the behavior occurring again. Example: being told thank you for holding the door open for another	The effect of the behavior is to decrease the chances of the behavior occurring again. Example: getting a ticket after speeding
	Positive punishment	Negative punishment
Undesired, aversive, disliked	The effect of the behavior is to decrease the chances of the behavior occurring again. Example: getting yelled at by your significant other for coming home late	The effect of the behavior is to increase the chances of the behavior occurring again. Example: having a headache go away after taking pain medication

schedule of reinforcement is an important principle of behavior; behaviors that are difficult to extinguish and occur at relatively high rate have been likely reinforced on an intermittent schedule. An intermittent schedule delivers reinforcement at unpredictable intervals, which encourages continued engagement due to the uncertainty of when a reward will occur.

If we were able to continuously observe the individual, then we would be able to understand a person's behavior and even predict when the behavior would occur given certain conditions. By knowing the antecedent, consequence, and function of a behavior, we also can alter or change the response by changing either the antecedent or the consequence. By changing the antecedent, the chances of the individual engaging in going to the water fountain can be changed. We can remove the water fountain, so she cannot engage in the behavior. We can make the room very warm and dry where the individual is working, thereby increasing her thirst by making her sweat more; we can increase the frequency of this behavior by increasing or decreasing the tediousness of the task that she is doing if she goes to the water fountain because of boredom. The rate of the person using the fountain can be altered by controlling when the water fountain delivers water when she goes to it. In summary, the behavior can be changed by observing the conditions when it occurs, becoming familiar with the antecedent conditions and manipulating the antecedent conditions and the consequences of going to the water fountain.

The response of going to the water fountain to get a drink can be replaced by teaching the new behavior of the individual asking for water, having scheduled breaks during which she can get a drink, provide water, or teach the individual to bring her own bottled water. All of these are replacement behaviors that serve the same functions—quenching thirst, decreasing boredom by having scheduled breaks, getting attention by asking for water. The replacement behaviors need to serve the same function as the behavior for which it is being replaced.

Skill building or teaching new behavior to take the place of a targeted behavior is essential in using ABA with people living with SMI (Bellack, 2004; Lyman et al., 2014; Pratt et al., 2017). It has been pointed out that some skills may have not been able to develop with the individual living with SMI depending on the onset of the SMI. The skills may have been learned but have not been reinforced since the onset of the SMI because of the situations in which the person living with SMI resides. Early onset of SMI may result in lack of opportunities to develop necessary skills to live and meet personal and other's expectations. There are deficits in MOs and EOs—MOs because of deficits in learning opportunities, EOs because of deficits in the limiting situations where the individual resides to display the appropriate behaviors; deficits in learning life skills may occur due to neurocognitive problems in SMI. There is a lack of naturally occurring reinforcers with behaviors if one is unsheltered, incarcerated or on a psychiatric unit. Many life skills that are expected from adults are not reinforced in the deprived environments in which many individuals living with SMI reside and at times are punished and extinguished by the environment.

Observing the targeted behavior will assist in gathering data about the dimensions of the targeted behavior for that individual. Individuals living with SMI may have the responses in their repertoires but the responses in one or more dimensions of the behavioral domain are not engaged in. If this is the scenario, then prompting the responses to occur and reinforcing the occurrence of the responses may alleviate the problem (Goldiamond, 2022). If the responses are lacking in the individual's repertoire, then a task analysis needs to be done to ascertain what responses are needed for the task to be accomplished. Depending on the steps in the task, skill building involves behavioral instruction for each step, role modeling, rehearsal, corrective feedback, prompting, and reinforcement. It is important that the responses for each skill be prompted and reinforced in the context in which the responses are to occur so that the antecedent conditions—the S^D and S_{delta}—will have control over the occurrence of the responses.

Assessment

ABA involves the individual from the beginning and views the person as center in the entire process—the person's behavior, situation, skills, likes, physical history, medications, success and failure, aspirations, and goals. It attempts to find out the antecedent conditions and environmental variables that affect the occurrence of the behavior; the ABA process focuses on the individual within the environment in which the behavior occurs and attempts to change the environment so that the challenging behavior no longer needs to occur—by changing the antecedents or context in which the behavior occurs, the behavior becomes unnecessary as the person no longer needs to engage in the behavior to get their needs communicated and met. ABA focuses on changing antecedent conditions and environmental variables to change the occurrence of challenging behaviors. The ABA process also looks for enduring changes in behaviors by assessing what skills the person may need to acquire so that the person can engage in adaptive behaviors without the use of artificially applied consequences. ABA looks to the natural social environment in which the individual resides as providing the consequences for adaptive prosocial behaviors so the more adaptive behaviors can be maintained.

The ABA service provider must first obtain data about the individual living with SMI, the dimensions of the problem behavior, and the environment in which the behavior is displayed. Initially the ABA service provider should observe the person and the behavior in the context in which it occurs to become aware of future challenges. A thorough review of available records should be undertaken to gather data about variables that may be significantly affecting the problem behavior; a few areas that should be investigated include medical history, academic and occupational history, history of trauma, admissions to facilities, legal problems, medications and their effects, side effects, cultural and spiritual background.

Functional Behavior Assessment

Functional Behavior Assessment (FBA) is a process for collecting information. The priority when conducting a functional behavioral assessment is on identifying significant, person-specific social, emotional, and/or environmental factors associated with the occurrence (and nonoccurrence) of specific behaviors.

All behaviors serve a function. Problem behaviors serve a function, or purpose, for the targeted individual in a specific context or situation. The FBA asks the question "why" the individual living with SMI is doing the behavior—what the purpose is, how is this challenging behavior serving the needs or wants of the person in the context. FBA assumes that challenging behavior is an individual's attempt to adapt to a specific situation. What the individual does (the behavior) and why the individual does it (the function) may be unrelated. Hitting another person may be the same behavior yet serve two very different functions in different settings. An individual living with SMI may hit another person to get out of a demand like going to a group, taking a shower or going to a discharge placement; the same individual may hit another to get attention from staff when the staff are busy with other residents. A person experiencing "paranoid delusions" that other people want to hurt him kicks a staff member; the consequence is that the staff will avoid that person living with SMI and not interact with him in the immediate future; according to his false belief, by engaging in aggressive behavior decreases the chances that he may get hit. The function of the behavior of hitting others is negatively reinforced (escaping from demands) in one setting but positively reinforced in another (getting attention). In the last example, the aggressive behavior of kicking is negatively reinforced as it removes—temporarily—a perceived threat and reduces the distress the person living with SMI may be experiencing. Once the function of the behavior is understood in different settings, adaptive replacement skill-oriented behaviors can be taught, prompted, and reinforced to replace the targeted challenging behavior.

In conducting an FBA, information is gathered that helps to understand how the behavior serves as a useful function for the targeted individual. In basic terms, an FBA is a process for collecting information to help determine why a problem behavior occurs and to serve as a basis for the development of a strategy to change the problem behavior. The data collected are used to help determine why problematic behaviors occur. The data will also help identify ways to address the behavior. Relevant studies analyzing the effectiveness of FBA provides convincing evidence of its utility for identifying functions of behavior and for developing effective interventions for challenging behaviors (Froján-Parga et al., 2019; Harvey et al., 2009).

FBAs also help to identify other variables that impact the person living with SMI, such as medical conditions, cultural and spiritual issues, language, sensory issues, neurocognitive functioning, academic, social, and occupational functioning. FBAs can provide the service provider with medications being prescribed as well as the side effects and the impact side effects have on the person living with SMI.

According to Cooper et al. (2020), the FBA aims to:

1. Define behavior in specific, objective, and measurable terms.
2. Determine what aspects of the environment or situation elicit the behavior.
3. Identify what consequences maintain the behavior.
4. Identify behaviors displayed that can be promoted and reinforced as an adaptive replacement.
5. Identify what behavioral skills the individual lacks or not displaying at an adequate rate.
6. Identify reinforcers that are available in the environment.

Once the function of the behavior is understood for the individual, then service providers assist the individual:

1. Change aspects of the situation or the context that are antecedents of the behavior.
2. Promote more adaptive behaviors that have the same function by teaching and the development of alternative behaviors and skills.
3. Modify the responses of other people to their behaviors.

Interviews

Important sources of information are from persons that are involved everyday with the individual living with SMI; these persons may include parents, group home staff, day program staff, staff in an institution, case managers, and other service providers who are familiar with the person living with SMI; these interviewees can be very familiar with the problem behavior being displayed, the functional capabilities of the person living with SMI, as well as the environmental variables and consequences impacting the problem behavior. Those interviewed should be knowledgeable about the person, their likes and dislikes, how the individual responds to certain situations, and the individual's routine.

An instrument that is used when conducting an FBA is the Functional Assessment Instrument—Mental Health Version (FAI-MH) (see Appendix A). This interview instrument guides the interviewee as to what areas need to be explored with the interviewer. The FAI asks the interviewee about:

(a) Specifics about the challenging behavior.
(b) Medications and health issues, diagnoses.
(c) The targeted individual's routine.
(d) What makes the behavior more and less frequent.
(e) Identification of general physical and environmental conditions that may be settings events and antecedent conditions.
(f) Identifications of possible functions of the behaviors and their relations to outcomes and consequences.
(g) How the indexed individual might respond in certain hypothetical situations so certain functions may be ascertained.

Once these data are collected, the interviewer may want to explore certain areas in depth using either more interview questions, instruments of observations, or rating scales. The data from the FAI is used as a "jumping off point" for further and more specific data collections. More than two people should be interviewed; the interviewees should be people who observe and interact with the individual in various settings and circumstances, so a range of observations are collected. The FAI also can be used to interview the individual. The FAI-MH is in the Appendix.

Another instrument is the Open-ended Functional Assessment Interview developed by Hanley (2012) (see Appendix B). It was originally developed for children with behavioral disturbances but can be easily adapted for adults. An edited version for adults living with SMI is available in the Appendix.

When conducting an interview-based FBA (Hanley, 2012), the ABA service provider should conduct an interview asking simple open-ended questions separately about variables. Responses to the questions can generate a "hunch"—hypothesis—to the ABA service provider about variables that influence the problem behavior; each of the hypotheses generated from the responses to the question can be analyzed and tested in a systematic fashion. Confirmed hypotheses can establish a baseline from which to assess a function-based intervention. It is important to ask simple questions about the variables that are most likely influencing behavior and initially test the variables that appear most important. Questions can be asked in more than one interview as well as other questions that develop over the course of the assessment as the FBA is flexible and individualized. He stated that no single analysis can determine all the environmental factors influencing a problem behavior and no analysis can test all the possible contingencies (Hanley, 2012). In conducting an assessment, Hanley suggested the following:

> Start with a structured, but open-ended, interview and a brief observation to discover potential factors that may be influencing problem behavior and then conduct a precise and individualized functional analysis based on the resultant information to examine the relevance of those discoveries. (2012, p. 58)

The FBA uses data from several sources, including records. Interviews can offer information, but the reliability and validity of the data received from interviews may be questionable given the problems with memory, attention, and speech that individuals living with SMI may display as well as other respondents. The interviewer needs to have skill in conducting clinical interviews. When conducting a clinical interview, it is imperative to establish rapport with the interviewee, have active listening skills, and be compassionate and humble during the interview. The interviewer is learning from the interviewee while conducting the FBA.

Direct Observations

It is imperative that data be collected from observing the behavior once it is clearly and operationally defined and hypotheses are derived from data obtained from the FBA. The responses on the FBA assist in making direct observations with the individual displaying the targeted behavior in the different settings in which the behavior is displayed. It is important to make observations in settings and times during which the challenging behavior has more and less of a chance of occurring. The responses from the FBA will provide data as to what to look for and where to start in observing the targeted behavior.

A "scatter plot" (see Appendix C) (Touchette et al., 1985) can make patterns of responding identifiable and, in turn, suggest environmental features that occasion undesirable behavior. The scatter plot can be used during the initial data collection to begin to understand some of the structure of the behavior—the when, where, and with whom. The data from the scatter plot can be used to determine when and where to observe the targeted individual to see what is occurring, how do others around the individual respond when the challenging behavior occurs and begin to make hypotheses about the purpose of the function of the challenging behavior. An example of a completed scatterplot is in Appendix D.

Other instruments that are used for observations include the ABC Log and the Maladaptive Behavior Rating Scale (MBRS).

ABC Log

The ABC log is used to observe observations of the pattern of antecedents and consequences that occur when the targeted behavior occurs. Observations should be conducted during those times that there are greater and lesser chances of the identified challenging behavior (usually derived from the scatterplot) so that the antecedents and consequences during those times can be contrasted; the ABC log addresses the questions as to what the differences in stimuli in those circumstances or situations are during which the challenging behavior does and does not occur. Using the ABC log, the observer records the date, time, the setting, and the person observing and recording; when the challenging behavior occurs, the observer records what was occurring immediately before and what occurred immediately after the identified behavior happened. The observer must be neutral during these observations and must act like a "camera"—just putting down what was seen and heard and no inferences, motivations, or other "private events" that are not actually seen or heard. The observer cannot record that the antecedent for slamming a bedroom door forcefully was that "Sean was angry because he was woken up" but simply, "Penelope (staff member) called Sean's name and touched his shoulder to awaken him; Sean rose out of bed and walked to door and slammed it forcefully 4 times." Using the same example, the consequence may be "Penelope loudly told him to stop and go to the bathroom 5 times before Sean stopped and walked to the bathroom"; it would be incorrect to record, "Sean was looking for attention and banged the door several times."

Below is an example of an ABC log for Peter who displays the behavior of "slapping others." From the ten observed incidents of Peter slapping others, one can calculate that six out of the ten occurrences of the identified behavior happened after Peter was told to "go back to work." Peter would be told to return to work, and he would slap staff. The observations showed that after Peter slapped staff, he would not return to work and would spend time away from the work situation or leave altogether (observation # 2). The consequence was that he was ignored and allowed to "escape" from doing the assigned task at the workstation. From the ABC log, a hypothesis could be made that the function of Peter slapping others is effective in that it allows him to escape from the work setting.

ABC LOG
Client Name: Peter__________________
Targeted behavior: slapping others with open hand

No.	Date	Time	Setting	Person recording	Antecedent	Behavior	Consequence
1	July 7	9:46 AM	Front of work shop	Fred	Fred instructed Peter to go back to workstation.	Slapped Fred (staff) on head	Fred said nothing; Peter hung around front door; did no go to workstation.
2	July 7	10:45 AM	Coffee room	Sue	Sue told Peter that break was over and that it was time to go back to work on sorting bolts.	slapped Sue (staff) across face	Peter continued to sit in chair, Sue asked him if he would like to go outside, he agreed and went outside with Sue.
3	July 7	1:47 PM	Workstation	Sue	Fred went over to ask Peter if needed any **help**.	Slapped Fred on chest	Fred didn't say anything and Peter stopped working for 10 minutes.
4	July 7	2:41 PM	Bathroom	Fred	Fred asked Peter to leave the bathroom and go back to work.	Slapped Fred on-chest	Fred repeated request and Peter went back to work station.
5	July 8	10:02 AM	Work station	Fred	Peter was getting up from his chair; Fred instructed Peter **to** stay in his seat and continue working.	Slapped Fred across chest	Peter got up and walked around the workshop for 15 minutes before returning to workstation.
6	July 8	10:50 AM	Coffee room	Fred	Fred told peter break was over and go back to work.	Slapped Sue who was walking by	Fred repeated request and Peter went back to work.
7	July 8	11:56 AM	Workstation	Sue	Sue told another client it was almost time for lunch.	Slapped Sue on back	Sue ignored Peter and she walked away. Peter got up and went to the bathroom.

No.	Date	Time	Setting	Person recording	Antecedent	Behavior	Consequence
8	July 8	1:30 PM	Lunchroom	Sue	Group told that lunch was over and to go back to workstations.	Slapped Fred on chest,.,	Fred repeated request directly to Peter; Peter remained in his seat for 15 minutes and then got up and wandered around lunchroom.
9	July 8	3:20 PM	Outside bath room	Sue	Sue walked by Peter.	Reached out arm and slapped Sue across back as she walked by	Sue ignored Peter and walked away. Peter got up and went to the bathroom for 10 minutes.
10	July 8.	3:45 PM	Outside	Sue	Sue said, "Goodbye, see you tomorrow" to Peter.	slapped Sue across chest	Sue ignored Peter; Peter got on the van.

The ABC log enables the observer to organize their observations when recording. Preferably at least 14 incidents of the targeted challenging behavior should be observed until consistent and accurate antecedents and consequences are shown. A blank copy of the ABC log is in Appendix E.

The data from the scatterplot helps to make the periods of observation more efficient in that the scatterplot helps to ascertain those times and setting during which the targeted behavior is most and least likely to occur. However, there are times when one is not able to conduct a scatterplot; archival records are not always readily available, especially if the FBA is conducted in the community. Service providers for individuals with challenging behaviors seldom keep reliable records or charts as recording naturalistic observations is a skill that needs to be taught and learned. There may be times when observations cannot be conducted as they may intrude on the privacy of others. The service provider then must rely on the observations of other people who are in contact with the person living with SMI and teach them how to conduct observations using observational instruments like the Scatterplot and the ABC log.

Maladaptive Behavior Rating Scale (MBRS)

Another way is to have the people observing the person displaying the targeted behavior record the data on the Maladaptive Behavior Rating Scale (MBRS). There are specific antecedents, behaviors, and consequences listed under each column. The examples for the antecedents, behaviors, and consequences are derived from reviewing any records available as well as conducting semi-structured interviews with the person living with SMI and those familiar with the person and the targeted behavior. The data collected from these sources using interviews, the MBRS is developed and given to those who will be observing and interacting with the individual living with SMI during a "routine" day in the setting in which the targeted behaviors occur. When one of the behaviors listed happens, the observer puts in the time and date and checks off what behavior occurred and the observed antecedent and consequence. For each incidence of behavior, there is one MBRS completed. The completed MBRS data cards are then collected in a specific location to analyze the data.

An example of a MBRS is below using the data from the ABC log on Peter. The completed MBRS form is based on the observation of Peter's slapping behavior at 3:20 PM. The MBRS is "tailored" to the data obtained from the FBA and other records and observations. A blank copy of a MBRS is in Appendix F.

Rating Scales

Rating scales are devices that are used to observe and record the occurrence of specific behaviors. Rating scales and checklists are used to obtain information from an individual living with SMI and service providers familiar with the person and their behaviors in various settings. Rating scales ask the respondent to "rate" their observations of the individual's occurrence of the identified challenging behaviors. For example, rating scales may ask the respondent if the targeted individual does the challenging behavior in a certain setting or situation and then requests the respondent to "rate" how frequently the behavior occurs in those situations from "none" to "all the time." Whereas direct observations record the relevant aspects and dimensions of the targeted behavior pertaining to when and where it occurs and the consequences of the behavior, rating scales ask the respondent to reconstitute or "think back" about the occurrences of the challenging behavior. As a result, rating scales have problems with valid and impartial reports of the problem behaviors as the ratings depend on the rater's recall of events. As was mentioned previously, personal feelings and opinions may at times "contaminate" retrospective reports of behaviors of the individual who is displaying the targeted behavior. Nevertheless, rating instruments are an important part of an FBA but are only one component of a comprehensive FBA, which includes observations, record reviews, and semi-structured interviews.

One instrument that has been used in conducting an FBA is the Questions About Behavior Functioning—Mental Ill version (QABF-MI) (Singh et al., 2006). The rating scale (see Appendix H) is a 25-item rating scale developed to identify the function(s) of one problem behavior displayed by individuals living with SMI. This rating scale asks the respondent—persons who are familiar with the individual in certain settings—to rate how frequently certain behaviors happen within certain situations, such as being alone and being physically ill. The rating scale ranges from

"0 = does not apply" to "4 = often." The responses are subsequently totaled based on the specific function each item is designed to assess. There are five functions which the questions attempt to assess—social attention; escape from demands (i.e., situations, tasks, demands); nonsocial (i.e., the individual is responding to auditory hallucinations, acting on delusions, changing environmental stimulation); physical (i.e., being ill or having medication side-effects such as disinhibition); and tangible (i.e., trying or getting an desired item or activity). As with any measure, it is important to get more than one respondent who is familiar with the individual displaying the targeted behavior in or across settings or situations. A QABF-MI should be completed for each challenging behavior; it is important to have at least 5–6 QABF-MIs completed for each behavior in each setting as the functions of the behaviors are different in each situation or setting. It is important to have additional QABF-MIs completed if there is a great deal of disagreement among the respondents in each situation or setting. The QABF-MI can be charted and graphed to give the ABA service provider a visual representation of the function of the behavior across antecedents and settings which helps in generating hypotheses about functions that can be strategically analyzed across various antecedent conditions.

The QABF-MI is a useful tool for determining the nature of the variables that maintain problem behavior exhibited by individuals living with SMI. However, it is only one tool and other sources of data from other methods—observations, record review, and interviews—must be obtained and utilized in developing hypotheses about the function of the problem behavior.

Human behavior is complex. As pointed out previously, no one assessment or analysis can determine all the variables that influence the display of behaviors by individuals. The best practice is to use multimodal/multimethod approach to conducting an FBA, be flexible, develop functional hypotheses and systematically analyze the hypotheses.

Replacement Behavior and Skill Building

Living organisms are always behaving. Even when at rest, the living organism is behaving along some dimension. There is an adage in behavior analysis: behavior abhors a vacuum. If one behavior decreases because of changes in the context, situation, antecedents or consequences, then another behavior will take its place. In the context of ABA intervention, if an adaptive behavior with the same function as the targeted maladaptive behavior is not specifically identified, prompted, and reinforced to replace the maladaptive behavior, there is a risk that a more problematic behavior may emerge as the frequency or intensity of the original maladaptive behavior decreases. An adaptive replacement behavior needs to be identified through functional analysis; a plan needs to be implemented to increase the occurrence following the same antecedent conditions as with the maladaptive behavior so that there is an available behavior to "replace" the targeted maladaptive behavior.

The ABA service provider intervenes with a problem behavior by setting up conditions to decrease the targeted behavior; but since behaviors are always occurring, an adaptive behavior with the same environmental functions under the specific antecedent conditions as the targeted problem behavior needs to be designated. The behavior can be identified and designated by conducting an FBA and analyzing the antecedents and consequences of the targeted behavior to determine the function. If the individual living with an SMI is emitting the replacement behavior—that is, the behavior is in their behavioral repertoire—then the replacement behaviors can be prompted and reinforced under the same antecedent conditions. There are times, however, when the replacement behavior is not displayed in the behavioral repertoire of the person living with SMI. This behavior represents the absence in a particular skill, necessitating targeted intervention for the development of an appropriate replacement behavior. Training and instruction are required to ensure the individual acquires the desired behavioral competencies. To achieve this, Behavioral Skill Training (BST) should be implemented.

After determining the functional replacement response, a task analysis should be conducted. A task analysis is the process of breaking down a task into smaller steps to understand how to complete it. It makes the acquisition of behavior easier to teach and learn as each step builds on the success of acquiring and correctly performing previous learned steps. The components of a task are taught by "chaining" with one step building on the next. Cooper et al. (2020) defined "chaining" as follows:

> A behavior chain is a linked sequence of responses leading to a terminal outcome. Each response produces a stimulus change which functions as conditioned reinforcement for that response and as a discriminative stimulus (S^D) for the next response in the chain. Reinforcement for the last response in the chain maintains the reinforcing effectiveness of the stimulus change produced by all the previous responses in the chain. (p. 558)

An aspect of BST for serious mental health challenges is the teaching of adaptive response chains. Using BST, the ABA service provider identifies specific target skills based on the individual's needs and wants that will be socially significant and improve the quality of life of the individual living with SMI. Providing skills training requires the ABA service provider to provide clear instructions, demonstrate the behavior through modeling, facilitate practice through role-playing, and give consistent positive feedback throughout the training process. The approach of training specific skills needs to be tailored to consider the neurocognitive abilities of the person living with SMI and ensuring a supportive and structured environment.

The sequence in BST is:

1. Assess and identify specific skills that would have a beneficial impact on the individual's daily functioning and quality of life.
2. Collaborate with the individual and other service providers to set realistic and achievable goals based on the individual's desires and needs.
3. Select the skill that would have a significant positive impact on the life of the individual living with SMI.

4. After selecting the skill, use task analysis (Cooper et al., 2020) to "chunk" the skill into smaller steps that can be learned. Make sure that all the steps that compose the skill are included.
5. Use clear and simple instructions; provide clear and concise verbal instructions explaining the target responses for the skill.
6. Provide training one step at a time and use modeling for each behavior; ask the person to imitate the modeled behavior.
7. Use graduated prompting—verbal, nonverbal, gestural, and physical guidance—to ensure that the individual living with SMI is displaying the correct responses.
8. Demonstrate the skill through role-playing, making the desired behavior clear to the person living with SMI.
9. Practice and rehearse through role playing. Encourage participation by having the individual practice the skill in a simulated situation through role-playing. Vary scenarios (i.e., antecedent conditions) promoting generalization to real-life situations.
10. Give corrective feedback and reinforcement, both verbal and tangible.
11. Provide immediate, specific, and positive feedback throughout practice sessions, highlighting areas of improvement. Providing frequent reinforcement is imperative to build novel responses. Use strategies like praise, encouragement, and positive reinforcement to motivate the individual.
12. Use gradual progression in teaching each skill component:

    (a) Begin with simple skills and gradually increase complexity as the individual demonstrates proficiency.
    (b) Incorporate real-life situations and practice opportunities to facilitate generalization to real-life contexts.
    (c) Identify positive consequences for displaying the skill in real-life situations.

There are important considerations when conducting BST with a person living with SMI. The ABA service provider should consider the following variables when training skills with the person living with SMI:

- Cognitive abilities: Adapt the training to the individual's cognitive abilities, using simple language and concrete examples. Frequent repetition of skills may be a necessary adaptation as frequent practice has been shown to facilitate the learning of new skills (Newell & Rosenbloom, 2013).
- Cultural aspects: Be aware of the person's culture and if the skill is culturally relevant and would be accepted in their culture. Modify the skill to fit the cultural needs of the person living with SMI.
- Motivation and engagement: Emphasize the importance of the skill and how it can improve the person's quality of life to maintain engagement.
- Pace and structure: Provide a structured and supportive environment, allowing adequate time for processing and practice.

- Collaboration: Work closely with the individual living with SMI, other service providers, family members, and support systems to reinforce the skills in daily life.

BST includes behavioral skills that are socially important, can improve the quality of life of the individual living with SMI and be utilized as replacement behaviors. Social and daily living skills are frequently the targeted skills that are provided to individuals living with SMI (Bellack, 2004). However, other important skills include what can be grouped together as self-control skills (Singh et al., 2007); this domain of skills include anger management skills (i.e., the identification of antecedents of anger, self-calming responses, stopping and thinking before acting, handling criticism, and avoiding and disengaging from explosive situations); and skills to manage the symptoms of living with SMI (i.e., recognize and modify unreasonable beliefs, thoughts and expectations; awareness of hallucinations as a symptom and engaging in alternative behaviors to reduce the distress of the hallucinations).

The initial step in any behavior change is to be aware of the occurrence of a behavior that is being displayed by the individual herself. Self-awareness means that a person responds discriminatively to her own externally observable behavior or products of the behavior (e.g., walking to a water fountain to get a drink of water) as much as the person differentiates observable actions of others (Skinner, 1953; Thompson, 2008). Self-awareness also means that the individual responds to her tendencies to display a behavior as well as actions that can be verified by others. The ability to be aware of variables that often exercise control over one's behavior is an important part of what is being self-aware. Self-awareness results in the generalization of inferences when similar behaviors to one's own are displayed. For example, seeing a person taking a drink from the water fountain for several seconds results in the inference that person is very thirsty; another inference may be that the person has not had any water for a long period of time or had done some strenuous activity. These are inferences as they are based on observable behaviors but without evidence to support the inference except what is observed; inferences are based on the experiences of the person and applied to the behavior of another person.

Self-awareness is necessary for behavior change to take place. Thompson (2008) suggested that self-awareness skills can be taught using the same BST paradigm as other skill domains. The first step would be teaching the individual observable aspects of another person using imitation and prompting, identification of common self-feeling states (e.g., hungry, tired, happy, sad, angry), and feeling states of others (e.g., hungry, tired, happy, sad, angry) with the associated observable collateral behaviors (e.g., facial expression, body posture). The training includes teaching generalization of antecedents including other persons and situations, teaching causal sequences, beginning with simple two-step sequences (e.g., if…then) and extending to more complex multistep scenarios. The final step is to teach events that are associated with feeling states building on previous causal sequence training (self, then others) (e.g., not eating for a long time, staying up late, receiving a present, having another person curse or make threatening statements, being criticized).

With an increase in self-awareness behaviors, teaching skills in the self-control domain can be facilitated. For example, a person initially is trained to recognize the experience of auditory hallucinations, associated collateral behaviors with the experience (e.g., talking and laughing to oneself, yelling, becoming distressed), recognize when others may be having similar experiences, the contexts when the hallucinations occur or change along dimensions such as intensity and frequency or the consequences of experiencing hallucinations. Using prompted problem-solving techniques, the individual experiencing hallucinations can develop alternative behaviors to when the hallucinatory behaviors occur such as getting involved in a card game, watching a program, listening to music, talking to another person, or taking a walk. With increases in self-awareness, the person living with SMI can self-monitor their behavior that they want to change. The result is that the person in recovery becomes the agent of their change in behaviors.

Self-awareness of the targeted behaviors also brings into awareness the antecedent and consequential conditions under which the targeted behavior occurs. The individual can self-monitor the targeted behavior and can initiate changing the conditions so that the problem behavior will be less likely to occur. As the individual living with SMI self-monitors his behaviors, other behavioral self-management skills can be used such as mindfulness, distress reducing skills, and assertiveness. With increase in self-awareness, the individual living with SMI can be their advocate and be able to institute rehabilitation goals.

Increased skills in self-awareness facilitates the therapies that have been found to be effective in the treatment of individuals living with SMI, in particular the cognitive behavior therapies (CBT) (Thase et al., 2014; Zhao et al., 2015). In CBT, awareness of one's internal experiences—self-talk (thoughts) and emotions (conditioned respondents) is a prerequisite; one must have the skill to be aware of one's thoughts and emotions to use the techniques that are offered in CBT to change behaviors that are causing distress for the individual (Fenn & Byrne, 2013). Variants of CBT have been used to effectively treat transdiagnostic mental health problems, including SMIs. To correct the cognitions and automatic thoughts that maladaptive "self-talk" generates, the individual must be aware of their internal experiences—private events—to change them. CBT can be used to reduce the distress of stigma and facilitate problem-solving for the rehabilitation and recovery efforts of the individual living with SMI.

Lack of awareness—"insight"—can be altered by prompting and reinforcing self-awareness on specific behaviors. For instance, a person can monitor how many cups of coffee he drinks; he can be reinforced with a preferred reinforcer for keeping within the limit. A person experiencing auditory hallucinations can be prompted and reinforced to recognize when the hallucinations occur and engage in other behaviors that may reduce the frequency or intensity of the hallucinations, including requesting "as needed" medications (PRNs). An individual living with an SMI who experiences "mood swings" can develop awareness of extreme changes in mood and become cognizant of situations that are antecedent conditions for the mood swings; the individual can then change those antecedent conditions when they occur (e.g., avoiding overstimulation) and reduce the probability of the problem behaviors occurring. Using BST, other socially important skills also can be taught to assist the person living with SMI to improve quality of life and contribute to progress with their rehabilitative efforts.

Summary

ABA is a scientific approach that applies the experimental principles of behavior derived from the scientific field of experimental analysis if behavior. ABA principles are utilized to improve significant behaviors that are socially important to improve the quality of life of individuals. ABA involves demonstrating cause-and-effect relationships between behavior and the environment. It uses data-based decision-making, functional behavioral assessments, and ongoing monitoring to ensure effective interventions. The three main components are real-life application, with the focus on observable actions, and demonstrating cause-and-effect relationships by altering environmental stimuli.

ABA focuses on observable behaviors rather than the inference of causality through "private events" such as self-esteem, emotions, thoughts, or physiological arousal that can only be accessed by self-report. ABA evaluates both antecedents—events preceding a behavior—and consequences—outcomes following the behavior—to discern its purpose or function. Through systematic analysis of these factors, ABA aims to accurately determine the function of specific behaviors.

Antecedents are the stimuli or events that occur before a behavior. Antecedents play a crucial role in understanding and modifying behavior. Antecedents are events or conditions that occur before a behavior. They set the context in which behavior is likely to occur. By identifying and understanding antecedents, practitioners can predict when a behavior might happen. Antecedents can act as triggers for specific behaviors. For example, a loud noise might trigger anxiety in an individual, or a specific instruction might prompt a person to start a task. By altering antecedents, practitioners can influence the likelihood of behavior occurring. This can involve modifying the physical or social environment to reduce triggers for maladaptive behavior; antecedent stimuli of visual, verbal, or physical prompts that helps guide the individual towards the targeted desired behavior; adjusting task demands to make them more manageable and decrease the chance of the individual displaying behaviors to escape the demand; and arranging activities at times when the individual is more likely to be successful in engaging in the adaptive targeted behavior. Antecedent conditions can be used to increase motivation for desired behaviors. Antecedent conditions that affect the individual's chance of engaging in a behavior to obtain or avoid a consequence are called motivating operations (MOs) as MOs impact the value of a consequence (e.g., ensuring that a child is hungry before a meal can increase the likelihood of eating). Establishing and ablative operations (EOs and AOs, respectively) are types of MOs that change the effectiveness of a reinforcing consequence that makes the consequence desirable thereby influencing the occurrence of the behavior. Antecedents also signal or cue the person if a previously available consequence will be presented after the behavior is displayed. A stimulus that means that the consequence will be available is called a discriminative stimulus (S^D) and an S delta (S^{delta}) when the consequence will not be available. By identifying, removing or modifying antecedents that influence and trigger problematic behaviors, ABA practitioners can decrease the chances of these behaviors occurring. Consequences are what happens in the environment after a behavior occurs, influencing whether the behavior will happen again in the future. There are two main types of consequences:

1. Reinforcement: This increases the likelihood of the behavior occurring again.
   - Positive reinforcement: Adding a pleasant or desired stimulus (e.g., being told "thank you" for holding the door open).
   - Negative reinforcement: Removing an unpleasant or desired stimulus (e.g., a headache going away after taking pain medication).
2. Punishment: This decreases the likelihood of the behavior occurring again.
   - Positive punishment: Adding an unpleasant or desired stimulus (e.g., getting yelled at for coming home late).
   - Negative punishment: Removing a pleasant or desired stimulus (e.g., losing recess time for speaking out of turn).

Extinction involves withholding the reinforcement that previously maintained a behavior, leading to a decrease in that behavior over time. Extinction leads to an initial increase in behavior (extinction burst), followed by a gradual decrease, and may involve temporary reappearances and emotional responses (e.g., frustration, anger).

Intermittent reinforcement occurs when a behavior is reinforced only some of the time, rather than every time it occurs. This type of reinforcement results in increased resistance to extinction with the behavior persisting even when reinforcement is no longer provided and high rates of behavior. Intermittent reinforcement makes behaviors more durable and harder to extinguish, which can be both beneficial and challenging depending on the context.

To change behaviors, ABA focuses on modifying antecedents, reinforcing desired behaviors, training skills, and using data-driven decision-making. The initial step is to determine the function of the targeted maladaptive behavior by conducting a Functional Behavioral Assessment (FBA). An FBA involves several systematic steps to identify the reasons behind problem behaviors and develop effective interventions. The key steps include:

1. Define the target behavior—clearly and specifically define the behavior to be assessed in objective and measurable terms. This ensures consistency in understanding and observation. Obtain a detailed description of the behavior, including its frequency, duration, intensity, and any pattern observed.
2. Gather information through descriptive assessment by reviewing records, obtaining medical, social, academic, and occupational history; cultural and

spiritual background; history of the behavior and interventions tried; the individual's strengths, skills, and abilities.

3. Conduct structured and semi-structured interviews and questionnaires from individuals familiar with the person (e.g., family, service providers, community support, friends) and the person living with SMI. The data collected should include the physical and social aspects of the environment that may affect behavior (such as noise levels, lighting, presence of specific individuals, availability of leisure activities); how the individual might respond in certain hypothetical scenarios to help identify potential functions of the behavior.
   - Ask questions related to antecedent conditions including what happens before the behavior occurs, including environmental conditions, interactions, and specific triggers.
   - Obtain information as to what happens immediately after the behavior, including reactions from others, changes in the environment, and any outcomes that may reinforce the behavior.
   - Identify potential reinforcers that are available in the environment and can be used to promote adaptive behaviors. It is important to ascertain the individual's daily routine, including typical activities, schedules, and any variations that might influence the behavior.
4. Direct observations—observe the individual in different settings and situations to gather real-time data on the behavior, including the antecedents (what happens before) and consequences (what happens after). Use tools like ABC logs, scatter plots, and rating scales to identify patterns and correlations between behavior and environmental factors.
5. Based on the collected data, develop hypotheses about the function of the behavior. Common functions include gaining attention, escaping tasks, obtaining tangible items, or fulfilling sensory needs.
6. Test hypotheses by systematically manipulating antecedents and consequences to see if the behavior changes as predicted by the hypotheses. This helps confirm or refine the understanding of the behavior's function.
7. Once the function of the behavior is understood, alternative and more adaptive replacement behaviors that serve the same function can be identified and taught. This helps in reducing the occurrence of the problem behavior.
8. Create a behavior support plan (BSP) based on the identified function of the behavior. The plan should include strategies to modify antecedents and consequences, teach alternative behaviors, and reinforce positive behaviors.
9. Put the intervention plan into action, ensuring that all stakeholders (e.g., family, community support people, service providers) are involved and understand their roles.
10. Continuously monitor the individual's behavior and the effectiveness of the interventions. Use data to make necessary adjustments to the intervention plan.
11. Regularly review the progress and revise the support plan as needed based on ongoing data and feedback.

Individuals living with SMI often exhibit challenging behaviors like hallucinations, delusions, aggression, and problems with social interactions and daily living skills that impact their social and occupational functioning. The use of ABA with people living with SMI has a history rooted in the principles of learning and the experimental analysis of behavior. The principles of ABA are based on the work of B.F. Skinner and his research on operant conditioning. Skinner began applying these principles in state psychiatric facilities as early as 1953 utilizing findings from the experimental analysis of behavior that focused on the components of complex behaviors and how they can be modified through reinforcement and punishment. Early applications of ABA in psychiatric settings focused on reducing psychotic behaviors and increasing functional behaviors in individuals with SMI. Studies demonstrated the effectiveness of ABA in these settings. The field of ABA was defined later and emphasized the application of behavior principles to improve specific behaviors and the importance of evaluating the effectiveness of these interventions. Research using ABA expanded to include a wide range of behaviors associated with SMI, such as delusional speech, hallucinatory behaviors, major depressive mental health problems, substance use, and social skills impairments. Studies showed that ABA could effectively reduce positive symptoms and increase functional behaviors by using the principles of reinforcement and building skills and replacement behaviors. ABA interventions focus on teaching adaptive skills and replacement behaviors to improve the quality of life for individuals with SMI.

ABA is effectively used to address various symptoms associated with SMI. ABA has been shown to effectively alter positive symptoms of SMI (e.g., hallucinations, delusions, incoherent nonsensical speech) as well as decreasing the occurrence of aggressive behaviors, substance use, and affective instability. Daily living skills, social skills, self-awareness, symptom awareness, and self-management and self-control skills have been taught using ABA principles. Negative symptoms or the absence of expected behaviors have been changed by the teaching, prompting, and reinforcement of adaptive alternative behaviors or skills that can replace maladaptive behaviors.

ABA emphasizes identifying the underlying functions of behaviors and implementing evidence-based interventions to replace maladaptive behaviors with adaptive alternatives, ultimately enhancing the quality of life for individuals living with SMI. The history of using ABA with individuals who live with SMI spans several decades, evolving from early experimental applications to a well-defined and empirically supported field that focuses on improving the quality of life for individuals with SMI through targeted behavioral interventions. ABA now involves a collaborative effort among service providers, family members, and the individuals themselves to create comprehensive and dynamic support plans.

References

Ayllon, T., & Azrin, N. H. (1965). The measurement and reinforcement of behavior of psychotics. *Journal of the Experimental Analysis of Behavior, 8*(6), 357–383. https://doi.org/10.1901/jeab.1965.8-357

Ayllon, T., & Michael, J. (1959). The psychiatric nurse as a behavioral engineer 1. *Journal of the Experimental Analysis of Behavior, 2*(4), 323–334. https://doi.org/10.1901/jeab.1959.2-323

Baer, D. M., Wolf, M. M., & Risley, T. R. (1968). Some current dimensions of applied behavior analysis. *Journal of Applied Behavior Analysis, 1*(1), 91–97. https://doi.org/10.1901/jaba.1968.1-91

Bellack, A. S. (2004). Skills training for people with severe mental illness. *Psychiatric Rehabilitation Journal, 27*(4), 375–391. https://doi.org/10.2975/27.2004.375.391

Bellus, S. B., Donovan, S. M., Kost, P. P., Vergo, J. G., Gramse, R. A., Bross, A., & Tervit, S. L. (2003). Behavior change and achieving hospital discharge in persons with severe, chronic psychiatric disabilities. *Psychiatric Quarterly, 74*, 31–42. https://doi.org/10.1023/A:1021353704062

Bellus, S. B., Vergo, J. G., Kost, P. P., Stewart, D., & Barkstrom, S. R. (1999). Behavioral rehabilitation and the reduction of aggressive and self-injurious behaviors with cognitively impaired, chronic psychiatric inpatients. *Psychiatric Quarterly, 70*, 27–37. https://doi.org/10.1023/A:1021189505212

Carey, M. P., & Carey, K. B. (1999). Behavioral research on the severe and persistent mental illnesses. *Behavior Therapy, 30*(3), 345–353. https://doi.org/10.1016/S0005-7894(99)80014-8

Cipani, E., & Schock, K. M. (2010). *Functional behavioral assessment, diagnosis, and treatment: A complete system for education and mental health settings*. Springer. https://www.springerpub.com/functional-behavioral-assessment-diagnosis-and-treatment-9780826170323.html

Cooper, J. O., Heron, T. E., & Heward, T. E. (2020). *Applied behavior analysis* (3rd ed.). Pearson. https://www.pearson.com/en-us/subject-catalog/p/applied-behavior-analysis/P200000000905/9780137477210

Fenn, K., & Byrne, M. (2013). The key principles of cognitive behavioural therapy. *InnovAiT, 6*(9), 579–585. https://doi.org/10.1177/1755738012471029

Froján-Parga, M. X., de Prado-Gordillo, M. N., Alvarez-Iglesias, A., & Alonso-Vega, J. (2019). Functional behavioral assessment-based interventions on adults' delusions, hallucinations and disorganized speech: A single case meta-analysis. *Behaviour Research and Therapy, 120*, 103444. https://doi.org/10.1016/j.brat.2019.103444

Goldiamond, I. (2022). *A programing contingency analysis of mental health*. Routledge. https://doi.org/10.4324/9781003260103

Hanley, G. P. (2012). Functional assessment of problem behavior: Dispelling myths, overcoming implementation obstacles, and developing new lore. *Behavior Analysis in Practice, 5*, 54–72. https://doi.org/10.1007/BF03391818

Harvey, M. T., Luiselli, J. K., & Wong, S. E. (2009). Application of applied behavior analysis to mental health issues. *Psychological Services, 6*(3), 212–222. https://doi.org/10.1037/a0016495

Hopko, D. R., Lejuez, C. W., Ruggiero, K. J., & Eifert, G. H. (2003). Contemporary behavioral activation treatments for depression: Procedures, principles, and progress. *Clinical Psychology Review, 23*(5), 699–717. https://doi.org/10.1016/S0272-7358(03)00070-9

Kazdin, A. E. (1982). The token economy: A decade later. *Journal of Applied Behavior Analysis, 15*(3), 431–445. https://doi.org/10.1901/jaba.1982.15-431

Kazdin, A. E. (2017). The token economy. In G. Davey (Ed.), *Applications of conditioning theory* (pp. 59–80). Routledge. https://www.routledge.com/Applications-of-Conditioning-Theory/Davey/p/book/9781138574946

Lattal, K. A., St. Peter, C., & Escobar, R. (2013). Operant extinction: Elimination and generation of behavior. In G. J. Madden, W. V. Dube, T. D. Hackenberg, G. P. Hanley, & K. A. Lattal (Eds.), *APA handbook of behavior analysis, Vol. 2. Translating principles into practice* (pp. 77–107). American Psychological Association. https://doi.org/10.1037/13938-004

Layng, T. J., & Andronis, P. T. (1984). Toward a functional analysis of delusional speech and hallucinatory behavior. *The Behavior Analyst, 7*(2), 139–156. https://doi.org/10.1007/bf03391897

Liberman, R. P. (1980). A review of Paul and Lentz's psychological treatment for chronic mental patients: Milieu versus social-learning programs. *Journal of Applied Behavior Analysis, 13*(2), 367. https://doi.org/10.1901/jaba.1980.13-367

Liberman, R. P., Derisi, W. J., & Mueser, K. T. (2001). *Social skills training for psychiatric patients*. Allyn&Bacon. https://www.pearson.com/store/p/social-skills-training-for-psychiatric-patients/P100000095637

Liberman, R. P., Teigen, J., Patterson, R., & Baker, V. (1973). Delusional speech in chronic, paranoid schizophrenics. *Journal of Applied Behavior Analysis, 6*(1), 57–64. https://doi.org/10.1901/jaba.1973.6-57

Lyman, D. R., Kurtz, M. M., Farkas, M., George, P., Dougherty, R. H., Daniels, A. S., Ghose, S. S., & Delphin-Rittmon, M. E. (2014). Skill building: Assessing the evidence. *Psychiatric Services, 65*(6), 727–738. https://doi.org/10.1176/appi.ps.201300251

Muyambi, K., Walsh, S., Bressington, D., Gray, R., Dennis, S., Brown, E., & Jones, M. (2023). Efficacy of behavioural activation in the treatment of negative symptoms in people with schizophrenia spectrum disorders: A systematic review. *International Journal of Nursing Studies Advances, 5*, 100132. https://doi.org/10.1016/j.ijnsa.2023.100132

Newell, A., & Rosenbloom, P. S. (2013). Mechanisms of skill acquisition and the law of practice. In J. R. Anderson (Ed.), *Cognitive skills and their acquisition* (pp. 1–55). Psychology Press. https://www.routledge.com/Cognitive-Skills-and-Their-Acquisition/Anderson/p/book/9781138875807

Öst, L., Melin, L., & Götestam, K. G. (1976). A token economy program for chronic schizophrenic patients. *Scandinavian Journal of Psychology, 17*(1), 272–282. https://doi.org/10.1111/j.1467-9450.1976.tb00285.x

Pavalonis, D., Shutty, M., Hundley, P., Leadbetter, R., Vieweg, V., & Downs, M. (1992). Behavioral intervention to reduce water intake in the syndrome of psychosis, intermittent hyponatremia, and polydipsia. *Journal of Behavior Therapy and Experimental Psychiatry, 23*(1), 51–57. https://doi.org/10.1016/0005-7916(92)90007-7

Pratt, S. I., Mueser, K. T., Wolfe, R., Santos, M. M., & Bartels, S. J. (2017). One size doesn't fit all: A trial of individually tailored skills training. *Psychiatric Rehabilitation Journal, 40*(4), 380. https://doi.org/10.1037/prj0000261

Preston, K. L., Kowalczyk, W. J., Phillips, K. A., Jobes, M. L., Vahabzadeh, M., Lin, J. L., Mezghanni, M., & Epstein, D. H. (2018). Before and after: Craving mood and background stress in the hours surrounding drug use and stressful events in patients with opioid-use disorder. *Psychopharmacology, 235*(9), 2713–2723. https://doi.org/10.1007/s00213-018-4966-9

Rutherford, A. (2003). Skinner boxes for psychotics: Operant conditioning at Metropolitan State Hospital. *The Behavior Analyst, 26*, 267–279. https://doi.org/10.1007/BF03392047

Singh, N. N., Lancioni, G. E., Winton, A. S. W., Adkins, A. D., Wahler, R. G., Sabaawi, M., & Singh, J. (2007). Individuals with mental illness can control their aggressive behavior through mindfulness training. *Behavior Modification, 31*(3), 313–328. https://doi.org/10.1177/0145445506293585

Singh, N. N., Matson, J. L., Lancioni, G. E., Singh, A. N., Adkins, A. D., McKeegan, G. F., & Brown, S. W. (2006). Questions About Behavioral Function in Mental Illness (QABF-MI): A behavior checklist for functional assessment of maladaptive behavior exhibited by individuals with mental illness. *Behavior Modification, 30*(6), 739–751. https://doi.org/10.1177/0145445506286700

Skinner, B. F. (1953). *Science and human behavior*. Simon and Schuster. https://www.amazon.com/Science-Human-Behavior-B-F-Skinner/dp/0029290406

Thase, M. E., Kingdon, D., & Turkington, D. (2014). The promise of cognitive behavior therapy for treatment of severe mental disorders: A review of recent developments. *World Psychiatry, 13*(3), 244–250. https://doi.org/10.1002/wps.20149

Thompson, T. (2008). Self-awareness: Behavior analysis and neuroscience. *Behavior Analysis, 31*(2), 137–144. https://doi.org/10.1007/BF03392167

Torrey, W. C., Drake, R. E., Dixon, L., Burns, B. J., Flynn, L., Rush, A. J., & Klatzker, D. (2001). Implementing evidence-based practices for persons with severe mental illnesses. *Psychiatric Services, 52*(1), 45–50. https://doi.org/10.1176/appi.ps.52.1.45

Touchette, P. E., MacDonald, R. F., & Langer, S. N. (1985). A scatterplot for identifying stimulus control of problem behavior. *Journal of Applied Behavior Analysis, 18*(4), 343–351. https://doi.org/10.1901/jaba.1985.18-343

Wallace, C. J., Liberman, R. P., Tauber, R., & Wallace, J. (2000). The independent living skills survey: A comprehensive measure of the community functioning of severely and persistently mentally ill individuals. *Schizophrenia Bulletin, 26*(3), 631–658. https://doi.org/10.1093/oxfordjournals.schbul.a033483

Wilder, D. A., Masuda, A., O'Connor, C., & Baham, M. (2001). Brief functional analysis and treatment of bizarre vocalizations in an adult with schizophrenia. *Journal of Applied Behavior Analysis, 34*(1), 65–68. https://doi.org/10.1901/jaba.2001.34-65

Whelan, R., & Barnes-Holmes, D. (2010). Consequence valuing as operation and process: A parsimonious analysis of motivation. *The Psychological Record, 60*, 337–354. https://doi.org/10.1007/BF03395711

Zhao, S., Sampson, S., Xia, J., & Jayaram, M. B. (2015). Psychoeducation (brief) for people with serious mental illness. *Cochrane Database of Systematic Reviews, 4*. https://doi.org/10.1002/14651858.CD010823.pub2

Chapter 4
Communicating Effectively, Developing Solutions, and Contracting for Adaptive Behaviors with Individuals Living with Serious Mental Illness

Introduction

Effective communication is foundational to therapeutic engagement with individuals living with serious mental illness (SMI), particularly when addressing behavioral challenges that impede recovery and quality of life. While pharmacological and diagnostic interventions remain central to psychiatric care, they are often insufficient for fostering adaptive behaviors, interpersonal trust, and collaborative problem-solving necessary for sustained rehabilitation. Individuals with SMI may experience cognitive, emotional, and social disruptions that complicate verbal and nonverbal communication, heighten vulnerability to stigma, and reduce responsiveness to traditional clinical approaches. In this context, person-centered communication strategies, grounded in behavioral science and therapeutic empathy, offer a pragmatic and ethically attuned framework for supporting behavioral change.

A range of evidence-based techniques designed to enhance communication and behavioral support planning for individuals with individuals living with SMI are presented and explained. Techniques discussed include motivational interviewing, active listening, and solution-focused methods that emphasize autonomy, dignity, and collaborative decision-making. Additionally, the use of behavioral contracting and token reinforcement systems as structured strategies for encouraging adaptive behavior through negotiated agreements and contingent rewards are analyzed. Each approach is contextualized within a broader framework of therapeutic alliance, highlighting the relational and environmental factors influencing engagement, trust, and goal alignment. By integrating behavioral principles with person-centered practices, these methods support service providers in managing complex interactions and collaboratively developing effective pathways to recovery.

The following chapter is organized into four sections. The first introduces the conceptual foundations of person-centered communication and its relevance to behavioral interventions in SMI. The second outlines core techniques—motivational

G. F. McKeegan, *Behavior Change Interventions for Serious Mental Illness*, Evidence-Based Practices in Behavioral Health,
https://doi.org/10.1007/978-3-032-18372-9_4

interviewing, active listening, and solution-focused dialogue—highlighting their empirical support and clinical utility. The third section presents behavioral contracting and token systems as tools for structuring and reinforcing adaptive behavior. The final section synthesizes these strategies within a collaborative problem-solving framework, offering practical guidance for service providers seeking to build therapeutic alliances and support individualized recovery goals. This framework enables the development of a comprehensive understanding of the intersection between communication and behavioral science as it pertains to enhancing outcomes for individuals living with SMI.

Communication and Person-Centered Approaches

Therapeutic approaches that are based on the applied principles of human behavior have been demonstrated to be effective in the treatment of people living with SMI. Programs that are based on the principles of learning have been shown to be the "treatment of choice" when treating individuals with persistent mental health problems when compared to treatment as usual (TAUs) programs including the psychopharmacological-based care routines that have become the standard of care provided to individuals living with SMI. Efforts at plans that are individualized and effective have been impeded by the lack of consistency in application by staff who often seemed unaware of, or unable to, implement the plans (Wong et al., 2004).

Effectively communicating with a person living with SMI is an essential component of any mental health intervention (Papageorgiou et al., 2017). Communication is more than just verbal behavior (i.e., talking) and the words used but also how the words are communicated to the individual. Communication includes verbal and nonverbal behaviors: what is said and how it is said. Verbal behaviors are the words used; nonverbal includes gestures, volume and tone of voice, tempo, eye contact, body stance, and facial expression. Attending to and comprehending what is being communicated is impacted by the nonverbal behavior displayed by the speaker as nonverbal behaviors send a message to the person living with SMI. Verbal and nonverbal skills allow a service provider to elicit and convey important information. Good communication fosters effective care, builds trust, establishes rapport, develops teamwork with the person living with SMI, and leads to successful outcomes and optimal therapeutic relationships. Poor communication leads to mistrust, inefficiency, ineffectiveness, and potentially negative outcomes for the support plan (Puscas et al., 2021). Communication is a reciprocal interaction (Nolan, 1999). Interactions involve both verbal and nonverbal behaviors but also listening. Being an empathetic, nonjudgmental listener, and conveying that the person is being heard and understood can make a potentially problematic interaction a safe and collaborative process that meets the goals of the person living with SMI and the service provider.

Communicating with individuals living with SMI presents challenges. People living with SMI may have experienced repeated interactions in which their statements have been dismissed, treated as if they are incompetent, inferior, or unrealistic. On some occasions, the individual living with SMI at times perceived the interactions as coercive and controlled by others. Living with SMI brings with it the stigma of having chronic and persistent mental health problems and experiencing prejudice, discrimination, and public perceptions of being devalued (Pescosolido et al., 2021). People living with SMI have lived with repeated frustrations and the lack of success in academia, occupations, and relationships; they may have been traumatized and rejected by others, including family and others in the community. The result is a person living with SMI brings to any interpersonal interaction an expectation of a negative outcome. Additionally, people living with SMI may experience cognitive problems that affect communication. Research has shown that persons living with SMI may have challenges with speaking intelligibly and problems in attending, comprehending, recall, and short- and long-term memory (Green et al., 2000; Harvey & Stassnig, 2012).

Skinner (1957) considered verbal behavior as social behavior that is shaped and maintained by the verbal community; while he recognized the separate roles of speaker and listener, he focused on how the speaker affects the listener's behavior, who in turn provides consequences to the speaker's behavior. Skinner hypothesized that verbal behavior is selected out by environmental and social contingencies and is shaped by individual's history of consequences during the occurrence of verbal behaviors. Certain topics are discussed with others due to past reinforcement through both verbal and nonverbal cues. For example, when discussing the latest football game with a friend, positive responses such as smiling, nodding, and reciprocal conversation act as reinforcing behaviors, supporting continued discussion. Conversely, topics like her job may be avoided because previous attempts have been met with aversive reactions, such as looking away, displaying negative facial expressions, or explicit verbal requests to change the subject. These responses function as aversive stimuli, leading to avoidance of the topic. If she does not respond to the subject, this may serve to extinguish the topic from future conversations. Ultimately, communication patterns are shaped by social contingencies established during interactions.

Verbal behaviors are displayed in situations in which the behaviors have a history of being reinforced. If the recent history of the individual living with SMI engaging in a specific class of behaviors—such as verbal interactions—have resulted in consequences that are punitive—or does not result in positive reinforcement—then the chances of the person engaging in that response class would decrease (e.g., extinction) (Goldiamond, 2022). The person living with SMI may not have opportunities to experience new situations or has "lost interest" in formerly reinforcing events because of not having the contexts or resources to engage in those activities, such as speaking with someone who engages in a mutually reinforcing communication (i.e., reciprocity, verbal content about topics of mutual interest). The result would be an absence of behaviors—speaking with others—in the context in which the behavior response class was not reinforced. If the interactions were punitive, in which the speakers were belittling, hostile, angry, or critical, then the person living with SMI may avoid interacting with people altogether. The absence of the expected behaviors would be labeled as the negative symptom of "asociality." The predominant communication that a person living with SMI has with others may be aversive and perceived as controlling, being criticized for either doing or not doing a behavior. Punitive interactions also may result in other behaviors such as aggression towards self and others as punitive interactions generate aversive emotional stimulation and perceptions. The person living with SMI may engage in an aggressive response class (e.g., yelling, cursing, threatening, hitting) to terminate and escape the aversiveness of the interactions.

Some symptoms of SMI, such as problems with concentration and attention, mood swings, memory problems, and delusions, can make it hard to participate in the "give and take" of a normal conversation. They can make it hard for the people living with SMI to express themselves and to understand what other people are saying. These challenges can frustrate both individuals living with SMI and their listeners during communication.

Communication Challenges Encountered

Some examples of possible challenges when communicating with an individual living with SMI are:

- The person talks about things that clearly are not real. A person who is living with SMI may have bizarre beliefs that are clearly unreal to other people and unsubstantiated by any fact. Because of symptoms associated with SMI, however, the person talks about them regardless of what other people think. For example, the person says that his food has been poisoned. He refuses all food and will only eat food that is bought in a sealed container.
- The person jumps from topic to topic. Even simple requests result in a strange response. The person is asked how they are doing, and the response is about another, unrelated topic, such as the weather. The topic quickly switches to talking about something else, such as asking what car is being driven by the listener. Sudden shifts in conversation may cause confusion and frustration for the listener, as the responses may not be coherent or relevant. It can be challenging to guide the individual back to the intended topic, which may ultimately lead to reduced social interactions with that person.
- Occasionally, verbal statements and comments may not elicit any response. The individual may display a blank stare without reacting to communication efforts or may mumble inaudible words while maintaining eye contact. While the person may appear physically well, this situation can be challenging for service providers. It may seem as though the individual is capable of responding but chooses not to do so.
- The person speaks rapidly and incessantly about topics that make no sense to the listener. Even when the topic changes, the person will continue with the same topic. There is no awareness that the topic has changed or moved on.

- The person becomes frustrated at attempts to communicate with her. It can be frustrating for a person living with SMI to have problems talking with other people. She can become frustrated and embarrassed at her inability to make herself understood by other people. When this is the case, she becomes angry at attempts to get her to talk.
- The quality of the conversation changes. The quality of the conversation varies; sometimes the person talks at a very rapid pace and is difficult to understand or the person talks over others, not giving anyone a chance to respond or ask a question. The conversation goes well at times but much more poorly at other times. To service providers, it appears that the person can do better. These fluctuations could reflect changes in the intensity of the problematic communication behaviors.

One complication of communication problems is that it is difficult to tell whether the problems are caused by problematic behaviors related to living with SMI. Just like anyone else, people living with SMI may "choose" when to listen and can respond appropriately when it is in their interest.

The bottom line is that communicating with a person who is living with SMI can be very challenging. Service providers cannot expect this will be "business as usual." Successful communication likely will require special attention and skills from the service provider. As stated above, good communication builds trust and is essential for collaboration with the person living with SMI. Whatever the reason, communicating effectively is something service providers should try to do. Communicating effectively does not solve all problems or make the person living with SMI well, but it will usually make interacting with the person living with SMI easier, especially regarding changing behaviors that impede success in rehabilitation and recovery.

Ineffective communication can result in other serious behaviors. For example, asking the person living with SMI, "Do you think you can make your bed?" may result in one of the following responses:

- "You're working with the people at the clubhouse to make me do things I don't want to do."
- Silence.
- "I don't think about the bed at all."
- "Of course I can make the bed." (But does not to start to make it.)
- "Why don't you get off my back before you get hurt!"

The outcome is that the bed goes unmade; the service provider is frustrated and angry with the person living with SMI. Effective communication can result in building the base of a relationship and alter the way the service provider and the person living with SMI interact to be successful.

The following section outlines key strategies that are essential for supporting individuals living with SMI. These are general strategies that are useful in a variety of situations faced by service providers. These strategies can be thought of as tools that service providers can use to help the person living with SMI overcome behavior challenges. Just as a person with a physical disability often requires aids to do more for himself (for example, a wheelchair and ramps help a person who is paralyzed below the waist to be more mobile and independent), these are tools service providers can use in assisting the individual living with SMI.

In later sections, the focus will be on several specific problems that service providers encounter on a frequent basis. To effectively work with such problems, service providers must become good behavior managers. What service providers do in response to problems can make a difference in how people living with SMI behave around others at their residence and in public. By understanding how to use the tools and strategies that are presented, service providers become better behavior managers. Using these tools requires considerable patience and effort from service providers. However, the results are usually beneficial.

Guidelines for Communicating More Effectively

Problems in communicating are often an important problem for a person living with SMI. Many symptoms or problematic behaviors related to living with SMI, such as concentration problems, mood swings, memory problems, and delusions, can make it hard to participate in the "give and take" of a normal conversation. They can make it hard for the person living with SMI to express himself or for him to understand what other people are saying. These challenges may render communication particularly challenging for individuals living with SMI as well as those around them. Pharmaceutical interventions have limited impact on enhancing effective communication skills. Consequently, service providers must adapt their approaches to accommodate the inherent limitations associated with SMI.

Effective communication is a process. The initial step is being mindful—fully aware—of the verbal and nonverbal behaviors of communication (Krasner & Epstein, 2010). Communication is determined by the behavior of the listener and the speaker as communication is reciprocal and interactive. What the service provider does will affect what the person living with SMI does and how the person living with SMI responds will be consequential to what the service provider does. A conversation is a chain of related behaviors with responses being the antecedent and the consequence for the verbal and nonverbal behaviors that follow.

The service provider ought to be aware of all aspects involved in communication, being aware of nonverbal and verbal behaviors when speaking and listening. It is not only important what is said but also how it is said. The service provider needs to be aware of facial expression, body position, proximity, volume, tone, and gestures. When listening, the service provider needs to give full attention to the speaker. If the service provider comes across a person living with SMI as disinterested, bored, angry, tense, demeaning, and belittling, then the person living with SMI may respond by becoming angry, anxious, or annoyed.

Below are some helpful ways to improve the effectiveness of communication:

- Match behavior to the message that is being given. When giving verbal praise to the person living with SMI, tone of voice should be pleasant, smiling facial expression, and relaxed posture (i.e., arms at side). When expressing displeasure with what the person has done, the voice should be low and firm, facial expression should be serious, and posture should be business-like. Even if giving a corrective response or a reprimand, the speaker needs to remain calm, but firm. Yelling, threatening, or lecturing the person living with SMI sets the conditions for the person getting angry, hostile, and rejecting what is being said by the service provider. If the service provider is angry, stands with clenched fists and arms crossed at the chest, points and shakes a finger or waves arms, these may be perceived as a threat to the person living with SMI. When threatened, most individuals do not listen well to the spoken message. They want to leave the person who is perceived as threatening, and they may threaten or engage in aggressive behavior.
- The speaker should be at eye level when communicating and not standing over the person living with SMI. If the individual living with SMI avoids direct eye contact, the speaker looks in the general area of the person's eyes to ensure that they have a chance to make eye contact; the person living with SMI is not forced to look at the speaker. Successfully making "eye contact"—even for a moment—increases the chances of effective communication.
- Before starting an interaction, the speaker ought to use the person's name to increase the chances that the person is attending.
- People living with SMI need as much help as possible to understand what is being communicated. Using simple gestures may help the person living with SMI understand what is wanted or requested. For example, pointing to the garbage can while asking the person to move it is an example of "total communication," which is a method for helping people with communication difficulties communicate in a way that works for them. Use gestures when making important points. Sometimes gestures can convey a message that words cannot. Simultaneously, too many gestures may distract the person living with SMI especially if done rapidly or excessively.
- Proximity is essential when communicating. Crowding a person, invading the person's personal space [i.e., 2–4 ft from the person (Wilson, 2000)] is perceived as intimidating and aggressive. Giving the person enough space is essential as the person living with SMI is sensitive to closeness, especially if that person has a history of physical trauma. The person living with SMI sometimes misinterprets physical closeness or reacts with anger or provocative behavior if the speaker is too close. Rule of thumb when interacting with a person living with SMI is to be at least an arm's length away when talking. Trauma sensitive general precautions—which is assuming that the person has experienced trauma—need to be taken.
- If the person living with SMI does not mind, a gentle touch on the arm or top of shoulder can focus attention and give reassurance, comfort, and be a pleasant experience to the person. This is especially important if the speaker wants to give a positive message to the person living with SMI.

- It is imperative to interact with the individual living with SMI in an area free from distraction. People living with SMI often have problems with focusing on what is important. Distraction may occur and attention to what is being said is attenuated if there is excessive stimulation around them, such as television or radio being on, phone ringing, or other people talking nearby. The environment should be as free as possible from potential distractions when talking or listening to a person living with SMI.
- Try to understand what the person living with SMI may be going through. People living with SMIs have feelings. These feelings can be distressful because they are associated with false beliefs, hearing voices, trauma, loss, disappointment. It is helpful to the person living with SMI to "label" the feeling that they are experiencing. The service providers should try to understand and communicate the feelings conveyed by the individual living with SMI, even though they are not having the same experiences. For example, if the person living with SMI tells the service provider that the voices in his head tell him that he is never getting well, then a response could be: "I don't know exactly what you're going through. If I heard what you are hearing, it would make me sad and depressed." This response gives the person a label for the feeling, validates the emotional experience, and expresses empathy from the service provider to what the person living with SMI is feeling.

Active Listening

Effective communication is rooted in attentive listening. When individuals living with SMI feel that they are being genuinely listened to by service providers, it facilitates the development of trust and rapport. This sense of being understood enhances their receptiveness to the information and guidance offered by service professionals.

"Active listening" was developed by Rogers and Farson in 1957. "Active listening" is not a passive process but one in which the listener is actively attempting to understand what the person is communicating; the listeners use verbal and nonverbal communication behaviors to make sure that both the content and the emotion behind what the person is saying is heard and understood.

Effective communication involves not only the skill of saying things clearly but also the ability to show that the service provider is listening by showing that they are trying to understand what the person living with SMI is saying. "Active listening" are behaviors that show the person living with SMI that they are being heard and understood (Rogers & Farson, 1957; Tennant et al., 2024; Waldron, 2024).

The following points help the service provider to more clearly show that they are listening and care about what the person living with SMI has to say.

- Focus attention on the person speaking. The service provider needs to stop all extraneous activity to listen. By focusing attention, the person living with SMI perceives that what they are saying is being listened to and not dismissed. This helps the individual living with SMI to more clearly see that the service provider is interested. Multitasking needs to be suspended so the person living with SMI perceives that what he is saying is important.

- The service provider looks at the person living with SMI when that person is trying to communicate. The service provider needs to attempt to maintain eye contact but not force it; an opportunity needs to be given to make eye contact by looking in the general area of the person's eyes.
- There are no assumptions or judgments when actively listening. Refrain from premature judgment. Observe the speaker's body language to gain insights into their attitudes toward the message that is being conveyed.
- Reflect and paraphrase. The service provider reiterates in her own words what she understood from the person living with SMI. Paraphrasing what the person living with SMI is saying demonstrates engagement to that person living with SMI and confirms the comprehension of the listener. For example, if the person living with SMI says that the other members of the clubhouse don't like him, the service provider might say, "I am hearing you say that the clubhouse members don't try to talk with you or ask you to do activities with them and that gives you the feeling they do not like you." This gives the person the opportunity to correct what the listener has said if there is any misunderstanding.
- Ask for clarification. Do not hesitate to ask if any part of the message remains unclear. This will ensure accurate understanding and prevent miscommunication.
- Maintain focus. If the sender veers off-topic, the conversation can be gently steered back to the original issue or concern.
- Avoid distractions and assumptions. Stay focused on the sender's words rather than letting thoughts wander or responding based on assumptions.
- Delay responding until the person living with SMI stops speaking. Ensure that the entire message is understood before responding. The service provider needs to clarify if there is a question as to the message being sent by the person living with SMI. Active listening is a two-way process.

However, it is counterproductive and potentially not beneficial to repeat delusional information. The service provider should paraphrase the information that is based on reality. Considerable time listening to clearly delusional topics should be avoided as it inadvertently reinforces the occurrence of delusional speech. If the person living with SMI is speaking rapidly or loudly, then the service provider should verbally and gesturally prompt the person to slow down or lower the volume of speech so that the person living with SMI is able to be heard and understood. If the person is not able to speak at a less rapid rate or more normal volume, then the service provider needs to politely and gently postpone the conversation for another time when the communication is more effective; the service provider should inform the person that the conversation can continue when he is able to "slow down" and "speak in a lower volume." Continuing with the conversation may reinforce the unintelligible speech. If the person living with SMI is displaying "hyperverbal speech" (i.e., rapid, pressured, excessive speaking), the service provider ought to prompt the person by saying "it is my turn to speak," and using a gestural prompt like a "time out" signal.

For example:

A person living with SMI may say:

The communists stopped me from going to the clinic because the bus was going to a labor camp.

The service provider can respond:

What I understand is that you did not go to the clinic because you were afraid to take the bus.

In this example, the service provider did not respond to the content of what they had just said. The service provider instead gave the person's feeling a name or label—that he was scared—though the feeling was because of an irrational and false belief or delusion. Although the reason for the person's feelings is irrational, the feelings that he is experiencing are not.

When listening to a person living with SMI, the service provider needs to avoid "reactive listening." The goal is to listen to understand and be compassionate about the experiences of the person living with SMI, instead of thinking of ways to convince the person to change his wrong beliefs or admit to problems with his behavior. It is imperative not to interrupt or criticize while listening. The service provider does not argue or defend what was done (or not done). The person living with SMI may be sensitized to any perception of rejection, negativity, and blame; the service provider ought to recognize that criticisms generally come from many disappointments with mental health service providers and the mental health system and not to take the negative feedback personally. The service provider needs to try to understand the experiences, perceptions, hopes, disappointments, and fears of the person living with SMI about himself and his situation. The goal is to understand reality from the point of view of the person living with SMI, even when the person experiences hallucinations, delusions, or mood swings. An aspect of living with SMI is a lack of awareness, insight or anosognosia about the behavior or symptoms of SMI. Arguing about what is real is not beneficial or productive.

However, there may be times that the service provider needs to set limits with the person living with SMI during an interaction. The service provider needs to be fully available so that active listening can take place and not multitask. The service provider should determine the appropriate timing, location, and duration of each interaction. These arrangements must be mutually agreed upon by both the service provider and the individual living with SMI. The service provider needs to follow through on what has been arranged. If a break is needed the service provider can say, "I'm sorry but I need to pause our talk. I know you probably have more to say, but I need to take a break now. How about we continue in about 30 minutes?" This type of limit setting role helps role model to the person living with SMI that it is fine to stop and pause during an interaction; just as importantly, the service provider needs to follow through and return to the interaction when it is time.

At times it is difficult to discuss topics that may be emotionally intense. If the person doesn't want to talk, the service provider may find that the person finds it easier if engaged in an activity with the service provider (e.g., taking a walk, playing cards, playing a board game). The service provider can arrange for the person living with SMI to talk to someone else if it is mutually agreeable.

It is easier to interact in a setting free of noise, commotion, other people, and bright lights; it is critically imperative that the service provider sets up a reinforcing environment. The interaction needs to begin with pleasantries; the service provider needs to be reinforcing and pointing out and praising the person living with SMI about progress made towards their goals and not beginning with what the person has not done or behavioral challenges. A person who lives with SMI often hears negative comments and complaints, not only from other people but from derogatory hallucinations. The saying "you can catch more bees with honey than with vinegar" applies universally to everyone. It is important to explicitly recognize the positive qualities and behaviors of the person living with SMI. It is often more effective to focus on creating a positive, supportive environment that prevents problems, instead of dealing with challenges after they arise.

Challenging Interactions

There are times, nevertheless, when the service provider needs to address a difficult topic and try to resolve a behavioral challenge with the person living with SMI. This interaction will occur more effectively if the service provider already has a trusting relationship with the person. If an individual living with SMI experiences difficulties with impulsivity and demonstrates aggressive behaviors when angry or frustrated, it is advisable to conduct interactions in open areas with nearby access to other people. A person's mood or concentration can change throughout the day. Some people are "morning people"; others are "night people." Individuals living with SMI may experience periods of increased alertness and comprehension throughout the day. Service providers should identify and utilize these times, particularly when interactions may be complex or demanding.

The service provider needs to be aware of the challenging behavior is the outcome of antecedent conditions that have not been recognized and ameliorated. Some challenging behaviors occur because of uncomfortable, overstimulating or under stimulating environments. Examples are too much noise, light, people, too little sleep, or sudden changes in the person's routines. For instance, certain individuals may experience discomfort due to heightened activity and the increased movement commonly observed during dinnertime or transitional periods (such as rising, retiring, mealtimes, or attending programs). Expectations beyond the capability of the person living with SMI can result in frustration and discouragement. This can lead to increases in problem behaviors. For example, if the person living with SMI prefers to stay by himself, it may be unrealistic to expect him to attend a clubhouse program for several hours every day of the week. If these expectations are pushed, more problems are likely to result. It is better to develop a solution for this than place the blame and responsibility on the person living with SMI.

There are difficulties and frustrations that almost everyone faces in living from day to day; the same is true for people living with SMI. Disagreements with other people, problems with money management, keeping up with maintenance in the home, are just a few examples of the many problems with which most people cope. For someone living with SMI, these problems of everyday life can be difficult, cause distress, and become "catastrophic." Sometimes, these "small" problems build up and worsen symptoms and problematic behaviors.

Below is an example of a solution which is a "win-win" for all:

> Janice was inconsistent with taking her shower and changing her clothes. The staff at her residence were frustrated because she refused to take a shower in the evening. When asked, she told them that she was angry and embarrassed that other residents had opened the bathroom door while she was showering. Janice and the service providers discussed the situation; service providers and Janice decided that she could shower every day in the morning while the other residents ate breakfast. This ensured her privacy. Janice asked the service providers to lay out her clothes and a clean towel the night before "to remind her." By changing the routine, the chances were greater that Janice would shower and change clothes regularly.

It is important to recognize that most problems or issues are not resolved after a single interaction. Instead, it usually takes a long series of interactions with service providers using active listening, having rapport and trust with the person living with SMI, and compassion and empathy towards the difficulties of the person living with SMI to solve problems. Also, behavioral change takes time and gradually occurs as the novel antecedents and consequences impact the occurrence of the requested behavior change. It takes time for most people to increase the amount of exercise they are doing, changing food for a diet, or stop smoking. Even after behavior begins to change, there will probably be incidences when the occurrence of the behavior that was desired does not occur, and the challenging behavior is emitted again because of individual variability and complexity (Cooper et al., 2020). Giving up after experiencing frustration due to impediments in progress is not the answer; it is best to review what has occurred, consider factors involved, and make changes.

When engaged in a challenging interaction, it is best to plan for the interaction. The service provider should be cognizant to speak to the person in an area with reduced stimulation and overcrowding. Only the people required to attend should be in the meeting with the person living with SMI; too many people participating in any interaction could be seen as threatening and confusing, especially if more than one person is speaking at the same time. People at the meeting with the person living with SMI ought to be mindful about attempting to pressure the person to agree to what others want; collaboration for the requested behavior change needs to be the goal. The service provider should speak to the person preferably at a time and place where the person living with SMI will have the best chance of paying attention and concentrating so that the person living with SMI can respond to the best of their abilities. If the service provider is making a request for a change in behavior, it is important to ask the person displaying the challenging behaviors if he is aware of the problem and what he believes he could do to change it. Do not ask a question about the behavior but make a clear and concise statement for the requested change. For example, instead of saying "Can you please get out of bed by 8 in the morning?", a simple clear statement is stated: "I would like for you to be out of bed by 8 o'clock in the morning." Asking a question about a requested behavior to occur instead of requesting for the behavior to occur confuses the person, is perceived as being treated "child-like" and offers an opportunity for the person to say "No!" to the request. Making a statement for the behavior to occur sets up the conversation to begin with discussing challenges that may be interfering with the behavior from occurring.

The service provider needs to speak slowly and in simple sentences. Many individuals living with SMI present with problems with attention; simple verbal statements will help with focusing. Speaking too quickly and using too many words will overwhelm the person living with SMI. The service provider needs to allow enough time between sentences so that what is said can be understood.

If the target of the conversation is asking the person living with SMI about his awareness about the dimensions of the challenging behavior, one question is asked at a time; the service provider needs to wait for a response before asking another question. If the person responds that he is not aware of any dimension or does not answer, the service provider can rephrase the question and allow extra time for him to answer the question. If the person does not respond, then do not keep pursuing the same question; the discussion may need to continue at another time. Don't provoke a problem by pushing the person living with SMI to engage in behaviors that he is not able to do.

If the person living with SMI has problems with answering questions, give clear alternatives, instead of open-ended questions. The person living with SMI will be more likely to understand and respond if the question requires a simple and short answer or even yes-no responses. Getting the individual living with SMI to verbally respond is the goal; asking for simple responses helps in getting the momentum started to speak. In addition, statements that have an expectation of the desired behavior are preferable. For example, "How are you getting to the clinic today?" gives the person living with SMI a chance to say "No, I am not going"; restating the request as "Are you going to the clinic by bus or van?" expects the person to go but asks how the person will get there.

To get the attention of a person living with SMI, use the name of the individual when beginning a conversation. The speaker needs to enable the person living with SMI to make eye contact to ensure that the person's focus is on the speaker.

If the conversation drifts off onto topics not reality-based, verifiable, or "off topic," distraction can be utilized to bring the conversation back to the topic at hand. Sometimes the person living with SMI talks about her "crazy" ideas and keeps on talking. Simply ignoring the "crazy" talk may make it worse. Instead, one could change the topic by using a compliment, recalling a situation when the person living with SMI accomplished something or using humor; if humor is used, ridicule or belittling statements are to be absolutely avoided with the person living with SMI as this will just make any future attempts at communication futile. When the person living with SMI responds to more reality-based topics, the person is reinforced and verbally praised about the conversation with her. It is very important to catch the person living with SMI doing something well and praise them for it.

After giving the person living with SMI a request for a behavior change, the person ought to be prompted to rehearse what they have heard and understood like giving someone a phone number to remember or an important date. Asking for them to paraphrase what was said will improve their ability to remember.

Requesting a Change in Behavior and Discussing Challenging Topics

As stated previously, discussing a challenging topic is best done where and when the time is right to maximize the chances that the person living with SMI will listen and collaborate with the service providers. If one or both parties are upset and angry, it is best to delay the discussion at a time when both service provider and the individual living with SMI are calm. When planning a conversation with an individual living with SMI, it is important to select an optimal setting. In many situations, a time and location free from interruptions and excessive external stimulation will be most appropriate.

Use "I-statements" to avoid demanding, accusatory, and blaming "you" statements (Gottman et al., 2013; Relationships Australia, 2024). When angry and frustrated, most people blame, criticize, and accuse. One way of communicating anger, disappointment, and frustration is by using the word "you." "You-messages" convey blame, criticism, and accusations. "You-statements" suggest blame, conveying judgment of the other person; using "you" in a statement presents opinions as facts and hinders any conversation; it results in the person living with SMI having difficulty in listening to what is being said and to respond calmly and not feeling intimidated. For example, consider how the listener would think and feel about the statements below:

- "You only think about yourself."
- "Can't you do anything for yourself?"
- "You are so helpless."
- "Why are you so stubborn and lazy? You want me to do everything for you!"

It is common for individuals to communicate messages like the above to others during periods of anger or frustration, and many have likely been recipients of such exchanges. The use of "You-statements" in these contexts often leads to hurt feelings for those receiving the message.

An alternative is using an "I-statement." "I-statements" help to convey feelings, telling the person how their behavior affects others including the speaker; "I-statements" give the person "feedback" on what to do to correct their behavior. By using "I-statements," the speaker states that they are responsible and in charge of their feeling and emotions. Instead of saying, "You disappoint me," the speaker says, "I feel disappointed" (Gottman et al., 2013).

When discussing challenging topics or asking for a change in the behavior of a person living with SMI, the service provider ought to use "I-statements." "I-statements" have a specific format that are listed below:

1. Describe the behavior. Do not blame. Put the behavior into observable words without using inferences or labels to blame, criticize, or demean the person living with SMI.

   For example: "When I see you smoking in your bed…"

2. State your feelings about the possible results of that behavior.

   For example: "I feel scared…"

3. State the consequences or results of that behavior.

For example: "Because you may fall asleep with a lighted cigarette and set the bed, yourself, and the house on fire."

4. State the behavior you want the person to do instead.

   For example: "Next time, I want you to smoke outside on the porch."
   Simply stated, "I-statements" take the following format:

   When…., I feel…, because… Next time, I want you to do…

   In summary, when speaking with a person living with SMI:

- Use a calm tone of voice and speaking style.
- Use "I-statements." Using "you-statements" often implies blame, which results in anger and frustration by the listener.
- Use brief, concise sentences as the person living with SMI may be hearing voices or have neurocognitive impairment, which can make it challenging to pay attention and process input.
- Be thoughtful about how the problem is described. Present a problem in a way that won't trigger emotional reactions that preclude reasonable discussion. Describe the specific problematic behavior without using labels, infer character flaws, or assumed motivations.
- Avoid terms such as "always" and "never."
- Allow time for the person to process what was said and respond.

If a change in behavior is considered, the service providers should focus on a single specific proposal. Find out what is reinforcing to the person living with SMI that serves as a motivator for the proposed change. Offering an activity or privilege she wants may appeal to her self-image, hopes, and aspirations in her recovery. For example, if the person living with SMI sometimes leaves the residence for several days, a family member or staff may be inclined to say:

> I'm so upset! You were missing for days, and I didn't know where you were. You're always so inconsiderate. You never think about my feelings. You just don't care except for yourself!

To improve the probability of having a beneficial conversation, the provider or family member can say:

> I get very worried when you're gone for several days, and I don't know where you are. I worry if you are safe. The next time, call the residence or your friend Charlie to let us know you are OK. Remember, you have your sister's wedding coming up and are looking forward to going. Do you have any suggestions about ways to let us know you are safe?

Be flexible in considering alternative solutions that may be a better compromise that meets the most important needs, goals, and aspirations of each person.

Emotions Affect Communication

People living with SMI have been exposed to negative interactions with family members, friends, acquaintances and health care providers since it was determined that they were living with an SMI. They have listened to criticism, negative, and hopeless statements for the duration of their mental health problem. People living with SMI have likely experienced repeated disappointment, rejection, and trauma. Because of feelings of frustration and hopelessness, family, friends, and service providers may have inadvertently communicated in a hostile and negative manner during times of behavioral crises. Repeated negative experiences "sensitizes" the person living with SMI to perceive that every interaction with others will be "just more of the same." The outcome may be that the person living with SMI will "turn off" chances of interacting and communicating with others in ways that could benefit both the person living with SMI and the service providers, family members, friends and acquaintances.

Expressed Emotionality

Expressed emotionality (EE) refers to affective attitudes and behaviors toward patients characterized by critical comments, hostility, and emotional overinvolvement. There is ample evidence of an association between living in environments with high EE and relapses, readmissions, nonadherence to medication, and poor outcomes in rehabilitation domains (Babbington & Kupiers, 1994; Berry et al., 2011; Ma et al., 2021; Manikandan & Raja, 2023; Marom et al., 2005). Training to reduce high EE has been effective in decreasing its deleterious impact on people living with SMI (Ma et al., 2021).

An aspect of expressed emotionality is the outcome of frustration with the behavior of the person living with SMI on the part of service providers, family members and others. Service providers and others who are concerned about the well-being of the person living with SMI can become intensely involved in trying to improve the lives of that person. At times, the desire to help the person living with SMI influences the person to persist at goals that are unrealistic or that are imposed against the desires and aspirations of the person living with SMI. The people who are overly involved expect more from the person living with SMI than what they can do. This sets up situations for increased frustrations and disappointments that are then communicated to the person living with SMI. Fostering a positive and supportive environment is a more effective approach to problem prevention than addressing issues after they have occurred. Individuals tend to perform optimally when they feel supported by their colleagues, while frequent criticism or anticipation of criticism can negatively impact performance. Service providers often notice shortcomings, but it's more beneficial to focus on what people who live with SMI do well. Maximizing success can help the person living with SMI feel that he is being supported by others with whom he interacts.

People living with SMI experience frequent negative interactions and outcomes. They are conditioned to expect criticism and negative comments. A person living with SMI may not be able to accurately appreciate intentions coming from others. It may take repeated positive interactions with service providers to undo the negative expectations that they have learned to expect.

Some people may perceive that they know what is best for the person living with SMI but have not discussed their concerns with the person. Others become "excessively" devoted to the welfare of the person living with SMI. The service providers, family members, partners and friends become overprotective and fail to allow the person living with SMI to use his capabilities to help himself. Success is cause for celebration; failures become antecedent for disappointment. This degree of emotional involvement may result in others reacting strongly, which can create a recurring pattern where individuals who live with SMI choose to distance themselves from these people. In response, service providers or family members may attempt to offer support, but the cycle continues. This situation can contribute to additional disappointment for the person who intensifies their over involvement with the person living with SMI.

Communication needs to be avoided when angry. There will be times when a behavioral emergency (e.g., mental health crisis) occurs with the person living with SMI; service providers need to respond even if emotionally stressed—but communication needs to be minimal and only enough to deal with the emergency. Any further communication needs to be done when everyone—including the person living with SMI—is calmer and less emotionally stressed. For example, service providers may need to tell a person living with SMI to stop hitting another person. The goal is to stop the behavior; any further communication about discussing the emergency and future interventions should be delayed until a future time to which all are in agreement.

To communicate effectively, avoid the following:

- Refrain from responding if angry or frustrated. Many of us tend to overreact when emotionally stressed. Anger and other intense emotions interfere with communicating rationally; effective communication to change a challenging behavior is impaired along with attempting to collaborate with the person living with SMI. The result could cause the service providers to respond with wrong and harmful statements. It is common to encounter emotionally charged situations in which statements are made impulsively, resulting in unintended consequences. Efforts may subsequently be made to mitigate the impact of such remarks; however, at times the damage cannot be easily reversed, and the effects of the statement persist.

- Intense emotions—or high emotionality—ought to be avoided when talking to a person living with SMI. If angry, the service providers need to be aware of their stressful emotions and avoid saying anything harmful. Taking a break, walking away from a tense situation, counting to ten, and deep breathing are some ways to calm down and consider a thoughtful response to communicate. During periods of emotional stress, it is advisable to refrain from speaking or attempting to resolve issues until emotions have subsided.
- It is advisable to manage any negative emotions that is being experienced prior to communicating with an individual living with SMI. Identify and deal with any anger, fears and concerns about communicating about a challenging behavior with a person living with SMI. It is important to reframe the perception of the challenging behaviors being displayed by the person living with SMI as an aspect of the mental health problems being experienced rather than unkind, thoughtless or manipulative actions on the part of the individual. Service providers may find it helpful to practice having a difficult conversation with the person living with SMI, focusing on the verbal message and how it will be communicated. Practice and feedback from another service provider can assist in communicating effectively and compassionately.
- Avoid demeaning, child-like communication. At times, the person living with SMI may need to be told what to do, even for simple expectations, such as taking a shower or changing clothes. The service provider may believe that the person living with SMI "does not know any better." There may be a tendency to think of the person living with SMI as a younger person. The result is talking to them like a child, using a sing-song tone of voice, talking about the person in front of them as if they cannot understand, nagging/lecturing the person about their behavior, being demeaning about the person and their skills, making inferences about the person's motivation. In addition, most people don't like to be ordered or "bossed around." Instead of "ordering" the person, it may be more helpful to get the person involved in trying to solve the problem behavior by using "I-statements" (presented above) and use techniques in solution-focused and problem-solving interventions. The goal is to encourage the person living with SMI to be their own agent of change.
- Avoid asking the person living with SMI why they are doing the problem behavior. People living with SMI could be unaware that their behavior is problematic and unacceptable and would stop the problem behavior if they could (i.e., lack of insight, anosognosia). People who do not experience mental health problems do things that are problematic, such as overeating or smoking. They often cannot come up with good reasons why they keep doing the behavior. Asking the person living with SMI "why" is just a frustrating experience for everyone involved. It

will not lead to any change in behavior. In fact, asking "Why?" may be perceived by the individual living with SMI as persistent questioning rather than as an act of helpfulness or support from the service provider.

At other times, the service providers may want to address a challenging topic and try to solve a problem. It may be necessary to postpone this type of conversation until a trusting relationship is established so the person living with SMI is willing to listen. Choosing a time when both parties are calm facilitates any discussion and problem-solving. Consider the most appropriate setting for engaging in conversation with individuals living with SMI. In certain situations, it may be beneficial to select a private time and location free from interruptions. Alternatively, some discussions may prove more effective in a semipublic environment.

Developing Solutions

To many service providers and families, the challenging behaviors that they confront daily with the person living with SMI may appear overwhelming. At times, the service providers and others feel that their backs are up against the wall in dealing with these problems. Feelings of hopelessness and helplessness are a leading cause of stress in service providers, especially if the person living with SMI is a family member (Acker, 2012; Laidlaw et al., 2002). When faced with a challenging behavior, many do nothing. It is hoped that the challenging behavior will "just go away" or that the person living with SMI is "just in a cycle," needs more or different medications, and nothing can be done about it. Others overreact with haste, anger, and criticism of the person living with SMI. As stated previously, high expression of emotionality around the person living with SMI has been shown to result in relapses, readmissions, and disruptions in the person's rehabilitation efforts.

Certain techniques have been proven successful in helping people solve their problems. Although nothing is perfect, the steps outlined below may help the service providers in coming up with possible solutions to the problem behaviors of the person living with SMI.

Solution-focused interventions (SFI) have wide applications in mental health care, in both inpatient and community settings. SFI has been utilized with victims of sexual abuse, eating disorders, relationship challenges and depression, as well as challenges associated with SMI. SFI successfully has been used with people who require ongoing support or with multiple challenges (Bedell et al., 1997; Webster, 2009).

SFI is a positive, person-centered approach. It places the person as the decision maker in their reality. It is oriented in the present, centering on what behavioral challenge the person is facing; it recognizes that change is inevitable across all situations and across the life span. SFI is strength based as it seeks competence in solving challenges and supports the person living with SMI. SFI accounts for the individual's language usage and skills, culture, and the present context in which the challenging behavior occurs. SFI supports and facilitates the person living with SMI as the expert regarding the situations, contexts, supports, and resources that are available to assist them in developing and implementing solutions for challenging behaviors (Corcoran & Pillai, 2009; Visser, 2013; Webster, 2009).

SFI assumes everyone's reality is always in flux; the result is that challenges and solutions change as the contexts and situations change. SFI uses the individual's perception of the presenting challenging behavior as the basis of change. This perception involves refining what the person living with SMI views as the problem, the extent the person is involved in the challenging behavior, and the awareness of solutions or changes that the person initiated to resolve other problems that had similar variables (e.g., similar antecedent conditions and consequences, dimensions of behaviors). The practitioner using SFI does not attempt to determine the source of challenging behavior by exploring the personal and family history, the identification of motives and inferences, mental health problems of the individual living with SMI. SFI is based on practical and relevant evidence of what works for the person. It focuses on asking if the challenging behavior changes what the change would accomplish for that person living with SMI. The practitioner of SFI assists the person living with SMI to identify meaningful goals and builds on the person's existing strengths and resources.

SFI uses a range of questions intended to develop an understanding of the individual living with SMI perspectives. The questions elicit responses from the person living with SMI about the perceptions of their realities. Practitioners of SFI ask the person living with SMI to retell their narrative stories to uncover and bring into awareness positive outcomes because of the solutions that they have enacted. By focusing on solutions, the user of SFI prompts the person living with SMI to consider how a change in the challenging behavior would impact their life in terms of the consequences of changing the behavior. SFI identifies the stimuli present when challenging behavior occurs and when it does not, highlighting these differences to help develop effective solutions.

SFI incorporates the "miracle question" into the strategy. The question asks the person living with SMI to project a possible future in which challenging behavior no longer exists. It asks what would be different in terms of the outcome, particularly what naturally occurring positive consequences would be available for the person living with SMI when the challenging behavior is no longer being displayed. For example:

> I'd like you to consider for a moment that when you go to sleep tonight a miracle happens while you are asleep. The challenges that concern you and others are gone. Since you were sleeping you would not know a miracle had happened; but when you awoke you would notice because things would be different. What is the first thing you notice that would be different? (Webster, 2009)

SFI recognizes that change is incremental, and progress comes in small steps. It accepts that changing behavior is difficult and that setbacks will occur. Using SFI when problem-solving with people living with SMI attempts to generate hopefulness by reinforcing the small successes when changing a challenging behavior. SFI attempts to motivate the person living with SMI by recognizing success and discussing future steps in the change process. It also generates a sense of mastery by asking about what the person living with SMI does that prevents the challenging problem from getting worse along one of the behavioral dimensions (i.e., frequency, intensity, generalization to similar contexts). Practitioners of SFI give active encouragement and are enthusiastic about successes based on progress towards the individual's goals of changing the challenging behaviors. Statements of support and verbal praise for progress not only offer support but can be the next question for clarifying how best to continue progress toward desired solutions.

SFI provides feedback on progress when requested by individuals living with SMI. If progress stalls, practitioners employ reframing strategies to clarify what aspects of challenging behaviors can and cannot be controlled during modification efforts. Additionally, SFI practitioners explain that changes in antecedents and contingencies do not always result in behavioral change, as these factors may lie beyond the person's control during the process of addressing challenging behaviors. Reframing is used to minimize blame for a lack of progress in altering the challenging behavior so as not to lose the focus of continuing with pursuing the individual's goal; the focus is shifted to the development of a novel solution if needed or refining some aspects of the present solution.

SFI practitioners model openness to new solutions and explore how and when the person living with SMI implements the solution. The practitioner is a helper and guide for the person living with SMI to solve the problem and implement the solution. For each new solution the focus using SFI is identifying the next steps in changing the challenging behavior, having the person living with SMI specify what difference it makes when the challenging behavior is changed and what difference it will make in the lives of the person living with SMI when the adaptive behavior continues over time.

SFI is a "tool in the therapeutic toolbox" when working with individuals living with SMI. Like any intervention, SFI has limitations as to whether it can be helpful changing a behavioral challenge with the person living. The service providers need to be flexible especially if the individual living with SMI displays neurocognitive problems, involved in legal problems, may be unable to make their own decisions (i.e., guardianship), and has problems with establishing trust after many years of disappointment and losses.

Again, SFI is client-centered; the goal is what the client has established, and the practitioner may need to help the person perceive that change can be beneficial in achieving what the individual aspires to and wants. Assessment of risk may appear counter to the principles of SFI. However, it is still necessary to protect the person living with SMI and other people being in proximity of the person. Assessing risk when using SFI must be carefully planned to protect everyone without undermining the focus on strengths, self-determination, and individuation. In cases where safety is a concern, practitioners of SFI need to state that safety is a goal but labeling it as the concern of the SFI practitioner if it is not identified as a goal by the person living with SMI (Webster, 2009).

In some circumstances, clients may have either life experience or access to information and resources that might be helpful to them. This is especially so when developing possible solutions in changing a behavioral challenge. The SFI practitioner can balance a need for giving further information with respect for the knowledge and experiences of the individual living with SMI. If the person living with SMI indicates a desire to have more options and choices, using modeling and role play helps to address the problem of developing and implementing solutions for behavioral challenges by providing modeling of replacement behaviors and roleplaying the behaviors in the contexts in which the challenging behavior occurs.

Service providers can use the steps below to work with the individual living with SMI to develop and implement solutions for behavioral challenges (Bellack, 2004; Fallon et al., 2007).

1. Define behavior that is challenging. The service provider needs to be clear and specific about what the challenging behavior is and what it is not; a topographical description is the shape or the form of the challenging behavior when it is displayed—basically what the observer is sensing (Cooper et al., 2020). This may be more difficult than it seems at first. It is common for individuals to use labels such as "uncooperative," "lazy," "disagreeable," or "mean as a snake." These descriptors reflect opinions about the character of a person living with SMI, rather than specifying observable behaviors during challenging situations. Identifying and agreeing upon the specific challenging behavior enables both service providers and individuals with SMI to address concerns more effectively. This collaborative approach allows for clearer identification of when and how frequently the behavior occurs. When both parties are clear about the problem, the solution also will likely be clearer. For example, the service provider may be told by other providers that a person living with SMI "sits around the house a lot." The service provider needs to clarify exactly what the behavior of "sitting around a lot" looks like to an observer. Questions include: What does "a lot" mean? What does "sitting" look like? Is the person sitting, lying in bed, in his room, talking with others? What is the frequency and duration of the behavior being displayed? In what context does the challenging behavior occur? What has been tried to rectify the challenge? When discussing the challenging behavior, the person living with SMI may identify that the problem is that he stays at the residence "as there is nothing to do." The solution might be to spend more time at the community mental health center's clubhouse, arrange for membership at the YMCA, join a club, or get a library card.
2. The next step is to refine the challenging behavior and the problem. Using the above example, the individual living with SMI may not have the resources to engage in activities that they like to do or the lack of opportunities as the individual may not be aware of what is available. The service provider and the person living with SMI can discuss their awareness about the dimensions of the behavior—the frequency of "sitting a lot" around, the antecedent and consequential stimuli when this challenging behavior is displayed. The service

provider can collaborate with the person as to what can be done so that the challenging behavior can be altered.

3. After the problem is defined and refined with the collaboration of the person living with SMI, different solutions can be developed. Brainstorm all the possible solutions for challenging behavior. At this stage, there is no discussion of what will or will not work. The goal is to generate as many solutions as possible. As much as possible, try to involve the person living with SMI to help come up with possible solutions. Using SFI techniques, focus on the strengths of the individuals living with SMI and what were previous solutions for similar challenging behaviors that may have been implemented.
4. Think about the possible results of each solution. The question at this point is "What will happen if…?" The service provider and the individual living with SMI discuss what might happen if each of the suggested solutions that were developed were tried. The person living with SMI and the service provider discuss the possible results—both positive and negative—for each solution. It may be helpful to have the individual living with SMI to "scale" the chances of each solution succeeding in resolving the challenging behavior.
5. Choose a solution to the challenging behavior: The best solution is the one that has more positive outcomes than negative ones. No solution will be perfect. Involving the person living with SMI in choosing a solution is helpful in that they are treated as an adult, an active participant, and are reinforced for mastery over their life and goals.
6. Implement the chosen solution: In this step, it is time to enact the chosen solution. The service provider and the individual living with SMI negotiate a time to enact the solution and follow through with it. Not all solutions will work to perfection and will not work right away. Implement the solution for a long enough time to see if it will work.
7. Decide whether the solution worked: The final step in solving a challenging behavior is to review whether the solution worked. Did the positive effects outweigh the negative? Did the challenging behavior improve? The person living with SMI and service provider reviews the data and the perception of the person living with SMI about the implementation of the solution. If it did work, the person living with SMI should be praised and reinforced for the success of the solution and for improvement in their behavior. If the selected solution did not work, review as to why the solution did not work, try the solution again, or try a different solution. Finally, another solution should be selected and tried until an effective one is found or generate new and different solutions from trying one that did not work. Enlist everyone's collaboration by involving all service providers, family members, and community resources in choosing the next solution.

The steps of problem-solving can be useful in many difficult situations faced by service providers. Below is an example of how the steps were applied to help Andre, who was discussed earlier.

Andre was a young man who was identified as living with schizophrenia spectrum mental health problem. After spending time at the state hospital, he was discharged to live with his parents. The family soon became frustrated with his "irresponsible" behavior. With help from the service providers, they were able to clarify that Andre's "irresponsible behavior" involved him not taking his medication the way he was supposed to, spending all day at home and smoking in the house. Andre, his family, and service providers thought of many possible solutions. Among these, they considered trying to get him back in the hospital because of the danger of smoking in the house. They found time when Andre was willing to talk with them about these problems. He talked about how he wanted to be able to smoke at home and simply could not remember how he was supposed to take his medications. Andre, his family, and the service providers worked out a contract (described below) that clarified what the family wanted to see Andre do more often and what Andre perceived as a problem. They worked with him to identify some incentives that would be available if Andre was successful in carrying out the solution. While this plan did not work perfectly during the first month, the family, Andre, and the service providers persisted, and the plan was successful with persistent effort.

Contracting for Desired Behaviors

Behavioral contracts (also known as contingency contracts) and written contracts that are like contracts for cellular service, bank loans, and college scholarships. Behavioral contracts are between the person living with SMI and service providers, family members, and community support (Houmanfar et al., 2008; Mann, 1972; Martin & Pear, 2019). Behavioral contracting has been applied to a wide variety of areas and settings such as classroom behavior, instructional design, addictive behaviors, staff management, delinquency, self-injurious behaviors, family relationships, anorexia, weight loss programs, and bedtime compliance (Houmanfar et al., 2008). Contracts define the terms to be followed by the individual living with SMI and the consequences to be carried out on the condition of compliance or noncompliance with following the terms put forth in the "quid pro quo" contract. The behavioral contract specifies the defined behaviors that the person needs to display so that the contingencies can be presented to the person living with SMI.

The foundations of behavioral contracts are based on the experimental analysis of behavior as described by Skinner (1953) and is the foundation for applied behavior analysis (ABA) (Cooper et al., 2020). Behavioral contracts are based on the A-B-C sequence for the occurrence of a behavior: there must be a situation (the antecedent) that sets up the conditions for the behavior to occur; this is then followed by the behavior, which in turn is followed by a result, a change, or a consequence in the environment that is around the person. The "A-B-Cs of behavior"—antecedent (A), behavior (B), and consequence (C)—is a widely recognized framework for understanding behavioral patterns. While all behaviors adhere to this sequence, it is important to recognize that they are often more complex than a straightforward A-B-C progression; typically, behaviors consist of extended chains of such sequences referred to as "behavioral chains."

ABA and behavioral approaches identify and modify antecedents to the target behavior, and change the consequences that shape, reinforce, and maintain behaviors. Since behavior is a function of its consequences, behaviors followed by positive or pleasant consequences are more likely to recur than behaviors followed by negative consequences. Behaviors that are influenced by a set of consequences can be changed either by withholding those consequences or imposing a new set of consequences. Accordingly, once challenging behaviors and their controlling consequences are identified, additional incentives such as points, cash, privileges, and other reinforcers as well as the loss of privileges can be implemented through behavioral contracting to change the existing contingencies. Behavioral contracting has the utility of precisely stipulating the contingencies and guidelines that have been mutually negotiated, so all parties are knowledgeable and responsible for the implementation of the contract.

Martin and Pear (2019) have outlined the functions of behavior contracting for the individual, service providers, family members, and community support:

1. Provide mutual agreement of the behaviors and goals.
2. Ensure that all individuals involved have access to the terms of the contract so that contingencies can be applied consistently.
3. Outline specific responsibilities of all individuals involved.
4. Accessible references of the behaviors displayed, and contingencies presented to monitor progress towards goals.
5. The costs of the program to everyone who needs to make sure the positive consequences get presented when the desired behavior is displayed in terms of time, effort, and money.

Impediments to the success of using behavior contracting begin when the behavioral challenge is not clearly identified and is confusing to the person living with SMI, the service provider, and family members. Clearly and concisely defining challenging behaviors has been emphasized as an essential and required initial step for any behavior change to occur. It may be necessary that functional assessment interviews (FAI) be conducted to be able to operationally define the challenging behavior and specify the dimensions of the challenging behavior; interviewees should include the person living with SMI who is displaying the challenging behaviors, service providers, family members, and community support people who have had frequent contact with the person.

The goals and the contingencies in the contract need to be agreed upon mutually by the individual living with SMI, service providers and other people involved who are responsible for the implementation and the monitoring of the contract. Behavior contracting is not successful when it is perceived by the person living with SMI as overly restrictive, punishing, demeaning, too rigid, and imposed upon the indexed person. Behavioral contracts ought to be negotiated with input from all parties. Vagueness of the terms of the contract, lack of vigilance to observe and monitor the fidelity by all parties following the contract and implementing the associated contingencies can impact on the effectiveness of the contract and attainment of the stated goals.

The behavioral contract needs to be written in the language and the reading level of the person living with SMI. Individuals living with SMI actively contribute to the development of the contract, collaboratively identifying both short- and long-term goals that are attainable and appropriate. When contractual objectives are excessively challenging, they are unlikely to be met; as a result, efforts by individuals who live with SMI to achieve the agreed-upon reinforcing outcomes may fall short, and the intended adaptive behaviors may not manifest or be reinforced, leading to noncompliance with the contract.

Providing reinforcing consequences is imperative for the completion of each small step toward the end goal. The specified replacement behaviors must be in the behavioral repertoire of the person living with SMI. Participation in skill training to acquire the defined behavioral skill can be a stipulation in the contract; participation in skill training can be reinforced as well as the display of the small steps in the shaping of the desired replacement behavior to enhance the completion of the contractual goal. This will increase treatment success for those individuals who do not present with the behavioral repertoire that is necessary to complete the end goal. The contract initially should specify relatively simple goals, ensuring that the individual living with SMI obtains access to the reinforcement. Once the client has achieved the desired level of the behavior, systematic increases in goal difficulty that are mutually agreed upon can be implemented with access to preferred reinforcement as a consequence of displaying the behavior in the next step.

The behavioral contract not only must identify specific target behaviors for change but behaviors that will be supported in natural environments once change occurs. It is important that the contract specifies the conditions under which target behaviors and access reinforcement occur, including times, frequency, and amount. The dates for review of the contract also should be established. The more specific the details of the contract are, the better the chances of all parties following the contract. Finally, signatures are acquired so that all individuals acknowledge the terms of the contract and increase chances of adherence.

Developing a "Token Economy" to Change Challenging Behavior

Token economies or point systems are behavioral interventions that use the principles of positive reinforcement with people or groups of people to reinforce expected appropriate adaptive behaviors (American Psychological Association, n.d.; Ayllon & Azrin, 1968). Contracts can be written so the person living with SMI can earn points for doing identified and adaptive replacement behaviors. The person living with SMI then can exchange points for certain rewards that have been agreed upon. The number of points determines what the person living with SMI can "earn" with his points. This is called a "token economy" as originally the person received tokens for the display of targeted adaptive behaviors; however, any stimulus can be used including points, fake money, and checkmarks.

Like the use of behavioral contracting, a token economy is a highly individualized, reinforcement-based, behavior change system, derived from the principles of operant conditioning and the experimental analysis of behavior (Ayllon & Azrin, 1968); reviews of the use and effectiveness of token economies have concluded that it is effective in altering both behavioral excesses and deficits in behaviors (Gholipour et al., 2012; McMonagle & Sultana, 2000). It has been utilized with changing behaviors in individuals living with SMI, autistic spectrum disorder, substance use, disorders of mood, and affective regulation. It has been effective in psychiatric hospitals, forensic settings, group homes, and academic and business settings and can be used with individuals or groups (Ayllon & Azrin, 1968; Dickerson et al., 2005; Glowacki et al., 2016; Kazdin & Bootzin, 1972; Lawrence et al., 2023).

The specific components of a token economy include (a) the identification of measurable and observable targeted behaviors (e.g., taking a shower, speaking without delusional content) by service providers, family members, and friends; (b) the presentation or giving of tokens (e.g., points, checkmarks, real or imitation money); and (c) the exchange of tokens by the individual for a variety of backup reinforcers (e.g., watching a movie, computer time, access to an activity) (Cooper et al., 2020). Tokens can be used to reinforce and strengthen identified replacement behaviors; consequences are most likely to influence subsequent behavior when they immediately follow the behavior rather than when there is a long interval between a behavior and its consequences.

The token stimulus becomes a generalized conditioned reinforcer when it is paired with a primary reinforcer. According to Skinner (1953), tokens can acquire properties of a reinforcer by repeated association with preferred reinforcers, such as food, clothing, activities, or time spent with a preferred person. A principle of the experimental analysis of behavior postulates that two stimuli will come to be associated with each other if they occur together temporally (Cooper et al., 2020). A neutral stimulus that is paired with a primary reinforcer will come to be a reinforcer through its association with reinforcing consequences. A common example is money, which has no inherent value except for the association it has with allowing the person possessing the money to be able to acquire preferred items (e.g., reinforcers) such as food, housing, and leisure activities. People will engage in many types of behavior—legal and illegal—to acquire money. The acquisition of money reinforces the behaviors and subsequent behaviors that are followed by access to money. Money is perhaps the best and greatest generalized reinforcer for humankind!

Advantages of a Point System

For ease of use, many practitioners of ABA have substituted points for tokens. Going forward in the chapter, point system will be in place of token economy but they are one and the same.

There are several advantages that a point system brings to changing behaviors. Points can be used like money. For example, just as people earn money for work, people can earn points for doing the behaviors that are in the contract. Also, just as money buys things that people want, points can be used to buy desired items and activities for the person living with SMI.

- Points are "portable." Points are easily portable and administered, giving points whenever and wherever a desired behavior occurs. Later, they can be exchanged for other incentives. Points represent items such as food or a trip to a preferred restaurant which cannot be immediately provided. Points also can represent privileges, such as allowing the person living with SMI to take his medications without supervision.
- The points represent a "bridge" to the actual reinforcers. While the points themselves will probably have little value for the person living with SMI, they knows that the points represent the opportunity to get other things that are wanted. The points help the person to remember what the reinforcers are and, in doing so, acquire value through pairing and association.
- A points system can be used to change behaviors if the person living with SMI needs more immediate and frequent reinforcement. If the replacement behavior is a new skill for the person to display, immediate reinforcement is needed as soon as possible after the adaptive behavior occurs.
- Points are flexible. They can be used to buy a wide variety of other incentives. Depending on the wants or desires of the person living with SMI, she may be able to buy from the point store make up, a movie, preferred food, clothing or many other items that are incentives to engage in the preferred behavior. This helps to keep the points from losing their value. The individual may lose her liking for videos or a favored food but she's not likely to lose her desire for all things that she can buy with the points.
- You can change the point exchange system to match the behavioral capabilities of the person living with SMI change. As the person living with SMI behavior changes, you can alter the point system to help her succeed. This means that your expectations can be lowered or raised to be more appropriate and in line with the capabilities of the person living with SMI by altering the amount or points earned for an identified behavior or increasing the number of points needed to acquire a preferred item (especially as behavior skills develop).
- For service providers, family and others providing the points, it is an opportunity to verbally praise and pay attention to the person living with SMI when they display an adaptive behavior. Changing behavior involves recognizing and acknowledging when an individual demonstrates adaptive behaviors.
- Giving points allows others a chance to compliment success. Compliments from other people are important incentives for everyone. It can be easy for many service providers to overlook opportunities to compliment the person living with SMI. A contract and point system help to remind service providers to identify successes and to compliment the person as well as give the points.
- The points provide a chance for the person living with SMI to compliment himself. It is important that the person living with SMI gives herself credit for her successes. By getting points and compliments from others, the individual living

Table 4.1 Example of a point sheet used for a person living with SMI in the community

Behaviors	Points	Mon	Tue	Wed	Thur	Fri	Sat	Sun
Take shower every morning	50							
Wash hair daily	50							
Eat meals with family	25							
Take medication	50							
Go to clubhouse Mon–Fri from 9 am to 3 pm	100							
Go to bed by 11 pm; midnight on weekends	10							

with SMI can begin to recognize her own success and reduce the negative impact of the stigma associated with SMI.

- The points provide a measure of success. By keeping track of the points that the person living with SMI is earning, service providers, family members, and community support people can track progress. The points are an objective way of measuring how well the person is doing in recovery.

Table 4.1 presents an example of a point sheet used for a person living with SMI in the community. The point sheet was used to increase her attendance at the day treatment center and independently doing her hygiene. With the points that she earned for the identified behaviors she can "purchase" a variety of things that she likes. The following are examples of number of points needed to get access to the preferred reinforcers:

1000 points = sleep late on weekends.
1200 points = choose a movie video on Friday.
1500 points = order pizza to be delivered.
4000 points = go to the restaurant of her choosing.

This was applied in Andre's case. As Andre improved and more easily met the criteria of his contract, his family adjusted the requirements of the contract. For example, a higher number of points (6000 instead of 4000) were required to go to his chosen restaurant. They adjusted other parts of the contract as well. Because Andre was improving and found it easier to meet his family's expectations, the increases in expectations didn't bother him (if he could still succeed in attaining enough points to get what he wanted).

Summary

The goal of effective communication with people living with SMI is to obtain collaboration with the individual to change a behavior that may be impeding their recovery journey. Good communication fosters effective care, builds trust, establishes rapport, develops teamwork with the person living with SMI, leads to successful outcomes and optimal therapeutic relationships. Communication involves both verbal and nonverbal behaviors but also listening. Being an empathetic, nonjudgmental listener, and conveying that the person is being heard and understood can make a potentially problematic interaction a safe and collaborative process that meets the goals of the person living with SMI and the service provider.

Communicating with individuals living with SMI presents challenges as the person living with SMI may have cognitive problems, bizarre beliefs, speech problems, and difficulty staying on topic. Active listening can enhance the effectiveness of the message being communicated when the service provider: (a) matches nonverbal behaviors to the verbal message being given; (b) maintains eye level contact and uses the person's name to ensure attention; (c) use simple gestures and avoid crowding the person; (d) communicate in a distraction-free environment; (e) shows empathy, validate the person's feelings, and avoids assumptions and inferences; and (f) asks for clarification to ensure understanding. Whether requesting a task to be done, conveying information or providing feedback to a person living with SMI, the speaker ought to use a calm tone, brief sentences, and clear statements. Allow time for the person to process and respond. Praise and reinforce positive behaviors and progress towards goals.

Emotions play a significant role in communication with individuals living with SMI. Expressed Emotionality (EE) occurs when high levels of criticism and hostility are communicated to the individual living with SMI; high EE has been shown to lead to poor outcomes. Interactions in which high EE is present can lead to mistrust and withdrawal. Service providers need to avoid communication with people living with SMI if angry or frustrated to avoid overreactions and harmful statements. Creating a supportive environment is more effective than dealing with problems after they arise.

To avoid the perception of blame and criticism by the person living with SMI, service providers need to communicate using "I-statements." The basic format of the type of "I-statement" is to say how the behavior is making the speaker feel when the person does an identified behavior. The speaker states what the person living with SMI can do the next time in the same context to change the outcome and the emotional impact on the speaker. When requesting a change in behavior, service providers should avoid reactive listening and attempt to understand rather than to respond, interrupt, criticize or argue. Limits should be set; if the discussion with the person living with SMI is not progressing, it should be continued at a future time and place. The discussion can be terminated if the person engages in delusional speech and does not respond to redirection. The discussion should be terminated as continuing may inadvertently reinforce the delusional behaviors. Establish mutually agreeable times and places for conversations and ensure to follow through on these arrangements.

A solution-focused approach is beneficial when discussing a behavior change with the person living with SMI. Solution-Focused Interventions (SFI) are positive, person-centered, strengths, competency-based and future-oriented; SFI views the people living with SMI as the decision-makers and experts in their reality by using their strengths and abilities to solve the challenging behavior. SFI focuses on current challenges and future solutions rather than past problems. It recognizes that change is gradual, and progress comes in small steps. SFI provides positive reinforcement and feedback, even if progress is slow, to maintain motivation and hope.

Hypothetical scenarios are developed using SFI with the individual living with SMI to help them to envision a future without the problem, identifying what would be different if the challenging behavior no longer occurred. Using reframing and feedback, SFI involves the individual in collaboratively setting meaningful and achievable goals. Emphasizing positive outcomes and solutions, SFI focuses on what works and how changes in behavior can lead to positive outcomes. Using reframing and feedback, the practitioner of SFI adjusts strategies based on the individual's unique context and needs. By utilizing collaboratively developed solutions with individuals living with SMI, service providers can establish and implement behavioral contracts designed to support desired behavioral change.

Behavior contracts are written agreements between the person living with SMI and service providers, family members, or community support that specify the behaviors to be performed and the consequences for compliance or noncompliance. The behavior contract clearly defines the targeted behaviors that need to be changed, making sure that the definition is specific, observable, and measurable to all. The contract should be written in a way that the person living with SMI can understand. All parties involved must mutually agree to the terms and goals of the contract, including using positive consequences for compliance and potential negative consequences when serious behavioral challenges such as aggression towards self or others occur. Short- and long-term goals need to be specified; goals should be reasonable and achievable, with incremental steps towards the ultimate desired change of behavior. Reviews are regularly scheduled to assess progress and make necessary adjustments. All parties sign the contract to acknowledge their commitment to the implementation of terms of the contract.

Another behavioral strategy that can be used to foster changes of challenging behaviors is the token economy. A token economy is a system where individuals earn tokens, points, or checkmarks for desired behaviors, which can be later exchanged for desired and preferred reinforcers. Advantages of using a token economy with a behavior change plan is that immediate reinforcement can be carried out; tokens or points are portable and can be used in various contexts and situations. Token economies provide flexibility as targeted behaviors can be added or removed. Points earned for each identified behavior can be easily increased or decreased depending on the objective measure of progress.

The initial step in any behavior change intervention is the clear identification and definition of target behaviors. The number of tokens or points for the occurrence of adaptive behavior must be specified and reinforcers that can be accessed through the earning of points need to be determined. An example would be earning points for taking a shower, attending a day program, and taking medications; points that are earned can then be exchanged for reinforcers such as movies, restaurant meals, takeout, and other privileges. Service providers can monitor points earned and spent and adjust as the targeted behaviors change. Regularly review of the token economy system ensures that it is effective as adjustments are made according to the outcome of the review.

By using behavioral contracts and token economies, service providers can create structured and motivating environments that encourage positive behavior changes in individuals living with SMI.

References

Acker, G. M. (2012). Burnout among mental health care providers. *Journal of Social Work, 12*(5), 475–490. https://doi.org/10.1177/1468017310392413

American Psychological Association. (n.d.). Token economy. In *APA Dictionary of Psychology*. https://dictionary.apa.org/token-economy

Ayllon, T., & Azrin, N. H. (1968). *The token economy*. Appleton-Century-Crofts. https://doi.org/10.1037/10627-000

Bebbington, P., & Kuipers, L. (1994). The predictive utility of expressed emotion in schizophrenia: An aggregate analysis. *Psychological Medicine, 24*(3), 707–718. https://doi.org/10.1017/S0033291700027860

Bedell, J. R., Hunter, R. H., & Corrigan, P. W. (1997). Current approaches to assessment and treatment of persons with serious mental illness. *Professional Psychology: Research and Practice, 28*(3), 217–228. https://doi.org/10.1037/0735-7028.28.3.217

Bellack, A. S. (2004). Skills training for people with severe mental illness. *Psychiatric Rehabilitation Journal, 27*(4), 375–391. https://doi.org/10.2975/27.2004.375.391

Berry, K., Barrowclough, C., & Haddock, G. (2011). The role of expressed emotion in relationships between psychiatric staff and people with a diagnosis of psychosis: A review of the literature. *Schizophrenia Bulletin, 37*(5), 958–972. https://doi.org/10.1093/schbul/sbp162

Cooper, J. O., Heron, T. E., & Heward, W. L. (2020). *Applied behavior analysis* (3rd ed.). Pearson Education. https://www.pearson.com/en-us/subject-catalog/p/applied-behavior-analysis/P200000000905/9780137477210

Corcoran, J., & Pillai, V. (2009). A review of the research on solution-focused therapy. *British Journal of Social Work, 39*(2), 234–242. https://doi.org/10.1093/bjsw/bcm098

Dickerson, F. B., Tenhula, W. N., & Green-Paden, L. D. (2005). The token economy for schizophrenia: Review of the literature and recommendations for future research. *Schizophrenia Research, 75*(2–3), 405–416. https://doi.org/10.1016/j.schres.2004.08.026

Falloon, I. R. H., Barbieri, L., Boggian, I., & Lamonaca, D. (2007). Problem solving training for schizophrenia: Rationale and review. *Journal of Mental Health, 16*(5), 553–568. https://doi.org/10.1080/09638230701494910

Gholipour, A., Abolghasemi, S. H., Gholinia, K., & Taheri, S. (2012). Token reinforcement therapeutic approach is more effective than exercise for controlling negative symptoms of schizophrenic patients: A randomized controlled trial. *International Journal of Preventive Medicine, 3*(7), 466–470. https://europepmc.org/article/PMC/3415186

Glowacki, K., Warner, G., & White, C. (2016). The use of a token economy for behaviour and symptom management in adult psychiatric inpatients. A critical review of the literature. *Journal of Psychiatric Intensive Care, 12*(2), 119–127. https://doi.org/10.20299/jpi.2016.009

Goldiamond, I. (2022). *A programing contingency analysis of mental health*. Routledge. https://doi.org/10.4324/9781003260103

Gottman, J. M., Katz, L. F., & Hooven, C. (2013). *Meta-emotion: How families communicate emotionally*. Routledge. https://www.routledge.com/Meta-Emotion-How-Families-Communicate-Emotionally/Gottman-Katz-Hooven/p/book/9780805849480

Green, M. F., Kern, R. S., Braff, D. L., & Mintz, J. (2000). Neurocognitive deficits and functional outcome in schizophrenia: Are we measuring the "right stuff"? *Schizophrenia Bulletin, 26*(1), 119–136. https://doi.org/10.1093/oxfordjournals.schbul.a033430

Harvey, P. D., & Strassnig, M. (2012). Predicting the severity of everyday functional disability in people with schizophrenia: Cognitive deficits, functional capacity, symptoms, and health status. *World Psychiatry, 11*(2), 73–79. https://doi.org/10.1016/j.wpsyc.2012.05.004

Houmanfar, R., Maglieri, K. A., Roman, H. R., & Ward, T. A. (2008). Behavioral contracting. In W. T. O'Donohue & J. E. Fisher (Eds.), *Cognitive behavior therapy: Applying empirically supported techniques in your practice* (2nd ed., pp. 53–59). Wiley. https://doi.org/10.1002/9780470228354.ch7

Kazdin, A. E., & Bootzin, R. R. (1972). The token economy: An evaluative review. *Journal of Applied Behavior Analysis, 5*(3), 343–372. https://doi.org/10.1901/jaba.1972.5-343

Krasner, M., & Epstein, R. (2010). Mindful communication: Bringing intention, attention, and reflection to clinical practice. *New York chapter of the American College of Physicians. Physicians Foundation for Health Systems Excellence, 103*. https://physiciansfoundation.org/wp-content/uploads/2017/12/NYACP_Mindful_Communication_Curriculum.pdf

Laidlaw, T., Coverdale, J., Falloon, I., & Kydd, R. (2002). Caregivers' stresses when living together or apart from patients with chronic schizophrenia. *Community Mental Health Journal, 38*(10), 303–310. https://doi.org/10.1023/A:1015949325141

Lawrence, K. C., Makhonza, L. O., & Aliya, M. S. (2023). The role of token economy therapy in reducing the psychological burden of formal caregivers. *The Open Public Health Journal, 16*(1), 1–7. https://doi.org/10.2174/18749445-v16-e230711-2022-190

Ma, C. F., Chan, S. K. W., Chung, Y. L., Ng, S. M., Hui, C. L. M., Suen, Y. N., & Chen, E. Y. H. (2021). The predictive power of expressed emotion and its components in relapse of schizophrenia: A meta-analysis and meta-regression. *Psychological Medicine, 51*(3), 365–375. https://doi.org/10.1017/S0033291721000209

Manikandan, S., & Raja, A. (2023). "Expressed emotion; a real thorn in the flesh": Addressing the role of expressed emotions (EE) in psychiatric illness outcome. *Journal of Emerging Technologies and Innovative Research, 10*(8), 558–563. https://www.jetir.org/papers/JETIR2308545.pdf

Mann, R. A. (1972). The behavior-therapeutic use of contingency contracting to control an adult behavior problem: Weight control. *Journal of Applied Behavior Analysis, 5*(2), 99–109. https://doi.org/10.1901/jaba.1972.5-99

Marom, S., Munitz, H., Jones, P. B., Weizman, A., & Hermesh, H. (2005). Expressed emotion: Relevance to rehospitalization in schizophrenia over 7 years. *Schizophrenia Bulletin, 31*(3), 751–758. https://doi.org/10.1093/schbul/sbi016

Martin, G., & Pear, J. J. (2019). *Behavior modification: What it is and how to do it* (11th ed.). Routledge. https://doi.org/10.4324/9780429020599

McMonagle, T., & Sultana, A. (2000). Token economy for schizophrenia. *Cochrane Database of Systematic Reviews, 2000*(3), Article CD001473. https://doi.org/10.1002/14651858.CD001473

Nolan, R. W. (1999). *Communicating and adapting across culture: Living and working in the global village*. Bergin & Garvey. https://doi.org/10.1007/978-0-313-37126-4

Papageorgiou, A., Loke, Y., Deane, K. H. O., & Fromage, M. (2017). Communication skills training for mental health professionals working with people with severe mental illness. *Cochrane Database of Systematic Reviews, 2017*(8), Article CD010006. https://doi.org/10.1002/14651858.CD010006

Pescosolido, B. A., Halpern-Manners, A., Luo, L., & Perry, B. (2021). Trends in public stigma of mental illness in the US, 1996–2018. *JAMA Network Open, 4*(12), e2140202. https://doi.org/10.1001/jamanetworkopen.2021.40202

Puscas, L., Kogan, J. R., & Holmboe, E. S. (2021). Assessing interpersonal and communication skills. *Journal of Graduate Medical Education, 13*(2), 91–95. https://doi.org/10.4300/JGME-D-20-00883.1

Relationships Australia. (2024, October 28). *How to use "I" statements instead of "You" statements during difficult conversations*. Relationships Australia NSW. https://www.relationshipsnsw.org.au/blog/i-statements-vs-you-statements/

Rogers, C. R., & Farson, R. E. (1957). *Active listening* (p. 84). Industrial Relations Center of the University of Chicago. https://doi.org/10.1080/08873267.2014.913247

Skinner, B. F. (1957). *Verbal behavior*. Appleton-Century-Crofts. https://doi.org/10.1037/11256-000

Skinner, B. F. (1953). *Science and human behavior*. Simon and Schuster. https://www.amazon.com/Science-Human-Behavior-B-F-Skinner/dp/0029290406

Tennant, K., Long, A., & Toney-Butler, T. J. (2024, January). Active listening. [Updated 2023 Sep 13]. In *StatPearls* [Internet]. StatPearls Publishing. https://www.ncbi.nlm.nih.gov/books/NBK442015/

Visser, C. F. (2013). The origin of the solution-focused approach. *International Journal of Solution-Focused Practices, 1*(1), 3–7. https://doi.org/10.14335/ijsfp.v1i1.10

Waldron, I. (2024, February). *Communicating with a loved one who has a mental illness.* National Alliance on Mental Illness (NAMI): Main Line PA. https://namimainlinepa.org/communicating-with-a-loved-one-who-has-a-mental-illness/#:~:text=Remember%20that%20a%20mentally%20ill,you%20and%20your%20loved%20one

Webster, D. (2009). Using solution-focused approaches. In P. Barker (Ed.), *Psychiatric and mental health nursing: The craft of caring* (2nd ed., pp. 377–383). Hodder Arnold. https://doi.org/10.1201/9781315382781

Wilson, T. D. (2000). Human information behavior. *Informing Science, 3*, 49–56. https://doi.org/10.28945/576

Wong, S. E., Wilder, D. A., Schock, K., & Clay, C. (2004). Behavioral interventions with severe and persistent mental disorders. In S. E. Wong (Ed.), *Using evidence in social work practice: Behavioral perspectives* (pp. 210–230). Routledge. https://doi.org/10.4324/9780203496396

Chapter 5
Collaboration and Ethical Considerations in the Treatment of People Living with Serious Mental Illness to Enhance Their Mental Health and Recovery

Introduction

The treatment of individuals living with serious mental illness (SMI) presents a complex interplay of clinical, ethical, and relational challenges that demand a nuanced understanding of recovery-oriented care. Following the preceding overview of the symptoms and functional impairments associated with SMI, this chapter shifts focus to the collaborative and ethical principles and dimensions of care that promote engagement, autonomy, and sustained recovery. As mental health professionals increasingly adopt person-centered frameworks, it becomes essential to examine how therapeutic relationships, interdisciplinary collaboration, and ethical decision-making shape outcomes for individuals navigating chronic psychiatric conditions.

The multifaceted barriers to engagement in treatment is explicated, including stigma, learned helplessness, neurocognitive deficits, and treatment discontinuation. It emphasizes the importance of fostering autonomy and shared decision-making through relationship-centered care (RCC), motivational interviewing (MI), and solution-focused practices. These approaches are not merely techniques but foundational strategies that reinforce agency, build trust, and counteract the passivity often observed in individuals with SMI. Ethical challenges—such as coercion, functional anosognosia, and risk-averse clinical practices—are addressed through applied behavioral and collaborative models that prioritize empowerment and respect for the lived experience of service users.

Structured around key themes—engagement, collaboration, RCC, MI, solution-focused practice, recovery, autonomy, stigma, ethical dilemmas, and interdisciplinary teamwork—this chapter provides a comprehensive framework for understanding how recovery-oriented systems of care can be implemented in real-world settings. Drawing on empirical evidence and clinical insights, it offers students a critical lens through which to evaluate their role in promoting wellness, preventing relapses, and

G. F. McKeegan, *Behavior Change Interventions for Serious Mental Illness*, Evidence-Based Practices in Behavioral Health,
https://doi.org/10.1007/978-3-032-18372-9_5

supporting meaningful participation in treatment. The goal is to equip future practitioners with the conceptual and relational tools necessary to navigate the ethical terrain of mental health care while honoring the dignity and preferences of those they serve.

Individuals living with SMI are known to have highly variable and heterogeneous behavioral problems, symptoms, onset, duration, and outcome of mental health problems and the need for extended treatment. Variables that determine outcomes of treatment include age of onset, premorbid functioning, and duration of the mental health problem, initial response to treatment, gender, race ethnicity, veteran status, family support, service availability, personality variables, co-occurring substance use, depression, neurocognitive performance, and certain genetic factors (Perkins et al., 2008). Poor outcomes and quality of life have been associated when the individual displays a preponderance of impairments in functional capacities (i.e., negative symptoms) (Fervaha et al., 2014; Rabinowitz et al., 2012). Negative symptoms are the absence or diminution of expected behaviors displayed by age-appropriate peers. The negative behaviors are heterogeneous and include challenges with basic activities of daily living and social roles, such as working, going to school, participation in leisure activities, and social and romantic relationships. It is estimated that up to 60% of individuals living with SMI have predominant negative symptoms that are clinically relevant and need intervention (Correll & Schooler, 2020). These functional impairments remain despite improvement in positive symptoms (i.e., the presence of problematic behaviors), such as hallucinations and delusions over the duration of living with an SMI. Additionally, there is the phenomena of loss of medication efficacy that results in a re-emergence of symptoms and possibly serious life-threatening behaviors. This phenomenon is estimated to contribute to 3.5% of relapses per month, yet it accounts for over 60% of psychiatric facility readmissions (Weiden & Olfson, 1995), ultimately disrupting the individual's recovery process.

Treatment discontinuation—dropping out of treatment—is a seminal factor that has plagued the treatment of people living with SMI. Treatment discontinuation results in an increase in positive symptoms and challenging behaviors, withdrawal from others, and readmissions to psychiatric facilities. Dangerous behaviors such as aggression and self-harm including suicide may re-emerge. Discontinuing treatment results in a worsened prognosis as formerly effective and beneficial medications may become ineffective, with resulting resistance to medications that were previously effective; discontinuation of treatment has also been shown to escalate health care costs. Variables involved in the discontinuation of treatment are persistent symptoms or side effects; lack of routines and community support; logistical problems (e.g., transportation, financial); homelessness; cognitive deficits; legal entanglements and incarcerations; and changes to dosing or medications due to side effects (Velligan et al., 2010).

Living with SMI is a long-standing mental health challenge; individuals living with SMI may require lifelong psychological and psychopharmacological treatment and interventions. People living with SMI often have difficulty engaging and remaining in treatment. Dropout rates from treatment are high and variable.

Manschreck and Boshes (2007) found that after 18 months, nearly a third of participants discontinued medications and treatment. In a study by Perkins et al. (2008), nearly half of the participants had discontinued treatment within a year. Other estimates are that 33–44% of individuals living with SMI discontinue treatment 6 months after onset of living with an SMI; by the first year after onset, it is estimated that 59% have dropped out of treatment (Jung et al., 2011). Research from Korea has shown that over 70% dropped out of treatment within 10 years after the initial recognition of living with an SMI. Whatever the duration of staying in treatment, discontinuing treatment can lead to serious consequences, including emergence of dangerous behaviors (e.g., suicide and aggression), and increased treatment resistance to pharmacological interventions (Jung et al., 2011).

People living with SMI often present to service providers as preferring a passive role in the decision-making process about their recovery, goal-making and interventions; they rely and depend on the service providers to be the expert and make the most beneficial choices for them.

Passivity in decision-making may be the result of the internalization of stigma of living with SMI, perceiving themselves as less competent and more dependent on others. The passivity may be reinforced by service providers who are risk averse about making any decisions that would increase the service providers' exposure to liability, legal involvement, and punitive reactions by institutional and professional boards of practice (Zisman-Ilani et al., 2021). People living with SMI probably have experienced more coercive interventions than in any other health care field (Zisman-Ilani et al., 2021). Decision-making is a skill that may not be appreciated, prompted for, and reinforced by mental health service providers and may result in aversive outcomes such as forced medications, involuntary commitment, and longer duration of hospitalizations.

In a study by Morán-Sánchez and his colleagues (Morán-Sánchez et al., 2021), 64.4% of service users living with SMI preferred to adopt a passive role in therapeutic relationships with service providers. The preference of playing a passive role in the decision-making process was significantly associated with older and disabled individuals. These service users perceived that their well-being depends on the actions and decisions of professional experts and were accustomed to being complaint with the service providers in their recovery.

One of the serious functional problems exhibited by individuals living with SMI is making decisions that result in adverse outcomes for the person. Mental health professionals assess the undesirable outcomes of decisions by people living with SMI as "poor judgment." Judgment is part of the mental status examination; it is defined as "the mental act of comparing choices between a given set of values in order to select a course of action" (Shahrokh & Hales, 2003, p. 106); a determination is made if the course of action from the decision-making is socially acceptable (Strub & Black, 1995). The problem in decision-making can contribute to challenging behaviors such as nonadherence to medications, refusing to attend recovery programs, nonattendance at outpatient appointments, failing to exercise, poor diet, excessive use of substances, or engaging in unprotected sex. Other consequences of poor decisions include worsening of symptoms and emergence of behavioral challenges, reduced life satisfaction, impaired daily and social functioning, rehospitalization, clashes with law enforcement, and impaired physical health; more tragic outcomes can include accidental death, homicide, or suicide. In some cases, flawed decision-making by individuals living with SMI is a product of neurocognitive problems, including impaired attention, working memory, and response inhibition (Cáceda et al., 2014). Emotional dysregulation—mood swings and lability—and impaired cognitive abilities due to altered mental states and intoxication from substance use contribute to impaired decision-making that would be described as "impulsive," often resulting in unfavorable and harmful outcomes for the individual (Oliani et al., 2021).

Decision-making for a problem is defined by the actions or options among which one must choose; the person making the decision must: (1) become aware of alternative behaviors or actions for the problem; (2) cognizant of the possible outcomes or consequences of the actions; (3) consider the contingencies or conditional probabilities that relate to the outcomes of each of the actions; and (4) a comparison of the accuracy and efficiency of each of these sets of consequences (i.e., chances of success).

Many people living with chronic physical or mental health challenges experience feelings of helplessness. "Learned helplessness" refers to the condition wherein behavior is consistent with the perception that actions do not impact outcomes, that someone feels unable to change or control a situation, even when presented with the opportunity to do so. This usually occurs after the person repeatedly experiences aversive and traumatic events. The person perceives that there is no avoiding or escaping traumatic and distressing events. The person perceives the events as uncontrollable and that she is powerless to affect the outcome. Behaviorally, one might fail to be proactive and active when opportunities to effect change exist (Morgan, 2020) as escape and avoidant behaviors are extinguished (i.e., the behaviors of escape and avoidance are not negatively reinforced by the cessation of the aversive event). Learned helplessness is more prevalent in people who consider their physical or psychological challenges as an adverse incident and experience powerlessness to alter its effects.

Learned helplessness also has a detrimental effect on behavior and physiological functions; people living with SMI commonly experience trouble completing activities and often display behavioral patterns of learned helplessness. Those individuals may possess unfavorable thoughts and perceptions concerning their capacity to engage in behaviors that would result in a beneficial outcome. Individuals living with SMI experience helplessness during involuntary treatment and medications over objections which significantly affect recovery (Mohamed et al., 2024).

Decision-making is a skill and uses the same steps as in problem-solving and solution-focused intervention (SFI) presented in Chap. 4. It is a routine process in life, occurring from when we wake up until we decide to go to bed. However, autonomous decision-making may not be a skill that can occur in settings in which people living with SMI reside; congregate living facilities for people living with SMI are mini-institutions that deprive the person living with SMI of being able to make basic daily decisions such as when to get up, what to wear, what to do, and what to eat. Consequently, individuals may have limited opportunities to engage in, practice, and refine decision-making skills that are influenced by environmental consequences, wherein effective choices are reinforced through positive outcomes. Developing sound decision-making abilities contributes to a sense of competence and personal control—attributes that directly counteract the development of learned helplessness.

Problems in displaying functional behaviors may occur as passivity, helplessness, and dependency on others that become learned behaviors as well. Neurocognitive problems that impact the functional capabilities of people living with SMI can be affected by side effects of psychiatric medications as well as the lack of stimulation and meaningful activities due to lack of opportunities and resources. Decision-making would be impacted if the person does not have options from which to choose, resulting in passivity, lack of socialization, and daily deficits in the availability of reinforcing stimuli. At times the only reinforcing stimulation individuals receive in settings in which they reside is from nicotine and caffeine in tobacco and coffee, respectively.

If a caretaker performs a task or activity for the person living with SMI, one will have to question as to why the person would do it himself. The law of least effort effects all organisms including humans; the law of least effort states that individuals will avoid putting effort into performing a task when the outcome is already determined as the effort to complete the task is perceived as not reinforcing (American Psychological Association, n.d.-c). Individuals frequently delegate routine tasks—such as cooking, laundry, childcare, or bill payment—to other household members, once they have already benefited from the outcomes of these activities (for instance, having meals prepared, access to clean clothing, avoidance of collection calls, or reduction of distress from children). The principle known as the "law of least effort" influences behavior broadly. When such patterns are observed in individuals with SMI, their actions may be interpreted as negative symptoms, specifically avolition and anergia, which refer to diminished motivation and energy required for carrying out daily responsibilities and routines.

Challenges with engaging in ongoing treatment individuals living with SMI may lead to discontinuation of treatment, resulting in symptoms, the return of challenging behaviors, rehospitalizations, disruptions in the recovery process, and poor clinical outcomes. Several variables impact the level of treatment engagement, including accessibility of care and the therapeutic alliance with service providers, including trusting that the service provider will address the unique goals and aspirations of the individual living with SMI. Establishing rapport with an individual living with SMI is an essential component of engagement in a therapeutic alliance during recovery.

Challenges to adherence to rehabilitation sometimes are the result of displayed behaviors by the person living with SMI that occur during participation in rehabilitative interventions. People living with SMI may be hesitant to engage in the recovery process because of past experiences of being treated as less competent and having perceptions as not having any control over their lives and futures (i.e., learned helplessness). Past service providers may have been authoritarian in the approach giving the message to the individual living with SMI that the service provider "knows what is best" for the individual. The person living with SMI also may be experiencing delusional suspicious beliefs about the service provider and the recovery interventions in general.

The stigma of living with SMI impacts the individual engaging in and participating in their recovery process. The stigma of living with SMI has been explained in terms of the cognitive and behavioral constructs of stereotypes, prejudice, and discrimination that contribute to social exclusion (McGinty et al., 2018). Discrimination reduces the belief of the individual in their abilities and strengths. The result of stigma is a lack of opportunities and decreases in self-esteem and self-efficacy (Avdibegović & Hasanović, 2017; Corrigan & Bink, 2016). Corrigan and Bink (2016) have outlined the various subtypes of stigmas including avoidance of the person because of the label of living with SMI; discriminatory behaviors from public and private institutions limiting and restricting access to options for the person living with SMI; and self-stigma when the individual believes and accepts the stereotypes of living with SMI. The effects of self-stigma include diminished confidence in an individual's abilities, the internalization of the "sick role," and the perception of oneself as incompetent. This may lead to a sense of reduced responsibility for one's actions and a belief that one cannot meet societal expectations for daily living and achievement. This perception by the person living with SMI results in loss of educational and employment opportunities, financial independence, self-sufficiency, supportive and intimate relationships, and opportunities to use innate talents and skills.

An individual living with SMI may give up trying because of a lack of confidence in their capabilities. The recovery interventions may not be consistent with the subjective experiences and/or the expressed desires of the person living with SMI. In addition, if the person living with SMI has neurocognitive challenges, he may not be able to participate and benefit from proposed recovery interventions. The above factors contribute to the person living with SMI having difficulty in engaging and being an active partner in their recovery and participating in beneficial interventions.

The concept of recovery-oriented care has been the focal point for people living with SMI for over three decades. The precise definition of what constitutes recovery has been elusive. Anthony (1993) has been credited with initially summarizing recovery in mental health as:

> …the process of changing one's attitudes, values, feelings, goals, and skills to live a satisfying life within the limitations caused by illness. A mental health service system based on the recovery concept incorporates the services of a community support system organized around the rehabilitation model's description of the impact of severe mental illness. Each service is examined in terms of amelioration of impairment, dysfunction, disability, and disadvantage. A recovery-based mental health system assumes that recovery can occur without professional intervention, requires support from an outside person, and can occur even though symptoms recur. Such a system also assumes that recovery can change the frequency and duration of symptoms, and that recovery is not a linear process. (p. 11)

The principles of recovery developed from a consensus of involved representatives from both recovery communities and other stakeholders were stated in 2010 by SAMHSA; this resulted in the following working definition of recovery for mental health and/or substance use disorders (SUD): Recovery is "a process of change through which individuals improve their health and wellness, live a self-directed life, and strive to reach their full potential" (SAMHSA, 2012).

Brown and Kandirikirira (2007) summarized recovery as:

> …being able to live a meaningful and satisfying life as defined by each person in the presence or absence of symptoms. It is having control over and input into your own life. Each individual's recovery, like his or her experience of mental health problems or illness, is a unique and deeply personal process. (p. 6)

However, the principles continue to have its detractors as well as supporters with some saying it ignored the impact of living with the identification of a mental health problem, medications and side effects, the behavioral challenges that continue to cause distress for individuals living with SMI, and a customary approach by many service providers that prioritizes symptom reduction and the assumption of normally accepted social roles by the person living with SMI (Davidson et al., 2021; Pilgrim & McCranie, 2013; Rose, 2014).

Despite the controversies, the defining statements of recovery offer several guiding principles. The recovery process prioritizes autonomy, empowerment and respect for the person receiving services for mental health problems (Corrigan, 1997). Recovery is individualized as the process is determined by the person receiving the services and not the service providers; the service user living with SMI defines the recovery services provided and is not defined by the services. Studies have shown that there are discrepancies between what service providers characterize as recovery for a person living with SMI and the person in recovery (Jung et al., 2011; Leonhardt et al., 2017). Recovery for service providers may encompass remission of symptoms and improvement of functioning, including independent living and employment; however, that may not be the case for the person living with SMI (Rose, 2014). Service users may desire harm reduction instead of complete remission of challenging behaviors; service users may have as their primary goal a life without side effects from medications or no medications at all. Service providers may see an end point in the recovery process but recovery for the individuals living with SMI is viewed as an evolving process as they continue in recovery (Bradstreet & Brierty, 2012; Davidson et al., 2021). As stated by Anthony (1993), recovery-based mental health systems assume that recovery can occur without professional intervention but requires support from outside persons in the community in that recovery can still occur despite symptoms and behavior challenges being displayed or recurring. By pursuing the goals established by the service user, the recovery team gives support and advocates for the person living with SMI who is recovering.

A treatment approach that uses the framework of recovery is "relationship-centered care" (RCC) (Beach et al., 2006). RCC includes the relationships of an individual with self and with others. RCC recognizes and appreciates the importance of relationships among all service providers, community support staff, and the person living with SMI. The concept of RCC is founded upon four principles:

> (1) relationships in health care ought to include the personhood of the participants; (2) affect and emotion are important components of these relationships; (3) all health care

relationships occur in the context of reciprocal influence; and (4) the formation and maintenance of genuine relationships in health care is morally valuable. (Beach et al., 2006, p. 53)

In RCC, the person-centered approach is described by the relationships between the service user and the service providers that is central; the relationships of clinicians with themselves, with each other and with the community are emphasized. As stated by Anthony (1993) recovery delineates a community of support for the person living with SMI. Decision-making is shared by the community of service providers, individuals in the social support network (i.e., teachers, activity directors, faith leaders) and the service user while focusing on the unique goals, life circumstances, and experiences of the recovering individual. Using the principles of RCC, the individual living with SMI who is recovering has the center seat at the table with the other members of the "recovery team" in determining their future.

The recovery team has the task of collaborating with each other. Collaboration is defined as "the process of two or more people, entities or organizations working together to complete a task or achieve a goal" (Merriam-Webster, n.d.).

Collaboration during the recovery process is accompanied by certain challenges (Scoular et al., 2020). The complexities associated with engaging individuals living with SMI have been previously addressed. The challenges may be an accumulation of negative experiences with service providers and ancillary staff, stigma, repeated trauma experiences, learned helplessness, and the display of behavioral challenges such as paranoid delusions, cognitive derailments while speaking, neurocognitive challenges, and lack of logistical and financial support. When a person living with SMI resists engagement with the recovery team, service providers may attribute these challenges to a lack of insight or awareness regarding their mental health condition or perceive the individual as unwilling or unable to change. Service providers will comment that the person is not ready for change even if the change will be beneficial.

Service providers on the recovery team must always be mindful about the assumptions, preconceptions, and pessimism that they may be bringing to the recovery team. Members of the recovery team must convey a message of hope and resilience when facing challenges with the recovery team. The recovery team in general conveys a message away from pathology, symptoms and illness to one of wellness, health, and strengths (Roe et al., 2018). Hope and optimism are central to recovery and can be enhanced by each person on the recovery team who assists the person living with SMI to have more active control over their life and making note of how others have found a way forward during recovery (Shepherd et al., 2008). On the recovery team, service providers no longer are experts but equal partners with the person living with SMI; the service providers on the recovery team serve as guides for the individual along the road to recovery; they provide information and knowledge to help the person in choosing the path that they decide to take on the journey of recovery. Recovery is about finding a sense of personal identity, which may or may not have been lost. The sense of identity and purpose is separate from illness or disability as the person living with SMI is no longer defined by the mental health problem (Roe et al., 2018). The team members must use language that supports the identity from the mental health problem (such as "living with schizophrenia" and not "being schizophrenic"; "service user" instead of "patient" or "client") to one of coping, problem-solving, adaptability, and flexibility. Recovery does not happen in isolation but with having opportunities to engage in preferred meaningful social and occupational roles within the macro and micro communities and cultures. Peer support and learning from other people living with SMI educate and benefits all members of the recovery team.

Members of the recovery team initially need to engage with each other and the person living with SMI. The team needs to agree that the principles of recovery guide the team. Some members of the recovery team may need to transition from the traditional illness-based medical model to a model of health and wellness; instead of focusing on defects, deficits and problems, the members need to focus on strengths, health and wellness, conveying a message of encouragement, hope, and optimism to the service user. The development of a recovery-based team emphasizes the personal qualities of staff as much as their formal qualifications. A sense of humor always helps! The team seeks to cultivate each other's capacities for hope, optimism, creativity, care, compassion, realism, and resilience. Family and other supporters are often crucial to recovery, and they should be included as members of the team wherever possible. Peers may be asked or requested to be a member of the team as well.

The RCR process begins by establishing rapport and trust in the relationships with each member of the recovery team—including the person living with SMI. The use of active listening facilitates laying the foundation of a trusting relationship with members of the recovery team as covered in Chap. 4. The keystones of active listening—eye contact, paraphrasing, reflective statements, empathy, using gestures, and other nonverbal communication behaviors—need to be utilized during any discussion with the person living with SMI (Karnieli-Miller & Salyers, 2011). Using the principles and techniques of active listening communicates with the individual living with SMI that the team members are paying respectful attention to the content and feeling expressed in their communication. Meeting with the team becomes a safe place to discuss concerns and issues; disagreements are not the end point of the discussion, but the beginning as active listening facilitates further discussion, leading to using solution-focused techniques (e.g., SFI) in resolving the differences.

When speaking with the person living with SMI, the team uses techniques to prompt and reinforce the person telling—narrating—her story. Using questions such as "tell me about yourself" will give the person the opportunity to pursue her own agenda in the discussion. The person living with SMI are "the experts" who have personal experiences; the experiences are subject to the individual perceptions and interpretations of the circumstances for each person living with SMI. Perceptions of the experiences of living with SMI have directed how the individual deals with her mental health problem including affective and emotional stability and behavioral and cognitive functioning (Swarbrick & Brandow 2025).

When engaged by members of the recovery team, each person living with SMI is encouraged to speak about her own life; the person is encouraged through active listening and open-ended questions to speak about herself; the team member can clarify and prompt further narrative by paraphrasing, the use of reflective statements, and motivational interviewing (MI) techniques. During each meeting, the team members systematically identify strengths, coping strategies, and reinforcing factors present within the narrative. The person living with SMI already displays strength by her abilities to survive the stigma and negative impacts of living with SMI. The focus of the meetings is to enable the person living with SMI to perceive that the outcome of the discussion with the team members will be positive, receiving messages of hope and possibilities. The person living with SMI has the capabilities of assuming personal responsibility to learn and apply self-care skills and routines which are important factors that can help the person achieve wellness, both physically and psychologically.

The service user identifies the goals of recovery during the meetings. Using MI techniques assists the person living with SMI to set goals and to participate in the endeavor (Hampson et al., 2015; Lawrence et al., 2023). Goals give direction and motivate people with SMI by providing something to work toward. Team members ask what changes the person is willing to make, how her life could improve, steps to start, resources needed, and potential challenges. Goal setting, like the recovery process, is not accomplished in one discussion; goals can be added, deleted, and modified as the RCR process continues.

When challenges occur, the individual living with SMI becomes involved in helping to solve the challenge with the team. SFI is used to incorporate her strengths and coping behaviors that have been used for prior challenges. SFI empowers the person living with SMI to become her own problem solver instead of relying on others; SFI encourages the person living with SMI to own the behavior challenges as well as the solutions. Using SFI encourages the service user to gain control through her actions and activities in solving behavioral challenges and replacing the perception of feeling misunderstood, powerless, and damaged by others (Swarbrick & Brandow, 2025). Solutions for behavioral challenges may require behavioral skill training (BST) and resources to reinforce the adaptive behaviors when they occur.

There is always the possibility of the individual living with SMI not engaging with the recovery team when a challenging behavior occurs; this is despite having worked before with service providers on the team when focusing on other aspects of recovery (e.g., setting goals, exploring resources and supports). The person may avoid or explicitly refuse to collaborate with the team, particularly the team members who would be responsible for developing an intervention for the behavioral challenge; this may be the ABA practitioner or another service provider who has expertise in assessing and changing behaviors using the principles of the applied analysis of behaviors.

The lack of awareness of behavior challenges is not an uncommon aspect of living with SMI. It has been postulated to be a negative symptom of SMI, labeled as "lack of insight"; like other negative symptoms, the use of psychiatric medications has little to no effect on the symptom. The lack of awareness or insight is at times referred to as "anosognosia," a symptom associated with a hemiplegia due to averse neurological events such as a cerebrovascular incident (CVA), closed brain injury (CHI), traumatic brain injury (TBI), and other insults to the brain such as surgery to remove a tumor (Acharya & Sánchez-Manso, 2023). Observable behaviors displayed by people experiencing anosognosia in people with neurological insult are comparable to what is observed in the individual living with SMI in that the person denies that a challenging behavior is occurring or denies features of the challenging behavior such as the setting, context, antecedents, and consequences. Although observable behaviors are similar, persons living with SMI may be denying the challenging behavior and the possibility of aversive consequences of the behavior to avoid criticism, blame, and embarrassment; generally, most people deny emitting certain behaviors if there is a probability of an unfavorable outcome (e.g., during a job interview, trying to impress another, speaking with a significant other that a bill was not paid). People living with SMI may be "repressing" awareness of challenging behaviors to avoid emotional distress. The denial of awareness has been termed "functional anosognosia" as the consequences of denying could result in the avoidance and escape from aversive private events (e.g., emotional distress) as mentioned above (Turnbull et al., 2014). The observed repression of awareness of behavioral challenges may be chiefly due to having experienced "high emotionality"—criticism, yelling, belittling—and punitive consequences imposed by others in the past for the occurrence of challenging behaviors and symptoms associated with SMI.

The hypothesis that the lack of awareness of behavioral challenges by people living with SMI is functional in nature has important implications for clinical practice and rehabilitation strategies as it would then be amenable to change through ABA. However, the recovery team still faces the complex responsibility of engaging and collaborating with individuals living with SMI, particularly if the individual does not acknowledge the presence of challenging behaviors. A service provider on the recovery team who has established rapport and a good relationship with the person living with SMI ought to attempt to have the person displaying the behavioral challenge to participate in shared decision-making and risk-taking with assessing and developing an intervention to least minimize the aversive consequences when the behavior occurs. Shared decision-making (SDM) has been proposed as a useful tool to facilitate self-determination, choice, and autonomy in the recovery process as it promotes joint decision-making by the person living with SMI and service providers on the recovery team (Zisman-Ilani et al., 2021).

The service provider using SDM presents to the individual living with SMI that decisions are not risk free for both parties. Risks are inevitable. Decisions are made together. The service provider uses active listening, MI, and SFI to discuss the risks and benefits of intervention with individuals who may deny their challenging behavior. The service provider opens the opportunity for the person displaying the challenging behavior to discuss the individual's worries and concerns about admitting to a behavior and collaborating on changing it with the hope of a beneficial outcome; the service provider models the process by speaking about the same from the perspective of the service provider, acknowledging the concerns and the hopes of the person displaying the behavior. Options are presented, the risks and benefits for each, and shared thoughts and feelings for the options. Using person-centered therapy skills, the service provider models and prompts the person living with SMI to express his thoughts and feelings about the choices and the process of decision-making as well. Perspective-taking techniques should be used to facilitate increased awareness of challenging behavior. An example would be the service provider discussing his concerns as if he was the individual displaying the challenging behavior and deciding whether: (1) a risk is worth taking when considering collaborating in developing and implementing an ABA intervention; and (2) the consequence or outcome of the change would be beneficial and helpful to the person in attaining her goals.

If the individual living with SMI is denying that the behavior occurs, the service provider ought to pursue having the individual be a third person observer of his behavior. Following along with this perspective-taking strategy, the service provider asks the person about his concerns if he observed another person manifesting the behavior. The discussion ought to include the hypothesized reactions by others, the consequences of the behavior when the behavior occurs, and the suggestion that he would give to the person displaying the behavior. The service provider acknowledges that through joint reflection, risks are given meaning in the context of the unique life and circumstances of the person living with SMI.

If behavioral challenges arise during the recovery process, team members explore and gather data about the dimensions of the challenging behaviors. Team members conduct interviews to assess the behavioral challenges, assessing the dimensions of the behaviors and stimuli associated with the occurrence of the behaviors. Interviews are conducted with the person displaying the challenging behaviors using the Functional Assessment Interview—Mental Health Version (FAI-MH) and the Open-ended Functional Assessment Interview. Interviewees include other team members (peers, family members, friends) that have observed the challenging behaviors or have expressed concern about the challenging behaviors and the possible negative outcomes due to the occurrence of the challenging behavior.

Collaborating with the person displaying the behavioral challenges, active listening, MI and SFI need to be employed as these approaches are strengths-based and person-centered. In all the approaches, the person is prompted and reinforced for being the responsible agent in her life in pursuing her aspirations and when resolving the challenges presented during the recovery process. Recovery is about building a meaningful and satisfying life, as defined by the person herself, whether there are ongoing or recurring symptoms or problems. Recovery represents a movement away from pathology, illness and symptoms to health, wellness, and competencies. Hope is identified as an element in recovery and may be supported by individuals gaining active control over aspects of their lives (agency) and by observing examples of others progressing in similar circumstances. Self-management is individualized, encouraged, facilitated, and reinforced by the recovery team. Using SFI, the person living with SMI and displaying behavioral challenges participates in the development and implementation of the intervention to change her behavior as well as others in her environment. The consequential responses of others will change as the challenging behaviors are altered using the interventions following the principles of ABA. For example, an individual living with SMI yells and threatens others when frustrated when asked to take a shower, saying he does not need one or took one already. As a consequence, individuals in the immediate environment limit their inquiries to matters such as personal hygiene and demonstrate reluctance to engage in broader social interactions. Additionally, his tendency to yell causes others to feel apprehensive, resulting in them maintaining a respectful distance. He also is labeled by others as "a difficult and aggressive person" which may affect his access to resources in society (e.g., job placement, social contacts). When the person changes his behavior and decreases the intensity and frequency of yelling, the anxieties for their safety experienced by others around him decrease; social interactions increase as avoidant behaviors are no longer negatively reinforced (i.e., staying away from him results in a reduction of anxiety and worries about safety).

The recovery team can incorporate the use of technology when developing the intervention. Monitoring by others as well as self-monitoring, automatic prompting to assist with following a routine by the individual (e.g., being prompted with text messages to shower, take medication, alarms on cell phones) may help with the person living with SMI become more autonomous and responsible for the implementation of the intervention—which is a goal in recovery. Access to technology could be used as a reinforcer once the behavioral criterion is met for a targeted behavior. Being creative and "thinking out of the box" by members of the recovery team facilitates doable and effective interventions.

Example of Engagement in Recovery

The following is an example of a recovery team and a service user engaged and collaborated to assist him in establishing and achieving his goals using resources and support in the family and the community.

Colin is a 25-year-old veteran who lives with his family. He is receiving services from the local Veteran's Administration (VA) outpatient facility. Colin had his first episode of SMI during his time in the service. He was stationed in Korea near the DMZ after boot camp and often participated in "war games" in case of an invasion from the North. He had a mental health crisis at his base in Korea when he believed that he had received a message from a higher power to save the prostitutes in the North. He left his base and attempted to enter the DMZ at night. He had to be rescued by his fellow soldiers as he and his rescuers were in danger of being shot by the North Korean guards. After being psychiatrically stabilized in a hospital in Japan, he was hospitalized at the local VA hospital. He was medically discharged and received full disability from the VA.

The recovery team at the VA reviewed his psychosocial history and interviewed Colin and his parents using person-centered techniques. Using active listening and MI techniques, Colin was able to give a narrative that he had a "normal childhood" with no traumatic events. He received B's and C's in school, was active in athletics, and had friends. Both parents worked and he has two younger siblings, both in school. He decided to join the military because he was usure of "what I want to do with my life"; he also was concerned about having debt as he would have to take out loans to go to college. With the support of his parents, he joined the military, believing it would give him "an opportunity to sort things out."

Colin had several short readmissions to the psychiatric ward at the VA since his discharge. The reason for the admissions was that Colin had stopped his medications; shortly after discontinuing medications, he experienced delusions that he was a famous rock star and later believed that he had to castrate himself to "keep my looks and my hair."

Colin reported that the medications made him "feel always tired and yawning" and would be asleep when his friends asked if he would meet them at a bar or club. He also experienced tremors in his legs and arms and added, "I felt embarrassed going out. I felt like an old man." He reduced the amount of the medications he was taking, and he noticed that "I had more energy; I was the life of the party; I could talk and joke with anyone. Talking to girls was not a problem. And I stopped yawning and shaking!" He later stopped the medications as he believed he no longer needed them as "I was doing OK and having fun."

Over several meetings, Colin told the service provider that he never had a girlfriend as "I was always shy, not knowing what to say if a girl talked to me. It is not like that when I am manic." He perceived that the episodes of mania helped him with interacting with others especially socially and "in way were good for me. I could pick up any girl at the club." He expressed concern that the medications would make him impotent and sterile as he was told that by some older vets when he was hospitalized. The service provider also explored with him his concerns about medications, side effects, and risks and benefits.

Colin was able to state that one of his goals was to help with his social skills and talking to young women. He also did not want to be seen as "a 'nut case' for the rest of my life. I want to get a good job, get married have kids, you know, like everyone else."

During meetings with the recovery team, Colin did discuss college and stated he still wanted to attend but did not know if any major interested him. Working with Colin, he decided that he should see if "I got what it takes to go to school; it has been a few years since I studied and took tests." The team members helped Colin access the local community college site and reviewed courses and majors. Colin and the service provider with whom he had established rapport and trust discussed auditing a required course initially to slowly shape the skills needed for college. Colin met with an academic advisor who assisted him with setting up auditing a class during the day.

Colin and the recovery team discussed the issue of medications. Colin agreed to talk to the psychiatric prescriber about the medications. Colin stated that he felt like the prescriber "just blows me off and he is handing me a script before I get a chance to say anything." He and the service provider discussed what he wanted to say with the prescriber. Colin and the team wrote down and practiced what he would discuss. The recovery team did ask the prescriber to schedule a longer time for Colin to discuss his concerns. Colin met with the prescriber, and both agreed to reduce the medication slowly until maximum benefit was reached. They agreed to meet every 2 weeks to follow up. In addition, Colin agreed to a low dose of side effect medication to help with the tremors. A contract was developed with Colin and the recovery team about the re-emergence of symptoms and thoughts of self-harm. His parents would assist the team to monitor Colin's safety.

The recovery teams worked with Colin to audit a class. Colin also enrolled in a remedial study skills class at the college during the day as Colin was educated that sleep was important as he understood that an early sign of relapse was not getting a full night's sleep.

His problems with social skills were also discussed and he agreed to participate in a group held by a recovery team member. During individual meetings with a member of his recovery team an intervention was developed to help him slowly teach and shape his ability and skills in speaking with young women in social interactions using instruction, role modeling, prompting, practice, and reinforcement. His social skills treatment plan was implemented. A major accomplishment was that he was able to identify someone who was an acquaintance that he knew from high school that lived nearby. He had communicated with her through social media. During the individual meeting with the service provider and the social skills group, Colin developed and practiced his own "social script" to ask her to meet face to face. He was able to ask her to meet for coffee and later developed a personal relationship with her.

Ethical Concerns and Challenges in the Treatment of the People Living with SMI

Mental health care with individuals living with SMI is characterized by an engaged and collaborative relationship between professional providers and consumers. Mental health care service professionals contribute specialized knowledge in human behavior while service users offer perspectives based on their individual experiences, preferences, and objectives pertaining to their individualized recovery. This partnership is anchored in ethical standards—most notably, beneficence and respect for autonomy—and frequently utilizes a shared decision-making approach (Hamann & Heres, 2014; Huang et al., 2020).

Collaboration commences with the exchange of concerns between the mental health service user and provider. The mental health care professional conducts an assessment in partnership with individuals living with SMI, focusing on issues that may be challenging, even if the current behaviors do not cause distress for the individual. Through constructive dialogue, both parties consider the nature of the problem, potential distress, and available treatment options. Ultimately, the consumer determines whether to pursue intervention or decline it; treatment is implemented only upon receiving the informed consent of the mental health service user (Herrings et al., 2020; Stallman & Gupta, 2025).

The collaboration between the service professional and service user is rooted in ethical principles. Morality, ethics, and law are the cornerstones of civilized society, shaping individual behavior, social interactions, and institutional frameworks. Their definitions overlap yet remain distinct, and their mutual influences are profound, creating a dynamic landscape for human conduct (Chadda & Agrawal, 2023; Lee, 1928; Floarea, 2022; Niemetz, 2008; Roberts et al., 2021).

Morals refer to the subjective beliefs and values regarding right and wrong that are held by individuals and communities (Chadda & Agrawal, 2023; Lee, 1928). These beliefs are deeply rooted in personal experience, cultural tradition, and historical context. Morality operates at both the common level—norms widely accepted across societies, such as prohibitions against harm—and where norms are specific to certain groups, professions, or cultures. Morals are inherently personal and internal, reflecting the intentions and beliefs of individuals (Floarea, 2022).

Ethics is the study and systematic evaluation of moral principles (Chadda & Agrawal, 2023; Lee, 1928). It seeks to critically analyze, rationalize, and universalize the guidelines by which actions are judged. Ethics is not directly regulatory but instead provides structured frameworks for interpreting and applying moral concepts. These frameworks support objective approaches to moral dilemmas, particularly in professional contexts such as medicine, business, and law (Niemetz, 2008). Ethics is thus both reflective and prescriptive, guiding decision-making through reasoned principles rather than custom alone (Cox, 2021).

However, certain principles have become statutory. Regulations have translated these moral obligations into legal requirements to ensure safety, quality of care, and adherence to standards in health care (McCradden et al., 2020). Nonadherence to certain ethical principles like non-maleficence, confidentiality, and autonomy could result in legal violations.

Law is the system of formal rules and regulations enacted by societies to govern external behavior (Floarea, 2022). It is considered the expression of objective ethics, designed to assess and manage the relationships and actions among individuals (Niemetz, 2008). While law is grounded in ethical principles, its primary focus is the enforcement and predictability of conduct, often through sanctions and remedies. Law is distinguished from both morals and ethics by its explicit codification and external application.

Morals, ethics, and the law have profound impacts on each other and are interdependent. The evolution of ethics is rooted in prevailing moral beliefs. Societal morality inspires the formulation of ethical theories, which in turn serve as the foundation for legal systems. A community's core values—such as justice, equality, and freedom—inform not only ethical discourse but also the development of legal codes (Lee, 1928). For example, the prohibition against causing harm is a moral principle that has been studied ethically and enshrined in legal statutes.

Ethics provides the rational scaffolding needed to evaluate and refine both moral beliefs and legal rules. It transcends cultural particularities, seeking universality and consistency, and often acts as a catalyst for legal reform. Ethical arguments have played crucial roles in landmark changes, such as the abolition of slavery, the recognition of human rights, and the reform of medical practices (Niemetz, 2008; Floarea, 2022). Moreover, ethical frameworks support professional standards and codes, particularly in medicine and law, advancing moral consistency in behavior and legal accountability.

Legal systems, by codifying certain behaviors as acceptable or unacceptable, influence societal morals over time. The enforcement of laws can lead to shifts in collective moral understanding, as seen in changing attitudes toward issues such as marriage equality or environmental protection (Floarea, 2022). Laws also reflect and reinforce ethical conclusions, bridging the gap between philosophical ideals and practical governance.

The interplay between morals, ethics, and law is cyclical and adaptive. Ethical inquiry clarifies and universalizes moral norms, which can inspire legal reform. In turn, legal changes recalibrate societal moral standards, influencing individual beliefs and conduct. This interdependence ensures the progress of society toward ideals of justice, equity, and human dignity (Niemetz, 2008).

Ethical decision-making stands as a cornerstone of high-quality mental health practice, underpinning integrity and trust which is essential to the therapeutic relationship and professional standards. The complexity of ethical dilemmas in mental health has demanded increasingly refined frameworks and models, evolving alongside advances in research, societal expectations, and legal landscapes. Mental health professionals regularly encounter complex ethical dilemmas that challenge not only what decisions are made, but why those decisions are justified (American Psychological Association, n.d.-b; Cox, 2021; Young, 2016). The field has responded by developing systematic models that offer both structure and flexibility, grounding ethical action in professional codes while accommodating the diversity of practice contexts and stakeholder interests.

The mental health care professions adhere to publicly articulated and codified ethical principles, which obligate their members to uphold fundamental ethical standards (Byrd & Winkelstein, 2014; Varkey, 2021). Disciplines subject to these codified ethics include psychiatry, psychology, nursing, social work, occupational and physical therapy, as well as other allied health professions. Ethical training is essential in mental health care, providing practitioners with the requisite knowledge, skills, and perspectives to address complex ethical challenges. This education enables mental health service professionals to understand and apply ethical principles, uphold professionalism, respect autonomy of the individual, maintain confidentiality, and demonstrate beneficence and non-maleficence. Central topics addressed include informed consent, therapeutic boundaries, stigma mitigation, cultural competence, and the administration of involuntary hospitalization and treatment. Ethical training actively promotes trust and effective therapeutic alliances, supports professionals in navigating dual roles and potential conflicts of interest, and reinforces compliance with legal and ethical frameworks in the provision of person-centered care (Roberts et al., 2021).

Mental health service providers need to be knowledgeable and follow ethical standards, such as autonomy, non-maleficence, beneficence, and justice, to ensure the welfare and safety of the individual living with SMI and uphold professional integrity. Key ethical considerations include informed consent, confidentiality, maintaining appropriate professional boundaries, and competence in their practice.

The four core principles related to the support of individuals living with SMI by service providers across all mental health professions include:

- Beneficence: The obligation to act in the individual's best interest, promoting his well-being and recovery. Ethical dilemmas occur when coercive measures are justified as beneficial but may harm the therapeutic alliance or the person's dignity (Byrd & Winkelstein, 2014; Laureano et al., 2024; Varkey, 2021). Beneficence has been postulated to be the cornerstone of ethical behaviors and decision-making (Glaser, 1994). Beneficence is present in the ethical domains of (a) the individual (what is good for the person); (b) the organization or institution (what benefits the organization in carrying out its mission); and (c) society (what is good for the well-being of the community) (Glaser, 1994). All three domains are involved in ethical decision-making by mental health service providers.

- Ethical decision-making within mental health is influenced by a range of contextual factors, including organizational culture, stakeholder interests, legal requirements, and societal norms (Liégeois & Van Audenhove, 2005; Suarez et al., 2023; Young, 2016). Ethical challenges may emerge when the best interests of individuals, institutions, or society come into conflict.
- Autonomy: The principle of respecting an individual's ability to make decisions about his treatment. Ethical concerns arise when treatment restricts autonomy, especially for people deemed capable of making informed decisions (Byrd & Winkelstein, 2014; Laureano et al., 2024; Liégeois & Van Audenhove, 2005; Varkey, 2021). A dilemma often occurs when a person living with SMI does not want certain information to be reported to others, including family. The duty of confidentiality is rooted in respecting autonomy but can conflict with stakeholder's involvement for what is in the best interest of the individual living with SMI (Hem et al., 2023).
- Non-maleficence: The principle of avoiding harm. Ethical concerns include whether coercive measures, such as involuntary hospitalization or administration of medication, cause more harm than good (Byrd & Winkelstein, 2014; Laureano et al., 2024; Varkey, 2021).
- Justice: Ensuring fairness and equity in treatment. Ethical concerns include potential discrimination against vulnerable and marginalized populations, such as ethnic and gender minorities or socioeconomically disadvantaged individuals (Byrd & Winkelstein, 2014; Laureano et al., 2024; Varkey, 2021).

In addition, other ethical principles that are related to and support the core ethical principles need to be considered in ethical behavior and decision-making by a mental health service provider:

- Human dignity: Protecting the inherent dignity of the individual (Laureano et al., 2024).
- Relational ethics: Emphasizing the importance of maintaining ethical relationships between the service user and mental health service providers, including engagement, collaboration, communication, respect, shared decision-making, and relational boundaries (Laureano et al., 2024).

- Informed consent: This is directly rooted in the principle of autonomy. Autonomy emphasizes that all individuals have intrinsic worth and the right to make rational decisions about their own bodies and health care (Varkey, 2021).
- Truth-telling: This supports autonomy and informed consent by providing service users with the information they need to make informed decisions about their health care (Varkey, 2021).
- Professional competence: The service professional requires specialist knowledge, training, skill, and experience and should not provide the service if the requisite skills and knowledge are lacking (American Psychological Association, 2017).
- Confidentiality: The principle of confidentiality refers to the ethical and legal obligation of mental health service professionals to protect the privacy of the individual's information (Hem et al., 2023). It ensures that personal and sensitive information shared by the person living with SMI during treatment is not disclosed to others without their consent. This principle is grounded in respecting the autonomy, privacy, and trust of the person, and it is a cornerstone of the therapeutic relationship between the service user and providers. Confidentiality must be balanced against other ethical principles, such as beneficence in all domains, the needs of stakeholders, and justice. In some cases, confidentiality may be breached, such as in crisis situations where the individual poses harm to themselves or others. However, overly rigid adherence to confidentiality can sometimes hinder the involvement of stakeholders, which may be beneficial for the individual's care and recovery (Hem et al., 2023).
- The principle of confidentiality is relational, involving the exchange of information between service professionals, the service user, and stakeholders. It requires careful consideration of the type of information being shared (e.g., general, personal, or sensitive) and the potential consequences of sharing or withholding information. Rigid adherence to confidentiality can be used as a "smoke screen" to avoid pursuing treatment that is in the best of the individual living with SMI (Hem et al., 2023).
- Least restrictive means: This principle emphasizes minimizing interference with individual autonomy in health interventions (Byskov, 2019). Mental health procedures and interventions should interfere with individual freedom to the least extent necessary. The least restrictive measures range from providing information, enabling choice, to mandatory interventions which require stronger justification due to increased infringement on individual freedom (Byskov, 2019).

Service providers often encounter ethical dilemmas regarding the protection of confidentiality. Balancing the need to safeguard the privacy of individuals living with SMI against the interests and involvement of stakeholders presents ongoing challenges. While strict adherence to confidentiality may leave stakeholders feeling excluded, sharing certain information can sometimes enhance recovery outcomes. Providers must carefully determine whether disclosing details to stakeholders supports the individual's well-being and recovery or if prioritizing confidentiality is warranted. These decisions require thorough ethical and legal consideration regarding what information can be shared. Trust between service users and providers remains essential, and confidentiality typically takes precedence when the therapeutic relationship could be compromised. However, strict confidentiality, while protecting privacy, may also limit collaborative support opportunities for service users (Hem et al., 2018, 2023).

Ethical decision-making is a process that typically commences when service providers sense an ethically significant issue, prompting further investigation (Suarez et al., 2023). An immediate detour may be required when legal or reporting obligations occur, such as mandatory safeguarding or compliance with statutory requirements.

Ethical challenges can take many forms. Mental health service providers have identified implicit challenges that are viewed as problems or discussions about what was right or good, while others emerged as professional issues with ethical undertones (Molewijk et al., 2015). Employees often grappled with emotionally challenging situations, where underlying values created inner tension. There are times when service staff openly questioned or reflected on what was ethically appropriate; in other cases, clear dilemmas arose when fundamental principles, such as safety and service user autonomy, were in conflict. Balancing legal requirements with ethical considerations can be a common struggle, as well as navigating disagreements over what constituted good care. Recovery teams have been found to vary in the way teams handled disagreements with some being managed poorly or disrespectfully that added to the ethical tension surrounding the issue. Staff reported experiencing challenges between loyalty to the recovery team or supervisors and fidelity to their own moral convictions, highlighting the complex landscape of ethical decision-making in their work (Molewijk et al., 2015).

Defining the ethical dilemma is a critical step, requiring that service providers clarify the nature and scope of the issue. Subsequently, a comprehensive information-gathering phase ensues. This involves the identification of affected parties, referencing professional and organizational codes of ethics, consulting legal and cultural guidelines, and evaluating person-specific contextual factors (Suarez et al., 2023).

Once sufficient information is collected, service providers systematically identify available options and potential courses of action, considering practical constraints and foreseeable consequences. These alternatives are then weighed, balancing risks, benefits, personal values, and professional standards (Suarez et al., 2023).

The synthesis and analysis of all relevant data lead to the selection of the most ethical course of action. Implementation follows, conducted with a commitment to transparency and fidelity. The final step in the process is a thorough follow-up, where service providers review the outcomes of their decisions to ensure satisfactory resolution and to inform future conduct (Suarez et al., 2023).

Cox (2021) distinguishes between descriptive ethical behavior ("what is right") and normative ethical behavior ("why it is right"), emphasizing that service providers often reach consensus on appropriate action while diverging in their justifications. This insight underscores the importance of not only clarifying recommended actions but also articulating the underlying values, theoretical frameworks, and rationales—be they deontological, consequentialist, or virtue-based. The personal values of mental health service providers frequently influence decision-making processes (Thomas, 2013). Individuals living with SMI and their families may experience exclusion from these processes, which can result in diminished dignity as well as increased disenfranchisement, marginalization, and stigmatization (Laureano et al., 2024).

Empirical investigations found substantial variability both within and across service providers regarding the theories invoked to justify ethical choices. This variability suggests that ethical decision-making in mental health is deeply influenced by individual learning histories, contextual cues, and the pluralistic nature of ethical reasoning (Cox, 2021).

Service users value having a say in decisions affecting their treatment and daily life. However, experiences vary; some users prefer to make decisions independently, while others seek involvement without full responsibility. Mental health service providers strive to involve users in care planning but face challenges such as time constraints and the impairments and problem behaviors presented by the service user (Herrings et al., 2020).

Informed Consent

Informed consent is a process in which an individual voluntarily agrees to participate in a specific activity, such as treatment, research, or a procedure, after being fully informed about its purpose, risks, benefits, and alternatives (American Psychological Association, n.d.-a; Herrings et al., 2020). This is directly rooted in the principle of autonomy. Autonomy emphasizes that all individuals have intrinsic worth and the right to make rational decisions about their own bodies and health care (Varkey, 2021).

For the person to give consent the person must demonstrate the ability to receive information about a specific matter, understand the information, to reason and deliberate, to maintain appropriate values and objectives, to appreciate one's situation, to comprehend provided information, and to make and communicate independent decisions (Herrings et al., 2020).

Consent is characterized as a legally binding agreement, granted by individuals with the recognized capacity and authority to make informed decisions (American Bar Association [ABA], 2018; Buchanan, 2004). The process of obtaining consent involves the provision of comprehensive information to the participant or their legal representative. This includes a clear explanation of the purpose of the procedure or intervention, the methods involved, potential risks and benefits, issues of confidentiality, and the explicit right to withdraw from participation at any stage without facing negative consequences. Only those individuals who possess the requisite neurocognitive ability (i.e., comprehension, memory, planning, flexibility) and legal standing may provide valid consent. The central tenet of consent is full comprehension; participants must demonstrate an understanding of all pertinent aspects of the research and their rights as participants before agreeing to take part (Herrings et al., 2020; Mead Jasperse et al., 2023).

In contrast, assent refers to the ethically significant expression of willingness to participate, offered by individuals who lack the legal capacity to provide informed consent. Assent is typically sought from minors or individuals with neurocognitive impairments. While not legally binding, assent is critical in affirming the autonomy and agency of those who cannot independently provide consent. The process does not require exhaustive understanding of every element of the proposed activity but rather centers on the voluntary indication—whether vocal or behavioral—that the individual is willing to participate (Mead Jasperse et al., 2023).

The assessment of decision-making capacity is pivotal in determining whether consent or assent is appropriate. Legal authority is inherently tied to consent, ensuring that the agreement carries legal weight and can be upheld if challenged. Conversely, assent, though not enforceable by law, carries important ethical weight; it signals respect for the individual's preferences and protects their welfare within the research context (Herrings et al., 2020; Mead Jasperse et al., 2023).

Obtaining consent and assent are distinct yet complementary processes that serve to safeguard the rights, dignity, and well-being of service users. Consent embodies a comprehensive, legally sanctioned agreement, while assent represents a meaningful, ethical affirmation of willingness from those without legal capacity. Together, these principles reinforce the ethical foundations by ensuring that all participants, regardless of age or cognitive ability, are accorded respect and protection throughout their involvement (Herrings et al., 2020; Mead Jasperse et al., 2023).

Summary

The chapter discusses the challenges and complexities faced by individuals living with serious mental illness and service providers. Lack of actively being in treatment, discontinuation of treatment, decision-making difficulties, and the impact of learned helplessness on behavior and recovery have been identified as factors that affect treatment outcomes. Lack of engaging and discontinuation of treatment by individuals living with SMI can lead to several detrimental consequences. Variables that contribute to a person living with SMI to either not start or quitting treatment and recovery are varied including the occurrence and worsening of positive and negative symptoms associated with SMI; persistence and intolerable side effects of medications; lack of routines and community support; logistical problems (transportation, financial constraints); legal entanglements resulting in authorities involved in treatment; changes to medications; homelessness; and cognitive deficits that impair remembering and abiding by treatment recommendation. Research shows that over a third discontinue treatment 6–18 months after diagnosis living with SMI and/or discharge from a psychiatric facility. The number increased over time with over 50% discontinuing treatment after a year and over 70% dropped out of treatment within 10 years.

Accessibility of care and service availability, family support, logistical support to get to appointments, and cultural and social factors contribute to challenges leading to a lack of engagement in recovery. At times, personality traits and co-occurring conditions result in behavioral challenges that can cause the person living with SMI to perceive that treatment would result in restrictions on his freedoms, goals, and aspirations so that the recovery process is not in his best interest. Challenges in cognitive and neurocognitive status add to difficulties if the individual living with SMI cannot remember appointments and meaningfully participate with service providers in the recovery process. Negative past experiences with service providers and the lack of a past or present therapeutic alliances with service providers can give rise to perceptions of a deficit in trust by the service user. Stigma and the internalization of the stigma of living with SMI impedes the recovery process in that stigmatization decreases hope and optimism about living with an SMI and access to opportunities.

Not engaging in or discontinuing treatment and recovery have serious consequences for the individual living with SMI. There is an increased chance of positive symptoms (hallucinations, delusions) and challenging behaviors (aggression, self-harm, suicide) re-emerging as well as social withdrawal and isolation. The likelihood of the recurrence of dangerous behavior, more frequent hospital admissions, worsened prognosis and medication resistance result in longer hospital stays and further disruption in the recovery process.

Recovery-orientation needs to be a part of the treatment approach and philosophy for the service providers who support and interact with people living with SMI. Recovery offers hope, optimism, peer support and community reintegration, and supports the direction of the treatment the person living with SMI wants for their life. The person living with SMI and the service providers are the recovery team, working together to create a supportive environment that promotes the individual's health, wellness, and ability to lead a self-directed life. Recovery stresses autonomy, individualization, respect, and compassion for the individual living with SMI. Recovery views the past and present coping behaviors of the person living with SMI as strengths and behaviors that can be used during recovery.

The role of the recovery team is to build trust and collaboration with each member of the recovery team, including the individual living with SMI. Team members coordinate care, promoting autonomy and active participation in recovery. Education involving family, peers, and community support staff are offered. Members work to engage, collaborate, and share decision-making with the person living with SMI and each other. The team recognizes that recovery is a nonlinear process. The recovery team provides support, focusing on strengths, and addressing barriers using person-centered, solution focused and motivational techniques to change behavioral challenges. Progress is monitored; alterations to the recovery plan occur as needed with the involvement of the entire recovery team.

Certain strategies have been found to be helpful when engaging individuals living with SMI. As people living with SMI have more than likely experienced discrimination, rejection, criticism, repeated trauma, and high emotionality from significant others, friends, or family, it is essential that the members of the team establish rapport and build trust with the individual living with SMI. Interactions with the person living with SMI ought to utilize active listening and other person-centered interviewing techniques, providing education and addressing barriers to recovery and establishing goals with the person living with SMI. The recovery team creates a supportive environment to counter stigma and foster hope in recovery. Follow-ups should be consistent and supported by using technology, such as automatic reminders, prompting through text and voice mail, and self-monitoring. It is common to encounter resistance from individuals who are not prepared or willing to change, regardless of the potential benefits. The recovery team addresses passivity and learned helplessness in individuals living with SMI, as these factors may affect their involvement in the recovery process.

During recovery, behavioral challenges will occur. Behavioral challenges may interfere with the recovery process and affect the quality of life for individuals living with SMI. Addressing these challenges requires the recovery team to adapt their strategies and consistently support the individual's recovery. Common behavioral challenges are nonadherence to medications, aggressive behaviors towards self and others, poor judgment, and excessive use of substances. Emotional dysregulation and lability, social withdrawal, functional impairments, and neurocognitive problems all impact a person living with SMI and their capabilities to adhere and follow a recovery plan.

The recovery team needs to address behavioral challenges as the outcome of the behaviors could be serious and negatively impact the individual living with SMI (e.g., involuntary hospitalization, legal involvement). At times, it is important to address the lack of awareness of the behavioral challenges that the service user is displaying. Service providers who have established rapport and built trust with the person displaying the behavioral challenges engage the service user in joint decision-making to manage and minimize the consequences of challenging behaviors. Techniques such as active listening, motivational interviewing (MI), and strengths-based approaches are recommended to facilitate engagement, self-determination, and autonomy. The person-centered assessment techniques of applied behavior analysis (ABA) are used, asking open-ended questions when conducting a functional assessment. The ABA practitioner collaborates with the recovery team and the service user displaying the behavior challenges in conducting assessments and developing interventions to promote recovery.

The recovery team needs to be mindful that recovery is defined as building a meaningful life despite ongoing symptoms. The goal is to enhance hope, self-management, and agency, leading to improved social interactions and reduced negative consequences of challenging behaviors.

Mental health care for individuals living with SMI relies on a collaborative relationship between service providers and users. The partnership is based on ethical standards, particularly beneficence and respect for autonomy. Shared decision-making is a key component, allowing consumers to determine their treatment options. Mental health professionals conduct assessments in collaboration with service users, focusing on their experiences and preferences. Informed consent is essential, requiring the user's agreement before any treatment is implemented.

Ethics, morals, and law are foundational to mental health practice, influencing behavior and decision-making. Morals are subjective beliefs about right and wrong, shaped by personal and cultural contexts. Ethics systematically evaluates moral principles, providing frameworks for professional conduct. Laws codify ethical principles into formal regulations, ensuring safety and quality in health care. The interplay between morals, ethics, and law is cyclical, influencing societal standards and legal reforms.

Four core ethical principles guide mental health service providers in supporting individuals with SMI including:

- Beneficence: Providers must act in the best interest of the individual, promoting well-being and recovery.
- Autonomy: Providers must respect the individual's right to make informed decisions about their treatment is crucial.
- Non-maleficence: Providers must avoid causing harm, particularly when considering coercive measures.
- Justice: Providers work to ensure fairness and equity in treatment, particularly for marginalized populations.

Other ethical principles complement the core principles in mental health practice.

- Human dignity: Protecting the inherent dignity of individuals is fundamental.
- Relational ethics: Emphasizes the importance of ethical relationships between service users and providers.
- Informed consent: Rooted in autonomy, it ensures individuals understand their treatment options.
- Confidentiality: Protecting the privacy of individuals is a cornerstone of the therapeutic relationship.
- Least restrictive means: Interventions should minimize interference with individual autonomy.

The ethical decision-making process is critical for mental health service providers facing dilemmas. It begins with identifying an ethically significant issue and gathering relevant information. Providers must consider affected parties, professional codes, and contextual factors. Available options are identified, weighing risks, benefits, and professional standards. The most ethical course of action is selected, implemented transparently, and followed up for evaluation.

Informed consent and assent are vital processes in mental health treatment and research. Informed consent requires individuals to understand the purpose, risks, and benefits of treatment. Assent is sought from those unable to provide consent, affirming their willingness to participate. Both processes protect the rights and dignity of service users, ensuring ethical involvement in care. Consent is legally binding, while assent carries ethical significance, emphasizing respect for individual preferences.

References

Acharya, A. B., & Sánchez-Manso, J. C. (2023). *Anosognosia*. In StatPearls. StatPearls Publishing. https://www.ncbi.nlm.nih.gov/books/NBK513361/

American Bar Association (ABA). (2018, December). *Assessment of older adults with diminished capacity: A handbook for psychologists*. American Bar Association Commission on Law and Aging; American Psychological Association. https://www.apa.org/pi/aging/resources/guides/diminished-capacity

American Psychological Association (APA). (n.d.-a). Consent. In *APA dictionary of psychology*. https://dictionary.apa.org/consent

American Psychological Association (APA). (n.d.-b). Ethical dilemma. In *APA dictionary of psychology*. https://dictionary.apa.org/ethical-dilemma

American Psychological Association (APA). (n.d.-c). Principle of least effort. In *APA dictionary of psychology*. https://dictionary.apa.org/principle-of-least-effort

American Psychological Association (APA). (2017). *Ethical principles of psychologists and code of conduct* (2002, amended effective June 1, 2010, and January 1, 2017). https://www.apa.org/ethics/code

Anthony, W. A. (1993). Recovery from mental illness: The guiding vision of the mental health service system in the 1990s. *Psychosocial Rehabilitation Journal, 16*(4), 11–23. https://doi.org/10.1037/h0095655

Avdibegović, E., & Hasanović, M. (2017). The stigma of mental illness and recovery. *Psychiatria Danubina, 29*(Suppl 5), 900–905. https://hrcak.srce.hr/264006

Beach, M. C., Inui, T., & Relationship-Centered Care Research Network. (2006). Relationship-centered care: A constructive reframing. *Journal of General Internal Medicine, 21*, 3–8. https://doi.org/10.1111/j.1525-1497.2006.00302.x

Bradstreet, S., & McBrierty, R. (2012). Recovery in Scotland: Beyond service development. *International Review of Psychiatry, 24*(1), 64–69. https://doi.org/10.3109/09540261.2011.650158

Brown, W., & Kandirikirira, N. (2007). The possibility of wellness. *Mental Health Today, 7*(7), 23–26.

Buchanan, A. (2004). Mental capacity, legal competence and consent to treatment. *Journal of the Royal Society of Medicine, 97*(9), 415–420. https://doi.org/10.1177/014107680409700902

Byrd, G. D., & Winkelstein, P. (2014). A comparative analysis of moral principles and behavioral norms in eight ethical codes relevant to health sciences librarianship, medical informatics, and the health professions. *Journal of the Medical Library Association: JMLA, 102*(4), 247. https://doi.org/10.3163/1536-5050.102.4.006

Byskov, M. F. (2019). Qualitative and quantitative interpretations of the least restrictive means. *Bioethics, 33*(4), 511–521. https://doi.org/10.1111/bioe.12548

Cáceda, R., Nemeroff, C. B., & Harvey, P. D. (2014). Toward an understanding of decision making in severe mental illness. *The Journal of Neuropsychiatry and Clinical Neurosciences*, 26(3), 196–213. https://doi.org/10.1176/appi.neuropsych.12110268

Chaddha, R., & Agrawal, G. (2023). Ethics and morality. *Journal of Orthopaedics and Injury Orthopaedics (JOIO), 57*, 1707–1713. https://doi.org/10.1007/s43465-023-01004-3

Correll, C. U., & Schooler, N. R. (2020). Negative symptoms in schizophrenia: A review and clinical guide for recognition, assessment, and treatment. *Neuropsychiatric Disease and Treatment, 16*, 519–534. https://doi.org/10.2147/NDT.S225643

Corrigan, P. W. (1997). Behavior therapy empowers persons with severe mental illness. *Behavior Modification, 21*(1), 45–61. https://doi.org/10.1177/01454455970211002

Corrigan, P. W., & Bink, A. B. (2016). The stigma of mental illness. In H. S. Friedman (Ed.), *Encyclopedia of mental health* (2nd ed., pp. 230–234). Academic Press. https://doi.org/10.1016/B978-0-12-397045-9.00182-1

Cox, D. J. (2021). Descriptive and normative ethical behavior appear to be functionally distinct. *Journal of Applied Behavior Analysis, 54*(1), 168–191. https://doi.org/10.1002/jaba.761

Davidson, L., Rowe, M., DiLeo, P., Bellamy, C., & Delphin-Rittmon, M. (2021). Recovery-oriented systems of care: A perspective on the past, present, and future. *Alcohol Research: Current Reviews, 41*(1), 1–11. https://doi.org/10.35946/arcr.v41.1.09

Fervaha, G., Foussias, G., Agid, O., & Remington, G. (2014). Impact of primary negative symptoms on functional outcomes in schizophrenia. *European Psychiatry, 29*(7), 449–455. https://doi.org/10.1016/j.eurpsy.2014.01.007

Floarea, T. (2022). The relationship between law and morality. *Scientia Moralitas: International Journal of Multidisciplinary Research, 7*(1), 94–100. https://econpapers.repec.org/RePEc:smo:journl:v:7:y:2022:i:1:p:94-100

Glaser, J. W. (1994). *Three realms of ethics: Individual, institutional, societal*. Sheed & Ward. https://openlibrary.org/books/OL1094951M/Three_realms_of_ethics

Hamann, J., & Heres, S. (2014). Adapting shared decision making for individuals with severe mental illness. *Psychiatric Services, 65*(12), 1483–1486. https://doi.org/10.1176/appi.ps.201400307

Hampson, M. E., Hicks, R. E., & Watt, B. D. (2015). Exploring the effectiveness of motivational interviewing in e-engaging people diagnosed with severe psychiatric conditions in work, study, or community participation. American Journal of Psychiatric Rehabilitation, 18(3), 265–279. https://doi.org/10.1080/15487768.2015.1053436

Herrings, M., van de Bovenkamp, H., Cardol, M., & Bal, R. (2020). Ethical dilemmas of participation of service users with serious mental illness: A thematic synthesis. *Issues in Mental Health Nursing, 41*(4), 283–295. https://doi.org/10.1080/01612840.2019.1667459

Hem, M. H., Molewijk, B., Gjerberg, E., Lillemoen, L., & Pedersen, R. (2018). The significance of ethics reflection groups in mental health care: A focus group study among health care professionals. *BMC Medical Ethics, 19*(1), 54. https://doi.org/10.1186/s12910-018-0297-y

Hem, M. H., Molewijk, B., Weimand, B., & Pedersen, R. (2023). Patients with severe mental illness and the ethical challenges related to confidentiality during family involvement: A scoping review. *Frontiers in Public Health, 10*, 960815. https://doi.org/10.3389/fpubh.2022.960815

Huang, C., Plummer, V., Lam, L., & Cross, W. (2020). Perceptions of shared decision-making in severe mental illness: An integrative review. *Journal of Psychiatric and Mental Health Nursing, 27*(2), 103–127. https://doi.org/10.1111/jpm.12246

Jung, S. H., Kim, W. H., Choi, H. J., Kang, M. H., Lee, J. S., Bae, J. N., & Kim, C. E. (2011). Factors affecting treatment discontinuation and treatment outcome in patients with schizophrenia in Korea: 10-Year follow-up study. *Psychiatry Investigation, 8*(1), 22–29. https://doi.org/10.4306/pi.2011.8.1.22

Karnieli-Miller, O., & Salyers, M. P. (2011). Clinical communication with persons who have serious mental illness. In A. Rudnick & D. Roe (Eds.), *Serious mental illness: Person-centered approaches* (pp. 155–167). Radcliffe Publishing. https://doi.org/10.1201/b13416

Laureano, C. D., Laranjeira, C., Querido, A., Dixe, M. A., & Rego, F. (2024). Ethical issues in clinical decision-making about involuntary psychiatric treatment: A scoping review. *Healthcare, 12*(4), 445. https://doi.org/10.3390/healthcare12040445

Lawrence, K. C., Makhonza, L. O., & Aliya, M. S. (2023). The role of token economy therapy in reducing the psychological burden of formal caregivers. *The Open Public Health Journal, 16*(1), 1–7. https://doi.org/10.2174/18749445-v16-e230711-2022-190

Lee, H. N. (1928). Morals, morality, and ethics: Suggested terminology. *The International Journal of Ethics, 38*(4), 450–466. https://www.jstor.org/stable/2377563

Leonhardt, B. L., Huling, K., Hamm, J. A., Roe, D., Hasson-Ohayon, I., McLeod, H. J., & Lysaker, P. H. (2017). Recovery and serious mental illness: A review of current clinical and research paradigms and future directions. *Expert Review of Neurotherapeutics, 17*(11), 1117–1130. https://doi.org/10.1080/14737175.2017.1378099

Liégeois, A., & Van Audenhove, C. (2005). Ethical dilemmas in community mental health care. *Journal of Medical Ethics, 31*(8), 452–456. https://doi.org/10.1136/jme.2003.006999

Manschreck, T. C., & Boshes, R. A. (2007). The CATIE schizophrenia trial: Results, impact, controversy. *Harvard Review of Psychiatry, 15*(5), 245–258. https://doi.org/10.1080/10673220701679838

McCradden, M. D., Joshi, S., Anderson, J. A., Mazwi, M., Goldenberg, A., & Zlotnik Shaul, R. (2020). Patient safety and quality improvement: Ethical principles for a regulatory approach to bias in healthcare machine learning. *Journal of the American Medical Informatics Association, 27*(12), 2024–2027. https://doi.org/10.1093/jamia/ocaa085

McGinty, E. E., Goldman, H. H., Pescosolido, B. A., & Barry, C. L. (2018). Communicating about mental illness and violence: Balancing stigma and increased support for services. *Journal of Health Politics, Policy and Law, 43*(2), 185–228. https://doi.org/10.1215/03616878-4303507

Mead Jasperse, S. C., Kelly, M. P., Ward, S. N., Fernand, J. K., Joslyn, P. R., & van Dijk, W. (2023). Consent and assent practices in behavior analytic research. *Behavior Analysis in Practice*, 1–16. https://doi.org/10.1007/s40617-023-00838-5

Merriam-Webster. (n.d.). Collaborate. In *Merriam-Webster.com dictionary.* Retrieved November 10, 2024, from https://www.merriam-webster.com/dictionary/collaborate

Mohamed, A. A., Sanad, H. S., & Abdel-Aziz, R. A. (2024). Effect of empowerment program on recovery and helplessness among patients with schizophrenia. *EKB Journal Management System*, 12(45), 63–74. https://doi.org/10.21608/asnj.2024.296250.1837

Molewijk, B., Hem, M. H., & Pedersen, R. (2015). Dealing with ethical challenges: A focus group study with professionals in mental health care. *BMC Medical Ethics, 16*(1), Article 4. https://doi.org/10.1186/1472-6939-16-4

Morán-Sánchez, I., de los Angeles Bernal-Lopez, M., Salmerón, D., & Pérez-Cárceles, M. D. (2021). Correlates of preferring a passive role in decision-making among patients with schizophrenia or bipolar disorder. *Patient Education and Counseling, 104*(5), 1125–1131. https://doi.org/10.1016/j.pec.2020.10.019

Morgan, T. A. (2020). Learned helplessness. In M. D. Gellman (Ed.), *Encyclopedia of behavioral medicine* (2nd ed., pp. 1277–1279). Springer. https://doi.org/10.1007/978-3-030-39903-0_1201

Niemetz, H. U. (2008). Understanding the difference between law, morals and ethics. In O. Steiger (Ed.), *Property economics: Property rights, creditor's money, and the foundations of the economy* (pp. 385–415). Metropolis-Verlag. https://www.metropolis-publisher.com/Understanding-the-Difference-Between-Law%2C-Morals-and-Ethics/11573/book.do

Oliani, S. M., Reichert, R. A., & Banaco, R. A. (Eds.). (2021). *Behavior analysis and substance dependence: Theory, research and intervention.* Springer International. https://doi.org/10.1007/978-3-030-71865-9

Perkins, D. O., Gu, H., Weiden, P. J., McEvoy, J. P., Hamer, R. M., & Lieberman, J. A. (2008). Predictors of treatment discontinuation and medication nonadherence in patients recovering from a first episode of schizophrenia, schizophreniform disorder, or schizoaffective disorder: A randomized, double-blind, flexible-dose, multicenter study. *Journal of Clinical Psychiatry, 69*(1), 106. https://doi.org/10.4088/JCP.v69n0114

Pilgrim, D., & McCranie, A. (2013). *Recovery and mental health: A critical sociological account.* Bloomsbury. https://www.bloomsbury.com/us/recovery-and-mental-health-9781137009319

Rabinowitz, J., Levine, S. Z., Garibaldi, G., Bugarski-Kirola, D., Berardo, C. G., & Kapur, S. (2012). Negative symptoms have greater impact on functioning than positive symptoms in schizophrenia: Analysis of CATIE data. *Schizophrenia Research, 137*(1–3), 147–150. https://doi.org/10.1016/j.schres.2012.01.015

Roberts, L. W., Kasun, M., & Termuehlen, G. (2021). Ethics, professionalism, and the field of mental health: An overview. In L. W. Roberts, M. Kasun, & G. Termuehlen (Eds.), *Professionalism and ethics: Q & A self-study guide for mental health professionals* (pp. 1–25). American Psychiatric Association. https://doi.org/10.1176/appi.books.9781615373617.ch01

Roe, D., & Davidson, L. (2018). Self and narrative in schizophrenia: Time to author a new story. In A. Rudnick (Ed.), *The Self in Health and Illness* (pp. 99–112). CRC Press. https://doi.org/10.1201/9781315381550

Rose, D. (2014). The mainstreaming of recovery. *Journal of Mental Health, 23*(5), 217–218. https://doi.org/10.3109/09638237.2014.928406

Scoular, C., Duckworth, D., Heard, J., & Ramalingam, D. (2020). Collaboration: definition and structure. *Australian Council for Educational Research.* https://research.acer.edu.au/ar_misc/3

Shahrokh N. C. & Hales, R. E. (Eds.) (2003). *American psychiatric glossary* (8th ed.). American Psychiatric Association

Shepherd, G., Boardman, J., & Slade, M. (2008). *Making recovery a reality* (pp. 1–3). Sainsbury Centre for Mental Health. https://www.centreformentalhealth.org.uk/publications/making-recovery-reality

Stallman, H. M., & Gupta, V. (2025, January 20). Involuntary commitment. In *StatPearls* [Internet]. StatPearls Publishing. https://www.ncbi.nlm.nih.gov/books/NBK557377/

Strub, R. L., & Black, F. W. (1995). *The mental status examination in neurology* (4th ed.). F.A. Davis Company. https://www.fadavis.com/product/mental-status-examination-neurology-strub-black

Suarez, V. D., Marya, V., Weiss, M. J., & Cox, D. (2023). Examination of ethical decision-making models across disciplines: Common elements and application to the field of behavior analysis. *Behavior Analysis in Practice, 16*(3), 657–671. https://doi.org/10.1007/s40617-022-00753-1

Substance Abuse and Mental Health Services Administration (SAMHSA). (2012). *SAMHSA's working definition of recovery: 10 guiding principles of recovery.* Author. https://library.samhsa.gov/sites/default/files/pep12-recdef.pdf

Swarbrick, M., & Brandow, C. L. (2025). The lived experience: Focus on wellness. In G. Thornicroft, R. E. Drake, O. Gureje, K. T. Mueser, & G. Szmukler (Eds.), *Oxford Textbook of Community Mental Health* (2nd ed., pp. 57–64). Oxford University Press. https://doi.org/10.1093/med/9780198898818.003.0006

Thomas, T. P. (2013). *The effect of personal values, organizational values, and person-organization fit on ethical behaviors and organizational commitment outcomes among substance abuse counselors: A preliminary investigation* [Doctoral dissertation, University of Iowa]. Iowa Research Online. https://doi.org/10.17077/etd.uzvjk997

Turnbull, O. H., Fotopoulou, A., & Solms, M. (2014). Anosognosia as motivated unawareness: The 'defence' hypothesis revisited. *Cortex, 61*, 18–29. https://doi.org/10.1016/j.cortex.2014.10.008

Varkey, B. (2021). Principles of clinical ethics and their application to practice. *Medical Principles and Practice, 30*(1), 17–28. https://doi.org/10.1159/000509119

Velligan, D. I., Weiden, P. J., Sajatovic, M., Scott, J., Carpenter, D., Ross, R., & Docherty, J. P. (2010). Strategies for addressing adherence problems in patients with serious and persistent mental illness: Recommendations from the expert consensus guidelines. *Journal of Psychiatric Practice, 16*(5), 306–324. https://doi.org/10.1097/01.pra.0000388626.98662.a0

Weiden, P. J., & Olfson, M. (1995). Cost of relapse in schizophrenia. *Schizophrenia Bulletin, 21*(3), 419–429. https://doi.org/10.1093/schbul/21.3.419

Young, G. (2016). A broad ethics model for mental health practice. *Ethics, Medicine and Public Health, 2*(2), 220–237. https://doi.org/10.1016/j.jemep.2016.03.005

Zisman-Ilani, Y., Lysaker, P. H., & Hasson-Ohayon, I. (2021). Shared risk taking: Shared decision making in serious mental illness. *Psychiatric Services*, 72(4), 461–463. https://doi.org/10.1176/appi.ps.202000544

Chapter 6
Problems with Delusional Behaviors in Individuals Living with Serious Mental Illness

Introduction

Delusional beliefs represent one of the most complex and clinically significant phenomena encountered in the assessment and treatment of serious mental illness (SMI). Defined as fixed, false beliefs held with strong conviction despite contradictory evidence and cultural norms, delusions are diagnostically central to schizophrenia spectrum and other psychotic disorders, and frequently observed across mood, anxiety, and neurocognitive conditions. Their persistence and resistance to counterargument pose substantial challenges to clinical engagement, functional recovery, and social integration. This chapter builds upon the foundational understanding of SMI symptoms by examining delusions not merely as diagnostic criteria but as multidimensional behavioral constructs shaped by neurocognitive, emotional, and environmental processes.

Traditional typologies, such as persecutory, grandiose, somatic, and erotomanic delusions, offer useful descriptive anchors but often fail to capture the dynamic interplay of factors that sustain delusional ideation. Drawing on contemporary dimensional models, this chapter explores the measurable attributes of delusional behavior, including conviction, preoccupation, distress, systematization, and behavioral disruption. These dimensions are contextualized within broader frameworks of associative learning, emotional dysregulation, and misattribution of salience, offering a detailed understanding of how delusions emerge, persist, and vary in intensity. Neurobiological substrates and environmental modulators, including trauma, stress, and social learning, are examined to underscore the multifactorial origins of delusional beliefs.

The chapter concludes by integrating these insights into a behaviorally informed approach to intervention. Emphasis is placed on individualized formulation, functional assessment, and the application of behavioral principles to reduce delusional speech and improve adaptive functioning. Case examples and clinical vignettes

G. F. McKeegan, *Behavior Change Interventions for Serious Mental Illness*, Evidence-Based Practices in Behavioral Health,
https://doi.org/10.1007/978-3-032-18372-9_6

illustrate the practical relevance of these concepts, while recommendations for future research and guideline development highlight the evolving landscape of delusion-focused care. By bridging categorical and dimensional perspectives, the chapter offers a comprehensive framework for understanding and addressing delusional behaviors in diverse clinical settings.

> My sister says things that are bizarre and believes things that are not part of reality. She says she is possessed, is a famous person, or can communicate telepathically. She believes she is married to a star and has 18 children. None of that is true, but she insists on talking about it to anyone who will talk with her.

The Case of Marie

Marie is residing at a group home and attends a day program. She has been living with schizophrenia spectrum mental health problems since the age of 18. Marie often talks about her belief that she is married to a well-known country singer, and he is coming to get her "any day now." She often interrupts conversations of others to ask if "my husband is here yet" and then continues talking about him and being married to him and having his children. If she is told this is not real, she becomes angry and curses the people who disagree with her. Other service users and providers avoid her at the day program as she talks about little else and changes the conversation back to false beliefs. Staff at the program become frustrated with Marie and avoid her because they don't feel that there is anything they can do to manage her delusional speech.

Definition and Characteristics of Delusions

Delusions are a prominent and core problematic behavior in the identification of a person living with severe mental health problems. A delusion is defined as a false belief resulting from an inaccurate interpretation of external reality, which is persistently upheld despite prevailing perspectives and clear, compelling evidence to the contrary. Typically, such beliefs are not shared by others within the individual's culture or subculture (American Psychiatric Association, 2022). Individuals experiencing delusions hold convictions that are not endorsed by those around them, are inconsistent with objective reality, and cannot be accounted for by religious or cultural factors (Munro, 1992; Shahrokh & Hale, 2003). In addition, people experiencing delusions will overinterpret ordinary events and experiences as having special meaning and significance (Holt et al., 2006). The individual living with a false belief perceives certain environmental stimuli as highly significant or puzzling due to heightened emotional reactivity. These stimuli, while task-irrelevant, acquire exaggerated emotional salience, prompting the subject to focus disproportionately on them (Petrolini, 2017). For instance, a store clerk smiles at a customer, and the customer interprets the smile as the clerk wanting a intimate relationship with her; a person experiences a thought or feeling and believes that the thought was put into his consciousness (i.e., "mind") by another person; experiencing a headache or sudden and brief pain in an extremity is perceived to be a sign of a cancer or that a body part has been removed by some known or unknown entity. The experiences of having delusions are frequently distressing and disabling for the person experiencing them.

Dimensions of Problematic Delusional Behavior

Delusions are multidimensional epiphenomena that result from a confluence of sensory experiences, perceptions, inferences, and decision-making. Delusions are constant in form in that the delusion is a false belief, and the person experiencing the delusion convincingly holds onto the false belief despite what others believe or know as true; ordinary events and circumstances are misperceived and overinterpreted in support of the false belief by the person experiencing the delusion (American Psychiatric Association, 2013; Kimhy et al., 2005). The presence of delusional behaviors is a necessary problem behavior to be identified to decide that a person is living with an SMI; the presence of delusions is transdiagnostic and is manifested in schizophrenia spectrum, bipolar, anxiety, and mood mental health problems, and delusional mental health condition (American Psychiatric Association, 2022; Manschreck, 1992).

Dimensions of symptoms and problematic behaviors that are displayed by people living with SMI, such as delusions, hallucinations, disorganized speech, and dysregulated affect, are defined as constructs representing observable and measurable behaviors (Morris & Cuthbert, 2012; National Institute of Mental Health [NIMH], n.d.). These constructs serve as fundamental aspects of functional behaviors. Dimensions are categorized under major domains, such as cognitive systems, social processes, and arousal, regulatory, and learning systems. Each dimension is assessed across multiple units of analysis, including genetic, neurological, physiological, behavioral, and self-report data. This multilevel approach facilitates a comprehensive perspective on the foundations of mental health problems.

There are multiple dimensions for each behavioral construct linked to an SMI. Each dimension of the construct needs to be "operationally defined," which is the description of something in terms of the actions or processes by which it could be observed and measured (American Psychological Association, n.d.-i). Each construct is multidimensional and multidirectional in that a change in one specific dimension can have notable impacts on other dimensions of the construct.

The core dimensions of behaviors that can be observed and measured are the quantifiable aspects of behavior used to define, observe, and measure a specific dimension once operationally defined (Cooper et al., 2020). These dimensions of behavior, as applied to delusion behaviors, are as follows:

- Topography: The physical form or shape of a behavior. Delusional behavior is a covert private event that can only be assessed by the overt display of delusional speech. The topography of delusional behavior is the content of the delusion that can be broadly categorized into themes and types of delusions.

- Frequency/rate: The number of times a behavior occurs within a specified time period.
- Count: A simple count of the number of times a behavior occurs.
- Temporal extent: The amount of time in which the person living with a delusion engages in delusional speech over a defined period (i.e., from the time the person engages in delusional behavior to the cessation of the defined behavior). It is a complex qualitative measure that evaluates how a delusion influences perceptions of past, present, and future behaviors.
- Duration: The total amount of time a delusional belief has been present. It is the total time from the beginning to the end of the amount of time the person has been experiencing a delusion. An example would be a person who daily stands on a street corner during the lunch hour and speaks to passersby about his belief that aliens have taken over the United Nations.
- Locus: The context and antecedent conditions that occur in relation to the person engaging in delusional behavior (e.g., speech and acting on the belief). Locus includes the environmental stimuli that are present when the delusional behavior is manifested; the pattern of the stimuli can assist in determining the antecedent stimuli that may "trigger" the individual to engage in delusional behavior. For instance, the person only speaks to his prescribing service provider about the thoughts that he believes are inserted into his consciousness.
- Temporal locus: The instance of delusional behavior that occurs at a specific point in time in relation to other events. This concept highlights the timing of the behavior and its position within a sequence of stimuli and events.
- Latency: The time between a stimulus (a triggering antecedent event) and the start of the delusional behavior.
- Interresponse time (IRT): The time between the end of one episode of delusional speech and the beginning of the next occurrence. One occurrence of delusional speech is operationally defined as the amount of time during which delusional speech occurs.
- Force/intensity: The magnitude or strength of a behavior.
- Conviction: Denotes the degree of certainty with which an individual holds a delusional belief. It is assessed by evaluating the strength and intensity with which the individual perceives the false notion as reality (Kendler et al., 1983; Kumari et al., 2013). Conviction reflects the magnitude or intensity of delusional thinking exhibited by the individual.
- Individuals experiencing delusions can vary as to the firmness and tenacity with which they/them holds onto the belief; studies have shown that grandiose and religious delusions are held more firmly than other delusional beliefs by the individuals experiencing the delusions (Appelbaum et al., 1999).
- Preoccupation: The extent to which the delusion occupies the individual's thoughts. This dimension can be assessed by evaluating the frequency and rate of delusional speech, the interresponse time (IRT), as well as the temporal locus and duration of the individual's engagement in delusional behavior. It may be

inferred that a higher occurrence of delusional speech indicates a greater preoccupation and magnitude of delusional thinking Kumari et al., 2013).

- External determinants: The influence of external factors on the dimensions of the delusion. External pressure in delusions refers to the influence of external or environmental factors that can trigger, shape, or intensify a person's false beliefs. While delusions are rooted in covert cognitive and biological processes, external pressures can exacerbate a person's vulnerability to manifestation of problematic behavior, alter the content of their beliefs, or drive their behaviors related to the delusion. Stressful life events, sensory impairments, trauma, over- and under-stimulation, and use of substances can have multidirectional impacts on the dimensions of delusional behaviors (Kumari et al., 2013).
- Implausibility and bizarreness: The degree to which the delusion conflicts with reality. Delusions vary in the dimensions of bizarreness, outlandishness, and eccentricity; some delusional beliefs are utterly implausible and impossible. Some delusional beliefs do have elements of reality, and although the beliefs may be possible, there is no supporting evidence to uphold or verify the beliefs (Kumari et al., 2013). Delusions are assessed as to the degree that the belief is clearly implausible, not understandable to others from the same culture, and not derived from ordinary experiences (American Psychiatric Association, 2022). Nonbizarre delusions realistically could occur, such as being cheated on, poisoned, or stalked by an ex-partner (American Psychiatric Association, 2022). A nonbizarre delusion is an individual seeing a police cruiser driving behind her at night and believing that the police are agents of the government that are trailing her and want to do her harm. A bizarre delusion is a person stating that she has had her brain removed by aliens.
- Distress: The emotional impact of the delusion on the individual. This dimension is defined as the amount and intensity of aversive emotional respondents that are related to the false belief, usually manifested as anger, shame, fear, and anxiety (Ali et al., 2011; Kumari et al., 2013). An individual experiencing a grandiose delusion (e.g., believing that she is a famous fashion designer) may experience positive emotions linked to the false belief, but if challenged, the person can become hostile and angry that her "exceptional talent" is not appreciated by others.
- Disruption to behavior: Disruption to behavior refers to the interference or impairment in an individual's ability to perform daily tasks or engage in normal activities due to the impact of delusional beliefs. This can manifest as difficulty concentrating, completing tasks, maintaining relationships, adhering to routines resulting from the distress, preoccupation, or emotional consequences caused by these symptoms (Kumari et al., 2013). For instance, an individual only washes in sinks in public bathrooms as he refuses to shower believing that aliens are watching and listening to him through the shower head.
- Extension: This dimension of delusional behavior refers to the breadth or scope of a delusional belief, describing how far the delusion expands and affects the individual's life beyond its initial core belief. A delusion with high "extension"

is one that is deeply interwoven with the person's life, impacting many different areas and thought processes, while a delusion with low "extension" is more contained and isolated (Kendall et al., 1983; Kumari et al., 2013). A delusion that is high on the dimension of extension would be if the individual remains in his apartment and refuses to leave as he believes that he is being targeted by foreign agents from a communist country.

- Systematization: It is the extent to which delusions are structured into a coherent, organized, monothematic, and logical framework. Systematized delusions are usually limited to a single false belief or theme with multiple variations or a group of false beliefs that a person relates to a single event or theme such that they/them believes that the event has caused all the problems that they/them is experiencing in their life and are consistent over time (American Psychological Association, n.d.-l; Munro, 2012). They are associated with a sense of reality and not associated with hallucinations (Bortolotti, 2016). Fragmentary delusions are disorganized, undeveloped false beliefs or a series of false beliefs that are disconnected, inconsistent, and illogical (American Psychological Association, n.d.-e; Bortolotti, 2016).
- Delusions are not isolated beliefs but are interconnected and structured in a way that they can form a consistent narrative or system. For example, a person with systematized delusions might weave various false beliefs into a detailed and elaborate story that appears internally logical, even though it is disconnected from reality. Delusion can be measured along this continuum of being coherent and organized into an understandable yet false narrative versus an incomprehensible verbal narrative of the belief (Kumari et al., 2013).
- Emotional commitment: Emotional commitment to a delusion refers to the extent of emotional investment or attachment an individual has toward a delusional belief (Kumari et al., 2013). Emotional commitment to delusions is marked by false beliefs held with unwavering conviction, often fueled by intense emotions such as fear or anger. While the beliefs themselves are unfounded, the emotional experiences accompanying them are authentic and profound, further entrenching the delusional state (Ghanem et al., 2023). This form of commitment indicates the degree to which a delusion impacts emotions, behaviors, and overall psychological functioning. Delusions held with strong conviction often persist despite contradictory evidence, and emotional commitment is a key factor in this resistance to change. Manifestations of this commitment can include distress, fear, anger, or other pronounced emotional responses associated with the delusional content, thereby intensifying the subjective reality of the belief. While the belief itself may be unfounded, the accompanying emotions are authentic and significant. The concept is commonly examined within a multidimensional framework for understanding delusions, considering elements such as conviction, preoccupation, and distress, all of which can interact and influence one another in a multidirectional fashion (Kumari et al., 2013). Research suggests that changes in negative emotions related to delusions correspond to shifts in both distress and the degree of preoccupation experienced by the individual (Leslie et al., 2025).

- Constancy of theme and content: Delusions are constant in form in that the delusion is a false belief and the person experiencing the delusion convincingly holds onto the false belief despite what others believe or know as true (American Psychiatric Association, 2013). In most circumstances, themes of delusional beliefs have been found to be constant (Grunfeld et al., 2024). Usually, the content of the delusion revolves around one theme, like believing that one is a billionaire and well-connected international soccer player. There are circumstances when the false beliefs do not encompass one predominant belief, or the predominant belief is not clearly articulated by the individual and is difficult to describe. These types are then labeled as mixed and unspecified types, respectively (American Psychiatric Association, 2022).
- Pressure: This is a subjective experience of having a forceful, urgent need to act on one's beliefs. This "realization pressure" is considered a prerequisite for a delusion to form and is seen as a component in the multidimensional nature of a delusion, alongside conviction, extension, and disorganization. It can indicate a severe level of the delusional experience, where the individual feels an intense urge to act upon their beliefs and is seriously bothered by them (Opjordsmoen, 2014).
- Delusions vary as to the risk that the person experiencing a delusional belief acts on the belief. A person experiencing delusional religious beliefs will be more likely to act on the beliefs than other types of delusions (Appelbaum et al., 1999; Munro, 2012). An example would be an individual firmly holding onto the belief that she is the mother of "the savior" and kidnaps an infant believing that the infant is her child as a higher power has sent her a message that the child is hers. People experiencing certain types of delusions have been known to act aggressively and be intimidating and hostile if the false beliefs are challenged in any way, which are predominant in individuals living with persecutory types of false beliefs (Teasdale et al., 2006). In cases of somatic delusions, there may be times when the person engages in aggressive behavior toward various medical personnel who are not complying with their demands for corrective treatment and intervention about complaints based on their false beliefs (e.g., a person violently attacking a surgeon who will not agree to operate on a delusion of some deformity or somatic complaint) (Munro, 2012). Unfortunately, the person acting on delusional beliefs may incur forensic complications (i.e., incarceration, probation, mandated treatment) as they are acting irrationally out of the belief that their behavior is correct; the behavior may be harassment, intrusiveness, violations of trespassing, and protective orders—with or without violence (Munro, 2012).
- The impact of delusions and the need to act are closely tied to the severity and nature of delusional beliefs. Behavior may be shaped by the delusional content,
- According to DSM-5-TR (American Psychiatric Association, 2022), the severity of delusions is rated on a scale from 0 (not present) to 4 (severe). Severe delusions are characterized by "severe pressure to act upon beliefs or being very bothered by beliefs." This indicates that individuals with intense delusions may feel compelled to act in ways consistent with their delusional beliefs, which can

lead to significant personal and social consequences, including litigious or criminal behavior.

- Delusions can serve defensive or dynamic functions, such as attempts to escape tension and anxiety through denial or blaming others. For some individuals, delusions become a way of living or assessing life, making counterarguments ineffective.
- Mood: Delusions also have been differentiated in the clinical literature along the dimensions of mood congruency; that is, the contents or themes of the false beliefs align with the mood of the person who is experiencing the delusions (American Psychiatric Association, 2022). Mood is defined as a "pervasive and sustained subjective emotion that colors the perception of the world" (American Psychiatric Association, 2013, p. 824). Examples of mood include depression, anxiety, anger and elation. Examples of mood (American Psychiatric Association, 2013) include:

  - Dysphoric: An unpleasant mood, such as sadness, irritability, and anxiety.
  - Elevated: An exaggerated feeling of well-being, euphoria, or elation.
  - Euthymic: Mood is in the normal range, with an absence of depressed or elevated mood.
  - Expansive: A lack of restraint in the expression of feelings by the person (e.g., affective response).
  - Irritable: Easily annoyed or provoked to anger.

  Affect, on the other hand, refers to the overt expression of mood, which can be incongruous to the individual's subjective assessment of their emotions.
- Delusions are assessed as to the congruency of the delusional content to the mood of the individual living with a delusion. The thematic content of mood incongruency delusions is consistent with the mood of the individual living with the delusion; mood incongruency occurs when the thematic content is not consistent with the mood of the individual (American Psychiatric Association, 2013). Mood-congruent delusions are beliefs that are consistent with a depressive or manic state, such as delusions of abandonment or persecution when depressed and delusions of superiority or fame when manic. Mood-incongruent delusions are not affected by a particular mood state. They may include delusions of nihilism (e.g., the world is ending) and delusions of control (e.g., an external force controls your thoughts or movements) but are not associated with either dysphoric or elated mood states (Junginger et al., 1992).
- Orientation of theme: The content and theme of delusional behavior can be assessed along the dimension of the belief being focused on external stimuli or internal stimuli. The focus on external stimuli would be attributing salience and importance to observed behavior by others and environmental events, such as believing that passersby are smiling at the individual as he is a famous rock star. Internal focus would be a person believing that she has committed a heinous sin or has had organs removed from her body while asleep.

Origins of Delusional Behaviors

Neurological Substrates of Delusional Behaviors

Delusions are a hallmark of several mental health problems and neurodegenerative conditions. The persistence of delusions in the face of contradictory evidence indicates impairments in neural systems involved in belief evaluation, reality testing, and emotional salience. Recent advances in neuroimaging and neuropathological research demonstrate that delusional beliefs may be shaped by dysfunction across multiple brain networks responsible for these functions. The neurobiological basis of delusions is thought to involve disturbances in networks associated with salience attribution, executive functioning, emotional regulation, and sensory integration. Neuroimaging and neuropathological findings have found consistent abnormalities in the anterior cingulate cortex (ACC), dorsolateral prefrontal cortex (dlPFC), insula (INs), amygdala (amyg), hippocampus (HC), and thalamus. These regions form the neurological pathways that result in disrupted cognitive-affective circuits that contribute to the formation and persistence of delusional beliefs; the findings reveal convergent neural mechanisms and shared pathophysiological processes across schizophrenia spectrum and bipolar disorder mental health problems and Alzheimer's and Parkinson's diseases.

Several core brain regions have been implicated in the presence of delusional behaviors:

- Anterior cingulate cortex (ACC): The ACC plays a central role in conflict monitoring, error detection, and cognitive control. Functional imaging studies consistently show reduced cerebral blood flow (CBF) and metabolic activity in the ACC among individuals experiencing delusions, particularly in schizophrenia spectrum mental health problems. These reductions impair the brain's ability to evaluate contradictory evidence and suppress erroneous and false beliefs, contributing to the persistence of delusional ideation (Rootes-Murdy et al., 2022; Zhu et al., 2016).
- Dorsolateral prefrontal cortex (dlPFC): The dlPFC is critical for executive functions such as working memory, planning, and cognitive flexibility. Structural and perfusion irregularities within this area are linked to deficits in reasoning abilities and challenges in adjusting beliefs when presented with conflicting information. In schizophrenia spectrum and bipolar mental health problems, dlPFC dysfunction correlates with the severity and complexity of delusional content, suggesting its role in the elaboration and maintenance of false beliefs (Rootes-Murdy et al., 2022; Zhu et al., 2016).
- Ventromedial prefrontal cortex (vmPFC): The vmPFC is crucial for evaluating self-relevant information and regulating emotion, and its dysfunction can contribute to delusions. Delusions often arise from failure to correctly assign personal value and significance to thoughts and external stimuli, a process heavily dependent on the vmPFC (Rootes-Murdy et al., 2022; Zhu et al., 2016).

- Insula: The insula integrates interoceptive signals and contributes to self-awareness and emotional salience (e.g., intensity of emotional respondents). Gray matter reductions and functional dysconnectivity in the insula are observed across schizophrenia spectrum and bipolar mental health problems and neurodegenerative conditions. These disruptions may lead to misattribution of internal experiences to external sources, a phenomenon central to many delusional themes (Rootes-Murdy et al., 2022; Zhu et al., 2016).
- Amygdala (amyg): The amygdala modulates emotional responses and threat detection. Atrophy and hypoactivation in this region are linked to impaired emotional regulation and heightened sensitivity to perceived threats, which may fuel persecutory delusions. Dysfunction of the amygdala is particularly evident in schizophrenia spectrum mental health problems and the condition of Alzheimer's (Rootes-Murdy et al., 2022; Zhu et al., 2016).
- Hippocampus (HC): The hippocampus supports memory consolidation and contextual processing. Delusions in Alzheimer's and schizophrenia spectrum conditions are associated with hippocampal atrophy and reduced connectivity with prefrontal regions. These deficits may distort autobiographical memory and contribute to confabulation and false belief formation (Rootes-Murdy et al., 2022; Zhu et al., 2016).
- Thalamus and superior temporal gyrus (STG): The thalamus acts as a relay center for sensory and cognitive information, while the STG is involved in auditory processing and language comprehension. Abnormalities in these regions are linked to misinterpretation of sensory input and language-based delusions, such as thought insertion or auditory hallucinations with delusional elaboration (Rootes-Murdy et al., 2022; Zhu et al., 2016).
- Transdiagnostic patterns: Although individuals living with delusions are identified through heterogeneous criteria, neuroimaging research consistently demonstrates convergent patterns of dysfunction. Gray matter reductions in the dlPFC, insula, amygdala, and hippocampus are recurrent across the schizophrenia spectrum, bipolar, and Alzheimer's mental health problems. These regions form part of the salience network and default mode network (DMN). DMN is the brain network that becomes active when the brain is at rest. It is crucial for processes like self-reflection, emotional processing, social interaction, and mental exploration. Dysregulation of DMN may underlie the aberrant assignment of significance to neutral stimuli (Azarias et al., 2025).

Environmental Influence on the Origins and Maintenance of Delusional Behaviors

Most living organisms strive to minimize uncertainty about future states and events by forming and maintaining a set of beliefs (i.e., self-statements or thoughts) about oneself and the environment through associative learning; that is, cause and effect which is a change in an independent variable (i.e., cause) and the sequential change in an independent variable (i.e., effect) (Skinner, 1953). Central to this explanation is that formal associative learning theory can provide an explanation for the development and persistence of delusions (Feeney et al., 2017).

Delusions involve the interplay of covert behaviors including cognitions (i.e., self-talk), emotional respondents, perceptions, and memory. Hohwy (2013) suggested that delusions arise from unusual or misperceived sensory experiences, not unlike experiencing illusions (i.e., a misperception of a real external stimuli (Shahrokh & Hales, 2003). The sensory experiences are accompanied by cognitive and heightened emotional respondents (i.e., fear, anxiety, joy). The person attempts to understand or make sense of the experience by inferring causality from the perceptions of the experience and the associated cognitive and emotional sequelae of the experience, as well as self-statements or beliefs that have been learned from "models" by observing and imitating others rather than solely through classical or operant conditioning. Through social interactions, learning occurs through social behaviors and covert processes like attention, memory, and motivation, which mediate whether an observed behavior is replicated (Farmer et al., 2018).

Social learning theory (American Psychological Association, n.d.-k) is based on observational learning and modeling, which are pervasive and powerful means of transmitting patterns of behavior. Once observers extract the rules and structure underlying the modeled activities, new patterns of behavior occur that conform to those properties and are extrapolated to other similar environmental stimuli and contexts.

The likelihood of an individual imitating modeled behaviors is shaped by a complex interplay of factors involving both the model and the observer (Farmer et al., 2018). People are more inclined to emulate models who exude competence, power, prestige, and attractiveness, especially when those models share similar characteristics such as age or gender. High-status individuals like celebrities or nurturing parental and authority figures are particularly impactful (Brauer & Tittle, 2012; Farmer et al., 2018).

On the observer's side, attributes like cognitive ability, motivation, prior knowledge, and confidence in certain abilities play crucial roles. Attention is key, as observers selectively focus on certain aspects of the modeled behavior, affecting what they learn and retain. The consequences witnessed during modeling, whether the model is rewarded or punished, also impact imitation or repetition of observed behavior. When individuals observe others receiving praise or reinforcement for a particular behavior, the likelihood of emulating that behavior increases; conversely, witnessing punishment reduces the propensity to replicate it. Additionally, if an observed behavior enables avoidance or mitigation of an overt or covert aversive consequence, this behavior is subject to negative reinforcement. For example, observing a respected authority figure lie about an event without facing adverse consequences raises the probability that the observer will also choose to lie under similar circumstances to prevent negative outcomes. This form of vicarious learning enables the efficient acquisition of behaviors while minimizing potential risks (Brauer & Tittle, 2012; Farmer et al., 2018; Fryling et al., 2011).

Finally, cognitive processes such as self-regulation, motivation, and rehearsal are integral to observational learning. Observers who mentally practice the behavior and have opportunities for real-world application are more likely to retain and successfully perform the modeled actions. In summary, the synergy between model characteristics, observer traits, emotional and attentional influences, behavioral consequences, and cognitive processes determines how and why modeled behaviors are adopted (Brauer & Tittle, 2012; Farmer et al., 2018; Fryling et al., 2011).

The result of social learning is rule-governed behavior (Barnes-Holmes & McEnteggart, 2015). Rule-governed behavior involves covert verbal self-statements that guide the behaviors of an individual based on an understanding of contextual stimuli and potential consequences of the emitted behavior following specific antecedent conditions; rules are acquired through observing and interacting with others instead of direct experience by manifesting the behavior. Repeatedly manifesting rule-governed behavior results in habit formation. Habits are behaviors that occur in specific situations and, over time, are performed with little or no conscious intent (American Psychological Association, n.d.-f; Lally & Gardner, 2013).

The formation of delusional behaviors can be postulated to arise from a confluence of environmental stimuli and consequences that result in heightened emotional experiences, an inability to regulate the emotional experiences, attempts to understand and control ambiguous and aversive emotional events, misattribution of environmental stimuli as contingencies on covert and overt behaviors, inflexible rule-governed behavior pertaining to one's behavior, and overt and covert consequences that reinforce the occurrence of delusional behaviors (e.g., decrease in aversive respondents and cognitions). Delusions are complex, transdiagnostic phenomena that reflect a dynamic interplay between emotional dysregulation and aberrant salience attribution, mediated by dysfunction in limbic-prefrontal circuits, heightened emotional reactivity, impaired regulatory control, and misattribution of significance to neutral stimuli contributing to the formation and maintenance of delusional beliefs.

Emotional experiences, when dysregulated, can distort perceptual and interpretive processes, leading to the erroneous assignment of significance to neutral or ambiguous stimuli. Emotional dysregulation refers to the impaired ability to modulate affective responses in accordance with contextual demands. It emphasizes that individuals exhibiting delusional behaviors often exhibit heightened emotional reactivity, particularly in response to perceived threats or uncertainty. This heightened arousal amplifies the subjective intensity of experiences, increasing the likelihood that emotionally charged interpretations will be encoded as fixed beliefs (Leslie et al., 2025).

Attribution of salience is the process by which the importance of stimuli is assigned. In delusional behaviors, this mechanism becomes distorted, leading to the erroneous elevation of neutral or irrelevant cues, resulting in inconsistencies between belief and reality. This misattribution is not merely a perceptual error but a failure of regulatory systems to suppress emotionally congruent but factually erroneous interpretations. This interaction fosters the development of delusions and sustains their resistance to disconfirmation, in which emotional dysregulation heightens the affective intensity of experiences, while salience misattribution distorts their interpretation (Holt et al., 2006).

If uncertainty is generated by environmental events—either because of ambiguous stimuli and covert self-statements that have been assimilated by social learning—beliefs begin to depart from reality and can manifest into delusions. Uncertainty caused by environmental events results in physiological stress (as defined by the "fight or flight" phenomenon and mediated by the release of stress-related hormones) and heightened emotional respondents and arousal. The competition for limited cognitive resources explains how strong emotional stimuli act as "negative distractors," undermining task performance and reinforcing delusional reasoning (Ghanem et al., 2023). Heightened emotional states linked to uncertainty and ambiguity in perceived environmental stimuli monopolize cognitive resources, impair executive functions, lead to attributing salience and importance to neutral stimuli, and lead to peculiar interpretations of reality. For instance, a minor change in a spouse's behavior or a burst of laughter may be erroneously construed as evidence of infidelity or ridicule, respectively.

Beliefs are constructed through associations between covert representations, such as those of cause and effect, by reducing uncertainty through new learning and the allocation of finite attentional processes (Feeney et al., 2017). When cognitive resources are exceeded, the capacity for attentional processes may be compromised, potentially resulting in inaccurate conclusions that, when repeatedly linked to certain events, can become habitual. "Cognitive resource theory" posits that individuals address problems, challenges, and choices by actively encoding, processing, and retrieving relevant information. However, these mental processes demand cognitive capacity, so substantial demands in one domain may diminish activity in another (American Psychological Association, n.d.-a).

Formal associative learning theory can provide an explanation for the development and persistence of delusions. Skinner (1953) defined associative learning paradigms that emphasized the importance of predictions and self-statements of control, predicting the effect of behavior on the environment (i.e., beliefs). Beliefs are self-statements that are conditioned through associations with perceptual stimuli. Beliefs are associations between the self-talk of cause and effect that are formed by minimizing uncertainty by way of new learning and attentional allocation. If uncertainty is generated through experiences, beliefs may begin to depart from consensual reality and can manifest into false beliefs or delusions by inferring causality instead of acknowledging the randomness of the events and therefore a lack of control. Further associative learning events can then lead to certainty of the inferential process, a belief that what one believes is true, through repeated "private event" associations (Skinner, 1984). Stimuli in the environment that are similar "trigger" further attentional processes of sensory experiences that reinforce the inferential conclusion resulting in ordinary events having special meaning for the person.

Attributing causality to stimuli is the covert process of sequencing the temporal association of a stimulus and an outcome. Repeated occurrences of a particular sequence result in attribution of causality. For instance, an individual eats a certain food and feels ill. He associates the food that was ingested with the physiological sensations of "not feeling well." By focusing attention on the detail of the ingested food—taste, texture, amount, where purchased, freshness—he attributes salience to certain aspects of the food. Depending on the history of ingesting that particular type of food, he attributes causality to one or more characteristics of what was eaten. When individuals experience heightened emotional arousal due to illness in the absence of effective emotional self-regulation, their causal inferences and resulting conclusions may be inaccurate. This misattribution arises because of attentional biases and emotional dysregulation within certain environmental contexts, compounded by a lack of strategies to manage arousal. Efforts to anticipate and control recurrent or similar stimuli can elicit covert self-statements, which may ultimately contribute to the development of delusional beliefs, such as the perception of being poisoned.

Delusional misattribution often arises when individuals repeatedly attribute causality based on temporal sequencing between a stimulus and subsequent events. For example, John eats a slice of pizza and becomes ill due to unknowingly being exposed to an intestinal virus from being on the subway beforehand. He has worries and anxiety about his illness and how this happened; he goes over the events leading up to the illness. He thinks about the clerk that sold him the slice of pizza and goes over the details of their interaction, attending to particulars of the interaction that result in uncertainties about the interaction. He begins to infer that the clerk did not say thank you or even greet John as he did during previous instances. He recalls that the clerk was a person of a minority status and recalls that his family had made repeated statements that minorities were not trustworthy, did not accept the predominant culture, and had hostile intentions to others, like John and his family; his family modeled racist and xenophobic behaviors to John and avoided interactions with minorities. His parents and others with whom he associates, as well as the social media he watches, make comments that reinforce his perceptions of minorities. John infers that the clerk does not like him and may have put something on his pizza that induced his illness and generates self-statements of worry and fear about his safety when in proximity to the clerk. When he perceives anything related to pizza, he experiences an internal sensation of nausea that is a trigger or discriminative stimuli to automatic cognitions associated with the pizza and stimuli associated with it, such as the clerk, and John's perceived allocation of negative feelings toward the clerk as conditioning can influence people to manifest specific behaviors, such as approach and avoidance behaviors (Sanvictores, Mahabadi, & Rehman, 2025). When John encounters narratives or accounts from others who report similar experiences, he engages in internal dialogue that covertly reinforces his adverse perceptions of the clerk. This pattern of negative self-talk and associated emotional respondents, particularly regarding individuals of minority status, subsequently is conditioned and generalized to other members of minority groups with whom he interacts, shaping his broader interpersonal attitudes and responses. Repeated self-statements and conditioned emotional respondents will reinforce the above association, and John begins to believe that the clerk attempted to poison him—and a paranoid delusion begins to develop as he avoids interacting and attributing salience to neutral stimuli associated with minorities.

Epidemiological Considerations

Little is known about the frequency and the specific prevalence of the various subtypes of delusions (Ertekin et al., 2021). Most are known from overt cases that are reported in the news media, the courts, and from hospitalized people; it is agreed that the prevalence is underreported. Many aspects and details of experiencing delusions are from case reports (Munro, 2012).

The prevalence of delusions in the general population varies significantly depending on the study and methodology used. Reported rates range from 3.0% endorsing at least one "delusional-like experience" to 91% endorsing at least one "delusion-like belief." This wide range reflects differences in assessment tools, the number of questions asked, and whether follow-ups by clinicians were conducted (Heilskov et al., 2020).

Experiences of delusions occur transdiagnostically. Delusions occur in several severe mental health problems, including schizophrenia spectrum, mood- and personality-related mental health problems, dementing conditions, and sequelae to adverse neurological events such as stroke or injury to the brain. Delusions can occur because of using psychoactive substances such as stimulants (e.g., amphetamines, cocaine, methamphetamines) and arise when experiencing symptoms of withdrawal, such as from alcohol.

Delusions can only be accessed and assessed through self-reports by the person experiencing false beliefs. Individuals experiencing delusions rarely seek assistance from health service providers independently, as they are convinced of the accuracy of their perceptions and beliefs despite contrary evidence and maintain these beliefs with strong conviction. Such individuals often avoid interactions with others who might challenge or dispute their beliefs. A person may be anxious and distressed about the potential negative outcome of a false belief—being followed by aliens, not being appreciated for their special abilities, believing that others see them as deformed—while others may experience satisfaction and elation in the belief that he is a genius, or the mother of 30 children. The prevalence of delusions remains largely speculative, as individuals experiencing such beliefs are unlikely to participate in research. This is due to their lack of recognition that their beliefs are false and their subsequent inability to identify with the criteria for research participation (Munro, 2012).

There is heterogeneity in how frequently people living with SMI experience a certain type of delusional belief (Ertekin et al., 2021; Munro, 2012; van der Vaart et al., 2024). The most frequently experienced delusion by individuals living with SMI is persecutory (i.e., a conviction that the person experiencing the delusion is being harassed, attacked, or conspired against by others), followed by grandiose delusions (i.e., exaggerated belief in one's fame, importance, abilities) (Brucato et al., 2017); however, research results have been as heterogeneous as the themes displayed in delusional beliefs (Ertekin et al., 2021; van der Vaart et al., 2024). The specificity of the content of the type of delusion being experienced is heterogeneous as content varies. The dimensions of tenacity and acting on delusional beliefs also vary and are difficult to predict.

Collin et al. (2023) conducted a meta-analysis of published literature examining the prevalence of various delusional themes. Their findings indicate that the most common types are persecutory (64.5%), reference (39.7%), grandiose (28.2%), control (21.6%), and religious (18.3%). These five delusional themes appeared with greater frequency in samples specifically restricted to individuals who live with SMI. The prevalence of these themes was not influenced by sociodemographic or cultural characteristics of the studied populations. The authors suggest that such delusional patterns may be indicative of underlying psychosocial mechanisms developed as adaptive responses to life challenges.

Culture Influences and Prevalence

Delusions, defined as firmly held false beliefs that persist despite clear contradictory evidence, constitute a central core feature of living with an SMI. However, their manifestation and prevalence are not globally uniform. The phenomenology and frequency of specific delusional themes exhibit substantial variation across cultural, ethnic, religious, and societal contexts. While the structural form of delusions is consistent across populations, the thematic content and epidemiological distribution differ markedly. As Spitzer (1990) notes, the types or contents of delusions remain broadly similar across cultures, yet their expression is modulated by contextual factors, resulting in variability in both thematic emphasis and prevalence. Recognition of these variations is essential for culturally sensitive assessment and intervention in clinical practice, ensuring that mental health service professionals can differentiate between culturally sanctioned beliefs and pathological delusions and provide appropriate care.

The types and prevalence of delusions across cultures are as follows:

- Persecutory delusions: These are the most prevalent type of delusion across global populations. Studies reveal high rates among Pakistanis-in-Pakistan (62%), British-Pakistanis (60%), and White-British individuals (48%). Within the South African Xhosa community, an astounding 86% believed that family or friends intended harm, often attributed to jealousy, black magic, or bewitchment. Latino populations also demonstrate high prevalence (76–82%), indicating a broad cross-cultural predominance of persecutory themes (Ghannem et al., 2023).
- Grandiose delusions: These involve beliefs in possessing exceptional abilities, being divine, or having a special mission. Prevalence is notably higher in Pakistanis-in-Pakistan (42%) compared to British-Pakistanis (23%) and White-British (14%). Among the South African Xhosa, two-thirds reported grandiose delusions, while European-Americans exhibited the highest rates (45%) compared to Latinos (25%) and African-Americans (35%) (Ghannem et al., 2023).

- Delusions of reference: This type of delusion, wherein individuals believe that innocuous events or remarks are specifically directed at them, is most prominent in White-British cultures (50%), markedly higher than in British-Pakistanis (26%) and Pakistanis-in-Pakistan (13%). White-British patients frequently describe delusions involving telepathic communication or themes related to technology (Ghannem et al., 2023).
- Religious delusions: Such delusions, characterized by beliefs of a special relationship with God or divine purpose, are evident among South African Xhosa people (26%), reflecting the integration of spiritual and religious concepts into delusional content.
- Somatic delusions: Focused on bodily sensations or health, somatic delusions are prevalent in the South African Xhosa group (37%), often centering on the head, skull, or brain (Ghannem et al., 2023).

Variations in prevalence have been found by certain population groups as follows:

- Pakistanis-in-Pakistan: High rates of both grandiose and persecutory delusions, suggesting societal factors such as economic and social class disparities may contribute to the prominence of these themes (Ghannem et al., 2023).
- White-British: Higher prevalence of delusions of reference and technology-related delusions, potentially reflecting increased exposure to modern communication and individualistic worldviews (Ghannem et al., 2023).
- South African Xhosa: Persecutory delusions predominate, but grandiose and somatic delusions are also common, often infused with local beliefs about witchcraft and spiritual harm (Ghannem et al., 2023).
- Latinos: Exhibit a greater prevalence of persecutory delusions compared to African-Americans and European-Americans, possibly reflecting community-oriented cultural frameworks (Ghannem et al., 2023).
- European-Americans: Demonstrate higher rates of grandiose delusions—twice as frequent as in Latinos and African-Americans—suggesting a cultural emphasis on individual achievement and uniqueness (Ghannem et al., 2023).

The observed variations in delusional content and frequency are shaped by a confluence of cultural, societal, and religious factors:

- Economic and social class disparities: These can intensify feelings of powerlessness and inferiority, fueling grandiose delusions as psychological compensation and avoidance of distressing private events, notably in Pakistani and African societies (Ghannem et al., 2023).
- Individualism versus collectivism: European-American cultures prioritize individualism, which may underlie the increased incidence of grandiose delusions, while collectivist Latino and African cultures tend toward persecutory themes (Ghannem et al., 2023).
- Technology exposure: Western societies' immersion in technology correlates with the emergence of technologically themed delusions, such as those involving telepathy or surveillance (Ghannem et al., 2023).

- Religious and spiritual beliefs: These beliefs are often reflected in the content of delusions, as seen in the prominence of religious delusions in societies where spirituality is central to daily life (Ghannem et al., 2023).

Types of Delusions

Delusions vary as to the content, theme, and orientation (i.e., external perceptions or self-perceptions) of the false belief. The themes of the delusions have been classified in the clinical literature but little research has been done due to the heterogeneity of the themes that are displayed (Ertekin et al., 2021); the key themes identified in the literature include paranoid or persecutory delusions, feelings of guilt or sin, grandiosity, religious ideation, somatic concerns, self-referential beliefs, experiences of being controlled, perceptions that one's thoughts are read or broadcast to others, and sensations of thoughts being inserted or withdrawn from one's consciousness. The content of some delusions may be difficult to classify as to a thematic category, such as the belief in ingesting buildings, as that peculiar belief may be thematically grandiose or somatic, although the content is bizarre and idiosyncratic.

Below are the types and subtypes of familiar and recognizable themes of various delusional content. The following are among the most reported types found in the mental health literature (Ertekin et al., 2021; Munro, 2012):

- Delusional jealousy: The belief that one's sexual partner is unfaithful. This phenomenon is also referred to as the "Othello delusion" (American Psychiatric Association, 2013; Shahrokh & Hales, 2003). Research indicates that it occurs more frequently in males, who typically express concerns regarding the potential loss of a partner. In contrast, when present in females, the primary concern is often the impact of infidelity on the relationship. At times, jealousy is usually expressed within a normal range with varying degrees of anger, but sometimes expressed as severe rage. There has been a demonstrated link between chronic alcohol abuse, as well as amphetamine and cocaine abuse and delusional jealousy (Munro, 2012).
- Persecutory delusions (delusion of persecution): Belief that the person is being persecuted, conspired against, harmed, harassed, or in other ways negatively impacted by another person, group of people, or organization (identified or not) such as the Federal Bureau of Investigation (FBI), Central Intelligence Agency (CIA), or the police (American Psychiatric Association, 2013; American Psychiatric Association, 2022; Shahrokh & Hales, 2003). Individuals exhibiting this delusion often demonstrate wariness, suspicion, hypervigilance, and anxiety; prominent features may include threatening behavior, which can sometimes lead to impulsive or premeditated acts of violence directed toward those whom the individual believes are involved in their persecution.
- Grandiose delusions refer to the belief that an individual possesses exceptional or exaggerated abilities, wealth, or notoriety (American Psychiatric Association,

2013). The content of these beliefs can vary widely, but they are strongly linked to the severity or intensity of the condition. Research indicates that grandiosity is frequently associated with a heightened sense of purpose, encompassing future-oriented goals and aspirations, as well as a strong conviction in one's understanding of personal experiences and life (Isham et al., 2021). This presentation is among the least thoroughly described variants of delusional mental health problems, partly because affected individuals are often persistently elated and may consider themselves too powerful or affluent to require assistance. Such individuals may exhibit aggressive behaviors when their perceived superiority is not recognized by others, potentially leading to frustration and anger. It is also common for individuals experiencing grandiose delusions to affiliate with political parties or religious organizations that affirm their beliefs regarding their own significance.

- Delusions of control (delusion of influence): The belief that private events of the individual, such as thoughts, feelings, and intentions, as well as actions and impulses, are imposed upon the person by an external force (American Psychological Association, n.d.-b; American Psychiatric Association, 2013; Shahrokh & Hales, 2003). It can also include the false belief that one's intentions or actions directly control external events or the thoughts and behavior of other people. Delusions of control are one of the first-rank symptoms of schizophrenia and are classified as Schneiderian delusions (Malinowski et al., 2020).
- Religious delusions: Beliefs that are associated with religion and encompass grandiose delusions with religious content. Delusional ideation frequently includes beliefs that the individual is a religious figure, such as a messiah or prophet, and that they possess extraordinary powers, such as the ability to cure illness (American Psychological Association, n.d.-j). Religious themes are common across delusional categories and types, with between a fifth and two-thirds of all delusions reflecting religious content. To be classified as a religious delusion, the belief must be idiosyncratic, rather than accepted within a particular culture or subculture. Strongly held beliefs that are shared within an existing religious or spiritual context, therefore, would not be a religious delusion. Speaking with a spiritual, all-powerful entity is acceptable and common among certain religious groups, so it is not considered a false belief. A person who believes that she is inhabited by spirits of multiple deities that are fighting among themselves and using her mind and body as their "battleground" would be considered delusional (e.g., demon possession) (Iyassu et al., 2014). The religious belief may be combined with other delusions, such as the delusion of control or grandeur and be related to experiencing auditory hallucinations, such as "hearing the voice of god." It may also be combined with erotic delusions in that the person believes that a higher power has "ordained" an intimate relationship to occur. Given the variety of religious beliefs, it is difficult to determine if the misperception is part of a faith-based belief or a symptom of living with SMI (Sofou et al., 2021).
- Delusions of guilt or sin: This refers to the person experiencing the misperception that they/them has done something seriously wrong and experiences unwar-

ranted and extreme feelings of remorse, shame, or debilitating dysphoria. As with religious delusions, this overinterpretation is difficult to determine whether it is an aspect of faith or a positive symptom of living with an SMI (Sofou et al., 2021).

- Delusions of poverty: The belief that one will be without any material possessions. The person is under the belief that they/them is about to become destitute, destined to fall into poverty, or impoverished despite evidence to the contrary (Shahrokh and Hales, 2003).
- Delusions of reference (also known as ideas of reference or delusions of influence): The belief that events, items, or other people in the immediate environment have a particular and unusually personal meaning for the person (American Psychiatric Association, 2013; Shahrokh & Hales, 2003). The event or object in the environment of the person having this belief may be a poster, song, advertisement, newscast, glance, or gesture that has a direct reference or a hidden meaning for the person. A person with this delusion may hear news on a podcast and perceive that what was being said was directed at them; a glance from another person at a public setting may have special significance for the person experiencing the delusion. The meaning that is being perceived may have negative or positive significance for the person. Delusions of reference are also known as ideas of reference and delusions of influence (American Psychological Association, n.d.-c).
- Nihilistic delusions: These involve the belief that oneself, aspects of oneself, other individuals, or even the world no longer exist. For example, an individual may be convinced that they do not have a brain or other vital organ. This type of delusion is also referred to as a delusion of nonexistence or delusion of negation (American Psychological Association, n.d.-h).
- Cotard delusions (originally negation delirium): Specific nihilistic delusions ranging from denial of the existence of certain body parts to denial that one is alive. The affected person holds the delusional belief that they/them is already dead, does not exist, is decaying or has decayed, or has lost their blood or internal organs (Debruyne et al., 2011; Sahoo & Josephs, 2018).
- Somatic delusions: The belief that there is a major problem with bodily functioning or personal health, that bodily organs are functioning improperly, or are diseased, injured, or altered (American Psychiatric Association, 2013). The somatic type of delusions can shade into the persistent conviction of illness in the absence of objective evidence with misinterpretation of ordinary bodily sensations as disease and with an inability to accept the responses from health care providers (DeSouza & McMichael, 2019); it may be difficult to differentiate between a systematized and congruent somatic delusion from the disorder of hypochondriasis (Munro, 2012) as both have similar content and themes.
- Dysmorphic delusions: The belief involving disturbance of body image that can vary in severity. A person experiencing a dysmorphic delusion presents with a perception that one is ugly or has a deformity; the expressed deformity may be a minor feature, such as the size or shape of one's nose; however, the person living with the delusions intensely complains and demands for alleviation of their dis-

tress by seeking corrective intervention that is out of proportion with expressions of being deformed. The delusion is systematized as the focus is usually a specific physical feature, such as an overly long nose, prominent ears, oversized or undersized breasts, dissatisfaction with the appearance of the genitalia, or skin blemish. People experiencing these types of delusions usually "doctor shop," going from surgeon to surgeon, demanding cosmetic procedures and being refused. Getting repeatedly refused may result in increased frustration and anger on the part of the person experiencing the delusion, and aggressive behaviors do sometimes occur toward the surgeon. In a limited subset of cases, individuals may perceive their entire body as abnormal and simultaneously present with both anorexia nervosa and bulimia nervosa (Munro, 2012).

- Delusional parasitosis (delusional infestation or Ekbom syndrome): The belief that there is a parasitic infestation of the skin, despite the absence of any medical evidence supporting the complaint (Reich et al., 2019). This delusion is rare in its occurrence. Delusions involving the skin seem to involve internal bodily sensations, just like muscle spasms, minor irritations, or rippling of muscles that are overly interpreted. Individuals experiencing these types of delusions believe that they are afflicted with a disease, with symptoms of crawling or stinging sensations; they believe that they have an insect or parasitic infestation, but examination finds none.
- Service providers disagree about the extent of considering complaints about sensation of the skin as delusional or an aspect of a rare but real dermatological disorder. An example is the disorder known as Morgellons disease (MD) (Middelveen et al., 2018). It is characterized by skin lesions that contain unusual filamentous threads or projections that spontaneously arise. The filaments are distinctive, in part due to their varied white, red, blue, green, or black colors; visually, they resemble microscopic textile fibers. Service providers believe that the filaments were intentionally embedded by the person with physical complaints and are an aspect of other mental health problems (e.g., Munchausen syndrome). Whether MD is a purely delusional mental health problem or a reality-based physical ailment is still undecided; it is listed in the ICD-11 (International Classiciation of Diseases 11th revision) (World Health Organization [WHO], 2022) as a delusional condition, and several studies have not found a direct link between an infectious agent and the symptoms; nevertheless, MD is linked to Lyme's disease, tick borne illnesses, and other pathogens. Middelveen et al. (2018) summarized the following regarding the research on MD:

  > Clinical studies supporting the hypothesis that MD is exclusively delusional in origin have considerable methodological flaws and often neglect the fact that mental disorders can result from underlying somatic illness. In contrast, rigorous experimental investigations show that this skin affliction results from a physiological response to the presence of an infectious agent (p. 71).

- Erotic delusions (also known as love delusion, erotomanic delusion, erotomania, erotic paranoia, de Clerambault's syndrome, and Simenon's syndrome): The belief and misperception that another person, usually famous or otherwise unavailable, is in love with or has had a sexual relationship with the person who is experiencing the belief (American Psychological Association, n.d.-d; American Psychiatric Association, 2013). A person experiencing this delusion may have strong erotic feelings associated with the love object. They may be persistent in contacting or trying to connect with the love object and, in fact, "stalk" the loved person. The person living with the false belief will offer "reasons" as to why they have not been together. Infrequently, the person who is the love interest does not exist (Munro, 2012).

- Delusions of smell (olfactory reference syndrome): The misperception that the whole body emanates an odor. As a rule, the odor is believed to be strong and repulsive enough to be noticed by everyone in the vicinity of the person living with the delusion. The character of the odor is often "nonbodily," likened to that of rotten eggs, garbage, human refuse, burning rubber, or ammonia. The person will state the odor is coming from their pores and orifices, has never experienced the odor themself, but knows that it is distasteful to others as gestures of disgust are perceived from others (Das et al., 2024). Some individuals experiencing this misperception also characterized the odor as excessive and strong flatulence, halitosis, or sweat. The individuals experiencing this belief are convinced that others smell the odor coming from them and will be humiliated or rejected. The condition causes significant distress, affecting daily activities, as the person experiencing this type of delusion will avoid social contact (Munro, 2012). They may also be experiencing olfactory hallucinations; olfactory hallucinations are perceptions of odors without identification of external stimuli. However, the person may have the delusion that the source of the odor that is being hallucinated is themselves.
- Delusions of transmitting nonsexual diseases: The belief that they/them is giving others a contagious disease. The person experiencing this delusion uses the over-interpretation of evidence by misperceiving sneezing or coughing by others nearby and attributing personal causality to the event (Munro, 2012). These beliefs can also be related to somatic delusions of having a contagious physical disease despite evidence to the contrary.
- Delusions of transmitting sexually transmitted diseases (STDs) (venereophobia): Refer to the unfounded belief that one has contracted a venereal disease despite the absence of any clinical evidence or history of risk-taking behavior (Munro, 2012). This type of delusion is observed more frequently in males. Individuals may repeatedly examine their genitalia for signs of disease, seek frequent testing for STDs, and avoid intimate relationships and physical contact (Mahajan & Shishak, 2017).
- Delusional procreational syndrome (DPS): DPS consists of a number of delusions, such as having a spouse, being pregnant, delusions of delivery (childbirth and labor), and being parents (paternity/maternity), as in the sequence of procreation (Johra & Uddin, 2024). The central misconception is that an individual experiencing this delusion is convinced she is pregnant, a condition referred to as "pseudocyesis" or "false pregnancy." In certain instances, women affected by pseudocyesis exhibit physical changes comparable to those observed in genuine pregnancies.

- DPS also includes the belief of having given birth and raising a child through the developmental stages, despite not having been pregnant or having a child (Manjunatha et al., 2010; Seeman, 2014). DPS could involve the belief of multiple pregnancies and children. Misidentification delusion, in which the person experiencing the delusion consistently misidentifies persons, places, objects, or events (Feinberg & Roane, 2005), could be an additional theme in DPS as the person misperceives that a child is his/hers (Munro, 2012; Seeman, 2014); although rare, the misidentification delusion of a child results in tragic events such as child kidnapping and violence (Silva et al., 1992).
- Denial of pregnancy: A rare false belief related to pregnancy that has been documented to occur in women who have other behaviors and symptoms of living with SMI. The women attribute the physical changes associated with pregnancy to other delusional themes (e.g., somatic, religious) (Velasco & Gerechter, 2023).
- Delusional misidentification syndrome (DMS): A group of complex, monothematic delusional phenomena in which a person holds the belief that the identity of a familiar person, object, location, or self has been altered or replaced (Christodoulou et al., 2009; Kim et al., 2022). DMS also includes the delusion of inanimate doubles (i.e., the belief that objects have been replaced by replicas), reduplicative paramnesia (i.e., the belief that a person or place has been duplicated) (Conners et al., 2014), and the delusional syndromes of intermetamorphosis, including Fregoli and Capgras syndrome (Leis et al., 2019). All these types of delusions are characterized by the belief that particular people have been physically and psychologically transformed into other people or replaced (American Psychological Association, n.d.-g). DMS impacts the abilities of the person experiencing this misperception to recognize familiar individuals, believing that the known person has changed physical characteristics (Feinberg & Roane, 2005; Munro, 2012).
- Misidentification also occurs as an illusion in other mental health problems, including schizophrenia spectrum and dementia-related problems; however, illusions are misperceptions of events that are real and verifiable by others observing the same event. The similarity between the two experiences is superficial in form in that events are misperceived and misinterpreted but are dissimilar in the conviction of the belief being real (Munro, 2012). Many individuals experiencing DMS are distressed and frightened about impending harm from the impostors. DMS often involves a limited number of familiar people but can be indiscriminate in the content of the delusion. It has been noted in the literature that aggressive behavior is often observed, aimed at alleged "doppelgangers" resulting from the anticipatory apprehensiveness and worry of being cheated and manipulated (Leis et al., 2019).
- Variants of DMS are metamorphosis and intermetamorphosis delusional syndrome. Delusional metamorphosis is when the individual believes that person A becomes person B and then can become person C, and so on. Intermetamorphosis syndrome is a misidentification syndrome characterized by delusions that particular people have been transformed both physically and psychologically into other people (American Psychological Association, n.d.-g).

- Capgras and Fregoli delusional syndromes are subtypes of DMS. A person experiencing a Capgras delusion falsely perceives that someone in his environment—usually a close service user or friend—has been replaced by an imposter having the exact visage and appearance (Munro, 2012). It is usually accompanied by hostile and negative feelings toward the other person. The negative emotions are attributed to the "imposter." The person experiencing a Capgras-type delusion can also believe that a favorite pet, coworker, or item has been replaced, usually for paranoid and nefarious intent (Ventriglio et al., 2020).
- Fregoli syndrome causes a person experiencing this delusion to believe that multiple people are a single person who is following the individual, repeatedly changing their appearance or in disguise. The alteration of appearance or disguise is to make their appearance resemble familiar people to prosecute, defraud, or somehow harm the person. This syndrome has been discussed in the mental health literature as a variant of the Capgras syndrome, but these two syndromes have different phenomenological structures (Mojtabai, 1994).
- Syndrome of subjected doubles (doppelganger syndrome): The belief that exact doubles exist, acquiring the physical characteristics identical with the person's own but having different personalities and psychological traits; the conviction is that the "doppelgangers" are leading a life of their own (Christodoulou, 1978). It is a subvariant of DMS and also intermetamorphosis delusional syndrome.
- Folie à deux ("madness for two"): Delusional content is communicated from a person who is living with SMI to another person who has no mental health problem. The delusional belief that is held by the person living with SMI is accepted as reality by the person without mental health problems. Folie à deux occurs in a close, intimate relationship and continues until the person without a mental health problem is no longer in the relationship (Munro, 2012).
- Folie à famille ("family madness"): The belief or abnormal behavior that is shared by multiple members of a family. The members of the family experiencing this phenomenon are usually closely associated proximally and have little social contact except with each other. They have a shared belief, depending on a predominant illusion of the family member living with SMI. This phenomenon can include convictions of delusions of persecution as well as other delusional themes (Munro, 2012). It is a rare delusional type.

People living with SMI often experience more than one theme of false beliefs. For example, a man breaks into a house early in the morning to "visit" a woman whom he believes is in love with him, believing that they have been married by a higher power, as he believes that he has been anointed to be the next prophet. This example shows that the contents of the delusions the man is experiencing can include delusions of grandeur, erotomania, and religion.

There are other delusional contents that are not easily categorized, such as the one mentioned previously, with the person being convinced that he eats brick and mortar buildings. These can be categorized as "miscellaneous delusional contents."

There are several types of delusions that have been grouped together as "Schneiderian delusions." These delusions are also known as mental health conditions of the self and are considered prominent symptomatic behaviors associated with SMI (Frith, 2005; Munro, 2012). Some research studies support the hypothesis that displaying these types of delusions is predictive of the seriousness of the mental health problem; prognosis is considered poor for the person experiencing these delusions (Munro, 2012). The occurrence of experiencing these delusions is associated more often with living with a schizophrenia spectrum mental health problem than mood-related mental health problems.

The delusions that are grouped as Schneiderian delusions are:

- Thought insertion: The person believes that someone has put thoughts from others into their awareness. The person experiencing this type of delusion believes that the inserted thoughts are from others familiar and/or unfamiliar to them (American Psychiatric Association, 2013).
- Thought withdrawal: The person believes that someone has removed their thoughts from consciousness (American Psychiatric Association, 2013).
- Delusion of control: The person believes that an outside force or agent is controlling their body or actions (American Psychiatric Association, 2013).

The content of the above list of delusions is comprised of false beliefs of being controlled and having thoughts withdrawn, broadcast, inserted, or read by others, which are part of the wider category of delusions of influence. Schneiderian delusions have been shown to be less related to themes that are influenced by the mood of the person experiencing the delusions (i.e., mood incongruent) (Junginger et al., 1992).

van der Vaart et al. (2024) assessed delusional types by analyzing data obtained using a reliable self-report instrument [i.e., Peters et al. Delusions Inventory (PDI-21, 2004)] that was completed by service users living with SMI and experiencing delusions. In addition, two instruments measuring the presence and severity of positive and negative symptoms associated with SMI (i.e., Positive and Negative Syndrome Scale [PANSS] (Kay et al., 1987) and Brief Psychiatric Rating Scale [BPRS] (Overall & Gorham, 1988)), completed by experienced service providers, were also analyzed together with the data from PDI-21. The data from the sample of service users clustered into four subtypes a subtype: (1) low-delusion, with low scores across all four factors of delusional behaviors; (2) grandiose-predominant delusions, (3) paranoid-predominant delusions, and (4) pan-delusion low-delusion, having high scores across all types. Paranoid-predominant form is the most distinctive and showed significantly higher prevalence of positive symptoms, along with service users clustering in the pan-delusion type. Service users in the low-delusion group showed the highest scores on negative symptoms and related absences or diminutions of expected behaviors. Using cluster analyses, the authors found four factors in delusional content: (1) paranoia, (2) grandiosity, (3) self-hood disruption or loss of self that pertains to the Schneiderian delusions mentioned above, and (4) low self-worth or negative self-evaluation, in which the person experiencing the delusion believes that they are viewed as "different" (van der Vaart et al., 2024). Perhaps the fourth factor is the outcome of stigma and the phenomenon of self-stigma, which is associated with living with an SMI, but further research is needed.

Delusions are transdiagnostic and are frequently associated with several mental health problems. Although they usually occur in schizophrenia spectrum conditions, they may also be an aspect of depression and bipolar mental health conditions, problems associated with dementia, and sequelae associated with several adverse neurological events. Delusions are not experienced by everyone living with SMI. If present, the frequency and intensity of the conviction may wax and wane, and the content of the delusion may change as well, although themes of delusional behavior appear to be constant in presentation (Grunfeld et al., 2024; Spitzer, 1990).

Behavioral Support Strategies for Delusional Behaviors

Delusions are false ideas that are believed to be real to the person living with SMI. These beliefs are held despite clear evidence that they are not true. Marie insisted that her famous husband was coming to get her, even though she was not married. Day in and day out, she continued to pack her clothes and tell others that he was coming, yet no one came.

Delusions are sometimes clearly odd, such as insisting that other people can read minds. In other cases, however, the person living with SMI may convincingly talk about being pregnant, even though it is not true. Using the example at the beginning of the chapter, Marie continued to tell other people that her husband was coming to get her, even though this repeatedly did not occur. It is unrealistic for service providers to expect themselves to convince the person with delusions that such beliefs are false. Several staff repeatedly tried to get Marie to understand that she was not married, but they consistently failed and were frustrated after Marie became angry and refused to talk to anyone for hours. Marie's delusion was very convincing, and many people not familiar with her were surprised to see her after she'd told them that she was leaving.

Existing treatments, both pharmacological and psychological, are only partially effective in reducing the frequency, intensity, conviction, and other dimensions of delusions (Freeman, 2011; Garety et al., 2011; Hughes et al., 2016; Opler et al., 1995). When the delusional problem is refractory to treatment, the psychiatric and psychological service providers need to further evaluate the underlying mental health or physical problems that may be contributing to the problem of delusional beliefs as delusions are transdiagnostic. Treatment should then be adjusted according to the findings of the evaluation.

There are, however, things that service providers can do to change when or how often the service user talks about these beliefs and how the beliefs affect other people's behaviors. The extent to which service providers may try to do this depends partly on how disruptive the delusion is and the negative impact it has on the service user. In many cases, some intervention must be tried before the impact of a false belief becomes a legal and forensic problem if acted upon. For example, one person with the delusion that neighbors are watching may call "911" and refuse to leave the house; the results for the person making the calls may be an altercation with authorities, arrest and incarceration. Another person with the same delusion may go to the clubhouse or go shopping with little problem. In this case, it may be more effort than it is worth trying to change the delusion of the service user.

Why Do Delusions Occur?

There is no straightforward answer to this question. It is likely that one or more of several factors contribute to the individual experiencing a false belief.

Part of the Reason May Be Biochemical or Physical

- Delusions are commonly associated with an imbalance of neurotransmitters believed to contribute to living with an SMI, although the specific mechanisms remain unclear. The reason why some individuals with SMI experience delusions while others do not is also not yet understood. Delusions may occur during withdrawal from drug intoxication, involving legal or illegal substances. Typically, these symptoms subside after the withdrawal period; however, they may persist beyond withdrawal due to the time required for brain structures to recover and return to normal functioning.
- Delusions may be due to neurological insults and damage that result from such events as severe head injuries, strokes, seizure and conditions of dementia, and infections of the central nervous system (CNS). These directly affect a person's ability to think clearly and act rationally on realistic perceptions and beliefs. Research has identified several areas of the brain that if damaged result in the person experiencing delusions. However, researchers are not clear as to how brain damage directly results in the person experiencing delusions.

Part of the Reason May Be Psychosocial

- What happens around the person living with SMI can also play a role. For example, when under stress, such as applying for a job or experiencing a family crisis, delusions will often be more likely to happen.
- Stress can result from interactions and situations in which high expressed emotionality (EE), such as criticism, humiliation, and yelling, is repeatedly experienced by the person living with SMI and delusions. Given that an individual experiencing a delusion is convinced that his belief is correct, arguing or attempting to reason with the person more than likely will result in frustration and annoyance on the part of the service user and provider.

- Errors in thinking due to faulty learning. Reasoning bias, misattribution of perceptions, jumping to conclusions, discarding contradictory evidence or data have been shown to be an aspect of the experience of delusions (Garety et al., 2011).
- Being exposed to role models early in life that display types of behaviors associated with experiencing delusions. Role modeling is a potent determinant of behaviors (Fryling et al., 2011). If exposed to suspicious behaviors, hearing others in the environment explain that events occurring are the result of beliefs that cannot be proven or are false and being prompted and reinforced to engage in similar private events (i.e., cognitions), the individuals may be predisposed to engage in similar behaviors as an adult.

Behavioral Strategies to Support Individuals Experiencing Delusions

Service providers can attempt to focus on three aspects of delusions:

1. Try to change the delusion itself. This may be what many service providers want to do. However, service providers must remember that delusions are firmly held beliefs that are extremely difficult to change. For some individuals living with SMI and experiencing delusions, psychopharmacological interventions may eliminate or at least decrease how firmly the false beliefs are held; however, this will not always be possible for some people living with SMI. Regardless of how much the medication helps, there is little likelihood that a service provider can talk the person out of the delusion. Trying hard to convince the person living with SMI that a delusion is not true often makes the situation worse, especially if it starts an argument. Many service providers became very frustrated trying to convince a person living with SMI that the delusion is not true.
2. Collaborate with the person experiencing the delusion and engaging in delusional talk. Discuss concerns about what happens when the person talks about false beliefs to others. A person may not want to change their false belief. A young man may not want to change the belief that he is a famous singer because “at least I believe I am important.” Although the person may not agree that the false belief is problematic, how others respond may be a problem, and less delusional talk would improve her quality of life.
3. Adjusting communication methods when interacting with individuals experiencing delusions can positively influence the expression of their beliefs. Engaging with a person living with SMI may present challenges; however, adopting effective response strategies can significantly impact outcomes. By learning evidence-based approaches to communication, one can facilitate more constructive and rewarding interactions. These improved communication skills may also enable individuals living with SMI to foster better relationships and enhance their social experiences.

4. It may be beneficial to consider modifying the impact that delusions have on essential behaviors. For instance, delusional beliefs can interfere with self-care, interpersonal relationships, or adherence to prescribed medication regimens. An individual experiencing delusions might perceive medications as harmful or believe that spiritual authority discourages certain personal hygiene practices. In some cases, such challenges can be mitigated indirectly using approaches outlined in other chapters, without addressing the delusions themselves directly.
5. It is important to clearly define the intended outcomes of any supportive intervention. Consider whether the goal is to address the delusional belief itself, reduce the frequency with which the individual discusses it, or mitigate other related effects. It may also be appropriate to pursue a combination of these objectives. Collaboratively establishing specific targets for change with the service user is recommended to ensure a focused and effective approach.
6. Before implementing any changes, it is important to determine whether intervention is necessary. The presence of delusional thinking does not automatically require service providers to intervene. Individuals experiencing delusions may maintain their personal appearance, physical health, and employment successfully. If these beliefs do not disrupt essential daily activities, it is worthwhile considering whether an intervention is appropriate or if tolerating the delusions may be a more pragmatic approach. Crucially, collaboration with the service user regarding the their perspectives and desired areas for change should be prioritized prior to planning and initiating any strategies.

When addressing challenges related to delusional experiences, the following recommendations may be beneficial. The choice of methods should align with the specific objectives being pursued. It is important to note that not all suggestions will be effective in every situation.

- Don't expect the delusions to stop completely. Remember, false beliefs are maintained despite evidence to the contrary. Avoid agreeing or disagreeing with the false belief. Above all, keep from trying to talk the person out of the delusion or arguing about it. This often makes the situation worse.
- Consider a review of medications. Consider seeking a review of medications by an experienced mental health service prescriber, including any over-the-counter (OTC) medications that the service user takes. Current medications may cause or worsen delusional behavior and may need changing. Listen to what the service user says about the medications. Ask the psychiatric service provider to explain the possible benefits and side effects to the service user.
- Ensure that prescribed medications are administered as directed. Prescriptions, regardless of their effectiveness, require correct usage to achieve optimal results. It is important to verify that the service user adheres to the prescribed regimen accurately. If there are problems, then review Chap. 16, which addresses problems with taking medications and following treatment recommendations for possible solutions. For example, if the service user has trouble swallowing pills or is simply reluctant to take them, a liquid or injectable form of the medication may help with compliance. A behavior contract or point system that prompts and

reinforces the behaviors of taking the medications may assist the service user. A person experiencing a delusion is likely to be concerned about why medications are needed as the person does not question the veracity of the false belief and will defend having the belief. Take time to explain any changes in medications and allow an opportunity for questions.

- Avoid the use of alcohol and other drugs. The use of alcohol and/or other drugs could make delusions more likely to occur, especially if the person is using stimulants. Help the service user to avoid the use of substances as much as possible as use of substances can contribute to a worsening of problematic behaviors in individuals living with SMI.
- Clearly identify statements made by individuals living with SMI that may be considered delusional. Some comments may obviously indicate delusions (e.g., "I receive messages from the president"), while others may be more ambiguous and could reflect legitimate concerns (e.g., "I had to wait three hours at the clinic. They're too busy to care about me."). These concerns may or may not stem from delusional thinking, as feelings of being mistreated or unfairly treated can occur without underlying false beliefs. When uncertainty exists, consult another service provider with expertise in assessing severe mental health conditions for further evaluation.
- Watch for circumstances that provoke the delusion. Try to become aware of what is happening in the environment when the service user begins talking about the delusion. Utilize the forms provided in the appendices to systematically observe and record instances of delusional behavior, aiming to identify any patterns related to timing, interpersonal interactions, or the emotional state of the individual with SMI. Establishing these connections can be instrumental in developing more effective behavioral management strategies. For instance, discussions about false beliefs may often arise during busy periods, such as meal preparation. In such situations, it may be beneficial to suggest that the service user spend some time alone in their room or engage in an alternative, distracting activity.

Strategies for Managing Conversations with Individuals Experiencing Delusions

- Change the topic of conversation: When a service user begins to engage in delusional talk, or even before such talk begins, redirect the conversation to a topic that is known to be real. Discuss subjects that both the service user and the person engaging in the conversation are usually interested in. If the service user can engage in this discussion, show genuine interest and continue the conversation. Should the service user attempt to revert to the delusional topic, introduce another alternative.
- End the conversation: Be prepared to politely but firmly excuse oneself when the service user begins discussing delusional beliefs. For example, one might say,

"excuse me; it is necessary to prepare dinner," or "excuse me, it is time to leave now." Practicing this approach and seeking guidance from a mental health professional may be beneficial. There is no need to feel guilty about declining to discuss delusional beliefs.

- Address implied feelings: Individuals living with SMI may express emotions such as fear, anger, or grief when discussing delusional beliefs. It may be helpful to address these emotions without engaging in the delusional content. For instance, one might say, "it seems that there is a lot of fear about this," in response to a delusion such as "the police have been following me." Continue this conversation only if the service user can discuss their feelings without reverting to the delusion. Remember that while the delusional content is false, the emotions experienced are real.
- Initiate "normal" conversations: If a service user frequently discusses delusions, there may be an inclination to avoid the individual. Instead, take time to engage in conversations about real topics, such as the weather or current events, that interest the service user. Initiate these conversations when the service user has not recently mentioned delusions. Show interest in these discussions and engage in everyday activities that the service user enjoys, such as grocery shopping, watching television, or playing cards.
- Seek support and advice: If efforts to change behavior are not successful, seek advice from other service providers and members of the recovery team experienced in behavioral interventions with individuals living with SMI. This will typically be a clinical psychologist trained in assessing problem behaviors and developing treatments based on functional behavioral assessments. Be prepared to discuss the service user's delusional statements, the frequency and context of these statements, and the strategies that have been employed.
- Maintain consistency: Consistency in responding to individuals experiencing delusions is crucial. These strategies should be tailored to the service user's responses and may not work equally well in all cases. Persistence, consistency, and reinforcement of adaptive behaviors are essential for success.

Conclusion for Behavioral Support Strategies

When delusions are a problem, consider the following steps:

1. Decide on the specific behavior related to delusional behavior to change, like the frequency of the person manifesting delusional speech, how the person communicates and interacts with others, or how it affects other behaviors with the person living with SMI and experiencing delusions?
2. Consider whether the problem is severe enough to make the effort.
3. Make sure medications are beneficial and are being taken as prescribed. Sometimes changing doses or adding a different class or medications can be helpful.

4. Be clear about what the service user says that is and is not delusional.
5. Watch to see if circumstances such as where, when, with whom, or what mood the person is experiencing at the time make a difference in predicting when the delusion talk occurs. It is just as important to reflect on when talking about the false belief does not occur as well. Use the monitoring forms and examples that are available in the appendices.
6. When the service user begins displaying delusional talk, change the topic of conversation, excuse oneself, or try to discuss the feelings that are being expressed.
7. Be alert for times that "normal talk" happens, and spend more time listening and talking with the service user at those times.
8. If delusional talk is a serious problem and efforts to change delusional behavior are unsuccessful, seek help from others.
9. Collaborate with the person experiencing the delusion. Find out if his recovery goals are in line with the goals of the support plan. Use all the listening tools and person-centered techniques that will assist in engaging and collaborating with the person living with SMI.

What About Marie?

Marie is residing at a group home and attends a day program. She has been living with schizophrenia since the age of 18. Marie talks often about her belief that she is married to a well-known country singer, and he is coming to get her "any day now." She often interrupts conversations of others to ask if "my husband is here yet" and then continues talking about him and being married to him and having his children. If she is told this is not real, she becomes angry and curses the people who disagree with her. Other service users and providers avoid her at the day program as she talks about little else and changes the conversation back to false beliefs. Staff at the day program become frustrated with Marie and avoid her because they don't feel that there is anything they can do to manage her delusional talk.

Several service providers decided to try something different. Because Marie seemed to enjoy talking with others so much, they didn't want to avoid her. However, they also didn't have time to listen to things that they knew were not real. Having tried to reason with Marie about her delusion in the past, they knew that this wouldn't change anything. They concluded that it would probably be better if they tried to change how they got along with her. They decided that when they saw Marie, they would take the initiative to begin talking about something that they knew was real (the weather, her clothes, a TV show). If the conversation remained on these "real" topics, they allowed the conversation to continue as long as they could. If she began talking about her "husband" coming to get her (or something else that they knew wasn't real), they politely excused themselves and left to do other things. When they did this consistently, Marie stopped talking to them about her "husband" coming to get her. They had many enjoyable (and lengthy) talks about other matters. Despite this, Marie still talked about the delusion with other staff who would listen to it. Many of these staff expressed frustration about her behavior as "nothing is working."

The way these service providers responded affected what Marie did. Some were able to increase her talk about real matters and decrease her talk about things that were not real. While she continued living with SMI (and continued to talk about delusions with those who would still listen), she demonstrated an ability to manage her behavior according to how other people behaved. With enough consistency by all staff members, it is likely that the delusional talk could be reduced to a low frequency as she was better able to get along with others.

In this example, the staff members:

1. Defined the problem as "She talks about a husband coming to get here even though she is not married."
2. Recognized that their behavior of listening and giving her attention was encouraging the delusional talk. They also recognized that talking with other people was something that she enjoyed (a reinforcer) and that if they began avoiding her, she would probably be disappointed, isolated, and become more involved in her delusional belief.
3. Identified some topics they knew were real.
4. When they saw her, the staff brought up the topics that they knew were real and attended to (reinforced) such talk as much as they had time to.
5. Excused themselves (stopped reinforcing the discussion) when Marie began talking about things that were delusional.

By following this plan, the staff decreased how much Marie talked about the delusional topic and increased how much she talked about other topics that they knew were real. This not only helped to make the problem manageable but also helped the staff to feel less frustrated because they had a plan to follow and had realistic expectations of what they could accomplish. While they did not "cure" the problem, Marie acted more "normal," had other people show interest in what she talked about, and they (the staff) felt more comfortable being around her.

Summary

Delusions are false beliefs held with strong conviction despite evidence to the contrary and cannot be explained by religion or culture. They are often distressing and disabling to the person experiencing the delusions. Delusions are an epiphenomenon that results from a confluence of sensory experiences, perceptions, inferences, and cognitive decision-making. Delusions have been hypothesized as developing from unusual or misperceived sensory experiences, not unlike experiencing illusions. The person attempts to understand the experience by inferring causality using the perceptions of the experience and the associated cognitive and emotional sequelae of the experience to exercise control and predictability of the environment. However, the result is a false conclusion and belief in explaining the ambiguous event. Acting on delusional beliefs can lead to legal issues, including incarceration and mandated treatment, stemming from irrational behaviors related to these beliefs.

To capture the complexity inherent in delusional phenomena, a multidimensional framework for assessment is essential. Delusions can be systematically evaluated through cognitive, social, and emotional dimensions, utilizing a multilevel approach that integrates genetic, neurological, and behavioral data.

Delusional behaviors can be understood through a multifaceted framework encompassing various dimensions that detail the frequency, duration, and impact of the occurrence of delusional behaviors. The topography dimension classifies delusions based on observable content, allowing for thematic categorization. Quantitative aspects such as frequency, rate, and count provide measures of how often delusional behaviors or expressions occur, while temporal extent and duration assess both the time spent engaging in delusional speech and the persistence of the underlying belief. Contextual factors are considered through locus and temporal locus, which examine the circumstances and timing associated with the onset of delusional phenomena.

Latency and interresponse time (IRT) focus on the delay between the presentation of an antecedent stimulus and the emergence of delusional behavior, as well as the intervals between episodes. The dimensions of force, intensity, and conviction capture the strength and certainty of the delusional belief. Preoccupation measures the dominance of delusional thoughts within an individual's cognitive landscape, inferred through frequency and duration of delusional speech. External determinants, such as environmental stressors and trauma, are recognized for their role in precipitating or exacerbating delusional thinking.

The dimension of implausibility and bizarreness assesses the extent to which delusions diverge from generally accepted reality, spanning a continuum from non-bizarre to bizarre beliefs. Distress assesses the emotional impact of delusions, including feelings of fear, anger, or anxiety, while disruption to behavior evaluates the degree to which delusional beliefs impair daily functioning. Extension looks at the breadth of a delusion's influence across different areas of life, and systematization distinguishes between organized, coherent delusional narratives and those that are fragmented.

Emotional commitment reflects the individual's level of emotional investment in delusional belief, often contributing to its persistence despite contradictory evidence. Constancy of theme and content evaluates the stability of delusional themes over time, and pressure describes the urgent compulsion to act on delusional beliefs, potentially leading to significant behavioral consequences. Delusions can be classified as mood-congruent, when they correspond with the individual's prevailing emotional state, or mood-incongruent, when they differ from it. Their focus may pertain to external factors, such as the perceived behaviors of others, or internal factors, including feelings of guilt or preoccupations with bodily integrity.

Delusions represent a defining feature of several mental health disorders as well as neurodegenerative diseases, with their persistence in the face of contradictory evidence reflecting fundamental disruptions in neural systems responsible for belief evaluation, reality testing, and emotional processing. Recent advances in neuroimaging and neuropathological studies have revealed that these disturbances are not confined to a single brain region but involve dysfunction across interconnected networks associated with salience attribution, executive function, emotion regulation, and sensory integration. Notably, consistent abnormalities have been identified in regions such as the anterior cingulate cortex (ACC), dorsolateral prefrontal cortex (dlPFC), ventromedial prefrontal cortex (vmPFC), insula, amygdala, hippocampus, thalamus, and superior temporal gyrus (STG). Each of these areas contribute to specific cognitive and affective processes implicated in the development and persistence of delusional beliefs.

For instance, the ACC is involved in conflict monitoring and cognitive control, with reduced activity in this region linked to an impaired ability to challenge false beliefs. Dysfunction in the dlPFC undermines reasoning and cognitive flexibility, correlating with the severity and complexity of delusional content. The vmPFC's role in self-referential processing and emotional regulation can lead to improper assignment of significance to thoughts and stimuli when disrupted. Disruption of the insula's role in integrating internal and external experiences may result in the misattribution of internal sensations to external sources, a phenomenon often observed in delusional states. Additionally, dysfunctions in the amygdala and hippocampus are linked to emotional dysregulation and memory distortion, respectively; these factors collectively contribute to the development and persistence of false beliefs. The thalamus and superior temporal gyrus, both essential for sensory processing and language comprehension, have been identified as contributing factors in cases of sensory misinterpretations and language-related delusions.

Neuroimaging studies across conditions such as schizophrenia spectrum and bipolar mental health problems, as well as conditions such as Alzheimer's and Parkinson's neurodegenerative diseases, consistently demonstrate convergent patterns of gray matter reduction and dysregulation within specific brain regions. These changes are particularly evident in the salience network and default mode network (DMN). Dysregulation of DMN, which plays a critical role in self-reflection and emotional processing, has been associated with the presence of delusions, potentially resulting in the misattribution of significance to neutral stimuli. Collectively, this body of evidence suggests a shared neurobiological substrate for delusional phenomena across a range of mental health and neurological conditions, emphasizing the need for integrated assessment and intervention strategies.

Environmental influences have a profound impact on the origins and maintenance of delusional behaviors through associative learning and emotional dysregulation. Delusions are complex phenomena resulting from a dynamic interplay of emotional dysregulation, misattribution of salience, and associative learning, highlighting the importance of understanding these processes in addressing delusional behaviors.

Delusions arise from the interplay of cognitive processes, emotional responses, and sensory experiences, often stemming from misperceived stimuli. Associative learning theory explains how beliefs, formed through self-statements and environmental interactions, can lead to delusions when uncertainty is present. Observational learning plays a crucial role, where individuals imitate behaviors from models perceived as competent or powerful, influenced by their own cognitive abilities and emotional states.

Emotional dysregulation can distort perception and interpretation, leading to the erroneous assignment of significance to neutral stimuli. Heightened emotional reactivity, particularly in response to perceived threats, amplifies the intensity of the experiences, fostering the development and persistence of delusions. Misattribution of salience occurs when individuals incorrectly elevate the importance of neutral cues, resulting in a disconnect between belief and reality. Cognitive resources are finite; when individuals experience overload, they may form inaccurate judgments, which can contribute to persistent delusional beliefs. The competition for cognitive resources allows salient emotional stimuli to serve as distractions, thereby compromising executive functions and reinforcing patterns of delusional reasoning.

Delusions are transdiagnostic, occurring in various mental health conditions, such as schizophrenia spectrum and mood mental health problems and in neurogenerative conditions; they can be triggered by substance use and withdrawal or neurological damage. Delusions are typically evaluated through self-report measures; however, individuals experiencing delusions seldom seek assistance independently, as they maintain a strong conviction in the accuracy of their perceptions.

Research indicates that the prevalence of core delusional themes, such as grandiose, religious, and control-oriented delusions, remains relatively stable across different sociodemographic and economic contexts. For example, grandiose delusions occur in 28.2% of cases, delusions of control in 21.6%, and religious delusions in 18.3%. Notably, these rates are elevated in samples consisting solely of individuals with psychotic-related conditions. Furthermore, the prevalence of delusional themes does not appear to be significantly affected by sociodemographic or cultural factors, nor by national characteristics such as individualism, power distance, or levels of atheism. Nonetheless, certain themes—specifically religious and control delusions—are observed with greater frequency in countries exhibiting higher income inequality.

Cultural influences emerge more prominently in the specific content of delusions rather than in the broad thematic categories. For instance, paranoid delusions among members of the South African Xhosa tribe frequently involve notions of bewitchment, whereas delusions of poisoning are more commonly reported in Germany than in Japan. This suggests that while the general themes of delusions are universal, the detailed content and subjective experience may be shaped by cultural and societal factors.

Delusional disorders represent a spectrum of false beliefs that profoundly affect how individuals perceive and interact with the world. These delusions are classified into various categories, each exhibiting unique features and behavioral consequences.

One common type is delusional jealousy, where individuals believe their partner is unfaithful, often observed more in males and associated with substance abuse. Persecutory delusions involve beliefs of being targeted or conspired against, leading to heightened suspiciousness and, in some cases, violent behavior. Grandiose delusions are characterized by an inflated sense of importance, abilities, or fame, which can provoke aggression if unacknowledged by others.

Other types include the delusion of control, where one feels manipulated by external forces (which is a core symptom of schizophrenia spectrum mental health problems) and religious delusions, involving beliefs of a special religious identity that deviate from cultural norms. Delusions of guilt or sin manifest as unwarranted remorse, while delusions of poverty involve fears of financial ruin without justification.

Delusions of reference cause individuals to assign personal significance to external events, and nihilistic delusions lead to the belief in the nonexistence of oneself or the world. Somatic delusions and dysmorphic delusions involve imagined physical disorders or deformities, often resulting in demands for medical intervention.

Additional variations include delusional parasitosis (belief of being infested with parasites), erotic delusions (belief that one is loved by another, often a public figure), and delusions of smell (belief in emitting a foul odor). Some individuals fear transmitting diseases without evidence, while others experience delusional procreational syndromes related to pregnancy and parenthood. Delusional misidentification syndromes involve misrecognition of familiar people or places, and folie à deux describes shared delusional beliefs.

The Schneiderian delusions, including thought insertion and withdrawal, are closely linked to schizophrenia spectrum mental health problems. Among those living with SMI, persecutory and grandiose delusions are most prevalent. Overall, the themes and content of delusions are diverse and may be challenging to categorize, reflecting the complex nature of these phenomena.

Behavioral interventions focus on changing the frequency of the person talking about the delusion, the interactions with the delusional person, or the impact of the delusion on other behaviors. Strategies include avoiding arguments, reviewing medications, monitoring substance use, identifying triggers, and prompting and redirecting conversations to reality-based themes. Consistency and collaboration with the person experiencing delusions are crucial for effective management of the problem behavior. Behavior contracting and point systems can be used to reinforce collaboration with the support plan and the self-monitoring of the occurrences of verbal behavior pertaining to the themes of false beliefs.

References

Ali, S., Patel, M., Avenido, J., Jabeen, S., & Riley, W. J. (2011). Hallucinations: Common features and causes. *Current Psychiatry, 10*(11), 22–29. https://cdn-uat.mdedge.com/files/s3fs-public/Document/September-2017/1011CP_Ali.pdf

American Psychiatric Association. (2013). *Delusion*. In *Diagnostic and statistical manual of mental disorders* (5th ed.). https://doi.org/10.1176/appi.books.9780890425596

American Psychiatric Association. (2022). Schizophrenia spectrum and other psychotic disorders. In *Diagnostic and statistical manual of mental disorders (DSM-5-TR)* (5th ed., text rev.). https://doi.org/10.1176/appi.books.9780890425787

American Psychological Association. (n.d.-a). Cognitive resource theory. *APA Dictionary of Psychology*. https://dictionary.apa.org/cognitive-resource-theory
American Psychological Association. (n.d.-b). Delusion of influence. *APA Dictionary of Psychology*. https://dictionary.apa.org/delusion-of-influence
American Psychological Association. (n.d.-c). Delusion of reference. *APA Dictionary of Psychology*. https://dictionary.apa.org/delusion-of-reference
American Psychological Association. (n.d.-d). Erotic delusion. *APA Dictionary of Psychology*. https://dictionary.apa.org/erotic-delusion
American Psychological Association. (n.d.-e). Fragmentary delusion. *APA Dictionary of Psychology*. https://dictionary.apa.org/fragmentary-delusion
American Psychological Association. (n.d.-f). Habit. *APA Dictionary of Psychology*. https://dictionary.apa.org/habit
American Psychological Association. (n.d.-g). Misidentification syndrome. *APA Dictionary of Psychology*. https://dictionary.apa.org/misidentification-syndrome
American Psychological Association. (n.d.-h). Nihilism. *APA Dictionary of Psychology*. https://dictionary.apa.org/nihilism
American Psychological Association. (n.d.-i). Operational definition. *APA Dictionary of Psychology*. https://dictionary.apa.org/operational-definition
American Psychological Association. (n.d.-j). Religious delusion. *APA Dictionary of Psychology*. https://dictionary.apa.org/religious-delusion
American Psychological Association. (n.d.-k). Social learning theory. *APA Dictionary of Psychology*. https://dictionary.apa.org/social-learning-theory
American Psychological Association. (n.d.-l). Systematized delusion. *APA Dictionary of Psychology*. https://dictionary.apa.org/systematized-delusion
Appelbaum, P. S., Robbins, P. C., & Roth, L. H. (1999). Dimensional approach to delusions: Comparison across types and diagnoses. *American Journal of Psychiatry, 156*(12), 1938–1943. https://doi.org/10.1176/ajp.156.12.1938
Azarias, F. R., Almeida, G. H. D. R., de Melo, L. F., Rici, R. E. G., & Maria, D. A. (2025). The journey of the default mode network: Development, function, and impact on mental health. *Biology, 14*(4), 395. https://doi.org/10.3390/biology14040395
Barnes-Holmes, Y., & McEnteggart, C. (2015). Behavior analysis and the treatment of human psychological suffering. In J. Luiselli, D. D. Reed, & J. S. Luiselli (Eds.), *Clinical and organizational applications of applied behavior analysis* (pp. 451–475). Academic Press. https://doi.org/10.1016/B978-0-12-420249-8.00018-6
Bortolotti, L. (2016). Epistemic benefits of elaborated and systematized delusions in schizophrenia. *British Journal for the Philosophy of Science, 67*(3), 879–900. https://doi.org/10.1093/bjps/axv024
Brauer, J. R., & Tittle, C. R. (2012). Social learning theory and human reinforcement. *Sociological Spectrum, 32*(2), 157–177. https://doi.org/10.1080/02732173.2012.646160
Brucato, G., Masucci, M. D., Arndt, L. Y., Ben-David, S., Colibazzi, T., Corcoran, C. M., Crumbley, A. H., Crump, F. M., Gill, K. E., Kimhy, D., Lister, A., Schobel, S. A., Yang, L. H., Lieberman, J. A., & Girgis, R. R. (2017). Baseline demographics, clinical features and predictors of conversion among 200 individuals in a longitudinal prospective psychosis-risk cohort. *Psychological Medicine, 47*(11), 1923–1935. https://doi.org/10.1017/S0033291717000319
Christodoulou, G. N. (1978). Syndrome of subjective doubles. *The American Journal of Psychiatry, 135*(2), 249–251. https://psycnet.apa.org/doi/10.1176/ajp.135.2.249
Christodoulou, G. N., Margariti, M., Kontaxakis, V. P., & Christodoulou, N. G. (2009). The delusional misidentification syndromes: Strange, fascinating, and instructive. *Current Psychiatry Reports, 11*(3), 185–189. https://doi.org/10.1007/s11920-009-0029-4
Collin, S., Rowse, G., Martinez, A. P., & Bentall, R. P. (2023). Delusions and the dilemmas of life: A systematic review and meta-analyses of the global literature on the prevalence of delusional themes in clinical groups. *Clinical Psychology Review, 104*, 102303. https://doi.org/10.1016/j.cpr.2023.102303

Conners, M. H., Langdon, R., & Coltheart, M. (2014). Misidentification delusions. In D. Bhugra, G. S. Malhi, & G. S. (Eds.), *Troublesome disguises: Managing challenging disorders in psychiatry* (pp. 167–185). John Wiley & Sons. https://doi.org/10.1002/9781118799574.ch13

Cooper, J. O., Heron, T. E., & Heward, W. L. (2020). *Applied behavior analysis* (3rd ed.). Pearson. https://www.pearson.com/en-us/subject-catalog/p/applied-behavior-analysis/P200000003382/9780134752556

Das, P., Singh, G. K., Arora, S., & Sapra, D. (2024). The delusion of odor: The olfactory reference disorder. *Journal of Marine Medical Society, 26*(1), 137–138. https://doi.org/10.4103/jmms.jmms_55_23

De Souza, B., & McMichael, A. (2019). A new somatic-type delusional disorder subtype: Delusion inversus. *Dermatology Online Journal, 25*(10), 1–6. https://escholarship.org/uc/item/20s9f78r

Debruyne, H., Portzky, M., Peremans, K., & Audenaert, K. (2011). Cotard's syndrome. *Mind and Brain: The Journal of Psychiatry, 2*(1), 67–72. https://www.proquest.com/docview/881273509

Ertekin, E., Ercis, M., Aliyeva, G., & Gürşahbaz, O. C. (2021). Clinical profile of delusional disorder and its subtypes: A descriptive study from Turkey. *Rivista di Psichiatria, 56*(6), 328–333. https://doi.org/10.1708/3713.37047

Farmer, H., Ciaunica, A., & Hamilton, A. F. D. C. (2018). The functions of imitative behaviour in humans. *Mind & Language, 33*(4), 378–396. https://doi.org/10.1111/mila.12189

Feeney, E. J., Groman, S. M., Taylor, J. R., & Corlett, P. R. (2017). Explaining delusions: Reducing uncertainty through basic and computational neuroscience. *Schizophrenia Bulletin, 43*(2), 263–272. https://doi.org/10.1093/schbul/sbw194

Feinberg, T. E., & Roane, D. M. (2005). Delusional misidentification. *Psychiatric Clinics of North America, 28*(3), 665–683. https://doi.org/10.1016/j.psc.2005.05.002

Freeman, D. (2011). Improving cognitive treatments for delusions. *Schizophrenia Research, 132*(2-3), 135–139. https://doi.org/10.1016/j.schres.2011.08.012

Frith, C. (2005). The self in action: Lessons from delusions of control. *Consciousness and Cognition, 14*(4), 752–770. https://doi.org/10.1016/j.concog.2005.04.002

Fryling, M. J., Johnston, C., & Hayes, L. J. (2011). Understanding observational learning: An interbehavioral approach. *Analysis of Verbal Behavior, 27*(1), 191–203. https://doi.org/10.1007/BF03393102

Garety, P., Freeman, D., Jolley, S., Ross, K., Waller, H., & Dunn, G. (2011). Jumping to conclusions: The psychology of delusional reasoning. *Advances in Psychiatric Treatment, 17*(5), 332–339. https://doi.org/10.1192/apt.bp.109.007104

Ghanem, M., Evangeli-Dawson, C., & Georgiades, A. (2023). The role of culture on the phenomenology of hallucinations and delusions, explanatory models, and help-seeking attitudes: A narrative review. *Early Intervention in Psychiatry, 17*(9), 843–863. https://doi.org/10.1111/eip.13449

Grunfeld, G., Lemonde, A. C., Gold, I., Paquin, V., Iyer, S. N., Lepage, M., Joober, R., Malla, A., & Shah, J. L. (2024). Consistency of delusion themes across first and subsequent episodes of psychosis. *JAMA Psychiatry, 81*(10), 1039–1046. https://doi.org/10.1001/jamapsychiatry.2024.2040

Heilskov, S. E. R., Urfer-Parnas, A., & Nordgaard, J. (2020). Delusions in the general population: A systematic review with emphasis on methodology. *Schizophrenia Research, 216*, 48–55. https://doi.org/10.1016/j.schres.2019.10.043

Hohwy, J. (2013). Delusions, illusions and inference under uncertainty. *Mind & Language, 28*(1), 57–71. https://doi.org/10.1111/mila.12008

Holt, D. J., Titone, D., Long, L. S., Goff, D. C., Cather, C., Rauch, S. L., Judge, A., & Kuperberg, G. R. (2006). The misattribution of salience in delusional patients with schizophrenia. *Schizophrenia Research, 83*(2–3), 247–256. https://doi.org/10.1016/j.schres.2005.12.858

Hughes, S., Stewart, C., & Stewart, I. (2016). A contextual behavioral approach to the study of (persecutory) delusions. *Journal of Contextual Behavioral Science, 5*(4), 235–246. https://doi.org/10.1016/j.jcbs.2016.09.002

Isham, L., Griffith, L., Boylan, A. M., Hicks, A., Wilson, N., Byrne, R., Emsley, R., Garety, P., Hardy, A., Jones, R., Kuipers, E., Peters, E., Sheaves, B., Waite, F., Waller, H., & Freeman, D. (2021). Understanding, treating, and renaming grandiose delusions: A qualitative study. *Psychology and Psychotherapy: Theory, Research and Practice, 94*(1), 119–140. https://doi.org/10.1111/papt.12260

Iyassu, R., Jolley, S., Bebbington, P., Dunn, G., Emsley, R., Freeman, D., Fowler, D., Hardy, A., Waller, H., Kuipers, E., & Garety, P. (2014). Psychological characteristics of religious delusions. *Social Psychiatry and Psychiatric Epidemiology, 49*, 1051–1061. https://doi.org/10.1007/s00127-013-0811-y

Johra, R. U., & Uddin, M. S. (2024). Delusion of maternity: Atypical symptom of schizophrenia in a Bangladeshi woman. *Psychiatry Research Case Reports, 3*(1), 100219. https://doi.org/10.1016/j.psycr.2024.100219

Junginger, J., Barker, S., & Coe, D. A. (1992). Mood theme and bizarreness of delusions in schizophrenia and mood psychosis. *Journal of Abnormal Psychology, 101*(2), 287–292. https://doi.org/10.1037/0021-843X.101.2.287

Kaur, A., & Ali, S. (2016). Hallucinations: Common features and causes. *Current Psychiatry, 15*(12), 12–18.

Kay, S. R., Fiszbein, A., & Opler, L. A. (1987). The positive and negative syndrome scale (PANSS) for schizophrenia. *Schizophrenia Bulletin, 13*(2), 261–276. https://doi.org/10.1093/schbul/13.2.261

Kendler, K. S., Glazer, W. M., & Morgenstern, H. (1983). Dimensions of delusional experience. *American Journal of Psychiatry, 140*(4), 466–469. https://doi.org/10.1176/ajp.140.4.466

Kim, E., Murphy, R., & Driscoll, M. (2022). Delusional misidentification syndrome or dead moneyman and sex offender? A case report of reverse Capgras syndrome. *Case Reports in Psychiatry, 2022*, 1–3. https://doi.org/10.1155/2022/9703482

Kimhy, D., Goetz, R., Yale, S., Corcoran, C., & Malaspina, D. (2005). Delusions in individuals with schizophrenia: Factor structure, clinical correlates, and putative neurobiology. *Psychopathology, 38*(6), 338–344. https://doi.org/10.1159/000089455

Kumari, R., Chaudhury, S., & Kumar, S. (2013). Dimensions of hallucinations and delusions in affective and nonaffective illnesses. *International Scholarly Research Notices, 2013*(1), 616304. https://doi.org/10.1155/2013/616304

Lally, P., & Gardner, B. (2013). Promoting habit formation. *Health Psychology Review, 7*(sup1), S137–S158. https://doi.org/10.1080/17437199.2011.603640

Leis, K., Mazur, E., Racinowski, M., Jamrożek, T., Gołębiewski, J., Gałązka, P., & Pąchalska, M. (2019). Delusional misidentification syndrome: Dissociation between recognition and identification processes. *Acta Neuropsychologica, 17*, 456–467. https://doi.org/10.5604/01.3001.0013.6551

Leslie, E., Weittenhiller, L. P., Sloan, A. F., & Sheffield, J. M. (2025). Delusional distress is associated with emotion dysregulation in schizophrenia-spectrum disorders. *Schizophrenia Bulletin Open, 6*(1), sgaf010. https://doi.org/10.1093/schizbullopen/sgaf010

Mahajan, B. B., & Shishak, M. (2017). An approach to venerophobia in males. *Indian Journal of Sexually Transmitted Diseases and AIDS, 38*(1), 103–106. https://doi.org/10.4103/0253-7184.203326

Malinowski, F. R., Tasso, B. C., Ortiz, B. B., Higuchi, C. H., Noto, C., Belangero, S. I., Bressan, R. A., Gadelha, A., & Cordeiro, Q. (2020). Schneider's first-rank symptoms as predictors of remission in antipsychotic-naive first-episode psychosis. *Brazilian Journal of Psychiatry, 42*(1), 22–26. https://doi.org/10.1590/1516-4446-2018-0237

Manjunatha, N., Sarma, P. K., Math, S. B., & Chaturvedi, S. K. (2010). Delusional procreation syndrome: A psychopathology in procreation of human beings. *Asian Journal of Psychiatry, 3*(2), 84–86. https://doi.org/10.1016/j.ajp.2010.02.001

Manschreck, T. C. (1992). Delusional disorders: Clinical concepts and diagnostic strategies. *Psychiatric Annals, 22*(5), 241–251. https://doi.org/10.3928/0048-5713-19920501-09

Middelveen, M. J., Fesler, M. C., & Stricker, R. B. (2018). History of Morgellons disease: From delusion to definition. *Clinical, Cosmetic and Investigational Dermatology, 11*, 71–90. https://doi.org/10.2147/CCID.S152343

Mojtabai, R. (1994). Fregoli syndrome. *Australian and New Zealand Journal of Psychiatry, 28*(3), 458–462. https://doi.org/10.3109/00048679409075874

Morris, S. E., & Cuthbert, B. N. (2012). Research domain criteria: Cognitive systems, neural circuits, and dimensions of behavior. *Dialogues in Clinical Neuroscience, 14*(1), 29–37. https://doi.org/10.31887/DCNS.2012.14.1/smorris

Munro, A. (1992). Psychiatric disorders characterized by delusions: Treatment in relation to specific types. *Psychiatric Annals, 22*(5), 232–240. https://doi.org/10.3928/0048-5713-19920501-08

Munro, A. (2012). Persistent delusional symptoms and disorders. In M. G. Gelder, N. C. Andreasen, J. J. Lopez-Ibor Jr., & J. R. Geddes (Eds.), *New Oxford textbook of psychiatry* (pp. 609–628). https://doi.org/10.1093/med/9780199696758.003.0082

National Institute of Mental Health (NIMH). (n.d.). Research Domain Criteria (RDoC). U.S. Department of Health and Human Services. https://www.nimh.nih.gov/research/research-funded-by-nimh/rdoc

Opjordsmoen, S. (2014). Delusional disorder as a partial psychosis. *Schizophrenia Bulletin, 40*(2), 244–247. https://doi.org/10.1093/schbul/sbt203

Opler, L. A., Klahr, D. M., & Ramirez, P. M. (1995). Pharmacologic treatment of delusions. *Psychiatric Clinics of North America, 18*(2), 379–391. https://doi.org/10.1016/S0193-953X(18)30061-3

Overall, J. E., & Gorham, D. R. (1988). The Brief Psychiatric Rating Scale (BPRS): Recent developments in ascertainment and scaling. *Psychopharmacological Bulletin, 24*(1), 97–99. https://psycnet.apa.org/record/2012-26630-001

Peters, E., Joseph, S., Day, S., & Garety, P. (2004). Measuring delusional ideation: The 21-item Peters et al. Delusions Inventory (PDI). *Schizophrenia Bulletin, 30*(4), 1005–1022. https://doi.org/10.1093/oxfordjournals.schbul.a007116

Petrolini, V. (2017). What makes delusions pathological? *Philosophical Psychology, 30*(4), 502–523. https://doi.org/10.1080/09515089.2017.1326275

Reich, A., Kwiatkowska, D., & Pacan, P. (2019). Delusions of parasitosis: An update. *Dermatology and Therapy, 9*(4), 631–638. https://doi.org/10.1007/s13555-019-00324-3

Rootes-Murdy, K., Goldsmith, D. R., & Turner, J. A. (2022). Clinical and structural differences in delusions across diagnoses: A systematic review. *Frontiers in Integrative Neuroscience, 15*, 726321. https://doi.org/10.3389/fnint.2021.726321

Sahoo, A., & Josephs, K. A. (2018). A neuropsychiatric analysis of the Cotard delusion. *The Journal of Neuropsychiatry and Clinical Neurosciences, 30*(1), 58–65. https://doi.org/10.1176/appi.neuropsych.17010018

Sanvictores, T., Mahabadi, N., & Rehman, C. I. (2025). Classical conditioning. [Updated 2024 Sep 5]. In: StatPearls [Internet]. StatPearls Publishing; 2025 Jan-. https://www.ncbi.nlm.nih.gov/books/NBK470326/

Seeman, M. V. (2014). Pseudocyesis, delusional pregnancy, and psychosis: The birth of a delusion. *World Journal of Clinical Cases, 2*(8), 338–344. https://doi.org/10.12998/wjcc.v2.i8.338

Shahrokh, N. C., & Hales, R. E. (Eds.). (2003). American psychiatric glossary (8th ed.). American Psychiatric Publishing.

Silva, J. A., Sharma, K. K., Leong, G. B., & Weinstock, R. (1992). Dangerousness of the delusional misidentification of children. *Journal of Forensic Sciences, 37*(3), 830–838. https://dl.astm.org/jofs/article/37/3/830/9828/Dangerousness-of-the-Delusional-Misidentification

Skinner, B. F. (1953). *Science and human behavior* (No. 92904). Simon and Schuster. https://www.bfskinner.org/product/science-and-human-behavior/

Skinner, B. F. (1984). Coming to terms with private events. *Behavioral and Brain Sciences, 7*(4), 572–581. https://doi.org/10.1017/S0140525X00027400

Sofou, N., Giannakopoulos, O., Arampatzi, E., & Konstantakopoulos, G. (2021). Religious delusions: Definition, diagnosis and clinical implications. *Psychiatriki, 32*(3), 224–231. https://doi.org/10.22365/jpsych.2021.014

Spitzer, M. (1990). On defining delusions. *Comprehensive Psychiatry, 31*(5), 377–397. https://doi.org/10.1016/0010-440X(90)90023-L

Teasdale, B., Silver, E., & Monahan, J. (2006). Gender, threat/control-override delusions and violence. *Law and Human Behavior, 30*(6), 649–658. https://doi.org/10.1007/s10979-006-9044-x

van der Vaart, A. D., Ma, Y., Chiappelli, J., Bruce, H., Kvarta, M. D., Warner, A., Goldwaser, E., Kippenhan, J., Powers, A., Buchanan, R. W., & Hong, L. E. (2024). Revisiting delusion subtypes in schizophrenia based on their underlying structures. *Journal of Psychiatric Research, 171*, 75–83. https://doi.org/10.1016/j.jpsychires.2023.12.025

Velasco, M. M., & Gerechter, I. R. (2023). Clinical management of psychotic pregnancy denial: What do we know? Case report and narrative review. *European Psychiatry, 66*(S1), S1128–S1129. https://doi.org/10.1192/j.eurpsy.2023.2400

Ventriglio, A., Bhugra, D., De Berardis, D., Torales, J., Castaldelli-Maia, J. M., & Fiorillo, A. (2020). Capgras and Fregoli syndromes: Delusion and misidentification. *International Review of Psychiatry, 32*(5–6), 391–395. https://doi.org/10.1080/09540261.2020.1756625

World Health Organization. (2022). *ICD-11: International classification of diseases* (11th revision). https://icd.who.int/

Zhu, J., Zhuo, C., Liu, F., Xu, L., & Yu, C. (2016). Neural substrates underlying delusions in schizophrenia. *Scientific Reports, 6*(1), 33857. https://doi.org/10.1038/srep33857

Chapter 7
Problems with Hallucinations in Individuals Living with Serious Mental Illness

Introduction

Hallucinations are among the most perplexing and clinically significant phenomena encountered in serious mental illness (SMI). They challenge conventional understandings of perception, cognition, and behavior, often presenting with profound emotional and functional consequences. While auditory hallucinations are the most frequently reported, individuals may experience perceptual anomalies across all sensory modalities, including visual, tactile, olfactory, gustatory, and somatic domains. These experiences are not monolithic; they vary in content, emotional valence, conviction, and controllability, demanding comprehensive assessment and individualized intervention. This chapter builds on the general introduction to SMI by examining hallucinations and related phenomena through a multidimensional lens that integrates clinical, behavioral, neurocognitive, and cultural perspectives.

To understand hallucinations in context, it is essential to differentiate them from closely related constructs such as illusions and pseudohallucinations. Illusions involve misinterpretations of real external stimuli, whereas pseudohallucinations are vivid perceptual experiences recognized by the individual as internally generated and not objectively real. These distinctions are not merely semantic; they carry implications for diagnosis, treatment planning, and the reduction of stigma. The nature of hallucination content, which may vary from neutral and benign to hostile and distressing, is discussed, and the interactions of the experience with emotional states, trauma histories, and environmental factors are considered. This examination of hallucinations in individuals who live with SMI also emphasizes the reinforcing aspects of hallucinatory experiences and discusses their influence on both treatment engagement and avoidance.

A central theme of this chapter is the dimensional nature of hallucinations. Rather than treating them as binary symptoms (present or absent), their variability is examined across dimensions such as frequency, intensity, emotional impact,

G. F. McKeegan, *Behavior Change Interventions for Serious Mental Illness*, Evidence-Based Practices in Behavioral Health,
https://doi.org/10.1007/978-3-032-18372-9_7

perceived origin, linguistic complexity, and degree of control. These dimensions offer a framework for clinical formulation and research inquiry, aligning with contemporary transdiagnostic models and person-centered care. The chapter also considers associative learning and signal detection theory as explanatory models, highlighting how cognitive biases and environmental cues may contribute to the emergence and persistence of hallucinatory experiences.

Associative learning, which explains how repeated associations between stimuli can lead to false perceptions, and signal detection theory, which describes how individuals may misinterpret ambiguous sensory information, are expounded as explanatory models. These frameworks highlight how cognitive biases, such as confirmation bias (the tendency to interpret evidence in a way that confirms existing beliefs), and environmental cues, like sensory deprivation or heightened stress, may contribute to the emergence and persistence of hallucinatory experiences. By examining these specific biases and environmental factors, an integrated approach to understanding the complex mechanisms underlying hallucinations is demonstrated.

Finally, the chapter addresses behavioral strategies commonly employed by individuals in response to hallucinations, including avoidance, safety behaviors, and social withdrawal. These responses, while often adaptive in the short term, may inadvertently reinforce distress and functional impairment. A functional analytic approach is proposed to assess the antecedents and consequences of hallucinatory behavior, guiding interventions that target maladaptive contingencies and promote coping, engagement, and recovery. By integrating phenomenology, neurobiology, behavioral science, and lived experience, a comprehensive understanding of hallucinations and their relevance to the broader aspects of SMI is explicated.

> The person for whom I care says she hears voices, but nobody else is around. I see her talking or whispering to herself a lot. When I ask who she is talking to, she either does not answer or says, "No one."

The Case of Marsha

Marsha is a 55-year-old woman who has been diagnosed as living with a schizophrenia spectrum condition since her early 20s. Before the onset of her mental health problem, she was trained as a concert pianist and attended a prestigious college. After being identified as living with a schizophrenia spectrum mental health problem, she had increased difficulty interacting with other people and taking care of her basic needs, such as getting up in the morning and dressing herself. She has been seen by many prescribers and has been prescribed 18 different psychiatric medicines, including several that are normally prescribed for schizophrenia spectrum and mood and anxiety conditions. Despite this, she has continued to have a variety of problems taking care of herself and being around other people.

One of Marsha's most important problems is the voices that she hears when she is around other people. Sometimes, when other people are around, she hears voices that curse and criticize her. In the past, when she heard these voices, she would yell at other people to stop cursing at her and calling her names. This scared people and they would avoid her. Other people sometimes tried to let her know that they didn't say anything to her. Unfortunately, this led to arguments that often resulted in her threatening to kill them if they didn't stop. Occasionally, she physically attacked other people; this behavior was considered intolerable and dangerous at her family's home and at several adult home placements in her community. Primarily because of this behavior, she has spent considerable time in hospitals. Presently, her parents are not able to support her at home. The hope is she can live with other residents of an adult home or similar placement in her community without engaging in behaviors that are distressing, disruptive, or dangerous to the other residents.

Definition and Characteristics of Hallucinations?

Hallucinations (also known as paracusia) (Ali et al., 2011) are perceptual experiences that occur in the absence of any external stimuli but are experienced as reality to the person having the experience (American Psychiatric Association, 2022a). An important component that differentiates a hallucination from other perceptual phenomenon is the absence of any external stimulus that is associated with the sensation in which the hallucination is experienced (e.g., there is no discernible sound or visual stimuli that is associated with auditory or visual hallucinations, respectively).

A comprehensive definition of hallucinatory experiences was reported by Slade and Bentall (1988); they defined a hallucination as a "perceptual-like" experience which:

a. Occurs in the absence of an appropriate stimulus
b. Has the same impact as real perceptions in that sensory area
c. Cannot be voluntarily controlled by the individual experiencing it

The Diagnostic and Statistical Manual of Mental Disorders (5th ed.) (DSM-5) (American Psychiatric Association, 2013) offers the following definition for hallucination:

> A perception-like experience with the clarity and impact of a true perception but without the external stimulation of the relevant sensory organ. The person may or may not have insight into the non-veridical nature of the hallucination. One hallucinating person may recognize the false sensory experience whereas another may be convinced that the experience is grounded in reality. (p. 822)

In addition, the hallucinatory experience must occur in a "clear sensorium" (i.e., being conscious and alert) and not related to onset of sleep (hypnagogic) or awakening (hypnopompic) (American Psychiatric Association, 2013).

Hallucinations are complex phenomena that are multidimensional, transdiagnostic, and heterogeneous (Benrimoh et al., 2019). The definitions by Slade and Bentall (1988) and in the DSM-5-TR (American Psychiatric Association, 2022b) fail to consider the multidimensional nature of the hallucinatory experience, which is researched and reported on in the literature. Slade and Bentall (1988) do not consider the awareness or lack of insight of the falsity of the experience, whereas the definition in the DSM-5-TR does not account for the dimension of control of the hallucinatory experience. Mental health assessments typically focus on identifying the presence or absence of specific behaviors, as well as evaluating the severity and the level of dysfunction related to problematic behaviors. While the nature of hallucinatory experiences is often documented, the broader dimensions that may affect individuals with SMI who experience hallucinations are seldom systematically assessed. Assessing other dimensions allows the service provider to engage with the service user and understand and appreciate the complexity of the behaviors that the person living with SMI is experiencing. Experiencing a problem behavior associated with SMI is not a discrete entity but heterogeneous, multidimensional, and multidirectional, with some behavioral dimensions impacting overall functioning and emotional outcomes positively or negatively. For example, a person living with SMI experiences auditory verbal hallucinations (AVH), but he does not experience them as distressing. He reports that he hears the voice of a guardian angel who tells him what to do. He refuses treatment for the hallucination. Further exploration by the service provider reveals that the person has little support in the community and is unsheltered for periods of time because of a co-occurring substance use problem. During the periods of homelessness, he finds the voice comforting in that "he tells me that I will be alright and to just keep on the straight and narrow. He keeps me company at night when it is pretty scary on the streets." He stated that he can control the voice as to how loud it is and perceives that it is coming from outside of himself, "like a guardian angel hovering over me." He has developed coping skills, such as listening to music if the voice is too distracting. His recovery goal is to find an apartment and to minimize his drug use, which he understands contributes to the behaviors associated with SMI.

Hallucinations occur in all sensory areas—visual, auditory, olfactory, tactile, gustatory (i.e., taste), and somatic (i.e., physical sensation on body, such as snakes crawling under one's skin) (Shahrokh and Hales, 2003). Hallucinations are experienced with a certain degree of clarity and have personal impacts as real perceptions. It may affect any of the senses, but auditory hallucinations (AHs) are most common, followed by visual hallucinations (VH). A high percentage of people living with SMI (60–80%) have both types of hallucinations. Having and responding to hallucinations are a common behavior problem and positive symptom associated with SMI; experiencing hallucinations is one of two symptoms (the other is experiencing delusions) that need to be present to determine that the individual is living with a schizophrenic spectrum disorder (American Psychiatric Association, 2022b). Hallucinations, however, are caused by a wide range of physical and psychiatric conditions resulting from substance use, neurological abnormalities, and other conditions (Ali et al., 2011; American Psychiatric Association, 2022a; American Psychological Association, n.d.-c; Shahrokh & Hales, 2003).

Hallucinations are and were viewed by some cultures as having religious significance. Historically, delusions and hallucinations with religious content that are associated with SMI have been of interest to mental health service providers and researchers for decades. The prevalence of these behaviors and symptoms varies across different time periods and cultures. Some religions induce hallucinations by using plant-based hallucinogens known as "entheogens" to connect with higher spiritual entities to send and receive messages for themselves and for other believers. The widespread use and importance of entheogens and the resulting hallucinatory experiences in different spiritual traditions and sacred contexts of other cultures are unquestioned, although presently forbidden by most major religions (Radenkova et al., 2011). The juxtaposition of religion, culture, symptoms, and behaviors indicative of mental health problems draws attention to religion and mental health interacting in complex ways.

Hallucinations have been recognized and studied as a human phenomenon of interest for centuries. It was a subject of philosophers such as Aristotle and Aquinas. Greek philosophers explained hallucinations as not due to superhuman entities (e.g., the voice of Zeus) but misperceptions of naturally occurring phenomenon during different types of consciousness, such as sleep (Harris, 2013). Philosophers in the Middle Ages (e.g., Augustine and Aquinas) tried to rectify the hallucinatory experience with errors in perception and metacognitions to naturally occurring events in attempts by the individual to make sense out of their existence; however, hallucinations also could be generated by higher powers for either good or evil intent for the individual having the hallucinatory experience.

The term "hallucination" was first used in 18485 by Jean-Étienne Dominique Esquirol, a French psychiatrist. The phenomenon and the term then became the purview of mental health providers of the time and have been ever since. Esquirol initially thought the hallucinatory phenomena as "involuntary exercise of memory and imagination" (Telles-Correia et al., 2015, p. 2). Over the decades, hallucinations have been described as a form of delusional thinking or have been explained as changes in the perceptual experiences through misperceptions. Others have taken into account the heterogeneity of hallucinations and their respective multiplicity of possible causes. To account for some of the forms, dimensions, and causes of hallucinations, other terms have been coined, including "pseudohallucination" and "hallucinosis," maintaining that illusions are an integral part of the concept of hallucination.

Since its introduction, the term pseudohallucination has been used with different meanings. The major characteristics associated with pseudohallucinations were the "lack of objectivity" and the "presence of insight" that differs from the definition of hallucinations (Telles-Correia et al., 2015). The phenomenon of pseudohallucination is defined as a vivid, sensory experience without corresponding external stimuli that the individual recognizes as not real; they are usually auditory or visual in modality. Pseudohallucinations are described as "subjective perceptions similar to hallucinations, with respect to their character and vividness, but that differ from those because these do not have objective reality" (López-Silva et al., 2022, p. 134).

Pseudohallucinations are distinguishable from hallucinations in certain dimensions. Pseudohallucinations are usually perceived by the person as originating internally (i.e., coming from within themselves), inconsistent with the environmental context, and the content related to their present emotional state (such as in extreme anxiety or dysphoria). They have been described as "inner speech," which is described as the silent expression of thought in a coherent linguistic form, the silent production of words in the mind of the person, or the activity of talking to oneself without any sound (López-Silva et al., 2022; Morin, 2012). Occasionally, the person reports "receiving" a message or meaning in the pseudohallucinatory experience. They are more prominently displayed in a person in acute distress, grieving, victims of trauma, and frequently present in a person living with a severe personality mental health problem. The term has become less commonly used due to its potential to create confusion among service providers, particularly when pseudohallucinations are treated with antipsychotic medications despite the likelihood that symptoms may subside as acute emotional distress resolves. In addressing the identification and management of pseudohallucinations, some mental health professionals have advocated for the use of "functional cognitive disorder" in place of the label of a schizophrenia spectrum condition, which can contribute to unnecessary trauma and stigma (Mustafa, 2020).

Illusions are generally understood as distortions of real objects in the environment that are perceived by the person. They are false sensory percepts. Illusions of the senses are the result of misinterpretation of sensory stimuli that are present in the environment of the individual. An example of a visual illusion would be the linear perspective in which parallel railroad track seems to meet in the distance or seeing mirages in the desert. "Aristotle's illusion" is the tactile perception that a single object is two objects when felt with the crossed index and middle fingers (American Psychological Association, n.d.-a). All of these illusions occur under ordinary conditions but can be experienced by individuals living with SMI and experiencing hallucinations as well (American Psychological Association, n.d.-e).

Hallucinosis is characterized by prominent and persistent hallucinations without alterations of consciousness (e.g., wakefulness, being alert) when caused by the direct physiological effects of a substance or associated with neurological factors such as Parkinson's disease and Lewy body dementia. Hallucinosis can be auditory, visual, tactile, olfactory, or a combination of sensory experiences. Visual sensory experiences are more common, with imagery of insects, animals, people, or disembodied heads. They may occur only with eyes being closed and tend to be fragmentary, lasting only minutes for each occurrence but lasting over several days. The person having hallucinosis generally considers it an abnormal experience and out of character; insight is intact, and the person is aware that the misperception is not real. The term was used in the description of substance misuse and withdrawal and described in the context of alcohol consumption (American Psychological Association, n.d.-d). The term is no longer used in DSM-5-TR (American Psychiatric Association, 2022a), and the present term for when experiencing false precepts during substance intoxication or withdrawal is "perceptual disturbances."

Dimensions of the Hallucinatory Experiences

Hallucinations are one of the key concepts and behavioral problems/symptoms in mental health but also one of the most puzzling and hardest to define and distinguish from other behavioral problems and concepts that occur in people living with SMI and other related mental health problems. Hallucinations are heterogeneous and transdiagnostic, which has led to competing definitions of the phenomenon. Moreover, a substantial minority of otherwise normal individuals report hallucinatory experiences. It is estimated that 10–20% of individuals in the general population with no known mental health problem experience hallucinations (Bentall, 1990; Blom, 2015; Upthegrove et al., 2016).

Hallucinations have been debated by mental health providers and researchers. Some suggest the possibility of multiple dimensions; others view the dimension of emotional distress and the resulting impact on the ability to function as a primary dimension that needs to be assessed and explored; other theorists and researchers argue that the hallucinations experienced by treatment-seeking and nontreatment-seeking individuals are fundamentally different (Janaki et al., 2017; Linscott & van Os, 2010; Powers, 2019). Studies have found that hallucinations in treatment-seeking and nontreatment-seeking individuals tend to be similar in the dimensions of loudness, location, and duration, but significantly differ along the dimensional characteristic of the person's perception of the origin of the hallucination (e.g., external or internal orientation), the ability of the person having the hallucinatory experience to engage and control the experience, and the negative content of the hallucinatory experiences (Swyer & Powers, 2020).

Most of the research on hallucinations has been with the auditory subtype (AH). AH includes auditory verbal hallucinations (AVH) in which the person experiences hearing a voice that has no identified external source in the environment, musical hallucinations (i.e., repeatedly hearing a tune or song with no nearby external source), echoes of reading, "exploding-head syndrome" (i.e., characterized by the perception of loud noises during sleep–wake or wake–sleep transitions) (Sharpless, 2015), and many other types of content (e.g., animal sounds, mechanical sounds, bells, static noise) (Bentall, 1990; Blom, 2015; Linn 1977). Infrequently, the content in AVH is a single word with no personal reference that is repeated (Linn, 1977) (e.g., repeatedly hearing the name of a common soy sauce).

Auditory hallucinations experienced by individuals living with SMI are usually sensed as coming from more than a single voice separate from the person and beyond their control. The voices are usually anonymous and not recognized by the person. Auditory hallucinations can be categorized as to the number of voices heard and whether the person experiencing the hallucination is being talked about directly or indirectly (Linn, 1977). Linn categorized this dimension as the following:

- First person: Infrequent in that the person hears voices talking about themselves and what they are doing in the moment.
- Second person: The most frequent type; the person experiencing is being addressed by the content of the hallucination using the pronoun "you."

- Third person: As if two or more people are overheard talking about the person in the first person.

People living with depression and mania generally experience hallucinations in the second person and mood-congruent in content (Janaki et al., 2017); a person experiencing mania may hear the voice exalting and praising him, making positive and exuberant statements (e.g., "you are a genius, you are the smartest person in the city"); a person living with a depressive type of SMI will usually hear derogatory and negative comments (e.g., "you have cancer," "everyone will die," "you have always been a loser") (Spence, 2009).

The preponderance of the content of auditory hallucinations experienced by individuals living with SMI is negative, hostile, disparaging, derogatory, critical, and accusatory, resulting in emotional distress ranging in degrees of severity with corresponding impact on the functioning of the person experiencing the hallucination. (Haddock et al., 1999; Linn, 1977; Telles-Correia et al., 2016). At times, the content varies from pleasurable to mundane to hostile, demeaning, accusatory, and critical (de Leede-Smith & Barkus, 2013).

Using only a sample of people who experience auditory hallucinations, McCarthy-Jones et al. (2014) concluded that 39% of participants reported that their voices appeared to be replays of memories of previous conversations they had experienced; 45% reported that the general theme or content of what the voices said was always the same; and 55% said new voices had the same content/theme as previous voices. The findings suggest that an aspect of the phenomenon of hallucinations needs to include memory and recall of previous perceptual events as an aspect of an explanatory model.

When considered from the perspective of memory, hallucinations frequently present as fragments or complete reenactments of previous conversations, experiences, or notable life events. These may include voices that resemble those of familiar individuals and can echo prior interactions, often accompanied by strong emotional responses—particularly those associated with negative or traumatic memories. In effect, the brain is "replaying" these memories as if they are occurring in real time, despite the absence of any external stimulus in the immediate environment (McCarthy-Jones et al., 2014).

McCarthy-Jones et al. (2014) have identified key features about hallucinations and memory:

- Personal relevance: The voices experienced by the person during AVH frequently relate to the person's history and relationships.
- Emotional intensity: The memories can reflect the emotions associated with the original event, whether positive or negative.
- Distorted perception: While the content might be based on real memories, the details may be distorted or exaggerated in the hallucinatory experience.
- Trauma connection: Individuals with a history of trauma may be more likely to experience hallucinations that are directly related to the traumatic experiences, such as hearing a deceased parent's voice giving critical comments; echoing past arguments; replaying of a traumatic event, including the sounds and voices that

were present at the time; and hearing a familiar voice from a past relationship saying hurtful things.

The preponderance of research on hallucinations focused on auditory hallucination, the negativity of the content that is heard, and the resulting emotional distress experienced by the person experiencing the hallucination. However, research has shown that some individuals experience neutral or pleasant hallucinations in auditory, visual, and olfactory modalities (Miller et al., 1993; Sanjuan et al., 2004). Voices perceived as "occasionally pleasurable" were endorsed by 26% of the participants, with 9% having very frequent pleasurable hallucinations. Pleasurable hallucinations showed negative associations with the amount and intensity of distress, degree of negative content, and loudness. Positive associations were found with the amount of time since initially experiencing the hallucination and perceived control over the voices. Pleasurable hallucinations were positively associated with experiencing other types of hallucinations, lower scores of emotional distress, and corresponding disruption of functioning in daily life. It appears that the longer an individual experiences hallucination, the more the person is able to exercise control of the experience and find the experience pleasurable. Pleasurable hallucinations were perceived as having positive effects on emotional well-being, self-concept, performance, and aspects pertaining to interpersonal relationships (Miller et al., 1993). The pleasurable hallucination was not distressful but helpful, and so the individual was not amenable to treatment. Individuals who placed value on hallucinatory experiences prior to undergoing treatment were more likely to continue experiencing hallucinations post treatment, as these experiences served as a reinforcing function. Miller et al. (1993) proposed that the reinforcing nature of hallucinations may contribute to individuals with serious mental illness opting out of treatment. The presence of olfactory hallucinations (OH), along with the ability to anticipate hallucinatory episodes linked to emotional states, showed a significant association with the perceived value of hallucinations. Miller et al. (1993) concluded that psychotropic medications may offer benefits not necessarily by reducing symptoms, but by alleviating the emotional distress associated with hallucinations and improving daily functioning.

The content of the percept during the hallucinatory experience varies according to the dimensions of complexity and novelty (Moseley & Mitrenga, 2022; Stephane et al., 2003). Some auditory hallucinations are experienced as various sounds, music, or a cacophony, with novel and repetitive sounds. The content of hallucinations can differ on syntactical and grammatical complexity and whether the ideas, information, and message are new or routine and repetitive. The complexity of the hallucination that is experienced is a dimension that is seldom clinically assessed but is of importance in determining the goals of treatment and engagement with the person experiencing hallucinations and living with SMI. Complexity as a dimension is complicated as it is comprised of several variables along other dimensions. The complexity of hallucinations is related to:

(1) Linguistic elements of the verbal percept
(2) Number of modalities (VH, AH, or other types) (Moseley & Mitrenga, 2022; Oorschot et al., 2012)

Oorschot et al. (2012) reported that 52% of a sample of participants living with SMI reported both AH and VH with 66% of the participants reporting both AH and VH being experienced simultaneously.

(1) Temporal synchronization of the experiences of different modalities of hallucinations
(2) Congruency of two or more hallucinatory experiences in different modalities with integration of identity and content

Stephane et al. (2003) identified dimensions of hallucinations as clustering along content, control, and location. The first cluster included auditory hallucinations with low linguistic complexity, repetitive content, attributed to self, located external to the person, and associated with different kinds of control strategies. The second cluster included hallucinations with high linguistic complexity, systematized content, multiple voices, attributed to others, and located originating internally. The results of multidimensional scaling analysis (in which data points are connected in space) identified three dimensions: linguistic complexity, self-other attribution, and internal–external location of perceived voice. The authors concluded that the results validated the description of the hallucination by the person experiencing it and suggested a language dysfunction according to the linguistic complexity of the experience. Further research using dimensions of hallucinations could assist in specific neural substrates for each dimensional characteristic of the hallucinatory experience (Stephane et al., 2003).

Additional dimensional matrices relevant to the assessment and research of hallucinations include the types and frequency of distinct voices, as well as the nature of messages conveyed by these voices, such as whether they are commanding, commenting, insulting, or interacting with each other. Furthermore, it is important to evaluate whether the individual experiencing the hallucination is being directly addressed or discussed across each content type.

Besides the dimensions of frequency, intensity, antecedent situational conditions (i.e., MO/EOs, S^D, S^{delta}) and the consequences of the occurrences of the hallucinations that are common to all behavioral challenges and symptoms associated with SMI, the definition by Slade and Bentall (1988) accounts for some of the additional dimensional variables associated with hallucinations such as the misattribution of stimuli, the impact of the experience on the individual (e.g., distress, humor, guilt), and the subjective perception of control over the experience (Badcock et al., 2011). In defining hallucinations, the DSM-5-TR (American Psychiatric Association, 2022a) adds the dimension of awareness or insight that the percept is not real as part of the definition of a hallucination.

Continuity of the hallucinatory experience is a dimension in which the content being perceived is continuous or episodic, with periods of no percept being experienced while conscious. Hallucinatory experiences have been described as discrete episodes of activity followed by episodes of inactivity, both with durations in the order of minutes for each duration (Blom, 2015). The dimension of continuity is: (1) total number of continuous and noncontinuous episodes of hallucinatory experiences; (2) the duration of each discrete episode of both activity and inactivity; (3) the total duration of the cumulative episodes within a specified period or antecedent condition; and (4) the range and other descriptive statistics of duration during the episodes of hallucinatory activity and inactivity. Further research is needed in this dimension for all the subtypes of hallucinatory experiences.

Only recently has the field of mental health investigated the dimension of control of hallucinations by the person experiencing them (Swyer & Powers, 2020). Not only has clinical literature reported on people being able to turn the experience on and off but also control other dimensions such as loudness, intrusiveness, and emotional impact. Control of hallucinations may be defined as the ability to voluntarily influence false perceptual experiences. Controllability has ranged from 17–20% of individuals having hallucinatory experiences being able to occasionally control the experience (de Leede-Smith & Barkus, 2013)

Control of hallucination is not a unitary phenomenon but a variety of abilities within a myriad of contexts. These abilities seem to fall into broad categories: direct control strategies and indirect control strategies. Indirect control strategies include those that influence the frequency or impact of the sensory percept by manipulating other related factors, like attention, concentration, metacognitive skills, and controlling the emotional impact of the hallucinations being experienced (Jenner et al., 2006). Metacognitive skills are any conscious cognitive or affective experiences that accompany and pertain to any intellectual enterprise by manipulating internal, private-event processes before, during, or after cognitive activity; metacognitive experiences are higher order skills related to executive functions such as verbal mediation, self-regulation, planning, judgment, and self-monitoring; they allow a person to be aware of beliefs, attitudes, and experiences and to relate those internal states to the external environment and events in order to construct meaning from information (American Psychological Association, n.d.-g; Flavell, 1979). Metacognition assists the person to analyze and assess the reality of the hallucinatory experience. Controlling the emotional experience of a hallucinatory experience is a combination of metacognition and behavioral and cognitive-behavioral skills to reduce emotional sequelae associated with the hallucinatory experience. Cognitive-behavioral techniques include reframing, challenging "prior" beliefs, irrational automatic self-statements, mindfulness exercises (e.g., soles of the feet technique (Singh et al., 2003)), and engaging in techniques to decrease physiological arousal such as relaxation training.

Direct control describes the ability to influence the onset and offset of these experiences by interacting with them more directly. The ability of some individuals to exercise indirect control of hallucinatory experiences by using cognitive strategies to manipulate the impact has been the basis for cognitive-behavioral approaches (Lincoln & Peters, 2019). The ability to directly control the onset and offset of the experiences of hallucinations still needs to be further researched for therapeutic strategies (Swyer & Powers, 2020).

Expanding on the dimensions of control includes a matrix of the efficacy of control and what dimensions of the hallucinatory experience are controlled by the individual. The dimensions of control of the hallucinatory experiences include the onset/offset of the experience, the intensity of the sensory experience, and the emotional impact of the experience. The type and degree of endorsed control in the individuals experiencing the subtypes of hallucinatory experiences should be defined carefully and specifically in future studies, as different types of control over the various dimensions of the subtypes are likely subserved by different cognitive and neural mechanisms and may drive the development of vastly different treatment strategies (Cho &Wu, 2013).

It has been cited in clinical literature that delusions and hallucinations are experienced simultaneously by some people living with SMI (Chen & Berrios, 1996; Telles-Correia et al., 2016). The temporal association of both phenomena occurring raises the question as to the relationship between the two. Scholars have questioned if reports of experiencing hallucinations are related to false beliefs but interpreted as a perceptual experience; on the other hand, are hallucinatory experiences interpreted as false beliefs? Although several authors have suggested the conceptual proximity between hallucinations and delusions, few empirical studies have been conducted to investigate the close relationship between the dimensions of hallucinations and delusions. The common cooccurrence of hallucinations and delusions associated with SMI is known in the mental health literature (Hustig & Hafner, 1990; Maher, 2006; Telles-Correia et al., 2016). However, the relationship between the two is less well known. It has been hypothesized that repeated hallucinatory experiences are linked to the development of delusions and have a direct causative role in the formation and continuation of delusional thinking and speech (Maher, 2006). Using self-report data from participants experiencing both hallucinations and delusions, Hustig and Hafner (1990) found a significant relationship between the loudness and intrusiveness of hallucinations and the intensity of delusional beliefs and the severity of averse emotional outcomes.

The directionality of a possible causative relationship between hallucinations and delusions is an ongoing debate. Telles-Correia et al. (2016) have postulated that both experiences can emerge simultaneously. The question is if the associated hallucination is a type or a consequence of the delusion. Given the relationship between hallucinations and delusions, a dimension of hallucinatory experiences is whether the experience occurs in conjunction with the presence of a delusion; furthermore, what subtypes of delusions are associated with the various dimensions of hallucinatory experiences. One approach is to assess whether somatic delusions are associated with, or coincide with, olfactory, tactile, or somatic hallucinations; alternatively, it may be considered whether both hallucinations and delusions stem from an unidentified underlying cause (Telles-Correia et al., 2016).

The mean age of onset of experiencing hallucinations determines the severity and impact that the experience has on the person. Daalman et al. (2011) have found the mean age of onset of experiencing hallucinations is 21 years, but Honig (1998) has found that 11% of individuals have the first hallucinatory experiences before age 12. Early onset and the degree of distress experienced by the individual during the hallucinatory experiences are correlated with the person living with SMI as an adult.

Instruments have been developed to assess and measure the multidimensional and heterogeneous nature of these complex phenomena that are hallucinations (Jenner & Van de Willige, 2002; Jenner et al., 2006; Steenhuis et al., 2019). The Psychotic Symptom Rating Scales (PSYRATS), developed by Haddock et al. (1999), evaluates the dimensions or characteristics of the experiences of hallucinations and delusions. The hallucination section was divided into four dimensional domains: (1) emotional characteristics—negative content and emotional impact; (2) physical characteristics—duration, frequency, intensity; (3) control; and (4) cognitive interpretation such as the source of the hallucinatory experience being generated internally or externally to oneself (Haddock et al., 1999). The 11 items of the subscale for hallucinatory experiences correspond to the following dimensions:

1. Frequency: How often does the experience occur.
2. Duration: How long does the experience last.
3. Intensity: The magnitude or intensity of the sensory perception of the hallucination. For auditory hallucinations, the intensity is the loudness of the sound; for somatic hallucinations, it would be the intensity of the internal sensation being experienced.
4. Location: The percept being experienced by the person as being outside or internal to oneself.
5. Beliefs reorigin: The belief of the person as to the source of the hallucination being generated from and by oneself or outside of oneself.
6. Amount of negative content: The amount of critical, threatening, or unpleasant themes that can significantly impact the individual's emotional state and overall well-being that is perceived during a hallucinatory episode.
7. Degree of negative content: The intensity of negative or distressing elements that are present in the content of the experienced hallucinations.
8. Amount of distress: How frequently the hallucinations cause distress to the individual.
9. Intensity of distress: severity or intensity of the distress
10. Disruption: The global impact on the person's functioning in daily life and society.
11. Control: The extent to which the person believes that they can manage or influence the occurrence and content of the hallucinations. Perceptions of not having the ability to manage or influence hallucinations lead to a greater degree of distress and result in disruptions in daily life.

Telles-Correia et al. (2016) analyzed data using PSYRATS from a clinical population of people living with SMI and the associated mental health problems of schizophrenia spectrum mental health problems. The sample of the clinical population showed that:

- Total 24% of people living with SMI did not show any hallucinations at the time of observation.
- Total 67% had auditory verbal hallucinations, and 9% had other types of hallucinations. During the AVH, 37% of the cases heard the voice in the first person,

58% in the second person, 52% in the third person, and in 43% of cases, only isolated words were present.

All individuals with auditory-visual hallucinations experienced delusions.

- Total 15% of individuals were nondelusional at the time of evaluation. Common delusion themes when present were persecutory (51%), followed by mystical/religious (31%) themes

Results showed that the variables that are determinants of the dimensions of hallucinations are:

- "Beliefs reorigin": Determined by a conviction of the belief of experiencing a hallucination as true; the frequency of experiencing the hallucinations; the perceived control of the experience of a hallucination; and the number of negative themes.
- Location: Determined by the "beliefs reorigin," control, and the amount of negative content.
- Disruption: Determined by "beliefs reorigin," amount of distress caused by negative content and themes, and years of living with an SMI.

Telles-Correia et al. (2016) proposed a model suggesting that the "beliefs reorigin" variable could mediate the relationship between "delusional conviction" (i.e., that the voices were real) and the location and disruption in the dimensions of hallucinations. More research needs to be done in this area of the hallucinatory experience.

Chen and Berrios (1996) have isolated 11 dimensions of the experiences of hallucinations that can be applied in clinical settings. There is an overlap between what is assessed with the PSYRAT and the scale suggested by Chen and Berrios (1996). The dimensions without overlap to the dimensions assessed by the PSYRAT are (1) vividness, detail, and clarity of the content; (2) complexity; (3) bizarreness; (4) situation (context/antecedents in which the hallucinatory experience occurs); and (5) attribution to specific events (such as experiences of trauma). Insight, localization, intensity, voluntary control, and constancy (frequency) have similar dimensions that are assessed on the PSYRAT. As noted previously, the dimension of attribution to specific events is more likely a component of pseudohallucinations, as traumatic events have been linked to the false perception that is being experienced

Origins of Hallucinations

Hallucinations are among the most severe and puzzling forms of symptoms and problem behaviors associated with SMI. They are also one of the most researched symptoms and behavior problems associated with SMI. Although usually regarded as first-rank symptoms of a schizophrenia spectrum mental health problem, they are found in a wide range of medical and psychiatric conditions including Parkinson's

Disease, dementia, diseases of the middle and inner ear, auditory nerve disease and lesions, CNS disorders, temporal lobe epilepsy (TLE), cerebrovascular accident (CVA), arteriovenous malformations, syncope, toxic metabolic disturbances, use of hallucinogens, and withdrawal of psychoactive drugs (Ali et al., 2011; Brust, 2014).

The origins of hallucinations are complex, probably involving genetic, neurological, cognitive, and environmental influences. Given the presence of hallucinations in conditions of the central nervous system (CNS), it stands to reason that there is a neurological substrate to the experience. Hallucinations are a prominent behavioral problem and symptom in several mental health problems, including schizophrenic spectrum, mood-, and personality-related mental health problems. Any genetic contribution to the origin of hallucinations is likely genotypically polygenic and heterogenous phenotypically; the stress-diathesis theory related to SMI, as well as the plasticity of the CNS, postulate that genes contribute a liability to develop problem behaviors and symptoms related to SMI, but that the environment influences the phenotypical display. However, no final common neurological pathway has been found. Studies about the cognitive and behavioral processes involved in the phenomenon of hallucinations have also not been able to determine a common process resulting in the experience of hallucinations.

Hallucinations occur in all areas of sensation: auditory, visual, olfactory, gustatory, tactile, and somatic hallucinations. Hallucinations are a phenomenon that results from a confluence of sensory experiences, perceptions, inferences, decision-making, attention, and memory (Larøi & Woodward, 2007). The sensory experiences associated with hallucinatory experiences are accompanied by cognitive and emotional respondents (i.e., fear, anxiety, joy, anger). The person attempts to understand or makes sense of the sensory experience by inferring causality using the perceptions of the experience, the associated cognitive and emotional sequelae of the experience, the use of covert verbal behavior, and the verbal behavior received from others. This covert process and its components are reinforced by stimuli that are available in the surrounding environment. Hallucinatory behaviors are maintained by changes in the behavior of a verbal community and can be classified as verbal behavior, like other verbal patterns. The behaviors associated with hallucinations are regarded as problematic not by the content but by the structure of the phenomenon—a percept without any external stimuli that is present (Layng & Andronis, 1984).

Therefore, the physical and the psychological contributions must be appreciated to fully understand and comprehend the origins of the hallucinatory experience. The mind-body dichotomy is outdated as research has shown that mind and body are interconnected and not separate entities; advancements in neuroscience and psychology demonstrate the direct influence of brain activity on mental states and vice versa.

Neurological Substrates

Research has centered on the neurological mechanisms underlying the phenomenon of hallucinations (Boksa, 2009; Braun et al., 2003; Lin et al., 2020). A description of what occurs in the brain during a specific hallucinatory experience is essential in attempting to comprehend the phenomenon since the assessment of a hallucination is by the person having the experience to verbally respond to questions concerning the occurrence of the hallucination. Given the nature of self-reports (especially on private events—cognitions, perceptions, emotions) and problems with metacognitive abilities (i.e., self-awareness, self-monitoring) associated with living with SMI, the validity of these reports can be an issue unless collateral observational data are available, such as a person mumbling, laughing, talking, and gesticulating to oneself when the person is reporting a hallucinatory experience. However, observational data may not be reliable as the hallucinatory experience is heterogeneous, and likewise, the behavioral response is idiosyncratic.

Brain scans have been used to study the architecture and metabolic activity of the various regions in the brain (Tracy & Shergill, 2006). Magnetic resonance imagery (MRI) uses the responses of hydrogen in tissue molecules of cells to strong magnetic impulses to form an accurate three-dimensional picture of body organs and tissues, including the brain (American Psychological Association, n.d.-f). Functional magnetic resonance imagery (fMRI) is a brain imaging technique using the same magnetic impulses, but it measures changes in blood flow and oxygenation to show which parts of the brain are active (American Psychological Association, n.d.-b) during a specific event, such as the reporting of the hallucination.

The results of various brain scans show that when hallucinations occur, brain areas like the superior and middle temporal gyri (primary auditory cortex), insula, hippocampus, amygdala, and the sensory cortex are typically activated, particularly in regions associated with the specific sense being hallucinated, like the visual cortex for visual hallucinations or the auditory cortex for auditory hallucinations; these areas are involved in processing sensory information and integrating it with memory and emotion, leading to the perception of a sensory experience without an external stimulus.

Below are key points from the results of brain activity during hallucinations:

- Sensory cortices: The primary sensory cortex for the relevant sense (e.g., visual cortex for seeing hallucinations, auditory cortex for hearing voices) shows increased activity during hallucinations.
- Limbic system: Areas like the amygdala and hippocampus, which are part of the limbic system responsible for emotions and memory, are often activated during hallucinations, potentially contributing to the emotional experience of the hallucination.
- Insula: This brain region is associated with integrating sensory information and bodily sensations; it is implicated in hallucinations across different sensory modalities.

- Anterior cingulate cortex: This area is involved in cognitive control and self-monitoring; this area may play a role in the abnormal perception of hallucinations.
- Thalamus: This subcortical structure is euphemistically known as the "switching station of the brain" as it relays sensory information from all sensory organs of the body to the sensory and association cortices. Abnormal activity in this area can contribute to hallucinations.

It is of interest that increased activity on fMRI scans in brain regions correlated with the auditory sense, speech production, and working memory were noted during a task in which the participants without mental health problems generated subvocal speech (Friedman et al., 1998). The areas of increased activity associated with the occurrence of hallucinations are like the results of increased activity during the occurrence of subvocalizations, which are equated with internal dialogue, self-statements, or self-talk (Spence, 2009).

There are important considerations that relate to the results of all psychological and neurological investigations of hallucinations. The operational definition of what is a hallucination—and what it is not—must be consistently applied across all studies. The debate as to whether pseudohallucinations, hallucinosis, and "perceptual disturbances" are hallucinatory experiences adds to the inconsistent results of the phenomenon being studied. The type, subtypes, and dimensions of the hallucinatory experiences also must be specified; statistical analyses need to take these variables into account as specific brain areas are activated depending on the type of hallucination (visual, auditory, tactile) and likely according to the dimensional experiences.

A preponderance of the imaging studies is on the experience of auditory hallucinations. More studies need to focus on the experience of having more than one type of hallucination (e.g., multimodal hallucinations) occurring sequentially or simultaneously since it appears to be a more frequent occurrence than previously thought by experts in the field (Montagnese et al., 2021).

Given that hallucinations are transdiagnostic, heterogeneous, and multidimensional, individual differences are expected to occur. Brain activity patterns during hallucinations can differ between individuals, even with similar experiences. Medications can also impact the activity of the various brain regions. Variables that can impact the results need to be minimized or controlled methodologically and statistically.

Finally, experiencing hallucinations is often associated with conditions like living with schizophrenia spectrum mental health problems; they also occur in other conditions associated with SMI, in addition to neurological conditions; it is hypothesized that abnormal activity in the brain is the causative factor for the associated observed symptoms and problem behaviors. Yet, the final common pathway for hallucinations—and other problem behaviors and symptoms associated with mental health problems—have not been found because of the many confounding variables involved.

Psychological and Behavioral Substrates

Hallucinatory behaviors—hearing voices, seeing things, feeling things on skin or proprioceptively, and smelling odors—are private events that can only be accessed through verbal self-reports by the individual having the experience. Hallucinations are verbal operants—self-generated covert talk—that are governed by consequences as are other behaviors.

Hallucinations are, in essence, a type of "false perception" but different from an illusion as there is no environmental stimulus present that is associated with the sensation. Perception is not simply the passive reception of inputs. It involves the inference as to the causes of the sensations. These inferences are influenced by our prior experiences. Prediction errors, the mismatch between prior experience and present inputs, contribute to an updating of attribution of causality. Attribution is the result of the role modeling of verbal behaviors (such as metaphorical language to explain causality) and a history of reinforcement of these private events. Hallucinations (percepts without external stimulus) may arise when there is a confluence of antecedent conditions involving previous perceptions and similarities of percepts but occurring in the absence of input in the immediate context.

Hallucinations are a phenomenon that results from a confluence of sensory experiences, perceptions, inferences, and decision-making. The sensory experiences are accompanied by cognitive and emotional respondents. The person attempts to understand or makes sense of the experience by inferring causality using the perceptions of the experience and the associated cognitive and emotional sequelae of the experience. Humans strive to minimize uncertainty about future states and events by forming and maintaining a set of beliefs (i.e., self-statements or thoughts) about oneself and the environment through associative learning; that is, cause and effect. Central to this explanation is that formal associative learning theory can provide an explanation for the development and persistence of hallucinations (Feeney et al., 2017) as well as behavioral operants.

Skinner (1953) defined associative learning paradigms that emphasized the importance of predictions and the self-statements of control; predicting the effect of behavior on the environment includes self-statements that are conditioned through associations with perceptual stimuli. Associations between the self-talk or subvocalizations of causes and effects are formed to minimize uncertainty by way of new learning and attentional allocation. For example, a person smells the odor of hamburgers being cooked as he walks past a newly opened restaurant. The smell is a perception and a stimulus that triggers an avalanche of subvocalizations, including past associations with the smell (memory), planning for dinner (including thinking if one has enough money), gustatory associations (that may trigger certain gastrointestinal sensation), temporal association with hamburgers, and emotional subvocalization that may vary on the degree of pleasantness. If the association with odor has been reinforcing, then the person may hesitate and decide to buy a hamburger to take home, given his past association of the odor associated with hamburgers has been reinforcing. But one can see how unpleasant association can likewise be triggered by a sensory experience, such as experiencing the odor of flowers used in funerals or the use of certain deodorizers and cleaning fluids used in courtrooms and jails

Subvocal speech may be involved in generating hallucinations (Burns et al., 1983). EMG studies show speech musculature activity during hallucinations. AHs may start with mishearing ambiguous auditory stimuli as "voices." To reduce uncertainty, a metacognitive error is made by attributing the ambiguous stimuli to a recognizable stimulus like a "voice." Subvocal behavior and intraverbal strengthening can lead to strings of unedited—and erroneous—covert verbal behaviors. The genesis of auditory hallucinations may be related to interactions of both subvocalizations and physiological stimuli (Burns et al., 1983).

Covert speech—what a person says to himself—is related to self-talk, self-control and monitoring, working memory, verbal rehearsal, utterances, self-verbalization, and statements—basically what the person is thinking at a point in time (Spence, 2009). What a person subvocalizes is based on verbal behaviors from others that have been role modeled and is repeated, or that has been experienced by other covert subvocalized speech, such as reading. If a person is training to run a marathon, she subvocalizes self-statements to engage in the behavior (motivating self-statements); on a cold and snowy day she may engage in self-statements pertaining to accessing positive reinforcement (e.g., "If I run today and get my miles in, I will beat my personal best") or avoid embarrassment (e.g., "If I don't run I may not finish the course and stay with my friend."). If she was a runner in college, she may "hear" (subvocalize) the words from her coach to run faster, be tough, and not give up. Although she may hear the voice of her coach saying the words, she attributes what she is experiencing not as external but as coming from an "internal dialogue" to which she has been exposed and perceived in a prior context. If the verbal behavior is associated with positive reinforcement in the past—winning races, compliments from others—there is a probability that she will emit the same behavior in the future in similar contexts or similar antecedent conditions. These behaviors can become an auditory verbal hallucination (AVH) if there is an error in attribution and the person perceives that the coach is speaking to her and reporting that she hears the voice of her coach talking to her. The AVH that she experiences may be adaptive if it is reinforced when she wins races, beats her previous times, and gets adulation from others. It also can become maladaptive if she cannot control the "voice" of her coach and she overtrains, gets hurt, loses races and results in emotional distress as the "voice" may become punitive and negative in that she hears that she is not tough enough and will never be good enough A predisposition to experiencing auditory hallucination in a person living with SMI is connected to failure in the activation of areas implicated in the normal monitoring of inner speech (McGuire et al., 1996).

Skinner (1953) postulated that repeated causally extended verbal responses evoked by a particular object, event, or property of an object or events may be among the fundamental bases for behavior that is the hallucinatory experience. Metaphorical words and phrases may tell us about the contingencies governing the behavior of others. In sports, a baseball player who excels in championship games may be called "a money player"—that is, his baseball skills improve when there is a great deal of money to be earned. Metaphors have been used and heard by people to explain events (e.g., "it is raining cats and dogs") as well as behaviors (e.g., "she must have gotten the devil in her") throughout the person's life; the individual may also use the same metaphors during periods of subvocal internal speech during self-reflection and self-awareness of one's own behaviors. If repeatedly told as a child that defiance of adults is because of "the devil," using the metaphor is reinforced by others in the person's community, then the metaphorical statement of "the devil made me do it" can result in subvocalizations and be triggered when confronted by sanctioned behaviors (i.e., illegal). Deficits in self-monitoring of self-talk could result in the person "hearing" a voice that is external to oneself. Behavior analysis could assist in uncovering the contingencies governing subvocalization of an individual and occurrences of hallucinations (Layng & Andronis, 1984).

Hallucinations are operant behaviors that operate under the principles of the experimental analysis of human behavior; studies have established that dimensions of hallucinations (e.g., frequency, intensity, antecedental and consequential conditions, self-monitoring) can be altered by the modification of reinforcing stimuli in the environment in which the behavior occurs (Burns et al., 1983; Layng & Andronis, 1984; Powers et al., 2017). A recent systematic review and meta-analysis of research using fMRI identified altered activation in brain regions and related brain networks that were associated with the effects of cognitive-behavior therapy (CBT) in people living with SMI (Yuan et al., 2022), showing the plasticity of the neurological substrates to therapeutic environmental manipulations. Given that hallucinations can be affected by the alteration of antecedental and consequential environmental stimuli (Burns et al., 1983; Lincoln & Peters, 2019), it is plausible that hallucinations can be functionally analyzed using the principles of ABA.

Ćurčić-Blake et al. (2017) summarized the four major hypotheses as to the causal phenomenon of auditory hallucinations: (1) memory intrusion into the processing of language; (2) disrupted self-monitoring and self-awareness of inner speech; (3) aberrant cerebral lateralization; and (4) disrupted top-down and bottom-up processing of incoming sensory information (i.e., sensory data coming from the sense organs to the brain and vice versa).

The available evidence suggests that hallucinations result from a failure of the metacognitive skills involved in discriminating between self-generated and external sources of information (López-Silva et al., 2022). Internal verbalizations of thought (i.e., endophasia) are postulated as subvocalizations pertaining to internal and external stimuli such as memories, sensations, and perceptions. Individuals experiencing hallucinations state that the hallucinatory experience is related to former sensory (e.g., seen, heard, felt) events that are recalled from memory. In a study of hallucinations, McCarthy-Jones et al. (2014) concluded that 39% of participants reported that their voices appeared to be replays of memories of previous conversations they had experienced; 45% reported that the general theme or content of what the voices said was always the same; and 55% said new voices had the same content/theme as previous voices. The findings suggest that an aspect of the phenomenon of hallucinations needs to include memory and recall of previous perceptual events as an aspect of an explanatory and causative model. What is experienced during a hallucination does not appear to be random perceptual events but is related to previous experiences with related stimuli.

Hallucinations are hypothesized as speech that is characterized as silent expressions of thought through the covert production of words in one's conscious awareness (López-Silva et al., 2022); it is the activity of talking to oneself in silence related to internal states and processes such as consciousness, self-awareness, self-regulation and higher order cognitive process such as comprehending and understanding the events that are occurring—to control and predict one's personal internal and external environment. It is likely that different aspects of these skills are implicated in different types of hallucinatory experiences (López-Silva et al., 2022). López-Silva et al. (2022) questions whether hallucinations are in fact an aspect of delusions that are reported as perceptions. During a mental health evaluation, hallucinations are assessed by asking the individual if they hear, see, smell, and feel a sensation that is not real (e.g., "Have you heard voices or other sounds that no one else can hear? How often do you hear them? What do the voices sound like? Do they seem to be inside or outside your head?"). The demand of the question sets up the conditions for the response to be a perceptually related experience; an alternative is that the internal private event may be a belief of the person that he is sensing something that is not there and is related to a covert self-statement about their experiences. Such a cognitive error may be related to problems in metacognition, in self-awareness, and attribution.

Attribution is a metacognitive skill involved in an individual's perception of the cause of events and behaviors (Davis et al., 2017). It is a covert probabilistic statement based on the history of reinforcement of an association between what is sensed and the outcome or consequence. It involves making decisions regarding causality based the four dimensions of attribution theory (Davis et al., 2017): (1) internality: the perceived source of the cause, whether internal or external; (2) stability: whether the cause is perceived to be permanent or transient; (3) controllability: whether and to what extent the cause is perceived to be controllable; and (4) globality: if the cause is perceived to affect many other situations. This theory helps explain how people attribute the reasons behind their own and others' behaviors. Problems with attribution skills can result if there are deficits in considering alternatives to initial perceptions and experiences, such as not considering other solutions and explanations to a problem or an experience.

Powers et al. (2017) conducted a study using classical conditioning to establish conditioned hallucinations in four groups of people with varying voice-hearing and treatment-seeking statuses. The conclusions were that people who hear voices were significantly more susceptible to conditioned hallucinations, regardless of whether they sought treatment. Participants experiencing frequent hallucinations endorsed significantly more conditioned hallucinations than those without. People who experienced hallucinations were more confident in the reality of the conditioned hallucinations. Both conditioned hallucinations and confidence in the reality of the conditioned hallucinations correlated with the severity of hallucinatory experiences in daily life. Participants experiencing hallucinations exhibited stronger perceptual beliefs about the hallucinatory experiences and were less sensitive to changes in contingencies during the conditioning. Functional neuroimaging and identified brain processes and circuits mediating conditioned hallucinations differentiated voice-hearers from nonvoice-hearers.

The results show that individuals who experience hallucinations have a "proneness" toward being conditioned about other false perceptions and attribute the conditioned experience to an actual percept in the absence of none—identical to the self-reports of experiencing hallucinations that are assumed to indicate a mental health problem or symptom. The question remains whether this difference is a learned response, an artifact of the demands of the psychiatric evaluation or a biologically determined problem in metacognitive skills. Being prone to being conditioned to other perceptual disturbances may be related to a finding by Lim et al. (2016). It was noted that there appears to be an additive progression of types of hallucinations in order of descending frequency to explain the considerable overlap between various types of hallucinations, and the finding that somatic/tactile and olfactory hallucinations were not reported by the participants without the appearance of auditory and visual hallucinations. Lim et al. (2016) speculated that the networks involved in the mediation of hallucinations may serve as points of origin in the perceptual network, which promotes the generation of other sensory modalities to mediate multimodal hallucinations. One component in this speculation could very well be a liability to condition related to other perceptual disturbances.

In a review of cognitive mechanisms related to auditory hallucinations, Bell et al. (2024) reported that auditory hallucinations are the perception of sound without external stimuli, often linked to inner speech or fragmented memories. Models suggest that auditory hallucinations involve difficulties in recognizing self-generated mental events, language processing, and weighing and judging of perceptual input. Cognitive mechanisms implicated in hallucinations include auditory signal detection, source monitoring, memory functions, attention modulation, language processes, and emotion detection. Meta-analyses show associations between auditory hallucinations and self-monitoring bias, externalizing source monitoring errors, and reduced left-hemispheric language lateralization.

Studies by Bell et al. (2024) and Bere et al. (2024) showed significant impairments in signal detection (i.e., making errors) when detecting targeted auditory stimuli among background noise, working memory, verbal fluency, and identifying the source of stimuli when distinguishing self from other stimuli (i.e., source monitoring), as well as the temporal context of when stimuli were presented. Conclusions were not able to be drawn (either due to insignificant, or inconsistent findings) with respect to recognition and recall memory (i.e., more basic measures of memory processes), attention, inhibition (i.e., the ability to block out irrelevant stimuli), emotional processing, language comprehension, and misattribution errors for form and spatial context (i.e., incorrectly recalling a stimuli or event for a different stimulus).

Using a sample of nearly 5000 individuals living with SMI and experiencing auditory hallucinations, Bell et al. (2024) found significant associations in nine out of 21 cognitive subdomains, including spatial context attribution, language comprehension, and working memory. Perceptual decision-making and imagery showed reduced sensitivity/accuracy for "signal to noise" discrimination and increased vividness/weighting of imagery in relation to the experience of hallucinations. Monitoring the source and context memory of the false percept indicated greater challenges in distinguishing temporal order, spatial location, and internal-external stimulus sources in relation to auditory hallucinations, which supports individuals experiencing hallucinations reporting that the hallucinated content was generated externally. General memory domains showed associations between auditory hallucination presence/severity and difficulties with the span of recall, recognition capacity, and working memory; verbal fluency and language comprehension capacity in relation to auditory hallucinations were also diminished. Executive functions and emotional processing domains underscored the reduced capacities in inhibition, attention, and accurate detection of emotional expressions in relation to hallucinations. Significant findings were found for difficulties in signal detection and monitoring for source of experience for both auditory and visual stimuli. The authors conclude that the generation and the experience of hallucinations were connected to the general cognitive challenges that have been faced by individuals living with SMI (Green, 2006; Wood et al., 2009).

In a recent systematic review of research specific to auditory hallucinations and cognitive mechanisms, findings have revealed significant impairments in signal detection (i.e., making errors when detecting targeted auditory stimuli among background noise) with individuals who experience auditory hallucinations (Bere et al., 2024). Signal detection theory (SDT) deals with the detectability of signals and controlling the criteria that are used for the detection of signals; that is, determining the threshold when a person attends to and registers sensory input. The theory of signal detection allows for the ability to separate the effects of stimulus detectability in experiments in which there is sensory input involving the occurrence of a behavior (Heeger, 2007). SDT has application in psychophysics and has similarities between signal detection and operant conditioning research and the immediate feedback of rewards and penalties among multiple schedules (Nevin, 1969).

It has been suggested that hallucinations are a result of the inability of an individual to distinguish if an object is real or if it is a product of the imagination. Hallucinations could be caused by a deficit in the metacognitive capacity of the assessment and discrimination of what percepts are real and what are not (Slade & Bentall, 1988). The hypothesis that people who experience hallucinations have impairments in the metacognitive skill of reality testing was tested using the methodology of signal detection theory (SDT). SDT is a concept that can be used to analyze the problem of whether auditory hallucinations arise from a sensory or judgmental disorder. Participants were assessed on a scale measuring a predisposition to experience hallucination and were then tested on an auditory SDT task. Participants more disposed to experience hallucinations significantly differed on a measure of perceptual bias from others. These results support the hypothesis that individuals prone to experience hallucinations are more liable to make errors in reality testing and to identify imaginary events as real (Bentall & Slade, 1985).

Experiments have applied the concept of SDT in the study of the hallucinatory phenomenon by calling for the participant to decide whether a voice was present in a burst of noise (Varese et al., 2012). In these tasks, individuals experiencing hallucinations tend to show a bias toward responding that a voice is present in the noise. Signal detection abnormalities were also evident in individuals who had a history of or were presently experiencing hallucinations. The SDT results were determined to not be a pathological dissociative symptom due to a history of trauma but a problem in metacognition (Varese et al., 2012). Ishigaki and Tanno (1999) used a visual continuous performance test (CPT) to investigate sensory discrimination ability (e.g., detecting signal from noise) and decision bias of individuals experiencing auditory hallucinations. These results suggest that hallucinations are characterized by a cognitive deficit of maintaining a relatively risk-taking decision bias despite decreased discriminating ability.

In a review of research on the cognitive characteristics of hallucinations across sensory modalities, other cognitive mechanisms have been studied, the most frequent being memory and perceptual processes. The findings were consistent with the existing literature on auditory hallucinations, which has seen a predominant focus on auditory source monitoring, context memory, the factors of auditory processes and the extent of processes of speech (Anthony, 2004; Upthegrove et al., 2016). Other cognitive mechanisms, such as attention, working memory, and inhibition, have been investigated but to a slightly lesser extent (Anthony, 2004; Upthegrove et al., 2016). Given the limited nature of the existing research on non-auditory hallucinations, future research needs to build on the current body of findings from the auditory hallucinations literature in exploring possible relationships among cognitive mechanisms such as source monitoring, signal detection, varying components of inhibition, and sensory processing in the hallucinatory experience in other modalities (Bere et al., 2024). Future research could focus on identifying whether hallucinations across different sensory modalities share global deficits, have cognitive determinants that are specific to a modality or a combination of both by understanding the interplay between modality-general and modality-specific processes for both cognitive and neural aspects of the hallucinatory experience (Fernyhough, 2019).

From a phenomenological perspective, hallucinations in individuals living with SMI are not primarily sensory-perceptual but rather a cognitive phenomenon arising from problems in certain functions of self-consciousness (i.e., self-awareness). Functions of self-consciousness are a feature of "metacognition"; metacognition is the process of thinking about one's own thinking, or the awareness and understanding of one's thought processes, which makes up self-awareness. It involves the actions people use to plan, monitor, and assess their understanding and performance and the awareness of one's own cognitive processes that involve a conscious attempt to control the processes (American Psychological Association, n.d.-h). It stands to reason that different types of hallucinations may be different in phenomenon than just the sensory experience, but the metacognitive events involved.

Delusional thinking and hallucinations occur concurrently for many people experiencing and living with SMI (Telles-Correia et al., 2015). There is an issue if delusions and hallucinations are part of the same processes. Hallucinations and delusional thoughts share phenomenological features, such as having a self-centered, autocentric, self-referential perspective that centers around oneself and relates everything back to one's own experiences, opinions, or interests (Humpston et al., 2019). Hallucinations and delusions share alterations in contextual dimensions and deviations from shared realities with others. This is manifested in "voices" that comment and/or make demands about an individual's behaviors, delusions about other people (such as erotomaniac delusions) or thought interference (e.g., delusions of control, thought insertion, thought withdrawal, and thought broadcasting), and in delusions of reference and persecution in which the person having the false belief is the referential "target." Recent empirical analyses indicate that hallucinations experienced by a person involve both cognitive and perceptual mechanisms. The experience during a hallucination is a percept that is internally generated, is not derived from any incoming sensory information, and is not in agreement with the reality of others. The delusional belief likewise is generated internally and is not in agreement with the beliefs and perceptions of others. One can question if this is the same process and whether hallucinations are a manifestation of delusions (Humpston et al., 2019).

In conclusion, hallucinations appear to be a phenomenon that is mediated by both neural substrates, various cognitive mechanisms, and experiential events. There is evidence that hallucinations are prominent symptoms of dysfunctions of the brain, in which there are biological substrates. Hallucinations occur in conditions that are associated with neurological insults and the resulting alterations of the neural connections and neurochemistry of the brain (Ali et al., 2011). However, hallucinations are a cognitive phenomenon that can only be assessed through formal verbal reports as to whether they are occurring or not; that is, there are no laboratory tests that can be done to confirm the presence of hallucinations. Hallucinations can be altered through environmental changes such as prompting and reinforcement, as well as training in self-monitoring and self-awareness skills that alter the dimensions of hallucinatory experiences. It has been noted that in auditory hallucinations, what is "heard" is related to experiences of the person having the hallucinations.

From the results of the research, hallucinations have both biological and environmental components. There are obvious organic and possibly genetic reasons for a person developing hallucinations, but the phenotypic display of the hypothesized genetic liability can be influenced by environmental factors. Using diabetes as an analogy, a person may be living with diabetes, which is caused by alterations and deficits in certain enzymes. Diabetes can have a genetic component, but having a genetic liability does not confirm with certainty that a person will develop the diabetic condition. The effects of diabetes can be ameliorated by environmental changes such as diet, exercise, and monitoring blood glucose. Type 2 diabetes mellitus (T2DM) is more influenced by the environment as obesity, sedentary lifestyles, smoking, use of alcohol, and stress impact the effects of T2DM. T2DM appears to have an inheritable genetic component, but the amount of the contribution is debatable. The adverse effects associated with the phenotypic expression of T2DM can be mitigated through targeted environmental and behavioral modifications. Based on insights from research into hallucinations, it appears that neurological, psychological, and behavioral interactions may exhibit comparable patterns.

A comprehensive understanding of the phenomenology of hallucinations is essential for developing accurate models of their causes but presently is lacking. The field is confronted with the use of a small sample size, methodological inconsistencies, lack of consistent operational definition of the hallucinatory phenomenon, control of dimensional factors in themselves or covariates, mental health conditions, and medications. There is a need for transdiagnostic and continuum-based research and better measurement of hallucinations across different sensory modalities. A multidimensional framework is recommended for understanding hallucinatory experiences, emphasizing transdiagnostic investigations at the symptom level.

Epidemiological Considerations

Hallucinations are a phenomenon that occurs in the general population, with a substantial minority of individuals without documented mental health problems reporting hallucinatory experiences (Bentall, 1990). Surveying a large sample of over 13,000 participants in three countries of the European Union, Ohayon (2000) reported that 38.7% had hallucinatory experiences, with over 92% of the experiences occurring during alterations in consciousness, such as periods just before awakening (6.6%) or falling asleep (24.8%) (known as hypnopompic and hypnogogic hallucinations, respectively (Shahrokh & Hales, 2003)) or using psychoactive substances. The median age for the people who reported hallucinations was 32 years, and over two-thirds were female (68.9%). Auditory hallucinations were the most frequently reported (29.4%), followed by visual (21.5%), tactile (19.9%), and olfactory hallucinations (17.3%). Reports of hallucinations were reported more frequently by younger females and respondents with lower educational attainment. Most participants experienced hallucinations less than once weekly, with the experience lasting only a few seconds, but some respondents reported daily occurrences, with the duration more than 10 min. Around half of the participants had experienced hallucinations for 10 years or longer, with a significant portion experiencing moderate emotional distress due to the occurrence. A small percentage of participants were convinced of the reality of their hallucinations, and some reported receiving commands from their hallucinations. The survey also revealed that delusions were more common among those with recent hallucinations, with delusions of paranoia, reference, and grandeur being the most frequent types (Ohayon, 2000; Stompe et al., 2007).

It should be noted that hypnopompic and hypnagogic hallucinations would not be included in the definition of hallucinations that is presently being used. They are classified as pseudohallucinations as defined by López-Silva et al. (2022) in that the percepts are usually vivid auditory or visual experiences without corresponding external stimuli that the individual recognizes as not real. The person also recognizes that the perceptual distortion is from an internal source (López-Silva et al., 2022). The term hallucination, as defined in the DSM-5 (American Psychiatric

Association, 2013), "is not ordinarily applied to the false perception that occur during dreaming, while falling asleep (hypnagogic), or upon awakening(hypnopompic)." (American Psychiatric Association, 2013, p. 822). Perceptual disturbances occurring during the use of substances were defined as hallucinosis in the DSM-5 (American Psychiatric Association, 2013); the present nomenclature for this condition is a substance use disorder with "perceptual disturbances."

Linscott and van Os (2013) have concluded that about 20% of individuals who experience hallucinations and have persistent occurrences are later classified as living with an SMI. Risk factors that significantly contribute to a conversion to SMI mental health problems are age when initially experiencing the hallucination, minority and migrant status, income, education, employment, marital status, alcohol use, cannabis use, stress, urbanicity, and family history of mental health problems. People who report having persistent hallucinations usually have a history of trauma and less awareness and control of the hallucinatory experiences (Swyer & Powers, 2020).

In general, researchers have found that between 60% and 80% of individuals living with SMI experience auditory-visual hallucinations, with a smaller proportion having visual hallucinations or other unimodal hallucinations (Lim et al., 2016; McCarthy-Jones et al., 2017). In a study investigating the prevalence and cooccurrence of hallucinations across different sensory modalities (auditory, visual, olfactory, and tactile) in individuals living with schizophrenia spectrum disorders, McCarthy-Jones et al. (2017) reported the following key findings:

- Lifetime prevalence: Auditory hallucinations are the most frequent type of hallucination, with 64–80% having experienced this type during the individual's lifetime followed by visual (23–31%), tactile (TH) (9–19%), and olfactory hallucinations (OH) (6–10%).
- Point prevalence (occurring in the past month): Experiencing a type of hallucination within the previous month occurs in the same order of frequency, with auditory hallucinations being most frequent (23–27%), followed by visual (5–8%), tactile (4–7%), and olfactory (2%).
- Cooccurrence: Most people report experiencing a hallucination in only one modality, predominantly auditory. About one-third experience hallucinations in two modalities, commonly auditory and visual. Visual hallucinations are highly likely to co-occur with auditory hallucinations (83–97%).
- Content of hallucinations: Auditory hallucinations often involve voices with religious or demonic themes. Visual hallucinations include seeing people change into vampires, flames, or religious figures. Tactile hallucinations involve sensations like burning or poking. Olfactory hallucinations include unusual smells like burning rubber or roses.
- Demographic factors: Age and gender did not contribute to the prediction of having a hallucinatory experience.

Dudley, Denton et al. (2023) and Dudley, Watson et al. (2023) reported that hallucinations across multiple sensory modalities are common in people with a first episode of experiencing psychotic symptoms, with visual and tactile hallucinations being reported by over half of participants. Multimodal hallucinations (MMH), where hallucinatory experiences occur simultaneously, are more frequent than multisensory hallucinations (MSH), which occur at different times and are unrelated. A greater number of hallucinations is associated with higher levels of delusional ideation and distress but not with reduced functioning. Current psychological treatments primarily focus on auditory hallucinations and may not adequately address the full range of sensory experiences reported by people living with a psychotic-type mental health problem. The results obtained by Dudley, Denton et al. (2023) are like previous results obtained by McCarthy-Jones et al. (2017), with auditory hallucinations being most frequently experienced (70–80%), followed by visual hallucinations (27%), tactile (9.3–19.3%), and olfactory (5.8–9.6%). In a transdiagnostic group of participants, 100% reported auditory type, 81.3% visual, 52.5% tactile, 35% olfactory, and 13.8% gustatory. Lifetime prevalence of experiencing a hallucination in two or more sensory modalities is twice as frequent (53%) as single sensory hallucinations (27%). Only 27.9% of participants reported experiencing only unimodal auditory hallucinations. Those with multiple hallucinations reported higher levels of anxiety.

Other studies have reported similar findings. Toh et al. (2019) found that 53% of a sample with symptoms associated with psychosis reported visual hallucinations, 46% tactile, 36% olfactory, and 18% gustatory hallucinations (GH). Isaacson et al. (2022) found high rates of hallucinatory experiences during the first episode of experiencing symptoms associated with SMI. Auditory types were experienced by 88% participants, 68% experienced visual type, 26% tactile, and 8% olfactory. Although the percentages differ across the studies mentioned, all the results are in accordance with the most to least frequently reported types of hallucinatory experience, with the auditory type being experienced most frequently, followed by visual, tactile, and olfactory. Although the gustatory type was not mentioned in the results, this type usually occurs simultaneously with olfactory hallucinations as a multimodal hallucinatory dimension. For example, unusual smells, such as burning flesh or rubber, may be accompanied by an epigastric sensation of "butterflies in the stomach" and facial flushing. An individual living with SMI who experiences the smell of burning flesh may have distressing associations (e.g., hell, the devil), while the depressed person smells her body rotting or giving off noxious fumes. The two types of hallucinations may occur simultaneously as these types are associated with temporal or frontal lobe pathology, particularly in the form of temporal lobe epilepsy (Spence, 2009).

Dudley, Watson, et al. (2023) reported that the median annual incidence of experiencing hallucinatory behaviors associated with SMI is 2.5%, with a lifetime prevalence of 7.2%. A greater frequency of experiencing hallucinations over time is associated with more traumatic adverse experiences and poorer clinical outcomes.

Cultural Considerations

Culture significantly influences the perception, symptoms, and problem behaviors associated with SMI; it is estimated that 15–40% of the variability in the frequency and dimensions of symptoms and behavior problems associated with SMI is attributable to cross-cultural differences (Ghanem et al., 2023). Lifetime prevalence rates of mental health problems associated with living with SMI are 1.5–3 times higher in Asian and African cultures compared to European-American counterparts (Ghanem et al., 2023). AHs are the most frequently reported type of hallucination experienced across cultures, with the highest 1-year prevalence at 74.8%, followed by visual hallucinations at 39.1%, cenesthetic (i.e., a subtype of somatic) at 28.9%, and tactile, olfactory, and gustatory types ranging from 1.3% to 6.6%. Auditory hallucinations were most prevalent in all countries, with the highest rates in Ghana (90.8%) and Nigeria (85.4%) and the lowest in Austria (66.9%) (Bauer et al., 2011). Although there were a higher number of male participants experiencing hallucinations, statistical analyses showed no significant sex differences in the prevalence of hallucinations (Bauer et al., 2011).

Visual hallucinations were most frequently reported by the West African participants (Nigeria, 50.8%; Ghana, 53.9%), but only 3.9% in Pakistani individuals. Cenesthetic hallucinations were most prevalent in Ghana, followed by European countries and Pakistan, with no significant differences found for tactile hallucinations. Olfactory and gustatory hallucinations were more common in European countries and relatively rare in non-European societies, except Nigeria. Individuals in Austria or Georgia showed significantly lower rates of auditory hallucinations, while those with an earlier age at onset of illness reported them more often. Visual hallucinations were more common in younger people and those of West African origins. Cenesthetic hallucinations were more prevalent after a long course of illness and in individuals living in Ghana or Austria (Bauer et al., 2011; Thomas et al., 2007).

The content of hallucinations differed across cultures, with Latinos reporting religious advisory-commanding voices, while European-Americans exhibited higher rates of grandiose delusions, reflecting cultural values of family interdependence in Latin cultures and individualism in Western cultures. Hallucinations are often attributed to religious-spiritual explanations and are prevalent in African, Asian, and highly religious Western cultures (Ghanem et al., 2023).

Visual hallucinations are reported significantly more frequently in non-Western cultures, specifically West African countries, where the experience occurs on average several times a year (Bauer et al., 2011; Ghanem et al., 2023). The content of the visual hallucination is sensitive to cultural interpretations such as "jinn" (i.e., spirits in Muslim demonology that inhabit the earth, assume various forms, and exercise supernatural powers (Merriam-Webster, n.d.) in Pakistani culture (Ghanem et al., 2023). Younger individuals reported a significantly higher prevalence of visual hallucinations. The significantly higher prevalence of visual hallucinations in non-Western societies may be due to cultural differences in perceptual and attentional processing (Bauer et al., 2011).

Types of Hallucinations

A hallucination is a perception (something seen, smelled, felt, or heard) in the absence of any stimulus to cause that perception. Hallucinations may be harmless, such as hearing odd noises or hearing a voice that repeats the same word. However, the hallucinations can also be tormenting, such as when the voices repeatedly say that the person living with SMI is evil, doesn't deserve to live, calls them names, and accuses the person of misdeeds, such as being a child abuser, murderer, or pedophile.

Hallucinations occur in all sensory modalities. Below are the types of hallucinations. Some occur more frequently in SMI than others.

- Auditory hallucinations (AH) are the most common type experienced by people living with SMI; lifetime prevalence is reported by 64–80% of people experiencing hallucinations; 23–27% of the participants report experiencing this type within the previous month (McCarthy-Jones et al., 2017). Auditory hallucinations involve hearing sounds, music, and voices. It is the perception of sound in the absence of an auditory stimulus or percept coming from the immediate environment (American Psychiatric Association, 2022a). The content of an auditory hallucination may be of accusatory or laudatory voices, recognizable or not, strange noises, and other nonverbal sounds. If voices occur, then the hallucination is an auditory verbal hallucination (AVH) (Garwood et al., 2015). Auditory hallucinations and auditory-visual hallucinations occur frequently in people living with schizophrenic spectrum disorders and other psychotic conditions but may be associated with other conditions as well (e.g., delirium, dementia, depression, posttraumatic stress disorder (PTSD), personality disorders) (Ali et al., 2011; American Psychiatric Association, 2022b). The content of what the person "hears" ranges from humorous to derogatory; at times the auditory hallucinations are described as "white noise," one word or a repeated phrase, or hearing a comment about what they is doing (Andrew, 2010). Auditory hallucinations are frequently described as "hearing voices"; sometimes the individual experiencing this type can identify the voice. The "voices" can be singular or multiple and speaks to the person experiencing the auditory hallucination in the first, second, or third person; at times, if multiple "voices" occur, the "voices" are heard to be conversing with each other. In their most serious form, the "voices" tells or "commands" the person living with SMI to engage in behaviors that are dangerous or offensive to others (e.g., "hit her" or "hurt her") or to hurt themselves (e.g., cut your arm). This type of hallucination is a "command hallucination" (Andrew, 2010). Command hallucinations are relatively common among individuals living with SMI, with reported prevalence rates among adult persons ranging from 18% to 89%, with a median of 53% (Buccheri et al., 2007; Rogers et al., 1990). People who experience command type of hallucinations respond with varying levels of compliance being reported, with the response typically being noncompliance or appeasement (Bucci et al., 2013). Prevalence rates for "dangerous or harmful" command hallucinations range from 7% to 70%, with a median of 48% (Shawyer et al., 2003). Experiencing a command hallucination, the frequency and the intensity of the hallucination, and the emotional distress of experiencing the command hallucination has been found to be a risk factor for future dangerousness in persons living with SMI (Monahan et al., 2001). The presence of command hallucinations often does not improve with treatment adherence (Andrew, 2010; Braham et al., 2004).

- Visual hallucinations (VH) are experienced as visual perceptions in the absence of any external stimulus. This type of hallucination may be unformed (e.g., shapes, colors) or complex (e.g., figures, faces, scenes) (American Psychiatric Association, 2013) involving seeing objects that are not in the immediate environment or extreme distortions of objects that are in the environment (Dudley et al., 2019). For example, the person may see bugs crawling all over the room. The lifetime prevalence of the reporting of the occurrence of visual hallucinations is approximately 23–31% of people living with SMI (Aynsworth et al., 2017; McCarthy-Jones et al., 2017), with 5–8% reporting the experience of visual hallucinations within the past month (McCarthy-Jones et al., 2017).
- Visual hallucinations may arise in association with lesions of the peripheral or central visual pathway or visual cortical areas, related to metabolic (e.g., withdrawal from alcohol, effects of some drugs) and neurodegenerative conditions, as well as seizures and other adverse neurologic events (Teeple et al., 2009). Visual hallucinations are often present in temporal lobe epilepsy and may appear during prolonged isolation (Ali et al., 2011; American Psychiatric Association, 2022b). Visual hallucinations are either elementary (e.g., simple streaks, patterns, or blurs of color) or complex (e.g., detailed images of animals or people). Typically, people see complex hallucinations, such as people, figures, or faces. Less commonly, people experience simple visual hallucinations, such as lines, dots, or flashes of light (Aynsworth et al., 2017). Visual hallucinations can also be geometric shapes and experienced as tunnels, funnels, spirals, lattices, or cobwebs (American Psychiatric Association, 2013; Dudley et al., 2019). Many people experiencing visual hallucinations report that they are aware that the hallucinations are not real and do not feel distressed that the hallucinations are threatening (Mocellin et al., 2006). Some authors have suggested that visual hallucinations can be experienced more frequently than auditory types (Delespaul et al., 2002).
- Tactile hallucinations (TH) are false sensations that occur in or to the body and are a type of somatic hallucination. A tactile hallucination is the perception of being touched or something moving under the skin. Tactile hallucinations are commonly experienced as electric shocks or something creeping or crawling under the skin. (American Psychiatric Association, 2022b). The lifetime prevalence of the reporting of the occurrence of tactile hallucinations is approximately 9–19% of people living with SMI (McCarthy-Jones et al., 2017), with 4–7% reporting the experience of this type within the past month (McCarthy-Jones et al., 2017). A subtype of tactile hallucination is a cenesthetic hallucination. This subtype is experienced as a burning sensation in the brain, a stinging sensation in the blood vessels, a cutting sensation in the bone marrow, a feeling of wires or coils in the oral region, or a tightening, burning, pressure, or tickling in somatic areas (Chaudhury, 2010). This subtype of hallucination is relatively rare

and is usually associated with a brain injury or a neurological problem such as a severe blow to the head, stroke, or seizure disorder.

- Olfactory hallucinations (OH) (phantosmia) involve the sense of smell and are a perception of an odor. It is usually experienced as a noxious odor such as burning or rotting flesh, brimstone, or decaying fish. The lifetime prevalence of the reporting of the occurrence of olfactory hallucinations is approximately 6–10% of people living with SMI (McCarthy-Jones et al., 2017), with 2% reporting the experience of olfactory hallucinations within the past month (McCarthy-Jones et al., 2017). Individuals living with a schizophrenic spectrum SMI may experience the odor as coming from an external source, whereas persons living with a depressive type of SMI may perceive the source as internal; they may perceive that they are the source of the offensive odor—a condition known as "olfactory reference syndrome"—and may engage in washing excessively, overusing deodorants and perfumes, or isolating from others as they are concerned about offending others because of the odor (Ali et al., 2011).
- Gustatory hallucination (GH) involves the perception of taste, which is usually unpleasant (American Psychiatric Association, 2013). Individuals having gustatory hallucination may experience salivation, sensation of thirst, or taste alterations. Olfactory and gustatory hallucinations often occur in conjunction with each other (Mueser et al., 1990). This phenomenon is not surprising given the close connection between the sense of smell and sensations of appetites and taste.
- Mood-congruent and mood-incongruent hallucinations involve the content of the hallucination and whether it is consistent with the overall mood of the person experiencing a hallucination (American Psychiatric Association, 2013). Mood congruency is the agreement between a particular expressed feeling and the general emotional context within which it occurs. Thus, the themes or contents of a hallucinatory experience are mood congruent if there is consistency between the expression of the characteristics or patterns of the hallucinatory experience and the exhibited mood of the person having the hallucination. Inconsistencies in the person's mood and the themes and content of the hallucination are described as mood incongruent (American Psychological Association, n.d.-i).

Hallucinations frequently occur in more than one sensory modality, either perceived simultaneously or sequentially, including those hallucinations that are or are not linked to the same identified source by the person experiencing the hallucinations (Moseley & Mitrenga, 2022). Hallucinations occurring in more than one sensory modality are labeled as multimodal hallucinations (MMH) and are also known as polymodal hallucinations, polysensual hallucinations, polysensory hallucinations, polysensorial hallucinations, intersensorial hallucinations, and fantastic hallucinations (Moseley & Mitrenga, 2022).

Multimodal hallucinations have been reported to be more prevalent than auditory hallucinations, with 27% of the participants reporting unimodal hallucinations and 53% reporting multimodal hallucinations (Dudley, Denton et al., 2023; Dudley, Watson et al., 2023). Twenty-nine percent of individuals experiencing hallucinations reported occurrences in two sensory modalities, while 7% experienced them in three modalities, and 8% in four modalities. Auditory hallucinations were the most commonly observed type among both unimodal (68%) and multimodal (88%) groups, followed by visual, somatic/tactile, and olfactory hallucinations (Moseley & Mitrenga, 2022).

Not all individuals identified as living with SMI experience hallucinations, and conversely, not everyone who hallucinates is living with SMI (Linszen et al., 2022). Hallucinations can also occur in those who are not affected by SMI but have been subjected to considerable stress, such as life-threatening situations. In these cases, the frequency of hallucinations typically diminishes as the stressful circumstances resolve, and the individual feels more at ease. Conversely, for individuals with SMI, hallucinations may persist even in calm environments when no apparent distress or troubling factors are present.

Additionally, individuals who experience hallucinations may not necessarily report or express concern about them. It is common for people living with SMI to exhibit responsive behaviors such as speaking to individuals not present, laughing or giggling without a clear external cause, or appearing to search for something that is not there, while displaying little or no distress regarding these experiences. Furthermore, such individuals may be unwilling or unable to acknowledge the presence of hallucinations when asked, which may stem from limited awareness or insight into their own behavior, or from efforts to avoid potential stigmatization.

Why Do Hallucinations Happen?

There is no singular, identifiable cause for the occurrence of hallucinations. It is probable that multiple factors interact to contribute to their manifestation.

Part of the Reason May Be Biochemical or Physical

- It is often assumed that hallucinations are a result of the chemical imbalance that results in the symptoms and problems associated with SMI. However, scientists have not yet discovered why and how this biochemical process happens. Explanations are lacking as to why hallucinations are not experienced by all people living with SMI who are experiencing extreme stress in their lives. Regardless, most researchers consider a biochemical imbalance in brain chemicals to be a major reason that hallucinations happen. The cause for the chemical imbalance may be due to genetic influence, aversive environmental conditions, neurological insult, substance use, or a combination of these factors.
- Hallucinations may also result from extended periods of malnutrition due to poor eating habits or poor fluid intake. These may result in a lack of what the brain needs to function normally.
- Some types of hallucinations, such as visual and olfactory hallucinations, are more likely to be experienced by people who have suffered some form of brain

injury. These include neurogenerative conditions such as Alzheimer's and Parkinson's, a severe blow to the head from an accident, long-term misuse of mood-altering drugs (including alcohol), and seizures.
- Hallucinations are more likely to happen if the person has sensory problems such as poor hearing or poor vision. This is an important concern if the person is older or in poor physical health. In such circumstances, a different treatment for the hallucinations may be indicated.
- Hallucinations also can be part of a physical illness, such as anemia or respiratory disease, which reduces the amount of oxygen delivered to the brain.

Part of the Reason May Be Environmental

- Environmental stress may play a role in the experience of hallucinations. Individuals living with SMI may experience hallucinations in environments with excessive noise or heightened excitement. Traumatic events, challenging life circumstances, and stressful situations—including job loss or interpersonal conflicts—can exacerbate behavioral manifestations and symptoms such as hallucinations.
- Excessive stimulation, such as heightened noise or excitement, may exacerbate existing mental health conditions; however, insufficient stimulation can also contribute to similar difficulties. Individuals may experience comparable levels of stress when faced with a lack of activity, as when overwhelmed by excessive demands. Research indicates that even individuals without SMI might develop hallucinations in environments deficient in stimulation, suggesting the brain compensates for insufficient external input. A key consideration for service providers is to accurately determine the optimal level of stimulation that individuals living with SMI can tolerate.

How to Change How Often Hallucinations Happen

- To change any behavior, the first step is to engage the person who is experiencing the hallucination in any behavior change plan that is developed. Is the behavior causing the person living with SMI distress, impeding progress in attaining what he wants to do, or impacting his daily functioning? The person experiencing hallucinations may not want the hallucination to be taken away, as the experience may be pleasant and rewarding to him. The individual needs to determine if they desire to change how often, when, and the intensity of the hallucinatory experience. The approach and likelihood of successful intervention will depend on the individual's desired changes and the practitioner's assessment of what can be realistically addressed. While complete elimination of hallucinations may not be feasible, it is possible to manage and modify certain dimensional aspects of hallucinatory behavior.

- Try to prevent or decrease the occurrence of hallucinations. This may be what most service providers want to do—to make them go away in certain situations. Unless you can identify and control the reasons that hallucinations happen, however, this may be an impossible task. If the hallucinations are primarily due to a biochemical imbalance in the brain, psychiatric medications may help in this regard. If external stress is involved, you may be able to keep the environment calm and, in doing so, keep the hallucinations from happening frequently. Often, however, it is impossible to make the hallucinations go away completely, although how often, how loud, how distressful, and when and where can be affected.
- Try to change how the hallucinations affect the person's ability to function daily, take care of himself, and other behaviors. Hallucinations can be highly distracting and challenging for individuals who experience them. Providing consistent support and encouragement is essential to help those living with hallucinations persevere despite their symptoms. Although medications may not eliminate hallucinations entirely, they can often reduce their impact sufficiently so that, with positive reinforcement, individuals living with SMI are able to manage or disregard hallucinations and continue performing necessary daily tasks. Many individuals experiencing hallucinations are still able to maintain routines such as waking on time, practicing good hygiene, adhering to medication schedules, socializing, shopping, and fulfilling other everyday responsibilities.

Behavioral Support Strategies

When focusing on problems that seem to be brought on by hallucinations, consider the following steps. Not all of these will apply in all cases. However, it is very likely that several of these can be used to improve the problems that are observed and help to improve the behavior of the person living with SMI.

- Hallucinations do not necessarily have to be eliminated or stopped completely. Occasionally, hallucinations are not a major problem and can be ignored by others. If the hallucinations do not upset the person who is experiencing them, don't interfere with necessary daily tasks, and do not disrupt other people, there may be no reason to try to stop them. The person who experiences hallucinations may want to acquire the ability to "turn the volume down" on hallucinations in certain situations.
- Consider a review of medications. An evaluation by an experienced psychiatric prescribing service provider can help to determine if medications (or a change in a medication) may be helpful in minimizing the problem behavior. It is generally accepted that a primary benefit of most antipsychotic medications (APs) is their effect on hallucinations either to stop or minimize them; in addition, the medica-

tions help in decreasing the emotional distress of the person having the hallucinatory experience. However, the wrong choice of medications or excessive dosages of medications may bring on hallucinations or other problems as well.

- Consider the general state of health of the person who is experiencing hallucinations. Consider seeking a medical evaluation to assess if various illnesses, infections, or other factors are occurring that may result in strange sensory experiences. This may include such conditions as dizziness, ringing in the ears, irritations of the skin, and inflammation of the joints. It may be helpful to have the person's hearing tested or a hearing aid serviced. With the elderly, poor hearing may lead to "hearing noises" that are difficult to identify clearly, and which can be mistaken for hallucinations. The psychiatric service provider who prescribes medications for the person living with SMI should be able to determine if this is worthwhile. This service provider or another provider may be able to have neurological tests performed to assess for any possible contributing neurological problem.
- Make sure that medications are being taken as prescribed. If medications have been prescribed and the behaviors continue, observe and determine that the medications are being swallowed. Consider whether the medications are being taken according to the prescribed schedule. It does happen that individuals use medications incorrectly; problems are even more likely if the person living with SMI has difficulties with attention or memory. If there continues to be a problem with taking medication on time, it may be possible to change to a form of medication that is active for a longer period (called long acting or LAs) and doesn't have to be taken as often. If the problem is in taking the medication, injectables form of medications and some mood stabilizers that are long acting are available.
- Define the behaviors that are observable evidence of hallucinations. Clearly identify behaviors exhibited by the service user that indicate hallucinations may be problematic. If uncertainty exists regarding whether hallucinations are contributing to concerning behavior, obtain an assessment from a qualified mental health professional. In some cases, the problem may be obvious, such as when the "voices" order or tell the person living with SMI to hit someone. In other cases, the problem behaviors may be less obvious, such as when the person experiencing hallucinations mumbles or has a conversation with other people who are not in the environment.
- Watch for circumstances and events that provoke hallucinatory behaviors to occur. Observe to see if there are any differences when the identified problem behavior occurs, where and with whom it occurs, and what was happening around the person at the time the hallucinations occurred. For example, the staff at the residences noticed that Marsha was more likely to hear voices when there was a lot of noise around her, such as when other people were talking or laughing loudly. Observing and using the forms in the Appendix to collect data greatly assists in identifying such circumstances. If circumstances can be identified, it is often the simplest and most realistic to avoid, decrease, or change the identified circumstances in the future.

What to Do When the Person Starts to Experience Hallucinations

- Remind the person who is having a hallucination that sometimes "your mind plays tricks on you." When the individual living with SMI is not hallucinating, help her to understand that what she is feeling and experiencing are behaviors and symptoms of her living with a mental health problem. If she can accept this, an agreement can be reached about what to do when the hallucinations begin. For instance, an individual living with an SMI may consent to receiving a designated prompt from service providers when hallucinations begin (e.g., "You're starting to giggle and talk to yourself. Remember that we have discussed how your mind can sometimes play tricks on you. Let's go play the piano."). This type of reminder communicates awareness of the hallucination and indicates an intention to support the individual in redirecting their attention toward an alternative, constructive activity.
- Try to get the person who is having the hallucination involved in some other activity. Distract the person from attending to the hallucination by getting him involved in some other activity, such as doing a household chore or going for a walk. Some people who experience hallucinations are easily able to be redirected to another activity, particularly if it is something that is enjoyable. After becoming involved in the other activity, the hallucinations will often stop or decrease in intensity so that the person can exercise some control over the hallucination. For example, Marsha stopped showing evidence of hallucinations when she played the piano. People living with SMI and "hearing voices" sometimes listen to music through some listening device (e.g., earbuds, headphones) to be distracted from the hallucination.
- Ignore it. This may be a realistic choice for many. The first two options may not work. People who experience hallucinations may argue and disagree with your attempts to correct them or get them involved in some other activity that might distract them; the person may deny that they hear voices. For some people living with SMI and hallucinating, more serious problem behaviors, such as arguing, getting angry, and perhaps aggression, may be provoked if an attempt is made to divert attention, and no agreement has been reached about dealing with the hallucinations. For these people, it does not mean to ignore everything that the person is doing. It is important to be clear about what the person living with SMI does correctly and competently. When the person is observed "doing something right," the preferred adaptive behaviors need to be complimented and reinforced. Research has shown that reinforcing any other adaptive behavior does result in decreases in problematic behaviors (Borrero & Vollmer, 2002).
- Simplify the environment. If hallucinations are a persistent problem, try to minimize changes in the environment as much as can be done. If it is necessary to make changes in the environment, try to include familiar objects from the old environment.

- Focus on what the person living with SMI continues to do well. Remember to focus on what the person can do competently. Competently engaging in tasks should not be taken for granted, thinking that "they should know better." Tasks others may perceive as simple may be challenging for the person living with SMI. For many people living with SMI, getting up on time, helping to prepare a meal, and taking medicine as prescribed are accomplishments that deserve recognition and praise. Even if the task can't be done without assistance, the effort merits a compliment.
- Encourage involvement in daily activities that are interesting but not stressful. Hallucinations will be more likely to occur if the person hallucinating has nothing to do and experiences long periods of boredom. Often, the behavior that is associated with hallucinations will be minimized simply by involving the person in preferred activities. Using the example of Marsha, she told other people that she never heard the voices when talking one on one with others or while playing the piano. Watch for activities that the person living with hallucinations seems to enjoy doing and try to make it easier for them to get involved in those activities.
- Prompt and reinforce any capacity for self-control in a person living with SMI. Some people experiencing hallucinations can ignore them and carry on with other activities. While they cannot keep the hallucinations from happening, many can adopt the attitude that it's "just my mental illness" and carry on with their normal daily activities. After some help from staff at the residence, Marsha was able to begin asking staff if they also heard something. She accepted their reply that nothing had been said and then was able to let them help her to become involved in other activities.
- Seek additional assistance if no progress is made. If the problem behavior has not responded to attempts to minimize it, consult an experienced service provider who is skilled in the application of applied behavior analysis (ABA) dealing with problem behaviors in persons living with SMI. While this will most frequently be a clinical psychologist, other mental health service providers may have such skills. Maintain records of observed behavior, noting its occurrence, context, and any variations such as timing, location, or individuals involved. that has been identified.

Conclusion for Behavioral Strategies

When you are trying to stop problems that happen because of hallucinations, consider the following steps:

1. Consult with the psychiatric service provider of the person having hallucinations to find the best medications and proper dosages for the problem.
2. Make sure that the person having hallucinatory experiences is taking the medication as prescribed. If there are concerns about the medications and side effects, consult with the prescriber and be specific about your concerns.

3. Engage with the person hallucinating and agree if the problem is serious enough to consider developing a plan to change a problem behavior that both service provider and user want to change.
4. Observe if circumstances such as where, when, with whom, or anything else seem to make a difference. This helps in developing either a formal or informal support plan on what to do when the problematic behavior occurs. For monitoring forms and examples, see the Appendix.
5. Help the person hallucinating to understand that when the voices start, it is a feature of a mental health problem. Encourage alternative activities in which to get involved. Be sure to compliment examples of cooperation and success.
6. Reinforce and give attention to the person living with SMI when the hallucinations are not happening, and not only when the hallucinations are occurring or causing a problem.
7. Seek consultation from service providers who have experience in behavioral consultation if the efforts to change the behaviors are not working or the behaviors are worsening.

What About Marsha?

At the residence, Marsha had to live with others with whom she was unfamiliar. This made it even more difficult for Marsha to control her hallucinations. She had to be around other people almost all the time and frequently accused the other residents and staff of talking about her. The staff was faced with the challenge of helping her to be around other people without accusing or threatening them. They could not identify the people who she accused or attacked more than other people. When asked by service providers, Marsha denied that she was hearing any voices. The staff at her residence consulted with community service providers knowledgeable in ABA and SMI; they decided that they would change their own behavior when Marsha started to accuse others. They identified several activities that she enjoyed, including playing the piano, talking about certain current events, and several other activities that she liked to do. They began using these activities at times when she wasn't accusing others of talking about her. They also explained to her that hearing voices was "part of her mental health problem." When the voices and accusations began, they reminded her that her mental health problem "makes your mind play tricks on you; it happens to everyone," and invited her to engage in one of the activities that they had identified with her.

The staff changed how they worked with her when she was doing well. They kept track of how long she was able to keep from accusing people or doing other things that seemed to be caused by her hallucinations. When she was able to keep herself "in control" for several hours, they offered to spend time with her and talk about current events or do something else that she wanted to do, like taking a walk or working in the flower garden. As she was able to do better at keeping herself "in control," they gradually increased the time that they expected her to stay in control before seeking her out. Because the change was very gradual, it didn't result in a worsening in Marsha's behavior.

To help Marsha, the staff did the following:

1. They clarified the problem behaviors that resulted from her hallucinations (accusing others of talking about her or cursing at her; hitting other people).
2. They identified several activities that she enjoyed doing (playing the piano, talking about current news events, taking walks, working in the garden).
3. When she was calm, they spent time with her to explain that mental health problems may sometimes make "your mind play tricks on you" and cause her to hear things that aren't real. They also minimized the stigma that exists with living with SMI by telling her that "everyone's minds play tricks every now and then. The key is how to control it."
4. They engaged Marsha in developing the plan and an agreement was reached that they would try to help her if her mind ever started "playing tricks" on her.
5. When Marsha began accusing others of talking about her, the staff suggested that it was "just your problem making you think that way" and offered to work with her on one of the preferred activities. If she agreed, they tried to spend as much time with her as they could.
6. They kept track of how long she was able to remain around other people without making accusations. When she was able to stay "in control" (not accuse or hit) for a specific length of time, they spent brief periods of time with her doing something that she enjoyed.
7. As Marsha was more successful at staying in control, they gradually increased their expectations before offering to spend time with her.

With this plan in place, Marsha accused and hit others less frequently. Although she still talked about hearing the voices, she stated that she can ignore what the voices are saying to her. She is now able to identify the voices as part of a mental health problem and can keep herself from accusing others or hitting them.

Summary

Hallucinations are perceptual experiences without external stimuli, experienced as reality, and are common in severe mental illness (SMI). According to definitions provided by Slade and Bentall (1988) and the DSM-5-TR (American Psychiatric Association, 2022a), hallucinations are characterized by the absence of external stimuli, significant functional impairment, and a lack of voluntary control. Hallucinations may involve any of the senses, with auditory hallucinations being the most prevalent, followed by visual hallucinations. It is estimated that 60–80% of individuals who live with SMI experience both auditory and visual hallucinations.

Hallucinations, pseudohallucinations, illusions, and hallucinosis are similar as they involve perceptual disturbances where a person experiences something that is not real or is a distorted perception of reality, often appearing very vivid and convincing to the individual experiencing it, even though it is not based on the reality of the external stimuli. Because these experiences are based on perceptions and false interpretations of what is perceived, the terms are often confused. Pseudohallucinations are vivid sensory experiences recognized as not real, often occurring in acute distress experienced by people living with mental health problems linked to personality difficulties. Illusions are misinterpretations of real sensory stimuli, while hallucinosis involves persistent hallucinations without consciousness alteration, often due to substance use or neurological conditions. Hallucinosis are perceptual disturbances occurring during substance use and withdrawal while the person is fully aware and conscious. The term "hallucinosis" in DSM-5-TR (American Psychiatric Association, 2022a) has been replaced with "perceptual disturbances" for perceptual abnormalities related to substance use.

Cultural and historical perspectives on hallucinations include religious significance across cultures and philosophical interpretations from Aristotle to Aquinas. The term "hallucination" was first used in 1845 by Jean-Étienne Dominique Esquirol, who viewed it as an involuntary exercise of memory and imagination.

Hallucinations are a multidimensional phenomenon, complex and transdiagnostic. Different types of hallucinations are experienced at different intensities, durations, and with emotional impacts by 10–20% of the general population who have no known mental health issues. Auditory hallucinations (AH) are the most researched subtype, often involving voices with no external source, and can be categorized by the number of voices and their content.

Auditory hallucinations in individuals living with SMI are typically negative, hostile, and emotionally distressing, impacting their daily functioning. Some individuals experience pleasurable hallucinations, which are associated with lower emotional distress and better control over the experience. The complexity of hallucinations includes linguistic elements, multiple modalities, and temporal synchronization, which are important for treatment and engagement. Research suggests that hallucinations may involve memory recall, with 39% of participants reporting voices as replays of past conversations. The DSM-5-TR includes awareness or insight that the percept is not real as part of the definition of hallucinations. Further research is needed on the dimensions of continuity, frequency, intensity, and the impact of hallucinatory experiences.

The field of mental health has recently begun studying the aspect of the control of hallucinations, with 17–20% of individuals occasionally able to control their experiences. Control strategies are categorized into direct and indirect, with indirect strategies involving metacognitive skills and cognitive-behavioral techniques. The relationships between hallucinations and delusions are complex, with some studies suggesting a causative link between repeated hallucinations and delusional thinking.

The Psychotic Symptom Rating Scale (PSYRATS) was used to assess various dimensions of hallucinations, including frequency, duration, intensity, and control in a sample of individuals living with schizophrenia spectrum mental health problems. The results showed that 67% of participants experienced hallucinations cooccurring with delusional thinking. Common delusion themes occurring and experiencing hallucinations include persecutory (51%) and mystical/religious

(31%) themes. Determinants of the dimensions of hallucinations included beliefs about the origin of hallucinations (internal or external), control, and the amount of negative content. More research is needed to understand the relationship between hallucinations and delusions and to develop effective therapeutic strategies.

Hallucinations have complex origins, substrates, subtypes, and cognitive-behavioral processes in various medical and mental health conditions. Hallucinations are severe symptoms found in various conditions, including schizophrenia spectrum mental health problems, Parkinson's disease, dementia, and other CNS disorders. Hallucinations are complex in origin with genetic, neurological, cognitive, and environmental influences, but no common neurological pathway has yet been identified. Hallucinations can occur in all sensory areas and are influenced by cognitive and emotional responses, as well as environmental stimuli, highlighting the interdependence of brain activity and mental states.

Research in understanding the experience of hallucinations involves neurological mechanisms, brain regions, and imaging techniques, emphasizing the need for consistent definitions and further research. Research focuses on the neurological mechanisms underlying hallucinations, with brain scans like MRI and fMRI used to study brain activity.

Key brain areas activated during hallucinations include the sensory cortices, limbic system, insula, anterior cingulate cortex, and thalamus. Increased activity in brain regions associated with auditory sensation, speech production, and working memory is noted during subvocal speech tasks similar to what is found in hallucinations. Consistent operational definitions of hallucinations are crucial for reliable research results, considering the debate over pseudohallucinations and perceptual disturbances.

Studies have predominantly focused on auditory hallucinations, but more research is needed on multimodal hallucinations (MMH) (i.e., hallucinatory experiences in more than one modality), which occur with moderate to high empirical probability by individuals living with SMI.

Hallucinations are transdiagnostic, heterogeneous, and multidimensional, often associated with schizophrenia spectrum mental health problems and other SMIs. The final common pathway for hallucinations and related symptoms remains unidentified due to numerous confounding variables. Individual differences in brain activity patterns during hallucinations are expected, influenced by factors like medications and specific mental health conditions.

Hallucinations are the result of a complex interplay between biological mechanisms and the environment, including cognitive mechanisms and learning. Hallucinations involve sensory experiences, perceptions, inferences, and decision-making, accompanied by cognitive and emotional responses. Hallucinations are private events accessed through self-reports and are considered verbal operants governed by consequences. They are false perceptions without external stimuli, influenced by prior experiences and prediction errors. Associative learning theory is used to explain the development and persistence of hallucinations, with self-talk and subvocalizations playing a significant role. Hallucinations are covert verbal operants that can be adaptive or maladaptive, influenced by reinforcement history and errors in self-monitoring.

Cognitive mechanisms implicated in hallucinations include signal detection, source monitoring, memory functions, and language processing. Studies show that individuals prone to hallucinations have impairments in testing the reality of perceptions in the environment and metacognitive skills, with significant associations found in nine out of 21 cognitive subdomains. Hallucinations have both biological and environmental components, and their understanding requires a multidimensional framework and transdiagnostic research.

Hallucinations are reported by a substantial minority of the general population, with 38.7% experiencing them, mostly during altered states of consciousness and/or substance use. Auditory hallucinations are the most common (29.4%), followed by visual (VH) (21.5%), tactile (TH) (19.9%), and olfactory (OH) (17.3%) hallucinations. Hallucinations are more frequently reported by younger females and those with lower educational attainment, with most experiences lasting only a few seconds. Persistent hallucinations are linked to SMI, with 60-80% of individuals with SMI experiencing auditory hallucinations, and a smaller proportion experiencing visual, tactile, and olfactory hallucinations. The median annual incidence of hallucinatory symptoms associated with SMI is 2.5%, with a lifetime prevalence of 7.2%. Co-occurrence of hallucinations in multiple sensory modalities is common (MMH), with auditory and visual types often occurring together. Hallucinations are associated with higher levels of delusional ideation and distress, but not necessarily reduced functioning. Psychological treatments primarily focus on auditory hallucinations, neglecting other sensory experiences reported by individuals with psychosis-related mental health problems.

Culture influences the prevalence, types, and intensity of emotional distress in the experience of hallucinations by individuals with SMI. It is estimated that 15–40% of symptom variability in epidemiological research with individuals living with SMI is attributable to cross-cultural differences. Lifetime prevalence rates of mental health problems are 1.5–3 times higher in Asian and African cultures compared to European-American counterparts. Auditory hallucinations are the most frequently reported type of hallucination across cultures, with the highest 1-year prevalence at 74.8% and the highest rates in Ghana (90.8%) and Nigeria (85.4%). Visual hallucinations are more common in West African participants, with 50.8% in Nigeria and 53.9% in Ghana, while cenesthetic, a rare type of somatic hallucination, is most prevalent in Ghana and European countries. The content of hallucinations varies culturally, with Latinos reporting religious advisory-commanding voices and European-Americans exhibiting higher rates of grandiose delusions, reflecting cultural values.

Types of hallucinations differ as to their prevalence, characteristics, and association with mental health problems corresponding to SMI. Hallucinations are perceptions without external stimuli; they can be harmless or tormenting and can occur in all sensory modalities. Auditory hallucinations are the most common, with a lifetime prevalence of 64–80% among people with SMI, and 23–27% of individuals experiencing auditory hallucinations in the past month. Experiencing visual hallucinations has a lifetime prevalence of 23–31% among people living with SMI, with 5–8% experiencing them in the past month. Tactile hallucinations are reported by 9–19% of people living with SMI, with 4–7% experiencing them in the past month, and include sensations like electric shocks, burning sensation, or crawling under the skin (i.e., cenesethetic hallucination). Olfactory and gustatory hallucinations are less common, with the olfactory type reported by 6–10%; the gustatory type often occur alongside olfactory hallucinations. Mood-congruent and mood-incongruent hallucinations depend on the consistency between the hallucination content and the person's mood. Multimodal hallucinations involve multiple sensory modalities, with 53% of people experiencing them, with the auditory type being the most prevalent. Hallucinations can occur in people not living with SMI under severe stress, but for those with SMI, they may happen even when calm and not in any distress.

Hallucinations likely result from multiple factors working together. Hallucinations are often linked to biochemical imbalances in the brain, potentially caused by genetics, environmental factors, neurological damage, or substance use. They can also result from malnutrition, brain injuries, sensory problems, or physical illnesses like anemia. Different treatments may be needed based on the underlying cause. Environmental stress and overstimulation can worsen the frequency and intensity of the hallucinatory experiences in people with SMI, while understimulation can also cause similar issues, as the brain may create its own "stimulation" in a lackluster environment.

Managing hallucinations that occur in individuals with SMI involve focusing on engagement, prevention, and functional impact of the experiences. To change hallucinatory behaviors, it is crucial to engage the person experiencing the hallucinations in any behavior change plan. The service user must determine if they want to change the frequency, timing, intensity, or other dimensions of the hallucinatory experiences. Preventing hallucinations entirely may be impossible, but various dimensions can be controlled through psychiatric medications and environmental adjustments. Encouragement and support can help individuals manage daily tasks despite hallucinations, even if medications do not eliminate them completely.

Strategies for managing hallucinations in individuals who live with SMI, including medication review, health assessment, and behavioral observation. Hallucinations do not always need to be eliminated if they do not cause distress and upset the person, interfere with daily tasks, or disrupt others. A review of medications by an experienced psychiatric service provider can help minimize hallucinations and emotional distress. Assess the general health of the person experiencing hallucinations, as various illnesses or conditions may contribute to strange sensory experiences. Ensure medications are taken as prescribed, considering long acting or injectable forms if adherence is an issue. Clearly define behaviors that indicate the individual is experiencing hallucinations and seek evaluation if there is doubt about the cause of problematic behavior. Observe circumstances that provoke hallucinatory behaviors and avoid or change these circumstances if identified.

When the individual living with SMI begins to experience hallucinations, the service providers ought to use prompting, distraction, and reinforcement. Remind the individuals experiencing hallucinations that their mind may be playing tricks on them and establish agreed-upon prompts for when hallucinations begin. Engage the person in other activities to distract them from hallucinations, such as household chores or enjoyable tasks and activities. If attempts to redirect fail, ignoring the hallucinations may be necessary, while still reinforcing any positive behaviors observed.

Simplify the environment to minimize changes and include familiar objects to reduce the persistence of hallucinations. Focus on and praise the tasks the person can competently perform, recognizing their efforts even if assistance is needed. Encourage involvement in daily activities that are interesting but not stressful to reduce the likelihood of hallucinations occurring. Prompt and reinforce any capacity for self-control, helping the person to carry on with normal activities despite hallucinations. Seek additional assistance from experienced service providers if the problem behavior does not improve, keeping detailed observational data for consultation.

References

Ali, S., Patel, M., Avenido, J., Jabeen, S., & Riley, W. J. (2011). Hallucinations: Common features and causes. *Current Psychiatry, 10*(11), 22–29. https://cdn-uat.mdedge.com/files/s3fs-public/Document/September-2017/1011CP_Ali.pdf

American Psychiatric Association. (2013). Glossary of technical terms. In *Diagnostic and statistical manual of mental disorders* (5th ed.). https://doi.org/10.1176/appi.books.9780890425787.x28_Glossary_of_Technical_Terms

American Psychiatric Association. (2022a). *Diagnostic and statistical manual of mental disorders* (5th ed., text rev.). https://doi.org/10.1176/appi.books.9780890425787

American Psychiatric Association. (2022b). Schizophrenia spectrum and other psychotic disorders. In *Diagnostic and statistical manual of mental disorders* (5th ed., text rev.). https://doi.org/10.1176/appi.books.9780890425787.x28_Glossary_of_Technical_Terms

American Psychological Association. (n.d.-a). Aristotle's illusion. In *APA dictionary of psychology*. https://dictionary.apa.org/Aristotle's-illusion

American Psychological Association. (n.d.-b). Functional magnetic resonance imaging (fMRI; functional MRI). In *APA dictionary of psychology*. https://dictionary.apa.org/fucntional-magnetic-resonance-imaging

American Psychological Association. (n.d.-c). Hallucination. In *APA dictionary of psychology*. https://dictionary.apa.org/hallucination

American Psychological Association. (n.d.-d). Hallucinosis. In *APA dictionary of psychology*. https://dictionary.apa.org/hallucinosis

American Psychological Association. (n.d.-e). Illusion. In *APA dictionary of psychology*. https://dictionary.apa.org/illusion

American Psychological Association. (n.d.-f). Magnetic resonance imaging (MRI). In *APA dictionary of psychology*. https://dictionary.apa.org/magnetic-resonance-imaging

American Psychological Association. (n.d.-g). Metacognition. In *APA dictionary of psychology*. https://dictionary.apa.org/metacognition

American Psychological Association. (n.d.-h). Mood congruent. In *APA dictionary of psychology*. https://dictionary.apa.org/mood-congruent

Andrew, E. M. (2010). *Command hallucinations and the risks of violence and self-harm: What distinguishes compliers from non-compliers?* [Doctoral dissertation, Cardiff University]. ORCA Cardiff University. https://orca.cardiff.ac.uk/id/eprint/54381/1/U584482.pdf.

Anthony, D. (2004). The cognitive neuropsychiatry of auditory verbal hallucinations: An overview. *Cognitive Neuropsychiatry, 9*(1–2), 107–123. https://doi.org/10.1080/13546800344000183

Aynsworth, C., Collerton, D., & Dudley, R. (2017). Measures of visual hallucinations: Review and recommendations. *Clinical Psychology Review, 57*, 164–182. https://doi.org/10.1016/j.cpr.2017.09.001

Badcock, J. C., Paulik, G., & Maybery, M. T. (2011). The role of emotion regulation in auditory hallucinations. *Psychiatry Research, 185*(3), 303–308. https://doi.org/10.1016/j.psychres.2010.07.011

Bauer, S. M., Schanda, H., Karakula, H., Olajossy-Hilkesberger, L., Rudaleviciene, P., Okribelashvili, N., Chaudhry, H. R., Idemudia, S. E., Gscheider, S., Ritter, K., & Stompe, T. (2011). Culture and the prevalence of hallucinations in schizophrenia. *Comprehensive Psychiatry, 52*(3), 319–325. https://doi.org/10.1016/j.comppsych.2010.06.008

Bell, A., Toh, W. L., Allen, P., Cella, M., Jardri, R., Larøi, F., Moseley, P., & Rossell, S. L. (2024). Examining the relationships between cognition and auditory hallucinations: A systematic review. *Australian & New Zealand Journal of Psychiatry, 58*(6), 467–497. https://doi.org/10.1177/00048674241235849

Benrimoh, D., Parr, T., Adams, R. A., & Friston, K. (2019). Hallucinations both in and out of context: An active inference account. *PLoS One, 14*(8), e0212379. https://doi.org/10.1371/journal.pone.0212379

Bentall, R. P. (1990). The illusion of reality: A review and integration of psychological research on hallucinations. *Psychological Bulletin, 107*(1), 82–95. https://doi.org/10.1037/0033-2909.107.1.82

Bentall, R. P., & Slade, P. D. (1985). Reality testing and auditory hallucinations: A signal detection analysis. *British Journal of Clinical Psychology, 24*(Pt 3), 159–169. https://doi.org/10.1111/j.2044-8260.1985.tb01331.x

Bere, M., Rossell, S. L., & Toh, W. L. (2024). Cognition in relation to non-auditory or multisensory hallucinations in schizophrenia-spectrum disorders: A scoping review. *Psychiatry Research*, 116268. https://doi.org/10.1016/j.psychres.2024.116268

Blom, J. D. (2015). Auditory hallucinations. In M. J. Aminoff, F. Boller, & D. F. Swabb (Eds.), *Handbook of clinical neurology* (Vol. 129, pp. 433–455). Elsevier. https://doi.org/10.1016/B978-0-444-62630-1.00024-X

Boksa, P. (2009). On the neurobiology of hallucinations. *Journal of Psychiatry & Neuroscience, 34*(4), 260–262. https://cdnsciencepub.com/doi/pdf/10.1139/jpn.0934

Borrero, J. C., & Vollmer, T. R. (2002). An application of the matching law to severe problem behavior. *Journal of Applied Behavior Analysis, 35*(1), 13–27. https://doi.org/10.1901/jaba.2002.35-13

Braham, L. G., Trower, P., & Birchwood, M. (2004). Acting on command hallucinations and dangerous behavior: A critique of the major findings in the last decade. *Clinical Psychology Review, 24*(5), 513–528. https://doi.org/10.1016/j.cpr.2004.04.002

Braun, C. M., Dumont, M., Duval, J., Hamel-Hébert, I., & Godbout, L. (2003). Brain modules of hallucination: An analysis of multiple patients with brain lesions. *Journal of Psychiatry and Neuroscience, 28*(6), 432–449. https://www.ncbi.nlm.nih.gov/pmc/articles/PMC2757708/

Brust, J. C. (2014). Acute withdrawal: Diagnosis and treatment. In E. V. Sullivan & A. Pfefferbaum (Eds.), *Handbook of clinical neurology* (Vol. 125, pp. 123–131). Elsevier. https://doi.org/10.1016/B978-0-444-62619-6.00010-2

Buccheri, R., Trygstad, L., & Dowling, G. (2007). Behavioral management of command hallucinations to harm in schizophrenia. *Journal of Psychosocial Nursing and Mental Health Services, 45*(9), 46–54. https://doi.org/10.3928/02793695-20070901-11

Bucci, S., Birchwood, M., Twist, L., Tarrier, N., Emsley, R., & Haddock, G. (2013). Predicting compliance with command hallucinations: Anger, impulsivity and appraisals of voices' power and intent. *Schizophrenia Research, 147*(1), 163–168. https://doi.org/10.1016/j.schres.2013.02.037

Burns, C. E., Heiby, E. M., & Tharp, R. G. (1983). A verbal behavior analysis of auditory hallucinations. *The Behavior Analyst, 6*, 133–143. https://doi.org/10.1007/BF03392392

Chaudhury, S. (2010). Hallucinations: Clinical aspects and management. *Industrial Psychiatry Journal, 19*(1), 5–12. https://doi.org/10.4103/0972-6748.77625

Chen, E., & Berrios, G. E. (1996). Recognition of hallucinations: A new multidimensional model and methodology. *Psychopathology, 29*(1), 54–63. https://doi.org/10.1159/000284972

Cho, R., & Wu, W. (2013). Mechanisms of auditory verbal hallucinations in schizophrenia. *Frontiers in* Psychiatry, *4*, Article 155. https://doi.org/10.3389/fpsyt.2013.00155

Ćurčić-Blake, B., Ford, J. M., Hubl, D., Orlov, N. D., Sommer, I. E., Waters, F., Allen, P., Jardri, R., Woodruff, P., David, N., & Aleman, A. (2017). Interaction of language, auditory and memory brain networks in auditory verbal hallucinations. *Progress in Neurobiology, 148*, 1–20. https://doi.org/10.1016/j.pneurobio.2016.11.002

Daalman, K., Boks, M. P., Diederen, K. M., de Weijer, A. D., Blom, J. D., Kahn, R. S., & Sommer, I. E. (2011). The same or different? A phenomenological comparison of auditory verbal hallucinations in healthy and psychotic individuals. *The Journal of Clinical Psychiatry, 72*(3), e245–e251. https://doi.org/10.4088/JCP.09m05797yel

Davis, M. L., Witcraft, S. M., Baird, S. O., & Smits, J. A. J. (2017). Learning principles in CBT. In S. G. Hofmann & G. J. G. Asmundson (Eds.), *The science of cognitive behavioral therapy* (pp. 51–76). Academic Press. https://doi.org/10.1016/B978-0-12-803457-6.00003-9

Delespaul, P., Devries, M., & van Os, J. (2002). Determinants of occurrence and recovery from hallucinations in daily life. *Social Psychiatry and Psychiatric Epidemiology, 37*(3), 97–104. https://doi.org/10.1007/s001270200000

de Leede-Smith, S., & Barkus, E. (2013). A comprehensive review of auditory verbal hallucinations: Lifetime prevalence, correlates and mechanisms in healthy and clinical individuals. *Frontiers in Human Neuroscience, 7*, Article 367. https://doi.org/10.3389/fnhum.2013.00367

Dudley, R., Aynsworth, C., Mosimann, U., Taylor, J. P., Smailes, D., Collerton, D., Dietrich, A., Hird, E., Knolle, F., & Urwyler, P. (2019). A comparison of visual hallucinations across disorders. *Psychiatry Research, 272*, 86–92. https://doi.org/10.1016/j.psychres.2018.12.119

Dudley, R., Denton, S., Mathewson, J., Pervez, S., Aynsworth, C., Dodgson, G., & Barclay, N. (2023). Prevalence of multisensory hallucinations in people at risk of transition to psychosis. *Psychiatry Research, 322*, 115091. https://doi.org/10.1016/j.psychres.2023.115091

Dudley, R., Watson, F., O'Grady, L., Aynsworth, C., Dodgson, G., Common, S., Brown, A., Steel, C., Spencer, H., & Fernyhough, C. (2023). Prevalence and nature of multi-sensory and multimodal hallucinations in people with first episode psychosis. *Psychiatry Research, 319*, 114988. https://doi.org/10.1016/j.psychres.2022.114988

Feeney, E. J., Groman, S. M., Taylor, J. R., & Corlett, P. R. (2017). Explaining delusions: Reducing uncertainty through basic and computational neuroscience. *Schizophrenia Bulletin, 43*(2), 263–272. https://doi.org/10.1093/schbul/sbw165

Fernyhough, C. (2019). Modality-general and modality-specific processes in hallucinations. *Psychological Medicine, 49*(16), 2639–2645. https://doi.org/10.1017/S0033291719002496

Flavell, J. H. (1979). Metacognition and cognitive monitoring: A new area of cognitive-developmental inquiry. *American Psychologist, 34*, 906–911. https://doi.org/10.1037/0003-066X.34.10.906

Friedman, L., Kenny, J. T., Wise, A. L., Wu, D., Stuve, T. A., Miller, D. A., Jesberger, J. A., Lewin, J. S., & Hyde, J. S. (1998). Brain activation during silent word generation evaluated with functional MRI. *Brain and Language, 64*(2), 231–256. https://doi.org/10.1006/brln.1998.1953

Garwood, L., Dodgson, G., Bruce, V., & McCarthy-Jones, S. (2015). A preliminary investigation into the existence of a hypervigilance subtype of auditory hallucination in people with psychosis. *Behavioural and Cognitive Psychotherapy, 43*(1), 52–62. https://doi.org/10.1017/S1352465813000714

Ghanem, M., Evangeli-Dawson, C., & Georgiades, A. (2023). The role of culture on the phenomenology of hallucinations and delusions, explanatory models, and help-seeking attitudes: A narrative review. *Early Intervention in Psychiatry, 17*(9), 843–863. https://doi.org/10.1111/eip.13449

Green, M. F. (2006). Cognitive impairment and functional outcome in schizophrenia and bipolar disorder. *Journal of Clinical Psychiatry, 67*(Suppl 9), 3–6. https://pubmed.ncbi.nlm.nih.gov/17017820/

Haddock, G., McCarron, J., Tarrier, N., & Faragher, E. B. (1999). Scales to measure dimensions of hallucinations and delusions: The psychotic symptom rating scales (PSYRATS). *Psychological Medicine, 29*(4), 879–889. https://doi.org/10.1017/S0033291799008661

Harris, W. V. (2013). Greek and Roman hallucinations. In W. V. Harris (Ed.), *Mental disorders in the classical world* (pp. 285–306). Brill. https://doi.org/10.1163/9789004252569_014

Heeger, D. (2007). *Signal detection theory* [PDF document]. Class Handouts Online. https://www.cns.nyu.edu/~david/handouts/sdt/sdt.html

Honig, A., Romme, M. A., Ensink, B. J., Escher, S. D., Pennings, M. H., & DeVreis, M. W. (1998). Auditory hallucinations: A comparison between patients and nonpatients. *The Journal of Nervous and Mental Disease, 186*(10), 646–651. https://doi.org/10.1097/00005053-199810000-00009

Humpston, C. S., Adams, R. A., Benrimoh, D., Broome, M. R., Corlett, P. R., Gerrans, P., Jardri, R., Larøi, F., Moseley, P., Raballo, A., Suzuki, T., Waters, F., & Linden, D. E. (2019). From computation to the first-person: Auditory-verbal hallucinations and delusions of thought interference in schizophrenia-spectrum psychoses. *Schizophrenia Bulletin, 45*(Supplement_1), S56–S66. https://doi.org/10.1093/schbul/sby073

Hustig, H. H., & Hafner, R. J. (1990). Persistent auditory hallucinations and their relationship to delusions and mood. *The Journal of Nervous and Mental Disease, 178*(4), 264–267. https://doi.org/10.1097/00005053-199004000-00006

Isaacson, M., Hazell, C. M., Cape, J., Hickson, E., Islam, F., Gill, A., Simon, K., Patel, R., Souray, J., & Raune, D. (2022). The cognitive–phenomenological assessment of delusions and hallucinations at the early intervention in psychosis service stage: The results of a quality improvement project. *Early Intervention in Psychiatry, 16*(12), 1345–1352. https://doi.org/10.1111/eip.13283

Ishigaki, T., & Tanno, Y. (1999). The signal detection ability of patients with auditory hallucination: Analysis using the continuous performance test. *Psychiatry and Clinical Neurosciences, 53*(4), 471–476. https://doi.org/10.1046/j.1440-1819.1999.00586.x

Janaki, V., Suzaily, W., Abdul Rahman, A. H., Hazli, Z., & Azmawati, M. N. (2017). The dimensions of auditory hallucination in schizophrenia: Association with depressive symptoms and quality of life. *IIUM Medical Journal Malaysia, 16*(2). https://doi.org/10.31436/imjm.v16i2.325

Jenner, J. A., & Van de Willige, G. (2002). *The auditory vocal hallucination rating scale (AVHRS)*. University Medical Center. https://www.rgoc.nl/wp-content/uploads/2020/02/AVHRS-english.pdf

Jenner, J. A., Nienhuis, F. J., van de Willige, G., & Wiersma, D. (2006). "Hitting" voices of schizophrenia patients may lastingly reduce persistent auditory hallucinations and their burden: 18-month outcome of a randomized controlled trial. *The Canadian Journal of Psychiatry, 51*(3), 169–177. https://doi.org/10.1177/070674370605100307

Larøi, F., & Woodward, T. S. (2007). Hallucinations from a cognitive perspective. *Harvard Review of Psychiatry, 15*(3), 109–117. https://doi.org/10.1080/10673220701401993

Layng, T. V. J., & Andronis, P. T. (1984). Toward a functional analysis of delusional speech and hallucinatory behavior. *The Behavior Analyst, 7*(2), 139–156. https://doi.org/10.1007/BF03392557

Lim, A., Hoek, H. W., Deen, M. L., Blom, J. D., Bruggeman, R., Cahn, W., de Haan, L., Kahn, R. S., Meijer, C. J., Myin-Germeys, I., van Os J., Wiersma, D., & GROUP Investigators. (2016). Prevalence and classification of hallucinations in multiple sensory modalities in schizophrenia spectrum disorders. *Schizophrenia Research, 176*(2–3), 493–499. https://doi.org/10.1016/j.schres.2016.06.010

Lin, X., Zhuo, C., Li, G., Li, J., Gao, X., Chen, C., & Jiang, D. (2020). Functional brain alterations in auditory hallucination subtypes in individuals with auditory hallucinations without the diagnosis of specific neurological diseases and mental disorders at the current stage. *Brain and Behavior, 10*(1), e01487, 1–12. https://doi.org/10.1002/brb3.1487

Lincoln, T. M., & Peters, E. (2019). A systematic review and discussion of symptom specific cognitive behavioural approaches to delusions and hallucinations. *Schizophrenia Research, 203*, 66–79. https://doi.org/10.1016/j.schres.2017.12.014

Linn, E. L. (1977). Verbal auditory hallucinations: Mind, self, and society. *Journal of Nervous and Mental Disease, 164*(1), 8–17. https://doi.org/10.1097/00005053-197701000-00003

Linscott, R. J., & van Os, J. (2010). Systematic reviews of categorical versus continuum models in psychosis: Evidence for discontinuous subpopulations underlying a psychometric continuum. Implications for DSM-V, DSM-VI, and DSM-VII. *Annual Review of Clinical Psychology, 6*(1), 391–419. https://doi.org/10.1146/annurev.clinpsy.032408.153506

Linscott, R. J., & van Os, J. (2013). An updated and conservative systematic review and meta-analysis of epidemiological evidence on psychotic experiences in children and adults: On the pathway from proneness to persistence to dimensional expression across mental disorders. *Psychological Medicine, 43*(6), 1133–1149. https://doi.org/10.1017/S0033291712001626

Linszen, M. M., de Boer, J. N., Schutte, M. J., Begemann, M. J. H., de Vries, J., Koops, S., van Dellen, E., van der Gaag, M., van Gasselt, S., van Lutterveld, R., & Sommer, I. E. (2022). Occurrence and phenomenology of hallucinations in the general population: A large online survey. *Schizophrenia, 8*(1), Article 41. https://doi.org/10.1038/s41537-022-00229-9

López-Silva, P., Cavieres, Á., & Humpston, C. (2022). The phenomenology of auditory verbal hallucinations in schizophrenia and the challenge from pseudohallucinations. *Frontiers in Psychiatry, 13*, 826654. https://doi.org/10.3389/fpsyt.2022.826654

Maher, B. A. (2006). The relationship between delusions and hallucinations. *Current Psychiatry Reports, 8*, 179–183. https://doi.org/10.1007/s11920-006-0021-3

McCarthy-Jones, S., Smailes, D., Corvin, A., Gill, M., Morris, D. W., Dinan, T. G., Murphy, K. C., & Dudley, R. (2017). Occurrence and co-occurrence of hallucinations by modality in schizophrenia-spectrum disorders. *Psychiatry Research, 252*, 154–160. https://doi.org/10.1016/j.psychres.2017.01.102

McCarthy-Jones, S., Trauer, T., Mackinnon, A., Sims, E., Thomas, N., & Copolov, D. L. (2014). A new phenomenological survey of auditory hallucinations: Evidence for subtypes and implications for theory and practice. *Schizophrenia Bulletin, 40*(1), 231–235. https://doi.org/10.1093/schbul/sbs156

McGuire, P. K., Silbersweig, D. A., Wright, I., Murray, R. M., Frackowiak, R. S. J., & Frith, C. D. (1996). The neural correlates of inner speech and auditory verbal imagery in schizophrenia: Relationship to auditory verbal hallucinations. *The British Journal of Psychiatry, 169*(2), 148–159. https://doi.org/10.1192/bjp.169.2.148

Merriam-Webster. (n.d.). "Jinn". In Merriam-Webster.com dictionary. Retrieved 12/21/2024, from https://www.merriam-webster.com/dictionary/jinn?src=search-dict-box

Miller, L. J., O'Connor, E., & DiPasquale, T. (1993). Patients' attitudes toward hallucinations. *American Journal of Psychiatry, 150*, 584–588. https://doi.org/10.1176/ajp.150.4.584

Mocellin, R., Walterfang, M., & Velakoulis, D. (2006). Neuropsychiatry of complex visual hallucinations. *Australian & New Zealand Journal of Psychiatry, 40*(9), 742–751. https://doi.org/10.1080/j.1440-1614.2006.01878.x

Monahan, J., Steadman, H. J., Silver, E., Appelbaum, P. S., Robbins, P. C., Mulvey, E. P., & Banks, S. (2001). Rethinking risk assessment: The MacArthur study of mental disorder and violence. Oxford University Press.

Montagnese, M., Leptourgos, P., Fernyhough, C., Waters, F., Larøi, F., Jardri, R., Bell, V., Smailes, D., Collerton, D., McCarthy-Jones, S., & Urwyler, P. (2021). A review of multimodal hallucinations: Categorization, assessment, theoretical perspectives, and clinical recommendations. *Schizophrenia Bulletin, 47*(1), 237–248. https://doi.org/10.1093/schbul/sbaa101

Morin, A. (2012). Inner speech. In W. Hirstein (Ed.), *Encyclopedia of human behavior* (Vol. 2, 2nd ed., pp. 436–443). Elsevier. https://doi.org/10.1016/B978-0-12-375000-6.00115-4

Moseley, P., & Mitrenga, K. (2022). The varieties and complexities of multimodal hallucinations in psychosis. In A. Woods, B. Alderson-Day, & C. Fernyhough (Eds.), *Voices in psychosis: Interdisciplinary perspectives [internet]* (pp. 66–73). Oxford University Press. Available from: https://www.ncbi.nlm.nih.gov/books/NBK593361/

Mueser, K. T., Bellack, A. S., & Brady, E. U. (1990). Hallucinations in schizophrenia. *Acta Psychiatrica Scandinavica, 82*(1), 26–29. https://doi.org/10.1111/j.1600-0447.1990.tb01350.x

Mustafa, F. A. (2020). Pseudohallucinations as functional cognitive disorders. *The Lancet Psychiatry, 7*(3), 230. https://doi.org/10.1016/S2215-0366(19)30517-6

Nevin, J. A. (1969). Signal detection theory and operant behavior: A review of David M. Green and John A. Swets' *Signal Detection Theory and Psychophysics*. *Journal of the Experimental Analysis of Behavior, 12*(3), 475–480. https://doi.org/10.1901/jeab.1969.12-475

Ohayon, M. M. (2000). Prevalence of hallucinations and their pathological associations in the general population. *Psychiatry Research, 97*(2–3), 153–164. https://doi.org/10.1016/S0165-1781(00)00227-4

Oorschot, M., Lataster, T., Thewissen, V., Bentall, R., Delespaul, P., & Myin-Germeys, I. (2012). Temporal dynamics of visual and auditory hallucinations in psychosis. *Schizophrenia Research, 140*(1–3), 77–82. https://doi.org/10.1016/j.schres.2012.06.010

Powers, A. R., III. (2019). Psychotic experiences in the general population: Symptom specificity and the role of distress and dysfunction. *JAMA Psychiatry, 76*(12), 1228–1229. https://doi.org/10.1001/jamapsychiatry.2019.2391

Powers, A. R., Mathys, C., & Corlett, P. R. (2017). Pavlovian conditioning-induced hallucinations result from overweighting of perceptual priors. *Science, 357*(6351), 596–600. https://doi.org/10.1126/science.aan3458

Radenkova, J., Saeva, E., & Saev, V. (2011). Psychoactive substances in different cultures and religious practices. *Acta Medica Bulgarica, 38*(1), 122–130. https://doi.org/10.2478/amb-2018-0020

Rogers, R., Gillis, J. R., Turner, R. E., & Smith, T. (1990). The clinical presentation of command hallucinations. *American Journal of Psychiatry, 147*, 1304–1307. https://doi.org/10.1176/ajp.147.10.1304

Sanjuan, J., Gonzalez, J. C., Aguilar, E. J., Leal, C., & Van Os, J. (2004). Pleasurable auditory hallucinations. *Acta Psychiatrica Scandinavica, 110*(4), 273–278. https://doi.org/10.1111/j.1600-0447.2004.00336.x

Shahrokh, N. C., & Hales, R. E. (2003). *American psychiatric glossary* (8th ed.). American Psychiatric Publishing. https://books.google.com/books/about/American_Psychiatric_Glossary.html?id=4p2vBAAAQBAJ

Shawyer, F., Mackinnon, A., Farhall, J., Trauer, T., & Copolov, D. (2003). Command hallucinations and violence: Implications for detention and treatment. *Psychiatry, Psychology and Law, 10*(1), 97–107. https://doi.org/10.1375/pplt.2003.10.1.97

Sharpless, B. A. (2015). Exploding head syndrome is common in college students. *Journal of Sleep Research, 24*(4), 447–449. https://doi.org/10.1111/jsr.12292

Singh, N. N., Wahler, R. G., Adkins, A. D., Myers, R. E., & Mindfulness Research Group. (2003). Soles of the feet: A mindfulness-based self-control intervention for aggression by an individual with mild mental retardation and mental illness. *Research in Developmental Disabilities, 24*(3), 158–169. https://doi.org/10.1016/S0891-4222(03)00026-4

Skinner, B. F. (1953). *Science and human behavior*. Simon and Schuster. https://books.google.com/books/about/Science_and_Human_Behavior.html?id=3rZ9AAAAMAAJ

Slade, P. D., & Bentall, R. P. (1988). *Sensory deception: A scientific analysis of hallucination*. Johns Hopkins University Press. https://www.press.jhu.edu/books/title/1166/sensory-deception

Spence, S. A. (2009). Psychopathology and consciousness. In W. P. Banks (Ed.), *Encyclopedia of consciousness* (pp. 245–271). Academic Press. https://doi.org/10.1016/B978-012373873-8.00066-9

Steenhuis, L. A., Pijnenborg, G. H. M., Visser, E., van de Willige, G., van Beilen, M., Nauta, M. H., Aleman, A., & Bartels-Velthuis, A.. A. (2019). The development, validity, and reliability of the auditory vocal hallucination rating scale questionnaire (AVHRS-Q). *Social Psychiatry and Psychiatric Epidemiology, 54*(8), 927–935. https://doi.org/10.1007/s00127-019-01692-z

Stephane, M., Thuras, P., Nasrallah, H., & Georgopoulos, A. P. (2003). The internal structure of the phenomenology of auditory verbal hallucinations. *Schizophrenia Research, 61*(2–3), 185–193. https://doi.org/10.1016/S0920-9964(03)00013-6

Stompe, T., Bauer, S., Karakula, H., Rudaleviciene, P., Okribelashvili, N., Chaudhry, H. R., Idemudia, E. E., & Gschaider, S. (2007). Paranoid-hallucinatory syndromes in schizophrenia—Results of the international study on psychotic symptoms. *World Cultural Psychiatry Research Review, 4*, 63–68. https://www.worldculturalpsychiatry.org/wp-content/uploads/2019/08/05-Paranoid-V02N2.pdf

Swyer, A., & Powers, A. R. (2020). Voluntary control of auditory hallucinations: Phenomenology to therapeutic implications. *Npj Schizophrenia, 6*, 19. https://doi.org/10.1038/s41537-020-0106-8

Teeple, R. C., Caplan, J. P., & Stern, T. A. (2009). Visual hallucinations: Differential diagnosis and treatment. *Primary Care Companion to the Journal of Clinical Psychiatry, 11*(1), 26–32. https://doi.org/10.4088%2Fpcc.08r00673

Telles-Correia, D., Moreira, A. L., Gama Marques, J., Saraiva, S., Moreira, C. A., Antunes, F., Almeida, C., & Rocha, N. B. (2016). The proximity between hallucination and delusion dimensions: An observational, analytic, cross-sectional, multicentre study. *Frontiers in Psychology, 7*, Article 1642. https://doi.org/10.3389/fpsyg.2016.01642

Telles-Correia, D., Moreira, A. L., & Gonçalves, J. S. (2015). Hallucinations and related concepts—Their conceptual background. *Frontiers in Psychology, 6*, Article 991, 1–9. https://doi.org/10.3389/fpsyg.2015.00991

Thomas, P., Mathur, P., Gottesman, I. I., Nagpal, R., Nimgaonkar, V. L., & Deshpande, S. N. (2007). Correlates of hallucinations in schizophrenia: A cross-cultural evaluation. *Schizophrenia Research, 92*(1–3), 41–49. https://doi.org/10.1016/j.schres.2007.01.017

Toh, W. L., McCarthy-Jones, S., Copolov, D., & Rossell, S. L. (2019). Have we overlooked the significance of multimodal hallucinations in schizophrenia? *Psychiatry Research, 279*, 358–360. https://doi.org/10.1016/j.psychres.2019.06.018

Tracy, D. K., & Shergill, S. S. (2006). Imaging auditory hallucinations in schizophrenia. *Acta Neuropsychiatrica, 18*(2), 71–78. https://doi.org/10.1111/j.1601-5215.2006.00129.x

Upthegrove, R., Broome, M. R., Caldwell, K., Ives, J., Oyebode, F., & Wood, S. J. (2016). Understanding auditory verbal hallucinations: A systematic review of current evidence. *Acta Psychiatrica Scandinavica, 133*(5), 352–367. https://doi.org/10.1111/acps.12531

Varese, F., Barkus, E., & Bentall, R. P. (2012). Dissociation mediates the relationship between childhood trauma and hallucination-proneness. *Psychological Medicine, 42*(5), 1025–1036. https://doi.org/10.1017/S0033291711001826

Wood, S. J., Allen, N. B., & Pantelis, C. (2009). *The neuropsychology of mental illness*. Cambridge University Press. https://doi.org/10.1017/CBO9780511642197

Yuan, S., Wu, H., Wu, Y., Xu, H., Yu, J., Zhong, Y., Zhang, N., Li, J., Xu, Q., & Wang, C. (2022). Neural effects of cognitive behavioral therapy in psychiatric disorders: A systematic review and activation likelihood estimation meta-analysis. *Frontiers in Psychology, 13*, 853804. https://doi.org/10.3389/fpsyg.2022.853804

Chapter 8
Problems with Affective Lability (Mood Swings) in Individuals Living with Serious Mental Illness

Introduction

Affective lability (AL) is characterized by rapid, intense, and unpredictable shifts in emotional states; it represents a transdiagnostic phenomenon that poses significant challenges to individuals living with serious mental illness (SMI). While mood variability is a normative aspect of human experience, affective lability exceeds typical fluctuations in both magnitude and frequency, often impairing psychosocial functioning, interpersonal relationships, and treatment engagement. This chapter examines affective lability as a multidimensional construct, integrating clinical, neurobiological, and behavioral perspectives to illuminate its role in the broader symptomatology of SMI.

The phenomenon of affective lability intersects with several core domains of emotional experience, including oscillation frequency, affective intensity, and perceived capacity for control. These fluctuations often span a wide range of affective poles, such as irritability, elation, anxiety, and dysphoria, and may occur independently of identifiable environmental triggers. Subthreshold syndromes, in which mood instability does not meet full diagnostic criteria yet contributes to functional impairment, further complicate assessment and intervention. Epidemiological data suggest a general population prevalence of approximately 13.9%, with markedly higher rates among individuals diagnosed with schizoaffective, bipolar, depressive, and trauma-related disorders.

This chapter is organized to provide a comprehensive understanding of affective lability within the context of SMI. It begins by defining key constructs including mood, affect, emotion, and lability and differentiating normative emotional variability from pathological instability. Subsequent sections explore the neurological substrates and environmental influences that contribute to affective dysregulation, including circadian rhythms, stress reactivity, and neurocognitive impairments. The dimensional features of affective lability, such as frequency, intensity, and

G. F. McKeegan, *Behavior Change Interventions for Serious Mental Illness*, Evidence-Based Practices in Behavioral Health,
https://doi.org/10.1007/978-3-032-18372-9_8

controllability, and reviews of validated instruments used in clinical assessment are addressed, focusing on psychometric instruments that are used.

Finally, the chapter outlines evidence-based behavioral strategies for managing affective lability, emphasizing psychoeducation, emotion regulation training, and individualized interventions. By integrating empirical findings with clinical insights, a nuanced understanding of affective lability and its implications for diagnosis, treatment, and recovery in serious mental illness is delineated.

> I work with a person who has changes in his moods for no apparent reason. One minute he is joking and smiling, and then he is crying; sometimes he begins to laugh hysterically or becomes angry and threatening. His moods quickly change and are unpredictable.

The Case of Juan

Juan is a 28-year-old man who was brought to a psychiatric hospital after the police found him wandering on a major highway. When they picked him up, he could not tell the police his name, where he was, or the date. He was performing a variety of odd behaviors. For example, he would frequently shake his head vigorously to dislodge a tumor that he said was growing behind his eye (no such tumor existed).

Juan had begun having psychiatric problems in high school. He was placed in special education classes because of unpredictable and dangerous behavior. Later, he dropped out of school. During these years, he began using illegal drugs. He frequently argued with his mother and was later hospitalized after hitting her. His mother obtained an order of protection from the court, and Juan was ordered to stay away from her. He spent several years living in supported housing shelters for the homeless and the mentally ill.

Since developing an SMI, he has been identified as living with a variety of mental health conditions. Eventually, it was determined that he was living with a schizoaffective mental health problem. In the hospital, many of Juan's symptoms and problematic behaviors responded to psychiatric medication. He made more sense when he talked and was able to spend time sitting quietly. While he continued to occasionally "shake the tumor out of my head," this happened less often, and he talked about it much less. However, he continued to be very unpredictable in his emotional behavior. He was soon discharged to a group home.

At the group home, the treating staff noticed that his emotions would quickly change. Some days he seemed pleasant and cooperative. However, he very quickly became frustrated and angry. He would pace the floor, complain that the staff was holding him against his will, and that they were refusing to do anything for him. Later, he would act discouraged, sit alone, not talk to anyone, and refuse to participate in any recovery programs, such as the clubhouse program.

Juan's unpredictable emotional behavior made it very difficult for the staff at the group home to work with him. They had the challenge of developing a strategy to adequately deal with his unpredictable emotions and behavior.

Definition and Characteristics of Affective Lability

A person displays periods of intense anger and irritability, yelling and cursing others, making threats, and accusing others of "cheating me" at work; within hours, the same person is laughing, is the "life of the party," and making others laugh with his infectious humor. By the end of the day, the same person is crying, making derogatory statements about himself, and is threatening to kill himself, saying, "I have nothing to live for!" This person is displaying affective lability, defined as fluctuations in a person's mood and affect over periods of time with repeated, rapid, and abrupt shifts in affective expression (American Psychiatric Association, 2013c). The fluctuations can occur within hours or days and occur repeatedly. The behavior becomes "abnormal" if the intensity or magnitude of the display of the behavior is high. Pinching oneself when in pain may not be a problem as some people pinch or rub in the place where the pain is felt; the behavior is abnormal when the behavior is displayed with high intensity, resulting in bruising, or the behavior occurs frequently. Research has shown that moods during the day fluctuate by time of day, physical status of the person, activities being performed, and anticipation of events (Dysinger, 1938; Stone et al., 1996). Most people have "good and bad days" depending on many factors that are often transient. "Bad days," or when mood is low, become a problem if the low mood lasts too long and interferes with the ability to get out of bed, interact with others, and function adaptively. A low mood becomes "abnormal" when the person remains isolated, does not take care of herself, and has dysregulation of appetite and sleep disturbances. If the "low mood" becomes so intense that the person keeps thinking that she is a burden to others, everyone would be better off if she were dead, has frequent and intense cognitions of committing suicide during periods of "low mood," and has difficulty decreasing the intensity and frequency of the suicidal thoughts, then her thoughts become "abnormal."

Marwaha et al. (2014) defined affective lability as:

> …frequent affective category shifts, disturbances in affect intensity, excessively rapid emotion rise-times and delayed return to baseline, excessive reactivity to psychosocial cues and overdramatic affective expression…. The term is used interchangeably with mood instability, affective instability, affective and emotional dysregulation and mood swings, by researchers and clinicians. (p. 3)

Affective lability (AL) is a problematic behavior present across mental health problems and is associated with suicidality and healthcare use (Marwaha et al., 2015). It has been shown that 13.9% of individuals living with SMI can be reliably diagnosed as experiencing affective lability (Marwaha et al., 2013a). It has been shown that a higher percentage of individuals with mental health problems experience this and have less control of emotional behaviors than those without a mental health problem (McDonald et al., 2017); intensity of the affective instability was not found to be a determining variable in differentiating between individuals with and without a mental health problem (Marwaha et al., 2013b). Researchers have called for focusing on treating affective lability in people living with SMI to improve psychosocial functioning and rehabilitation efforts (McDonald et al., 2017).

Affective lability refers to changes of mood or feelings that are greater and/or more frequent than those experienced by most people. Affective dysregulation is considered a risk factor for poor clinical and functional outcomes (Høegh et al., 2020). It is characterized by frequent, intense, and wide-ranging changes in affective states that result in adverse consequences for the individual experiencing it (Contardi et al., 2018).

Høegh et al. (2022) have found that affective instability is more prevalent with fluctuations between anxiety and depression than between affective states of anger and elation. Positive associations between affective lability, social functioning, and indicators of quality of life were also shown.

Everyone experiences some degree of emotional variability (e.g., normal "ups and downs"). For instance, many people feel a "let down" around midafternoon; to deal with it, the person may get coffee or take a break from whatever task was being performed. Moods and physiological states are affected by diurnal cycles or rhythms (circadian or biological rhythm) (American Psychological Association, n.d.-b). There are periodic variations in physiological or behavioral activity that repeat at approximately regular intervals and affect energy level, sexual desire, and menstruation; the intervals are usually 24 h in duration, such as the sleep–wake cycle. Such rhythms can be linked to cyclical changes in environmental cues, such as daylength or change of seasons (American Psychological Association, n.d.-b). Cyclical changes in mood are found regarding moods (e.g., happy, tired), activities (e.g., discourse, thinking), and locations (e.g., home, work). Diurnal cycles in most moods were strongly associated with activities and location; yet diurnal cycles of some moods (e.g., rushed, sad, and tired) were not dependent on these factors (Stone et al., 1996).

Affective lability (or commonly called "mood swings") can be extreme and happen so suddenly that they clearly interfere with the ability to carry out normal daily functioning. It may be difficult to identify anything going on around the person to account for the "mood swing." Even when a situation that brought on the emotion can be identified, the emotional reaction often seems "over the top." The person can become extremely angry, depressed, or happy (i.e., elated), and he cannot control himself while others believe that he should be better able to control himself. However, someone with these problems often cannot. Juan would sometimes raise his voice and start pacing when the staff was not able to give him permission to see his mother, despite being reminded that legally he could not see her.

Affective lability is defined as unstable emotional experiences and frequent changes in mood. It refers to the frequency, speed, and range of changes in the expression of experienced emotions (i.e., affective states) (Oliver & Simons, 2004). Affective lability are emotions that are easily aroused, intense, and/or disproportionate to events and circumstances (National Institute of Health [NIH], 2024). According to the Diagnostic and Statistical Manual of Mental Disorders (fifth ed., text rev.) (DSM-5-TR) (American, Psychiatric Association, 2022a), affective lability refers to rapid mood changes occurring over short periods of time, including alterations among states such as euphoria, dysphoria, and irritability. Affective lability is defined as distinct periods of elevated mood (mania or hypomania) alternating with periods of depressed mood. The DSM-5-TR (American Psychiatric Association, 2022a) describes "severity" as the temporal speed of the occurrence of the shifts to different moods and the impact on functioning sometimes requiring close supervision of the person experiencing the rapid shifts of affect. Impairment in functioning is determined by adverse consequences on social roles, social interactions, school and work, effective communication, and cognitive skills such as attending, organizing, planning, and remembering.

Definitions of affective lability often lack specificity and are not tied to a particular theoretical framework (Marwaha et al., 2014). Affective lability is a poorly understood, but common, mental health problem in the general population (Marwaha et al., 2013b). In a survey of households in the United Kingdom, the occurrence of "mood instability" in the adult population was 13.9% (responding affirmatively to a question about whether the respondent ever had "mood swings"). The high rate of occurrence was related to the prevalence in Gulf War veterans exposed to war trauma and living with posttraumatic stress disorder (PTSD). Rates of "mood instability" were high, with more than 49% of individuals who were living with a range of behavioral health problems responding affirmatively to having an occurrence of "mood swings" (Marwaha et al., 2013b). Affective lability has been found to be a risk factor for suicidal behavior in the general population (Marwaha et al., 2013a), particularly with the cooccurrence of sleep disturbance (McDonald et al., 2017). Affective lability is transdiagnostic, being present in mental health problems associated with SMI, including schizophrenia spectrum, bipolar, depressive, personality, and severe anxiety-related mental health problems (Marwaha et al., 2014; Patel et al., 2015). Affective lability can occur independently of living with SMI but has been found to be a precursor to the occurrence of other mental health problems related to living with SMI (McDonald et al., 2017).

Mood, affect, emotions, and lability are four characteristics that are at the center of the definition and understanding of the phenomenon of affective lability:

- Mood: It is defined as a pervasive and sustained emotion that impacts the perception of the environment or context of the person experiencing the mood. It permeates the entirety of the individual (American Psychiatric Association, 2022b; Shahrokh & Hales, 2003). Mood is defined as a disposition to respond emotionally in a particular way that may last for hours, days, or even weeks, perhaps at a low level and without the person knowing what prompted the state (American Psychological Association, n.d.-f).

- Moods differ from emotions in that moods lack a stimulus to which cause is attributed; for example, the emotion of joy can be aroused by the birth of a child, but a joyful mood (i.e., elation) may arise when one does not know the reason for being joyful or elated and is not aware of any stimulus or event that elicited the feeling.
- Affect: It is the fluctuating changes in demeanor due to changes in experienced emotion and the objective expression of that feeling or emotion (American Psychological Association, n.d.-a). Affects are behaviors that express a covertly or subjectively experienced emotion (Shahrokh & Hales, 2003). Affects can

range from suffering to elation, from the simplest to the most complex sensations of feeling, and from the most normal to the most pathological emotional reactions. It is often described in terms of positive or negative and appropriate or inappropriate affect. Both mood and emotion are considered affective states (American Psychological Association, n.d.-a). Affect and mood can differ in congruency. Affect can differ from the self-reports of a person's mood (a subjective private event). A person can be yelling and threatening others (a behavioral expression of anger) but reports "feeling" elated and happy.

- Lability: It is rapidly shifting unstable mood over brief periods of time (American Psychiatric Association, 2022b; Shahrokh & Hales, 2003).
- Emotions: These are complex reaction patterns involving subjective experiences and perceptual, cognitive, behavioral, and physiological elements. A specific type of emotion is determined by aspects of environmental stimuli by which an individual attempts to deal with events, cognitively and physiologically. Emotion typically involves feelings. Emotion differs from feeling in having an overt or implicit engagement with the world. Feelings are a phenomenon that is completely covert and private, whereas emotions are observable responses to the covert experiences of feelings (American Psychological Association, n.d.-d).

Many terms have been used when discussing affective lability, including emotional instability, mood changes, mood swings, emotional lability, emotional instability, emotionally labile, labile in mood, emotional dysregulation, variable or changeable mood, unstable mood, and labile mood. A common term used by mental health service providers and users to describe affective lability is "mood swings." Affective lability is a behavior problem and symptoms that have psychophysiological components, including emotional overreactivity that is transdiagnostic and observed in mental health problems in children (e.g., depressive-type problems and attention deficit/hyperactivity disorder (ADHD). It is a complex construct that encompasses (1) primary emotions, or affects, and secondary emotions, with each category having its own dimensional characteristics, including intensity, frequency, antecedental and consequential stimuli, and duration; (2) rapid shifting from ranges including neutral affect to intense affect; and (3) incapacity to adaptively modulate emotions (Renaud & Zacchia, 2012).

The nomenclature surrounding affect or mood includes valence (positive or negative), intensity, frequency of shifts, how rapidly affect and mood change and return to baseline, reactivity to psychosocial cues (e.g., impulsivity), and the intensity of emotional expression (Renaud & Zacchia, 2012). The research literature spans psychiatry, psychology, neurology, and neuroscience, and multiple terms are used to describe the same or related phenomena, including affective instability, emotional dysregulation, mood swings, and emotional impulsiveness with overlapping dimensions, definitions, and measurements.

Marwaha et al. (2014) have used the term affective instability (AI) in their review of the definition and measurement of behavioral health problems related to mood and affect. They found the following terms used to define "affective instability" (AI) in the research literature, listed from being most to least frequently mentioned: affective lability, emotional dysregulation, emotion regulation, mood instability, mood lability, affective dysregulation, emotional lability, and mood swings. In a review of the research on the phenomenon, the concepts associated with the terms showed considerable overlap in features, finding 24 distinct variables that were identified (Marwaha et al., 2014).

Affective lability is widely described in the mental health literature, but there is a lack of agreement and consistency in definitions in clinical and research settings (Broome et al., 2015; Marwaha et al., 2014). Marwaha et al. (2014) categorized the definitions that have been used in the research in this area as primarily measuring one of four dimensions of affective lability: (1) oscillation, (2) intensity of affect, (3) ability to regulate the affective change triggered by the environment, or (4) measuring general emotional regulation. These dimensions need to be operationally defined and assessed simultaneously to more precisely measure the phenomenon that is being studied to have consistency across research findings. With lack of a consensual operational definition of what is affective lability, the findings and conclusions from the studies may be applicable only to the singular event for which it is defined; despite this weakness, research findings are generalized across affective lability in the mental health field. Without an agreed-upon operational definition of affective lability, treatments and outcomes may be impacted by this mental health problem.

Marwaha and others (Broome et al., 2015; Marwaha et al., 2014) have suggested the following definition for affective lability: "rapid oscillations of intense affect, with a difficulty in regulating these oscillations or their behavioural consequences" (Marwaha et al., 2014, p. 2). This definition considers the dimensions of a temporal aspect (rapidity), intensity, and perceptions of controllability. Other temporal aspects that need to be operationalized are periods between the oscillations, frequency, and durations of the phases that fluctuate and fluctuations between specific affective poles. It is important to determine between which emotional or affective poles these fluctuations occur, and whether they consistently involve the same poles or vary over time. A multidimensional approach is required for a comprehensive understanding of affective lability.

Dimensions of Affective Lability

Affective lability is one of the key symptoms and behavioral problems/symptoms in mental health; many terms and definitions have been used in research literature and in the assessment of the phenomenon (Marwaha et al., 2014; Broome et al., 2015). A clear and precise operational definition has been elusive, adding to the puzzle that is affective lability. Affective lability has proven to be difficult to define and clearly separate from other behavioral problems and concepts that occur in people living with SMI and other related mental health problems. Affective lability is heterogeneous and transdiagnostic and may have led to other definitions of the concept in the literature in the mental health fields of psychiatry, psychology, and neuroscience, as affective lability may be radically different in origin and presentation across mental health problems. Multiple terms are used to describe the same or related phenomena, including affective instability, emotional dysregulation, mood swings, emotional impulsiveness, and affective lability. The nomenclature surrounding affect or mood includes valence, intensity, frequency of shifts, rapidity of rise-times and return to baseline, reactivity to psychosocial cues, and the extent to which there is an extreme behavioral expression (e.g., dressing bizarrely during a manic mental health event) (Broome et al., 2015). Collating the main overlapping dimensions, definitions, and the measurement scales, a recent systematic review proposed that mood instability is "a rapid oscillations of intense affect, with a difficulty in regulating these oscillations or their behavioural consequences" (Marwaha et al., 2014, p.12). The presence of these various elements mandates a multidimensional approach to the assessment of mood instability.

The dimensions of frequency, intensity, antecedent situational conditions, and the consequences of the occurrences are common to all behavioral challenges and symptoms associated with SMI; the definition promulgated by Marwaha et al. (2014) accounts for some of the additional dimensional variables associated with affective lability. The four core dimensions of affective lability are (1) rapid oscillation and intensity of affect; (2) a subjective sense of the capacity to control the affect; (3) sense of controlling the behavioral consequences of the affective state; and (4) whether the change in affect is triggered in response to environment stimuli or not (e.g., time of day, season of the year). A dimension assessing the degree of conviction of the person in having a belief that the experienced affective state can be modulated and controlled, as well as the consequences of the state (i.e., to what degree is the affective state beneficial to the person) needs to be considered in the operational definition of affective lability. An additional dimension is whether the rapid change is triggered by behavioral variables such as lack of sleep or experiencing aversive and stressful situations. As in other behavioral health problems associated with SMI, the dimension of the emotional impact of oscillation and the affective state ought to be considered a dimension of affective lability for future research. Individuals living with a bipolar mental health problem often report "enjoying" the feelings of boundless energy, being quick witted and being creative and sociable that are correlates of a manic mental health episode; the individuals find the affective and mood state of mania to be beneficial at times, and this does not change until the negative outcomes of the affective state result in altercations with authorities and family such as impulsive risk-taking behaviors.

Instruments have been developed to assess and measure the multidimensional and heterogeneous nature of this complex phenomenon of affective lability. The Affective Liability Scale (ALS) was developed by Harvey et al. (1989) to measure affective lability; it is a 58-item questionnaire measuring oscillations among euthymia and four affect states (i.e., depression, elation, anger, and anxiety) with the goal of identifying patterns of mood instability. Scales measuring lability among shifts in euthymia, anxiety, depression, anger, and hypomania and labile shifts between anxiety and depression and hypomania and depression were constructed. Oliver and Simons (2004) considered the 58-item ALS as too lengthy and developed an 18-item short form (ALS-18) consisting of at least two items from each affective state dimension of the ALS. Confirmatory factor analysis supported the adequacy of a three-factor structure composed of changeability between the affective poles of euthymia-anxiety/depression, euthymia-depression/elation, and euthymia-anger (Contardi et al., 2018).

The Mood Spectrum Structured Interviews (SCI-MOODS) were developed to discriminate between people living with mood-related mental health problems receiving treatment by outpatient service providers and two control groups without any mental health problems and between individuals living with unipolar depressive and bipolar mental health problems (Fagiolini et al., 1999). The self-report version (MOODS-SR) was developed by the same authors; the intent of MOODS-SR is to obtain a picture of the dimensions and domains of affective lability during the previous month (i.e., point prevalence) (Benvenuti et al., 2015).

SCI-MOODS is composed of 140 items grouped into four domains, mood (50 items), energy (21 items), cognition (46 items), and rhythmicity and vegetative functions (23 items). The first 3 domains are each divided into two subdomains, depressive and manic; the "mood" domain assesses the individual's experience of mood lability and the impact of the affective changes pertaining to interest in family, social and romantic relationships, work, and leisure activities. Questions in the "energy" domain require the presence of periods when there are changes in energy levels that are noticed by the respondent; the items assess changes in everyday activities, with focus on behaviors related to work, leisure activities, and social and romantic life; the "cognition" domain inquiries about changes in cognitive facets such as memory, attention, and planning that are connected with energy or mood fluctuations. "Rhythmicity and neurovegetative functions" are evaluated by exploring routine daily changes in mental and physical efficiency, mood changes, and energy and physical well-being related to the weather, seasons (or the change of season), and shifts in mood associated with changes in appetitive functions such as eating, sleep habits, and sexual activities; this domain also assesses variations and oscillations in problem behaviors that are experienced by a person living with mood-related SMIs (Fagiolini et al., 1999). MOODS-SR follows the same organization as SCI-MOODS, being composed of the same four domains: neurovegetative, energy levels, mood, and the cognitive domains (Benvenuti et al., 2015). SCI-MOODS has been found sensitive to change in the "depression" and "rhythmicity and neurovegetative functions" domains (Cassano et al., 2002; Miniati et al., 2009).

The two moods assessment instruments rely on the self-reports of individuals who are living with mood-related mental health problems. The questions asked in SCI-MOOD and MOOD-SR are based on the criteria in the DSM-5 (American Psychiatric Association, 2013b) for depressive- and manic-related mental health problems. The criteria in DSM-5 for mania and depressive-related mental health problems (DSM-5, 2013b, pp. 124–125) assessed by the instruments are listed according to the four domains in Table 8.1.

Several of the criteria for affective poles of mood-related mental health problems possibly overlap in the domains. For example, the criteria for less than 3 h sleep for manic-related mental health problems are listed under the "neurovegetative/rhythmicity" domain but could be part of the "energy" domain as well; the depressive

Table 8.1 DSM-5 criteria for manic- and depressive-related mental health problems according to domains in SCI-MOOD/MOOD-SR

Mania				Depressive			
Rhythmicity	Mood	Energy	Cognition	Rhythmicity	Mood	Energy	Cognition
Decreased need for sleep less than three hours	Inflated self-esteem or grandiosity	Increase in goal-directed activity at work/school and sexual behaviors; increase in psychomotor agitation	Flight of ideas or subjective experience that thoughts are racing	Significant weight loss, lack of appetite	Feelings of worthlessness, excessive or inappropriate guilt	Psychomotor agitation or retardation, Fatigue, loss of energy	Decreased ability to think or concentrate
		Purposeless nongoal-directed activity	Attention too easily drawn to irrelevant external stimuli	Insomnia or hypersomnia	Depressed mood	Markedly diminished interest or pleasure in all or almost all activities for most of the day or nearly every day	Indecisiveness
		Excessive involvement in activities that have a high potential for painful consequences	Distractibility				Repeated thoughts of death
		More talkative than usual or pressure to keep talking					Suicidal ideation

criterion/symptom of repeated thoughts of death and suicidal ideation that is a feature of the "cognitive" domain could overlap with the "mood" domain since feelings of despair, hopelessness, and depressed mood are correlated with morbid thinking.

The regulation of emotions has been defined as the basic processes by which individuals influence which emotions they have, when they have them, and how they experience and express these emotions (Victor & Klonsky, 2016). Gratz and Roemer (2004a) expanded on this concept by proposing multidimensionality in assessing the concept. To be successful in regulating one's emotions, the individual must (1) be aware and accept the experience of the emotion; (2) have the ability to change the experience of the emotion to achieve the stated goals of the individual; and (3) have the ability to control behavior when being faced with negative emotions. Emotional dysregulation is defined as the absence of or deficits in any of these abilities (Victor & Klonsky, 2016).

To assess the concept of emotional regulation, Gratz and Roemer (2004b) developed the "Difficulties in Emotion Regulation Scale" (DERS). It is a 36-item self-report instrument that assesses the dysregulation of emotions; individuals are to respond on a Likert-type scale for each item, ranging from "Almost Never" to "Almost Always"; some items are reversed scored. The 18-item short form of the DERS (DERS-18) (Victor & Klonsky, 2016) also placed a numerical percentage of the likelihood that the person would engage in the behavior of corresponding item for each Likert scale item as follows: almost never (0–10%); sometimes (11–35%); about half the time (36–65%); most of the time (66–90%); almost always (91–100%) (Victor & Klonsky, 2016).

Factor analyses identified 6 factors from the DERS, which were translated into six subscales (Gratz & Roemer, 2004a; Hallion et al., 2018); below are examples of item content for each of the dimensional subscales (reverse scoring is the second example):

1. Lack of emotional awareness (factor name: awareness). Examples of item contents are "I have no idea how I am feeling" and "I pay attention to how I feel."
2. Lack of emotional clarity (factor name: clarity). Examples of item contents are "I have difficulty making sense out of my feelings" or "I know exactly how I am feeling."
3. Difficulty regulating behavior when distressed (factor name: impulse). Examples of item contents are "When I'm upset, I become out of control" and "When I'm upset, I feel like I can remain in control of my behaviors."
4. Difficulty engaging in goal-directed cognition and behavior when distressed (factor name: impulse). Examples of item contents are "When I'm upset, I have difficulty getting work done" and "When I'm upset, I can still get things done."
5. Unwillingness to accept certain emotional responses (factor name: nonacceptance). Examples of item contents are "When I'm upset, I become angry at myself for feeling that way" and "When I'm upset, I believe that my feelings are valid and important."
6. Lack of access to strategies for feeling better when distressed (factor name: strategies). Examples of item contents are "When I'm upset, I believe there is noth-

ing I can do to feel better" and "When I'm upset, I know that I can find a way to eventually feel better."

Two additional dimensions of affective lability are average affect and affective variability (Dejonckheere et al., 2019; Hossain & Kangas, 2020). Average affect is defined as the average level of emotions someone felt throughout the day or for a specified duration. Affective variability is commonly defined as the deviations from a person's typical emotions. Affective variability can be used to measure the range of fluctuations, whereas affective instability is defined as the changes in affective intensity between periods of time. Affective bipolarity is defined as the correlation between positive and negative affect at any given point of assessment.

The different assessments of affective lability cite different dimensions of affective lability but do not incorporate all the possible dimensions that make up the experiences of affective lability. Directions for future research on affective lability ought to explore all the dimensions to determine the contribution of each to the impact and the experience of affective lability for the individual.

Summarizing the multidimensionality of affective lability that is present in the literature, the following dimensions need consideration in a comprehensive operational definition and assessment of affective lability:

1. Awareness: Cognizant of emotions, moods, and feelings and when oscillations of affective states occur.
2. Impact: The impact and disruption of the affective states and oscillations have on the person's capabilities to function in various personal and social roles.
3. Frequency: The recurrences of affective states during a defined period. Any assessment needs to assess the lifetime prevalence and point prevalence occurrences of affective lability. Lifetime prevalence refers to the number of occurrences of affective lability during a person's lifetime; point prevalence refers to the number of oscillations, affective states, and other dimensions of affective lability that have occurred within a specified period.
4. Duration: The temporal lengths of each affective state (e.g., mania, depressive, euthymic) and the temporal durations between durations of oscillations among specified affective states.
5. Average affect: It is defined as the average level of perceived emotions someone felt throughout the day or during a specified duration. Average affect is the baseline from which all variability can be determined.
6. Range of affective states: This dimension is also known as affective variability (Dejonckheere et al., 2019). It is imperative to determine the mood and affective states that result from the repeated oscillations in mood and affect. The range of affective variability is determined by deviations from a person's perceived typical affective state over a certain duration. There is a need for future research into the relation and oscillations of manic and depressive mental health problems to more precisely define the criteria of affective and emotional states such as frustration, anger, and impatience to the concept of affective lability (Moore et al., 1997).

7. Intensity: This is the magnitude or intensity of the affective states; in the research literature, it has been labeled as "severity." For affective lability the intensity is the subjective intensity of the internal sensation of the emotion being experienced. For example, individuals experiencing a manic type of mental health problem sometimes describe their emotional experience as "being on top of the world" or "never felt better."
8. Amount of emotional distress: How frequently do oscillations cause distress to the individual experiencing rapid changes.
9. Origin: This is the perception of the person as to the source of the cause of the oscillation of affective states, whether being caused by environmental conditions (e.g., time of day, seasons), behavioral causes (e.g., sleep, stressful events, medications, substances), or random occurrences.
10. Control: This is the extent to which the person believes that they can manage or influence the occurrence, duration, intensity, and impact of the affective lability and the corresponding affective states. Perceptions of not having the ability to manage or influence the dimensions of affective lability and the resulting affective states lead to a greater degree of distress and result in disruption of daily life.

SMI is heterogeneous and transdiagnostic in problem behaviors and symptoms. Multidimensionality recognizes that people with the same mental health problem can present with varying experiences, behavioral problems, and perceptions of living with a certain mental health problem.

By having a multifaceted viewpoint of mental health, a multidimensional approach can inform the development of specific and effective treatments that address the individual's needs across various domains of each dimension of the mental health problem. By considering various dimensions, researchers can gain a more nuanced understanding of the complex mechanisms underlying mental health conditions. Recognizing the multifaceted nature of mental illness can help destigmatize mental health issues by avoiding simplistic "all or nothing" explanations of mental health problems.

Origins of Affective Lability

Affective lability involves emotions, moods, and affective responses. Human emotions and affective responses based on emotions and moods are intrinsic to behavior, yet there is no consensus on their definition, elemental nature, or cause. Research endeavors span the fields of behavioral genetics, neuroimaging, psychopharmacology, behavioral neuroscience, behavioral and cognitive learning paradigms, and psychology (Roxo et al., 2011; Šimić et al., 2021).

Neurological Substrates

Moods, emotions, and affective responses are postulated to be functions of the limbic system of the central nervous system (CNS). Emotions are defined as cerebral functions resulting from states of reward and punishment, influencing behavior to seek satisfaction and avoid harm; yet there is little agreement as to an operational definition for emotions since it is a private event and can only be accessed through self-report that may or may not be reliable (Bilderbeck et al., 2014; Roxo et al., 2011) because of problems of valid reporting, difficulty in understanding what is being asked, and problems in recall. Bilderbeck et al. (2014) recommend the use of collateral information and data obtained from others in the respondents' support systems. The limbic system (also known as the visceral brain) (Shahrokh & Hales, 2003) is a widespread group of brain structures and nuclei. It includes portions of the cerebral cortex (especially the prefrontal cortex [PFC]), thalamus, and certain cortical and subcortical structures, such as the hippocampus, amygdala, and septal area, to form a network that is involved in autonomic and visceral processes and mechanisms of emotion, memory, learning, and goal-directed behaviors that change according to emotion and mood being experienced by the individual (Shahrokh & Hales, 2003).

An important part of the limbic system is the temporo-amygdala-orbitofrontal network (Catani et al., 2013). The network is dedicated to the integration of visceral sensations and emotions with semantic memory and behaviors. The anatomical components of this network include:

- Temporal lobe: Specifically, the anterior part of the temporal lobe, including the temporal pole and the parahippocampal gyrus.
- Amygdala: A key structure involved in processing emotions. The amygdala plays a central role as the subcortical emotional brain structure that constantly evaluates and integrates a variety of sensory information from the internal and external environments of an individual and assigns them values of emotional dimensions, such as valence, intensity, and approachability (e.g., assessment of threat). The amygdala participates in the regulation of autonomic and endocrine functions, decision-making, and adaptations of instinctive and motivational behaviors to changes in the environment through associative learning, changes in short- and long-term synaptic plasticity, and activation of the fight-or-flight response via efferent projections from its central nucleus to cortical and subcortical structures (Šimić et al., 2021).
- Orbitofrontal cortex (OFC): Located in the frontal lobe, this area is involved in decision-making and the integration of sensory input with emotional responses. The prefrontal cortex (PFC) plays a crucial role in emotions and affect by regulating and integrating emotional responses with cognitive processes. The PFC, particularly the ventromedial prefrontal cortex (vmPFC) and dorsolateral prefrontal cortex (dlPFC), helps in modulating emotional responses. It exerts top-down control over subcortical structures such as the amygdala, thereby regulating the intensity and expression of emotions. The vmPFC and dlPFC use what it has

learned from environmental consequences to mediate the emotional responses from the amygdala and communicate to other cerebral regions to respond affectively to the contextual stimuli that are presently occurring. The vmPFC is involved in decision-making processes that require evaluating emotional outcomes. It helps in anticipating the emotional consequences of different actions and making choices that align with long-term goals, social norms, role modeling, and consequences of emotional responses (Šimić et al., 2021).

- Prefrontal cortex (PFC): It is essential for understanding and interpreting social cues and emotions in others. It contributes to empathy, moral reasoning, and the ability to navigate complex social interactions. The PFC is involved in the cognitive appraisal of emotional stimuli, which includes assessing the significance of an event and determining an appropriate emotional response that is based on associative learning experiences and role models. The PFC interacts with the hippocampus and amygdala to influence the storing and retrieval of emotionally charged memories. This interaction helps in learning from past experiences and applying that knowledge to future situations. Overall, the PFC integrates emotional and cognitive information, enabling individuals to respond to their environment in an adaptive manner based on the integration of present sensory input and past experiences. Dysfunction in the PFC can lead to impaired emotional regulation that is displayed in depressive, anxious, and impulsive mental health problems (Šimić et al., 2021).
- The vmPFC and dlPFC are thought to regulate amygdala activity by monitoring fear-inducing stimuli and its termination in the environment. The vmPFC integrates emotional and cognitive information and has an important role in decision-making and behavioral choices at different time periods, whereas the dlPFC is critical to carry out working memory, especially in remembering previous sensory events as well as sustaining attention and planning responses to emotional stimuli. The vmPFC has an inhibitory effect on the amygdala and reduces the reaction to the stressor/stressful event and excessive emotional reactivity. Greater vmPFC activity means greater conscious effort and suppressed activity of the amygdala, along with a tendency to positively evaluate external experiences. Optimal regulation of emotions is thought to arise from the balance between the PFC and amygdala activity. Stress negatively affects this activity of the PFC, which explains why a strategy of cognitive reappraisal in adverse real-life situations is often ineffective (Šimić et al., 2021).
- Uncinate fasciculus: It is a white matter tract that connects the anterior temporal lobe with the orbitofrontal cortex, facilitating communication between these regions (Catani et al., 2013). It is a bundle of axons that connect the amygdala to the vmPFC and play a role in the development and maturation of emotional processing and decision-making. This connection is essential for the generation of secondary emotions from primary ones, as the vmPFC receives information about primary emotions via the uncinate fasciculus (Šimić et al., 2021). These components work together to integrate visceral sensations and emotions with verbal memory and behavior. This network involves connections through the uncinate fasciculus and is engaged in tasks that involve naming, single-word comprehension, response inhibition, face processing, and monitoring of out-

comes (Catani et al., 2013). The maturation of the uncinate fasciculus as other neuronal structures and connections in the PFC continues up to 30 years of age, correlating with its prolonged development throughout adolescence (Šimić et al., 2021) and an explanation for the emotional storm that is a feature of adolescence. Damage to this network can manifest cognitive and behavioral symptoms characteristic of temporal lobe epilepsy (TLE), traumatic brain injury (TBI), neurodegenerative syndromes, and personality- and mood-related mental health problems (Catani et al., 2013).

- Dorsomedial prefrontal context (dmPFC): Another area that is involved in the regulation of emotion and affective responses in the dorsomedial prefrontal cortex (dmPFC) (Šimić et al., 2021). It is hypothesized to play a significant role in the higher-order theory of emotion that emphasizes the role of cortical processing in the conscious experience of emotions, integrating information from subcortical first-order networks (i.e., amygdaloid circuits) to create a subjectively coherent emotional experience, especially in the context of fear and anxiety (Šimić et al., 2021). The dmPFC, along with the ventromedial prefrontal cortex (vmPFC) and orbitofrontal cortex (OFC), contributes to the regulation of emotional responses and the processing of social cognition, such as recognizing emotional facial expressions and attributing mental states to oneself and others. The dmPFC is also implicated in working memory and higher cognitive functions, which are essential for managing emotional and social behaviors (Šimić et al., 2021). The vmPFC seems to play a crucial role across various mental functions, particularly (1) reward- and value-based decision-making; (2) generation and regulation of negative and distressful emotion (e.g., fear, anxiety); and (3) social cognition (e.g., emotional facial recognition and metacognitive capabilities) (Dixon et al., 2017; Hiser & Koenigs, 2018).

Disorders that are associated with disruptions in the activity of the dmPFC show problems in autobiographical memory, introspective self-directed thinking, and other cognitive functions (Catani et al., 2013). Disorders linked to the dmPFC network include:

1. Major depressive mental health problems: Altered activation of the network has been observed in people living with major depressive mental health problems (Catani et al., 2013).
2. Schizophrenia spectrum mental health problems: Functional magnetic resonance imagery (fMRIs) have reported altered activation of this network (Catani et al., 2013).
3. Autism spectrum disorder (ASD): The social and communication deficits observed in ASD have been attributed to abnormalities in the dmPFC (Catani et al., 2013).
4. Alzheimer's disease (AD): fMRIs show reduced metabolism and activation of the dmPFC in individuals living with AD and mild cognitive impairment (MCI) (Catani et al., 2013).

The neurological substrates for affective lability directly involve the mesolimbic dopamine (ML-DA) system, which plays a major role in regulating emotional states and affective responses (Alcaro & Panksepp, 2011). The ML-DA system connects the midbrain and forebrain nuclei, influencing the expression of exploratory and approach behaviors, goal-directed activity, and positive excitement. Affective lability, characterized by rapid and intense changes in emotional states and changes in intensity and frequency of goal-directed behaviors, can be linked to the dysregulation of the ML-DA system. This system's activity is modulated by both tonic (normal or restorative) and phasic (change in stimulus conditions) releases of endogenous dopamine, which influences the overall emotional tone and responsiveness to environmental stimuli. Abnormalities in dopamine transmission, such as excessive or deficient dopamine levels, can lead to the occurrence of affective lability (Alcaro & Panksepp, 2011).

In conditions like a depressive mental health problem, the system's abnormal expression is evident as the activation of the ML-DA system is reduced, with decreased goal-directed behaviors and positive excitement, leading to the behavior problems of anhedonia, anergia, avolition, dysphoric mood, and helplessness present in persons living with SMI. The ML-DA system's role in modulating affective states, its dysregulation in mental health problems, including mental health problems characterizing SMI, and the neural connections to the temporo-amygdala-orbitofrontal network highlight its importance as a neurological substrate for affective lability (Alcaro & Panksepp, 2011).

The findings suggest that while both disorders exhibit similar patterns of neural activity in the lateral prefrontal cortex (lPFC), they differ in the dorsomedial PFC (dmPFC) and amygdala (amyg) activity, which may explain the distinct clinical features of each distinct mental health problem.

Affective lability and difficulties with emotional regulation are central to the clinical presentation of individuals living with certain characterological mental health problems, such as the condition of borderline personality disorder (BPD) (Edwards et al., 2021). The behaviors that are commonly exhibited in people living with BPD include problems in the ability to successfully engage in self-directed and meaningful short-term goals; excessive emotional reactions to stresses, frustrations, and disappointments; variable and intense emotions and self-regulation difficulties impacting functioning and interpersonal relationships and well-being; maladaptive attempts at self-soothing and emotional regulation that include suicide threats, self-harm, and angry behavior; and problems in intimacy and empathy (American Psychiatric Association, 2022c).

Research on the amygdala and people living with BPD shows reduced amygdala volumes and poorer white matter integrity in tracts connecting the amygdala to prefrontal regions, indicative of less density of neural connections within that area compared to others that do not display the problem behaviors. Studies show varied results on amygdala responses in individuals living with BPD, with some indicating exaggerated responses and others showing blunted amygdaloid responsivity (Silvers et al., 2016). The study hypothesized that affective lability correlates with amygdaloid responses during emotional responding in people living with BPD. Emotion regulation strategies like reappraisal involve prefrontal cortex (PFC) regions, with

BPD individuals showing different PFC and amygdala activation when compared to others with no mental health problem (Silvers et al., 2016).

Using an fMRI paradigm, Silvers et al. (2016) assessed individual differences in a large sample of women living with BPD and matched females with no known mental health problems. Affective Lability Scale (ALS) and Difficulties in Emotion Regulation Scale DERS scores were significantly higher than published norms for the group with no known mental health problems. Greater affective lability, as measured on the ALS and DERS, correlated positively with amygdala activation during exposure to aversive versus neutral stimuli.

Difficulties in emotional regulation were associated with less inferior frontal gyrus (IFG) activation during regulation, particularly with difficulty engaging in goal-directed behavior and impulse control difficulties. Activation of the IFG is associated with response inhibition, attention, social cognition, planning, and problem-solving functions. IFG activation during emotion regulation was associated with greater regulation success but not related to amygdala activation during emotional reactivity. The results support the conclusion that affective lability in individuals living with BPD is correlated with increased amygdala activation, while difficulties with emotion regulation were linked to reduced left IFG activation. These two results were found to be unrelated, suggesting different features for affective lability and emotional regulation in different problem behaviors associated with BPD. Greater activation in the IFG area was associated with greater regulatory success. The findings suggest that fMRI may be more sensitive than self-report measures for probing individual differences in BPD on emotion regulation paradigms. The authors (Silvers et al., 2016) concluded that future research should examine the connectivity between brain regions and the role of individual differences.

Emotional regulation involves the fronto-limbic network (FLN) with input coming from lower and higher cortical areas (Malhi et al., 2013). Disturbances in the FLN are hypothesized to produce affective lability exhibited by people living with SMI, particularly BPD- and bipolar-related mental health problems (BD) (Malhi et al., 2013). Individuals living with either BD or BPD showed reduced neural activity in the dlPFC and increased activity in the right ventrolateral PFC (vlPFC) compared to results on fMRI scans from people with no mental health problems. The individuals living with BD exhibited heightened dmPFC activity, while those living with BPD showed diminished amygdaloid activity while doing an emotion-related task. Analyses revealed that emotion regulation difficulties were associated with reduced left dlPFC activation and increased right vlPFC activation, showing a greater need for inhibition to control emotional responsivity (Malhi et al., 2013; Ojha et al., 2024).

Psychological Substrates

Learning plays a significant role in emotions and affective responses by shaping how individuals respond based on past experiences and outcomes to external and internal stimuli (Thompson, 2019). The regulation of emotions and affective behaviors impacts social adjustments by the management of emotional experiences, so the individual can achieve desired goals.

Emotions are not just innate responses but are influenced by social (i.e., role modeling) and associative learning as the brain creates and stores memories about the relationships and parameters of experiential events. The learning of emotions involves the attention to and modification of emotional states and reactions as well and is a skill that begins in childhood and is crucial for interactions with family and peers, educational success, and psychological health. Learning emotions and affective responses is a process that involves both covert private events and external environmental experiences such as cultural expectations and parenting styles (Sezgin et al., 2023). For example, fear conditioning involves associating a neutral stimulus with an aversive event, leading to a conditioned emotional response. Once established, the individual can engage in cognitive and behavioral strategies that have been learned to manage the emotional response (i.e., cognitive restructuring, exposure gradients, modulating physiological arousals). Emotions are behavioral patterns reinforced or diminished through life experiences (Ewen, 2014).

Emotions play a significant role in everyday behaviors. They are not just internal experiences but observable behaviors in response to stimuli. This perspective allows for a tangible way to assess emotions through the actions that are provoked (Ewen, 2014). Emotions translate into physical actions that differ as to the degree of observability, prominence, and subtlety; some of the behaviors can only be observed by psychophysiological assessments. For example, finger temperature, blood pressure, and heart rate are all behaviors that indicate responses to certain emotional contexts, such as anxiety, stress, fear, and relaxation.

Pharmacologic and behavioral interventions were found to be equally effective in reducing the occurrences of affective lability (Agapoff et al., 2023). CBT-based interventions such as dialectical behavior therapy (DBT) have been found effective in reducing "emotional dysregulation," which has been defined as the extreme or inappropriate emotional response to a situation (such as temper outbursts, aggressive behaviors, and self-harm) (American Psychological Association, n.d.-c). Deliberate self-harm is a behavior that has been reinforced as a mediator of the intensity of averse respondents originating from private events such as traumatic memories triggered by both behavioral and emotional cues that are similar to the traumatic experience. DBT has demonstrated efficacy in stabilizing and controlling self-destructive behavior and improving adherence to treatment (Panos et al., 2014). Modifying behaviors associated with emotions can alter emotional responses (Ewen, 2014).

Emotions are dynamic and can be influenced by situational learning. Emotions are not static but can change and adapt based on new experiences and contexts. They can rise from certain innate feelings such as happiness, sadness, anger, fear, disgust, and surprise. These emotions are considered innate as they are expressed similarly in people around the world, including isolated areas where there had been little contact with others and little opportunity for emotional expressions to have been learned and culturally transmitted (LeDoux, 2012). The different emotions that are experienced are derived from the basic emotions through associative conditioning (respondent or classical conditioning) to the context or situation, including subvocalizations associated with the emotional contexts. Emotions can take on different forms depending on the specific situations in which they are experienced and learned. According to learning-based theories, emotions are the result of the assembly of perceptual, cognitive, interoceptive, and motor processes that are experienced and have positive and negative consequences according to the outcome of the experience (Lebois et al., 2020). People accumulate different populations of emotional standards or prototypes for emotional categories. Consequently, when people categorize the same situation as an instance of an emotional category, different emotional prototypes become active to interpret the situation, thereby producing different emotional states in the individuals.

Learning is fundamental in establishing the adaptive and maladaptive emotional styles of individuals. When, for example, an individual experiences a dysfunctional and distressful situation frequently, cognitive and behavioral processes that are closely connected to the contextual environments in which they take place become entrenched in memory; the behavioral and cognitive strategies that are used have the goal of mitigating the negative impact of the distressful situation. The strategies are active efforts that an individual engages in to deal with a difficult situation through problem-solving, emotional regulation, or other means; they are deliberate behaviors and subvocal thought processes that an individual utilizes to manage or reduce stress arising from a perceived challenging or threatening situation. The behavioral and cognitive strategies become available for producing emotion in other situations, perhaps inappropriately, through "stimulus generalization" (Cooper et al., 2020), in which the response occurs to situations that are like the stimuli in the primary situation in which the responses were conditioned.

The context in which the emotion and the behavioral responses to the emotion occur is conditioned and reinforced as other behavioral responses. The context and the resulting emotions are antecedent conditions for the display of behaviors associated with the emotions and the context. Emotion is an antecedent condition of the behavioral response that impacts the internal and external environments of the person. The impact on the environment is the consequence of the emotional behavioral response that is reinforced or punished and increases or decreases the chance of that behavioral response being emitted to the contextual antecedent conditions in the future.

Emotions and the associated learned responses are tailored to the context. How emotion is experienced is the result of modifications of the basic emotions through associative and social learning. For example, an emotion is experienced differently while facing physical harm (such as an oncoming car driving the wrong way) and involves different private events and processes than the same emotion that is experienced (such as going into a major exam unprepared). The experience of the emotion is impacted by subvocal speech— thoughts, cognitions—about the perceptions of the situation based on previous experiences. The subvocal speech that is emitted is derived from memories of overt experiences of similar situations or from associative learning from role modeling.

Role modeling in emotional learning occurs due to observation, imitation, and social interactions with others in the environment. Social learning involves acquiring new knowledge or skills by watching others, with factors such as similarity, empathy, social status, and the expectancy of the magnitude of reinforcer contingent on engaging in the observed behavior influencing the efficacy of learning (Gregorová et al., 2024; Joiner et al., 2017). Behavior is developed and regulated by external stimulus events, such as the influence of other individuals, and by external reinforcement, such as praise, blame, and reward. Through role modeling, the observer can determine the contingencies underlying the modeled activities, generate patterns of behavior that conform to the stimulus conditions and the contingencies of the observed behaviors, acquiring behaviors and skills without having to go through the process of learning by consequences to responses.

During childhood, individuals observed others in the environment that have confronted stressful situations. The stimulus conditions, behaviors that are emitted, and the consequences are observed by the individual and are consolidated into memory to be used in similar situations. When similar antecedent stimulus conditions occur, what has been observed is then "replayed" as part of behavioral chains that are associated with the emotional contextual situation.

However, what is "replayed" may be the memories of observed maladaptive responses to emotional situations. The person then engages in maladaptive behaviors that result in desired and undesired consequences. The consequences can result in alterations of what is replayed, but the changes depend on the frequency of the modeled behavioral situation and the schedule of reinforcement of the responses; intermittent reinforcement, in which only some of the responses are reinforced, results in behaviors that are difficult to change (Cooper et al., 2020).

Behavioral chains can occur when a contextual cue triggers an action, or the cognitive representation of an action (e.g., thought, subvocal speech), that has been performed repeatedly in that context that is occurring. The behaviors can be a "habitual response" as the behavior is an automatic or nearly automatic reaction to a situation or cue, triggered by a previously learned pattern of goal-directed behavior that occurs repeatedly in similar contexts, often without conscious thought or decision-making involved; essentially, an emotional and affective response has become a habit through repetition (Papies et al., 2022).

Additionally, researchers have found that repetitive traumatic, unstable, distressful, and abusive experiences result in increases in amygdala activation in conjunction with diminished activation of the inferior frontal gyrus (IFG) network, which is correlated with an aspect of executive control referred to as response inhibition (Hampshire et al., 2010). The result is difficulties in emotion regulation as greater activation in the IFG area has been associated with greater regulatory success (Silvers et al., 2016). A combination of neurological substrates that are hyperreactive to perceptions of threat due to environmental experiences and flawed learned maladaptive responses to emotions and their contexts could possibly result in affective lability and emotional dysregulation.

For instance, a child spills milk in front of a parent. The parent screams at the child for spilling the milk and may threaten or strike the child; the child reacts by crying, withdrawing, or other behaviors showing distress. Spilling milk behavior occurs again shortly thereafter, but this time the parent laughs and smiles, joking about the spilled milk and saying "accidents happen," and the child reacts with laughter and smiles; the third time the behavior occurs, the parent wails and cries about how her life has been ruined, and the spilling of milk is just an example of how awful life is and how hard she tries with the child reacting with sadness, guilt, and shame about causing the parent to feel so badly. The child has emitted emotional respondents to the behaviors that the parent has emitted and has observed prototypes of responses to emotional contexts. The responses and observed parental behaviors and the emotional contexts associated with the behaviors are incorporated into memory. The more frequently is the occurrence of the behaviors outlined above the stronger is the consolidation of the memories and the easier to retrieve these memories as repetition grows the brain's neural network (Schmelzer, 2015). Repetition of occurrences of behaviors result in habitual behavioral and emotional responses that are automatic reactions to a situation or cue, often without conscious thought or decision-making involved (Papies et al., 2022). If repeated, the maturing child replays these maladaptive behaviors that are associated with similar emotional contexts and situations. The observed inconsistent emotional affective responses by Person A as consequences to the behaviors of Person B and the conditioned emotional respondents of Person B to the inconsistent affective responses by Person A result in labile emotional reactions (AL) by Person B in the future.

The hypothesis that emotions and affective displays are impacted by environmental stimuli is supported by studies that looked at the effect of childhood trauma and emotional abuse on affective lability and emotional dysregulation. Findings support that childhood trauma has an impact on affective lability. Specifically, body image dissatisfaction and being bullied affect the relationship between emotional abuse and affective lability (Wu et al., 2023). Dysfunctional cognitive structures that are learned from environmental interactions often underlie the mental health problems that are evident in SMI, and restructuring (or disabling) them is central to successful treatment (Beck & Dozois, 2011).

Epidemiological Considerations

Mood instability is a common experience. In the Adult Psychiatric Morbidity Survey (APMS), with over 7400 individuals living in England participating, 13.9% of respondents were found to experience affective lability (Marwaha et al., 2013b). It was more common in women than men, with the highest prevalence in the age range of 16 to 24 years and gradually declining with age, with 7% of 65- to

74-year-olds reporting unstable mood. Mood instability is reported in 40–60% of those with depressive, anxiety-related, posttraumatic stress, and obsessive–compulsive mental health problems, associated with increased health service use and suicidal ideation, and not associated with other mental health problems such as substance use and personality-related mental health problems.

Patel et al. (2015) documented affective lability in 12.1% of individuals seeking mental healthcare. It was most frequently documented in people with bipolar-related mental health problems (22.6%) but was common in people with personality-based mental health problems (17.8%) and schizophrenia spectrum mental health problems (15.5%). Affective lability was associated with a greater number of days spent in hospital, frequency of admissions, higher incidence of involuntary admissions, and an increased likelihood of the individuals being prescribed antipsychotics or mood stabilizing medications. The results showed that affective lability occurs in a wide range of mental health problems and is not limited to affective mental health problems. It is generally associated with relatively poor clinical outcomes.

Mood-related mental health problems have varying prevalence rates globally (Merikangas et al., 2011). These include major depressive (Marwaha et al., 2015), bipolar, and subthreshold mental health conditions (Merikangas et al., 2011). The concept of subthreshold (subsyndromal) mood-related mental health problems has received attention in recent decades. Individuals living with mood-related mental health problems may be experiencing affective lability and other problems more than 60% of the time, but the problem behaviors and symptoms are at a subthreshold level of intensity, with each symptom level representing a different phase of the intensity, frequency, duration, and other dimensions of the problem behaviors, such as affective lability (Juruena, 2012). Juruena (2012) proposed an operational definition of subsyndromal mood-related mental problems that included two or more simultaneously occurring behavioral problems and symptoms that are present most of the time for at least 2 weeks in duration. The occurrence of mental health problems such as affective lability is correlated with diminished capabilities in daily and social functions and increased personal distress by the individual.

Under the auspices of the World Health Organization (WHO) Mental Health Survey Initiative (Kessler et al., 2006), face-to-face, household surveys were conducted with over 6000 adults in 11 countries in the Americas, Europe, and Asia. The participants were living with bipolar-type spectrum mental health problems in their home communities. The lifetime prevalence and point prevalence (12 months) of affective lability experienced by the participants were as follows:

- Lifetime prevalence: Affective lability as a feature of living with bipolar type I (BP-I) or bipolar type II (BP-II) mental health problems was experienced by 0.6% and 0.4% of the individuals, respectively. Affective lability was experienced by 1.4% of individuals living with subthreshold bipolar spectrum mental problems (SBD), and 2.4% of people living with all types of bipolar spectrum mental health problems (BSP) experienced affective lability over a lifetime (Merikangas et al., 2011).

- Point prevalence for 12 months: Affective lability as a feature of living with BP-I and BP-II was experienced by 0.4% and 0.3% of people, respectively. Affective lability was experienced by 0.8% of individuals living with SBD. Affective lability occurred in 1.5% of people living with any type of BPS (Merikangas et al., 2011).
- Country-specific prevalence: The United States had the highest lifetime prevalence (4.4%) and 12-month point prevalence (2.8%) of BPS. India had the lowest lifetime and 12-month point prevalence of BPS (both 0.1%), followed by Japan with a lifetime prevalence of affective lability (0.7%) and 12-month point prevalence of affective lability at 0.2% despite being a high-income country. Colombia was found to have a high lifetime prevalence of affective lability associated with BPS of 2.6% (Merikangas et al., 2011).
- Major depressive–related mental health problems are generally more prevalent than BPS. The World Health Organization (WHO) estimates that depression-related problems affect more than 264 million people worldwide (Merikangas et al., 2011).
- The study found that lifetime rates of BP-I and BSP were higher in males, while females had higher rates of BP-II. Marital status and employment status were significantly associated with BPS, but family income was not. The mean age at onset was 18.4 years for BP-I, 20.0 years for BP-II, and 21.9 years for subthreshold BP (Merikangas et al., 2011).

Epidemiologic studies show that mood-related mental health problems are comparatively rare among children, but common among adolescents, with up to 25% lifetime prevalence by the end of adolescence for a depressive mental health problem and an approximate 2% lifetime prevalence for manic-related mental health problems by the end of adolescence (Beauchaine, 2015). Subthreshold mood behavioral problems and symptoms are reportedly more common, but data are inconsistent (Kessler et al., 2001). Retrospective reports about the age of onset in adult studies suggest that at least 50% of young people living with depressive-related mental health problems and 90% of those living with manic type of mental health problems continue to have adult recurrences (Kessler et al., 2001).

The prevalence of mood conditions in children and adolescents varies across different countries and cultures. Specific findings indicated that depression-related mental health problems occurred in 1.0–3.3% of children and adolescents within a 3- to-12-month point prevalence in the United States and 0.6–2.5% in Great Britain. The results cannot be compared due to methodological variations in the studies and cultural differences in the magnitude of childhood mood problems (Merikangas et al., 2009). In addition, manic-related mental health problems and affective lability were not included in any of the studies.

In a study involving nearly 2600 high school–age students (median age 16.4 years) in Thailand, the prevalence of mood swings among participants was 26.4%, with the highest rate (55.9%) having problematic social media use involving bullying. Bullying involvement increased the likelihood of mood swings by more than twice. Participants with a family history of mental health problems and high expressed emotionality (high EE) were associated with experiencing mood swings (Angsukiattitavorn et al., 2020).

Cultural influences significantly impact emotional dysregulation by determining what is learned and expected from individuals in a particular culture. Cultural expectations and parenting styles shape whether individuals are motivated to regulate their emotions. Culture affects the motivation to regulate emotions by influencing how emotions are perceived and valued within a cultural context (Weiss et al., 2022). The regulation strategies used in different cultures are learned behaviors and differ in adaptiveness, given the situational context. This cultural orientation can influence the adaptiveness of emotion regulation strategies (Ford & Mauss, 2015). Lack of learned adaptive emotional regulation strategies has been shown to result in variability in emotions and affective responses (Dejonckheere et al., 2019; Hossain & Kangas, 2020).

Cultures that promote interdependence, such as East Asian cultures, often view emotions as potentially disruptive to social harmony and thus encourage emotion regulation strategies such as suppression (Ford & Mauss, 2015; Weiss et al., 2022). Suppression is a conscious effort to push disturbing thoughts and experiences from awareness, or to control and inhibit the expression of unacceptable impulses and feelings (American Psychological Association, n.d.-g). Suppression is often linked to worse psychological and social functioning in independent cultural contexts but may be less harmful or even beneficial in interdependent cultures as an expression of emotions as a form of individuality in independent cultures.

Individuals in these interdependent cultures are more motivated to regulate their emotions to maintain group cohesion and avoid conflict (Ford & Mauss, 2015). Asian individuals reported more difficulties in overall potential for emotion regulation compared to White and Black individuals (Weiss et al., 2022). Research indicates that individuals from interdependent cultures, such as Asian Americans, report using emotion regulation more frequently and have a stronger preference for controlling their emotions compared to European Americans. Therefore, individuals from independent cultures—such as European countries—may be less motivated to regulate their emotions, as expressing emotions is seen to assert one's unique identity and personal views (Weiss et al., 2022). This cultural orientation toward emotion regulation is not solely based on cultural group membership but also on the extent to which individuals endorse the values of their respective cultures.

Types of Affective Lability

Affective lability is a complex term that encompasses: (1) primary emotions or affects and secondary emotions, with each category having its own dimensions; (2) rapid shifts from neutral or positive and negative affective states to very intense affect; and (3) dysfunctional modulation and control of emotions (Renaud & Zacchia, 2012). The types of affective lability are defined by the affective shifts and if the affect is consistent with the mood of the person.

The DSM-5 defines affect as a "pattern of observable behaviors that is the expression of a subjectively experienced feeling state (emotion)" (American Psychiatric Association, 2013a, p.817). The DSM-5 lists four types of affects, which are (Shahrokh & Hales, 2003):

1. Blunted affect: A great reduction in the expected range and intensity of the expression of an emotion (Shahrokh & Hales, 2003).
2. Constricted or restricted affect: A mild to moderate reduction in the expected range and intensity of the expression of an emotion (Shahrokh & Hales, 2003).
3. Flat affect: The absence of any behaviors associated with an emotional expression (Shahrokh & Hales, 2003).
4. Inappropriate affect: A significant and evident difference between the affective expression and what is the context of the situation (e.g., laughing when speaking about the loss of a spouse). Inappropriate affect is the same as incongruent affect where there is an observed mismatch between a person's expressed emotion and affective display (Shahrokh & Hales, 2003).
5. Labile affect: Abnormal variation if affect characterized by repeated, rapid, and abrupt shifts in affective expression (Shahrokh & Hales, 2003).

(The types of affect responses that are observed in people living with SMI are no longer included in the DSM-5-TR (American Psychiatric Association, 2022a).

Affective lability is described by many service providers as shifts between various poles of emotional and affective states, such as happiness and sadness, intense laughing or crying at inappropriate times, from affectionate to rage and anger, exaggerated emotional responses (uncontrollable laughter or crying that goes beyond the situation), and unpredictable mood swings.

Why Does Affective Lability Happen?

Part of the Reason May Be Biochemical or Physical

Swings of mood are most obvious in bipolar-related mental health problems, commonly called bipolar disorder (in the past it was called "manic-depressive illness"). Most clinicians agree that this mental health problem appears to have irregularities in chemical and neuronal connections in certain areas of the brain that are important in the expression and control of emotional behaviors, such as the temporo-amygdala-orbitofrontal network (Catani et al., 2013). The neurological irregularities result in extreme fluctuations of emotional and affective responses.

In some other mental health problems, less severe but still troublesome swings of mood may occur. SMI may involve some disturbance of the person's ability to stay calm and engage in emotional regulation skills and strategies. This may happen with people living with schizophrenia spectrum mental health problems. For example, a person living with thoughts of paranoia may become uncontrollably angry from time to time. People living with a schizophrenia spectrum mental health problem of "schizoaffective disorder" may show a combination of symptoms associated with a schizophrenia spectrum mental health problem and symptoms usually seen in a mood-related mental health problem, such as bipolar. Additionally, those who have sustained trauma or brain injury may encounter challenges in regulating their emotional states.

Problems with emotional lability and swings of mood may also happen because of alcohol and other substance use and misuse. Some drugs, called "mood-altering drugs," affect emotions and mood. Alcohol, for example, can strongly affect a person's mood. Cocaine will usually make the user feel more energetic. The effect of these drugs is presumed to happen because the drug changes the chemistry of those areas of the brain that are important in managing and controlling emotional behavior. For people who already have problems managing their emotions and mood, the use of such mood-altering drugs will make their moods and affective response more unpredictable and extreme. People taking psychiatric medications are cautioned to not use such drugs. Prescribed medications sometimes bring unexpected problems with emotions and mood. While these medications are prescribed to help with such problems, the effect that they have can be difficult to predict. Sometimes the medications may make problems with emotions and mood worse instead of better. They may also have another side effect, such as interfering with sleep, which can also contribute to problems with emotional control. This is why the use of such medication should be closely monitored by a qualified prescribing service provider.

Unfortunately, individuals living with SMI have histories of repeated trauma. Related traumatic experiences impact the neuronal connections of the brain, resulting in certain brain structures overreacting to certain environmental stimuli.

Part of the Reason May Be Psychosocial

Swings of mood may also happen because of the effects of stress in the person's life. Like people not living with SMI, a person living with SMI will sometimes react to difficult situations with emotional responses that are difficult to control. In some mental health problems, the person may overreact to minor stressful situations; faced with difficult situations, the person may literally lose emotional control. Unfortunately, people living with SMI will likely face more stressors in their lives because of living with an SMI. The demands made on their ability to cope will, therefore, often be greater and more frequent than other people experience.

Mood swings may also be affected by the personality features of a person living with SMI. For example, many people living with SMIs may have lowered capabilities due to their mental health problems. At the same time, they may feel inadequate when they cannot meet expectations set by themselves or others. Over time, an individual will become self-critical and discouraged, not willing or able to engage in adaptive behaviors because of perceptions of being helpless and incompetent. Aversive emotional experiences during maturation interfere with the learning of adaptive emotional and affective regulation skills by interfering with the learning process involving attention, memory, and concentration (Alcaro & Panksepp, 2011; Silvers et al., 2016).

The quality of the environment can affect emotional control and mood. Most people who must spend a lot of time in a place that is loud, chaotic, or crowded will be more likely to become frustrated and have more difficulty controlling their emotions and mood. A person living with SMI will probably have less choice about where they spend waking hours. Unfortunately, many individuals living with SMI must spend time in a place that will contribute to, rather than help with, problems with emotional control.

Behavioral Support Strategies for Affective Lability, Emotional Dysregulation, and Mood Swings

There are a variety of steps that service providers can take to minimize problems related to emotional lability and mood swings. While not all of these will apply in all cases, some of the following suggestions will likely be helpful if the service user encounters this problem.

- Be clear about what the problem is. An important first step toward helping someone with emotional lability—or "mood swings"—is to clearly identify what the person does that leads you to identify extreme changes in emotions/moods as a problem. Some people living with SMI will experience changes in mood that are more frequent than normal. Many others will experience less frequent but more severe changes in mood. Some people will be disabled by their moods, while others may be able to carry on with what they need to do. This will help you to focus your efforts. If you seek professional help, a clear definition of the problem will likely be the first question that an experienced service provider will ask.
- Watch for circumstances that provoke "mood swings" or emotional problems. "Mood swings" may be tied to time of day, type of situation, who is around the person living with SMI when the "mood swings" occur, as well as other influences that can only be identified through observation and recording what is observed. Such information may be very important in devising effective strategies to help the person experiencing mood swings engage in a plan to learn self-management skills and behaviors. There were certain problems that Juan would get upset about, such as wanting clear information about visiting family members. When he did not get the answer he wanted, he became "irritable," would stare at and talk angrily to others, pace around the group home, and show other problems that frightened the other residents.
- Consider seeking a review of current medications. Emotional liability can be an indication that the current medication needs to be reviewed. It is also possible that certain medications can be prescribed for times when the loss of emotional control begins to happen. These medications can be used as needed and can be

taken in addition to scheduled medications. This is called "pro re nata (PRN)" medication or "as needed" according to certain criteria when problem behaviors are occurring. Juan was encouraged to ask for a specific kind of medication when he felt that he was getting upset. Also, the hospital service providers were instructed to remind him about taking the "PRN" if they noticed behaviors that indicated that he was getting upset. When he did ask, he was praised by staff for his awareness that he may have been losing control and asked for assistance to remain in control.

- Remain calm and patient. Avoid becoming "swept up" with the emotion. This is likely to make the situation worse. You may become impatient and want to tell the person exhibiting "emotional dyscontrol" to just "cut it out and get a grip on yourself!" This is understandable, but a perceived critical response may result in more serious behaviors such as physical aggression. High expressed emotionality in terms of critical comments and statements will often exacerbate an already tenuous situation. Avoid reacting in a way that excites or upsets the person living with SMI and exhibiting the problem behavior of affective lability and dysregulation. Getting excited or upset may trigger the person having problems with affective lability to do likewise as they do not have sufficient capabilities to modulate emotions. In situations where the service provider becomes distressed, it may be appropriate to relocate to another area in order to regain composure before engaging with an individual displaying affective lability. Juan sometimes became angry and paced in the group home. While this was scary to watch, there were staff that could remain calm. Because they remained calm, they were able to approach him and tell him that he was getting upset and either go outside or to his room to relax. Reacting angrily or frustrated when Juan was angry would be like "putting gasoline in a fire."
- In most cases, focus on the behavior that is observed. While the problem may be an "emotional" or "mood" problem, it is usually best to try to change what is observed; that is, the behavior of the service user that is being perceived. Keep two things in mind: (1) encourage those behaviors that help mood to improve; and (2) avoid doing those things that seem to worsen the mood problem. Encouraging the service user to engage in activities that promote relaxation when they are agitated, or increased activity when they are experiencing low mood, can positively impact their emotional state. Juan frequently paced back and forth and stared at other people. The staff thought he was angry and wanted to help him. Rather than ask him if he was angry, they focused on getting him to sit down and do something that he enjoyed, such as word games. In other words, they focused on changing the behavior that they saw and reinforced him with an activity he preferred.
- It is advisable to promote the use of coping strategies that have been previously introduced. In cases where emotional lability has presented challenges, a mental health professional may have instructed the individual on specific coping mechanisms, such as relaxation techniques or participation in preferred activities, which can be employed upon recognition of diminished emotional control. Members of the recovery team should become acquainted with effective methods for supporting the individual's emotional regulation and actively encourage their

use. If coping skills have not been addressed, consultation with a qualified mental health provider is recommended to identify appropriate interventions.

- Encourage the use of coping skills with an agreed-upon signal or statement. Try using a special signal, such as holding your hand up as in a "Stop" sign, or a statement, such as "I hear what you are saying but you need to get a back in control now before this can be handled," as a shorthand method telling the person living with affective lability that he needs to stop what he's doing and use his coping skills. Meet with the person who is experiencing affective lability when he is calm and agreeable, and try to agree on what this "signal" should be. Service providers and recovery team members need to agree and give the same signal or make the same statement when noticing the person who is experiencing affective lability is beginning to lose control. Juan had a preferred chair to sit in to "chill out." When a staff member suggested that it was "time to chill out," he would usually begin to argue. However, if the other person walked away (and didn't keep talking to him), he would usually pace for a few minutes, then go to "his chair." It may be helpful to develop a behavioral contract or point system with the person who experiences dysregulation of mood and affect that specifies what behavior should be practiced and used as self-control and self-calming strategy when the signal is given. Praise, compliment, and reinforce the willingness of the service user to follow directions, even if the attempt at emotional self-control does not always work.
- When talking to the person living with affective lability, communicate in areas of low stimulation. If stimulation in the environment (such as the noise level) seems to contribute to the loss of emotional control, identify a relatively quiet or otherwise less stimulating area to which the person living with SMI can go. For example, it may be helpful to set aside a specific room in the living area for relaxation. Encourage the use of this room when early signs of a worsening mood are observed.
- Consider redirecting the person to specific activities that have a calming effect. Watch for preferred activities that are helpful in calming the person who experiences affective lability when they begin to lose control. Encourage these activities when the early signs of losing control are noticed. There will often be a variety of activities that a person enjoys and can help him to gain more emotional control. These may include reading a preferred magazine, watching a preferred TV program, or taking a walk. Sometimes these activities can be unique to a person. For example, the person may enjoy watching certain kinds of videos. If the service provider is familiar with the person living with emotional dysregulation, the service provider can probably be effective at helping to identify unique activities that might work for the person.
- Maintain realistic expectations for the person who experiences affective lability. Immediate mood changes in the person living with affective lability are unlikely, and self-control cannot be achieved quickly. Instead, remain patient and encourage those activities that seem to be helpful in reducing the excited state. Be supportive as they try to calm down and carry out a relaxing task. It often took Juan several hours before he was calm enough to talk with other people.

- Avoid discussions with the service user experiencing affective lability until calm has been achieved. For problems of emotional decontrol and dysregulation, the primary goal is to encourage the person living with SMI to calm down by whatever method seems useful at the time. Service providers can encourage the use of such skills but should allow the person living with SMI an opportunity to be alone. Later, after stability has been achieved, compliment the person for successfully calming down and offer to discuss the circumstances that seemed to have brought on the change in mood. It is usually not helpful to try to reason with the individual until after they have calmed down. When Juan was pacing and staring, the staff focused on helping him to change that behavior by sitting in his chair to be away from others and beginning the calming process. Later, after he was calm and more reasonable, a staff member would sit with him and try to identify what may have provoked that behavior. At this time, the staff would try to help Juan identify ways that he could calm himself before he started pacing.
- The person experiencing affective lability ought to avoid alcohol and other mood-altering drugs. Many of these drugs are a problem specifically because they affect the person's mood. For someone who is already challenged to engage in emotional control, these drugs will make the problem worse. In almost all cases, alcohol and other mood-altering drugs should be avoided, except those prescribed by a psychiatric service provider.

Conclusion for Behavioral Support Strategies

When emotional lability and "mood swings" are a problem, there are several suggestions that may help. While not all of these will be helpful in every case, it is likely that a number of these suggestions will be appropriate for the situation that is being faced:

1. Check with a psychiatric service provider to make sure that the current medications are the most appropriate for the person living with SMI and affective lability. Most medications can affect a person's mood. Moodiness and irritability can be helped or worsened by medications.
2. Service providers should utilize their own stress management skills. Working with someone who is moody and irritable can be very frustrating and discouraging. Service providers need to work on their abilities to remain patient and compassionate. Recognize personal limits and know when a break is needed.
3. Work with the person living with SMI and affective lability and discuss developing methods that the person prefers to use to calm down. Working together, develop a reminder signal or a prompt to signal "time out" as a reminder that self-calming strategies should be used if other service providers and recovery team members observe the signs of emotional dysregulation and affective lability.

4. Minimize possible sources of stimulation when interacting with the person living with SMI. For example, talk and discuss issues in an area that is quiet (without distractions by TV or radio) and has a minimal number of people around.
5. Do not continue conversations or activities with the person experiencing affective lability unless an acceptable level of calm has been achieved. Forcing such conversations or activities will likely only cause things to worsen.

What About Juan?

Juan's unpredictable behavior and emotions were very frustrating for the people who had to work with him. When he acted friendly and cooperative, the service providers were encouraged. When he acted angry, threatening, and complaining, they became scared and sometimes angry with Juan. When he acted discouraged and depressed, they became worried and felt bad about having been angry at him. Some of them began to wonder if he was manipulating and changing his behavior to get back at them. These staff wanted to start being firmer with him and get him to "shape up."

The service providers were first cautioned to avoid getting swept up in the emotions of Juan. They were instructed to remain calm regardless of his emotions and behaviors. Beyond this, the service providers were cautioned to avoid acting based on the frustration that Juan's changeable behavior aroused in them. They were instructed to encourage Juan's participation in activities regardless of his behavior but to accept the response that he gave to their invitation. When he was sociable and was willing to interact with others, they were to make sure that they showed interest in what he was doing. If he declined to interact or participate, they briefly reminded him that he was welcome to join the activity. If he continued to refuse, they showed respect for his right to refuse to be involved. If he complained about the program, service providers were to show respect for his opinion but avoid arguing with him. Regardless of these problems, they were to continue to watch for any indication of cooperation by Juan and be sure to briefly state their appreciation for this cooperation.

Over time, Juan behaved in a more emotionally stable manner. He complained and argued less frequently and attended the clubhouse on a regular schedule. He also began to volunteer for extra duties at the group home. This gave the staff extra opportunities to compliment him. While Juan continued to show evidence of several unusual behaviors, such as his "head shaking," he was less moody and irritable with other people and was better able to get along with them. His mother heard of his improvement from relatives and eventually removed the protection order so he could visit her. The visits were incorporated into a contract for desired behavior with Juan that stipulated that he had to show a defined behavioral criterion of "in control behavior" for 3 days before he could visit his mother.

In this example, the staff made several adjustments to how they worked with him to support him in managing his moods.

1. The staff recognized that Juan's medications could have a potentially beneficial effect on his ability to keep his mood and affect stable. They made every effort to encourage him to keep his mood and affect under control. They encouraged him to consistently take his medication. For Juan, it was important that he felt that he was calling "the shots" for his treatment. When he refused to take his medication, the staff briefly stated their concern and avoided arguing with him about it. When he took it, they acknowledged his medication adherence by briefly commenting on his commitment to doing what he needs to do to recover and emphasizing his progress toward his goals.
2. They recognized that Juan's changes in mood were very frustrating. There were also many long periods of time when his mood was stable and when he acted very friendly toward others.
3. They also recognized that it was easy for them to get frustrated with him. They decided that when they started to become angry at him, they would do something else and let another staff member interact with him and "handle the situation."
4. They knew that Juan could participate in all the activities available at the clubhouse. They made a point to give him a brief reminder about the activities for the day. If he refused to go, they accepted this and went on about their duties.
5. They were aware of the times when Juan cooperated with what they asked him to do. They always made a point to briefly acknowledge his cooperation and state their appreciation. They did not try to keep the conversation going, however, unless it appeared that Juan wanted to.

As this plan progressed, the staff helped Juan to act in a more stable manner. Because there were fewer arguments and other conflicts with the staff, Juan became better able to talk about how his moodiness and irritability caused problems for him and other people. He recognized that many of the problems that he faced with other people were because of changes in mood and how this impacted other people.

Summary

Affective lability (AL) refers to rapid and intense fluctuations in mood and affect over short periods, often leading to significant impairment in daily functioning. It is characterized by frequent, intense, and wide-ranging changes in emotional states, often disproportionate to the triggering events; the emotions and affect are more likely to fluctuate between anxiety and depressive affective states, involving both primary and secondary emotions. It is transdiagnostic and is linked to a range of mental health concerns, such as suicidality and serious mental illness (SMI), including conditions on the schizophrenia spectrum, bipolar conditions, and mental health challenges related to personality difficulties. Definitions of affective lability often lack specificity and consistency, leading to challenges in research and treatment. Research literature uses various terms to describe affective lability, leading to overlap in dimensions as multiple terms pertaining to affective lability are used to describe similar phenomena; affective lability or mood swings are used interchangeably along with mood instability, affective instability, and emotional dysregulation.

Affective lability is a poorly understood mental health concept that commonly occurs, impacting a significant portion of the general population and those individuals with mental health problems. Affective lability may manifest independently of living with an SMI, yet research indicates it can serve as a precursor to SMI development. The prevalence of affective lability among individuals with SMI is 13.9%, which is notably higher than that observed in the general population. Affective lability is a risk factor for poor clinical and functional outcomes and is associated with significant impairment in social roles, interactions, and cognitive skills. Treating affective lability in people with SMI can improve psychosocial functioning and rehabilitation efforts.

A multidimensional approach is required for a comprehensive understanding of affective lability. Affective lability is a complex and multidimensional concept that often overlaps with other behavioral problems associated with living with SMI. Instruments such as the Affective Liability Scale (ALS) and Mood Spectrum Structured Interviews (SCI-MOODS) assess some of the dimensions of affective lability including frequency, intensity, and impact on daily life. The Affective Liability Scale (ALS) assesses mood changes across depression, elation, anger, and anxiety. Mood Spectrum Structured Interviews (SCI-MOODS) assess mood-related mental health problems across four domains: mood, energy, cognition, and rhythmicity/vegetative functions. The self-report version, MOODS-SR, follows the same structure as SCI-MOODS.

Emotional regulation is crucial for managing affective lability. Emotional regulation involves awareness, acceptance, and control of emotions to achieve personal goals. The Difficulties in Emotion Regulation Scale (DERS) measures emotional dysregulation across six subscales: awareness, clarity, impulse, goals, nonacceptance of emotional experiences, and strategies.

Like other mental health problems that are prevalent among people living with SMI, affective lability is multidimensional. Affective lability can be measured in several dimensions including: (1) awareness: cognizance of emotions during mood oscillations; (2) impact: effect of mood changes on personal and social roles; (3) frequency: recurrence of mood changes over time; (4) duration: temporal lengths of each mood state; (5) average affect: baseline level of emotions over a specified period; (6) range of affective states: variability in mood states; (7) intensity: magnitude of emotional experiences; (8) amount of emotional distress: frequency of distress caused by mood changes; (9) origin: perceived source of mood changes, whether due to internal or external events; (10) control: belief in managing or influencing mood changes.

Affective lability seems to be mediated by interactions between neurological substrates and learning from experience. The limbic system, including the prefrontal cortex, thalamus, hippocampus, amygdala, and septal area, is crucial for emotions, memory, learning, and goal-directed behaviors (American Psychological Association, n.d.-e). The temporo-amygdala-orbitofrontal network integrates visceral sensation and emotion with semantic memory and behavior, involving the temporal lobe, amygdala, orbitofrontal cortex, and uncinate fasciculus. The prefrontal cortex (PFC), particularly the ventromedial (vmPFC) and dorsolateral (dlPFC) prefrontal cortex, regulates emotional responses, decision-making, and social cognition, with dysfunction leading to mental health issues such as depression and anxiety. The dorsomedial prefrontal cortex (dmPFC) is involved in higher-order emotion processing, social cognition, and working memory, with disruptions linked to mental health conditions such as major depression, schizophrenia spectrum, ASD, and Alzheimer's disease. The mesolimbic dopamine (ML-DA) system regulates emotional states and affective responses, with dysregulation leading to affective lability and mental health problems such as depression.

Individuals experiencing mental health conditions related to personality disorders often demonstrate emotional dysregulation and behavioral challenges. Functional MRI (fMRI) studies have indicated that such individuals may exhibit reduced amygdala volumes, diminished white matter integrity, and altered activation in both the prefrontal cortex and the amygdala. Emotional regulation involves the fronto-limbic network (FLN), with disturbances linked to affective lability in people living with SMI. Research indicates that fMRI may be more sensitive than self-report measures for assessing emotion regulation, highlighting the need for future studies on brain connectivity and individual differences.

Learning significantly influences emotional and affective responses, shaping how individuals react to stimuli based on past experiences. Emotions are not just innate but are influenced by social factors, role modeling, and associative learning. The regulation of emotions impacts social adjustments and is crucial for interactions, educational success, and psychological health. Emotions can be modified through cognitive-behavioral strategies and are reinforced or diminished through life experiences. Behavioral interventions like CBT and DBT are effective in managing emotional dysregulation.

Emotions are dynamic and can change based on new experiences and contexts. They are influenced by both innate feelings and learned responses. Childhood trauma and emotional abuse can impact affective lability and mental health. Role modeling and social learning play a significant role in emotional development. Repetitive traumatic experiences can lead to changes in brain activation resulting in emotional dysregulation.

Mood instability is a common experience, with varying prevalence across different demographics and mental health conditions. It is more common in women and younger individuals and is associated with a range of mental health problems and issues, increased health service use (e.g., more hospital days, frequent admissions, and higher likelihood of being prescribed antipsychotics or mood stabilizers), suicidal ideation, and poor clinical outcomes. Affective lability is reported in 40–60% of those with mental health related problems associated with depression and anxiety related problems (e.g., PTSD, and OCD). It is documented in 12.1% of individuals seeking mental healthcare, most frequently by those with mental health problems related to bipolar conditions (22.6%), personality (17.8%), and schizophrenia spectrum (15.5%).

Affective lability is associated with mood-related mental health problems, having varied global prevalence rates. Surveys in 11 countries by the World Health Organization (WHO) show lifetime prevalence of affective lability in bipolar related mental health problems ranging from 0.6% to 0.4%; the prevalence is 1.4% for subthreshold mental health problems (involving symptoms and behavioral problems present for at least 2 weeks and leading to diminished daily functioning and increased personal distress) and 2.4% for all bipolar spectrum mental health problems. Point prevalence (12 months) of affective lability ranges from 0.4% to 0.3% for bipolar related mental health problems and 0.8% for subthreshold and 1.5% for all bipolar spectrum mental health problems. The United States has the highest lifetime prevalence of bipolar spectrum mental health problems (4.4%) and 12-month point prevalence (2.8%), while India has the lowest (0.1% for both). Lifetime rates of bipolar spectrum mental health and subthreshold problems are higher in males, while depressive related mental health problems are higher in females. Marital and employment status are associated with occurrences of affective lability.

Mood disorders are rare in children but common in adolescents, with up to 25% of lifetime prevalence for depressive problems and 2% for manic-related problems by the end of adolescence. Prevalence of mood-related mental health problems in children and adolescents varies by country and culture, with depressive problems affecting 1.0–3.3% of children and adolescents in the United States and 0.6–2.5% in Great Britain. A study in Thailand found a 26.4% prevalence of mood swings among high school students, with higher rates linked to problematic social media use and bullying.

Cultural influences significantly impact emotional regulation strategies and their adaptiveness. Cultural influences shape emotional regulation strategies, with interdependent cultures (e.g., East Asian) promoting suppression to maintain social harmony, while independent cultures (e.g., European and American) value emotional expression for individuality. Suppression is linked to worse psychological and social functioning in independent cultures but may be less harmful or beneficial in interdependent cultures.

Affective lability involves primary and secondary emotions with distinct dimensions. It includes rapid shifts from neutral or positive to intense negative states. Dysfunctional modulation, exaggerated emotional responses, and lack of control of emotional responses are key aspects of affective lability. The DSM-5 defines affect as observable behaviors expressing emotions and lists various types of observable affective responses, including: (1) blunted affect: significant reduction in emotional expression; (2) constricted or restricted affect: mild to moderate reduction in emotional expression; (3) flat affect: absence of emotional expression behaviors; (4) inappropriate affect: mismatch between emotional expression and context.

Future research should address multiple facets of affective lability to advance effective treatment strategies and mitigate stigma. Such an approach acknowledges the diverse experiences and perspectives of individuals living with similar mental health conditions. The overarching aim is to foster a nuanced understanding of mental health challenges, thereby reducing stigma by moving beyond simplistic explanations and supporting the creation of more targeted and efficacious interventions.

Managing emotional lability and mood swings in individuals with SMI and affective lability ensures medications are appropriate by having current medications reviewed as emotional lability may indicate a need for adjustment or additional PRN medications. Service providers need to encourage the service user who displays affective lability and emotional dysregulation to avoid alcohol and mood-altering drugs as these may exacerbate the problem behaviors.

Service providers should use stress management skills and self-calming skills to remain calm during times when the service user displays affective lability and emotional dysregulation; it is imperative to minimize stimulation, avoiding forcing conversations and interactions of high expressed emotionality until the person is calm and in control.

Strategies for service providers to help individuals with emotional lability and mood swings begin with clearly identifying the behaviors that indicate emotional lability or mood swings to focus efforts effectively. Observe and record circumstances that provoke mood swings to devise effective self-management strategies with the service user. Service providers need to remain calm and patient to avoid escalating the situation and encourage the person to use coping skills. Focus on changing observable behaviors and encourage activities that improve mood. Service providers ought to employ agreed-upon signals or statements to prompt the use of coping skills and maintain realistic expectations for mood changes. Communicate in environments with minimal stimulation and redirect the individual to calming activities at the earliest indication of escalating distress. Refrain from addressing the problematic behavior until the individual is calm and has regained self-control. Interactions characterized by heightened emotional expression are likely to intensify emotional dysregulation and exacerbate the problematic behavior.

References

Agapoff, J. A., Chong, Z., Meek, M., & van Schalkwyk, G. I. (2023). Pharmacologic and nonpharmacologic interventions for emotional lability: A meta-analysis. *Neuroscience and Biobehavioral Reviews, 149*, 105184. https://doi.org/10.1016/j.neubiorev.2023.105184

Alcaro, A., & Panksepp, J. (2011). The SEEKING mind: Primal neuro-affective substrates for appetitive incentive states and their pathological dynamics in addictions and depression. *Neuroscience & Biobehavioral Reviews, 35*(9), 1805–1820. https://doi.org/10.1016/j.neubiorev.2011.03.002

American Psychiatric Association. (2013a). *Glossary of technical terms.* In Diagnostic and statistical manual of mental disorders (5th ed.). https://doi.org/10.1176/appi.books.9780890425787.x28_Glossary_of_Technical_Terms

American Psychiatric Association. (2013b). *Diagnostic and statistical manual of mental disorders* (5th ed.) (DSM-5) https://doi.org/10.1176/appi.books.9780890425596

American Psychiatric Association. (2013c). Schizophrenia spectrum and other psychotic disorders. In *Diagnostic and statistical manual of mental disorders* (5th ed.). https://doi.org/10.1176/appi.books.9780890425787.x02_Schizophrenia–Spectrum_and_Other_Psychotic_Disorders

American Psychiatric Association. (2022a). *Diagnostic and statistical manual of mental disorders* (5th ed., text rev). https://doi.org/10.1176/appi.books.9780890425787

American Psychiatric Association. (2022b). Bipolar and related disorders. In *Diagnostic and statistical manual of mental disorders* (5th ed.). https://doi.org/10.1176/appi.books.9780890425787.x03_Bipolar_and_Related_Disorders
American Psychiatric Association. (2022c). Personality disorders. In *Diagnostic and statistical manual of mental disorders* (5th ed., pp. 645–684).
American Psychological Association. (n.d.-a). Affect. In *APA dictionary of psychology*. https://dictionary.apa.org/Affect
American Psychological Association. (n.d.-b). Biological rhythm. In *APA dictionary of psychology*. https://dictionary.apa.org/Biological-rhythm
American Psychological Association. (n.d.-c). Dysregulation. In *APA dictionary of psychology*. https://dictionary.apa.org/Dysregulation
American Psychological Association. (n.d.-d). Emotion. In *APA Dictionary of Psychology*. https://dictionary.apa.org/emotion
American Psychological Association. (n.d.-e). Limbic system. In *APA dictionary of psychology*. https://dictionary.apa.org/Limbic-system
American Psychological Association. (n.d.-f). Mood. In *APA dictionary of psychology*. https://dictionary.apa.org/Mood
American Psychological Association. (n.d.-g). *Suppression*. In APA dictionary of psychology. https://dictionary.apa.org/Suppression
Angsukiattitavorn, S., Seeherunwong, A., Panitrat, R., & Tipayamongkholgul, M. (2020). Prevalence and distribution pattern of mood swings in Thai adolescents: A school-based survey in the central region of Thailand. *BMC Psychiatry, 20*, 1–12. https://doi.org/10.1186/s12888-020-02605-0
Beauchaine, T. P. (2015). Future directions in emotion dysregulation and youth psychopathology. *Journal of Clinical Child & Adolescent Psychology, 44*(5), 875–896. https://doi.org/10.1080/15374416.2015.1038827
Beck, A. T., & Dozois, D. J. (2011). Cognitive therapy: Current status and future directions. *Annual Review of Medicine, 62*(1), 397–409. https://doi.org/10.1146/annurev-med-052209-100032
Benvenuti, A., Miniati, M., Callari, A., Giorgi Mariani, M., Mauri, M., & Dell'Osso, L. (2015). Mood spectrum model: Evidence reconsidered in the light of DSM-5. *World Journal of Psychiatry, 5*(1), 126–137. https://doi.org/10.5498/wjp.v5.i1.126
Bilderbeck, A. C., Saunders, K. E., Price, J., & Goodwin, G. M. (2014). Psychiatric assessment of mood instability: Qualitative study of patient experience. *The British Journal of Psychiatry, 204*(3), 234–239. https://doi.org/10.1192/bjp.bp.113.128348
Broome, M. R., Saunders, K. E. A., Harrison, P. J., & Marwaha, S. (2015). Mood instability: Significance, definition and measurement. *The British Journal of Psychiatry, 207*(4), 283–285. https://doi.org/10.1192/bjp.bp.114.158543
Cassano, G. B., Frank, E., Miniati, M., Rucci, P., Fagiolini, A., Pini, S., Shear, M. K., & Maser, J. D. (2002). Conceptual underpinnings and empirical support for the mood spectrum. *Psychiatric Clinics Of North America, 25*(4), 699–712. https://doi.org/10.1016/S0193-953X(02)00025-4
Catani, M., Dell'Acqua, F., & De Schotten, M. T. (2013). A revised limbic system model for memory, emotion and behaviour. *Neuroscience & Biobehavioral Reviews, 37*(8), 1724–1737. https://doi.org/10.1016/j.neubiorev.2013.07.001
Contardi, A., Imperatori, C., Amati, I., Balsamo, M., & Innamorati, M. (2018). Assessment of affect lability: Psychometric properties of the ALS-18. *Frontiers in Psychology, 9*, 427., 1–8. https://doi.org/10.3389/fpsyg.2018.00427
Cooper, J. O., Heron, T. E., & Heward, W. L. (2020). *Applied behavior analysis* (3rd ed.). Pearson. https://www.pearson.com/store/p/applied-behavior-analysis/P100000688401
Dejonckheere, E., Mestdagh, M., Houben, M., Rutten, I., Sels, L., Kuppens, P., & Tuerlinckx, F. (2019). Complex affect dynamics add limited information to the prediction of psychological Well-being. *Nature Human Behaviour, 3*(5), 478–491. https://doi.org/10.1038/s41562-0190555-0

Dixon, M. L., Thiruchselvam, R., Todd, R., & Christoff, K. (2017). Emotion and the prefrontal cortex: An integrative review. *Psychological Bulletin, 143*(10), 1033–1081. https://doi.org/10.1037/bul0000096

Dysinger, D. W. (1938). The fluctuations of mood. *Psychological Record, 2*, 115–123. https://doi.org/10.1007/BF03393214

Edwards, E. R., Rose, N. L., Gromatsky, M., Feinberg, A., Kimhy, D., Doucette, J. T., & Hazlett, E. A. (2021). Alexithymia, affective lability, impulsivity, and childhood adversity in borderline personality disorder. *Journal of Personality Disorders, 35*(Supplement A), 114–131. https://doi.org/10.1521/pedi_2021_35_513

Ewen, R. B. (2014). *An introduction to theories of personality*. Psychology Press. https://www.routledge.com/An-Introduction-to-Theories-of-Personality/Ewen/p/book/9781848725923

Fagiolini, A., Dell'osso, L., Pini, S., Armani, A., Bouanani, S., Rucci, P., Cassano, G. B., Endicott, J., Maser, J. D., Katherine Shear, M., Grochocinski, V. J., & Frank, E. (1999). Validity and reliability of a new instrument for assessing mood symptomatology: The structured clinical interview for mood Spectrum (SCI-MOODS). *International Journal of Methods in Psychiatric Research, 8*(2), 71–82. https://doi.org/10.1002/mpr.58

Ford, B. Q., & Mauss, I. B. (2015). Culture and emotion regulation. *Current Opinion in Psychology, 3*, 1–5. https://doi.org/10.1016/j.copsyc.2014.12.004

Gratz, K. L., & Roemer, L. (2004a). Multidimensional assessment of emotion regulation and dysregulation: Development, factor structure, and initial validation of the difficulties in emotion regulation scale. *Journal of Psychopathology and Behavioral Assessment, 26*(1), 41–54. https://doi.org/10.1023/B:JOBA.0000007455.08539.94

Gratz, K. L., & Roemer, L. (2004b). *Difficulties in emotion regulation scale (DERS)* [Database record]. *APA PsycTests*. https://doi.org/10.1037/t01029-000

Gregorová, K., Eldar, E., Deserno, L., & Reiter, A. M. (2024). A cognitive-computational account of mood swings in adolescence. *Trends in Cognitive Sciences, 28*(4), 290–303. https://doi.org/10.1016/j.tics.2024.02.006

Hallion, L. S., Steinman, S. A., Tolin, D. F., & Diefenbach, G. J. (2018). Psychometric properties of the difficulties in emotion regulation scale (DERS) and its short forms in adults with emotional disorders. *Frontiers in Psychology, 9*, 539., 1–12. https://doi.org/10.3389/fpsyg.2018.00539

Hampshire, A., Chamberlain, S. R., Monti, M. M., Duncan, J., & Owen, A. M. (2010). The role of the right inferior frontal gyrus: Inhibition and attentional control. *NeuroImage, 50*(3), 1313–1319. https://doi.org/10.1016/j.neuroimage.2009.12.109

Harvey, P. D., Greenberg, B. R., & Serper, M. R. (1989). The affective lability scales: Development, reliability, and validity. *Journal of Clinical Psychology, 45*(5), 786–793. https://doi.org/10.1002/1097-4679(198909)45:5<786

Hiser, J., & Koenigs, M. (2018). The multifaceted role of the ventromedial prefrontal cortex in emotion, decision making, social cognition, and psychopathology. *Biological Psychiatry, 83*(8), 638–647. https://doi.org/10.1016/j.biopsych.2017.10.030

Høegh, M. C., Melle, I., Aminoff, S. R., Laskemoen, J. F., Büchmann, C. B., Ueland, T., & Lagerberg, T. V. (2020). Affective lability across psychosis spectrum disorders. *European Psychiatry, 63*(1), e53. https://doi.org/10.1192/j.eurpsy.2020.44

Høegh, M. C., Melle, I., Aminoff, S. R., Olsen, S. H., Lunding, S. H., Ueland, T., & Lagerberg, T. V. (2022). Affective lability and social functioning in severe mental disorders. *European Archives of Psychiatry and Clinical Neuroscience, 272*(5), 873–885. https://doi.org/10.1007/s00406-022-01380-1

Hossain, S., & Kangas, M. (2020). Association between emotion regulation and psychopathology: The role of culture. *Mental Health Literacy, Emotion Regulation and Psychological Wellbeing: An Exploration in Australian and Bangladeshi Adults, 40*(103), 104. https://doi.org/10.1007/s00406-022-01380-1

Joiner, J., Piva, M., Turrin, C., & Chang, S. W. (2017). Social learning through prediction error in the brain. *npj Science of Learning, 2*(1), 1–9. https://doi.org/10.1038/s41539-017-0009-2

Juruena, M. F. (2012). Understanding subthreshold depression. *Shanghai Archives of Psychiatry, 5*, 292–293. https://doi.org/10.3969/j.issn.1002-0829.2012.05.009

Kessler, R. C., Haro, J. M., Heeringa, S. G., Pennell, B. E., & Üstün, T. B. (2006). The World Health Organization world mental health survey initiative. *Epidemiology and Psychiatric Sciences, 15*(3), 161–166. https://doi.org/10.1017/S1121189X00004395

Kessler, R. C., Avenevoli, S., Ries, K., & Merikangas, K. (2001). Mood disorders in children and adolescents: An epidemiologic perspective. *Biological Psychiatry, 49*(12), 1002–1014. https://doi.org/10.1016/S0006-3223(01)01129-5

Lebois, L. A., Wilson-Mendenhall, C. D., Simmons, W. K., Barrett, L. F., & Barsalou, L. W. (2020). Learning situated emotions. *Neuropsychologia, 145*, 106637. https://doi.org/10.1016/j.neuropsychologia.2018.01.008

LeDoux, J. E. (2012). Evolution of human emotion: A view through fear. *Progress in Brain Research, 195*, 431–442. https://doi.org/10.1016/B978-0-444-53860-4.00021-0

Malhi, G. S., Tanious, M., Fritz, K., Coulston, C. M., Bargh, D. M., Phan, K. L., Ivanovski, B., & Das, P. (2013). Differential engagement of the fronto-limbic network during emotion processing distinguishes bipolar and borderline personality disorder. *Molecular Psychiatry, 18*(12), 1247–1248. https://doi.org/10.1038/mp.2013.22

Marwaha, S., Balbuena, L., Winsper, C., & Bowen, R. (2015). Mood instability as a precursor to depressive illness: A prospective and mediational analysis. *Australian & New Zealand Journal of Psychiatry, 49*(6), 557–565. https://doi.org/10.1177/0004867415579920

Marwaha, S., He, Z., Broome, M., Singh, S., Scott, J., Eyden, J., & Wolke, D. (2014). How is affective instability defined and measured? A systematic review. *Psychological Medicine, 44*(9), 1793–1808. https://doi.org/10.1017/S0033291713002407

Marwaha, S., Parsons, N., & Broome, M. (2013a). Mood instability, mental illness and suicidal ideas: Results from a household survey. *Social Psychiatry and Psychiatric Epidemiology, 48*, 1431–1437. http://link.springer.com/article/10.1007%2Fs00127-013-0653-7

Marwaha, S., Parsons, N., Flanagan, S., & Broome, M. (2013b). The prevalence and clinical associations of mood instability in adults living in England: Results from the adult psychiatric morbidity survey 2007. *Psychiatry Research, 205*(3), 262–268. https://doi.org/10.1016/j.psychres.2012.09.036

McDonald, K. C., Saunders, K. E., & Geddes, J. R. (2017). Sleep problems and suicide associated with mood instability in the adult psychiatric morbidity survey, 2007. *Australian & New Zealand Journal of Psychiatry, 51*(8), 822–828. https://doi.org/10.1177/0004867416687398

Merikangas, K. R., Jin, R., He, J. P., Kessler, R. C., Lee, S., Sampson, N. A., Zarkov, Z., Lepine, J. P., Huang, Y., Hu, C., Karam, E. G., Mneimneh, Z., Medina-Mora, M. E., Borges, G., Kessler, R. C., Nakamura, Y., & Andrade, L. H. (2011). Prevalence and correlates of bipolar spectrum disorder in the world mental health survey initiative. *Archives of General Psychiatry, 68*(3), 241–251. https://doi.org/10.1001/archgenpsychiatry.2011.12

Merikangas, K. R., Nakamura, E. F., & Kessler, R. C. (2009). Epidemiology of mental disorders in children and adolescents. *Dialogues in Clinical Neuroscience, 11*(1), 7–20. https://doi.org/10.31887/DCNS.2009.11.1/krmerikangas

Miniati, M., Rucci, P., Frank, E., Oppo, A., Kupfer, D. J., Fagiolini, A., & Cassano, G. B. (2009). Sensitivity to change and predictive validity of the MOODS-SR questionnaire, last-month version. *Psychotherapy and Psychosomatics, 78*(2), 116–124. https://doi.org/10.1159/000201937

Moore, S. R., Gresham, L. S., Bromberg, M. B., Kasarkis, E. J., & Smith, R. A. (1997). A self-report measure of affective lability. *Journal of Neurology, Neurosurgery & Psychiatry, 63*(1), 89–93. https://doi.org/10.1136/jnnp.63.1.89

National Institute of Health (NIH). (2024). *Emotional lability. U.S. Department of Health and Human Services*, National Institutes of Health. Retrieved December 30, 2024, from https://www.ncbi.nlm.nih.gov/medgen/39319

Ojha, A., Jones, N. P., Henry, T., Versace, A., Gnagy, E. M., Joseph, H. M., Molina, B. S. G., & Ladouceur, C. D. (2024). Altered lateral prefrontal cortex functioning during emotional interference resistance is associated with affect lability in adults with persisting symptoms of attention-deficit/hyperactivity disorder from childhood. *Biological Psychiatry: Cognitive Neuroscience and Neuroimaging, 9*(6), 588–596. https://doi.org/10.1016/j.bpsc.2024.02.003

Oliver, M. N., & Simons, J. S. (2004). The affective lability scales: Development of a short-form measure. *Personality and Individual Differences, 37*(6), 1279–1288. https://doi.org/10.1016/j.paid.2003.12.013

Panos, P. T., Jackson, J. W., Hasan, O., & Panos, A. (2014). Meta-analysis and systematic review assessing the efficacy of dialectical behavior therapy (DBT). *Research on Social Work Practice, 24*(2), 213–223. https://doi.org/10.1177/1049731513503047

Papies, E. K., Barsalou, L. W., Claassen, M. A., Davis, T., Farrar, S. T., Gauthier, E., Gawronski, B., Genschow, O., Hofmann, W., Kruglanski, A. W., Scholer, A. A., & Werner, J. (2022). Grounding motivation for behavior change. In J. M. Olson (Ed.), *Advances in experimental social psychology* (Vol. 66, pp. 107–189). Academic Press. https://doi.org/10.1016/bs.aesp.2022.04.002

Patel, R., Lloyd, T., Jackson, R., Ball, M., Shetty, H., Broadbent, M., Stewart, R., Dobson, R., & Taylor, M. (2015). Mood instability is a common feature of mental health disorders and is associated with poor clinical outcomes. *BMJ Open, 5*(5), e007504. https://doi.org/10.1136/bmjopen-2014-007504

Renaud, S. M., & Zacchia, C. (2012). Toward a definition of affective instability. *Harvard Review of Psychiatry, 20*(6), 298–308. https://doi.org/10.3109/10673229.2012.747798

Roxo, M. R., Franceschini, P. R., Zubaran, C., Kleber, F. D., & Sander, J. W. (2011). The limbic system conception and its historical evolution. *The Scientific World Journal, 11*(1), 2427–2440. https://doi.org/10.1100/2011/157150

Schmelzer, G. (2015, January 11). Understanding learning and memory: The neuroscience of repetition. *Journey through trauma: A trail guide to the 5-phase cycle of healing repeated trauma.* https://gretchenschmelzer.com/blog-1/2015/1/11/understanding-learning-and-memory-the-neuroscience-of-repetition

Sezgin, E., Bilge, Y., Çelik, B., & Sevük, E. N. (2023). The mediating role of emotion lability and emotion regulation in the relationship between social-emotional adaptation with behavior regulation and social skills among preschool children. *Yaşam Becerileri Psikoloji Dergisi, 7*(14), 161–183. https://doi.org/10.31461/ybpd.1373592

Shahrokh, N. C., & Hales, R. E. (2003). *American psychiatric glossary* (8th ed.). American Psychiatric Publishing. https://doi.org/10.5555/appi.books.9781615373758.db23Glossary

Silvers, J. A., Hubbard, A. D., Biggs, E., Shu, J., Fertuck, E., Chaudhury, S., Koenigsberg, H. W., & Stanley, B. (2016). Affective lability and difficulties with regulation are differentially associated with amygdala and prefrontal response in women with borderline personality disorder. *Psychiatry Research: Neuroimaging, 254*, 74–82. https://doi.org/10.1016/j.pscychresns.2016.06.009

Šimić, G., Tkalčić, M., Vukić, V., Mulc, D., Španić, E., Šagud, M., Babić, L., Borovečki, F., & Hof, P. R. (2021). Understanding emotions: Origins and roles of the amygdala. *Biomolecules, 11*(6), 823. https://doi.org/10.3390/biom11060823

Stone, A. A., Smyth, J. M., Pickering, T., & Schwartz, J. (1996). Daily mood variability: Form of diurnal patterns and determinants of diurnal patterns. *Journal of Applied Social Psychology, 26*(14), 1286–1305. https://doi.org/10.1111/j.1559-1816.1996.tb01781.x

Thompson, R. A. (2019). Emotion dysregulation: A theme in search of definition. *Development and Psychopathology, 31*(3), 805–815. https://doi.org/10.1017/S0954579419000282

Victor, S. E., & Klonsky, E. D. (2016). Validation of a brief version of the difficulties in emotion regulation scale (DERS-18) in five samples. *Journal of Psychopathology and Behavioral Assessment, 38*, 582–589. https://doi.org/10.1007/s10862-016-9547-9

Weiss, N. H., Thomas, E. D., Schick, M. R., Reyes, M. E., & Contractor, A. A. (2022). Racial and ethnic differences in emotion regulation: A systematic review. *Journal of Clinical Psychology, 78*(5), 785–808. https://doi.org/10.1002/jclp.23284

Wu, S., Liu, J., Xue, Z., Xu, J., Lin, L., Sun, Y., Wang, Y., Zhang, Y., & Lu, J. (2023). Association between childhood trauma and affective lability among adolescents: A moderated mediation model. *Journal of Affective Disorders, 338*, 21–31. https://doi.org/10.1016/j.jad.2023.05.092

Chapter 9
Problems with Disorganized Thinking and Motoric Behaviors in Individuals Living with Serious Mental Illness

Introduction

Disorganization in thought and behavior represents a core domain of psychopathology in serious mental illness (SMI), particularly within schizophrenia spectrum and related disorders. These disturbances manifest in a range of cognitive, linguistic, and motoric anomalies that can profoundly impair communication, goal-directed activity, and social functioning. Unlike mood or psychotic symptoms, disorganized features often present as diffuse, unpredictable, and difficult to interpret, posing unique challenges for diagnosis, treatment, and daily support. For clinicians, educators, and researchers, understanding the nature and structure of disorganization is essential to improving care and advancing theoretical models of mental illness.

This chapter explores the multifaceted construct of disorganization through its two principal expressions: disorganized speech and disorganized motor behavior. Disorganized speech, conceptualized as formal thought disorder, includes disruptions in coherence, logic, and syntax that compromise verbal expression and comprehension. Disorganized motor behavior encompasses a spectrum from purposeless agitation to catatonia, a syndrome marked by psychomotor immobility, rigidity, or excessive motor activity. These phenomena are not merely symptomatic but reflect underlying neurocognitive and neurobiological dysfunctions, often shaped by environmental stressors and developmental trajectories.

To provide a comprehensive framework, this chapter is organized into several key sections. It begins with definitional clarity and clinical examples of disorganized speech and motor behavior, followed by a review of formal thought disorder and catatonia as distinct but overlapping constructs. Next, it examines dimensional models of disorganization and their relevance to assessment, including rating scales and observational tools. This chapter then addresses neurological substrates and environmental influences, integrating findings from neuroimaging, pharmacology,

G. F. McKeegan, *Behavior Change Interventions for Serious Mental Illness*, Evidence-Based Practices in Behavioral Health,
https://doi.org/10.1007/978-3-032-18372-9_9

and psychosocial research. Finally, it presents typologies of disorganized behavior and outlines behavioral strategies for clinical management and support.

A detailed understanding of disorganization in SMI, including its various manifestations, underlying mechanisms, and the implications these have for clinical practice, is presented. This comprehensive knowledge forms the foundation for developing care approaches that are both empathic and grounded in evidence. Additionally, it supports the cultivation of deeper insight into the lived experiences of individuals who are navigating the challenges posed by these complex symptoms.

> When my brother talks to me, I can't follow what he says. He jumps from one topic to another and rambles about stuff that does not make any sense. When you try to tell him that it is hard to follow him, he just keeps on talking fast or becomes angry.

The Case of Matthew

Matthew is a 35-year-old man who was admitted to a psychiatric hospital when he began to neglect his daily hygiene, stopped bathing, stayed alone whenever possible, and had difficulty keeping a conversation going for more than a few sentences. When other people tried to ask him about something, he had difficulty clearly answering the question. It usually appeared that he didn't understand what the other person was asking. These problems became so serious that hospitalization was necessary.

Matthew did not have unusual problems during his childhood. While his parents described him as a "loner" during his school years, he did not show serious psychiatric or behavioral problems during that part of his life. He began having more serious problems during college, particularly during his second year. He began to spend more time by himself and stopped going to class. He began wearing the same clothes for several days in a row without bathing or washing the clothes. He began having difficulty understanding what others were saying to him and keeping a conversation going with them. His family petitioned that he be involuntarily admitted to a psychiatric hospital.

He had received several psychiatric conditions, but it was finally determined that he was living with schizophrenia spectrum mental health problem. While he improved with some medications, he continued to have difficulty with the same problem behaviors but at a much less serious level. Often, when another person tried to talk with him, he had trouble staying on the topic. What he said usually came close to the topic, but it was usually confusing enough to make it difficult for the other person to understand what he meant. Sometimes, the other person thought that Matthew misunderstood what was said and would repeat what was said. Before long, it became clear that Matthew couldn't keep the conversation going. Other people around Matthew usually became frustrated and began to complain that Matthew couldn't follow what was being discussed. Others became frustrated and stayed away from him, calling Matthew "crazy" or "brain damaged." After a while, Matthew would sit in a corner and cover himself with his shirt or a jacket. Because many people had tried and failed to carry on a conversation with him, they stopped trying.

Definition and Characteristics of Confused and Disorganized Thinking and Motoric Behaviors in Individuals Living with SMI

Behaviors that are determined as "problematic" in mental health are not problematic in general; the behaviors listed as "symptoms" by mental health service providers are displayed to some degree by everyone (e.g., talking to oneself when a cell phone is misplaced, sometimes not taking prescribed medications, drinking too much, forgetting what one was saying). The behavior being displayed is labeled as "symptomatic" if it results in an unfavorable outcome or consequence for the person emitting the behavior and has a negative impact on others as well. Many behaviors that are displayed by people living with SMI are not dangerous but make others feel uncomfortable; the behaviors may be annoying or cause other individuals to be distressed. Behaviors can be labeled as "abnormal" if the behavior is displayed too often, too intensely, in the wrong settings, or has deleterious impacts on the daily functioning of the person living with SMI. The behaviors that become problematic may not be under the control of setting events; that is, the behaviors that are displayed in the wrong setting lack adequate stimulus control. Behavior is under stimulus control when the behavior appears more often in the context of the presence of a certain class of stimuli and not in the absence of that class of stimuli (Cooper et al., 2020). Behaviors lacking in stimulus control occur in settings or contexts in which the behaviors should not occur. People do not take off their clothes in public places if their clothes get wet after a rainstorm; they wait until they get home or change in private settings. The behavior of "taking off wet clothes" becomes "abnormal" when the behavior occurs in settings where it should not occur. Behavior lacking stimulus control is displayed in situations where behavior should not be displayed such as urinating in public or speaking or laughing loudly during a funeral. The behavior of any person becomes "abnormal" when the behavior interferes with the display of other adaptive behaviors.

Behaviors are multidimensional in terms of frequency, magnitude, settings, and effect or outcome. Behaviors also differ on how the behaviors can be assessed. Some behaviors are known as "private events" or "covert events" because they are known only to the individual experiencing the behavior such as thoughts, feelings, perceptions, and sensations (Dougher, 2013). The "private events" can be accessed through self-reports from the individual or sometimes inferred from other observable behaviors. At times, assessing "private events" is unreliable and invalid; for instance, the person may be exaggerating or minimizing the pain they are experiencing and report the pain differently depending on the setting and the anticipated consequence. People are usually not aware of what they are thinking, especially if they are asked to recall what they thought in the past. Additionally, language, cultural, and social differences can affect any verbal question and responses.

Another source of assessing private events is whether the behaviors have collateral sources of observation. Collateral sources can be reports from others about what the person is experiencing or behaviors that are associated with each other. For example, pain is a covert private behavior or event. The person experiencing pain can inform others about where the pain is, how often it occurs, the intensity, and what decreases the intensity and frequency. There are, however, other collateral behaviors that can be used to assess the pain. These may be facial expressions of discomfort, absence or slowness of physical movement, and behavior changes observed by others familiar with a person experiencing pain (e.g., no longer performing some leisure activities). There are assessments during which the person is asked to perform certain movements, called range of motion (ROM); the ease of and fluidity of performing the movements can be used to assess how pain may be impacting the person's ability to function. The person experiencing the covert behavior is asked to communicate it to others but having collateral observable data aids in any assessment.

However, these measures are not predictive of actual "real life" functioning (Harvey & Strassnig, 2012). Social functioning, such as interpersonal perception and interactions, has a better predictive value for adaptive functioning than scores on neuropsychological performance tests (Docherty, 2005). Domains of social cognition including emotional recognition, in both visual and auditory modalities, inference of other's impressions of oneself, judgment of intentions, and other related domains appear to impact functional capacities in everyday life (Green, 1996; Harvey & Strassnig, 2012). These domains of social functioning are part of a person's metacognitive capabilities; that is, being aware of one's own cognitive processes and often involves an overt attempt to control them (American Psychological Association, n.d.-k).

The problem behaviors of disorganized thinking and behaviors are assessed in two ways: (1) as a cluster of problem behaviors or (2) by specifically assessing the speech of the person for evidence of disorganization. Disorganized thinking is typically inferred from the individual's speech (Myers et al., 2024) and is considered a positive symptom according to cluster analysis of scores (Bell et al., 1994) on the Positive and Negative Symptoms Scale (PANSS) (Kay et al., 1987). It is characterized by the individual switching from one topic to another (i.e., derailment or loose association). The person experiencing confused and disorganized thought processes answers questions marginally or completely unrelated to the topic (i.e., tangentiality). If the thought processes are extremely disorganized, the person may be incomprehensible in what they are saying, at times speaking incoherently using words and phrases that are linguistically or semantically unrecognizable (American Psychiatric Association, 2022).

When measured as a cluster (i.e., a group of similar things such as problem behaviors associated with mental health), a wide range of behaviors are assessed including disorganized speech and behavior (Harrow et al., 2003; Myers et al., 2024). When measured on its own, disorganized speech is frequently assessed by examining loose associations between ideas (Kay et al., 1987) because mild and disorganized speech is common in the general population (Hirjak et al., 2024; Myers et al., 2024). The dimensions of speech must be severe and frequent enough to substantially impair effective communication to be considered a symptom or behavior problem of living with SMI (American Psychiatric Association, 2022).

The problems associated with disorganized speech include the following dimensions:

1. Cognitive derailment (thought derailment): the frequent abrupt shifting of thoughts or associations so that they do not follow one another in a logical sequence. Speech is often disconnected and fragmented, with the individual jumping from one idea to another unrelated or indirectly related idea. It is also known as loose associations; the association may be so unconnected and unrelated that the speech is not understandable (American Psychological Association, n.d.-e).
2. Flight of ideas: a nearly rapid, continuous succession of superficially related thoughts and ideas, usually based on understandable associations, distracting stimuli, or playing on words. It is manifested behaviorally as "hurried" speech (e.g., increased rate of word production) with frequent abrupt shifts in topic (American Psychological Association, n.d.-h; Shahrokh & Hales, 2003).
3. Tangentiality: responding to a question in an oblique or irrelevant way (Shahrokh & Hales, 2003). It is verbal behavior that repeatedly diverges from the original subject. It may be the result of disorganized thought processes or a diminished ability to focus attention; the verbal digressions may continue until the original topic is no longer the focus of the conversation (American Psychological Association, n.d.-p).
4. Circumstantiality: a pattern of speech that is indirect and delayed in reaching its goal because of excessive or irrelevant detail or parenthetical remarks. The speaker does not lose the point as is characteristic of loosening of associations, and clauses remain logically connected, but to the listener, it seems that the end will never be reached (Shahrokh & Hales, 2003). Speech is often indirect and circuitous in which the individual gives unnecessary and often irrelevant details before arriving at the main point. Circumstantiality differs from tangentiality in that the main point is never lost but rather accompanied by a large amount of nonessential information. (American Psychological Association, n.d.-d).
5. Word salad (jargon aphasia): a mixture of words and phrases in speech and writing that lack comprehensive meaning or logical coherence (Shahrokh & Hales, 2003); the associations and connections may be so fragmented as to be virtually incomprehensible. The person's associations appear to have little or no logical connection (American Psychological Association, n.d.-q).
6. Neologism: unintelligible speech containing a mixture of new words or inappropriately condensed combination of several words and bizarre expressions of speech to communicate a highly complex idea not readily understood by others (American Psychological Association, n.d.-l; Shahrokh & Hales, 2003).

It is important to clarify whether assessment methods that focus on disorganized speech are detecting the same phenomenon as those that measure disorganized behaviors more broadly, questioning if the separate but related or the same constructs are being assessed (Myers et al., 2024).

Harrow et al. (2003) reported that disordered speech on cognitive psychological tests also shows strange nonverbal behavior and unrealistic ideas. Harrow and colleagues concluded that the obtained results support the framework that disorganized dimensions of speech exhibited by people living with schizophrenia spectrum mental health problems are not a speech disorder. The problem that underlies confusing and disorganized aspects of speech is the result of problems in thought processes, including bizarre behavior, unrealistic ideas, and disordered thinking.

Disorganized motoric behavior is a problem behavior exhibited by people living with SMI. Disorganized motoric behaviors are movements that can range from childlike silliness (e.g., making faces, giggling) to unpredictable agitation (e.g., yelling, running with no purpose, pushing others) and aggressive behaviors; it can be exhibited as repetitive purposeless movements of arms or legs (Torres, 2024).

Catatonia is defined as a state of muscular rigidity or other disturbances of motor behaviors, extreme overactivity, or adoption of bizarre postures; it is classified as a negative symptom in people living with SMI since it is the absence of purposeful behaviors to a goal that can be acknowledged by others (Jain & Mitra, 2023). When exhibited, it can obstruct the performances of activities of daily life as the problem behaviors interfere with the initiation and completion of daily tasks; at times, the person experiencing catatonia does not respond to requests or prompts, appearing as if in a daze or does not respond to environmental cues (e.g., fire alarms).

Catatonia is characterized by extremes in motoric under- and overactivity. Underactivity in motoric behaviors are decreases in reactivity to the environment ranging from motiveless resistance to instruction and attempts to be moved (i.e., "negativism"), reduction in spontaneous movements, lack of responsiveness to and awareness of the environment, and at times assuming and maintaining a rigid, inappropriate, or bizarre posture. It can be exhibited as a complete lack of verbal and motor responses (mutism and stupor). Catalepsy is defined as long periods of extreme irresponsiveness during which the person is in a state of unresponsiveness usually in a fixed body posture. During these periods, the person can be placed in poses or positions by others that are maintained by the person. It is also termed "catatonic rigidity," "flexibilitas cerea," and "waxy flexibility" (American Psychological Association, n.d.-c; Shahrokh & Hales, 2003).

The overactive motoric behavior observed in a person experiencing catatonic behavior is purposeless excessive motor activity not influenced by any observed external stimuli and seemingly without observed cause (i.e., catatonic excitement); other features of catatonic excitement can be repeated stereotype movements, staring, grimacing, and the echoing of speech (American Psychological Association, n.d.-c; Shahrokh & Hales, 2003).

As with other problem behaviors that people living with SMI exhibit, the problematic behaviors of disorganization in speech and behavior are transdiagnostic and multidimensional. The dimension of disorganization includes bizarre behavior, nonsensical and difficult to comprehend speech, and inappropriate affect (Hardy-Baylé et al., 2003). Disorganized speech and behaviors occur in several mental health problems associated with SMI including schizophrenia spectrum, affective/mood, and anxiety-based mental health problems and problems associated with neurological problems, such as dementia related conditions, traumatic brain injury, infectious processes, and metabolic and degenerative conditions (e.g., Parkinson's disease). The problem of disorganized thought processes and behaviors is composed of separate domains: (1) problems in speaking coherently so that others in the environment can understand what is said, and (2) motoric behaviors that are intentional, purposeful, and goal directed. Each domain varies in independence from each other as the domains can occur simultaneously in the same or other contexts (Hardy-Baylé et al., 2003).

The dimensions of the domains of disorganized speech and motoric behaviors include the frequencies of occurrences and nonoccurrences, magnitude/severity of the behaviors, and temporal aspects of the displayed behaviors (e.g., duration of the occurrences and nonoccurrences, time between occurrences), the degree of the awareness and controllability of the displayed behavior by the person, the amount of distress that results during the occurrence of the behaviors in addition to other dimensions of behaviors such as contextual, antecedental and consequential conditions of the behaviors. The domains have behavioral dimensions that refer to that specific domain of disorganization.

Dimensions of Disorganized Speech and Motoric Behaviors

Disorganized Speech

Disorganized speech is a critical barrier to recovery in living with SMI; disorganized speech has profound negative impacts on the capabilities of a person living with SMI to engage with the environment. There has been limited research regarding the dimensional aspects of disorganized speech; the outcome of the limited research is a lack of existing effective treatments in addressing the problem behavior.

Andreasen (1986) developed a scale that identified 20 different dimensions of disorganization and abnormalities in rate of speech that are presumed to be a function of thought disorganization, known in the psychiatric literature as formal thought disorder (FTD). The "Thought, Language and Communication" (TLC) scale emphasizes the importance of assessing language behavior that is directly observable during verbal interactions. The ratings for the 18 dimensions are based on the frequency of occurrences during a standard mental health interview and are rated on an ordinal scale from absent (0) to extreme or frequent (3 or 4).

The specific dimensions that are rated and the operational criteria for the items are:

- Poverty of Speech: Restriction in spontaneous speech; rated from 0 to 4.
- Poverty of Content of Speech: Speech is adequate in amount but conveys little information; stereotyped and meaningless repetition of words (i.e., verbigeration); rated from 0 to 4.

- Pressure of Speech: Increased amount and speed of speech; difficult to interrupt; long duration before responding to question; rated from 0 to 4.
- Distractible Speech: Speech gets interrupted by nearby stimuli; rated from 0 to 4.
- Tangentiality: Replies are oblique or irrelevant; rated from 0 to 4.
- Derailment: Ideas slip off track, also known as loose associations; rated from 0 to 4.
- Incoherence: Speech is incomprehensible usually because of a preponderance of word salad (schizophasia), "jargon aphasia" (speaking fluently but incomprehensible), or "paragrammatism" (in which portions of coherent sentences may be observed during a sentence that is incoherent as a whole); rated from 0 to 4.
- Illogicality: Conclusions do not follow logically; conclusions are reached by inferring relatedness between 2 or more unrelated statements; rated from 0 to 4.
- Clanging: Word choice is governed by sounds rather than meaning; punning and rhyming may substitute for logic (Shahrokh & Hales, 2003); rated from 0 to 4.
- Neologisms: New word formations; rated from 0 to 3.
- Word Approximations: Old words which are used in a new and unconventional way, or new words which are developed by conventional rules of words; rated from 0 to 3.
- Circumstantiality: Speech is indirect and delayed; rated from 0 to 3.
- Loss of Goal: Failure to follow thought to conclusion; sometimes observed in conjunction with derailment; rated from 0 to 3.
- Perseveration: Repetition of words or ideas; rated from 0 to 3.
- Echolalia: The individual repeats words or phrases from the speaker; rated from 0 to 3.
- Blocking: A sudden obstruction or interruption of normal flow of speech before a thought has been completed; the person is unable to return to topic as unable to recall what the topic was (Shahrokh & Hales, 2003); rated from 0 to 3.
- Stilted Speech: Excessively stilted or formal quality. Speech appears outdated, pompous, overly polite. Rated from 0 to 3.
- Self-Reference: Repeatedly referring subjects back to oneself; rated from 0 to 3.

Two additional dimensions of speech and communication problems are included in the TLC: 1) Paraphasia (Phonemic): Recognizable mispronunciation of a word because sounds or syllables have slipped out of sequence (rated from 0 to 3); and 2) Paraphasia (Semantic): Substitution of inappropriate words with different meaning (rated from 0 to 4). Paraphasia is included in the TLC scale because it is considered a language usage disorder. Specifically, paraphasia refers to the production of unintended syllables, words, or phrases during speech, which can result in speech that is difficult to understand. This type of language disturbance is often observed in individuals with conditions such as aphasia, which can result from neurological injuries and disorders. Including paraphasia in the TLC scale helps to assess and diagnose various language and communication problems more accurately (John, 2019); paraphasia is not included in the final scoring of the TLC and is not categorized as domains or areas to include in either FTD or disorganization of speech.

The ratings are summed up to obtain a global rating of the severity of the dimensions, or the service provider can provide a global rating based on the subjective impression of the totality of the disorganized communication following the criteria below:

- No TLC disorder (score = 0): Occasional instances of the less problematic forms and no more than one instance of the more problematic form (which is felt in context to be clinically insignificant) (Andreasen, 1986).
- Mild TLC disorder (score = 1): Occasional instances of a TLC problem that are felt in context to be mild but clinically significant (Andreasen, 1986).
- Moderate TLC disorder (score = 2): Significant and unquestionable impaired verbal output, which leads to a moderate disturbance in communication at least from time to time (Andreasen, 1986).
- Severe TLC disorder (score = 3): Problem is significant enough to impair communication for a substantial part of the interview; many instances of the more problematic manifestations of TLC (Andreasen, 1986).
- Extreme TLC disorder (score = 4): Problem is so severe that communication is difficult or impossible most of the time (Andreasen, 1986).

The TLC can be scored using an alternate method in which the dimensions that suggest severe disorganization are summed and multiplied by 2 indicating more dysfunction and disorganization in speech. The following dimensions have been identified by Andreasen (1986) as being indicative of "more pathological" (p. 281): (a) poverty of speech; (b) poverty of content of speech; (c) pressure of speech; (d) distractible speech; (e) derailment; (f) tangentially; (g) incoherence; (h) illogicality; (i) clanging; (j) neologisms; and (k) word approximations.

Andreasen (1986) categorized the 18 dimensions into three main areas:

1. Thought disorders: "The concept of thought disorder comprises only those disorders in which thinking alone seems aberrant: poverty of speech (aberrant because thought seems not to occur) and illogicality (aberrant inferential processes)" (Andreasen, 1986, p. 474).
2. Language usage disorders: These involve the dimension in which the speaker does not follow the syntactical and semantic conventions that govern language usage including incoherence, clanging, neologisms, and word approximations (Andreasen, 1986).
3. Communication disorders: These include the dimensions in which the speaker fails to take the various needs of the listener into account. According to this definition, the failure to communicate effectively includes the dimensions of poverty of content of speech, pressure of speech, distractible speech, tangentiality, derailment, stilted speech, echolalia, self-reference, circumstantiality, loss of goal, perseveration, and blocking (Andreasen, 1986).

The TLC scale describes 18 dimensions of speech disorganization that are hypothesized to reflect "thought," "language," and "communication" problematic conditions (Roche et al., 2015). However, this division may not accurately reflect the factor structure of FTD. Data from scores on the TLC have identified 7 different domains of FTD with 42–78% variance accounted for by 3 domains: the "disorganization domain," "negative domain," and the "verbosity/productivity domain." The disorganization domain is characterized by dimensional items such as tangentiality, derailment, incoherence, illogicality, circumstantiality, and loss of goal. The negative domain comprises the items assessing poverty of speech and content with or without perseveration. This domain is distinct from disorganized speech and may be better classified as alogia (Roche et al., 2015), which is "negative symptom" characterized by a significant reduction of speech content, fluency, and spontaneity (Shahrokh and Hales, 2003). The verbosity/productivity domain includes items on the dimension of pressure of speech and poverty of speech, often loading inversely on the factor structure, as the more the individual speaks, the more content and less restriction on the occurrence of spontaneous speech.

Andreasen (1986) originally proposed a dichotomous structure of FTD, with "negative" (poverty of speech and poverty of content) and "positive" (pressure of speech, tangentiality, derailment, incoherence, and illogicality) subtypes. Results from factor analyses have shown that these subtypes are weakly correlated and have distinct clinical associations (Roche et al., 2015).

Overall, the TLC scale's factor structure highlights the complexity and multidimensional nature of disorganized speech and the presumed association with FTD, with disorganization, negative, and verbosity domains being commonly identified.

As stated above, disorganized speech is a major domain of disorganized symptoms, which includes problems in verbal behaviors like tangentiality, derailment, and incoherence, that impact functioning in all spheres of daily life. It represents a severe form of disorganization, with individuals facing added social challenges, impeding their recovery. Negative affect—shame, distress, guilt, dysphoria, anger, worry—has been identified as a potential antecedent conditions or triggers for the occurrences of disorganized speech, with studies showing increased disorganized speech in response to induced negative affect (Bettis et al., 2024). Previous research by Leonhardt et al. (2017) found that themes of inadequacy and vulnerability often precede disorganization, but these findings were limited to psychotherapy transcripts from a single case.

Bettis et al. (2024) analyzed 30 narrative interview transcripts to identify themes preceding disorganized speech using "inductive thematic analysis." Inductive thematic analysis is a qualitative research method used to identify, analyze, and report patterns or themes within data.

The themes are derived from the data itself without the influence of preexisting theories or frameworks. The approach allows researchers to remain open to new ideas and themes that emerge from the data, making it particularly useful for exploratory research where the goal is to develop new theories or insights (Naeem et al., 2023).

Bettis et al. (2024) identified four main themes preceding the display of disorganized speech: alienation, interpersonal tension, personal benchmarks, and adverse experiences, each with two subthemes. Relationship tension was the most frequent topic preceding disorganization followed by alienation related to illness, social alienation, past hardships, and inadequacy. Missed important personal events (e.g., life passage events, such as graduations, marriages, births, death) that often led to self-criticism or disappointment, with recognizing missed potential and inadequacy being key subthemes indicating that social dynamics and self-assessment can trigger disorganized speech. Adverse experiences, including past hardship and grief, were significant precursors to disorganization. The authors concluded that disorganization of speech may be a response to the distress that was experienced by the participants living with SMI and that treatment ought to focus on building awareness of alienation triggers, especially in individuals living with SMI displaying extremely disorganized speech.

Another scale assessing disorganization of behavior in the domains of language, affectivity, and motor behavior in individuals living with SMI is the Bern Psychopathology Scale-Revised (BPS-R) (Strik et al., 2010). The scale includes qualitative, quantitative, and subjective judgment dimensions to rate the severity of problems in each domain; most of the qualitative items are in the scale assessing affective behaviors. The BPS-R items are rated on a three-point scale: −1 (pathologically inhibited), 0 (normal), and 1 (pathologically disinhibited). The global assessment of each domain's severity is rated on a seven-point scale, from −3 (severely inhibited/anxious) to 3 (severely disinhibited/elated). Three factors were consistently identified from data using the BPS-R: language, affectivity, and motor behavior (Strik et al., 2010).

The operational definitions for the items on the BPS-R refer to behavioral observations and subjectively judged phenomena and constructs on the part of the observer; the items are not based on theoretical content. For instance, instead of relating to the concept of psychomotor retardation or agitation, speed of thought and speed of movements are observed separately reflecting thought/cognitive and motor behaviors. Each of the two speed functions is further rated as increased, normal, or decreased over a defined time span considering temporal dimension of the observed behaviors (Strik et al., 2010).

The BPS-R for speech and motor scales are structured as follows:

- Speech scale: composed of 15 items, each describing an inhibited and disinhibited occurrence of specific language and speech features divided into quantitative and qualitative abnormalities, having 6 and 5 items, respectively. "Subjective experiences" has four items that are related to thoughts that are expressed verbally but judged by the observer. Each item is rated on a three-point scale: −1 (pathologically inhibited), 0 (normal), and 1 (pathologically disinhibited) (Strik et al., 2010).
- Motor scale: composed of 10 items describing inhibited and disinhibited motor behaviors; divided into quantitative and qualitative aspects, having 5 and 3 items, respectively. Subjective perception has two items. Each item is rated on a three-point scale: −1 (pathologically inhibited), 0 (normal), and 1 (pathologically disinhibited) (Strik et al., 2010).

- Global assessment: For each domain, the global rating is calculated by considering the individual scores of the symptoms within that domain. The overall global rating for each domain is then summarized as: a) Negative: scores ranging from −3 to −1; b) Normal: score of 0; c) Positive: Scores ranging from +1 to +3. Each domain is rated on a seven-point scale: −3 (severely inhibited/anxious), −2 (moderately inhibited/anxious), −1 (mildly inhibited/anxious), 0 (normal), 1 (mildly disinhibited/elated), 2 (moderately disinhibited/elated), 3 (severely disinhibited/elated) and is indicative of the overall problematic psychological and behavioral state of the individual living with SMI (Strik et al., 2010).

The language scale on the BPS-R assesses various aspects of language and speech, categorized into negative, normal, and positive symptoms. The items in each qualitative and quantitative category are:

- Quantitative
  - Spontaneity to speak: reduced or increased spontaneity to talk.
  - Speech pauses: more or fewer spontaneous pauses.
  - Speech rate: decelerated or accelerated speech rate.
  - Ideas: lack of ideas or inventiveness.
  - Latency of responses: prolonged or shortened latency of responses.
- Qualitative
  - Mistaking identity: false negative or false positive whereby the patient incorrectly identifies someone or something as not being what it is or engages in mistaken identity.
  - Coherence: thought blocking or interruptions of coherence by changing the subject.
  - Interruptions: omissions or intrusions of speech (including neologisms).
  - Attribution of terms (naming): ongoing questioning of terms or hasty, playful attribution of terms.
  - Comprehension of meaning: to wonder verbally in an agonizing and seeking way or speaking in an attempt to persuade the listener.
- Subjective experiences
  - Stream of thoughts: loss of thoughts or insertions of thoughts, noisy thoughts (including auditory-verbal hallucinations).
  - Quantity of thoughts: poverty of thoughts or pressure of thoughts.
  - Clarity of thoughts: perplexity or confusion.
  - Need to talk: lack of need to talk or an urge to talk.

Each item is rated on a scale from −3 (negative) to +3 (positive), with 0 indicating normal behavior.

The global subjective behaviors in the language scale of the BPS-R are rated by the judgment of the observer based on what is observed during the assessment period. They are:

1. Stream of thoughts: loss of thoughts or insertions of thoughts, noisy thoughts (including auditory verbal hallucinations being experienced by the individual during the observational period).
2. Quantity of thoughts: poverty of thoughts or pressure of thoughts.
3. Clarity of thoughts: perplexity or confusion.
4. Need to talk: lack of need to talk or an urge to talk.

Each item is rated by the observer on a scale from −3 (negative) to +3 (positive), with 0 indicating normal behavior.

The Positive and Negative Symptom Scale (PANSS) is a commonly used dimensional scale for assessing symptoms and problem behaviors exhibited by people living with SMI. Each item of the PANSS is rated with 1 to 7 points ranging from absent to extreme (Kay et al., 1987). Large-scale factor analysis studies on the PANSS have yielded five dimensions of problem behavior in people living with SMI: positive symptoms and behaviors, negative symptoms and behaviors, behavioral disorganization, behavioral excitement, and emotional distress (van der Gaag et al., 2006). Using a sample of consecutively admitted individuals to inpatient psychiatric care at a large European urban hospital, Lang et al. (2016) compared scores obtained on the PANSS and the BPS-R. The results showed some overlap between the system-specific approach of the BPS and the five-factor PANSS model. The positive factor of the PANSS was associated with the affect domain (inhibition and disinhibition), while the negative factor was associated with inhibition on all three BPS domains (i.e., affect, language, and motor). PANSS excitement factor was associated with inhibition of affect and disinhibition of language and motor domains.

Anderson et al. (2015) reanalyzed data from the PANNS using a different factor analytic method whereby every PANSS item was assigned to exactly one domain based on the maximal average cross-validated pretreatment matrix. The results supported the following factor structure and the dimensional items on each factor:

- Negative: Dimensional items included Blunted Affect, Emotional Withdrawal, Poor Rapport, Passive Apathetic, Social Withdrawal, Lack of Spontaneity and Flow of Conversation, Motor Retardation, and Active Social Avoidance.
- Positive: Dimensional items included Delusions, Unusual Thought Content, Hallucinatory Behavior, Suspiciousness Persecution, and Grandiosity.
- Disorganized: Dimensional items included Conceptual Disorganization, Poor Attention, Mannerisms and Posturing, Difficulty in Abstract Thinking, Disturbance of Volition, Preoccupation, Disorientation, Stereotyped Thinking, and Lack of Judgment and Insight.
- Excited: Dimensional items include Excitement, Poor Impulse Control, Hostility, and Uncooperativeness.
- Anxiety: Dimensional items include Anxiety, Tension, Depression, Guilt Feelings, and Somatic Concern.

A review of the PANSS items shows that there is some direct correspondence between the various operationalized dimensions of disorganized speech and motor behaviors that are displayed by individuals living with SMI on the various assessment instruments. Specifically, the items and their definitions directly and tacitly related to disorganization of speech are:

- Conceptual disorganization: a disorganized process of thinking characterized by disruption of goal-directed sequencing (e.g., circumstantiality, loose associations, tangentiality, gross illogicality, or thought block) (Positive and Negative Syndrome Scale [PANSS] for Schizophrenia, 2024).
- Poor rapport: a lack of interpersonal empathy, openness in conversation, and sense of closeness, interest, or involvement with the interviewer. This is evidenced by interpersonal distancing and reduced verbal and nonverbal communication (Positive and Negative Syndrome Scale [PANSS] for Schizophrenia, 2024).
- Difficulty in abstract thinking: an impairment in the use of the abstract-symbolic mode of thinking, as evidenced by difficulty in classification, forming generalizations, and proceeding beyond concrete or egocentric thinking in problem-solving tasks (Positive and Negative Syndrome Scale [PANSS] for Schizophrenia, 2024).
- Lack of spontaneity and flow of conversation: a reduction in the normal flow of communication associated with apathy, avolition, defensiveness, or cognitive impairment. This is manifested by diminished fluidity and productivity of the verbal interactional process (Positive and Negative Syndrome Scale [PANSS] for Schizophrenia, 2024).
- Stereotyped thinking: decreased fluidity, spontaneity, and flexibility of thinking, as evidenced in rigid, repetitious, or barren thought content (Positive and Negative Syndrome Scale [PANSS] for Schizophrenia, 2024).
- Disorientation: a lack of awareness of one's relationship to the milieu, including person, place, and time, which may be due to confusion or withdrawal (Positive and Negative Syndrome Scale [PANSS] for Schizophrenia, 2024).

As evidenced, disorganized speech is multidimensional. The various dimensions of the disorganized speech displayed by individuals living with SMI need to be operationalized and precisely defined to have a complete and comprehensive understanding of the phenomenon. Only in this manner can the problem behavior of disorganized speech be adequately assessed and treated.

The dimensions of disorganized speech that need to be included in assessment and treatment include:

1. Frequency: How often disorganized speech occurs and does not occur.
2. Magnitude/severity: the intensity or severity of disorganized speech; frequency and durations of periods when the person is not displaying disorganized speech.
3. Contextual, antecedental, and consequential conditions: the conditions surrounding the behavior, including what happens before and after the occurrence of disorganized.
4. Temporal aspects: duration of occurrences and nonoccurrences of disorganized speech over defined periods and the time between occurrences. Latency of verbal behaviors in response to questions.

5. Rate and pace of speech and thoughts: the rate of word usage by the person varying from rapid and intense to slow and delayed with long latencies between sentences/thoughts.
6. Spontaneity of speech and thoughts: speaking without long delays and need for prompts to continue speaking.
7. Awareness and controllability: the degree to which the person is aware of and can control the display of disorganized speech.
8. Distress: The amount of distress displayed by the person during the occurrences of disorganized speech.
9. Mistaking identity: The speaker incorrectly identifies someone or something as not being what it is.
10. Incoherence, tangentiality, "flight of ideas": interruptions of speech by insertions of thoughts or displaying loose association (e.g., changing the subject), including the speaker responding to auditory verbal hallucinations while speaking. The flow of speech content is uneven and disconnected.
11. Stream of thoughts: loss of thought, unable to return to thought, thought blocking.
12. Illogicality: Content of speech is illogical, impractical.
13. Interruptions: omissions or intrusions of speech (including neologisms, clanging, word approximations).
14. Attribution of terms (Naming): ongoing questioning of terms or hasty, playful attribution of terms.
15. Quantity of thoughts: poverty of speech and thoughts or pressure of speech and thoughts.
16. Clarity of thoughts: perplexity or confusion while speaking.
17. Comprehension of meaning: defined as the person wondering and puzzling in a distressing manner while speaking. Seeming unsure as to what they are saying makes sense and is being understood.
18. Need to talk: lack of need to talk or an urge to talk. Frequently interrupting and talking over the other person.

These dimensions provide a comprehensive understanding of disorganized speech, aiding in the assessment and treatment of individuals with SMI. However, the dimensions need to be precisely and clearly operationally defined with concrete examples given for each dimension so further research in this area can be pursued.

Disorganized Motoric Behaviors

The domain of disorganized or atypical motoric behaviors is movements that can range from childlike silliness, inappropriate giggling, and grimaces to unpredictable agitation; it can be manifested as repeated movements without purpose, pacing or wandering aimlessly, social withdrawal, inability, and/or refusals to complete tasks and emotionless expressions or mannerisms (Mayo Clinic, 2024). When the behavior is severe, it can cause problems in the performance of activities of daily life and activities to maintain health and wellbeing, such as not eating or drinking.

Disorganized motoric behavior includes the behavioral dimensions of catatonia; catatonia is manifested when a person appears as if in a daze with little movement or response to the surrounding environment (stupor) (American Psychiatric Association, 2025). It is characterized by motor, affective, and cognitive-behavioral signs including disorganization of motor behavior such as immobility, rigor, and dyskinesia, affective signs (anxiety, aggression), and cognitive-behavioral signs including mutism, echolalia, and automatic obedience (Hirjak et al., 2024; Rasmussen et al., 2016).

The DSM-5-TR (American Psychiatric Association, 2022) criteria for catatonia are based primarily on problems with motor behaviors, requiring the presence of three or more of the following 12 psychomotor dimensions:

1. Stupor: no psychomotor activity; not actively relating to or engaged with the environment (p. 135).
2. Catalepsy: passive induction of a posture held against gravity (p. 135).
3. Waxy flexibility: slight and uniform resistance to positioning by the examiner (p. 135).
4. Mutism: very little or no verbal responses (excluding aphasia) (p. 135).
5. Negativism: opposition or no response to instructions or to external stimuli (p. 135).
6. Posturing: spontaneous and active maintenance of a posture against gravity (p. 135).
7. Mannerism: odd, circumstantial caricature of normal actions (p. 135).
8. Stereotypy: repetitive, abnormally frequent, purposeless movements (p. 135).
9. Agitation: state of increased but typically purposeless and repetitious activity not influenced by external stimuli (American Psychological Association, n.d.-a; American Psychiatric Association, 2022, p. 135).
10. Grimacing: facial contortions (p. 135).
11. Echolalia: mimicking another's speech (p. 135).
12. Echopraxia: mimicking another's movement (p. 135).

Disorganization of motoric behaviors displayed by people living with SMI is multidimensional and idiosyncratic. There are a variety of motoric behaviors that compose the disorganization of the motoric behavior domain. Although possible, it is highly unlikely that a person living with SMI who displays disorganized motoric behaviors will exhibit all dimensions of this domain; it is more likely that a person will display a few disorganized motoric behaviors that are distinctive or characteristic for them.

The first step in changing any challenging problem behavior is to ascertain what operationally defined behaviors are being exhibited by the person living with SMI (Sarkar et al., 2016; Sienaert et al., 2011). The Positive and Negative Symptom Scale (PANSS) is a commonly used dimensional scale for assessing symptoms and problem behaviors exhibited by people living with SMI (Kay et al., 1987). Reanalyzing data by assigning every PANSS item to exactly one domain based on the maximal average cross-validated pretreatment loading matrix (called the "Full

Model"), Anderson et al. (2015) found two factors that conceptualized disorganized behaviors displayed by individuals living with SMI—"disorganized" and "excited." The disorganized factor was composed of the following items from the PANSS: (a) Conceptual Disorganization; (b) Poor Attention; (c) Mannerisms and Posturing; (d) Difficulty in Abstract Thinking; (e) Disturbance of Volition; (f) Preoccupation; (g) Disorientation; (h) Stereotyped Thinking; (i) Lack of Judgment; and (j) Insight. The factor termed "Excited" is composed of the following items that pertain to motoric behaviors: (a) Excitement; (b) Poor Impulse Control; (c) Hostility; and (d) Uncooperativeness (Anderson et al., 2015). The content of the items on the PANSS are as follows:

- Excitement: hyperactivity as reflected in accelerated motor behavior, heightened responsivity to stimuli, hypervigilance, or excessive mood lability (Positive and Negative Syndrome Scale [PANSS] for Schizophrenia, 2024).
- Mannerisms and posturing: unnatural movements or posture as characterized by an awkward, stilted, disorganized, or bizarre appearance (Positive and Negative Syndrome Scale [PANSS] for Schizophrenia, 2024).
- Motor retardation: reduction in motor activity as reflected in slowing or lessening or movements and speech, diminished responsiveness to stimuli, and reduced muscle tone (Positive and Negative Syndrome Scale [PANSS] for Schizophrenia, 2024).
- Uncooperativeness: active refusal to comply with the requests of significant others, including the interviewer, hospital staff, or family, which may be associated with distrust, defensiveness, stubbornness, negativism, rejection of authority, hostility, or belligerence (Positive and Negative Syndrome Scale [PANSS] for Schizophrenia, 2024).
- Disturbance of volition: disturbance in the willful initiation, control, and the continuation of one's thoughts, behavior, movements, and speech (Positive and Negative Syndrome Scale [PANSS] for Schizophrenia, 2024).
- Poor impulse control: disordered regulation and control of action or impulses, resulting in sudden, unmodulated, arbitrary, or misdirected discharge of tension and emotions without concern about consequences (Positive and Negative Syndrome Scale [PANSS] for Schizophrenia, 2024).
- Hostility: verbal and nonverbal expressions of anger and resentment, including sarcasm, passive-aggressive behavior, verbal abuse, and assaultiveness (Positive and Negative Syndrome Scale [PANSS] for Schizophrenia, 2024).
- Disorientation: lack of awareness of one's relationship to the milieu, including persons, place, and time, which may be due to confusion or withdrawal (Positive and Negative Syndrome Scale [PANSS] for Schizophrenia, 2024).

A qualitative content analysis focusing on the themes of the items featuring motoric behaviors of the items that compose the two factors found by Anderson et al. (2015) shows that the motoric items include "Mannerisms and Posturing" and "Disturbance of Volition" on the "Disorganized" factor; the "disorientation" item on the disorganized factor may be included as an item assessing disorganized motoric behaviors if it entails the person engaging in purposeless behaviors, such as pacing and wandering aimlessly. On the "Excitement" factor, all the items pertain to behaviors that are displayed motorically.

The Bern Psychopathology Scale (BPS-R) (Bracht et al., 2013; Strik et al., 2010; Walther & Strik, 2016; Walther et al., 2014) assesses various dimensions of motor behavior on the Motor Behavior Scale. The items are categorized into negative, normal, and positive. They include:

1. Spontaneous movements: amount and frequency of spontaneous movements.
2. Spontaneous rest: amount and frequency of pauses in movement.
3. Velocity: rate of movement (accelerated/decelerated).
4. Movement quality: monotonous, repetitive, or playful diversity of movements.
5. Excitability: sparse or lively reactions in motor behavior.
6. Motion sequence: blockages or parakinesia (i.e., awkwardness or clumsiness of movement (American Psychological Association, n.d.-m) and dyskinesia (i.e., involuntary or unintended movement, such as a tic or spasm; denotes distorted or impaired voluntary movement (American Psychological Association, n.d.-f).
7. Volition: negativism or automatic obedience/echolalia/echopraxia/verbigerations.
8. Functionality of movements: rituals/stereotypies or mannerisms; purposefulness of displayed motoric behaviors.
9. Decision-making: ambivalence or excessive self-will.
10. Motor drive: lacking energy to move or an urge to move.
11. Motor pleasure: idleness or a desire for moving.

Each item is rated on a scale from −3 (negative) to +3 (positive), with zero indicating normal behavior.

The dimensions of motoric behaviors on the BPS-R account for the presence or absence and the frequency and rate of motoric behaviors but do not specify any temporal aspect on the dimensions. For example, amount and frequency of spontaneous movements and lack of movement (pauses) do not assess the duration of the movements and "pauses" when they occur. A temporal duration would offer greater precision of the dimension being defined and measured.

The Bush-Francis Catatonia Rating Scale (BFCRS) (University of Rochester Medical Center, Collaborative Care and Wellness Center, 2025) is a tool used to assess the presence and frequency of the dimensions of catatonia in a person exhibiting disorganized motor behaviors over a specified period. It includes 23 items, each rated on a scale from 0 (not present), 1 (occasional), 2 (frequent), and 3 (constant) during a defined duration (usually during the length of the assessment) with higher scores indicating more severe symptoms based on frequency of occurrences. Each item is accompanied by a video example to aid in the assessment.

The items cover a range of dimensions of motoric behaviors and physical signs, including:

1. Excitement: extreme hyperactivity.
2. Immobility/stupor: extreme hypoactivity and minimal responsiveness.
3. Mutism: minimal or no verbal response.
4. Starring: fixed gaze with little visual scanning.

5. Posturing/catalepsy: spontaneous maintenance of posture(s), including mundane (e.g., sitting/standing for long periods without reacting) (Bush-Francis Catatonia Rating Scale (BFCRS), 2025).
6. Grimacing: odd facial expressions.
7. Echopraxia/echolalia: mimicking movements or speech.
8. Stereotypy: repetitive, non-goal-directed motor activity.
9. Mannerisms: odd, purposeful movements. Performing actions at inappropriate times (e.g., saluting), displaying an odd gait (e.g., tiptoeing), and/or exaggerated politeness.
10. Verbigeration: repetition of a word, phrases or sentences.
11. Rigidity: maintenance of a rigid position. A subvariety is known as "psychological pillow" described as the person maintaining a reclining posture, with their head a few inches above the bed surface for prolonged periods (Rajagopal, 2007).
12. Negativism: resistance to instructions or attempts to move.
13. Waxy flexibility: during re-posturing, individual offers initial resistance before allowing himself to be repositioned, similar to that of a bending candle (Bush-Francis Catatonia Rating Scale (BFCRS), 2025).
14. Withdrawal: refusal to eat, drink, or make eye contact.
15. Impulsivity: sudden inappropriate behavior.
16. Automatic obedience: exaggerated cooperation with examiner's request or spontaneous continuation of movement requested (Bush-Francis Catatonia Rating Scale (BFCRS), 2025).
17. Mitgehen: arm-raising in response to light pressure. An extreme form of *mitmachen* in which very slight pressure leads to movement in any direction, also called the "anglepoise" effect or "anglepoise lamp sign." This movement occurs despite instructions to resist the pressure, as individuals with this condition often experience even slight pressure as forcible grasping and pushing (Glossary of Psychiatry, 2024).
18. Gegenhalten: resistance to passive movement, which is proportional to strength of the stimulus, appears automatic rather than willful (Bush-Francis Catatonia Rating Scale (BFCRS), 2025).
19. Ambitendency: indecisive, hesitant movement. The individual appears motorically "stuck" in indecisive, hesitant movements (Bush-Francis Catatonia Rating Scale (BFCRS), 2025). It is a pattern of incomplete motor responses in anticipation of voluntary action. It is a type of psychomotor retardation in which the individual appears motorically stuck and exhibits hesitant, indecisive motions in the absence of voluntary movement (American Psychological Association, n.d.-b).
20. Grasp reflex: neurological reflex. This is an involuntary grasping by an individual of anything that touches the palm (American Psychological Association, n.d.-i).
21. Perseveration: repeatedly returning to the same topic or movement.
22. Combativeness: striking out in an undirected manner, with no, or only a facile explanation afterwards (Bush-Francis Catatonia Rating Scale (BFCRS), 2025).

23. Autonomic abnormality: abnormalities in temperature, BP, pulse, respiratory rate, or diaphoresis.

The BFCRS has the most items that assess the dimensions of disorganized motoric behaviors; the behaviors in each dimension are observed and rated during the period of assessment. The dimensions are rated if the specified behaviors occur during the period of the examination but do not account for the frequency or rate of the behavior (e.g., how many times per hour), the duration during each discrete occurrence, or the duration when the behavior does not occur. The rating of the frequency is based on the subjective judgment of the observer/examiner. The individual's awareness of the behaviors being displayed, the dimension of perceived and actual controllability (e.g., successfully ceasing the behavior after being asked to control the behavior), and the degree of distress that accompanies the display of the behavior should be included in any comprehensive evaluation of the disorganized motoric behavioral dimensions. As with other operant behaviors that are displayed by people living with SMI, the "three pillars" of behavior—antecedent, precisely defined behavior, and consequence—need to be part of any assessment so that there is a better understanding of the phenomena of disorganized motoric behaviors and effective treatment.

A combination of all the cited dimensions would assist in developing a robust assessment tool when assessing disorganized motoric behavior displayed by individuals living with SMI. Using the BFCRS as a base (as having the most comprehensive multidimensional assessment), a proposed expanded version would include:

1. Frequency or rate of behavior (e.g., how many times per hour).
2. Duration of each discrete occurrence.
3. Duration when the behavior does not occur.
4. Awareness of the behaviors being displayed: individuals' awareness of the behavior that is displayed.
5. Perceived controllability: perception of self-control of behavior by the individual.
6. Actual controllability: successfully ceasing the behavior by the person after being asked to control it.
7. Degree of distress: negative emotions that accompany the display of the behaviors.
8. Antecedent: the event or stimulus that precedes the displayed behavior and elicits or sets the occasion for the behavior or response.
9. Consequence: an event, situation, stimulus, or circumstance that follows from the behavior being displayed.
10. Excitement: extreme hyperactivity and over-responsiveness to minimal stimuli (e.g., yelling that arm is hurting if touched by another).
11. Immobility/stupor: extreme hypoactivity and minimal responsiveness.
12. Mutism: minimal or no verbal response.
13. Starring: fixed gaze with little visual scanning.

14. Posturing/catalepsy: spontaneous maintenance of posture(s), including mundane (e.g., sitting/standing for long periods without reacting) (Bush-Francis Catatonia Rating Scale (BFCRS), 2025).
15. Grimacing: odd facial expressions and contortions (e.g., suddenly sticking tongue out).
16. Echopraxia/echolalia: mimicking movements or speech or another person.
17. Stereotypy: repetitive, non-goal-directed motor activity (e.g., repetitively tapping teeth).
18. Mannerisms: odd, purposeful movements: performing actions at inappropriate times (e.g., saluting), displaying an odd gait (e.g., tiptoeing), and/or exaggerated politeness (e.g., genuflecting to others).
19. Verbigeration: repetition of a word, phrases or sentences.
20. Rigidity: maintenance of an unusual rigid position (e.g., bent over from waist).
21. Negativism (uncooperative): resistance to instructions or attempts to move.
22. Waxy flexibility: individual offers initial resistance when being re-postured before allowing himself to be repositioned, like bending a wax candle (Bush-Francis Catatonia Rating Scale (BFCRS), 2025).
23. Withdrawal: refusal to eat, drink, or make eye contact.
24. Impulsivity: sudden inappropriate, random behavior (e.g., throwing food into air).
25. Automatic obedience: exaggerated cooperation with examiner's request or spontaneous continuation of movement requested (Bush-Francis Catatonia Rating Scale (BFCRS), 2025).
26. Mitgehen: raising of an extremity in response to light pressure. An extreme form of "mitmachen" in which very slight pressure leads to movement in any direction, also called the "anglepoise" effect or "anglepoise lamp sign." This movement occurs despite instructions to resist the pressure, as individuals with this condition often experience even slight pressure as forcible grasping and pushing (Glossary of Psychiatry, 2024).
27. Gegenhalten: resistance to passive movement, which is proportional to strength of the stimulus; it appears automatic rather than willful (Bush-Francis Catatonia Rating Scale (BFCRS), 2025).
28. Ambitendency: indecisive, hesitant movement. Individuals appear motorically "stuck" in indecisive, hesitant movement (Bush-Francis Catatonia Rating Scale (BFCRS), 2025).
29. Grasp reflex: neurological reflex. This is an involuntary grasping by an individual of anything that touches the palm (American Psychological Association, n.d.-i).
30. Perseveration: repeatedly returning to the same topic or movement.
31. Combativeness: striking out in an undirected manner, with no, or a superficial explanation afterwards (Bush-Francis Catatonia Rating Scale (BFCRS), 2025).
32. Decision-making: ambivalence (i.e., uncertainty and indecisiveness regarding a decision because of the coexistence of contradictory ideas, emotions, attitudes, and desires in an individual) (Shahrokh & Hales, 2003) or excessive self-will

(i.e., stubborn and uncompromising adherence to one's own desires and ideas) (Merriam-Webster Dictionary, n.d.).

33. Motor drive: lacking energy to move or urge to move; has difficulty initiating moving or unable to remain still for a duration of time.
34. Velocity: rate of movement (accelerated/decelerated).
35. Motion sequence: smooth uninterrupted motoric behaviors taking note of blockage, hesitancies, or parakinesia (i.e., awkwardness or clumsiness of movement (American Psychological Association, n.d.-m) and dyskinesia (i.e., involuntary or unintended movement, such as a tic or spasm. Denotes distorted or impaired voluntary movement (American Psychological Association, n.d.-f).

Problem behaviors displayed by people living with SMI are not one-dimensional experiences but rather involve a complex interplay of various aspects of the problem behaviors, which should be considered together for a comprehensive understanding and treatment approach. A multidimensional approach goes beyond just the behaviors listed in the DSM-5-TR (American Psychiatric Association, 2022) that are observed and that a person reports. By taking a multidimensional perspective, clinicians can develop more tailored treatment plans that address the various aspects contributing to a patient's mental health concerns. There is a need for interventions beyond psychiatric medications, given the impact that disorganized speech and motor behaviors have on outcomes and their persistence in some people living with SMI despite compliance with medication regimens.

Origins of Disorganization in Speech and Motor Behaviors

Disorganized speech and motor behaviors are typically associated with individuals living with SMI. The neural and cognitive/behavioral substrates collectively contribute to the cognitive and behavioral problems observed in people living with SMI.

Neuronal Substrates of Disorganization in Speech and Thought Processes

Disorganized thinking can only be accessed and observed through overt speech and motor behaviors; disorganized thinking or FTD is inferred from the observed dimensions of disorganized speech. The neural substrates of disorganized thinking are the substrates of overt and observable behavioral dimensions that compose the domains of speech and language.

Recent research has found that the problem behaviors of disorganization in speech involve dysfunction within the prefrontal cortex (PFC), particularly the dorsolateral prefrontal cortex (DLPFC), alongside abnormalities in connections between the PFC and other brain regions like the thalamus, hippocampus, and anterior cingulate cortex (ACC), leading to impaired executive function and difficulty with thought and speech organization (Krajcovic et al., 2019).

Key regions of the brain that are influential in the display of disorganized thinking and speech include:

- Prefrontal cortex (PFC): This region is crucial for cognitive control, goal selection, planning, response inhibition, performance monitoring, and working memory, all of which are disrupted in disorganized thinking and speech. Dysfunction in the PFC is linked to impairments in working memory and cognitive flexibility (Krajcovic et al., 2019; Viher et al., 2018).
- Dorsolateral prefrontal cortex (DLPFC): The DLPFC is implicated in higher-order cognitive functions like reasoning and decision-making, and its dysfunction is strongly linked to disorganized thought and speech processes. Neuroimaging findings show reduced activity in the DLPFC. Studies using fMRI often show decreased activation in the DLPFC during tasks requiring cognitive control in individuals experiencing disorganized thinking and speech (Krajcovic et al., 2019).
- Thalamus: This structure acts as a relay center for information across the brain, and abnormalities in its connections to the prefrontal cortex (PFC) can contribute to the display of problem behaviors. Studies using neuroimaging have also revealed disrupted functional connectivity between the PFC and other brain regions, indicating problems with information integration (Krajcovic et al., 2019).
- Hippocampus (HPC): Though primarily associated with memory, the hippocampus is also involved in spatial navigation and can play a role in the organization of thoughts, making its dysfunction relevant to disorganized thinking. The HPC is essential for representing contextual information and supporting flexible behavior. HPC-PFC interactions are crucial for adaptive behavior. Discoordination in the HPC-PFC circuitry is associated with cognitive and behavioral disorganization (Krajcovic et al., 2019; Viher et al., 2018).
- Anterior cingulate cortex (ACC): This region is involved in monitoring conflict in cognitions and error detection, which are crucial for maintaining coherent thought processes (Krajcovic et al., 2019).
- Superior temporal gyrus (STG): N-methyl-d-aspartate (NMDA) receptor activity within the STG is important for processing auditory information, including speech sounds, and contributes to the neural mechanisms underlying language comprehension. Alterations in NMDA receptor functions within the STG have been implicated in various conditions, including SMI, where individuals often exhibit difficulties in language comprehension and speech (Roche et al., 2015).

Some research suggests that disorganized thinking and speech may be associated with alterations in gamma brainwave activity, which is thought to be involved in neural communication (Krajcovic et al., 2019). GABAergic system abnormalities in GABAergic interneurons may contribute to the disorganization of neuronal activity as these interneurons are crucial for maintaining the balance of excitation and inhibition in neural circuits (Viher et al., 2018).

Disordered functional connectivity within and between large-scale brain networks affects cognitive functions and complex behaviors. Discoordination at the level of neuronal ensembles, where the precise timing of neuronal spikes is crucial for information processing, is observed in persons living with SMI. This discoordination can lead to cognitive impairment and behavioral disorganization.

The dimensions of disorganized speech that compose FTD are associated with structural and functional abnormalities in the left STG and middle temporal gyrus, angular gyrus, inferior operculum, and orbito-frontal cortex (OFC). Abnormalities in white matter (i.e., nerve fibers allowing different areas of the brain to communicate in language-related pathways) in these areas have been linked to linguistic deficits in individuals living with SMI, but the relationship between white matter and disorganized speech is not well understood (Viher et al., 2018). Results from MRI studies focusing on white matter microstructures link abnormalities of white matter in the left fronto-temporal language network to FTDs and disorganized speech (Kim et al., 2010). The fiber tracts associated with FTDs include the left uncinate fascicle, superior and inferior longitudinal fascicle, and the inferior fronto-occipital fascicle. The different dimensions of disorganized speech assessed by the BPS-R are related to differences in white matter microstructure values in language tracts indicating distinct neuronal substrates for the behavioral dimensions of disorganized speech (Viher et al., 2018).

Disorganized thinking and speech are likely due to a complex circuitry and interplay between multiple brain networks and not a dysfunction in a single brain region (Kim et al., 2010). However, the specific neural correlates of disorganized thinking and speech can vary depending on the individual, the dimensions of disorganized speech being displayed and the frequency and intensity of the occurrences of the problem behaviors.

While the underlying causes are not yet fully understood and may vary between individuals, the severity of disorganized speech as described by derailment, tangentiality incoherence, and distractible speech is associated with reduced gray matter in the superior temporal and inferior frontal cortices and abnormal activation in superior temporal cortex (Hitczenko et al., 2021). People living with SMI who produce fewer complex sentences showed weaker activation in the right temporal cortex and left PFC; FTD is associated with gray matter reductions in the orbital frontal cortex (OFC) and insular cortex. Lack of prosody and affective behaviors during speech and problems in emotional processing is associated with reduced activity in the amygdala, parahippocampal gyrus, as well as multiple regions of the left PFC (Hitczenko et al., 2021).

Neuronal Substrates of Disorganization in Motoric Behaviors

The neurobiology of motor behavior is well established, providing a basis for assessing brain networks related to SMI. Motor dysfunction is a critical physiological pathway in people living with SMI, involving basic motor processing and control. Aberrant motor functioning in schizophrenia has been noted since early clinical descriptions of SMI, including dyskinesia, psychomotor slowing, and catatonic behaviors (Ariza-Salamanca et al., 2022). Delayed motor development in childhood has been identified as a risk factor for the development of SMI, indicating a potential vulnerability marker. Estimates of motor dysregulation range from 50% to 65% in people living with SMI (Abboud et al., 2017).

Key brain regions associated with both higher-order and basic motor functions include the dorsal anterior cingulate cortex (dACC), basal ganglia, and cerebellum. Motor problems displayed in SMI can be categorized into neurological soft signs, abnormal involuntary movements, and catatonia. The observed motor dysregulation in the motor system affects structure, function, and connectivity of brain regions (Abboud et al., 2017).

Individuals living with SMI exhibit hyper-activation in the premotor cortex (PMC) during finger sequence learning, indicating impaired motor control efficiency, but hypo-activation of motor cortices is observed in non-learning tasks, suggesting task-specific dysfunctions. Structural MRI studies show reduced size of the pre-supplementary motor cortex (pre-SMA). The pre-SMA holds a cognitive or abstract role in the performance of complex tasks, preparation for movement, motor selection, acquisition of new motor skills, and higher-order aspects of speech; dysfunction in this area correlates with impaired motor sequencing. Decreased volume in the dACC is linked to executive dysfunction and precedes the onset of behaviors associated with SMI. There are noted structural deviations in cerebellar structure (i.e., decreased Purkinje cell size) and connectivity that contribute to motor dysfunction (Abboud et al., 2017).

Impaired coordination between motor regions and altered neurotransmitter systems is critical in understanding motor dysfunction in SMI especially since Parkinsonian motor dysregulation is linked to deficits in dopamine in the neural circuits. The dopamine hypothesis posits a causal connection between dopamine overproduction or receptor overstimulation and the development of behaviors associated with SMI. Increased presynaptic dopamine synthesis and storage were found in the striatum, and excessive dopamine (D2) receptor stimulation correlates with the severity of behaviors in SMI (Abboud et al., 2017). Studies indicate increased levels of dopamine metabolites with periodic catatonia, suggesting dopaminergic excess (Mohandas & Rajmohan, 2008). Antipsychotic medications reduce dopamine receptor density in the striatum, impacting motor control, as evidenced by slower finger-tapping speeds (Abboud et al., 2017).

The motor system in persons living with SMI and displaying motor dysregulation is subject to neurobiological alterations as shown with various imaging techniques including diffusion tensor imaging, functional magnetic resonance imaging (fMRI), structural MRI, and perfusion MRI (Bracht et al., 2012). However, the pathobiology of motor symptoms is still poorly understood, and findings have been inconsistent. This may be an effect of the current concepts that cover a wide range of behavioral dimensions, clinical course, and outcomes. Most of the previous studies investigated people living with SMI who display a wide range of disorganized motoric behaviors. This limits the comparability of results and may contribute to inconsistent findings. Identifying individuals living with SMI with specific behavioral dimensions might enable the investigation of significant behavior problems displayed in SMI and their underlying neuronal substrates (Bracht et al., 2012).

Neuropsychological studies indicate that people displaying catatonic and disorganized motor behaviors perform poorly on visual-object-space and perception tests, particularly related to the function of the right parietal lobe. Dysfunction in the right inferior parietal cortex is proposed to underlie the catatonic behavior of posturing. Movement-related cortical potentials show that while initiation of movements is normal in individuals displaying catatonic behaviors, the termination of movements is significantly delayed (Mohandas & Rajmohan, 2008).

Structural imaging reveals cortical enlargement in the left frontoparietal area of individuals displaying catatonic behaviors, with hypoperfusion in the right parietal cortex correlating with impaired visuospatial abilities as seen in neuropsychological studies. fMRIs show decreases in the activation of the right lateral orbitofrontal area during working memory tasks, indicating deficits in spatial movement monitoring and abnormal orbitofrontal connectivity with motor areas, potentially explaining symptoms like mutism and stupor observed in catatonic behaviors (Mohandas & Rajmohan, 2008). Overall, these findings highlight significant neuroanatomical and functional substrates that are correlated with the display of catatonic and disorganized motor behaviors (Mohandas & Rajmohan, 2008).

Lorazepam and other benzodiazepines effectively alleviate the occurrence of catatonic behaviors, highlighting the role of GABA receptors, which show significantly lower binding in specific brain areas (Mohandas & Rajmohan, 2008; Rajagopal, 2007). A "top-down modulation" of the basal ganglia due to deficiency of cortical GABA, the primary inhibitory neurotransmitter of the brain, may explain the catatonic motor behaviors. This explanation might account for the dramatic therapeutic effect of benzodiazepines, which cause an increase in GABA activity (Rajagopal, 2007). Similarly, hyperactivity of glutamate, the primary excitatory neurotransmitter, has also been suggested as an underlying neurochemical dysfunction (Rajagopal, 2007). Catatonia may improve with NMDA glutamate antagonists like amantadine and memantine, indicating a secondary involvement of the glutamatergic system. The findings suggest that the interaction of multiple neurotransmitters and neural systems contributes to the development of catatonic and disorganized motor behaviors (Mohandas & Rajmohan, 2008).

Psychological and Behavioral Substrates of Disorganized Speech and Motoric Behaviors

Neurocognitive impairments on neuropsychological performance measures have been shown in different domains in people living with SMI; impairments have repeatedly been shown with significant differences in the cognitive domains of attention and memory in people living with SMI from persons not having any serious mental health problems (De la Torre et al., 2021). People living with SMI have typically performed around one standard deviation below the level of controls in specific cognitive domains. Seven cognitive domains affected in SMI are: (a) processing speed; (b) attention; (c) working memory; (d) verbal learning and memory; (e) visual learning and memory; (f) reasoning; and (g) social cognition (McCutcheon et al., 2023). Further dimensionality reduction suggests that these domains be grouped into larger parent domains of (1) processing speed, (2) attention/working memory, and (3) learning (McCutcheon et al., 2023).

Disorganized Speech

There are similarities between disorganized speech displayed by people living with SMI and developmental language disorder (DLD) in children (National Institute on Deafness and Other Communication Disorders [NIDCD], 2023). Behaviors associated with DLD include the following: limited use of complex sentences and phrases, problems in finding the right words, difficulty understanding figurative language and abstract concepts, disorganized narratives, frequent grammatical and syntactical errors, and reading problems (NIDCD, 2023). DSM-5-TR (American Psychiatric Association, 2022) states that language disorders are highly heritable, and family members are more likely to have a history of language impairment.

Although genetics may be involved, there is also an environmental component as a child will role model and repeat what is heard from others in his daily environment, including errors in speech. The developing speaker will receive naturally occurring consequences from others for what they say (e.g., receiving what is requested, smiles). "Verbal behavior" is a type of behavior that is reinforced through the actions of another person, meaning language is learned and maintained through social interaction where responses are reinforced by others. Verbal behavior is a social act where the meaning of a word is derived from its function in a given situation, with different types of verbal behaviors categorized as "verbal operants" based on the stimuli that control them, such as "mands" (requests), "tacts" (labels), "intraverbals" (responses to questions), and "echoics" (repeating heard words) (Sundberg, 2020). It is logical inference that if correct speech is learned, then incorrect verbal behaviors—including disorganized speech—can likewise have a learning component.

Processing speed is often the most affected domain with individuals living with SMI typically performing around one standard deviation below the level of individuals with no mental health problems. Deficits in processing speed are the strongest predictor of general cognitive performance in individuals living with SMI. Because processing speed is a component of many other cognitive functions, deficits in this domain may reflect impairments in other higher-order functions (McCutcheon et al., 2023). For example, people living with SMI may approach processing speed tests with less strategic planning. Impairments in lower-level domains such as reaction time could contribute detrimentally to the scores in higher-order domains such as memory, learning, and cognitive flexibility (McCutcheon et al., 2023).

Clinically rated formal thought disorder (FTD) in people living with SMI is linked to semantic processing deficits, with over 40% variance explained by specific tests (Myers et al., 2024). Dougherty and Goldberg et al. (1998) postulated that disorganized speech displayed by people living with SMI is more highly related to speech disorders measured as communication failures than speech disorders as the presence of FTD and disorganization. Dougherty (2009) tested samples of people living with SMI and living without any mental health problem for sustained attention, sequencing, and conceptual sequencing ability. Speech was also rated for communication failures, thought disorder, and conceptual disorganization. Attention and sequencing impairments explained a substantial percentage of the variance in the communication measure of speech disorder but little of the variance in FTD or conceptual disorganization. The conclusion was that impairments in attention and sequencing abilities contribute substantially to the impaired communication in people living with SMI. It is important to consider lower-level cognitive "third variables" when examining higher-level cognitive components of speech disorder (Dougherty, 2009) such as attention, memory, executive functioning (planning, problem-solving), reasoning, language comprehension, pragmatics (social communication skills), and self-awareness of communication difficulties.

Goldberg et al. (1998) assessed individuals living with SMI using the Peabody Picture Vocabulary Test (PPVT). The scores correlated with illogicalities in speech, suggesting a lack of semantic knowledge that contributes to inferring formal thought disorder (FTD). Significant differences in verbal fluency scores were observed, indicating difficulties in accessing semantic items among patients with moderate to severe FTD. Performance on semantic tests predicted positive thought disorder but not negative thought disorder, indicating different underlying mechanisms. A semantic priming task (American Psychological Association, n.d.-o) in which meaningfully related stimuli are presented during processing revealed that individuals living with SMI showed a lack of priming for closely related words, indicating aberrant semantic activation. The findings from the study suggested that FTD may be linked to a fundamental misunderstanding of semantics, affecting both language and behavior (Goldberg et al., 1998).

Impairments in semantic memory and working memory or executive functions have been shown to predict clinical language disturbances. This has led to the hypothesis that language dysfunction in people living with SMI can be explained by dual deficits in these systems (Kuperberg, 2010). Semantic memory dysfunction may result in disorganized speech from impairments in the structure and function of semantic memory. Semantic memory refers to a type of long-term memory that involves the storage and retrieval of general knowledge about the world, including concepts, facts, and meanings of words. It is distinct from episodic memory, which involves the recollection of personal experiences and specific events. Semantic memory allows individuals to understand language, recognize objects, and comprehend abstract concepts without needing to recall the specific context in which the information was learned. Dysfunction in semantic memory suggests that individuals living with SMI experience a more rapid and widespread automatic activation within semantic memory. This phenomenon contributes to the loosening of associations observed in disorganized speech, where a sequence of semantically related words is used without forming a coherent narrative (Kuperberg, 2010).

Context impairments attribute language dysfunction to difficulties in building up and using context, often linked to poor working memory (WMem) or general executive function deficits. WMem is the neurocognitive ability to hold and manipulate information over short periods. General executive functions are a set of cognitive processes that are essential for controlling and managing cognitive abilities and behaviors. These functions are crucial for goal-directed behavior and include:

- Cognitive flexibility: the capacity to switch between thinking about different concepts or to adapt behavior to new, changing, or unexpected events.
- Inhibitory control: the ability to suppress automatic, impulsive responses in favor of more appropriate actions.
- Planning and organization: the ability to create and maintain a plan to achieve a goal.
- Problem-solving: the ability to identify solutions to complex or novel situations.
- Self-monitoring: the ability to track and assess one's own performance and behavior.

These functions are often associated with the prefrontal cortex (PFC) of the brain and are critical for tasks that require attention, decision-making, and the regulation of emotions and actions. The data suggested that people living with SMI have trouble maintaining and manipulating contextual information, which affects their ability to produce coherent speech. Both theories are supported by studies showing correlations between clinical language measures, such as the severity of FTD, and individuals' performances on tasks probing semantic memory, WMem, and executive processes (Kuperberg, 2010).

Two cognitive anomalies are considered central mechanisms of the observed disorganization in speech in people living with SMI: impairments in the ability to integrate contextual information and impairments in the Theory of Mind (ToM) (Hardy-Baylé et al., 2003).

ToM refers to the ability to understand and infer the mental states of others, including their intentions, beliefs, desires, and emotions. It involves recognizing that others have thoughts, feelings, beliefs, and knowledge that are different from one's own and using this understanding to predict and interpret behaviors of oneself and others during verbal and nonverbal social interactions. These covert cognitive capabilities are crucial for effective social interactions and communication, as it enables individuals to empathize with others, understand social cues, and navigate complex social situations. Social cognition includes recognizing and interpreting facial expressions, body language, and vocal tones. ToM uses this information to infer what others might be thinking or feeling. It enables a person to understand another person's perspective and recognizing emotional states are essential for empathetic interactions (Cotter et al., 2017).

Impairments in Theory of Mind (ToM) lead to challenges in social cognition and interactions. Social cognitive impairments are common across a wide range of mental health, neurological, and developmental conditions. These deficits are significant and consistent across almost all clinical groups examined (Cotter et al., 2017). The severity/magnitude of social cognitive deficits is broadly like other cognitive impairments such as memory, processing speed, and executive functions. In specific conditions, the deficits in facial emotion recognition and ToM are comparable in magnitude to other neurocognitive impairments. Individuals living with SMI present with wide variation in the severity of impairments, potentially due to variability in the identification, operational definition, and assessments of the dimensions of the mental health problems being studied (Cotter et al., 2017).

Despite their importance, social cognitive assessments are not widely used in clinical practice. There is a need to integrate these measures into large-scale, longitudinal studies to better understand their potential as predictors of clinical and functional outcomes and to develop effective interventions in people living with SMI.

Experimental evidence supports the link between these cognitive deficits and disorganization (Hardy-Baylé et al., 2003). Lexical decision-making tasks have been used to assess the integration of contextual information in individuals living with SMI (Hardy-Baylé et al., 2003). In lexical decision-making tasks, the participant is presented with strings of letters and is required to determine whether each string spells a word. The reaction time required to make the decision is usually measured (American Psychological Association, n.d.-n). Studies using lexical decision tasks show deficits in integration of contextual information in people living with SMI who display disorganized speech (Hardy-Baylé et al., 2003).

Neurocognitive impairments demonstrated by people living with SMI affect abilities like processing speed, executive functioning, and social cognitive functioning. Neurocognition is often impaired in people living with SMI and is linked to both disorganized behaviors and metacognition (Myers et al., 2024). Social cognitive functioning involves metacognitive impairments that range from recognizing specific thoughts and feelings to integrating complex representations of oneself and others. Adequate neurocognition is necessary but not sufficient for effective social cognition and metacognition (Minor et al., 2015). Disorganized behaviors displayed by people living with SMI are more strongly related to cognitive processes than reality distortions or negative symptoms/diminution of socially accepted behaviors (Ventura et al., 2013). Conceptual disorganization weakens the connections between neurocognitive abilities and social/metacognitive tasks (Minor et al., 2015). In a meta-analysis of metacognition and disorganized verbal behaviors, Myers et al. (2024) reported a large negative relationship between metacognitive capacity and disorganized symptoms.

Assessing conceptual disorganization, neurocognition, social cognition, and metacognition, Minor et al. (2015) studied the severity level of conceptual disorganization that disrupts the influence of neurocognition on social cognition and metacognition. Conceptual disorganization was found to be significantly associated with social cognition but not with neurocognition or metacognition and did not moderate the relationship between neurocognition and social cognition. No disorganized behavioral domain significantly influenced the link between neurocognition and social cognition. The effect of neurocognitive abilities on metacognition was no longer present when conceptual disorganization was minimal or mild. The results indicated that the severity of conceptual disorganization changes how cognitive processes relate to each other. This study also implied that addressing conceptual disorganization may help strengthen the link between neurocognitive and metacognitive difficulties in individuals living with SMI.

Correlates for neurocognitive, neural, and functional speech impairments have been found for the occurrence of disorganized speech. Nevertheless, disorganized speech is an operant behavior and operates under the principles of behaviors. Disorganized speech does not randomly occur; it is under the influence of a learning history of the individual, environmental stimuli, antecedent conditions (e.g., MOs, EOs, S^D, S^{delta}), and consequences. Bettis et al. (2024) explored conversational themes that preceded disorganized speech in persons living with SMI, highlighting alienation, interpersonal tension, personal benchmarks, and adverse experiences. Themes of alienation were a significant theme, showing more frequent occurrences preceding disorganized speech. Interpersonal tension and personal benchmarks were also key themes, indicating that social dynamics and self-assessment can trigger disorganized speech. Adverse experiences, such as past hardships and grief, were found to lead to disorganized speech, supporting the idea of disorganization as a possible "coping" mechanism (Bettis et al., 2024) as it may decrease the adverse respondents associated with traumatic content in speech by "diverting" from the distressing topic.

Using an ABA approach, future studies could explore the function of disorganized speech. Disorganized speech could be negatively reinforced as social interaction is terminated when the person engages in disorganized speech and the distressful emotions associated with the themes associated with the social interaction are likewise terminated; that is, the display of disorganized speech results if the escape by the individual from an adverse situation. Interventions should focus on building awareness of alienation triggers, especially in people engaging in disorganized behaviors (Bettis et al., 2024).

Disorganized Motoric and Catatonic Behaviors

Correlations for neurocognitive and neural impairments have been documented for the occurrence of disorganized motoric behaviors, but no common pathway has been delineated. One possible explanation is that multiple pathways and substrates are involved with specific dimensions of disorganized motoric behaviors. Nevertheless, disorganized motoric behaviors do not occur randomly as they are operant behaviors that are affected by the principles of behaviors and influenced by environmental events.

Persistent fear is a significant psychological factor in catatonia, influencing behaviors and mental states of affected individuals. Fink and Shorter (2017) reviewed historical description and explanation of disorganized and catatonic behaviors. The review found that people who show disorganized movements or catatonic behaviors often experience ongoing fears and anxieties. The authors questioned whether, during catatonia, individuals are simply in a "stupor" with reduced responsiveness (Shahrockh & Hales, 2003), or if they are actively focused on negative emotions and responses (Fink & Shorter, 2017).

Signs of disorganized motoric and catatonic behaviors may be adaptations to persistent fear, like tonic immobilizations that are seen in other mammalian species (Fink & Shorter, 2017). Tonic immobility is a temporary state of motor inhibition believed to be a response to situations involving extreme fear. In humans, it is believed to occur during sexual assault, and there have been reports of fear-induced freezing in the contexts of combat and other traumatic disasters (Abrams et al., 2009). Significant positive correlations were found between responses to a questionnaire about tonic immobility and measures of posttraumatic symptoms, dissociation, anxiety sensitivity, and preoccupied by cognitions and emotions associated with the traumatic experiences. Tonic immobility may represent an extreme behavioral expression of trauma-induced behavioral disconnection from emotions and thoughts (i.e., subvocal speech) associated with the trauma, providing immediate but temporary relief from aversive emotional respondents such as fear and anxiety (Abrams et al., 2009).

Not engaging in goal-directed behaviors could be a response to avoid adverse consequences. Research has shown that response-punisher associations result in little autonomic disturbances and are more typically associated with abortive responses (e.g., terminating response early) (Jean-Richard-Dit-Bressel et al., 2018). The inclusion of an unpunished behavior in an experimental decision task results in the suppression of responding in the unpunished situation and correlates strongly with expression of defensive behaviors such as "freezing" and reflects Pavlovian fear conditioning (Jean-Richard-Dit-Bressel et al., 2018)—basically uncertainty of a possible adverse consequence results in tonic immobility and other behaviors associated with response suppression. Further research and more well-defined operational definition of the dimensions of disorganized motor and catatonic behaviors are needed.

Epidemiological Considerations

Disorganized Speech

The DSM-5-TR (American Psychiatric Association, 2022) describes disorganized behaviors that are displayed by persons living with SMI as composed of disorganized thinking, speech, and motor behavior that are multidimensional. Disorganized thinking is described in the mental health literature as jumbled or incoherent speech that is difficult to follow because of switching topics and responding with an unrelated topic while speaking. Incoherence, use of unrecognizable words (e.g., word salad), illogical inferences, violation of rules of grammar and syntax, and repetition of phrases and sentences, constitute disorganized speech; odd facial expressions, repetition of movements, unusual postures, random and unpredictable behaviors not related to context, extremes of smoothness and speed of movement, constitute disorganized motor behavior. Disorganized behaviors can make it difficult to communicate, perform daily tasks, and function in social relationships. Given that thought processes can only be accessed and assessed by verbal behaviors (e.g., speaking), formal thought disorder (FTD) is inferred from the result of observations by a service provider of the facets of the speech and motoric behaviors by an individual living with SMI.

As assessed by the Thought, Language, and Communication scale (TLC) (Andreasen, 1986), FTD is characterized by 18 different behavioral problems in speech rate and organization, reflecting a cluster of cognitive, linguistic, and affective disturbances (Roche et al., 2015). The prevalence of FTD (and disorganized speech and motoric behaviors) is estimated to range between 50.39% and 72.7% of people living with SMI with differences in presentation between early onset and late-onset mental health problems; the dimensions of FTD and disorganized speech and motoric behaviors are more severe and deleterious in persons with early onset SMI. The prevalence of FTD and the associated disorganized problem behavioral domains varies with age, being more common in early onset schizophrenia spectrum mental health problems (27.4%) compared to late-onset (10.4%) (Roche et al., 2015). Longitudinal studies show that FTD and the associated problem behaviors persist or worsen over time (Roche et al., 2015). Co-occurring substance use is associated with more severe FTD. FTD negatively impacts social functioning, with verbal underproductivity predicting poor social skills and disconnected speech affecting social behavior. FTD and related disorganized problem behaviors predict longer hospital stays and less awareness of problem behaviors.

Not all individuals living with SMI exhibit these problems in speech and language production; one study found that 32% of individuals with no known mental health problems exhibited "tangentiality" in 50 min of speech vs 50–60% of people living with SMI (Hirjak et al., 2024).

Disorganized Motoric and Catatonic Behaviors

Problematic motor functions and disorganization displayed by individuals living with SMI have been one of the characterizations of problematic behaviors in people living with SMI. These motoric problems can be categorized into neurological soft signs, abnormal involuntary movements, and catatonic behaviors. People living with SMI who display problematic motor functions and disorganization experience less favorable outcomes and more severe side effects from antipsychotic medications, whereas neurological soft signs predict elevations in problematic behaviors associated with diminution in functional capabilities (e.g., negative symptoms), highlighting the importance of motor function in recovery outcomes. There appears to be a connection between motor functions and cognitive processes (Abboud et al., 2017), suggesting that thinking is an active motor process, supporting the behavioral definition of thinking as subvocal speech.

Disorganized motoric behaviors are likewise multidimensional and transdiagnostic. An aspect of disorganized motoric behaviors is catatonic behaviors that were first described in 1874 by Kahlbaum as a "brain disorder" and later associated with schizophrenia spectrum mental health problems by Kraepelin (Dhossche et al., 2016). Prevalence of catatonic behaviors in acute psychiatric inpatients ranges from 7% to 17%, with most cases linked to mood-related mental health problems. Approximately 10–25% of people living with SMI exhibit disorganized motoric behaviors that at times meet the criteria for catatonia according to diagnostic criteria in the DSM-5 (American Psychiatric Association, 2013). Studies show, however, that this can be an underreporting of disorganized motoric behaviors. It was postulated that nonspecific sociocultural changes and historical classification decisions may have contributed to the under-recognition and decreased interest in catatonia and related disorganized motoric behaviors in the mental health field (Dhossche et al., 2016). The prevalence of catatonic-related disorganized behaviors was reported to be between 19.5% and 50% in the early 1900s; however, this rate has substantially declined following the introduction of psychotropic medications. For instance, in two Polish hospitals where catatonia diagnoses were approached conservatively, the incidence decreased by a factor of 190 from 1929 to 1999 and by a factor of 36 from 1963 to 1999 (Ungvari et al., 2023).

By the mid-1900s, mental health service providers believed catatonia was disappearing; this was supported by some epidemiological studies reporting a decline in prevalence from 6% to less than 1% in London in 1950 (Ungvari et al., 2023). The development and subsequent use of operationalized behavior rating scales for disorganized behaviors—including catatonia—revealed more disorganized motoric behaviors displayed by individuals living with SMI than was recognized previously (Ungvari et al., 2023). Recent studies show an average of 10% of individuals presenting with acute SMI display catatonic behaviors. However, present-day mental health practices may overlook catatonia-related disorganized behaviors due to the brief interactions during assessment that occur with individuals living with SMI leading to inaccuracies in prevalence. In addition, antipsychotic medication-induced motoric behaviors may obscure disorganized motoric behaviors that is an aspect of living with SMI (Ungvari et al., 2023). The rate of prevalence of disorganized motoric behaviors and catatonic behaviors has ranged from 0.7% to 31.1%; many studies have reported the rate to be in the range of 5 to 10% (Sarkar et al., 2016). The use of different behavioral assessments of disorganized motoric and catatonic-like behaviors results in varying rates of frequency (Sarkar et al., 2016) as the number and type of behavioral dimensions vary on each scale.

These problematic motor functions and disorganization can include Parkinsonian syndrome (i.e., a group of disorders that share similar symptoms to Parkinson's disease), including abnormal involuntary movements (dyskinesia), psychomotor slowing, problems with coordination and sensory-motor tasks (neurological soft signs (NSS)), and catatonia (i.e., rigid posturing, grimacing, and mannerisms). Studies indicate that problematic motor functions in individuals living with SMI begin in childhood with delayed motor development. These deficits tend to aggregate in families of people living with SMI, suggesting that problematic motor development in childhood is a risk factor to develop SMI in adulthood (Abboud et al., 2017).

Estimates suggest that problematic motor functions and disorganization are present in 50–65% of individuals living with SMI, compared to about 5% in people with no mental health problem (Abboud et al., 2017). The prevalence of catatonia in people living with SMI recently admitted to psychiatric inpatient facilities ranges from 7% to 17%, with most cases linked to mood disorders (Dhossche et al., 2016). Studies show that catatonic like behaviors in person living with schizophrenia spectrum and bipolar mental health problems are under-recognized with a significant percentage of individuals living with persistent schizophrenia spectrum mental health problems exhibiting more frequent catatonic related behaviors (Dhossche et al., 2016). Catatonic behaviors affect 5–18% of individuals living with SMI who are hospitalized in a psychiatric facility and 3.3% of medical inpatients; catatonia often goes unrecognized, leading to serious complications for the person displaying the behaviors. Studies show a low global incidence of catatonia at about 10 per 100,000 person-years, with varying prevalence across different physical and mental health conditions (Hirjak et al., 2024).

Among people living with mental health problems, the prevalence of catatonia varies widely with 9% of inpatients and outpatients exhibiting catatonic signs. Among individuals living with different mental health problems, catatonic behaviors occur in 71% of people living with mood-related mental health problems, 67% of people living with schizophrenia spectrum mental health problems, and 46% among those with general medical illnesses (Hirjak et al., 2024). Catatonic behaviors were present in 26% of individuals with delirium. In older adults, the prevalence of catatonic behaviors in psychiatric units ranges from 6.2% to 39.6%, depending on the criteria used. Catatonic and disorganized motor behaviors occur across mental health problems and are associated with various medical conditions, including autoimmune encephalitis, systemic lupus erythematosus, thyroid disease, epilepsy, and drug intoxications or withdrawals (Hirjak et al., 2024). The prevalence also differed based on the treatment setting, with the highest prevalence in nonpsychiatric outpatient or inpatient services (15.8%) and the lowest in psychiatric outpatient services (3.2%). Additionally, the prevalence was higher in the presence of medical or neurological illness with no comorbid psychiatric condition (20.6%) and lower in mixed psychiatric samples (5.7%) (Solmi et al., 2018). Catatonia can occur throughout the entire lifespan, including in children, adolescents, and older adults, and affects both genders equally.

Cultural Considerations

Reports show a significant variability in prevalence of reported disorganized motoric behaviors across cultures, ranging from 1% in Nigeria, 3.7% in Mexico, 38% in Greece, 50% in Belgium, and 68% in the United States (Ungvari et al., 2023). Multiple studies conducted in India have investigated the phenomenology and prevalence of disorganized motoric behaviors and catatonia among recently admitted patients to mental health units, reporting rates ranging from 4.8% to 37.2% (Chalasani et al., 2005).

Chalasani et al. (2005) compared the prevalence of disorganized motoric behaviors of recently admitted individuals to mental health units in both India and Wales. The frequency of disorganized motoric behaviors as assessed by a standardized behavior rating scale was 13.5% in India and 9.6% in Wales. The difference in frequency and severity was not statistically significant. However, the type of behaviors exhibited were significantly different on the assessment scale with items related to a slowing down of thought processes and physical movements (e.g., posturing, catalepsy, staring, and stupor) more commonly displayed in India (12.5%) than by individuals in Wales; frequency of items describing excitability, impulsivity, hyperkinesis, pacing and aggressive behaviors were equally common in the samples from both countries.

The prevalence of catatonic behaviors varies significantly by country and study, thereby indicating a wide range of prevalence rates, reflecting differences in practices in identification, awareness, and possibly socio-cultural factors (Chalasani et al., 2005). Cross-cultural differences in the prevalence of catatonia have been observed. A systematic review by Solmi et al. (2018) found that more than half of the 74 studies included a European population. The highest prevalence was observed in Uganda (48.5%) and the lowest in Mexico (1.9%). Zingela et al. (2022) reported a prevalence of 47.7% among the South African population. It is of interest to note that using the criteria for catatonia in the DSM-5 identified only 6.6% of the cases that were identified by using the Bush-Francis Catatonia Rating Scale (BFCRS), and that the "missed cases" still required treatment for catatonic and disorganized motor behaviors (Zingela et al., 2022).

These differences highlight the variability in assessment tools and the heterogeneity in behaviors and criteria across different regions and populations, emphasizing the need for further studies using consistent operationally defined behaviors of the dimensions of the phenomenon to understand the epidemiology of catatonic and motor disorganization displayed by individuals living with SMI.

Types of Disorganized Behaviors

Disorganized Speech and Language

Hitczenko et al. (2021) have identified three main types of disturbances of speech and language in people living with SMI: (1) disorganized speech (inferred positive thought disorder), (2) poverty of speech (inferred negative thought disorder), and (3) speech and conversation (e.g., flat affect, aspects of voice, pausing).

1. Disorganized speech I (DS-I): The involved dimensions are semantic and working memory (WMem), atypical semantic associations between words, attention, and other executive functions, possibly resulting in impairments to incorporate linguistic context. These facets have been found to correlate with other positive symptoms and problem behaviors displayed in SMI, primarily delusions (Hitczenko et al., 2021). It is associated with impairments in lexicosemantic retrieval as well as WMem impairments.
2. Disorganized speech II (DS-II): The dimensions involved are atypical use of referential markers and illogicality. It is associated with similar impairments found in DS-I.
3. Negative thought disorder (NTD): (Poverty of speech/content and reduced syntactic complexity): This type of disorganized speech appears related to NTD (Nickl-Jockschat et al., 2023), which is associated with the dimensions of reduced amounts of speech production and content, slowing and paucity of speech and thought (by inference), concrete thinking (an inability to think abstractly), and an over-literal interpretation of proverbs (Hitczenko et al., 2021). This type of disorganized language and speech correlates with other negative symptoms and is a "negative symptom" (i.e., alogia which is a lack of spontaneity and content in speech and diminished flow of conversation (Shahrockh & Hales, 2023)). It is commonly predictive of early onset of living with a SMI. It is prognostic of future outcomes and social role functioning. NTD occurs more persistently in people living with SMI than DS-I (Hitczenko et al., 2021).

Additionally, DS-I, DS-II, and NTD need not co-occur in individuals living with SMI. Studies investigating the co-occurrences of these types of disorganizations of speech and thought have found weak and sometimes inverse correlations. As a result, the authors suggest that these abnormalities should be approached dimensionally rather than as a discrete variable (categorically present or absent) (Hitczenko et al., 2021).

4. Speech and conversation: The dimensions involved in this type of speech disorganization involve "flat affect" and pausing and not abiding by turn taking during conversations. "Flat affect"—total or near absence of appropriate emotional responses to situations and events (American Psychological Association, n.d.-g)—predicts the course and outcome of the illness and is associated with worse

quality of life and poorer social functioning. Flat affect has been shown to correlate with other negative symptoms, including NTD. (Hitczenko et al., 2021).
5. Lexical abnormalities: The dimension of disorganized speech involved in this type is differences in use of part of speech and use of neologisms and word approximations (Hitczenko et al., 2021).

Hitczenko et al. (2021) have differentiated some of the dimensions of disorganized speech and language that are displayed in individuals living with SMI into 5 broad categories. Below are the descriptions of the dimension of disorganized speech and examples of the observed dimension during problematic language and speech production.

1. Disorganized Speech-I (DS-I) (Hitczenko et al., 2021, p. 346):

   - Derailment: progressively moving off-topic.

     Example: "I always liked geography… There are also blue and grey eyes and other sorts, too…"

   - Tangentiality: providing oblique or irrelevant answers.

     Example: Q: "What city are you from?" A: "Well that's a hard question to answer…"

   - Incoherence: essentially incomprehensible speech.

     Example: "They're destroying too many cattle and oil just to make soap…"

   - Distractible speech: abrupt topic shifts.

     Example: "Then I left San Francisco and moved to… where did you get that tie?"
2. Disorganized Speech-II (DS-II) (Hitczenko et al., 2021):

   - Abnormal use of referential markers: ambiguous references.

     Example: "They let him go, so why not me?"

   - Illogicality: nonlogical conclusions.

     Example: "Parents are the people that raise you. Anything that raises you can be a parent. Parents can be anything, material, vegetable or mineral that has taught you something."
3. Poverty of speech and speech content (Hitczenko et al., 2021):

   - Poverty of speech content: non-substantive, vague speech.

     Example: "… I happen to be quite pleased with who I am or how I am and many of the problems I have and have been working on are difficult for me to handle or to work on because I am not aware of them as problems which upset me personally."

4. Poverty of speech:

   - Minimal responses.

   Example: Q: "Do you think there's a lot of corruption in the government?" A: "Yeah, seem to be."

   - Reduced syntactic complexity: higher percentage of simple sentences.

   Example: "I jumped at the sound of his voice." Complex sentences and clauses are used less frequently.
5. Lexical abnormalities: differences in use of speech.

   - Decreased use of adjectives, possessive pronouns (e.g., his, her, mine), and determiners (that, what).
   - Neologisms (new words); increased approximation use and creating new words or using unusual terms.

   Example: "I got so angry I picked up a dish and threw it at the geshinker."
6. Flat affect and pausing:

   - Flat affect: monotonous, emotionless speech.

   Example: speech that is monotonous, emotionless, slow, and lacking in prosody (i.e., rhythm, stress, pitch, inflection, and tone of voice)

   - Abnormal turn-taking: more frequent and/or longer pauses, interrupting, especially when turn-taking.

The observable dimensions of disorganized speech and by inference thought processes can be categorized into other broad categories based on the excess or distortion of average functions (such as hallucinations and delusions) and the diminution or loss of normal functions, such as reduced emotional expression and lack of motivation; these are termed positive and negative symptoms, respectively. Disorganized speech falls under the positive symptoms category and is specifically assessed under the "Conceptual Disorganization" item if disorganized speech and language are assessed using the PANSS (Kay et al., 1987). However, operationally behavioral definitions of the dimensions in the assessment of problematic behaviors would result in more precise descriptions and understanding of the phenomena as behaviorally defined problems have been undervalued in accuracy in mental health, as shown in studies comparing different assessment methods (Ungvari et al., 2023).

Disorganized Motoric and Catatonic Behaviors

Two subtypes of disorganized and catatonic behaviors have been described: retarded and excited. Behaviors correlated with the retarded type are associated with behaviors reflecting a paucity of movement, including immobility, staring, mutism, rigidity, withdrawal, and refusal to eat, along with more bizarre features such as posturing, grimacing, negativism, waxy flexibility, echolalia or echopraxia, stereotypy, verbigeration, and automatic obedience. The excited type is characterized by severe psychomotor agitation and excesses of purposeless motoric behaviors, potentially leading to life-threatening autonomic dysfunction. This so-called "malignant" or "lethal" catatonia can be fatal if not appropriately treated (Rassmussen et al., 2016).

Walther et al. (2019) categorize the dimensions of disorganized and catatonic behaviors rated by the items on the Bush-Francis Catatonia Rating Scale (BFCRS) into three main types of psychomotor activity: increased, abnormal, and decreased. The types and the behaviors in each type are listed below:

- Increased psychomotor activity: agitation/excitement (combined item), impulsivity, and combativeness.
- Abnormal psychomotor activity: grimacing, stereotypy, mannerism, posturing, perseveration, echolalia, echopraxia, verbigeration, automatic obedience, waxy flexibility, catalepsy, rigidity, *gegenhalten*, and *mitgehen*.
- Decreased psychomotor activity: stupor, ambitendency, staring, negativism, mutism, withdrawal, and grasp reflex.

Additionally, autonomic abnormality (e.g., tachycardia, hypertension, fever) is noted but is not categorized under psychomotor activity.

Subramaniyam et al. (2020) assessed a random sample of 300 individuals who were admitted to a psychiatric inpatient facility using the BFCRS (Bush et al., 1996). Cluster analysis followed by discriminant analysis was conducted; three subtypes were found and labeled retarded, excited and "aberrant volitional." The aberrant volitional dimension comprises behaviors that need to be elicited rather than passively observed. Using a qualitative thematic review of operationally defined behaviors of the items of the BFCRS (2025), many of the "aberrant volitional" behaviors in the study by Walther et al. (2019) corresponded to items that were assessed and found by interview or physical exam as the behaviors in this subtype need to be elicited by interacting verbally and/or physically with another person. These BFCRS (2025) items for the subtype of "aberrant volitional" of disorganized and catatonic behaviors include echolalia, echopraxia, verbigeration, automatic obedience, waxy flexibility, catalepsy, rigidity, *gegenhalten, mitgehen*, grasp reflex, negativism, mutism, and withdrawal.

What Kinds of Problems with Confusion and Disorganization Might Happen?

Sometimes, the service provider will have difficulty following what the person living with SMI is saying and will take the conversations in directions that were not intended. With Matthew, a comment about what he was wearing might get an answer that focused on the importance of the color of his clothing, where it was made, what clothes he wore in school, or some other topic that was unintended by the person asking the question. Sometimes confusion could be so bad that the person living with SMI will not know where he is, who other people are or even the time of the year; this is called "disorientation." SMI can result in disorganization or confused thinking that is inferred from the speech of the person living with SMI. Disorganized or confused speech shows itself in a variety of ways. Some of these are:

- "Loose associations," also known as "derailment," refers to a problem in which the ideas that are being expressed by the person living with SMI keep shifting from one subject to another. These ideas are often completely unrelated or very poorly related at best. The other person will quickly become confused (and often very frustrated) because it is difficult to see the link from one subject to another. When other people asked Matthew about a picture he drew, he might reply "I used blue; like the sky; makes you feel sad; like the other day and I could not get a hamburger. I love hamburgers, especially McDonald's. I worked there once and met a girl." and on and on. Many of the hospital staff began to avoid Matthew because they couldn't keep track of what he was saying. The person living with SMI will usually show little or no awareness of the poor link between the topics they are talking about.
- "Flight of ideas" refers to an almost continuous flow of rapid speech that changes suddenly from one topic to another. In loose associations, the ideas will have little relation to each other. In flight of ideas, there will usually be an understandable link between the topics. However, it will usually be difficult and frustrating for the other person to try to keep up with what the person living with SMI is talking about. The person might quickly say: "Let's go to the mall. We can take the car or we can walk. We need to have time so we'd better take the car. As long as there's enough gas so we don't have to stop to get some. That way we'll have enough time to look around. I can smoke in the car, can't I?" The other people will usually want to tell the person living with SMI to slow down so they can keep track of what he's saying and think about it.
- "Disorientation" involves confusion about what is happening around you (recognizing who familiar people are, what day of the week it is, and where you are). Consequently, the person appears very disorganized. In most cases, this is very frustrating for both the person and the service provider. It can contribute to fear and anxiety, problems with attention and memory, and may provoke delusions and/or hallucinations.

Why Do Problems with Confusion and Disorganization Happen?

Part of the Reason May Be Biological or Physical

- Problems such as these may be the result of biochemical imbalance in the brain that results in problem behaviors displayed by people living with SMI. Flight of ideas is usually part of the emotional excitement and hyperactivity of a "manic episode" in a person identified with bipolar mental health problem. Loose associations may occur with several types of SMIs but are most frequently associated with a schizophrenic spectrum mental health problem. Disorientation may also occur because of a bad reaction to current medication, a serious physical problem, substance abuse, or a recent head injury. As a person living with SMI ages, the body will have more difficulty adjusting and processing forms of medication and disorientation is more likely to happen.

- Problems with confusion and disorganized speech may be the result of drug use or the use of certain medications. These drugs or medications may create a biochemical imbalance that brings on or worsens some problem behaviors. Even "safe" drugs such as caffeine can bring on confusion or disorganization if used excessively.
- These problems may happen if there has been damage to the brain in an accident. While problems resulting from brain damage may improve quite a bit during the weeks and months after such an accident, they will often continue at a less severe level.

Part of the Reason May Be Psychosocial

- A busy and chaotic environment—characterized by multiple simultaneous conversations, rapid movement, or fast-paced speech—can be disorienting for most individuals. For example, after disembarking from an aircraft, people are often confronted with a multitude of sounds, announcements, conversations, and individuals moving in various directions, which can make it challenging to immediately orient themselves. While many individuals eventually regain their sense of direction, those living with SMI may experience ongoing difficulty establishing their bearings in such environments. If a person is living with SMI, they will be more likely to have difficulty tolerating a noisy, busy, chaotic environment. A person living with SMI who may do fine in a quiet, calm setting may become easily confused or excited in a busy over-stimulating setting. Matthew had much more difficulty communicating with other people when there was a lot of activity happening around him. If he could, he would try to leave the area.
- Many people who experience stress that won't go away (such as feeling a lot of pressure at work, frequent arguments at home, or experiencing trauma) will often begin to have problems with their ability to think clearly. A person living with SMI will probably face more stressful situations in life than most other people. This person may have more difficulties with the job (or be jobless), may not have a place to live, have less money to buy things, or may not even know how to cook. All of these contribute to stress and make it more difficult to think clearly.

Behavioral Support Strategies for Confusion and Disorganized Behaviors

- Consider seeking a review of current medications. Problems such as these are very serious and, in many cases, will require a review of current medications. Be prepared to identify all medications being taken for any reason. Remember that some medications taken for problems other than mental health problems can cause problems such as confusion and disorganized thinking. Some medications for physical problems such as high blood pressure, when used together with medications for treating the symptoms of SMI will bring confusion or disorganized speech and motor behaviors, such as tremors, or slow movements. Seek the opinion of an experienced prescribing service provider as to whether the current medications can be changed to more effectively manage these problems.
- Consider a consultation with a medical service provider. Disorganized behaviors are associated with several physical and neurological disorders. It is best to make sure it is not related to one of these.
- Clearly define the problematic behavior. Specify the actions and statements exhibited by the individual living with SMI that are considered concerning. Outline your responses when these behaviors occur and describe how the individual reacts to supportive interventions from others. Establishing an objective understanding of these aspects of behaviors is an essential initial step toward accurately assessing the situation and determining appropriate strategies for intervention.
- Watch for circumstances that provoke the problem. Use the forms in the Appendices to monitor the problem behavior and to record when these problems occur during the day, with whom they occur, where they happen, or other ways in which the problems may vary. Ask the question in what context does the disorganization occur and what is happening and not happening when it does occur.
- Try to be clear about anything that seems to help the person living with SMI to do better. Such information will likely be important in devising support strategies to minimize the problem and improve their behaviors. The example of Matthew clearly showed that his difficulties increased in crowded and noisy settings. Conversely, he could communicate more effectively with specific staff members when the environment was quieter and less populated.
- Hold conversations in environments with minimal distractions. Assisting individuals living with SMI becomes more effective when attention is not divided by external activities or disturbances. Consider relocating discussions to settings devoid of potential distractions, such as other people, televisions, or music, to facilitate focused communication.
- Communicate in a calm, patient manner. When faced with these behaviors, maintain a calm, matter of fact, noncritical approach to the person living with SMI. The interaction may be very frustrating for the listener, but it is important to avoid looking frustrated, impatient, or critical. If the problem is "flight of ideas," gently remind the person living with SMI that he is talking too fast and he

needs to slow down so you can understand. Regarding loose associations, calmly and nonjudgmentally inform the person living with SMI that it is difficult to understand how the ideas relate to each other when he starts to move from one topic to another. Ask them to slow down and so he can be understood. It may be helpful to paraphrase or summarize what the person was saying before the conversation was "derailed." It may take coaching and practice to be able to do this in a patient, clear, noncritical, and matter-of-fact fashion. Advice from an experienced mental health service provider may be required to do this effectively.

- Start conversations on a topic that the person living with SMI has good knowledge of. The person living with SMI probably will be better able to stay on topic if he is interested in and knowledgeable about the topic. Develop awareness of how the person living with SMI spends his time and what his interests are. Set time aside to ask him about such topics. For example, because Matthew had an interest (and talent) in art, staff took time to ask him about his work with the art therapist. Even if the person living with SMI requires help from other service providers (such as reminding him to slow down), he is more likely to succeed if the topic interests him. Conversations such as these can build the skills necessary to improve conversations on other topics.
- Be aware of what the person living with SMI does during the day and focus the conversations on them. It can be helpful to talk about the most important things that happen to the person living with SMI during the day. The topic may be as simple as what he had for lunch or how long he had to wait for the bus. For Matthew, the staff knew that he was scheduled for the art room every day because it was something that he enjoyed doing. After the art session, they made sure to ask him about it and tried to keep a brief conversation going on it.
- Try "rewording" what the person living with SMI has said. Become familiar with what the person living with SMI likes to talk about; by knowing the person's interests and routines, it may be easier to understand what he is trying to say when most other people can't. If this is the case, it is helpful to "fill in the blanks" for the person living with SMI when disorganized and confusing speech occurs. If the staff commented on Matthew's art and he replied by commenting on the blue of the sky and went on about the weather or other topics, they might reply: "The blue in your picture is a lot like the sky on a clear day. How did you mix the color?" This may help him to bring his focus back to the topic and keep the conversation going. This is more than just repeating back to the person what he has just said. Try to restate what he has said in a clear and simple way. This is a basic skill for mental health service providers and consultation with an experienced and knowledgeable service provider could assist in improving abilities to do this.
- Focus on the feelings that are implied by the communication of the person living with SMI. Even though there may be difficulty in understanding what the person living with SMI is trying to say, it is important to clearly see when he is angry, nervous, or discouraged. In some cases, it is helpful to talk about the feeling and change the efforts to understand exactly what the person living with SMI has been saying. If emotional distress is worsening the person's problems with communicating, then focusing on that experienced emotion may help to calm him

down and make it easier for communication to succeed. In most cases, emotions should be discussed patiently and supportively. Matthew and service providers recognized that his communication problems were worse when he was nervous. They agreed that when his nervousness was making things worse, they would allow him to go off by himself to calm down. After he calmed down, they tried again, and Matthew usually did much better.

- Sometimes it will be best to just be patient and listen. Sometimes the person living with SMI simply needs another person to patiently listen to him. When this seems to be a priority for him, the situation may be made worse by trying to correct him to improve his conversational skills. At such times, it may be best to just patiently listen to him even though there are difficulties in understanding what he is trying to say. By being familiar with the needs, moods, and concerns of the person living with SMI, service providers are better able to decide how to respond. Sometimes it will be best just to listen rather than try to help solve problems or actively work on improving his skills.
- Assist the person living with SMI to speak in a slow, clear manner. Encourage the person living with SMI to slow down and explain the connections between ideas to help him make himself understood to others. In dealing with loose associations, it may be helpful to assist the person living with SMI in reviewing what has been said over the past few minutes. Ask the person who has problems with communicating clearly to "help me understand what you just said" and paraphrase what was said to assist the person "make the connection." Remember to compliment them for their ability to slow down and be more understandable in what he is saying.
- Learn to stop the conversation when it is needed. Service providers probably want to improve communication with the person living with SMI, but sometimes service providers will need a break from their efforts. There will almost certainly be times when the service provider does not have the time or effort to improve disorganized behavior. At such a time, the service provider needs to be able to stop the conversation and go on about what they need to do; saying something like, "I can't keep talking now, we'll have to talk again later" will sometimes be the best thing to do. This can be more difficult to do than it seems. Discuss it with other service providers at a support group meeting, seek advice from an experienced and knowledgeable service provider to be more effective, and decide when it is best to work on improving the communication of the person living with SMI.
- Model the behavior that is being encouraged in the person living with SMI. Be brief and clear in how the preferred behavior is "modeled" or the person living with SMI. When speaking, stand in front of the person living with SMI, make eye contact (but don't force it), speak slowly, use short and simple sentences, and pronounce the individual words clearly. Avoid making sudden or distracting movements. Try to avoid appearing rushed or frustrated. A patient, nonthreatening, and noncritical approach, with few gestures, is likely to help maintain the attention of the person living with SMI. When talking with Matthew, the staff were instructed to make sure that they had at least 15 min that they could spare,

move to a relatively quiet area of the ward, and speak slowly and clearly to him so that there was a better chance of him paying attention and understanding.

Conclusion of Behavioral Support Strategies

When confusion and/or disorganized speech interfere with the ability of the person living with SMI to communicate with others, the following suggestions might help:

1. Have the medications reviewed by an experienced and knowledgeable psychiatric provider to see if any changes could help the problematic behaviors.
2. Be clear about what the person living with SMI does that leads to identifying confusion or disorganized behaviors as a problem. This helps focus efforts in observing the behaviors and determining what can be done about the problem. Descriptions need to be clear and avoid the use of labels and inferences; examples of what the definition means are an important part of describing the behavior.
3. Watch for circumstances (such as time of day, what the person is trying to talk about) that seem to affect the person's ability to think and speak in a clear and understandable manner. Developing an idea as to the context in which disorganized behaviors occur assists in changing some of these conditions.
4. When talking with the person living with SMI, do it in a way that helps the person living with SMI to think and speak clearly. Do it in a quiet area, speak slowly and clearly to the person, and talk about things that the person is interested in or knows about.
5. Be patient. Try to meet the person living with SMI at the level that they can succeed.
6. Start conversations on topics that the person living with SMI likes or is familiar with. This helps the person to focus on the topic and talk with confidence.
7. Be prepared to just listen. Sometimes this will be the best that can be done.
8. Practice doing things that help the person living with SMI to slow down and be clear.
9. Stay calm. Occasionally, restate what the person living with SMI is saying. Let her know that she needs to slow down as it may be difficult to keep up with what she is saying.
10. Don't be afraid to seek help. Most of these suggestions are easier said than done. An experienced mental health service provider may be able to help by putting these suggestions into action.

What about Matthew?

The staff at the hospital tried several strategies to communicate with Matthew. First, they made sure that he was taking the proper medications. Because Matthew had been inconsistent in taking his medication properly in the past, he was prescribed a long-acting form of antipsychotic medicine. Next, they identified a few activities that Matthew preferred and scheduled those at different times of the day. They left plenty of free time in between these activities so he could spend time by himself. They also agreed that they would encourage but not force Matthew to be involved in these activities. If he stayed for only a few minutes, they accepted that limit and praised him for attending.

When in the activities, they did not force Matthew to talk with them. When they did talk with him, they tried to make sure the topic was related to what he was doing. For example, Matthew enjoyed doing art projects. When working on such a project, the staff tried to start conversations on the colors that he was using or similar topics. This helped Matthew to stay on topic, and it helped the other people to make sense of what he was saying to them. If they could not understand what he said, they would patiently ask him to repeat. When talking to him, they refrained from talking fast, kidding around, or otherwise doing something that Matthew might have difficulty in understanding. Sometimes Matthew would stay in the room, sitting in a corner and cover himself with a jacket. The staff would invite him to participate but would allow him to stay in the corner if he declined.

Outside of the group, the staff also tried to have short conversations with him. They tried to make sure it was on a reality-based topic, such as the weather or what was served for lunch, so he and others were more likely to understand what each other was saying. If the conversation seemed to be going well, staff tried to keep it going if they reasonably could.

Gradually, Matthew's ability to stay with other people and engage in conversation with them improved. Over a period of several months, he stopped leaving group situations and became better able to maintain longer conversations, if only for 5 min. He also began talking with some staff about his difficulty being with other people and his frustration at trying to communicate with them when his "thoughts jumble together." He was also much more willing to take his medications because he understood that it was important in helping him to do all this. Because of this, he was much better prepared to live in a community setting.

In this example, the staff members took several steps to help Matthew improve at being able to keep his focus on one topic of conversation:

1. They recognized that Matthew had to improve his consistency at taking his medication. Without consistency, the problems with confusion were much worse. The psychiatric mental health service provider prescribed a long-acting form of medication that could last for a month. This helped other strategies to be more successful.
2. They recognized that Matthew was better able to keep his focus on one topic when there was something around him that reminded him of the topic. The staff

identified several activities that he preferred and arranged for his involvement in them. They respected his right to refuse to do them. When he did participate, however, they offered to help and started conversations about what he was doing. If Matthew could keep his focus on that topic, they kept the conversation going as long as reasonably possible.

3. They recognized that Matthew became very frustrated when he had difficulty keeping track of a conversation. If he became frustrated and wanted to leave, they allowed him to leave. If he stayed in the room but covered himself with a jacket, they invited him to participate but accepted whatever response he gave. They avoided pushing him beyond his capability.
4. They recognized that Matthew's difficulty in keeping the focus of conversations would always be a challenge for him. They accepted the fact that he would continue to have problems in this area and set their goal for him in accordance with this reality. The hospital staff met with the staff of a community-supported living placement to let them know what interventions worked most effectively with him.

By following these steps, the staff helped Michael to become involved in more group activities and to talk more frequently with other people. This helped him to get along better with others in his community placement.

Summary

Problematic behaviors in mental health are often common human behaviors that become symptomatic when they lead to negative outcomes such as disorganized speech and motoric behaviors. Disorganized behaviors are transdiagnostic and can occur in various mental health conditions, including schizophrenia spectrum and mood-related mental health problems. The assessment of disorganized behaviors includes both observable actions and self-reported experiences, highlighting the complexity of these symptoms. Dimensions of disorganized behaviors include frequency, severity, awareness, and the distress caused during occurrences. Understanding these behaviors requires a multidimensional approach, considering both speech and motoric behaviors in individuals with SMI.

Disorganized speech must be severe and frequent enough to impair effective communication to be considered a problem behavior in SMI; these behaviors are assessed in various dimensions, including cognitive derailment, flight of ideas, and tangentiality. Disorganized speech significantly impairs recovery in individuals with SMI and affects the person's engagement with others in their environment.

Several assessment instruments have been developed with overlaps as to the dimensions that are assessed. The Positive and Negative Symptom Scale (PANSS) categorizes behaviors into five dimensions, including behavioral disorganization and emotional distress. The Thought, Language and Communication (TLC) scale identifies 18 dimensions of disorganized speech, rated from 0 to 4 based on the frequency of occurrence for each dimension. Factor analyses of the TLC scale reveal three main domains: disorganization, negative symptoms, and verbosity/productivity, accounting for 42% to 78% of variance. The Bern Psychopathology Scale–Revised (BPS-R) assesses disorganization in language, affectivity, and motor behavior, rated on a three-point scale based on the judged severity of the displays of the behavioral dimension.

Comprehensive assessment of disorganized speech should include frequency, severity, context, and awareness, among other dimensions. The dimensions of disorganized speech that have been studied in the research literature include:

1. Cognitive derailment (thought derailment): frequent abrupt shifting of thoughts or associations, leading to disconnected and fragmented speech.
2. Flight of ideas: rapid, continuous succession of superficially related thoughts and ideas, often resulting in hurried speech with frequent topic shifts.
3. Tangentiality: responding to questions in an oblique or irrelevant way, diverging from the original subject.
4. Circumstantiality: indirect and delayed speech with excessive or irrelevant detail, eventually reaching the main point.
5. Word salad (jargon aphasia): mixture of words and phrases that lack comprehensive meaning or logical coherence.
6. Neologism: creation of new words or inappropriately condensed combinations of words that are not readily understood by others.
7. Poverty of speech: restriction in spontaneous speech.
8. Poverty of content of speech: adequate amount of speech that conveys little information.
9. Pressure of Speech: increased amount and speed of speech, difficult to interrupt.
10. Distractible speech: speech interrupted by nearby stimuli.
11. Incoherence: incomprehensible speech due to a preponderance of word salad or jargon aphasia.
12. Illogicality: conclusions that do not follow logically from the preceding statements.
13. Clanging: word choice governed by sounds rather than meaning, often involving punning and rhyming.
14. Word approximations: old words used in a new and unconventional way or new words developed by conventional rules.
15. Loss of goal: failure to follow thought to conclusion.
16. Perseveration: repetition of words or ideas.
17. Echolalia: repetition of words or phrases from the speaker.
18. Blocking: sudden obstruction or interruption of normal flow of speech before a thought is completed.
19. Stilted speech: excessively formal or outdated speech.
20. Self-reference: repeatedly referring subjects back to oneself.

These dimensions provide a comprehensive understanding of disorganized speech, aiding in the assessment and treatment of individuals living with SMI, but no instrument assesses all identified dimensions of disorganized speech.

A sub-domain of disorganized behaviors is motoric behaviors in individuals living with SMI. Disorganized motoric behaviors have been categorized as including childlike silliness, agitation, and purposeless movements, impacting and at times impeding daily life activities. One aspect of disorganized motoric behavior is catatonia, which is characterized by stupor and motor disorganization. The DSM-5-TR outlines 12 psychomotor dimensions for assessing catatonia, requiring at least three to be present for a determination of the condition.

Several assessment instruments have been developed for disorganized motoric and catatonic behaviors with overlaps as to the dimensions that are assessed. The Positive and Negative Symptom Scale (PANSS) identifies two factors of disorganized behaviors: "disorganized" and "excited," with specific items linked to each. The Bern Psychopathology Scale (BPS-R) assesses motoric behavior dimensions, categorizing them into negative, normal, and positive, but lacks temporal measurement. The Bush-Francis Catatonia Rating Scale (BFCRS) is the most widely used scale and includes 23 items to evaluate the frequency and presence of catatonic behaviors. Any proposed expanded assessment tool ought to incorporate frequency, duration, awareness, controllability, and distress related to disorganized motoric behaviors.

The dimensions of disorganized motor and catatonic behaviors that have been studied in the mental health research literature include:

- Excitement: extreme hyperactivity and over-responsiveness to minimal stimuli.
- Immobility/stupor: extreme hypoactivity and minimal responsiveness.
- Mutism: minimal or no verbal response.
- Starring: fixed gaze with little visual scanning.
- Posturing/catalepsy: spontaneous maintenance of posture(s), including mundane (e.g., sitting/standing for long periods without reacting).
- Grimacing: odd facial expressions and contortions.
- Echopraxia/echolalia: mimicking movements or speech of another person.
- Stereotypy: repetitive, non-goal-directed motor activity.
- Mannerisms: odd, purposeful movements, performing actions at inappropriate times, displaying an odd gait, or exaggerated politeness.
- Verbigeration: repetition of a word, phrases, or sentences.
- Rigidity: maintenance of an unusual rigid position.
- Negativism: resistance to instructions or attempts to move.
- Waxy flexibility: slight, even resistance to positioning by the examiner.
- Withdrawal: refusal to eat, drink, or make eye contact.
- Impulsivity: sudden inappropriate, random behavior.
- Automatic obedience: exaggerated cooperation with examiner's request or spontaneous continuation of movement requested.
- *Mitgehen*: raising of an extremity in response to light pressure, despite instructions to resist.
- *Gegenhalten*: resistance to passive movement, proportional to the strength of the stimulus.
- Ambitendency: indecisive, hesitant movement, appearing motorically "stuck."

- Grasp reflex: involuntary grasping of anything that touches the palm.
- Perseveration: repeatedly returning to the same topic or movement.
- Combativeness: striking out in an undirected manner, with no or only a superficial explanation afterward.
- Decision-making: ambivalence or excessive self-will.
- Motor drive: lacking energy to move or an urge to move.
- Velocity: rate of movement (accelerated/decelerated).
- Motion sequence: smooth uninterrupted motoric behaviors, noting blockages, hesitancies, or parakinesia (awkwardness or clumsiness of movement) and dyskinesia (involuntary or unintended movement).

These dimensions provide a comprehensive understanding of disorganized motor and catatonic behaviors, aiding in the assessment and treatment of individuals living with SMI.

The neuronal substrates of disorganized speech and thought processes involve several key brain regions and their connections:

- Prefrontal cortex (PFC): crucial for cognitive control, goal selection, planning, response inhibition, performance monitoring, and working memory. Dysfunction in the PFC is linked to impairments in working memory and cognitive flexibility.
- Dorsolateral prefrontal cortex (DLPFC): implicated in higher-order cognitive functions like reasoning and decision-making. Reduced activity in the DLPFC is associated with disorganized thought and speech processes.
- Thalamus: acts as a relay center for information across the brain. Abnormalities in its connections to the PFC can contribute to disorganized behaviors.
- Hippocampus (HPC): involved in memory and spatial navigation, playing a role in the organization of thoughts. Discoordination in the HPC-PFC circuitry is associated with cognitive and behavioral disorganization.
- Anterior cingulate cortex (ACC): involved in monitoring conflict in cognitions and error detection, crucial for maintaining coherent thought processes.
- Superior temporal gyrus (STG): important for processing auditory information, including speech sounds. Alterations in N-methyl-D-aspartate (NMDA) receptor functions within the STG are linked to difficulties in language comprehension and speech.
- White matter (WM) abnormalities: structural and functional abnormalities in the left STG, middle temporal gyrus, angular gyrus, inferior operculum, and orbitofrontal cortex (OFC) are associated with disorganized speech. MRI imaging links WM abnormalities in the left fronto-temporal language network to disorganized speech.

Disorganized thinking and speech are likely due to a complex interplay between multiple brain networks rather than dysfunction in a single brain region. The specific neural correlates can vary depending on the individual and the dimensions of disorganized speech being displayed.

Correlations exist between neurocognitive impairments and disorganized motoric behaviors, but no common pathway has been identified. Multiple pathways may be involved, indicating specific dimensions of disorganized motoric behaviors.

The motoric behaviors displayed are observable operants and influenced by environmental events. Psychological factors have been identified that are correlated with disorganized and catatonic behaviors. It has been found that persistent fear significantly impacts behaviors and mental states in individuals displaying catatonic behaviors. Tonic immobility (TI) is a hypothesized origin of some of the dimensions of disorganized motoric and catatonic behaviors. Tonic immobility is a temporary state of motor inhibition in response to extreme fear, observed in both humans and other mammals. In humans, tonic immobility can occur during traumatic events like sexual assault or combat. Positive correlations exist between tonic immobility responses and posttraumatic symptoms, dissociation, and anxiety sensitivity. Avoiding goal-directed behaviors may be a response to prevent adverse consequences. Research indicates that response-punisher associations lead to little autonomic disturbance, often resulting in defensive behaviors like "freezing." Uncertainty about potential adverse consequences can trigger tonic immobility and other response suppression behaviors that are topographically like disorganized motor and catatonic behaviors. More research is needed to define the dimensions of disorganized motoric catatonic behaviors operationally.

Disorganized behaviors associated with SMI include disorganized thinking, speech, and motor behavior, affecting communication and daily functioning. Disorganized thought processes (e.g., formal thought disorder (FTD)) are inferred from the observation of the dimensions of disorganized speech and motoric and catatonic behaviors. The prevalence of FTD ranges from 50.39% to 72.7% among individuals living with SMI, with more severe cases in early onset conditions. FTD is more common in people living with early onset SMI (27.4%) compared to late-onset (10.4%), and these behaviors tend to persist or worsen over time. Co-occurring substance use is linked to more severe FTD, which negatively impacts social functioning and leads to longer hospital stays.

Problematic motor functions in individuals living with SMI include neurological soft signs, abnormal involuntary movements, and catatonic behaviors. Approximately 10% to 25% of individuals with living SMI exhibit disorganized motoric behaviors that may meet criteria for catatonia.

The prevalence of catatonic behaviors in acute psychiatric inpatients ranges from 7% to 17%, primarily linked to mood disorders. Historical data shows a significant decline in diagnosed catatonia, with rates dropping from 19.5% to 50% in the early 1900s to less than 1% by the mid-1900s.

Current estimates suggest that 50–65% of individuals with living SMI experience problematic motor functions, compared to about 5% in the general population. Catatonic behaviors affect 5–18% of hospitalized individuals living with SMI, often going unrecognized and leading to serious complications. The prevalence of catatonic behaviors varies widely among different mental health conditions, with 71% in mood mental health problems and 67% in schizophrenia spectrum disorders.

Catatonic behaviors can occur across the lifespan and affect both genders equally, with higher prevalence in nonpsychiatric settings (15.8%).

Across cultures and countries, reports indicate significant variability in disorganized motoric behaviors, with prevalence rates ranging from 1% in Nigeria to 68% in the United States. In India, the prevalence of disorganized motoric behaviors among recently admitted individuals to mental health units ranged from 4.8% to 37.2%. A comparison between India and Wales showed a prevalence of 13.5% in India and 9.6% in Wales, with significant differences in the types of behaviors exhibited. A systematic review found the highest prevalence of catatonia in Uganda (48.5%) and the lowest in Mexico (1.9%), highlighting the need for consistent assessment tools.

Research has shown that disorganized speech can be categorized into three types: disorganized speech I (DS-I), disorganized speech II (DS-II), and negative thought disorder (NTD). DS-I includes the dimensions of derailment, tangentiality, incoherence, and distractible speech. DS-II involves abnormal use of referential markers and illogicality, sharing impairments with DS-I. NTD is characterized by poverty of speech/content, reduced syntactic complexity, and correlates with negative symptoms like alogia. Flat affects and lexical abnormalities are also noted, impacting emotional expression and language use.

Researchers have identified different subtypes of disorganized catatonic behaviors, noting that the characteristics of disorganized and catatonic actions often overlap. The subtypes are labeled as "retarded" and "excited" and increased, abnormal and decreased motoric behaviors. The "retarded" subtype includes immobility, mutism, rigidity, and bizarre features like posturing and echolalia; "excited" subtype is marked by severe psychomotor agitation, which can lead to life-threatening conditions. The subtype on increased psychomotor activity includes agitation; abnormal activity includes grimacing and stereotypies, and decreased activity includes stupor and extreme withdrawal.

The strategies for managing disorganized behaviors in individuals with SMI include:

- Medication review: Review current medications to identify those causing confusion or disorganized thinking. Consult experienced psychiatric providers for potential medication adjustments. A medical examination may be needed if there are any signs that the disorganized behaviors are due to possible biological factors.
- Clarifying problem behaviors: Clearly define the specific problematic behaviors exhibited by the individual. Document responses to interventions to understand the issues better.
- Monitoring provoking circumstances: Use monitoring forms to track when and where problems occur. Identify environmental factors that exacerbate disorganized behaviors, such as noise, crowding, and distressful emotions.
- Minimizing distractions: Conduct conversations in quiet areas to reduce distractions. Focus on clear communication to enhance understanding.

- Calm communication: Maintain a calm, patient demeanor during interactions. Gently remind the individual to slow down if they are speaking too quickly or are not understood.
- Engaging topics of interest: Start conversations on topics the individual is knowledgeable about. Use interests to facilitate better communication and engagement.
- Focus on daily activities: Discuss daily events to keep conversations relevant and engaging.
- Encourage sharing about enjoyable activities, like art sessions, news, sports, and music.
- Rewording and clarifying: Become familiar with the individual's interests to aid understanding. Restate their thoughts in clear, simple terms to maintain focus.
- Emotional awareness: Recognize and address the emotions behind communication difficulties. Allow time for the individual to calm down if they are anxious.
- Active listening: At times, it's important to just listen and not attempt to change or steer the discussion. Pay close attention to what the person needs and how they are feeling.
- Encouraging clear speech: Assist the individual in speaking slowly and clearly. Provide positive reinforcement for improved communication efforts.
- Knowing when to pause: Recognize when to end a conversation if it becomes unproductive.
- Communicate the need to pause respectfully and plan to revisit later.
- Modeling desired behavior: Demonstrate clear communication techniques through your own behavior. Use eye contact, simple sentences, and a calm approach to engage effectively.

References

Abboud, R., Noronha, C., & Diwadkar, V. A. (2017). Motor system dysfunction in the schizophrenia diathesis: Neural systems to neurotransmitters. *European Psychiatry, 44*, 125–133. https://doi.org/10.1016/j.eurpsy.2017.04.004

Abrams, M. P., Carleton, R. N., Taylor, S., & Asmundson, G. J. (2009). Human tonic immobility: Measurement and correlates. *Depression and Anxiety, 26*(6), 550–556. https://doi.org/10.1002/da.20462

American Psychiatric Association. (2013). *Diagnostic and statistical manual of mental disorders* (5th ed.). https://doi.org/10.1176/appi.books.9780890425596

American Psychiatric Association. (2022). *Diagnostic and statistical manual of mental disorders* (5th ed., text rev). https://doi.org/10.1176/appi.books.9780890425787

American Psychiatric Association. (2025). *What is Schizophrenia?* Psychiatry.org. https://www.psychiatry.org/patients-families/schizophrenia/what-is-schizophrenia#:~:text=Disorganized%20or%20abnormal%20motor%20behavior,of%20activities%20of%20daily%20life

American Psychological Association. (n.d.-a). Agitation. In *APA dictionary of psychology*. https://dictionary.apa.org/Agitation

American Psychological Association. (n.d.-b). Ambitendency. In *APA dictionary of psychology*. https://dictionary.apa.org/Ambitendency

American Psychological Association. (n.d.-c). Catatonia. In *APA dictionary of psychology*. https://dictionary.apa.org/Catatonia

American Psychological Association. (n.d.-d). Circumstantiality. In *APA dictionary of psychology*. https://dictionary.apa.org/Circumstantiality

American Psychological Association. (n.d.-e). Cognitive derailment. In *APA dictionary of psychology*. https://dictionary.apa.org/Cognitive-derailment

American Psychological Association. (n.d.-f). Dyskinesia. In *APA dictionary of psychology*. https://dictionary.apa.org/Dyskinesia

American Psychological Association. (n.d.-g). Flat affect. In *APA dictionary of psychology*. https://dictionary.apa.org/Falt-affect

American Psychological Association. (n.d.-h). Flight of ideas. In *APA dictionary of psychology*. https://dictionary.apa.org/Flight-of-ideas

American Psychological Association. (n.d.-i). Grasp reflex. In *APA dictionary of psychology*. https://dictionary.apa.org/Grasp-reflex

American Psychological Association. (n.d.-j). Lexical decision. In *APA dictionary of psychology*. https://dictionary.apa.org/Lexical-decision

American Psychological Association. (n.d.-k). Metacognition. In *APA dictionary of psychology*. https://dictionary.apa.org/Affect

American Psychological Association. (n.d.-l). Neologism. In *APA dictionary of psychology*. https://dictionary.apa.org/Neologism

American Psychological Association. (n.d.-m). Parakinesia. In *APA dictionary of psychology*. https://dictionary.apa.org/Parakinesia

American Psychological Association. (n.d.-n). Reaction time. *APA Dictionary of Psychology*. https://dictionary.apa.org/reaction-time

American Psychological Association. (n.d.-o). Semantic priming. In *APA dictionary of psychology*. https://dictionary.apa.org/Semantic priming

American Psychological Association. (n.d.-p). Tangentiality. In *APA dictionary of psychology*. https://dictionary.apa.org/Tangentiality

American Psychological Association. (n.d.-q). Word salad. In *APA dictionary of psychology*. https://dictionary.apa.org/Word-salad

Anderson, A., Wilcox, M., Savitz, A., Chung, H., Li, Q., Salvadore, G., Hsu, J., Tu, P. C., & Bilder, R. M. (2015). Sparse factors for the positive and negative syndrome scale: Which symptoms and stage of illness? *Psychiatry Research, 225*(3), 283–290. https://doi.org/10.1016/j.psychres.2014.12.025

Andreasen, N. C. (1986). Scale for the assessment of thought, language, and communication (TLC). *Schizophrenia Bulletin, 12*(3), 473. https://doi.org/10.1093/schbul/12.3.473

Ariza-Salamanca, D. F., Corrales-Hernández, M. G., Pachón-Londoño, M. J., & Hernández-Duarte, I. (2022). Molecular and cellular mechanisms leading to catatonia: An integrative approach from clinical and preclinical evidence. *Frontiers in Molecular Neuroscience, 15*, 993671. https://doi.org/10.3389/fnmol.2022.993671

Leonhardt, B. L., Huling, K., Hamm, J. A., Roe, D., Hasson-Ohayon, I., McLeod, H. J., & Lysaker, P. H. (2017). Recovery and serious mental illness: A review of current clinical and research paradigms and future directions. *Expert Review of Neurotherapeutics, 17*(11), 1117–1130. https://doi.org/10.1080/10503307.2016.1219421

Bell, M. D., Lysaker, P. H., Milstein, R. M., & Beam-Goulet, J. L. (1994). Concurrent validity of the cognitive component of schizophrenia: Relationship of PANSS scores to neuropsychological assessments. *Psychiatry Research, 54*(1), 51–58. https://doi.org/10.1016/0165-1781(94)90064-7

Bettis, R. J., Faith, L. A., Beard, A. M., Whan, B. A., Hegwood, C. M., Monette, M. A., McCleery, A., Harvey, P. D., Nuechterlein, K. H., Carroll, J. M., Keefe, R. S. E., Burdick, K. E., Goldberg, T. E., Ardila, A., Ostrosky, F., McCutcheon, R., Schaefer, J., Baggetta, P., Alexander, P., et al. (2024). Narrative forewarnings: A qualitative analysis of the themes preceding disorganized speech in schizophrenia. *Behavioral Sciences, 14*(3), 212. https://doi.org/10.3390/bs14030212

Collaborative Care and Wellness–Department of Psychiatry–University of Rochester Medical Center. (2025). *BFCRS–Bush-Francis Catatonia Rating Scale. Rochester.edu.* https://

www.urmc.rochester.edu/psychiatry/divisions/collaborative-care-and-wellness/bush-francis-catatonia-rating-scale/bfcrs#:~:text=Exaggerated%20cooperation%20with%20examiner's%20request,Autonomic%20Abnormality

Bracht, T., Heidemeyer, K., Koschorke, P., Horn, H., Razavi, N., Wopfner, A., Federspiel, A., Wiest, R., Dierks, T., Strik, W., & Walther, S. (2012). Comparison of objectively measured motor behavior with ratings of the motor behavior domain of the Bern psychopathology scale (BPS) in schizophrenia. *Psychiatry Research, 198*(2), 224–229. https://doi.org/10.1016/j.psychres.2011.12.038

Bracht, T., Schnell, S., Federspiel, A., Razavi, N., Horn, H., Strik, W., Stegmayer, K., & Walther, S. (2013). Altered cortico-basal ganglia motor pathways reflect reduced volitional motor activity in schizophrenia. *Schizophrenia Research, 143*(2–3), 269–276. https://doi.org/10.1016/j.schres.2012.12.004

Bush, G., Fink, M., Petrides, G., Dowling, F., & Francis, A. (1996). Catatonia. I. Rating scale and standardized examination. *Acta Psychiatrica Scandinavica, 93*(2), 129–136.

Chalasani, P., Healy, D., & Morriss, R. (2005). Presentation and frequency of catatonia in new admissions to two acute psychiatric admission units in India and Wales. *Psychological Medicine, 35*(11), 1667–1675. https://doi.org/10.1017/S0033291705005453

Cooper, J. O., Heron, T. E., & Heward, W. L. (2020). *Applied behavior analysis* (3rd ed.). Pearson. https://www.pearson.com/en-us/subject-catalog/p/applied-behavior-analysis/P200000003465/9780134752556

Cotter, J., Granger, K., Backx, R., Hobbs, M., Looi, C. Y., & Barnett, J. H. (2017). Social cognitive dysfunction as a clinical marker: A systematic review of meta-analyses across 30 clinical conditions. *Neuroscience and Biobehavioral Reviews, 80*, 365–371. https://doi.org/10.1016/j.neubiorev.2017.11.014

De la Torre, G., Doval, S., López-Sanz, D., García-Sedeño, M., Ramallo, M., Bernal, M., & González-Torre, S. (2021). Neurocognitive impairment in severe mental illness. Comparative study with Spanish speaking patients. *Brain Sciences, 11*(3), 389. https://doi.org/10.3390/brainsci11030389

National Institute on Deafness and Other Communication Disorders. (2023, May 8). *Developmental language disorder*. NIDCD. https://www.nidcd.nih.gov/health/developmental-language-disorder#:~:text=Developmental%20language%20disorder%20(DLD)%20is%20a%20communication%20disorder%20that%20interferes,lack%20of%20exposure%20to%20language

Dhossche, D. M., Wachtel, L. E., Goetz, M., & Sienaert, P. (2016). *Catatonia in psychiatric illnesses*. In *the medical basis ofpsychiatry* (pp. 517–535). https://doi.org/10.1007/978-1-59745-252-6_27

Docherty, N. M. (2005). Cognitive impairments and disordered speech in schizophrenia: Thought disorder, disorganization, and communication failure perspectives. *Journal of Abnormal Psychology, 114*(2), 269–278. https://doi.org/10.1037/0021-843X.114.2.269

Dougher, M. J. (2013). Behaviorisms and private events. Behavior. *Analysis, 36*(2), 223–227. https://doi.org/10.1007/BF03392308

Fink, M., & Shorter, E. (2017). Does persisting fear sustain catatonia? *Acta Psychiatrica Scandinavica, 136*(5), 441–444. https://doi.org/10.1111/acps.12796

Glossary of Psychiatry. (2024, December 20). Mitgehen. In Wikipedia. Accessed Jan 30, 2025, from https://en.wikipedia.org/wiki/Glossary_of_psychiatry#:~:text=mitgehen,as%20forcible%20grasping%20and%20pushing

Goldberg, T. E., Aloia, M. S., Gourovitch, M. L., Missar, D., Pickar, D., & Weinberger, D. R. (1998). Cognitive substrates of thought disorder, I: The semantic system. *American Journal of Psychiatry, 155*(12), 1671–1676. https://doi.org/10.1176/ajp.155.12.1671

Green, M. F. (1996). What are the functional consequences of neurocognitive deficits in schizophrenia? *The American Journal of Psychiatry, 153*(3), 321–330. https://doi.org/10.1176/ajp.153.3.321

Hardy-Baylé, M. C., Sarfati, Y., & Passerieux, C. (2003). The cognitive basis of disorganization symptomatology in schizophrenia and its clinical correlates: Toward a pathogenetic approach to disorganization. *Schizophrenia Bulletin, 29*(3), 459–471. https://doi.org/10.1093/oxfordjournals.schbul.a007019

Harrow, M., O'Connell, E. M., Herbener, E. S., Altman, A. M., Kaplan, K. J., & Jobe, T. H. (2003). Disordered verbalizations in schizophrenia: A speech disturbance or thought disorder? *Comprehensive Psychiatry, 44*(5), 353–359. https://doi.org/10.1016/S0010-440X(03)00113-5

Harvey, P. D., & Strassnig, M. (2012). Predicting the severity of everyday functional disability in people with schizophrenia: cognitive deficits, functional capacity, symptoms, and health status. *World Psychiatry, 11*(2), 73–79. https://doi.org/10.1016/j.wpsyc.2012.05.004

Hirjak, D., Rogers, J. P., Wolf, R. C., Kubera, K. M., Fritze, S., Wilson, J. E., Sambataro, F., Fricchione, G., Meyer-Lindenberg, A., Ungvari, G. S., & Northoff, G. (2024). Catatonia. *Nature Reviews Disease Primers, 10*(1), Article 49. https://doi.org/10.1038/s41572-024-00534-w

Hitczenko, K., Mittal, V. A., & Goldrick, M. (2021). Understanding language abnormalities and associated clinical markers in psychosis: The promise of computational methods. *Schizophrenia Bulletin, 47*(2), 344–362. https://doi.org/10.1093/schbul/sbaa141

Jean-Richard-Dit-Bressel, P., Killcross, S., & McNally, G. P. (2018). Behavioral and neurobiological mechanisms of punishment: Implications for psychiatric disorders. *Neuropsychopharmacology, 43*(8), 1639–1650. https://doi.org/10.1038/s41386-018-0047-3

John, J. (2019). *Thought, language and communication (speech): Concepts, clinical assessment & neurobiology [pdf]*. D. Y. Patil PG lecture series 13 September 2019 Sion hospital and Lokmanya Tilak medical college, Mumbai University. Accessed Jan 26, 2025, from https://pgpsychlectureseries.com/wp-content/uploads/2021/07/thought-language-and-communication-concepts-clinical-assessment-neurobiology.pdf

Kay, S. R., Fiszbein, A., & Opler, L. A. (1987). The positive and negative syndrome scale (PANSS) for schizophrenia. *Schizophrenia Bulletin, 13*(2), 261–276. https://doi.org/10.1093/schbul/13.2.261

Kim, J. H., Lee, J. M., Jo, H. J., Kim, S. H., Lee, J. H., Kim, S. T., Seo, S. W., Cox, R. W., Na, D. L., Kim, S. I., & Saad, Z. S. (2010). Defining functional SMA and pre-SMA subregions in human MFC using resting state fMRI: Functional connectivity-based parcellation method. *NeuroImage, 49*(3), 2375–2386. https://doi.org/10.1016/j.neuroimage.2009.10.016

Krajcovic, B., Fajnerova, I., Horacek, J., Kelemen, E., Kubik, S., Svoboda, J., & Stuchlik, A. (2019). Neural and neuronal discoordination in schizophrenia: From ensembles through networks to symptoms. *Acta Physiologica, 226*(4), e13282. https://doi.org/10.1111/apha.13282

Kuperberg, G. R. (2010). Language in schizophrenia part 1: An introduction. *Language and Linguistics Compass, 4*(8), 576–589. https://doi.org/10.1111/j.1749-818X.2010.00216.x

Lang, F. U., Mueller-Stierlin, A. S., Walther, S., Stegmayer, K., Becker, T., & Jaeger, M. (2016). Dimensional approaches to schizophrenia: A comparison of the Bern psychopathology scale and the five-factor model of the positive and negative syndrome scale. *Psychiatry Research, 239*, 284–290. https://doi.org/10.1016/j.psychres.2016.03.032

Jain, A., & Mitra, P. (2023). Catatonic schizophrenia (archived). In StatPearls. StatPearls Publishing. https://doi.org/10.13140/RG.2.2.22841.24161

Mayo Clinic. (2024). *Schizophrenia–Symptoms and causes*. Mayo Clinic. https://www.mayoclinic.org/diseases-conditions/schizophrenia/symptoms-causes/syc-20354443#:~:text=Extremely%20disorganized%20or%20unusual%20motor,not%20want%20to%20follow%20instructions

McCutcheon, R. A., Keefe, R. S., & McGuire, P. K. (2023). Cognitive impairment in schizophrenia: Aetiology, pathophysiology, and treatment. *Molecular Psychiatry, 28*(5), 1902–1918. https://doi.org/10.1038/s41380-022-01975-9

Merriam-Webster. (n.d.). Self-will. In *Merriam-Webster.com dictionary*. Retrieved January 30, 2025, from https://www.merriam-webster.com/dictionary/semantics

Minor, K. S., Marggraf, M. P., Davis, B. J., Luther, L., Vohs, J. L., Buck, K. D., & Lysaker, P. H. (2015). Conceptual disorganization weakens links in cognitive pathways: Disentangling neurocognition, social cognition, and metacognition in schizophrenia. Schizophrenia Research, 169(1–3), 153–158. doi:https://doi.org/10.1016/j.schres.2015.09.026.

Mohandas, E., & Rajmohan, V. (2008). Neural correlates of catatonia. *Delhi Psychiatry Journal, 11*(1) https://delhipsychiatryjournal.org/archives/vol11-issue1/neural-correlates-of-catatonia/

Myers, E. J., Abel, D. B., Mickens, J. L., Russell, M. T., Rand, K. L., Salyers, M. P., Luther, L., & Minor, K. S. (2024). Meta-analysis of the relationship between metacognition and disorganized symptoms in psychosis. *Schizophrenia Research, 264*, 178–187. https://doi.org/10.1016/j.schres.2023.12.009

Naeem, M., Ozuem, W., Howell, K., & Ranfagni, S. (2023). A step-by-step process of thematic analysis to develop a conceptual model in qualitative research. *International Journal of Qualitative Methods, 22*. https://doi.org/10.1177/16094069231205789

Nickl-Jockschat, T., Sharkey, R., Bacon, C., Peterson, Z., Rootes-Murdy, K., Salvador, R., Pomarol, E., Karuk, A., Homan, P., Ji, E., Omlor, W., Homan, S., Georgiadis, F., Kaiser, S., Kirschner, M., Ehrlich, S., Dannlowski, U., Grotegerd, D., Goltermann, J., et al. (2023). Neural correlates of positive and negative formal thought disorder in individuals with schizophrenia: An ENIGMA schizophrenia working group study. *Research Square*. https://doi.org/10.21203/rs.3.rs-3179362/v1

Positive and Negative Syndrome Scale (PANSS) for Schizophrenia. (2024). *MDCalc. https://www.mdcalc.com/calc/10414/positive-negative-syndrome-scale-panss-schizophrenia*

Rajagopal, S. (2007). Catatonia. *Advances in Psychiatric Treatment, 13*(1), 51–59. https://doi.org/10.1192/apt.bp.106.002360

Rasmussen, S. A., Mazurek, M. F., & Rosebush, P. I. (2016). Catatonia: Our current understanding of its diagnosis, treatment and pathophysiology. *World Journal of Psychiatry, 6*(4), 391–398. https://doi.org/10.5498/wjp.v6.i4.391

Roche, E., Creed, L., MacMahon, D., Brennan, D., & Clarke, M. (2015). The epidemiology and associated phenomenology of formal thought disorder: A systematic review. *Schizophrenia Bulletin, 41*(4), 951–962. https://doi.org/10.1093/schbul/sbu129

Sarkar, S., Sakey, S., Mathan, K., Bharadwaj, B., Kattimani, S., & Rajkumar, R. P. (2016). Assessing catatonia using four different instruments: Inter-rater reliability and prevalence in inpatient clinical population. *Asian Journal of Psychiatry, 23*, 27–31. https://doi.org/10.1016/j.ajp.2016.07.003

Sienaert, P., Rooseleer, J., & De Fruyt, J. (2011). Measuring catatonia: A systematic review of rating scales. *Journal of Affective Disorders, 135*(1–3), 1–9. https://doi.org/10.1016/j.jad.2011.02.012

Solmi, M., Pigato, G. G., Roiter, B., Guaglianone, A., Martini, L., Fornar, M., Monaco, F., Salcuni, S., Favaro, A., Ostinelli, E. G., Papola, D., Brambilla, P., Fusar-Poli, P., De Hert, M., Stubbs, B., Carvalho, A. F., & Correll, C. U. (2018). Prevalence of catatonia and its moderators in clinical samples: Results from a meta-analysis and meta-regression analysis. *Schizophrenia Bulletin, 44*(5), 1133–1150. https://doi.org/10.1093/schbul/sbx157

Strik, W., Wopfner, A., Horn, H., Koschorke, P., Razavi, N., Walther, S., & Wirtz, G. (2010). The Bern psychopathology scale for the assessment of system-specific psychotic symptoms. *Neuropsychobiology, 61*(4), 197–209. https://doi.org/10.1159/000297737

Subramaniyam, B. A., Muliyala, K. P., Suchandra, H. H., & Reddi, V. S. K. (2020). Diagnosing catatonia and its dimensions: Cluster analysis and factor solution using the Bush Francis catatonia rating scale (BFCRS). *Asian Journal of Psychiatry, 52*, 102002. https://doi.org/10.1016/j.ajp.2020.102002

Sundberg, M. L. (2020). Verbal behavior. In J. O. Cooper, T. E. Heron, & W. L. Heward (Eds.), *Applied behavior analysis* (3rd ed., pp. 412–449). Pearson. https://www.pearson.com/en-us/subject-catalog/p/applied-behavior-analysis/P200000003465/9780134752556

Torres, F. (2024). "What is schizophrenia?" *American Psychiatric Association*, www.psychiatry.org/patients-families/schizophrenia/what-is-schizophrenia

Ungvari, G. S., Caroff, S. N., Csihi, L., & Gazdag, G. (2023). Catatonia: "Fluctuat nec mergitur.". *World Journal of Psychiatry, 13*(5), 131–137. https://doi.org/10.5498/wjp.v13.i5.131

van der Gaag, M., Hoffman, T., Remijsen, M., Hijman, R., de Haan, L., van Meijel, B., van Hemert, A. M., Beekman, A., & Wiersma, D. (2006). The five-factor model of the positive and negative syndrome scale II: A ten-fold cross-validation of a revised model. *Schizophrenia Research, 85*(1–3), 280–287. https://doi.org/10.1016/j.schres.2006.03.021

Ventura, J., Wood, R. C., & Hellemann, G. S. (2013). Symptom domains and neurocognitive functioning can help differentiate social cognitive processes in schizophrenia: A meta-analysis. *Schizophrenia Bulletin, 39*(1), 102–111. https://doi.org/10.1093/schbul/sbr067

Viher, P. V., Stegmayer, K., Giezendanner, S., Federspiel, A., Bohlhalter, S., Wiest, R., Schmitt, A., Strik, W., & Walther, S. (2018). White matter correlates of the disorganized speech dimension in schizophrenia. *European Archives of Psychiatry and Clinical Neuroscience, 268*, 99–104. https://doi.org/10.1007/s00406-016-0753-y

Walther, S., & Strik, W. (2016). Catatonia. *CNS Spectrums, 21*(4), 341–348. https://doi.org/10.1017/S1092852916000274

Walther, S., Ramseyer, F., Horn, H., Strik, W., & Tschacher, W. (2014). Less structured movement patterns predict severity of positive syndrome, excitement, and disorganization. *Schizophrenia Bulletin, 40*(3), 585–591. https://doi.org/10.1093/schbul/sbt038

Walther, S., Stegmayer, K., Wilson, J. E., & Heckers, S. (2019). Structure and neural mechanisms of catatonia. *The Lancet Psychiatry, 6*(7), 610–619. https://doi.org/10.1016/S2215-0366(18)30474-7

Zingela, Z., Stroud, L., Cronje, J., Fink, M., & Van Wyk, S. (2022). A prospective descriptive study on prevalence of catatonia and correlates in an acute mental health unit in Nelson Mandela Bay, South Africa. *PLoS One, 17*(3), e0264944. https://doi.org/10.1371/journal.pone.0264944

Chapter 10
Problems with Cognitive Impairments (Memory and Concentration) in Individuals Living with Serious Mental Illness

Introduction

Cognitive impairments are increasingly recognized as core features of serious mental illness (SMI), transcending diagnostic boundaries and exerting profound influence on functional outcomes. While traditional psychiatric models have emphasized symptomatology such as hallucinations, delusions, and mood disturbances, contemporary research underscores the pervasive and enduring nature of neurocognitive deficits—including impairments in memory, attention, executive functioning, and processing speed—as integral to the lived experience of SMI. These deficits often preceded the onset of overt symptoms, persisted across illness phases, and contributed substantially to disability, social disengagement, and reduced quality of life.

This chapter examines neurocognitive functioning as a multidimensional construct, emphasizing its relevance to assessment, intervention, and prognosis in individuals living with SMI. Drawing on empirical findings and clinical observations, we explore the structure and measurement of neurocognitive domains using standardized neuropsychological performance measures. Particular attention is given to executive functions, working memory, and processing speed, which are frequently impaired and closely linked to adaptive functioning.

The idiographic and nomothetic approaches to understanding cognitive profiles are addressed, highlighting the need for culturally sensitive and behaviorally anchored assessments. Beyond core neurocognitive domains, the role of social cognition, including theory of mind (ToM), as a critical mediator of interpersonal functioning and community integration is considered. Impairments in emotion recognition, perspective-taking, and inferential reasoning are discussed in relation to their impact on social outcomes and their complex interplay with broader neurocognitive deficits. The limitations of current assessment tools and the challenges of linking test performance to real-world behavior are critically evaluated, with emphasis on the need for operational clarity and ecological validity.

G. F. McKeegan, *Behavior Change Interventions for Serious Mental Illness*, Evidence-Based Practices in Behavioral Health,
https://doi.org/10.1007/978-3-032-18372-9_10

Offering a framework linking cognitive impairment models with real-world support, practical behavior support strategies are outlined to enhance functional capacity, covering compensatory techniques that help individuals adapt to cognitive impairments and environmental modifications such as simplifying tasks, organizing spaces, and providing cues to reduce barriers in daily life. Integrative interventions are also discussed, emphasizing the use of neuropsychological insights and person-centered cognitive profiles and support planning that underscores the value of individualized, evidence-based care in clinical practice, research, and policy.

> My relative sometimes doesn't listen and forgets things we tell him. He forgets to take his medications and what days he has appointments. I asked him to help with chores, and he does not do it. I asked him what happened, and he said that he forgot but I told him only 10 min ago.

The Case of Donald

Donald is a 48-year-old man who was hospitalized after he began complaining about being constantly nervous and fearful, unable to sleep, wanting to stay alone, and having thoughts of suicide. He was admitted to a psychiatric facility. Upon being admitted, he refused to speak to anyone, ate very little, and sat in a corner so nobody could "sneak up" on him. He had difficulty finding his way around the ward and could not remember much of what he was told.

Donald had been previously hospitalized it was determined that he was living with "paranoid schizophrenia." He recovered quickly during that hospitalization and returned to his job as a supermarket clerk. During this hospitalization, he was diagnosed as severely depressed and was given antidepressant medication. Because he stayed in his room and could not remember much of what other people said to him, the staff was also concerned that he might be showing early signs of a dementing illness. They referred him to a neuropsychological assessment. This revealed a variety of mild cognitive problems and a serious impairment with his ability to remember information.

After a few weeks, Donald began to talk to other people more often, attended more groups, and was able to find his way around the ward and the hospital with fewer problems. However, the staff noticed that he continued to have problems with his memory and concentration. For example, he had difficulty remembering when family was scheduled to visit. In addition, he could talk to staff about general things that happened during mealtimes but could not remember what food had been served. While this improved a little with continued medication, it was still an obvious problem and one that would make it very difficult for Donald to take care of himself outside of the hospital. The staff decided that they needed to find a way to help him do more for himself despite his problems with memory and concentration.

Definition and Characteristics of Cognitive Impairments in Individuals Living with Serious Mental Illness

The concept of severe mental illness (SMI) is used to refer to a certain group of people with specific difficulties in personal and social functioning, derived from living with severe and persistent mental health problems. The concept of SMI is transdiagnostic; it is heterogeneous in problem behaviors emitted by people and is not related to a specific cluster of problem behaviors. An individual who experiences a persistent mental health condition resulting in considerable functional impairment, which substantially restricts major life activities, is classified as living with an SMI. The multiplicity and severity of the problems encountered when living with SMI impact the person's capabilities in social, family, educational, and occupational functioning.

According to the Diagnostic and Statistical Manual of Mental Disorders (fifth ed., text rev.) (American Psychiatric Association, 2022), neurocognitive impairments in people living with SMI:

> ... are common and strongly linked to vocational and functional impairments. These deficits can include decrements in declarative memory, working memory, language function, and other executive functions as well as slower processing speed. abnormalities in sensory processing and inhibitory capacity as well as reductions in attention are also found (p. 116).

Neurocognitive impairment affects 50–80% of individuals living with SMIs, impacting development and treatment strategies (McCleery & Nuechterlein, 2019). A high percentage of people living with SMI show poor performance in different aspects of neurocognitive abilities, such as processing speed, attention, working memory, verbal and learning skills, reasoning, and social cognition (O'Carroll, 2000; Keefe & Harvey, 2012; McCleery & Nuechterlein, 2019). In addition, these impairments predate the onset of the problem behaviors and symptoms that are linked to living with SMI and are persistent. They are an intrinsic part of the mental health problem of living with SMI (O'Carroll, 2000). Neurocognitive functioning has been shown to be moderately to severely impaired in people living with SMI; efforts to explain core features of SMI as a consequence of specific neuropsychological performance impairments have been disappointing as the studies find that the total composite scores on neuropsychological performance test batteries are the sole correlated index with other problems behaviors and symptoms of living with SMI (O,Carroll, 2000). The impairments found in neurocognitive domains have been hypothesized to be the prime driver of the significant disabilities in occupational, social, and economic functioning in people living with SMI and should be an important target of treatment (Green et al., 2000; Keefe & Harvey, 2012; Réthelyi et al., 2012).

Neurocognitive functioning is determined by the evaluation of dimensions of a domain using neuropsychological performance measures or tests. For example, the dimensions of verbal memory in the neurocognitive domain of memory can be assessed using the California Verbal Learning Test (CVLT). The task demands of the CVLT require the examinee to learn a 16-word list that is read to them by the examiner and then is asked to recall the words. The number correctly recalled is then compared to a sample of people who are representative of a larger group. This "normative group" is used to establish what is considered normal or average for a particular test or measure. The task demands of the CVLT implicitly measure dimensions in other neurocognitive domains such as attention to verbal stimuli, comprehension of verbal presented instructions, and the planning and execution of learning the words. Neuropsychological performance measures tap into the capacities of dimension in other domains than the intended domain. The performance tests typically measure the examinees current "abilities" on a dimension of a "capacity" in a specified neurocognitive domain.

"Ability" is the current overtly or covertly displayed skill, while capacity is the potential to develop the skill. Capability is the assessed proficiency for a defined end (amastyleinsider, 2011). Although these words are used interchangeably, one must consider what is being assessed and whether the observed neurocognitive impairment on a neuropsychological performance measure is the current ability in a dimension or future capability to acquire proficiency in that dimension (Hoffman, 2023).

Neurocognitive impairments in people living with SMI are defined as obtained scores on neuropsychological performance measures in certain neurocognitive domains that are lower when compared to a normative group based on sex, age, and educational level. Neuropsychological performance tests (American Psychological Association, n.d.-e) are clinical instruments for assessing impairment in dimensions of neurocognitive domains, including those measuring memory, language, learning, attention, and visuospatial and visuo-constructive functioning (Burdick & Goldberg, 2008). A comprehensive neuropsychological testing battery is usually used; it is a compendium of different evaluative techniques that is used to assess the functioning and integrity of various neurocognitive capabilities of an individual (Ardila & Ostrosky, 2022; McCleery & Nuechterlein, 2019). People living with SMI have typically performed between one and two standard deviations below the level of the normative sample in specific neurocognitive domains (McCutcheon et al., 2023).

Standard neuropsychological performance measures continue to demonstrate the greatest sensitivity to functionally relevant neurocognitive impairments (Keefe & Harvey, 2012). Neurocognitive impairments on neuropsychological measures are found in different domains in people living with SMI. Impairments have repeatedly been shown with significant differences in the neurocognitive domains of attention and memory in people living with SMI when compared to results from people not having any serious mental health problems (De la Torre et al., 2021). Other studies showed that impairments in reaction time, processing speed, and episodic memory show the largest differences compared to individuals with no mental health problem and possibly impact overall performance on many other neuropsychological tests (Barrett et al., 2009; McCutcheon, 2023; Schaefer et al., 2013). According to reviews (McCleery & Nuechterlein, 2019), the largest and significant effect sizes on neuropsychological performance measures have been shown to be on the neurocognitive domains of memory, processing speed, attention/vigilance, working memory, verbal learning and memory, and visual learning. Results on measures of reasoning and problem-solving show less impairment compared to other domains but are still significant.

Executive function (EF) is composed of an array of neurocognitive skills, such as task initiation, organization, flexibility, setting priorities, problem solving, working memory, and control of impulsivity and emotions (Baggetta & Alexander, 2016). EF is crucial for self-regulation and goal-directed behavior. Individual differences in EF are linked to academic performance, interpersonal issues, substance use, and both physical and mental health. Impairments in this neurocognitive domain are associated with various mental health problems and predict intrusive and repeated worrying and poor emotion regulation strategies (Snyder et al., 2015).

Executive function (EF) (Shahrockh & Hales, 2003) consists of distinct neurocognitive processes, including cognitive flexibility (i.e., capacity for objective appraisal and appropriate flexible action (American Psychological Association, n.d.-c), inhibition, updating, and working memory (WM) (American Psychological Association, n.d.-o). Impairments in EF are prevalent across various mental health problems corresponding to SMI, with the largest deficits observed in individuals living with schizophrenia spectrum mental health problems followed by bipolar and major depression mental health problems. Impairments in EF are linked to behavioral disinhibitions and various externalizing behavior problems, such as ADHD, substance use, and personality disorders (Snyder et al., 2015). However, EF is difficult to define operationally and measure due to non-specificity of assessment tasks and overlapping neurocognitive processes that compose EF.

The neurocognitive impairments that are found in people living with SMI are consistent across various studies and meta-analyses, indicating a broad and significant impact on neurocognitive functioning in people living with SMI (McCleery & Nuechterlein, 2019); in addition, the impairments are relatively stable over time, with no significant progressive decline in most cases (McCleery & Nuechterlein, 2019).

Despite these impairments being consistently found, no associations have been demonstrated between impairments of performances on specific neuropsychological measures and observed problem behaviors and symptoms (both positive and negative) in individuals living with SMI. Research has shown that the relationships between scores on neuropsychological measures and functional behaviors are often not specific, with multiple neurocognitive domains often contributing to functional difficulties, making it challenging to pinpoint a single neurocognitive impairment as the sole cause of a functional deficit (Harvey et al., 2006; Harvey & Strassnig, 2012). Evidence suggests that there are certain functional domains (such as social outcomes) that are more strongly predicted by impairments other than neurocognition, including social skill deficits and certain problem behaviors and symptoms (i.e., blunted affect and apathetic social withdrawal) (Leifker et al., 2009). The term neurocognition will be used in this chapter to denote objective, performance-based operations related to the uptake and manipulation of information, whereas cognition will be defined as the subjective, self-reported, private event that is related to problems with thinking, beliefs, and perceptions.

Neurocognitive impairments in people living with schizophrenic spectrum mental health problems are phenotypically similar to other severe mental health problems but differ in magnitude of the impairment (McCutcheon et al., 2023). There appear to be nonlinear relationships between dimensions of symptoms and behavior problems related to living with a SMI and neurocognitions; this suggests that neurocognitive domain impairments may impact functioning but only beyond a certain level of severity (McCutcheon et al., 2023).

Problems in the functional domains of neurocognition must be considered for a complete picture of the individual's problems in psychosocial functioning. Demonstrated impairments on assessments of long- and short-term memories, planning, vigilance, psychomotor speed, and executive functioning appear to be positively correlated with levels of functional capacities in certain domains (Green, 1996; Heinrichs & Zakzanis, 1998) but lack specificity in how neurocognitive impairment affects the performance of a particular behavioral function. The lack of consistent operational definitions of functional behaviors, the heterogeneity of neurocognitive and functional impairments in individuals living with SMI and the use of composite scores from neuropsychological test batteries with large samples deter the identification of specific neurocognitive impairments being linked to specific behavioral deficits or excesses in defined problem behaviors. Future research needs to aim at improving behavioral and neuropsychological assessments and integrating both with operational definitions of the dimensions of problem behaviors exhibited by people living with SMI.

Individuals living with SMI show impairments in social cognition. Social cognition refers to domains of abilities that are neurocognitive but directly linked to the skills required for social functioning, such as interpersonal perception and interactions. Domains of social cognition include visual and auditory modalities of recognition of emotions, inference of other's impressions of oneself, judgment of intentions, and other related domains (Green et al., 2019; Hugenberg & Wilson, 2013).

Several reviews suggested that social cognition has consistent correlations with social functioning, including social milestones such as marriage and developing and maintaining stable relationships with others. One of the issues associated with social cognition, however, is that its definition and measurement are not as advanced in neuropsychological performance measures or defining functional capacity. There is very little known about the psychometric properties of these measures, and many of them have been modified by individual research groups, leading to reduced comparability across studies related to more standardized neuropsychological assessment methods. Furthermore, there has been very little research examining the contribution of social cognition to other functional domains such as employment, where social abilities are required to acquire and maintain employment (Cotter et al., 2017; Leifker et al., 2009). Nevertheless, adequate neurocognitive abilities are necessary but not sufficient for effective social cognition and higher-order metacognitive abilities (i.e., awareness of and ability to think about one's own thinking processes (Minor et al., 2015).

A component of social cognition is the theory of mind (ToM). ToM includes the ability to infer the intentions of other people (Thomas, 2010). It has been hypothesized that individuals living with SMI have impairments in ToM based on impairments in social skills and social neurocognitions (Myers et al., 2024; Roncone et al., 2002); one possible result of this impairment is that the person living with SMI attends to and interprets irrelevant stimuli as meaningful and causative leading to erroneous decisions, deleterious interpersonal behaviors, and social maladjustment (e.g., misinterpreting a person's accidental contact in a crowded subway as a physical threat). One can see how an impairment in the social cognition of recognizing emotions in faces of others can lead to other symptoms and problem behaviors displayed by people living with SMI, like delusions.

Correlations have been shown between ToM tasks and neurocognitive functions like sustained attention, verbal fluency, and psychomotor speed. Global neurocognitive impairments significantly correlate with ToM impairments (Roncone et al., 2002). Neurocognitive impairment differences exist, but their specific impact on ToM performance has not been thoroughly analyzed. IQ correlates with ToM task performance but adding IQ as a variable does not add to any prediction of social functioning (Mitchell & Young 2016). A review of research examining Theory of Mind (ToM) task performance suggests that individuals diagnosed with schizophrenia spectrum conditions frequently demonstrate more pronounced impairments compared to those with bipolar mental health problems. Furthermore, people living with schizophrenia spectrum conditions face heightened difficulties in comprehending social cues (Mitchell and Young, 2016). Studies indicate that differences in neurocognitive functions, including verbal and working memory, co-exist with ToM impairments. Overall, the findings suggest a complex interplay of factors influencing performances on ToM measures (Mitchell & Young, 2016).

However, these measures are not predictive of actual "real life" functioning (Harvey & Strassnig, 2012). Social functionings, such as interpersonal perception and behavioral interactions, have a better predictive value for adaptive functioning than scores on neuropsychological tests. Performance on tests associated with domains of social cognition, such as emotion recognition (in both visual and auditory modalities), inference of other's impressions of oneself, and judgment of intentions of others, is inferred to impact functional capacities in everyday life (Green, 1996; Harvey & Strassnig, 2012); however, significant correlations have not been found. Causal relationships between neuropsychological test scores and behavioral functions would be more difficult to obtain due to the complexity of the variables involved.

It has been acknowledged by academics and researchers that a broad spectrum of neurocognitive impairments accompanies the phenomenon of SMI. There is a question whether the neurocognitive impairments seen in individuals living with SMI are the core features of the mental health problems related to SMI and if the mental health problems linked to SMI are best characterized by the neurocognitive impairments and problems (Elvevag & Goldberg, 2000; Green & Nuechterlein, 1999). Furthermore, do specific profiles of neurocognitive impairments assist in determining treatments and outcomes? Yet despite the acknowledgment of neurocognitive impairments as being a serious problem resulting in compromised functioning, it is not a diagnostic criterion for a determination of any mental health problems associated with SMI (Galderisi & Marder, 2024) but is an associated feature (American Psychiatric Association, 2022). Neurocognitive impairments associated with living with SMI are not included in the DSM-5 (American Psychiatric Association, 2022) or ICD-11 (World Health Organization [WHO], 2019) criteria for any mental health problems associated with SMI. The neurocognitive impairments that have been researched are heterogeneous and independent of other domains of problem behaviors and symptoms and are observed across all stages of living with SMI (Galderisi & Marder, 2024).

Dimensions of Neurocognitive Capabilities and Impairments

Neurocognitive capabilities such as memory, attention, problem-solving, and decision-making are crucial in determining an individual's functional status. Neurocognitive impairments can affect rehabilitation outcomes, functional independence, and quality of life. Comprehensive assessment tools that include neurocognitive components are necessary to accurately evaluate functional status, especially in populations with neurocognitive impairments (Knight, 2000).

Neurocognitive abilities and impairments can be defined as mental processes of learning and knowing, including domains in awareness, perception, reasoning, memory, and judgment. Neuropsychology focuses primarily on assessing aspects of neurocognition by using a variety of computerized and pencil-and-paper tests to assess these functions of a person's neurological system (Burdick & Goldberg, 2008). Neurocognitive capability is a complex construct with individual processes interdependently contributing to the person's performance on an individual test. Studies using imaging techniques have shown that multiple neuroanatomical substrates subserve distinct neurocognitive functions that are activated while a person is engaged in performing on a specific neuropsychological test that assesses one dimension of neurocognitive capabilities (Ardilia & Ostrosky, 2022; Burdick & Goldberg, 2008).

Neurocognitive domains—such as memory—are composed of dimensions that exist on a continuum rather than distinct categories. A dimensional focus recognizes that problems displayed by people living with SMI can vary in intensity and frequency across a spectrum, rather than being simply present or absent in all contexts (i.e., categorical approach). A dimensional perspective unifies normal functioning and behaviors and impairments on an underlying continuum. Neurocognitive abilities and impairments are demonstrated by scores obtained on standardized neuropsychological tests; results are then compared to normative scores of a specified population. Impairments are defined when the scores on neuropsychological performance measures are statistically significantly lower than would be expected or when compared to scores from a normative group. The scores on neuropsychological tests are influenced by age, gender, and education of the person taking the test. The demands of the testing items also influence the score. For example, some test items have strict time limits that impact the successful completion of the items so slower response time will negatively impact the person's score.

The Positive and Negative Symptom Scale (PANSS) is a commonly used dimensional scale for assessing symptoms and problem behaviors exhibited by people living with SMI. Each item of the PANSS is rated with 1 to 7 points ranging from absent to extreme (Kay et al., 1987). Nielsen et al. (2014) explored the relationship between "cognitive factors" on the PANSS and neuropsychological test performances in persons living with SMI. The findings indicated variability in neurocognitive performance, with certain indices falling within normal limits, whereas others, particularly those associated with speed, were markedly diminished. The rating from the PANSS showed nonspecific associations with neurocognitive indices related to performance speed, accuracy, problem-solving, and executive functioning (EF) (Bell et al., 1994; Rèthelyi et al., 2012). No discriminant validity, which is the degree to which a test or measure does not correlate with another measure whose underlying construct is conceptually unrelated to it (Kaplan & Saccuzzo, 2010), for neurocognitive factors was found, but the PANSS cognitive factors reflected verbal IQ but not memory, attention, or speed. Nielsen et al. (2014) concluded that neurocognitive test performances correlated with PANSS overall scores of problem behaviors and symptoms but in a nonspecific manner. The PANSS cognitive subscale appears to be reflective of over-learned verbal skills rather than specific neurocognitive impairments in people living with SMI.

Performance on four key neurocognitive tasks was used to search for subtypes in neurocognitive impairment in a sample of people living with SMI (Heinrichs & Awad, 1993). The neuropsychological instruments used were the Wisconsin Card Sorting Test (WCST) to assess executive functioning (EF), the California Verbal Learning Test (CVLT) to measure verbal memory function, the Purdue Pegboard (Lafayette Instrument Company, n.d.) to index fine motor bilateral function, and the IQ from the Wechsler Adult Intelligence Scale-Revised (WAIS-R) to measure general neurocognitive functioning. The description, task demands, and neurocognitive domains assessed by each neurocognitive test used were as follows:

- WCST: requires the examinee to decide from verbal feedback (right vs. wrong) how to sort a series of cards depicting different geometric shapes in various colors, shapes, and quantities. Once the examinee has identified the initial underlying sorting solution (e.g., by color) and correctly sorts 10 consecutive cards, the solution is changed without being explicitly told but still getting verbal feedback as to the correctness of their solution. The task requires the examinee to change the concept to continue to correctly solve the sorting task. The sorting rule changes several times throughout the test, and the participant must adapt their strategy accordingly. The test is scored as to the number of correct sorts, the number of perseverative (repeating an incorrect sorting rule despite feedback) and non-perseverative errors (making a new, incorrect sorting rule), and number of categories completed (American Psychological Association, n.d.-n). Although the task involves many aspects of brain function, it is primarily considered a test of EF particularly abstract reasoning, working memory (WM), planning and problem-solving, and cognitive flexibility in response to external changes.
- CVLT: is a verbal word-list learning test consisting of 16 items belonging to one of four categories. The test assesses immediate free call in which the examiner is asked to recall as many words from a list following each of five learning trials as

well as an interference trial. Free recall and cued recall (recalling the word after being given a semantic cue) are also assessed following a short-term delay (immediately after the interference trial) and a long-term 20-min delay. Finally, long-term recognition is assessed using distractors that vary in their likelihood of eliciting false positive errors. CVLT measures short- and long-term verbal memory as well as verbal learning strategies (American Psychological Association, n.d.-b).

- Purdue peg board: is a test of manual dexterity and fine motor speed in which the participant—first with the dominant hand, then with the nondominant hand, and finally with both hands—inserts pegs in a series of holes as rapidly as possible. (American Psychological Association, n.d.-f). The results are the number of pegs inserted in the time-period for each hand (Lafayette Instrument Company, 2025).
- WAIS-R: is a test of intellectual abilities. The test yields separate verbal, performance, and overall IQ. The test includes verbal subtests (information, comprehension, arithmetic, similarities, digit span, vocabulary) and performance subtests (digit symbol, picture completion, block design, picture arrangement, object assembly, symbol search). It also gives index scores on four domains of neurocognitive abilities—verbal comprehension, perceptual organization, processing speed, and WM (American Psychological Association, n.d.-m).

Data were analyzed using cluster analyses, and five clusters were found. Cluster 1 was comprised of individuals with EF impairment; cluster 2 suggested neurocognitive functioning within the average range; cluster 3 involved persons with EF and neurocognitive motor impairments; cluster 4 suggested general and multifocal impairments; and cluster 5 consisted of people living with SMI with selective motor and coordination impairments (e.g., tremors, involuntary movements, slurred speech) (Heinrichs & Awad, 1993). The clusters significantly differed in age, duration of illness, and extent of hospitalization. There were trends in gender composition and anti-Parkinsonian medication patterns. The authors (Heinrichs & Awad, 1993) concluded that the cluster analyses of the scores on the neurocognitive tasks has the possibility in reducing and clarifying the heterogeneity of neurocognitive impairments in persons living with SMI; however, the results also supported the heterogeneity of neurocognitive impairments obtained on neuropsychological testing given that the number of persons in each cluster of impairments were roughly equivalent, ranging from 19 to 25.

McCutcheon et al. (2023) found that seven neurocognitive domains were affected in persons living with SMI: (a) processing speed; (b) attention; (c) working memory (WM); (d) verbal learning and memory; (e) visual learning and memory; (f) reasoning; and (g) social cognition. Further dimensionality reductions suggest that these seven domains can be grouped into larger parent domains of (1) processing speed; (2) attention/WM; and (3) learning (McCutcheon et al., 2023). Processing speed is often the most affected domain with individuals living with SMI typically performing around one standard deviation (SD) below the level of individuals with no mental health problems. Deficits in processing speed are the strongest predictor of general cognitive performance in individuals living with SMI. Because processing speed is a component of many other cognitive functions, deficits in this domain may reflect impairments in other higher-order functions (McCutcheon et al., 2023). For example, people living with SMI may approach processing speed tests with less strategic planning. Impairments in lower-level domains such as reaction time could contribute detrimentally to the scores in higher-order domains such as memory, learning, and cognitive flexibility (McCutcheon et al., 2023).

There are a variety of neuropsychological tests that are aimed at measuring various domains of neurocognitive functioning. For example, there are at least four different tests of learning and memory to assess this neurocognitive domain including logical memory (LM); California Verbal Learning Test (CVLT); Verbal Paired-Associate Learning (VAL); and digit span (DS) (Silva et al., 2012). There are three frequently used comprehensive neurocognitive performance batteries, four brief neurocognitive performance batteries; and two interview-based measures of neurocognition that differ on correlated reports from other individuals familiar with the behavior of the person living with SMI. The neurocognitive performance measures and batteries differ on the domains assessed and the length of time needed to complete the evaluation (Nasrallah, 2023).

In an effort to standardize the assessment of neurocognitive functions in people living with SMI, the National Institute of Mental Health–Measurement and Treatment Research to Improve Cognition in Schizophrenia (NIMH-MATRICS) (Marder & Fenton, 2004) collaborated with researchers and academics to develop an initiative dedicated to enhancing research on the neurocognitive impairments exhibited by people living with SMI and the development of effective neurocognitive-enhancing medications for these mental health problems. The initiative developed a standard neuropsychological test battery to assess neurocognition in people living with SMI (MATRICS Consensus Cognitive Battery (MCCB)). The primary aim for the MATRICS is that neurocognitive impairments as assessed with neuropsychological performance measures should be linked to the daily activities of individuals living with SMI; that is, what specific neurocognitive impairments impact on what specific functional capabilities of the person living with SMI (Green et al., 2004). Adoption of the MCCB in studies of neurocognition in individuals living with SMI facilitates replication to confirm research findings (Nasrallah, 2023).

The MATRICS initiative agreed on a battery of seven major neurocognitive functions that often show impairments in individuals living with SMI (Green et al., 2004). The seven major neurocognitive dimensions that were identified in the NIMH-MATRICS endeavor include:

1. Speed of processing: Processing speed is the speed at which an individual identifies, manipulates, and responds to information. Processing speed encompasses "active" and "automatic" activities. Processing speed is the ability to identify, discriminate, integrate, and decide about information using both visual and verbal information. Response processes for speeded tests are typically motoric (e.g., written response, check a response) or oral (e.g., saying an object's name, reading numbers or letters aloud).

2. Attention/vigilance: It is a state in which neurocognitive resources are focused on certain aspects of the environment rather than on others, and the central nervous system (CNS) is in a state of readiness to respond to stimuli (American Psychological Association, n.d.-a).
3. Working memory (WM): WM comprises a phonological loop (repeating short string of verbal information) for temporarily manipulating and storing speech-based information and a "visuospatial sketchpad" that performs a similar function for visual and spatial information. Both are monitored by a limited capacity in EF (American Psychological Association, n.d.-o).
4. Verbal learning and memory: Process of learning verbally presented stimuli and responses and the capacity to remember and recall what was previously learned (American Psychological Association, n.d.-k).
5. Visual learning and memory: The process of learning visually presented stimuli and responses and the capacity to remember and recall what was previously learned (American Psychological Association, n.d.-l).
6. Reasoning and problem-solving: Higher-order neurocognitive domains in which logical processes of an inductive or deductive character are used to draw conclusions from facts or premises to overcome difficulties, achieve plans that move from a starting situation to a desired goal, and reach conclusions (American Psychological Association, n.d.-h).
7. Verbal comprehension (VC): It is an individual's ability to understand the language used by others (American Psychological Association, n.d.-j).

Although identified as a major neurocognitive domains and whose impairments are significantly related to neurocognitive and adaptive functioning in people living with SMI Nasrallah, 2023), VC was not included in the MCCB due to its resistance to change; it was not considered appropriate for a neurocognitive battery intended to be sensitive to change, (Nuechterlein et al., 2004; Nuechterlein et al., 2008). A measure of social cognition was included in the final version of the MCCB (Nuechterlein et al., 2004; Nuechterlein et al., 2008).

The MCCB is composed of neuropsychological tests whose aim is to obtain a score that is indicative of seven domains of neurocognitive functioning that have been reported to impact overall functioning in people living with SMI (Green et al., 2004). The seven domains were chosen using empirical evidence for neurocognitive performance dimensions in people living with SMI, emphasizing factor analytic studies (Burton et al., 2013; Nuechterlein et al., 2004). A summary of the tests in the MCCB to assess dimensions associated with neurocognitive domains and performance indices is as follows (McCleery & Nuechterlein, 2019):

1. Speed of processing

   Tests: BACS Symbol Coding, Category Fluency Test (Animal Naming Fluency), Trail Making Test (TMT) (Part A).

   Performance indices: total number correct, total number of animals named in 60 seconds, time to completion
2. Attention/vigilance

   Test: Continuous Performance Test (Identical Pairs) (CPT-IP)

Performance index: overall performance

3. Working memory

   Tests: Wechsler Memory Scale Third Edition Spatial Span (WMS-III), Letter-Number Span Test (LNS).

   Performance indices: sum of raw scores for forward and backward conditions, number of correct trials

4. Verbal learning and memory

   Test: Hopkins Verbal Learning Test-Revised (HVLT-R).

   Performance index: total number of words recalled correctly over three learning trials.

5. Visual learning and memory

   Test: Brief Visuospatial Memory Test-Revised (BVMT-R)

   Performance index: total recall score over learning trials

6. Reasoning and problem solving

   Test: Neuropsychological Assessment Battery (NAB) Mazes Subtest (NAB Mazes).

   Performance Index: total raw score

7. Social Cognition

   Test: Mayer-Salovey-Caruso Emotional Intelligence Test (MSCEIT) Managing Emotions (DeTore et al., 2018).

   Performance index: standard score across all responses.

The CogState Schizophrenia Battery is a brief computerized neurocognitive test battery designed to assess neurocognitive impairment in individuals with SMI. The battery is designed to be brief, taking approximately 40 min to complete, and is administered using a computerized format to ensure standardized presentation of stimuli and recording of responses. The tasks are selected and modified from established neurocognitive and experimental psychological paradigms to be sensitive to neurocognitive changes and to minimize practice effects. The battery assesses the same identified neurocognitive domains as the MATRICS (Pietrzak et al., 2009). The computerized neuropsychological performance tasks included in the battery are listed as follows:

- Detection task (detect): measures speed of processing by assessing the average speed of correct responses.
- Identification task (Ident): measures attention/vigilance by assessing the average speed of correct responses.
- One-back memory task (one-back): measures WM by assessing the proportion of correct responses.
- Two-back memory task (two-back): measures WM by assessing the proportion of correct responses.
- Visual learning task (vis-learn): measures visual learning by assessing the proportion of correct responses.
- International Shopping List Task (ISLT): measures verbal learning by assessing the number of words recalled across three learning trials.

- Groton Maze Learning Task (GMLT): measures reasoning and problem solving by assessing the number of errors made across five learning trials.
- Social Emotional Cognition Task (SECT): measures social cognition by assessing the proportion of correct responses.

Pietrzak et al. (2009) compared the scores on the MATRICS and the CogStat battery and found that both batteries equally detected neurocognitive impairments in individuals living with SMI. The study used a functional capacity assessment instrument: the University of California at San Diego (UCSD) Performance-based Skills Assessment (UPSA) (Patterson et al., 2001). The UPSA was used to determine the impact of neurocognitive impairments on functional abilities in daily life. The UPSA assesses the ability to perform everyday tasks and activities that are necessary for independent living using role plays that simulate everyday activities. The UPSA includes role-plays of functional tasks in the following domains:

- Household chores: creating a grocery shopping list based on a recipe.
- Managing finances: writing a check to pay a bill or reading a bank statement and asked to identify possible errors or budget concerns.
- Communicating with others: calling to make or reschedule a doctor's appointment or having a phone conversation with a landlord to discuss a repair issue.
- Transportation: planning a trip using public transportation using a bus schedule.
- Planning and organizing recreational activities: getting tickets for a show.

The role plays on the UPSA are a limited sample of functional capacities yet complex domains of functional capacities are inferred from the results based on the assessment of role plays. Not surprisingly, evidence supports that functional capacity is strongly related to neuropsychological performance scores, but only moderately to real-world scores (Bowie & Harvey, 2006).

There has been a historic overlap in the neuropsychological test performance demands and neurocognitive abilities and the domains being assessed. The overlap has been found in the patterns of positive correlations among diverse neurocognitive tests. The numerous positive correlations have been described as a general factor, or "g" (for general intelligence) in the literature, a process overlap theory in which neurocognitive tests tap into domain-general executive functioning (EF) processes (identified primarily in research on WM), or more domain-specific processes. EF processes are tapped into more frequently across many neurocognitive tests than domain-specific ones (Kovacs & Conway, 2016).

Research is needed to assess the relationships among the behavioral task domains of functional capacities and the results on the specific neuropsychological performance measures in the neurocognitive domains being assessed for individuals living with SMI; research results have shown variability on neuropsychological performance scores across individuals but more importantly intraindividual differences across performance scores (Casaletto & Heaton, 2017).

Neuropsychological performance batteries differ widely in content, duration, procedures, and implementation. The limited generalizability of neurocognitive findings across studies has reduced the ability of clinicians and researchers to make clear conclusions about the relative impact of the various interventions, dimensions of neurocognitive domains, and the relationship to functional behavioral capacities in people living with SMI (Keefe et al., 2004). The NIMH-MATRICS agenda was to identify neurocognitive domains and a battery of neuropsychological performance tests both to increase standardization aiming to increase sensitivity to improvement from interventions, most notably for neurocognitive training interventions (Green et al., 2014). In this way, specific impairments in both the neurocognitive and functional behavioral domains can be targeted and effective interventions developed.

Neurocognitive improvements are linked to better functional outcomes, but neurocognitive performance alone does not directly predict real-world success. Factors such as motivation and negative symptoms (i.e., the diminution of expected behaviors) also influence functional performance. Comprehensive treatment strategies targeting skill acquisition and behaviors that are related to decreased display of behavioral skills are essential for improving real-world outcomes (Bowie & Harvey, 2006).

The neuropsychological performance measures on the MCCB to assess the identified neurocognitive domains were chosen by consensus decision of a panel of experts in the field (Nuechterlein et al., 2004; Nuechterlein et al., 2008). However, other valid and reliable neuropsychological performance measures have been used to assess the neurocognitive domains assessed by the MCCB. Using a sample of participants living with multiple sclerosis, Eilam-Stock et al. (2021) validated the Cognitive Assessment Interview (CAI), an interview-based measure of cognitive impairment (Ventura et al., 2010). The CAI is composed of 10 items that are administered to both the person living with SMI and another individual familiar with their daily functioning. Ventura et al. (2010) reported that the CAI was validated by examining the relationship between the CAI and objective measures of neurocognitive functioning, intermediate measures of neurocognition, and functional outcomes. Table 10.1 presents the interview items on the CAI, the neurocognitive domain related to the item, and the neuropsychological performance measures used by Eilam-Stock et al. (2021). The results found that the CAI ratings were moderately correlated with self-reported neurocognitive difficulties by the sample of people living with MS but only mildly correlated with objective neuropsychological measures (Eilam-Stock et al., 2021; Giordano et al., 2022) showing that the social and construct validity of the CAI when used with a people living with a neurological health problem may be lacking. Studies following the experimental method of Eilam-Stock et al. (2021) should be used with samples of individuals living with SMI and differentiation on other significant variables including scores of measures of adaptive functioning.

The Brief Assessment of Cognition in Schizophrenia (BACS) was developed for clinical use as the length of administration is 35 min as compared to primary neuropsychological performance batteries that require up to 2 h. BACS was found to be sensitive to neurocognitive impairments in people living with SMI as a standard primary battery. In addition, the domains of neurocognitive functions that are assessed by the BACS are those found in the research literature to be consistently impaired and related to outcomes in individuals living with SMI (Keefe et al., 2004).

Table 10.1 CAI item number, item, neurocognitive domain, and the neuropsychological performance measures used by Eilam-Stock et al. (2021)

CAI #	Item	Neurocognitive domain	Neuropsychological performance measure
1	Difficulty maintaining newly learned information in mind for brief periods (long enough to use)	Working memory	Wechsler adult intelligence scale, fourth edition (WAIS-IV): Digit span backward and letter–number sequencing subtests
2	Difficulty performing "on the spot" mental manipulations or computations	Working memory	
3	Problems sustaining concentration over time (without distraction)	Attention/ concentration	WAIS-IV: Digit span forward
4	Difficulty focusing on select information (if there is not obvious distraction)?	Attention/ concentration	
5	Trouble learning and remembering verbal material?	Verbal learning and memory	Selective reminding test (SRT); brief visuospatial memory test—Revised (BVMT-R)
6	Difficulty recalling recent events?	Verbal learning and memory	
7	Lack of flexibility in generating alternate plans when needed?	Reasoning and problem solving	Delis-Kaplan executive function system (D-KEFS); trail making test-B (alternating numbers and letters condition)
8	Problems in situations requiring judgment?	Reasoning and problem solving	
9	Performs tasks slowly?	Speed of processing	Paced auditory serial addition test (PASAT)
10	Difficulty appreciating another person's intentions/ point of view?	Social cognition	Symbol digit modalities test (SDMT)

The domains assessed in the BACS are reasoning and problem solving, verbal fluency, attention, verbal memory, working memory (WM), and motor speed. The neurocognitive domain, the neuropsychological performance measures to assess the domain, and a description of the task demands on the BACS are listed below:

- Verbal memory: list learning test. The examinee is presented with 15 words and then asked to recall as many as possible. This procedure is repeated five times. The outcome measure is the total number of words recalled. There are two alternate forms (Keefe et al., 2004).
- WM: digit sequencing task. The examinee is presented with numerical clusters of increasing length and is asked to tell the experimenter the numbers in order, from lowest to highest. The trials increase in difficulty, and the outcome measure is the total number of correct items.

- Motor speed: token motor task. The examinee is given 100 plastic tokens and asked to place them into a container as quickly as possible for 60 seconds. The outcome measure is the total number of tokens placed in the container.
- Semantic fluency: category instances test. The examinee is given 60 seconds to name as many words as possible within the category of supermarket items. The outcome measure is the total number of unique words generated.
- Letter fluency: controlled oral word association test. In two separate trials, the examinee is given 60 seconds to generate as many words as possible that begin with the letters F and S. The outcome measure is the total number of unique words generated.
- Reasoning and problem solving: Tower of London Test. The examinee looks at two pictures simultaneously. Each picture shows three different-colored balls arranged on three pegs, with the balls in a unique arrangement in each picture. The examinee is told about the rules of the task and is asked to provide the least number of times the balls in one picture would have to be moved to make the arrangement of balls identical to that of the opposing picture. The outcome measure is the number of trials on which the correct response is provided. There are two alternate forms.
- Attention and processing speed: symbol coding. The examinee is asked to write numerals 1–9 as matches to symbols on a response sheet as quickly as possible for 90 seconds. The outcome measure is the total number of correct responses.
- Composite Score. A composite score is calculated by comparing the examinee's performance on each measure to the performance of a comparison group.

The Cambridge Neuropsychological Test Automated Battery (CANTAB) (Sahakian & Owen, 1992) is neuropsychological performance battery that has been developed over two decades; it consists of eight computerized tests assessing the same neurocognitive domains as MCCB (Nuechterlein et al., 2008). A primary computerized neuropsychological performance battery to assess neurocognition in people living with SMI is advantageous as the use of a computerized version reduces the variability in administration of the tests (e.g., instructions and timing are standardized). The CANTAB has been found to have similar properties to the MCCB to assess impairments in the dimensions of neurocognitive domains in people living with SMI (Barrnett et al., 2010).

The tests on the CANTAB battery are described along with the neurocognitive processes it measures, and the approximate duration for administration to the examinee is summarized below (Barrnett et al., 2010):

Attention/Vigilance (sustained attention, signal detection, impulsivity).

Rapid visual information processing (RVP): a continuous performance test of sustained attention where examinees monitor a stream of single digits for a sequence of three-digit numbers.

Duration: 9 min.

WM (WM, strategy use).

Spatial working memory (SWM): self-ordered search task based on foraging behavior, where participants search an array for tokens without returning to previous token locations.
Duration: 10 min.

Visual learning (associative learning, short-term visual memory).

Paired associates learning (PAL): object-location associative learning test where participants learn to associate patterns with locations on the screen.
Duration: 10 min. .

Speed of processing (processing speed, motor speed, divided attention).

Simple and five-choice reaction time (RTI): human analogue of the five-choice serial reaction time task (5-CSRTT), measuring reaction time and movement time separately. This test is employed extensively to measure attention in nonhuman species in the laboratory. The task involves animals trained to respond to a brief, unpredictable visual stimulus presented in one of five locations. The effects of experimental manipulations on response speed and choice accuracy are measured, and each related to attentional performance. The 5-CSRTT is also used to measure motor impulsivity (Higgins & Silenieks, 2017).
Duration: 5 min.

Verbal learning (verbal learning, immediate recall, recognition, and delayed recognition).

Verbal recognition/recall Memory (VRM): Verbal list learning task with delayed recognition after 20 min, available in multiple languages.
Duration: 7 min.

Social cognition (emotion recognition, decision latency).

Emotion Recognition Test (ERT): facial emotion labeling task where participants choose between six primary emotions and neutral.
Duration: 10 min.

Reasoning/problem solving (rule learning, rule reversal, attentional set shifting).

Intra/extra-dimensional set-shifting (IED): test of cognitive flexibility analogous to the Wisconsin Card Sort Test (WCST), with multiple stages segregating neurocognitive processes.
Duration: 10 min.

Visual planning (visual planning, reasoning, impulsivity).

One-Touch Stockings of Cambridge (OTS): visual planning task based on the Tower of London and the CANTAB Stockings of Cambridge (One Touch Stocking of Cambridge (OTS)—Cambridge Cognition, 2023). The Stockings of Cambridge presents three colored balls. The stacks of colored balls held in stockings or socks are suspended from a beam. The examinee is required to move the balls in the lower display to copy the pattern in the upper display. After completing one demonstration problem, requiring one move, the examinee must then complete three further problems, one each requiring two moves, three moves, and four moves. Next, the examinee is shown further problems and must work out how many moves the solutions require and then select the appropriate box at the bottom of the screen to indicate their response (One Touch Stocking of Cambridge (OTS) - Cambridge Cognition, 2023).

Duration: 9 min.

As with other neuropsychological performance batteries, there is an overlap in the dimensions of the neurocognitive domains that the individual tests in the battery are measuring. For example, the test that is used to assess the domain of speed of processing on the CANTAB also measures the dimensions of processing speed, motor speed, divided attention, and impulsivity as the task used also measures impulsiveness in lower animals in experimental procedures (Higgins & Silenieks, 2017).

The CogState Schizophrenia Battery is a brief computerized self-administered neurocognitive performance test battery that assesses the same cognitive domains as the MCCB (Pietrzak et al., 2009): speed of processing, attention/vigilance, working memory (WM), verbal learning, visual learning, reasoning and problem solving, and social cognition. Table 10.2 summarizes the details of the tasks and scoring criteria for the assessed neurocognitive domains. .

Pietrzak et al. (2009) found that both the MCCB and CogState batteries equally detected neurocognitive impairments in individuals living with SMI. The authors also found positive correlations using the scores from a functional behavioral capacity measure (i.e., UPSA) and the composite scores on both batteries that support the link between neurocognitive and functional performances. Limitations included potential fatigue effects from test order.

The UPSA is a brief measure of functional behavioral capacities (Patterson et al., 2001); it uses short role plays in simulated situations to assess the proficiency and correctness of behaviors in five dimensions in the functional domain of daily adaptive behaviors—housekeeping, communication, finance, transportation, and planning a recreational activity. The authors state that there is a need for further research on other functional capacity measures. Specifically, more research is needed to determine which specific neurocognitive domains—and specific dimensions in neurocognitive domains—are associated with behavioral functional capacity outcomes. This can help tailor interventions to target the neurocognitive impairments that significantly impact daily functioning. Future studies should include a variety of functional behavioral capacity measures beyond the UPSA to validate the findings and explore the relationships between neurocognitive functions and different aspects of functional capacity. The influence of cultural, ethnic, and demographic factors on neurocognitive performance and functional capacity needs to be considered and researched to ensure the generalizability of the findings (Pietrzak et al., 2009).

A study by Gold et al. (2018) theorized that people living with mental health problems associated with SMI demonstrate impairments on neuropsychological tests for selective attention, working memory (WM), and executive functioning

Table 10.2 Computerized neurocognitive tasks, domains, outcome score, and task completion criteria on the cogstate schizophrenia battery developed by Pietrzak et al. (2009)

Computerized neurocognitive tasks	Task description	Neurocognitive domain	Outcome score	Task completion criteria
Detection task (detect)	Speed of response to a simple stimulus	Speed of Processing	Average speed of correct responses	75% of trials completed
Identification task (ident)	Assesses ability to identify stimulus and respond accurately and quickly.	Attention/ Vigilance	Average number of correct responses	75% of trials completed
One-Back memory task (one-back)	Ability to remember and respond to a stimulus that appeared one step earlier in a sequence	Working memory	Proportion of correct responses	75% of trials completed
Two-Back memory task (two-Back)	Ability to remember and respond to a stimulus that appeared two steps earlier in a sequence.	Working memory	Proportion of correct responses	75% of trials completed
Visual learning task (Vis-learn)	Ability to learn and recall visual information.	Visual Learning	Proportion of correct responses	75% of trials completed
International shopping list task (ISLT)	Ability to learn and recall a list of words presented verbally.	Verbal Learning	Number of words recalled across three learning trials	Recall on third trial attempted
Groton maze learning task (GMLT)	Ability to learn and navigate a hidden pathway in a maze, measuring problem-solving skills and learning efficiency.	Reasoning And problem solving	Number of errors made across five learning trials	Five learning trials completed
Social emotional Cognition task (SECT)	Ability to understand and respond to social and emotional cues.	Social Cognition	Proportion of correct responses	75% of trials completed
Composite score (computer composite)	Measure of cognitive function by combining scores from the various tasks	General cognitive function	Composite standardized score	None specified

(EF) that could explain impairments in other neurocognitive domains. After administering neurocognitive tasks to people living with SMI and volunteers with no mental health problems, the authors found that WM and EF independently contribute to neurocognitive impairments in individuals living with SMI. The finding suggests that these two functions are separable features of the observed neurocognitive impairments in SMI, supporting that distinct impairments on neurocognitive performance measures are manifestations of a possible higher-order impairment in one domain (e.g., EF).

As stated previously, Nuechterlein et al. (2004) found seven domains of neurocognitive functioning that are common to people living with SMI using factor analyses. McCutcheon et al. (2023) reported that dimensionality reduction of the seven domains to parent domains of processing speed, attention/WM, and learning. Some reports indicated that processing speed is the most affected neurocognitive domain in people living with SMI (and the most sensitive to side effects from psychiatric medications), and that processing speed impairments are the strongest predictor of general neuropsychological performances. Processing speed is a component of many neurocognitive functions and neuropsychological performance demands. Impairments in this domain may reflect impairments in other higher-order functions. For example, people living with SMI may approach processing speed tests, such as symbol-coding, with impaired strategic planning and problem solving than people with no known mental health problem. Likewise, impairments in lower-level domains such as reaction time could contribute to deficits in higher-order domains (e.g., social cognitions, EF). Given the existence of impairments of low-level neurocognitive processes across many domains, there is support that neurocognitive impairments in people living with SMI could be conceptualized as a generalized impairment. However, there are limitations of existing neuropsychological tests that may not be able to isolate specific neurocognitive dimensional processes and more specific neurocognitive impairments. Tests that can examine more specific neurocognitive and perceptual processes may be more sensitive to the non-generalized components of neurocognitive impairments observed in people living with SMI (McCutcheon et al., 2023).

Lahera et al. (2017) studied the relationship between the neurocognitive functions of processing speed, reaction time, attention, and social functioning in individuals living with SMI. Processing speed was evaluated by measuring performance in three tests:

(a) a symbol coding subtest used in the Brief Assessment of Cognition in Schizophrenia (BACS). Symbol coding is a paper-and-pencil test that evaluates the ability to match symbols to numbers within a short time limit; number of errors is scored. It is used to assess attention, planning, and memory (Galvin et al., 2020).
(b) the Trail Making Test—A (TMT-A). It is used to measure several functions, particularly cognitive flexibility, alternating attention, sequencing, visual search, and motor speed (Kaplan & Saccuzzo, 2010).
(c) a verbal fluidity test in which the person was required to name the animal in a picture.

Reaction time was evaluated by having the individual observe a fixed green circle displayed on a computer screen; the individual is required to respond by pressing a key when a visual stimulus in the form of a red circle appears (i.e., simple reaction time). A figure in the form of a square then appears at random in the center, right, or left of the screen, requiring that certain keys had to be pressed depending on the position of the square figure; this was a measure of elective reaction time. Capacity for sustained attention or vigilance was evaluated using the Continuous Performance Test (CPT). The CPT is a computer-based neuropsychological test that presents several series of single visual stimuli (usually letters) projected at brief intervals. Participants must respond when a letter was preceded by a designated target letter (Cullum, 1998). Emotional processing was evaluated using the Facial Emotions Identification Test (FEIT). This test includes 19 photographs of faces presented on a monitor expressing one of six basic emotions: happiness, sadness, anger, fear, surprise, or shame. The task consists of identifying the emotion expressed by each face (Lahera et al., 2017).

Results showed emotion recognition impairments in the participants living with SMI, showing difficulties in recognizing fear and anger. This result correlated with measures of processing speed and attention, indicating that processing speed, sustained attention, and elective reaction time were significantly associated with social-emotional functioning as measured by the FEIT. The study highlights the importance of processing speed and emotional recognition in understanding functional outcomes in people living with SMI. The recognition of emotional expression on faces is one aspect of the wide array of behaviors that correspond to social functioning. However, the study infers social functioning from the recognition of facial expressions of basic emotions and does not evaluate the overt behaviors that are related to the domain of basic social competencies, such as eye contact and conversational turn taking.

As with other neurocognitive studies, the neuropsychological performance tasks demonstrate overlap with neurocognitive domains other than the domain intended for assessment. For example, the symbol coding task cited by Lahera et al. (2017) is related to executive functioning (EF), which includes attention, planning, and switching of problem-solving sets (i.e., cognitive flexibility). Studies using symbol and number coding tasks show moderate-to-strong correlations with other neuropsychological measures, particularly those with EF components such as attention, judgment, decision making, and problem solving (Galvin et al., 2020).

Self-report measures of neurocognitive impairment have been developed as adjuncts to clinical assessment when time is limited. An interview-based reliable measure such as the Schizophrenia Cognition Rating Scale (SCoRS) may be appropriate (Jeon et al., 2020a, 2020b) for ongoing assessment of neurocognitive domains during treatment. The SCoRS consists of 20 items assessing neurocognitive impairments and their impact on daily functioning. Items were developed by a team including psychologists and research assistants with experience in neurocognitive assessments (Jeon et al., 2020a, 2020b; Keefe et al., 2006a, 2006b). Neurocognitive domains assessed include attention, memory, reasoning, working memory (WM), language production, and motor skills. Each item is rated on a 4-point scale, with higher ratings indicating greater impairment, and can include a "not applicable" option. The assessment includes interviews with both the patient and an informant who is familiar with the daily functioning of the person living with SMI. Keefe et al. (2006a, 2006b) found that informant ratings are more reliable than self-reports of the person living with SMI in determining neurocognitive deficits with significant variability between the two probably as a result of "social desirability" which is a "bias or tendency of individuals to present themselves in a manner that will be viewed favorably by others" (American Psychological Association, n.d.-i).

The SCoRS correlates strongly with neurocognitive performance measured by the BACS (Keefe et al., 2006a, 2006b; Jeon et al., 2020a, 2020b). It also showed a strong relationship with adaptive functioning, as measured by the Independent Living Skills Inventory (ILSI) and scores obtained on the UPSA (Keefe et al., 2006a, 2006b; Menditto et al., 1999). The ILSI is a standard functional capacity assessment instrument designed to measure the extent to which individuals can competently perform a broad range of skills important for successful community living. The ILSI includes 89 items covering 11 subscales: personal management, hygiene and grooming, clothing, basic skills (e.g., remembering a personal phone number), interpersonal skills, home maintenance, money management, cooking, resource utilization, general occupational skills, and medication management. Data are obtained from an interview with the person being assessed, who provides information about their performances. Each item is rated based on the individual's self-reported ability to perform a skill and the extent of assistance or guidance required. Keefe et al. (2006a, 2006b) noted "that real-world functioning (as measured by the ILSI) was stronger than the relationship of the cognitive performance score (BACS) or a performance-based measure of functional capacity (UPSA)" (p. 431). Unfortunately, no collateral data were obtained using the ILSI from an informant familiar with the person living with SMI given the unreliability of self-reported neurocognitive impairments cited by the authors (Keefe et al., 2006a, 2006b).

Jeon et al. (2020a, 2020b) and Keefe et al. (2006a, 2006b) analyzed the correlations between the neurocognitive domains measured on the neuropsychological performance measures on the MATRICS Consensus Cognitive Battery (MCCB) and each item of the SCoRS to identify the domains and items most associated with each other when the measures are conjointly used. The strongest association was with the total score on the SCoRS and composite score on the MCCB but was statistically weak ($r = -0.35$) (Keefe et al., 2006a, 2006b). Correlation showed weak to no correlations on most items on the SCoRS, while a few had multiple correlations with more than one neurocognitive domain on the MCCB. It was noted that there was variability among the correlations (Jeon et al., 2020a, 2020b). The item ratings based solely on the reports from the person living with SMI had either weak or no correlations indicating that individuals living with SMI are less reliable in reporting their own neurocognitive performances when compared to their neuropsychological dimensional performances. Keefe et al. (2006a, 2006b) noted that the information obtained by the interviewer from the familiar informant improved the correlation with the MCCB compared to only using self-reports from the person living with SMI.

An essential conclusion is that awareness of functioning in people living with SMI may be unreliable. There is a need for collateral data either from familiar informants or from objective behavioral observation of the targeted behaviors of the dimension in functional and neurocognitive performance domains and less reliance on other similar interview-based assessments of neurocognitive functioning in domains that are reported to be essential for competent and adaptive daily functioning.

Origins of Problems in Memory and Concentration and Neurocognitive Impairments

Neurological Substrates

Neurobiological factors—genetic, metabolic, immunological, and neurochemical—and their correlated mechanisms collectively contribute to the neurocognitive impairments observed in people living with SMI, highlighting the complexity of the various problems displayed by people living with SMI (Wang et al., 2022).

Neurocognitive domains are complex in functioning and their relationships to various neuroanatomical areas of the brain. The relationships are listed below and are divided into three main neurocognitive domains: attention, memory, and executive functioning (EF). The dimension of the neurocognitive domain is followed by the neurological structures to which that dimension is linked (Burdick & Goldberg, 2008).

- Attention:
  - Vigilance: locus coeruleus (LoC)
  - Alerting: posterior parietal lobe, superior colliculus
  - Detection/conflict: anterior cingulate, ventral prefrontal cortex (vPFC)
  - Inhibition/decision-making: orbitofrontal cortex, anterior cingulate cortex (ACC)
  - Spatial/verbal WM: superior parietal lobe, dorsolateral prefrontal cortex (dlPFC)
  - Verbal fluency: prefrontal cortex (PFC)
  - Facial affect discrimination: Amygdala (Amyg), dlPFC
  - Motor speed/skill: subcortical ganglia, basal ganglia (BG)
- Memory:
  - Encoding: hippocampus (HP), PFC
  - Storage: HP
  - Retrieval: ventromedial prefrontal cortex (vmPFC), temporoparietal junction
- Executive function (EF):
  - Logical reasoning: left frontal cortex, temporal cortex
  - Cognitive control: ventrolateral prefrontal cortex (vlPFC), dlPFC, ACC
  - Set shifting (cognitive flexibility): cerebellum (CERB), left dlPFC, BG

By reviewing the structures associated with the dimensions of the neurocognitive domains, one can see that there is a lack of a clearly defined area of the brain associated with a specific dimension; dimensions are associated with more than one neuroanatomical region, and neuroanatomical regions are linked to more than one dimension. Achieving an average score on a neuropsychological performance measure requires competent and adequate functioning in multiple distinct anatomical regions, each associated with specific neurocognitive domains and related dimensions. A neurological insult or defect in one area of the brain may trigger cascading negative effects on other regions and their respective functions, leading to neurocognitive impairments.

Mental health problems linked to living with SMI are associated with various genetic factors and mechanisms. Genome-wide association studies (GWAS) have identified multiple genetic loci linked to neurocognitive functions in people living with SMI. Specific polymorphisms in genes have been associated with neurocognitive impairment in SMI (Morozova et al., 2022).

Epigenetic changes, such as DNA methylation and other modifications, may play a role. Decreased expression of histone deacetylase (HDAC) in the dlPFC and regulation of N-methyl-D-aspartate (NMDA) receptors correlate with neurocognitive impairment (Morozova et al., 2022).

Disruption of neurotransmitter systems, with particular emphasis on glutamate and GABA, plays a critical role in the biological foundations of SMI. Evidence indicates NMDA receptor hypofunction, notable changes in GABAergic neurotransmission such as reduced levels in the prefrontal cortex, and mitochondrial dysfunction arising from genetic deletions that impact neuronal functions including synaptic transmission and neuroplasticity. These factors are closely associated with neurocognitive deficits (Morozova et al., 2022).

Neuroinflammatory processes and cerebral vascular functioning are likewise implicated. Elevated levels of inflammatory biomarkers are associated with neurocognitive impairment with microglial activation and cytokine production playing a role (Morozova et al., 2022; Wang et al., 2022). Cerebral vascular problems have been found in studies of people living with SMI with links to microvascular abnormalities and brain hypoperfusion of blood. Vascular endothelial growth factor (VEGF) is involved in brain perfusion and synaptic plasticity, with altered VEGF levels correlated with neurocognitive impairment (Morozova et al., 2022; Wang et al., 2022).

Goodkind et al. (2015) conducted a meta-analysis of structural neuroimaging studies across multiple mental health problems. The study found a transdiagnostic pattern of gray matter loss in the anterior insula and dorsal ACC (dACC) among individuals with mental health problems linked to SMI. The decrease in gray matter in these regions correlates with impairments executive functioning (EF) domains in participants with no known mental health problems. The neurocognitive domain of EF is composed of neurocognitive dimensions, such as task initiation, organization, flexibility, setting priorities, problem solving, working memory (WM), and control of impulsivity and emotions (Baggetta & Alexander, 2016). EF is crucial for self-regulation and goal-directed behavior. Individual differences in EF are linked to academic performance, interpersonal issues, substance use, and both physical and mental health. Impairments in this neurocognitive domain are associated with various mental health problems and predict intrusive and repeated worrying and poor emotion regulation strategies (Snyder et al., 2015). Impairments in EF are prevalent across various mental health problems corresponding to SMI, with the largest deficits observed in individuals living with schizophrenia spectrum mental health problems followed by bipolar and major depressive mental health problems.

The findings suggest that cortical thinning and gray matter loss in the anterior insula, fronto-temporal regions, and dACC may contribute to functional impairments in EF and WM rather than specific symptoms (Goodkind et al., 2015; Huang et al., 2025). Effects related to specific mental health problems were observed only in participants with schizophrenia-spectrum and major depressive mental health problems. No significant effects of medications or comorbid health problems were found on gray matter volume.

The researchers (Goodkind et al., 2015) concluded that there are neurological commonalities across mental health problems contrasting with previous studies related to specific mental health problems; future research should explore how gray matter loss relates to the severity, chronicity, and dimensions of symptoms and behavior problems linked to specific mental health problems as the findings suggest shared neural substrates and structural brain changes for mental health problems, particularly those corresponding to SMI.

Psychological and Behavioral Substrates of Neurocognitive Impairments

The impairments in the dimension of neurocognitive domains that have been the focus of research and clinical intervention are based on the results on neurocognitive performance measures. The findings suggest that the behavioral challenges observed in individuals who live with SMI, specifically in adaptive functional behaviors, may be attributable to deficits across multiple neurocognitive domains. Difficulties in adaptive functional behaviors observed in individuals living with SMI are attributed to either an excessive or diminished frequency of these behaviors within appropriate contexts, corresponding to positive or negative symptoms, respectively. Nevertheless, substantial correlations between neuropsychological test performance and adaptive functional outcomes have not been consistently established (Harvey & Strassnig, 2012).

It has been found repeatedly that people living with SMI show impairments in neuropsychological performance measures that evaluate dimensions in the neurocognitive domains of attention, memory (especially WM), processing speed, executive function (EF), and social cognition. Research has indicated that individuals with SMI exhibit intra-individual variability in neuropsychological performance scores. This variability is believed to reflect random errors in neurocognitive functioning associated with underlying neurocognitive impairments and has been hypothesized to correlate with white matter integrity in the corpus callosum (Ahn et al., 2019).

The scores on the neurocognitive performance measures across people living with SMI have been found to be consistently heterogeneous in studies focusing on neurocognitive impairments. There are complex interactions among various brain structures and regions that have been identified as being involved in the neurocognitive impairments observed on neuropsychological performance measures, but no common "pathway" or structure has been found to account for the impairments.

Impairments in one or even a few neurocognitive dimensions and domains assessed by neuropsychological performance measures have been taken to be conclusive evidence as to "general" cognitive impairments in people living with SMI. Studies have found that only composite scores on the neuropsychological test batteries to be consistently lower in people living with SMI and that there was minimal evidence for specificity of relationships between dimensional scores in domains and indices of adaptive behavioral functioning that suggest global instead of specific dimensional relationships (Harvey et al., 2020); however, composite scores are a number that combines multiple data points from obtained scores (including scores within the average range) on the various neurocognitive dimensions measured by the individual performance tests for neurocognitive domain. Future research should study the associated functional socio-behavioral dimensions of living with SMI in people obtaining scores within the average range.

Neurocognitive functioning involves tasks on neurocognitive dimensions for the targeted domains that require mental effort, including memory, attention, and executive functions (EF); these tasks differ in complexity requiring greater effort and attention. Environmental conditions such as heat, cold, and hypoxia can negatively impact neurocognitive performance through interrelated psycho-physiological pathways (Bratman et al., 2012). Environmental stressors related to trauma and stress due to socio-behavioral variables also impact neurocognitive performance and are linked to living with SMI (Adams et al., 2015; Mauritz et al., 2013).

A systematic review examining interpersonal trauma and trauma-related issues among individuals living with SMI identified prevalence rates of 47% for physical abuse and 37% for sexual abuse. Compared to the general population, those with SMI exhibited significantly higher rates of trauma-related disorders, with physical abuse reported at 47% versus 21% and sexual abuse at 37% versus 23%. The data also indicated that women experienced a higher prevalence of abuse across mental health conditions associated with SMI. Additionally, exposure to traumatic events was found to correlate with earlier onset and increased severity of symptoms in individuals determined to be living with SMI (Mauritz et al., 2013).

Adams et al. (2015) assessed a random sample of individuals living with SMI, focusing on stressful events, traumas, and discrimination. Over 95% reported experiencing at least one childhood adversity, with 52.4% hospitalized for a major illness. Neighborhood problems were prevalent, with 45% citing heavy traffic and 37% reporting drug and alcohol issues where they lived. Everyday discrimination was reported by 17.7% who felt perceived as "not smart" and 16.5% reported feeling inferior; these were linked to higher rates of depression and lower quality of life. Chronic stress was reported by 86%, with 41% facing serious illness and 36% losing a close friend in the past year.

People living with SMI have experienced trauma in the past and continue to experience stress and trauma due to living with SMI (Adams et al., 2015; Mauritz et al., 2013). The impact of stress on neurocognitive functions and mental health problems highlights treatment gaps and interventions.

Stress significantly contributes to many mental health problems corresponding to SMI. Neurocognitive impairments, such as cognitive flexibility, working memory (WM), and behavioral inhibition, are common across stress-related conditions and people living with SMI. When experiencing stress, the neuroendocrine stress response is activated and releases glucocorticoids, affecting neurocognitions. Elevated glucocorticoids, such as cortisol, can impair neurocognitive functions, particularly in memory tasks as approximately 83% of people living with Cushing's Syndrome (i.e., chronic overproduction of corticosteroid hormones (APA Psych, n.d.-d)) report memory issues.

Chronic stress may be implicated in the neurocognitive impairments in dimensions and domains that are obtained on neuropsychological performance measures. Chronic stress models in animal studies show behavioral and neuronal changes that mimic symptoms of mood and anxiety mental health problems in humans. Studies indicate that repeated stress can cause neuronal remodeling in the prefrontal cortex (PFC) and hippocampus (HC), affecting neurocognitive functioning in those structures (Girotti et al., 2024).

Chronic stress affects several neurocognitive domains (Girotti et al., 2024), including:

- Cognitive flexibility: the ability to adapt behavior to changing environments or suppress old information to learn new information. Chronic stress can lead to perseverance of behaviors that are no longer beneficial and impair the ability to learn new rules and switch problem-solving strategies (Girotti et al., 2024).
- Behavioral inhibition: the ability to restrain a response in a specific context. Chronic stress can increase impulsivity, leading to difficulties in inhibiting inappropriate actions.
- Working memory (WM): the temporary storage and manipulation of information used for neurocognitive tasks such as language comprehension, learning, and reasoning. Chronic stress can impair WM, affecting tasks that require the retention and manipulation of information (Girotti et al., 2024).
- Prenatal factors: Complications and infections during gestation are linked to disruptions in brain development, resulting in lower IQ and lifelong neurocognitive impairments. Prenatal adversities put the person at risk of developing a mental health problem linked to SMI (Girotti et al., 2024). .
- Urban environment: Growing up in urban areas is associated with a higher incidence of living with a SMI and potentially impaired neurocognitive development. Factors such as socioeconomic deprivation, pollution, lack of green spaces, overcrowding, and stress related to urban living (e.g., noise, crime, inferior housing) may contribute to these outcomes (Girotti et al., 2024).
- Socioeconomic deprivation: Lower socioeconomic status (SES) is associated with poorer educational attainment and neurocognitive performance. Lower SES

is related to lifestyles that place a person at risk for developing other risk factors (i.e., smoking, exposure to toxins such as lead paint). Individuals from deprived backgrounds may have less resources and finances to access stimulating environments and educational resources, which can hinder neurocognitive development (Girotti et al., 2024).

- Childhood trauma: Exposure to trauma during childhood is linked to both an increased risk of developing mental health problems and lower neurocognitive performance. Traumatic experiences can lead to stress-related changes in the brain, affecting neurocognitive functions such as memory, attention, and executive functions (EF) (e.g., cognitive flexibility) (Girotti et al., 2024).
- Substance use: Acute and chronic cannabis use is associated with neurocognitive impairments. Cannabis use can affect brain regions involved in neurocognitive processes, leading to deficits in memory, attention, and executive function (Girotti et al., 2024).
- Ethnic minority status: Ethnic minority status is a strong risk factor for developing a serious mental health problem. It is also associated with poorer educational attainment. Factors such as socioeconomic deprivation, exposure to racism, and cultural stressors can negatively impact neurocognitive development and function (Girotti et al., 2024).
- Physical health: Poor physical health, including conditions like smoking, obesity, and hyperglycemia, can adversely affect cognitive function. These health issues can lead to cerebrovascular problems and other complications that impair neurocognitive abilities (Girotti et al., 2024).

These environmental factors interact with each other, and genetic predispositions contribute to the neurocognitive impairments observed in individuals living with SMI.

Results from studies show that environmental stimuli impact neurocognitive processes and problem behaviors in SMI. The display of disorganized speech (from which a formal thought disorder (FTD) is inferred) has been shown to change in frequency related to antecedent conditions. Research by Leonhardt et al. (2017) found that themes of inadequacy and vulnerability often preceded the display of disorganized behaviors in people living with SMI. Bettis et al. (2024) identified four main themes preceding the display of disorganized speech by people living with SMI: alienation, interpersonal tension, personal benchmarks, and adverse experiences. Relationship tension was the most frequent topic preceding disorganization followed by alienation related to illness, social alienation, past hardships, and inadequacy. The finding showed that socio-behavioral stimuli can trigger disorganized speech. Adverse experiences, including past hardship and grief, were significant precursors to the occurrence of disorganized speech. The authors concluded that disorganization of speech may be a response to the distress that was experienced by the participants living with SMI.

Emotion recognition impairments have been found in individuals living with SMI (Green et al., 2019). The recognition of facial expressions of emotions is a dimension of social cognition and Theory of Mind (ToM); a study by Lahera et al.

(2017) found that people living with SMI had difficulty in recognizing facial expressions of fear and anger. This result correlated with measures of processing speed and attention, indicating that processing speed, sustained attention, and elective reaction time were significantly associated with social-emotional functioning. The study highlights the importance of processing speed and emotional recognition in understanding functional outcomes in people living with SMI. The recognition of emotional expressions on faces is an aspect of a wide array of behaviors that correspond to socio-behavioral functioning. Childhood trauma, particularly neglect, has been found to have a significant impact on social neurocognitions in individuals living with SMI. Green et al. (2019) reported that studies suggest that social neurocognitive impairments on neuropsychological performance measures are more closely related to experiences of neglect than other types of adversity. The conclusion is that early adverse experiences can have long-lasting effects on neurocognitive functions related to social interactions (Green et al., 2019).

As can be seen, the display of neurocognitive processes as measured by neuropsychological tests can be altered by environmental stimuli. Adverse stimuli have modified and continue to alter the displays of behaviors corresponding to neurocognitive dimensions during neuropsychological performance testing. All overt and covert behaviors are the product of brain activity. From a behavioral perspective, results or scores on neuropsychological performance measures are observable behaviors and the consequences of complex behaviors including motor behaviors and subvocal speech (i.e., thinking, reasoning, and other neurocognitive processes) (Thomas, 2010). The results on neuropsychological performance measures are a "snapshot" of a person's strengths and weaknesses in certain identified neurocognitive dimensions and domains. However, the scores obtained and the behaviors of the examinee during the neuropsychological performance measure are the outcome of the person's actions and functioning, rather than inferred underlying brain pathology or neurological mechanisms.

Hoffmann (2023) formulated a neuropsychological model of human behavior. This model serves to systematically analyze, interpret, and potentially guide human behavioral patterns. The goal of every person is to satisfy all basic needs and to achieve subjective psychological and physical well-being. The basic needs for attachment, security, orientation and control, for self-esteem, and for the enjoyment and avoidance of displeasure are at the center of all behaviors, including test-taking behaviors. If basic needs are not met consistently or the person has a learning history containing adverse experiences (i.e., being punished for not completing task demands on tests), the person may experience stress in similar contexts, which then impacts performance on neurocognitive tasks. Perceptions from the environment lead to negative or positive emotional experiences and, accordingly, to an avoidance or approach strategy (motivational (MO) and evocative (EO) operations) based on prior experiences.

Neuropsychological performance measures of neurocognitive domains may not always accurately reflect real-world abilities and functioning in daily life situations. Neurocognitive domains, like social cognition or higher-level executive functions (EFs), may not be adequately assessed by neuropsychological performance measures, and overinterpretation of results needs to be avoided. Skinner (1953) summarized the problem with testing for covert processes as follows:

> Certain variables in the history of the individual and in the current environment are responsible for the behavior in the test situation and they also determine their behavior in the larger situation. The prediction is not from cause to effect but from one effect to another. This is shown by the fact that we use tests as a basis for prediction without knowing what variables are responsible for the score obtained or for the behavior predicted. It is shown by the fact that we extend the test without limit, adding more and more items, it eventually coincides with the behavior to be predicted. No true prediction then survives (p. 199).

Neurocognitive impairment in people living with SMI is multifaceted and varies among individuals (Huang et al., 2025). Research in impairments in neurocognitive dimensions and domains in people living with SMI has traditionally relied on nomothetic methods, which aggregate data from groups (Barlow & Nock, 2009). The nomothetic approach (i.e., the study of interindividual variation) dominates analyses of research data on neurocognitive impairment, even though its assumption of homogeneity across people and time is often violated. The idiographic approach (i.e., the study of intraindividual variation) is best suited for analyses of heterogeneous data (Beltz et al., 2016); it focuses on the intraindividual variations in results on neuropsychological performance measures in people living with SMI. The reliance on the nomothetic approach has resulted in limitations in flexibility and generalizability of the findings of the research and their use in clinical practice (Barlow & Nock, 2009).

The studies of neurocognitive impairments are based on comparing scores obtained on neuropsychological performance measures by participants living with SMI and normative samples. Normative data for some neuropsychological tests are based on small samples or have limited validity or reliability data (Howieson, 2019). The normative samples are based on individuals with no known mental health problems. Normative data of performance scores on neuropsychological performance measures with samples of people living with SMI based on onset and duration of living with SMI, functional behaviors, and frequency of occurrences, and the severity of problem behaviors would be a more meaningful comparison and would lead to more detailed information and the development of effective interventions. Normative data may not capture the nuances and complexities of SMI, potentially leading to inaccurate or misleading conclusions about an individual's mental health. Using norms based on clinical clusters will allow for individual-level statistical inferences about deviations from normative patterns, accommodating diverse outcome pathways (Marquand et al., 2019). Research and assessment in SMI need to shift focus to understanding the specific experiences, strengths, and challenges for the individual rather than comparing them to a "norm." Additionally, there is a lack of performance measures and interrelationship for high-level neurocognitive and social skills (Howieson, 2019).

The behavioral view of neuropsychological testing is an idiographic approach to analyzing the data from the use of performance measures of neurocognitive dimensions. Idiographic research focuses on the intensive study of individuals, offering a more efficient and flexible alternative to group comparisons (Barlow & Nock,

2009). The behavioral approach to neuropsychological testing incorporates observations of an examinee's behavior during testing, including task strategies, effort, frustration level, and response to cues. The goal is to translate test findings into meaningful information regarding an individual's functional abilities and limitations in everyday life to minimize any deleterious effect on a person's everyday functional ability. A purely neuroanatomical view primarily focuses on interpreting test results based on which brain region is likely affected by a "disease process," without sufficient emphasis on how the impairment manifests in daily functional behaviors. Behavioral perspective is particularly important for treatment planning, as it helps identify specific areas of behavioral adaptation needed to address impairments in daily functioning that could impede the recovery of a person living with SMI. For example, an individual living with SMI performs poorly on a neuropsychological performance measure in memory. During the assessment, the examiner observes that the individual frequently interrupts the instructions to ask clarifying questions, suggesting difficulties with attention and comprehension rather than a primary memory impairment. This observation indicates that the individual's memory difficulties might be partially due to problems with executive function (attention and planning) and verbal comprehension which could be addressed through specific behavioral strategies like providing clear instructions, breaking tasks into smaller steps, rehearsal, using teach-back (i.e., asking a person to explain in their own words what a health provider has just told them (Talevski et al., 2020)). In conclusion, neuropsychological performance measures of neurocognitive domains and dimensions are another source of observable behavioral data that can be used in functional assessments and analyses of problem behaviors in people living with SMI.

Epidemiological Considerations

Approximately 60–80% of individuals living with mental health problems corresponding to SMI exhibit significant impairments on results on neuropsychological performance measures assessing neurocognitive domains and dimensions that impact functional recovery as measured by adaptive functional behaviors (i.e., Independent Living Skills Inventory (ILSI); UCSD Performance-based Skills Assessment (UPSA)). Impairments in certain domains such as memory and processing speed have a negative cascading effect on other neuropsychological performance measures since tasks on neuropsychological performance measures require both neurocognitive domains (McCleery & Nuechterlein, 2019).

Neurocognitive impairments are common during the initial phase of living with SMI, impacting daily functioning and outcomes in recovery. Studies show that 70–80% of individuals living with SMI exhibit neurocognitive impairments in dimensions of neurocognitive domains on results from neuropsychological performance measures. Up to 32% of people being treated for major depressive mental health problems showed impairments of up to two SDs below people with no mental health problems. A study found 78.6% of people living with a major depressive mental health problem had neurocognitive impairments when defined as greater than one SD below healthy controls on two neuropsychological performance measures (Stainton et al., 2023).

Cultural Considerations

A review concluded that there is scant research on neurocognitive impairments exhibited by people living with SMI in other countries, particularly non-Western countries and cultures (Kline et al., 2019). One study found that 62% of people in Uganda living with the initial phase of SMI had cognitive impairments defined as greater than two SDs below individuals with no known mental health problems (Stainton et al., 2023).

One contributing factor is the limited availability of psychometric data for neurocognitive performance measures validated in individuals with SMI residing in low- and middle-income countries. The study reviewed 28 studies and identified 23 distinct measures, none originating from low-income regions. While most of these measures were validated in populations living with SMI and included assessments of group, convergent, and divergent validity, most studies exhibited questionable methodological quality due to small sample sizes and insufficient validation procedures (Haile et al., 2022).

The main challenges in adapting neurocognitive performance measures for non-Western low- and middle-income countries (LMICs) include:

- Cultural differences: Neurocognitive tests developed in Western countries may not be culturally relevant or appropriate. Cultural practices and interpretations can significantly influence test results.
- Language barriers: Many LMICs are linguistically diverse, with multiple languages spoken within a single country. It is challenging to adapt tests to different languages while maintaining their validity and reliability given the nuances of language like dialects.
- Educational disparities: The average educational level in many countries is often lower than in high-income countries. Neurocognitive tests that require a certain level of literacy and familiarity with specific content may not be suitable for populations with limited educational opportunities.
- Economic factors: Economic constraints can affect the availability of resources needed to administer neurocognitive tests, such as trained personnel and testing materials. Additionally, some assessment instruments may have economic implications that are not relevant in the contexts of other countries (e.g., need for laptop computers, Internet access). Neurocognitive tests need to be feasible and practical to administer in other settings, considering factors like time, cost, and the availability of trained professionals.
- Lack of norms: There is often a lack of normative data for neurocognitive tests in other countries, making it difficult to interpret test results accurately.

The authors (Haile et al., 2022) concluded that the following neuropsychological performance measures should be considered when assessing neurocognitions for clinical and research use with people living with SMI across cultures and countries: The Brief Assessment of Cognition in Schizophrenia (BACS), Cognitive Assessment Interview (CAI), MATRICS Consensus Cognitive Battery (MCCB), and CogState Schizophrenia Battery (CSB).

The prevalence of neurocognitive strengths in SMI has not been previously studied, highlighting a gap in research. There is a need for assessing both neurocognitive impairments and strengths in individuals living with SMI by using comprehensive neurocognitive profiles to inform interventions and resource allocation in clinical services.

Stainton et al. (2023) studied a large sample of 1286 participants across three clinical groups living with mental health problems and one group with no mental health problem; the participants lived in different European countries. One clinical group was defined as "at risk" of developing a psychotic type of mental health problem, and another group was individuals living with "recent onset" of living with an SMI (i.e., psychosis); the third clinical group was people living with a recent onset of a depressive mental health problem.

These neuropsychological performance measures were chosen to provide a comprehensive evaluation of neurocognitive functioning across various domains, including memory, attention, processing speed, and executive functions (EFs); the domains follow the MATRICS guidelines in assessing neurocognitive domains of neuropsychological functioning in people living with SMI (Nuechterlein et al., 2008). All participants were evaluated using the following neuropsychological performance measures for the neurocognitive domains as in the guidelines:

1. Trail Making Test (TMT) Parts A & B:

   Outcome of dimension: total reaction time.
   Domain: assesses processing speed and cognitive flexibility.

2. Phonetic Verbal Fluency (PVF) and Semantic Verbal Fluency (SVF):

   Outcome of dimension: total number of correct words.
   Domain: measures verbal fluency and EF.

3. Continuous Performance Task (CPT):

   Outcome of dimension: d-Prime Sensitivity Index: based on the hit rate (correctly identifying the signal) and the false alarm rate (incorrectly identifying noise as the signal).
   Domain: evaluates sustained attention and vigilance.

4. Rey Auditory Verbal Learning Test (RAVLT):

   Outcome of dimension: sum of trials 1 to 5.
   Domain: assesses verbal learning and memory.

5. Rey-Osterrieth Complex Figure (ROCF):

Outcome of dimension: total score at immediate recall.
Domain: measures visuospatial constructional ability and visual memory.

6. Self-Ordered Pointing Task (SOPT):

   Outcome of dimension: total errors.
   Domain: evaluates WM and EF.

7. Auditory Digit Span Task:

   Outcome of dimension: number of correct trials forwards (FDS) and backwards (BDS).
   Domain: assesses working memory (WM).

8. Digit-Symbol Substitution Test (DSST):

   Outcome: total score of the number correct minus the number of errors.
   Domain: measures processing speed and WM.

9. Diagnostic Analysis of Nonverbal Accuracy (DANVA):

   Outcome of dimension: total number of correct faces identified.
   Domain: evaluates nonverbal emotion recognition.

10. Wechsler Abbreviated Scale of Intelligence (WASI):

    Outcome of dimension: vocabulary and matrix reasoning subscales.
    Domain: assesses general cognitive ability.

All scores of the participants in the clinical group on the 10 neuropsychological performance measures were compared to scores of the participants with no mental health problems. The operational definitions of impairment on the tested dimensions were as follows: moderate impairment was a score of up to two SDs below on at least two of the performance tests, and severe impairment was greater than two SDs below in at least two neuropsychological tests (Stainton et al., 2023).

Results of the recent onset group showed 88.3% with moderate impairments, while 45.1% showed severe impairments; in the at-risk group, 71.2% were moderately impaired and 22.4% were severely impaired; in the group living with depression mental health problems, 61.6% were moderately impaired and 16.2% severely impaired. The average number of tests showing moderate or severe impairment was significantly different among the groups, with the recent onset group showing the highest rates of impaired performances (Stainton et al., 2023).

Strengths in the dimensions of the neurocognitive domains tested were operationally defined as having performed in at least two neuropsychological performance tests as follows: "above average" when scores were one to two SDs above; and "extremely high level" when scores were greater than two SDs. The recent onset group showed that 16.1% obtained "above average" scores, and the clinically at-risk group showed 36.1% and 1.4% obtaining "above average" or at "extremely high level" scores, respectively. The results of the group living with depression mental health problems were 40.5% and 1.8% obtaining at "above average" or "extremely high levels" scores, respectively (Stainton et al., 2023).

It is worth noting that the group with no mental health problems had the following results: 48.6% showed moderate impairments, while 6.7% showed severe impairment; 52.3% performed "above average," while 2.2% performed at "extremely high level" (Stainton et al., 2023).

The results found that working memory (WM), processing speed, and verbal learning were the most impaired neurocognitive domains across all clinical groups. A significant proportion of individuals in the clinical groups demonstrated above-average cognitive performance, suggesting areas of neurocognitive strengths that could be leveraged in treatment (Stainton et al., 2023).

Types of Neurocognitive Impairments

Neurocognitive impairment in people living with SMI is a complex and multifaceted construct. Research has identified several subgroups of neurocognitive impairments in individuals living with SMI, each characterized by different neurocognitive profiles and associated neurological substrates.

An unresolved issue is whether there are distinct domains of neurocognitive impairment in people living with SMI, or whether the deficits are better viewed as a global measure. This issue parallels the debate over whether the neurological substrates of mental health problems corresponding to SMI involve specific areas of brain dysfunction or a system-level disruption. Factor analyses of results on the MATRICS-MCCB test battery identified seven neurocognitive domains: processing speed, attention, working memory (WM), verbal learning and memory, visual learning and memory, reasoning, and social cognition. Further dimensionality reduction suggests that these seven domains can be reduced to three parent domains of processing speed, attention/WM, and learning (McCutcheon et al., 2023).

Studies have consistently shown that neurocognitive impairment is a common feature in people living with SMI, affecting up to 75–80% of individuals living with SMI (Huang et al., 2025). Previous research has identified multiple neurocognitive domains affected in mental health problems corresponding to SMI, including memory, attention, executive functions (EFs), and motor skills. These impairments have been hypothesized to impact social and functional outcomes. In addition, Huang et al. (2025) identified significant gradient characteristics of brain structures across neurocognitive subgroups, with variations in cortical thickness and gray matter volume in regions such as the fronto-temporal areas, hippocampus (HC), and insula, providing a more nuanced picture of the relationship between types of neurocognitive impairment and brain structures in people living with SMI.

Huang et al. (2025) found impairments across multiple neurocognitive domains, with specific subgroups showing distinct profiles of neurocognitive impairments, supporting the multiple findings that neurocognitive impairment in people living with SMI is multifaceted and heterogeneous among individuals. Huang et al. (2025)

identified four distinct cognitive subgroups or subtypes on neurocognitive impairments, highlighting the heterogeneity of the impairments displayed on neuropsychological performance measures by people living with SMI:

1. Multidomain-intact: This subtype shows relatively intact neurocognitive function across multiple domains, including memory, attention, and EF. This subtype exhibits the most intact brain structure compared to individuals with no mental health problems.
2. Executive-preserved: Individuals in this subtype have preserved EF but show impairment in other neurocognitive domains. Neurological substrate changes are observed in the posterior cingulate cortex (PCC).
3. Executive-deteriorated: This subtype is characterized by significant impairments in EF, while other neurocognitive domains may be less affected. Morphological features include changes in the fronto-temporal regions, HC, and insula.
4. Multidomain-deteriorated: People in this subtype exhibit widespread neurocognitive impairments across multiple neurocognitive domains. The people in this subtype show the most extensive changes in neurological substrates, particularly in younger individuals.

The findings of Huang et al. (2025) are similar to the findings from the study by Heinrich and Awad (1993) in that EF appears differentially impacted in some groups; it should be noted that both Heinrich and Awad (1993) and Huang et al. (2025) found a cluster of people living with SMI with relatively intact neurocognitive functioning. Heinrich and Awad (1993) found that cluster analyses of neurocognitive task scores have the potential to reduce and elucidate the heterogeneity of neurocognitive impairments among individuals who live with SMI; nonetheless, their findings also affirmed the persistent diversity of such impairments.

Clustering individuals into subtypes of neurocognitive impairments is an idiographic technique that may enhance understanding more than group-level models (e.g., nomothetic) when people differ in defined observable behaviors, such as results on neuropsychological performance measures (Arizmendi & Gates, 2024; Heinrich & Awad, 1993). To improve this, clustering methods could group individuals with similar performances and patterns, helping researchers discover if there are subtypes with shared performances, differentiating groups in terms of strengths and impairments (Arizmendi & Gates, 2024). This approach also examines if different patterns point to the same underlying construct of neurocognitive impairments in people living with SMI that can assist in focusing on personalized interventions to address the specific neurocognitive deficits experienced by individuals (Huang et al., 2025).

What Are Memory and Concentration Problems?

Problems with the ability to pay attention and remember information frequently occur among people who live with SMI. Sometimes, these problems are short term and will improve as the problem behaviors linked to living with SMI improve. However, these may also be persistent and show little improvement. Regardless, the ability to attend to and remember information is important for carrying out daily activities, and problems in this area may cause problems with many important daily routine skills.

There are several kinds of memory problems that may affect someone living with SMI. Sometimes, the amount of time that has passed since something happened may make a difference in whether the person can remember it. A person may have problems remembering something that happened earlier in the same day (a problem with recent memory) but still be able to remember things that happened many years ago (suggesting that remote memory may not be affected). In other cases, the kind of information that the person is trying to remember can make a difference. For example, a person may have difficulty remembering information that he was told that morning (indicating a problem with verbal memory) but easily describe things that he had seen or done that morning (suggesting that his visual memory or what he sees may not be a problem). Any of these types of memory can be impaired while other aspects of memory are unaffected. Because of this, memory problems can be different for people. When this happens, it may appear to a service provider that the person living with SMI isn't trying hard enough, is "lazy," or does not want to do what they are asked to do. Understandably, this can be very frustrating for the service provider and the person living with SMI and may lead to worse reactions on the part of all involved.

Why Do Problems with Memory, Concentration, and Learning Happen?

Part of the Reason May Be Biological or Physical

- Problems with attention, memory, learning, and concentration may be a direct result of the neurological and biochemical impairments in the brain that are part of living with SMI. This is particularly true for a person living with schizophrenia spectrum mental health problems.
- Many people living with SMIs will have a history of incidents that involve severe or repeated blows to the head, such as being subdued by police, falling when dizzy, unsteady, or off balance. Such incidents may result in damage to certain areas of the brain that will impair the ability to attend, concentrate, and remember information. Similar problems may also be due to brain damage from long term effects of excessive use of alcohol and other drugs.

- Medications that are prescribed for SMI are potent and do have side-effects. While they may help to minimize psychiatric symptoms and problem behaviors such as delusions or hallucinations, they may also interfere with the ability to attend to information, concentrate on tasks, and remember information.
- Medications for a variety of other medical problems, such as high blood pressure or heart conditions, may also interfere with a person's ability to concentrate and remember information. This is particularly true if the person is taking several kinds of medicine or is not taking the appropriate dosage.

Part of the Reason May Be Psychosocial

- The environment can influence the ability to attend and concentrate. Having too much or too little stimulation in the environment will often interfere with these abilities. If the service provider talks quickly, tries to say too much, or says something in a place where there are a lot of distractions (noise, movement), the person living with SMI will have trouble attending and remembering.
- Problems with remembering information are more likely to happen if the person is upset about something. One common example of this is when the person living with SMI feels that he is being forced to do things that he doesn't want to do. When this is the case, the person living with SMI may become upset and not think about what has been said making it more likely that he will not remember.
- An individual living with SMI may not have had the opportunity to learn certain aspects of neurocognitive skills. Many skills that are expected from functional adults are learned in mid-to-late adolescence. If the onset of living with SMI occurs during this period of adolescence, the person may not have chances to learn necessary skills. The young person living with SMI may have disruptions in her life due to being admitted to psychiatric facilities, entanglements with legal authorities, placements outside of the home and family, and problems with school attendance If the young person living with SMI may be experiencing neurocognitive problems in memory, attention, and planning, they will have fewer opportunities to engage in meaningful and practical skill acquisitions to improve quality of life. The results are the persistent and pervasive functional problems that are common across many contexts for the person living with SMI including remembering and understanding. For example, most people when young are reminded to write things down or repeat information given to them such as a phone number of a friend. A person living with SMI who displays problems in memory may not have had the opportunity to engage in memory-enhancing skills or had role models for such behavioral skills.

Behavioral Support Strategies for Memory and Concentration Problems

- Be clear about what the problem is. Try to be as clear as possible about what the person living with SMI does that makes you consider that he has problems with concentrating and remembering. Does he forget to do things that he is asked to do? Does he start tasks and fail to finish them? Does he forget to put on a coat when it is cold outside? Does he spend his money in a short period of time without thinking about the consequences for the rest of the week? Time (recent and remote memory) or the kind of information (verbal or visual memory) to be remembered and recalled may make a difference. Messages that are clear about what behavior is expected and when it is to occur will help the person to understand what he needs to do and when. "Chunk information" when talking to the person; "chunking" means to break down a large piece of information into smaller, more manageable units or "chunks" which makes it easier to remember and process. Clear and chunked information may help if concentration and memory are problems.
- Watch for circumstances that affect the ability to concentrate and remember information of the person living with SMI. Carefully consider the current abilities of the person living with SMI to attend to various tasks. Regardless of the cause, the abilities to attend and remember will often differ considerably from task to task or according to the time of day. Sometimes the problem will only happen with certain people. For example, Donald was much more likely to complain about bad nerves and problems with his memory when the hospital ward was crowded and loud. This would happen at predictable times of the day, such as at a change of shift for the staff or during an emergency with another individual.
- Seek a review of current medications. The medications that are prescribed for SMI are powerful. Even when they are effective in reducing such problem behaviors as delusions and hallucinations, they may interfere with the ability to concentrate and remember. If there are persistent problems with attention and memory, consider having the medications reviewed by an experienced prescribing service provider. It is possible that another medication may be just as effective for the delusions, hallucinations, and other problem behaviors/symptoms while not interfering with the ability to pay attention and remember information. The assessment should also include medications that the person living with SMI is taking for other physical problems. These can also affect the person's ability to remember information.
- Begin with realistic goals and increase your expectations slowly. The initial expectations should be close to what the person living with SMI is currently successful in doing. Avoid setting expectations that are beyond the capability of the person living with SMI. Expectations that are set too high are likely to frustrate him and will make matters worse. When trying to improve memory or increase the attention span of the person living with SMI, try to provide simple and clear directions about what is expected to be done and when. Ask the person

to repeat or rehearse what has been said to him (i.e., teach back). Complex tasks or information should be broken down into small parts that can be more easily understood and remembered (e.g., chunking). Ask the person to complete one step before giving another. The following is what can be said to the person living with SMI when giving instructions to make his bed, clean his room, and do his laundry:

Good morning. Before you eat breakfast, I want you to make your bed.

After he has made his bed, say the following:

Good job, you made your bed. Now I want you to pick the trash off the floor and put it in the container (pointing to the trash container).

When he picks up the trash, follow by saying:

Great, you picked up the trash. Now I want you to carry your laundry basket downstairs to do your laundry.

Once he accomplishes that, thank the person and praise him.

- Respect the limitations of individuals living with SMI. Service providers often face challenging decisions regarding when to persist in encouraging behavioral change and when to pause and allow the individual some respite. At times, continued efforts may lead only to increased frustration for the person with SMI; in these cases, further attempts to elicit compliance may be ineffective. For example, Donald could not remember when his family was going to visit. The staff accepted that no matter how often they repeated this information to him, and he repeated it, he would have trouble remembering it. So instead of trying to get him to keep remembering the dates of the visits, they helped him to write the dates on the calendar in his room and prompted him to frequently check the calendar. He soon stopped asking the staff and relied on the calendar.
- Emphasize structure and predictability in the daily routine. The person living with SMI will probably be able to concentrate and remember information if the daily routine is consistent and predictable. Try to set a daily schedule that is consistent throughout the days of the week. If roughly the same events happen at the same time each day (get up at 7 a.m., eat lunch at noon, go to the clubhouse at 1 p.m.), then the schedule will be easier to remember. With Donald, the hospital staff made up a schedule for him each day so he would know what was going to happen throughout the day. The staff tried hard to avoid making sudden changes to the routine.
- Allow for frequent breaks from difficult and complex tasks. When trying to improve attention or memory skills, allow for frequent breaks as the task gets more difficult or complex. It is advisable not to wait until an individual living with SMI exhibits signs of frustration before providing a rest break. A qualified occupational therapist or behavioral psychologist can collaborate with the individual to determine appropriate intervals for breaks, utilizing observational assessment during task performance to guide this decision.

- Reduce possible distractions in the environment. In trying to increase attention span or memory of the person living with SMI, minimize distractions (such as television, radio, and activities of others in the environment). Distractions will make it more difficult for the person living with SMI to succeed. Donald had much more difficulty concentrating and remembering things if there was noise around him. When it was noisy on the ward, the staff would ask Donald to walk with them to a quiet area to talk.
- When necessary, remind the person living with SMI of what needs to be done. In many cases, the person living with SMI may make modest improvements in his ability to remember information. Reminders at the appropriate times will usually help the person living with SMI to do what he is asked to do. If these reminders are necessary, it will be a significant challenge to remember and manage time so the person living with SMI ought to be reminded, or "prompted" to do what needs to be done. During his first week on the hospital ward, Donald could not remember where he was supposed to be and when he was supposed to be there. The staff decided that they would structure their time so they would be able to go see him about 5 min before an activity was scheduled. They reminded him of what was about to happen and offered to walk him to that location. This way, Donald was able to be where he was supposed to be.
- When communicating, talk slowly and clearly and give brief, simple "chunks" of information. Be sure that the person living with SMI is paying attention when asking him to do something. Calling the person's name and making eye contact with the person to ensure that he is attending and then giving the information is helpful. Give the directions in a very simple manner but be specific about what the person living with SMI is to do. Instead of telling him that "It's time to do your chores now," tell him "First, I want you to pick up the clothes around your bed." This can be much harder to do than it sounds. If it is difficult doing this, a professional mental health service provider can help.
- Consider repeating information to ensure that it is understood. Repeat information or request that the person living with SMI repeat what was said to him if necessary. This helps to check whether he understood what was said. This may require considerable patience, especially if the person living with SMI becomes angry or frustrated with being asked to request to repeat what was said; if asking to repeat results in verbal or physical threats then re-consider doing this and seek help from other service providers.
- Encourage the person living with SMI to use memory aids, such as a small notebook to record information. It may be helpful to have the person living with SMI to carry a notebook in which to record information such as "things to do today." Another example is to record important events and appointments on a calendar in the bedroom. Donald frequently asked about events that were important to him, such as weekend passes. The staff helped him to use a calendar in his room to keep track of when a relative planned to visit. Then they helped him to check his calendar when he began asking if anyone would be visiting soon. Donald also became bored and complained that he couldn't think of anything to do. The staff helped to make a list of things that he could do. The activities included such

things as going to the library, checking his activity list in his bedroom, or asking the staff if he could help them with anything. When he became bored, they reminded him to check the list in his bedroom. With practice, he began to check it on his own.
- Recognize successful maintenance of memory and attention. It is important not to disregard the individual's current capabilities in task attention and information recall, particularly for those living with SMI. The individual may recollect details that are easily overlooked due to their routine nature; acknowledging and positively reinforcing these behaviors is especially beneficial when notable effort is demonstrated.
- Seek assistance from experienced service providers in assessing the problem. Memory and concentration problems can be extremely difficult to clearly define and develop support strategies. If the strategies outlined above don't seem to work well, consider seeking a professional assessment by a clinical psychologist or neuropsychologist of the person's ability to concentrate and remember information. These professionals are qualified to administer tests of memory, learning, planning, and other neurocognitive functions. The neuropsychological test results are compared to those of individuals with similar age and education as the person with SMI. This way, the psychologist can tell what types of memory abilities are impaired. This will help clarify what is causing the problem and how serious it is. Such a detailed assessment of the neurocognitive capabilities (ability to attend, concentrate, and remember) of the person living with SMI may be required to accurately identify the problems and develop support strategies to improve them. For example, the assessment may find that the person living with SMI has severe problems with information verbally given to him but does better with written information. This will have implications for the type of information that the person living with SMI is likely to forget and the strategies used to minimize the problem and improvement functioning.

Conclusion

When persistent problems with memory and concentration interfere with the ability of the person living with SMI to take care of herself, the following suggestions may be helpful:

1. If the medications prescribed to the individual with serious mental illness have not been reviewed by a psychiatric service provider recently, it is recommended to schedule an appointment for evaluation and potential adjustment to enhance their well-being.
2. Be clear about what the person living with SMI does, which causes one to think that she has problems with memory and concentration. This will help focus efforts on determining the extent of the problems and what interventions to consider.

3. Watch for circumstances (such as time of day and the kind of information that is forgotten) that seem to affect the abilities of attending, remembering, and concentrating for the person living with SMI. This information will likely be useful in developing a plan to improve the problem.
4. Make sure that expectations for improvement are realistic. For people living with SMI, lower the expectations and increase them slowly as success is achieved, no matter how small.
5. Try to establish a structure of daily activities that is predictable. The more routine and predictable the routine is, the more likely the person living with SMI will be able to remember.
6. If there are new activities or the person living with SMI has been inconsistent about remembering daily activities, plan on giving a brief reminder shortly before the activity begins.
7. When giving information, minimize possible distractions, talk slowly and clearly, chunk information and if necessary, repeat the information. Try having the person living with SMI repeat what was said and what she heard and understood.
8. Use lists, signs, and notes as memory aids. Set up an "information center" which lists important things to remember. Work with the person living with SMI to get her to frequently check the list or look at the signs in places she will be using, such as the mirror in the bathroom/bedroom.
9. Don't be afraid to seek help. Many of these suggestions are much easier said than done. Expect difficulty in putting these suggestions into action. An experienced professional service provider may be able to help develop an intervention to achi*eve success.*

What About Donald?

While Donald's behavior had improved in many ways with antidepressant medication, he continued to have trouble remembering information. Because of this, he was inconsistent in attending group activities and other important meetings in the hospital program. The staff recognized that because he was so quiet and didn't cause any major disruption on the ward, it was easy for them to forget about him. They also recognized that they would have to think about ways that they could structure Donald's environment to help him remember important information.

The staff took several steps to accomplish their goal. They recognized that Donald became easily confused and nervous when his environment was chaotic or if there weren't clear expectations for what he was supposed to do. They decided that they would have to make sure that they spoke to Donald at an appropriate pace and avoided appearing rushed when telling him something. They made sure that they set a time during the day when they could sit with him and patiently ask how he felt things were going. This gave him an opportunity to talk with someone else in a quiet setting. If he declined to talk, they would accept this and try again later.

Because Donald had difficulty remembering which activities he was supposed to go to and when these activities were held, the staff made sure to give him a reminder about the activity and offered to escort him to the room where it would be held. If Donald declined to go, they accepted this but continued to remind him of future activities. They made sure to frequently show him the place on the ward where the schedule for all groups was posted. With repetition and prompted practice, Donald began to check this list by himself. The staff also made a calendar and message board for his room, listing any information which they felt would be important to him, such as the date and time of his wife's next visit. They helped him to change the date after getting out of bed and to check it frequently for information.

With these steps and continued medication, Donald was better able to remember important information and required fewer reminders from the staff. While he continued to have problems remembering information, he and his wife had learned ways to help him remember, and his memory difficulties were less of a problem.

In this example, the staff members took several steps to help Donald improve his ability in concentrating and remembering information:

1. They recognized that Donald had limited capabilities to concentrate and remember information and that it was even worse when things were hurried and chaotic in the environment. As much as possible, they tried to be patient when talking with him.
2. They recognized and accepted that Donald frequently became discouraged and socially withdrawn. They set time to seek him out and talk with him away from noise and other distractions. If he said that he didn't feel like talking, they accepted this but tried again at another time.
3. They took steps to help him recall his daily routine. Every day, they posted his group and activity schedule in an area that he could easily check. They reminded him several times during the day to check his schedule. Until he became accustomed to doing this, they made sure to give him a brief reminder about 5 min before each of his appointments.
4. Because he frequently asked about other important events, such as visits by relatives, they set up a calendar in his room that listed when these events would happen. Every day, they would make a mark to show which day it was and reminded him to check his calendar to see if he was asking when his next visit would be. After a while, Donald began marking the days off with no reminding.

They also recognized that, after discharge, he would still have problems remembering things such as when to take his medication. They worked with his family to help them set up a routine at home with lists like the one used in the hospital. They also set up a schedule for taking medication and advised the family how to remind him of this.

With this assistance, Donald improved during his impatient stay and, despite having continuing problems with his memory, adjusted well at home after leaving the hospital.

Summary

The concept of SMI refers to individuals with significant functional impairments due to persistent mental health problems. It is transdiagnostic and heterogeneous, affecting various adaptive behavioral domains including social, educational, and occupational functioning.

A significant problem behavior associated with SMI is neurocognitive impairments on various dimensions of neurocognitive domains that are displayed and assessed on neuropsychological performance tests. Neurocognitive deficits are common in 50–80% of individuals living with SMI. Although neurocognitive impairments are a significant area of concern in the mental health field, neurocognitive impairments are not a diagnostic criterion for SMI-related mental health problems.

Neurocognitive impairments have been found in the neurocognitive domains that include memory, attention, processing speed, working memory, executive functioning, psychomotor speed, and social cognitions; these impairments have been found to often predate the onset of mental health problems and behaviors that correspond to SMI and may persist despite improvements in other problem behaviors or symptoms.

Neuropsychological performance measures assess various dimensions of neurocognitive domains. Individuals living with SMI typically score one to two standard deviations (SD) in neurocognitive domains below individuals with no mental health problems. Neurocognitive capabilities are essential for functional status and quality of life in individuals with SMI. Impairments in executive functioning (EF) and social cognitions impact many areas of daily functioning. EF includes skills like task initiation, organization, and problem-solving (American Psychological Association, n.d.-g), which are crucial for self-regulation. Social cognition involves skills necessary for interpersonal interactions, including recognition of emotion and theory of mind (ToM) that are essential in self-awareness and social behaviors. Impairments in dimensions of social cognition correlate with dimensions of social functioning but are not well-defined or standardized. Difficulties with social cognition are better predictors of social outcomes than other types of neurocognitive impairments. In individuals living with SMI, particular neurocognitive impairments do not reliably forecast certain behavioral difficulties, including those required for everyday functioning. Future research needs to integrate neuropsychological assessments with operational definitions of behavioral problems for more effective treatment outcomes. Comprehensive assessment tools are necessary to evaluate neurocognitive impairments, which can affect rehabilitation outcomes.

The Positive and Negative Syndrome Scale (PANSS) assesses behavior problems and symptoms linked to living with SMI. Five clusters of problem behaviors were identified in a study of individuals living with SMI, highlighting the heterogeneity of problem behaviors and symptoms. Results of factor analysis of scores from the PANSS show nonspecific associations with neurocognitive performance and have found the neurocognitive impairments to be an independent factor contributing to the overall scores on the PANSS but not to specific clusters.

The National Institute of Mental Health (NIMH) Measurement and Treatment Research to Improve Cognition in Schizophrenia (MATRICS) initiative was started to investigate neurocognition in individuals living with SMI and develop effective treatments (Marder & Fenton, 2004). The initiative focused on addressing barriers to drug development and promoting consensus on neuropsychological performance measures and treatment targets. Empirical evidence and factor analytic studies guided the selection of neurocognitive domains to be assessed by the MATRICS Consensus Cognitive Battery (MCCB), emphasizing their impact on overall functioning in living with SMI. Analyses of studies of impairments on neuropsychological tests found seven neurocognitive domains that consistently were affected in people living with SMI who typically obtain scores one to two SDs below the normative sample for each specific neuropsychological performance measure.

The Measurement and Treatment Research to Improve Cognition in Schizophrenia (MATRICS)-MATRICS Cognitive Census Battery (MATRICS-MCCB) is a standardized neuropsychological battery that includes 10 tests that assess the seven domains of neurocognitive functioning, excluding verbal comprehension due to its resistance to change. Empirical evidence and factor analytic studies guided the selection of neurocognitive domains in the MCCB.

The assessed domains and the tests on the MCCB are:

1. Speed of processing: Tests include Brief Assessment of Cognition in Schizophrenia (BACS) Symbol Coding, Animal Naming Fluency, and Trail Making Test-Part A (TMT-A) with performance metrics. Processing speed has been found to be consistently impaired in people living with SMI, impacting overall neuropsychological performance.
2. Attention vigilance: Test includes the Continuous Performance Test (Identical Pairs) (CPT-IP).
3. Working memory (WM): Tests used are the Wechsler Memory Scale (third ed) (WMS-III) and Letter-Number Span.
4. Verbal learning and memory: Test includes the Hopkins Verbal Learning Test-Revised (HVLT-R) with total number of words recalled correctly over three learning trials as performance index.
5. Visual learning and memory: Test is the Brief Visuospatial Memory Test-Revised (BVMT-R). Performance index is total recall score over learning trials.
6. Reasoning and problem solving: Test used is the Neuropsychological Assessment Battery (NAB) Mazes Subtest (NAB Mazes) with the performance index being the total raw score.
7. Social cognitions: Test used is the Mayer-Salovey-Caruso Emotional Intelligence Test (MSCEIT) Managing Emotions. Performance index is the standard score across all responses.

Various neurocognitive assessment tools have been developed. The CogState Schizophrenia Battery assesses cognitive impairment in individuals living with SMI and takes approximately 40 min to complete. The Brief Assessment of Cognition in

Schizophrenia (BACS) is a 35-min test sensitive to neurocognitive impairments, assessing domains like reasoning, attention, and memory. A computerized battery of performance measures is the Cambridge Neuropsychological Test Automated Battery (CANTAB). Eight computerized performance tests are used to measure similar neurocognitive domains as the MATRICS. Self-report measures like the Schizophrenia Cognition Rating Scale (SCoRS) and the Cognitive Assessment Inventory (CAI) are used for ongoing assessment, showing strong correlations with other standard neurocognitive performance batteries.

Studies have been conducted to correlate results on neuropsychological performance measures and their relationship to functional capacities in individuals living with SMI using measures of basic adaptive functional behaviors. The measures that have been used include the University of California at San Diego Performance-Based Skills Assessment (UPSA) and the Independent Living Skills Inventory (ILSI). The UPSA evaluates functional capacities through role plays in five domains, including household chores and managing finances. The ILSI assesses real-world functioning. Results have found that neurocognitive performance scores alone do not predict daily living success as measured by these assessments. Research indicates a strong relationship between neuropsychological performance scores and functional capacity, but only a moderate correlation with real-world outcomes.

Neurocognitive impairments in SMI have been linked to neurological substrates, genetic factors, and structural brain changes. Neurocognitive impairments arise from complex interactions of neurobiological factors. Key neurocognitive domains including attention, memory, and executive functions (EFs) have correspondence to multiple structural brain regions that are activated during neurocognitive activities, such as emotion recognition or working memory (WM). Damage or structural change to one brain area can negatively impact others, leading to neurocognitive impairments.

Genetic factors, including specific polymorphisms, are linked to neurocognitive function in people living with SMI. Certain environmental and lifestyle factors change how genes are expressed and correlate with neurocognitive impairments. Dysfunction in neurotransmitter systems, particularly glutamate and GABA, is central to neurocognitive impairments in people living with SMI. Other biological factors that contribute to these impairments in people living with SMI include certain neuroinflammatory processes. Elevated inflammatory biomarkers and microglial activation are associated with impairments. Cerebral vascular issues, including microvascular abnormalities and brain hypoperfusion, and altered levels of vascular endothelial growth factor (VEGF) correlate with the impairments.

Structural neuroimaging findings have been found to be related to neurocognitive impairments. A meta-analysis of MRIs found gray matter loss in anterior insula and dorsal anterior cingulate cortex among individuals living with SMI. Decreased gray matter in these regions correlates with impaired EF. Future studies should explore the relationship between gray matter loss and severity of symptoms and problem behaviors in people living with SMI. Shared neural substrates and structural brain changes are evident across different mental health problems corresponding to SMI. Impairments in EF are prevalent across various mental health problems, especially in schizophrenia spectrum mental health problems.

Many individuals with SMI show impairments in attention, memory, processing speed, executive function (EF), and social cognition. However, there is a demonstrated intra-individual variability in neuropsychological performance. It has been hypothesized that this intra-individual variability reflects random errors by the examinee and is linked to white matter integrity. Composite scores on neuropsychological tests are consistently lower in people living with SMI, suggesting global neurocognitive impairments rather than specific deficits.

Environmental factors have been shown to be strong determinants of neurocognitive impairments in people living with SMI. Environmental stressors, including trauma and socioeconomic deprivation, significantly affect neurocognitive performance in SMI. There is a high prevalence of childhood adversity in people living with SMI with 95% reporting at least one childhood trauma and 47% experiencing physical abuse. Chronic stress from living conditions and trauma can impair neurocognitive functions, particularly memory and EF. Chronic stress results in the release of glucocorticoids, such as cortisol. Individuals living with persistent elevated levels of glucocorticoids (such as Cushing's syndrome) have impairments in neurocognitive flexibility, behavioral inhibition, and working memory (WM). Animal studies show that repeated stress causes neuronal changes mimicking mood and anxiety disorders.

Socio-behavioral dimensions such as trauma exposure correlate with earlier onset and more severe behaviors in individuals living with SMI. Childhood neglect has a significant impact on impairments of social neurocognitive functions in emotion recognition; the impairments are more prevalent in recognizing fear and anger. These problems in recognizing facial emotions of fear and anger are linked to problems in processing speed and attention.

It has been questioned whether performance on neuropsychological tests accurately reflects real-world functioning. A behavioral perspective on neuropsychological testing uses an idiographic approach, focusing on individual variations; the behavioral approach views behaviors during testing as a sample of behaviors that can provide valuable insights and data that can be used to assess and develop effective interventions. Observations during testing can reveal underlying issues, such as attention problems, that may contribute to perceived memory deficits. The behavior approach to neuropsychological performance testing offers a more flexible analysis of neurocognitive impairments and interventions.

Reviews of the available research have found challenges that highlight cultural considerations, assessment difficulties, and the need for comprehensive evaluations of both impairments and strengths across different populations.

Studies have shown that the prevalence of neurocognitive impairments is displayed by approximately 50–80% of individuals with SMI, particularly with impairments in the domains of memory and processing speed. The neurocognitive impairments are heterogeneous in the different mental health problems that correspond to SMI. Prevalence of people living with a schizophrenia spectrum mental health problems have a higher rate of prevalence of neurocognitive impairments compared to people living with a major depressive or bipolar type of mental health problems.

Challenges have been found when researching prevalence and types of neurocognitive impairments in individuals living with SMI across different cultures. Research is limited, especially in non-Western countries but one study in Uganda found that 62% of individuals with recent onset of living with SMI exhibited neurocognitive impairments greater than two SDs below healthy individuals, which is the same found in high income western countries. Common challenges in adapting neurocognitive tests include cultural differences, language barriers, educational disparities, and economic factors. Twenty-three unique neurocognitive measures were identified from 28 studies, with none validated in low-income settings. The authors recommend using specific neuropsychological performance measures, including Brief Assessment of Cognition in Schizophrenia (BACS), Cognitive Assessment Interview (CAI), MATRICS Consensus Cognitive Battery (MCCB), and CogState Schizophrenia Battery (CSB), for assessing neurocognition in SMI.

There is a notable gap in research regarding the prevalence of neurocognitive strengths in individuals living with SMI. A study involving participants across Europe evaluated neurocognitive functioning in various domains that followed the MATRICS guidelines. The study found both strengths and impairments in the neurocognitive domains that varied as to the recency of onset of living with SMI. The degree on impairment was defined as the number of SDs below the norms used for each neuropsychological performance measure. Moderate impairment was defined as one to two SD below the norms and severe impairment defined as greater than two SDs below. In total, 88% of individuals with recent onset of living with SMI exhibited moderate neurocognitive impairments, while 45.1% were in the severe range of impairments on neuropsychological performance measures. Other results found that 71.2% of the people in the at-risk group (displaying behaviors that could potentially result in living with SMI) demonstrated moderate neurocognitive impairment, while 22.4% showed severe impairments; the group of individuals living with depressive mental health problems showed 61.6% with moderate impairments and 16.2% with severe impairments.

Cognitive strengths were defined as "above average" and "extremely high level" when the obtained score on neuropsychological tests was one and two SDs above the norm, respectively. Over 16% of people in the recent onset group performed above average, compared to 36.1% in the at-risk group and 40.5% in the depressive mental health group. In the group without mental health problems, the results indicated that 48.6% had moderate impairments and 52.3% performed above average. The results indicated that people living with SMI display heterogeneity on neurocognitive performance measures in addition to the strengths and weaknesses in the neurocognitive domains that the tests are inferred to measure.

Neurocognitive impairments are a complex construct, affecting up to 80% of individuals living with SMI. They are complex, multifaceted, and characterized by distinct neurocognitive subtypes and brain structure variations. Factor analyses identified seven neurocognitive domains that appear to have significant impact on people living with SMI. The seven neurocognitive domains are processing speed, attention, working memory (WM), verbal learning, visual learning, reasoning, and social cognition but these domains can be reduced to three "parent" domains processing speed, attention/WM, and learning. These three "parent" domains explain much of the variance in the outcomes on neuropsychological performance measures.

Distinct neurocognitive subtypes have been identified by researchers. The subtypes include individuals with intact functioning across multiple neurocognitive domains with neurological structure being relatively intact. Other subtypes show degrees of impairment in EF with correlated cortical changes. The final clustering is individuals displaying widespread impairments across neurocognitive domains with extensive neurobiological changes, especially in younger individuals.

Studies on the neurocognitive performances of people living with SMI have been numerous and well supported. However, despite the plethora of research, no conclusive evidence has been found linking specific neurocognitive impairment with specific symptoms and problem behavioral profiles displayed by individuals living with SMI; the result is a lack of development of cutting-edge treatment for the remediation of the neurocognitive impairments. Future research should consider new approaches including clustering of individuals living with SMI into subtypes that may enhance the understanding of neurocognitive impairments beyond group-level models. Personalized interventions can be developed by focusing on specific neurocognitive deficits experienced by individuals with SMI using an idiographic approach to the neurocognitive impairments that are displayed on neuropsychological performance measures.

Individual strategies to assist individuals living with SMI in improving concentration and memory can be developed and implemented. Clear identification of memory and concentration issues is essential, including specific behaviors that indicate problems. "Chunking" information into smaller units can help individuals living with SMI to process and remember tasks more effectively. Consistent daily routines and predictable schedules enhance the ability to concentrate and remember information. Frequent breaks during complex tasks can prevent frustration and improve attention span. Reducing environmental distractions, such as noise, can significantly aid concentration for individuals living with SMI. Utilizing memory aids, such as notebooks and calendars, can help individuals track important tasks and events. Acknowledging and rewarding successes in memory and attention can motivate individuals to continue improving their skills. Professional assessments by psychological service providers can clarify memory issues and guide effective strategies for improvement.

References

Adams, R. E., Ritter, C., & Bonfine, N. (2015). Epidemiology of trauma: Childhood adversities, neighborhood problems, discrimination, chronic strains, life events, and daily hassles among people with a severe mental illness. *Psychiatry Research, 230*(2), 609–615. https://doi.org/10.1016/j.psychres.2015.10.012

Ahn, J. I., Yu, S. T., Sung, G., Choi, T. K., Lee, K. S., Bang, M., & Lee, S. H. (2019). Intra-individual variability in neurocognitive function in schizophrenia: Relationships with the corpus callosum. *Psychiatry Research: Neuroimaging, 283*, 1–6. https://doi.org/10.1016/j.pscychresns.2018.11.005

amastyleinsider. (2011, July 5*). Ability, capacity, capability. AMA Style Insider*. Retrieved March 2, 2025 from https://amastyleinsider.com/2011/07/05/ability-capacity-capability/#:~:text=Ability%20=%20Actual%20skill%2C%20either%20mental,incorrect.%E2%80%94Phil%20Sefton%2C%20ELS

American Psychiatric Association. (2022). *Diagnostic and statistical manual of mental disorders* (5th ed., text rev.). doi:https://doi.org/10.1176/appi.books.9780890425787

American Psychological Association. (n.d.-a). Attention. In *APA dictionary of psychology*. https://dictionary.apa.org/attention.

American Psychological Association. (n.d.-b). California Verbal Learning Test. In *APA dictionary of psychology*. https://dictionary.apa.org/california-verbal-learning-test

American Psychological Association. (n.d.-c). Cognitive flexibility. In *APA dictionary of psychology*. https://dictionary.apa.org/Cognitive -flexibility

American Psychological Association. (n.d.-d). Cushing's syndrome. In *APA dictionary of psychology*. https://dictionary.apa.org/cushings-syndrome

American Psychological Association. (n.d.-e). Neuropsychological test. In *APA dictionary of psychology*. https://dictionary.apa.org/Neuropsychological-test

American Psychological Association. (n.d.-f). Pegboard test. In *APA dictionary of psychology*. https://dictionary.apa.org/pegboard-test

American Psychological Association. (n.d.-g). Problem solving. In *APA dictionary of psychology*. https://dictionary.apa.org/problem-solving

American Psychological Association. (n.d.-h). Reasoning. In *APA dictionary of psychology*. https://dictionary.apa.org/reasoning

American Psychological Association. (n.d.-i). Social desirability. In *APA Dictionary of Psychology*. https://dictionary.apa.org/social-desirability

American Psychological Association. (n.d.-j). Verbal comprehension. In *APA dictionary of psychology*. https://dictionary.apa.org/verbal-comprehension

American Psychological Association. (n.d.-k). Visual learning. In *APA dictionary of psychology*. https://dictionary.apa.org/visual-learning

American Psychological Association. (n.d.-l). Visual memory. In *APA dictionary of psychology*. https://dictionary.apa.org/visual-memory

American Psychological Association. (n.d.-m). Wechsler Adult Intelligence Scale (WAIS). In *APA dictionary of psychology*. https://dictionary.apa.org/wechsler-adult-intelligence-scale

American Psychological Association. (n.d.-n). Wisconsin Card Sorting Test (WCST). In *APA dictionary of psychology*. https://dictionary.apa.org/wisconsin-card-sorting-test

American Psychological Association. (n.d.-o). Working memory. In *APA dictionary of psychology*. https://dictionary.apa.org/working-memory

Ardila, A., & Ostrosky, F. (2022). What do neuropsychological tests assess? *Applied Neuropsychology: Adult, 29*(1), 1–9. https://doi.org/10.1080/23279095.2019.1699099

Arizmendi, C. J., & Gates, K. M. (2024). Clustering individuals based on similarity in idiographic factor loading patterns. *Multivariate Behavioral Research*, (1), –25. https://doi.org/10.1080/00273171.2024.2374826

Baggetta, P., & Alexander, P. A. (2016). Conceptualization and operationalization of executive function. *Mind, Brain, and Education, 10*(1), 10–33. https://doi.org/10.1111/mbe.12100

Barlow, D. H., & Nock, M. K. (2009). Why can't we be more idiographic in our research? *Perspectives on Psychological Science, 4*(1), 19–21. https://doi.org/10.1111/j.1745-6924.2009.01088.x

Barnett, J. H., Robbins, T. W., Leeson, V. C., Sahakian, B. J., Joyce, E. M., & Blackwell, A. D. (2010). Assessing cognitive function in clinical trials of schizophrenia. *Neuroscience and Biobehavioral Reviews*. https://doi.org/10.1016/j.neubiorev.2010.01.012

Barrett, S. L., Mulholland, C. C., Cooper, S. J., & Rushe, T. M. (2009). Patterns of neurocognitive impairment in first-episode bipolar disorder and schizophrenia. *The British Journal of Psychiatry, 195*(1), 67–72. https://doi.org/10.1192/bjp.bp.108.054874

Bell, M. D., Lysaker, P. H., Milstein, R. M., & Beam-Goulet, J. L. (1994). Concurrent validity of the cognitive component of schizophrenia: Relationship of PANSS scores to neuropsychological assessments. *Psychiatry Research, 54*(1), 51–58. https://doi.org/10.1016/0165-1781(94)90084-1

Beltz, A. M., Wright, A. G. C., Sprague, B. N., & Molenaar, P. C. M. (2016). Bridging the nomothetic and idiographic approaches to the analysis of clinical data. *Assessment, 23*(4), 447–458. https://doi.org/10.1177/1073191116648209

Bettis, R. J., Faith, L. A., Beard, A. M., Whan, B. A., Hegwood, C. M., Monette, M. A., Myers, E. J., Abel, D. B., Mickens, J. L., Russell, M. T., Rand, K. L., Salyers, M. P., Luther, L., & Minor, K. S. (2024). Narrative forewarnings: A qualitative analysis of the themes preceding disorganized speech in schizophrenia. *Behavioral Sciences, 14*(3), 212. https://doi.org/10.3390/bs14030212

Bowie, C. R., & Harvey, P. D. (2006). Cognitive deficits and functional outcome in schizophrenia. *Neuropsychiatric Disease And Treatment, 2*(4), 531–536. https://doi.org/10.2147/nedt.S24531

Bratman, G. N., Hamilton, J. P., & Daily, G. C. (2012). The impacts of nature experience on human cognitive function and mental health. *Annals of the New York Academy of Sciences, 1249*(1), 118–136. https://doi.org/10.1111/j.1749-6632.2011.06400.x

Burdick, K. E., & Goldberg, T. E. (2008). Chapter 1. Overview and introduction: Dimensions of cognition and measures of cognitive function. In *Cognitive dysfunction in bipolar disorder: A guide for clinicians* (pp. 1–22). American Psychiatric Publishing. https://doi.org/10.1176/appi.books.9781615377756.lg01

Burton, C. Z., Vella, L., Harvey, P. D., Patterson, T. L., Heaton, R. K., & Twamley, E. W. (2013). Factor structure of the MATRICS consensus cognitive battery (MCCB) in schizophrenia. *Schizophrenia Research, 146*(1–3), 244–248. https://doi.org/10.1016/j.schres.2013.02.026

Cambridge Cognition. (2023, June 19). *One Touch Stockings of Cambridge (OTS)*. Cambridge Cognition. https://cambridgecognition.com/one-touch-stockings-of-cambridge-ots/

Casaletto, K. B., & Heaton, R. K. (2017). Neuropsychological assessment: Past and future. *Journal of the International Neuropsychological Society, 23*(9–10), 778–790. https://doi.org/10.1017/S1355617717001060

Cotter, J., Granger, K., Backx, R., Hobbs, M., Looi, C. Y., & Barnett, J. H. (2017). Social cognitive dysfunction as a clinical marker: A systematic review of meta-analyses across 30 clinical conditions. *Neuroscience and Biobehavioral Reviews, 80*, 365–371. https://doi.org/10.1016/j.neubiorev.2017.11.014

Cullum, C. M. (1998). Neuropsychological assessment of adults. In A. S. Bellack & M. Hersen (Eds.), *Comprehensive clinical psychology* (Vol. 4, pp. 303–347). Pergamon. https://doi.org/10.1016/B0080-4270(73)00227-3

De la Torre, G., Doval, S., López-Sanz, D., García-Sedeño, M., Ramallo, M., Bernal, M., & González-Torre, S. (2021). Neurocognitive impairment in severe mental illness: Comparative study with Spanish speaking patients. *Brain Sciences, 11*(3), 389. https://doi.org/10.3390/brainsci11030389

DeTore, N. R., Mueser, K. T., & McGurk, S. R. (2018). What does the managing emotions branch of the MSCEIT add to the MATRICS consensus cognitive battery? *Schizophrenia Research, 197*, 414–420. https://doi.org/10.1016/j.schres.2018.02.018

Eilam-Stock, T., Best, P., Sherman, K., Shaw, M. T., Ventura, J., Krupp, L. B., & Charvet, L. E. (2021). An interview-based assessment of the experience of cognitive impairment in multiple sclerosis: The cognitive assessment interview (CAI). *Frontiers in Neurology, 12*, 637895. https://doi.org/10.3389/fneur.2021.637895

Elvevag, B., & Goldberg, T. E. (2000). Cognitive impairment in schizophrenia is the core of the disorder. *Critical Reviews in Neurobiology, 14*(1). https://doi.org/10.1615/CritRevNeurobiol.v14.i1.10

Galderisi, S., & Marder, S. R. (2024). Cognitive impairment associated with schizophrenia: New research agenda. *Schizophrenia Bulletin Open, 5*(1), sgae023. https://doi.org/10.1093/schizbullopen/sgae023

Galvin, J. E., Tolea, M. I., Moore, C., & Chrisphonte, S. (2020). The number symbol coding task: A brief measure of executive function to detect dementia and cognitive impairment. *PLoS One, 15*(11), e0242233. https://doi.org/10.1371/journal.pone.0242233

Giordano, G. M., Palumbo, D., Mucci, A., Ventura, J., Giuliani, L., Perrottelli, A., Bucci, P., Rocca, P., Rossi, A., Bertolino, A., Rucci, P., Galderisi, S., Maj, M., & Italian Network for Research on Psychoses. (2022). The cognitive assessment interview (CAI): Association with neuropsychological scores and real-life functioning in a large sample of Italian subjects with schizophrenia. *Schizophrenia Research.* https://doi.org/10.1016/j.schres.2022.01.029

Girotti, M., Bulin, S. E., & Carreno, F. R. (2024). Effects of chronic stress on cognitive function–from neurobiology to intervention. *Neurobiology of Stress*, 100670. https://doi.org/10.1016/j.ynstr.2024.100670

Goodkind, M., Eickhoff, S. B., Oathes, D. J., Jiang, Y., Chang, A., Jones-Hagata, L. B., Ortega, B. N., Zaiko, Y. V., Roach, E. L., Korgaonkar, M. S., Grieve, S. M., Galatzer-Levy, I., Fox, P. T., & Etkin, A. (2015). Identification of a common neurobiological substrate for mental illness. *JAMA Psychiatry, 72*(4), 305–315. https://doi.org/10.1001/jamapsychiatry.2014.2206

Gold, J. M., Robinson, B., Leonard, C. J., Hahn, B., Chen, S., McMahon, R. P., & Luck, S. J. (2018). Selective attention, working memory, and executive function as potential independent sources of cognitive dysfunction in schizophrenia. *Schizophrenia Bulletin, 44*(6), 1227–1234. https://doi.org/10.1093/schbul/sbx155

Green, M. F., & Nuechterlein, K. H. (1999). Should schizophrenia be treated as a neurocognitive disorder? *Schizophrenia Bulletin, 25*(2), 309–319. https://doi.org/10.1093/oxfordjournals.schbul.a033380

Green, M. F. (1996). What are the functional consequences of neurocognitive deficits in schizophrenia? *The American Journal of Psychiatry, 153*(3), 321–330. https://doi.org/10.1176/ajp.153.3.321

Green, M. F., Harris, J. G., & Nuechterlein, K. H. (2014). The MATRICS consensus cognitive battery: What we know 6 years later. *American Journal of Psychiatry, 171*(11), 1151–1154. https://doi.org/10.1176/appi.ajp.2014.14070936

Green, M. F., Horan, W. P., & Lee, J. (2019). Nonsocial and social cognition in schizophrenia: Current evidence and future directions. *World Psychiatry, 18*(2), 146–161. https://doi.org/10.1002/wps.20624

Green, M. F., Kern, R. S., & Heaton, R. K. (2004). Longitudinal studies of cognition and functional outcome in schizophrenia: Implications for MATRICS. *Schizophrenia Research, 72*(1), 41–51. https://doi.org/10.1016/j.schres.2004.09.009

Green, M. F., Kern, R. S., Braff, D. L., & Mintz, J. (2000). Neurocognitive deficits and functional outcome in schizophrenia: Are we measuring the "right stuff"? *Schizophrenia Bulletin, 26*(1), 119–136. https://doi.org/10.1093/oxfordjournals.schbul.a033430

Haile, Y. G., Habatmu, K., Derese, A., Gouse, H., Lawrie, S. M., Cella, M., & Alem, A. (2022). Assessing cognition in people with severe mental disorders in low- and middle-income countries: A systematic review of assessment measures. *Social Psychiatry and Psychiatric Epidemiology, 57*(3), 435–460. https://doi.org/10.1007/s00127-021-02120-x

Harvey, P. D., & Strassnig, M. (2012). Predicting the severity of everyday functional disability in people with schizophrenia: Cognitive deficits, functional capacity, symptoms, and health status. *World Psychiatry, 11*(2), 73–79. https://doi.org/10.1016/j.wpsyc.2012.05.004

Harvey, P. D., Horan, W. P., Atkins, A. S., Stevens, H., Welch, M., Yuan, J., Ventura, J., Kegeles, S., Burdick, K. E., & Keefe, R. S. E. (2020). Factor structure of cognitive performance and functional capacity in schizophrenia: Evidence for differences across functional capacity measures. *Schizophrenia Research, 223*, 297–304. https://doi.org/10.1016/j.schres.2020.08.010

Harvey, P. D., Koren, D., Reichenberg, A., & Bowie, C. R. (2006). Negative symptoms and cognitive deficits: What is the nature of their relationship? *Schizophrenia Bulletin, 32*(2), 250–258. https://doi.org/10.1093/schbul/sbj011

Heinrichs, R. W., & Awad, A. G. (1993). Neurocognitive subtypes of chronic schizophrenia. *Schizophrenia Research, 9*(1), 49–58. https://doi.org/10.1016/0920-9964(93)90009-8

Heinrichs, R. W., & Zakzanis, K. K. (1998). Neurocognitive deficit in schizophrenia: A quantitative review of the evidence. *Neuropsychology, 12*(3), 426–433. https://doi.org/10.1037/0894-4105.12.3.426

Higgins, G. A., & Silenieks, L. B. (2017). Rodent test of attention and impulsivity: The 5-choice serial reaction time task. *Current Protocols in Pharmacology, 78*(1), 5.49.1–5.49.17. https://doi.org/10.1002/cpph.27

Hoffmann, C. (2023). Neuropsychological model of human behavior. In *Brain-adapted leadership: Effective leadership according to neuropsychological findings* (pp. 71–103). Springer Berlin Heidelberg. https://doi.org/10.1007/978-3-662-65841-3_4

Howieson, D. (2019). Current limitations of neuropsychological tests and assessment procedures. *The Clinical Neuropsychologist, 33*(2), 200–208. https://doi.org/10.1080/13854046.2018.1549259

Huang, Y., Wang, W., Hei, G., Shao, T., Li, L., Yang, Y., Wang, X., Long, Y., Xiao, J., Peng, X., Song, C., Cai, J., Song, X., Xu, X., Gao, S., Huang, J., Kang, D., Wang, Y., Zhao, J., … Wu, R. (2025). Subgroups of cognitive impairments in schizophrenia characterized by executive function and their morphological features: a latent profile analysis study. *BMC Medicine, 23*(1), Article 13. https://doi.org/10.1186/s12916-024-03835-9

Hugenberg, K., & Wilson, J. (2013). Faces are central to social cognition. In D. E. Carlston (Ed.), *The Oxford Handbook of Social Cognition* (pp. 167–193). Oxford University Press.

Jeon, D. W., Jung, D. U., Kim, S. J., Oh, M., Moon, J. J., & Kim, Y. S. (2020a). Correlation between performance-based and interview-based cognitive measurements in patients with schizophrenia. *Schizophrenia Bulletin, 46*(Suppl 1), S257. https://doi.org/10.1093/schbul/sbaa029.629

Jeon, D.-W., Jung, D.-U., Oh, M., Moon, J.-J., Kim, S.-J., & Kim, Y.-S. (2020b). Correlation between performance-based and interview-based cognitive measurements in patients with schizophrenia. *Psychiatry Investigation, 17*(7), 695–701. https://doi.org/10.30773/pi.2020.0085

Kaplan, R. M., & Saccuzzo, D. P. (2010). *Psychological testing: Principles, applications, and issues* (7th ed.). Wadsworth. https://www.cengage.com/c/psychological-testing-principles-applications-and-issues-7e-kaplan/9780495602203

Kay, S. R., Fiszbein, A., & Opler, L. A. (1987). The positive and negative syndrome scale (PANSS) for schizophrenia. *Schizophrenia Bulletin, 13*(2), 261–276. https://doi.org/10.1093/schbul/13.2.261

Keefe, R. S. E., Poe, M., Walker, T. M., Kang, J. W., & Harvey, P. D. (2006a). The schizophrenia Cognition rating scale: An interview-based assessment and its relationship to cognition, real-world functioning, and functional capacity. . *American Journal of Psychiatry, 163*(3), 426–432. https://doi.org/10.1176/appi.ajp.163.3.426

Keefe, R. S., Goldberg, T. E., Harvey, P. D., Gold, J. M., Poe, M. P., & Coughenour, L. (2004). The brief assessment of Cognition in schizophrenia: Reliability, sensitivity, and comparison with a standard neurocognitive battery. *Schizophrenia Research, 68*(2–3), 283–297. https://doi.org/10.1016/j.schres.2003.09.011

Keefe, R. S., Poe, M., Walker, T. M., & Harvey, P. D. (2006b). The relationship of the brief assessment of cognition in schizophrenia (BACS) to functional capacity and real-world functional outcome. *Journal of Clinical and Experimental Neuropsychology, 28*(2), 260–269. https://doi.org/10.1176/appi.ajp.163.3.426

Keefe, R. S. E., & Harvey, P. D. (2012). Cognitive impairment in schizophrenia. In M. Geyer & G. Gross (Eds.), *Novel Antischizophrenia treatments. Handbook of experimental pharmacology* (Vol. 213, pp. 11–37). Springer. https://doi.org/10.1007/978-3-642-25758-2_2

Kline, E., Hendel, V., Friedman-Yakoobian, M., Mesholam-Gately, R. I., Findeisen, A., Zimmet, S., DeRosse, P., Malin, M. A., Galatzer-Levy, I. R., & Seidman, L. J. (2019). A comparison of neurocognition and functioning in first episode psychosis populations: Do research samples reflect the real world? *Social Psychiatry and Psychiatric Epidemiology, 54*, 291–301. https://doi.org/10.1007/s00127-018-1631-x

Knight, M. M. (2000). Cognitive ability and functional status. *Journal of Advanced Nursing, 31*(6), 1459–1468. https://doi.org/10.1046/j.1365-2648.2000.01459.x

Kovacs, K., & Conway, A. R. (2016). Process overlap theory: A unified account of the general factor of intelligence. *Psychological Inquiry, 27*(3), 151–177. https://doi.org/10.1080/1047840X.2016.1153946

Lafayette Instrument Company. (n.d.). *Purdue pegboard test: Model 32020A user's manual.* Lafayette Instrument Company. Retrieved February 22, 2025, from https://www.limef.com/downloads/MAN-32020A-forpdf-rev0.pdf

Lahera, G., Ruiz, A., Branas, A., Vicens, M., & Orozco, A. (2017). Reaction time, processing speed and sustained attention in schizophrenia: Impact on social functioning. *Revista de Psiquiatría y Salud Mental (English Edition), 10*(4), 197–205. https://doi.org/10.1016/j.rpsm.2017.04.001

Leifker, F. R., Bowie, C. R., & Harvey, P. D. (2009). Determinants of everyday outcomes in schizophrenia: The influences of cognitive impairment, functional capacity, and symptoms. *Schizophrenia Research, 115*(1), 82–87. https://doi.org/10.1016/j.schres.2009.09.004

Leonhardt, B. L., Huling, K., Hamm, J. A., Roe, D., Hasson-Ohayon, I., McLeod, H. J., & Lysaker, P. H. (2017). Recovery and serious mental illness: A review of current clinical and research paradigms and future directions. *Expert Review of Neurotherapeutics, 17*(11), 1117–1130. https://doi.org/10.1080/10503307.2016.1219421

Marder, S. R., & Fenton, W. (2004). Measurement and treatment research to improve cognition in schizophrenia: NIMH MATRICS initiative to support the development of agents for improving cognition in schizophrenia. *Schizophrenia Research, 72*(1), 5–9. https://doi.org/10.1016/j.schres.2004.09.010

Marquand, A. F., Kia, S. M., Zabihi, M., Wolfers, T., Buitelaar, J. K., & Beckmann, C. F. (2019). Conceptualizing mental disorders as deviations from normative functioning. *Molecular Psychiatry, 24*(10), 1415–1424. https://doi.org/10.1038/s41380-019-0441-1

Mauritz, M. W., Goossens, P. J., Draijer, N., & Van Achterberg, T. (2013). Prevalence of interpersonal trauma exposure and trauma-related disorders in severe mental illness. *European Journal of Psychotraumatology, 4*(1), 19985. https://doi.org/10.3402/ejpt.v4i0.19985

McCleery, A., & Nuechterlein, K. H. (2019). Cognitive impairment in psychotic illness: Prevalence, profile of impairment, developmental course, and treatment considerations. *Dialogues in Clinical Neuroscience, 21*(3), 239–248. https://doi.org/10.31887/DCNS.2019.21.3/amccleery

McCutcheon, R. A., Keefe, R. S. E., & McGuire, P. K. (2023). Cognitive impairment in schizophrenia: Aetiology, pathophysiology, and treatment. *Molecular Psychiatry, 28*(9), 1902–1918. https://doi.org/10.1038/s41380-023-01949-9

Menditto, A. A., Wallace, C. J., Liberman, R. P., Wal, J. V., Jones, N. T., & Stuve, P. (1999). Functional assessment of independent living skills. *Psychiatric Rehabilitation Skills, 3*(2), 200–219. https://doi.org/10.1080/10973439908408384

Minor, K. S., Marggraf, M. P., Davis, B. J., Luther, L., Vohs, J. L., Buck, K. D., & Lysaker, P. H. (2015). Conceptual disorganization weakens links in cognitive pathways: Disentangling neurocognition, social cognition, and metacognition in schizophrenia. Schizophrenia Research, 169(1–3), 153–158. doi:https://doi.org/10.1016/j.schres.2015.09.026.

Mitchell, R. L. C., & Young, A. H. (2016). Theory of mind in bipolar disorder, with comparison to the impairments observed in schizophrenia. *Frontiers in Psychiatry, 6*, 188. https://doi.org/10.3389/fpsyt.2015.00188

Morozova, A., Zorkina, Y., Abramova, O., Pavlova, O., Pavlov, K., Soloveva, K., Volkova, M., Alekseeva, P., Andryshchenko, A., Kostyuk, G., Gurina, O., & Chekhonin, V. (2022). Neurobiological highlights of cognitive impairment in psychiatric disorders. *International Journal of Molecular Sciences, 23*(3), 1217. https://doi.org/10.3390/ijms23031217

Myers, E. J., Abel, D. B., Mickens, J. L., Russell, M. T., Rand, K. L., Salyers, M. P., Luther, L., & Minor, K. S. (2024). Meta-analysis of the relationship between metacognition and disorganized symptoms in psychosis. *Schizophrenia Research, 264*, 178–187. https://doi.org/10.1016/j.schres.2023.12.009

Nasrallah, H. A. (2023). The Cognition self-assessment rating scale for patients with schizophrenia. *Current Psychiatry, 22*(3), 30–34. https://doi.org/10.12788/cp.0335

Nielsen, R. E., Lindström, E., Telléus, G. K., & Levander, S. (2014). Is the PANSS cognitive scale measuring cognition? *Nordic Journal of Psychiatry, 68*(8), 573–578. https://doi.org/10.3109/08039488.2014.898790

Nuechterlein, K. H., Barch, D. M., Gold, J. M., Goldberg, T. E., Green, M. F., & Heaton, R. K. (2004). Identification of separable cognitive factors in schizophrenia. *Schizophrenia Research, 72*(1), 29–39. https://doi.org/10.1016/j.schres.2004.09.007

Nuechterlein, K. H., Green, M. F., Kern, R. S., Baade, L. E., Barch, D. M., Cohen, J. D., Essock, S., Fenton, W. S., Frese, F. J., Gold, J. M., Goldberg, T., Heaton, R. K., Keefe, R. S. E., Kraemer, H., Mesholam-Gately, R., Seidman, L. J., Stover, E., Weinberger, D. R., Young, A. S., et al. (2008). The MATRICS consensus cognitive battery, part 1: Test selection, reliability, and validity. *American Journal of Psychiatry, 165*(2), 203–213. https://doi.org/10.1176/appi.ajp.2007.07010042

O'Carroll, R. (2000). Cognitive impairment in schizophrenia. *Advances in Psychiatric Treatment, 6*(3), 161–168. https://doi.org/10.1192/apt.6.3.161

Patterson, T. L., Goldman, S., McKibbin, C. L., Hughs, T., & Jeste, D. V. (2001). UCSD performance-based skills assessment: Development of a new measure of everyday functioning for severely mentally ill adults. *Schizophrenia Bulletin, 27*(2), 235–245. https://doi.org/10.1093/oxfordjournals.schbul.a006870

Pietrzak, R. H., Olver, J., Norman, T., Piskulic, D., Maruff, P., & Snyder, P. J. (2009). A comparison of the CogState schizophrenia battery and the measurement and treatment research to improve Cognition in schizophrenia (MATRICS) battery in assessing cognitive impairment in chronic schizophrenia. *Journal of Clinical and Experimental Neuropsychology, 31*(7), 848–859. https://doi.org/10.1080/13803390802592458

Réthelyi, J. M., Czobor, P., Polgár, P., Mersich, B., Bálint, S., Jekkel, É., Molnár, K., Kovács, G., Fekete, S., Elek, L., & Bitter, I. (2012). General and domain-specific neurocognitive impairments in deficit and non-deficit schizophrenia. *European Archives of Psychiatry and Clinical Neuroscience, 262*, 107–115. https://doi.org/10.1007/s00406-011-0224-4

Roncone, R., Falloon, I. R., Mazza, M., De Risio, A., Pollice, R., Necozione, S., Tansella, M., & Casacchia, M. (2002). Is theory of mind in schizophrenia more strongly associated with clinical and social functioning than with neurocognitive deficits? *Psychopathology, 35*(5), 280–288. https://doi.org/10.1159/000067062

Sahakian, B. J., & Owen, A. M. (1992). Computerized assessment in neuropsychiatry using CANTAB: Discussion paper. *Journal of the Royal Society of Medicine, 85*(7), 399–402. https://doi.org/10.1177/014107689208500716

Schaefer, J., Giangrande, E., Weinberger, D. R., & Dickinson, D. (2013). The global cognitive impairment in schizophrenia: Consistent over decades and around the world. *Schizophrenia Research, 150*(1), 42–50. https://doi.org/10.1016/j.schres.2013.07.009

Shahrokh, N. C., & Hales, R. E. (2003). *American psychiatric glossary* (8th ed.). American Psychiatric Publishing. https://doi.org/10.5555/appi.books.9781615373758.db23Glossary

Silva, D., Guerreiro, M., Maroco, J., Santana, I., Rodrigues, A., Bravo Marques, J., & de Mendonça, A. (2012). Comparison of four verbal memory tests for the diagnosis and predictive value of mild cognitive impairment. *Dementia and Geriatric Cognitive Disorders Extra, 2*(1), 120–131. https://doi.org/10.1159/000336224

Skinner, B. F. (1953). *Science and human behavior.* Macmillan. https://psycnet.apa.org/record/1954-05139-000

Snyder, H. R., Miyake, A., & Hankin, B. L. (2015). Advancing understanding of executive function impairments and psychopathology: Bridging the gap between clinical and cognitive approaches. *Frontiers in Psychology, 6*, 328. https://doi.org/10.3389/fpsyg.2015.00328

Stainton, A., Chisholm, K., Griffiths, S. L., Kambeitz-Ilankovic, L., Wenzel, J., Bonivento, C., Brambilla, P., Iqbal, M., Lichtenstein, T. K., Rosen, M., Antonucci, L. A., Maggioni, E., Kambeitz, J., Borgwardt, S., Riecher-Rössler, A., Andreou, C., Schmidt, A., Schultze-Lutter,

F., et al. (2023). Prevalence of cognitive impairments and strengths in the early course of psychosis and depression. *Psychological Medicine, 53*(12), 5945–5957. https://doi.org/10.1017/S0033291723001770

Talevski, J., Wong Shee, A., Rasmussen, B., Kemp, G., & Beauchamp, A. (2020). Teach-back: A systematic review of implementation and impacts. *PLoS One, 15*(4), e0231350. https://doi.org/10.1371/journal.pone.0231350

Thomas, M. V. (2010, January). What is mind?: A neuropsychological perspective. *Seminar on mind, brain, and consciousness*, 159–163. Retrieved from https://vpmthane.org/Publications/MindBrainAndConsciousness/Tomas%20M.V.pdf.pdf

Ventura, J., Reise, S. P., Keefe, R. S. E., Baade, L. E., Gold, J. M., Green, M. F., Nuechterlein, K. H., & Bilder, R. M. (2010). The cognitive assessment interview (CAI): Development and validation of an empirically derived, brief interview-based measure of cognition. *Schizophrenia Research, 121*(1–3), 24–31. https://doi.org/10.1016/j.schres.2010.04.016

Wang, Y., Meng, W., Liu, Z., An, Q., & Hu, X. (2022). Cognitive impairment in psychiatric diseases: Biomarkers of diagnosis, treatment, and prevention. *Frontiers in Cellular Neuroscience, 16*, 1046692. https://doi.org/10.3389/fncel.2022.1046692

World Health Organization (WHO). (2019). *International statistical classification of diseases and related health problems* (11th ed.). https://icd.who.int/

Chapter 11
Problems with Anger and Aggression in Individuals Living with Serious Mental Illness

Introduction

Anger and aggression are among the most complex and consequential behavioral phenomena encountered in clinical mental health practice. While often conflated in everyday discourse, these constructs are distinct in origin, expression, and impact, particularly within the context of serious mental illness (SMI). Anger, a fundamental human emotion, serves adaptive functions in signaling perceived injustice or threat and mobilizing goal-directed action. Aggression, by contrast, refers to behaviors intended to harm or intimidate others, whether physically, verbally, or passively. In individuals living with SMI, the dysregulation of anger and the emergence of aggressive behaviors pose significant challenges to assessment, treatment, and community integration, often exacerbating stigma and complicating care.

This chapter examines the multidimensional nature of anger and aggression in SMI, beginning with definitional clarity and theoretical distinctions. It explores the neurophysiological substrates and environmental contingencies that shape these behaviors, emphasizing the role of impulsivity, trauma, and social learning. Drawing on DSM-5-TR diagnostic criteria, this chapter highlights conditions in which anger and aggression are core features, such as intermittent explosive disorder, borderline personality disorder, and disruptive mood dysregulation disorder, while also addressing their transdiagnostic relevance across schizophrenia spectrum and bipolar disorders. This chapter further considers passive-aggression and other forms of maladaptive expression, underscoring the importance of context-sensitive interpretation.

A central focus is placed on dimensional models and psychometric approaches to assessing anger and aggression. Key instruments are reviewed, including the Multidimensional Anger Inventory (MAI) and the Dimensions of Anger Reactions (DAR-5), and synthesizes recent factor analytic research that identifies overlapping domains such as anger-arousal, rumination, frustration-discomfort, regulation, and

G. F. McKeegan, *Behavior Change Interventions for Serious Mental Illness*, Evidence-Based Practices in Behavioral Health,
https://doi.org/10.1007/978-3-032-18372-9_11

socially constituted anger. Limitations in construct validity and cultural sensitivity are critically examined, with attention to how these gaps affect clinical decision-making and intervention planning. The overlap between emotional experience and behavioral expression is examined through behavioral analytic frameworks, including motivating operations and stimulus control.

Evidence-informed strategies for behavioral support and intervention are outlined. These include functional assessments, collateral observation, and contingency-based approaches that differentiate normative emotional responses from clinically significant dysfunction. Emphasis is placed on the need for individualized, multidimensional treatment planning that accounts for neurobiological, psychological, and environmental influences. By integrating empirical findings with clinical pragmatism, a nuanced understanding of anger and aggression in SMI, fostering both diagnostic precision and therapeutic empathy, is articulated.

> The person for whom I care gets frustrated over little things; he yells at me and others if anything does not go the way he wants it to go; he has threatened to hurt others. He has been kicked out of group homes because others are afraid of him

The Case of Charles.

Charles is a young man in his 20's who is diagnosed as having an "intermittent explosive disorder" or IED. This mental health condition was given because he had difficulty managing his frustrations and associated emotions, particularly anger. It was assumed that this problem was due to an abnormality in his brain, but no specific abnormality could be found. He had episodes of extreme anger and aggression that had no clear cause. Because of his difficulty with anger and aggressive behaviors, Charles was frequently suspended during his school years and had to attend special schools during adolescence. During one home visit, he became angry at his sister and chased her with a knife. After this incident, he was hospitalized. Since returning home, he has had episodes of anger and aggression, which have resulted in police involvement and emergency hospitalizations.

Charles does not experience delusions, hallucinations, or other symptoms of severe mental health problems. However, he occasionally starts to complain about something that happened to him (e.g., "She told me I had to clean my room." or "He called me stupid."). Once this begins, it is very difficult for him to calm down. When others try to reason with him, Charles often gets louder and starts threatening to hurt the other person (e.g., "I'm a man. They can't do this to me. I'll punch their lights out."). Often, the more people try to reason with him, the worse he gets. This is very frustrating and frightening for those around him. Many have learned to stay away from him and just let him get worse until he does something that requires them to call the police. Frustrated and scared caregivers have yelled back at him and made the situation worse when they really were only trying to help. Charles blows up over minor incidents. Even something as minor as another person bumping into him will result in him attempting to punch the other person or throw furniture around the room. The frustration and fear that many other people feel around Charles have led many of them to consider him beyond help.

Definitions and Characteristics of Anger and Aggressive Behaviors by Individuals Living with Serious Mental Illness?

Anger and aggressive behavior play a prominent role in the mental health field. Anger is one of four basic emotions that include happiness, sadness, fear, and anger. Emotions are essential to adaptive functioning across all human behaviors. The basic emotions are associated with three environmental contingencies: reward/reinforcement (happiness), punishment (sadness), and stress (fear and anger) (Gu et al., 2019).

Emotions differ along various dimensions of behavior, including frequency of occurrences, intensity or magnitude, stimulus control, context, and antecedental and consequential conditions. Behaviors differ on how they can be assessed. Some behaviors are known as "private events" or "covert events" that are known only to the individual experiencing the behaviors such as thoughts, feelings, perceptions, and sensations (Tourinho, 2006). The "private events" can be accessed through verbal self-reports from the individual, which are verbal responses that operate under environmental contingencies (Tourinho, 2006). At times, assessing "private events" is unreliable and invalid. For example, the person may be exaggerating or minimizing the emotion that they are experiencing and vary the details of the experience of the emotion as to the setting and the consequence. Sometimes the person may not be aware of the expression of emotion. For example, a person may be angry, have a scowl on her face, talking loudly but deny that she is angry. People are usually not aware of what they are thinking or feeling, especially if what is being recalled is in the past. Additionally, language, cultural, and social differences can affect any verbal exchange.

An additional method for evaluating private events involves determining whether behaviors have collateral sources of observation. Collateral sources may include reports from others regarding an individual's experiences or observable behaviors that are interrelated. For instance, pain is a private and covert event; the individual experiencing pain can communicate details such as location, frequency, intensity, and factors influencing its severity. Beyond self-reporting, collateral behavioral indicators, such as facial expressions of discomfort, reduced or slowed physical movement, and noticeable changes in activities previously enjoyed, can further inform assessments. Observers, especially those familiar with the individual, may detect these behavioral changes. Moreover, assessment tools such as range of motion (ROM) tests, which require the individual to perform specific movements, allow evaluators to observe ease and fluidity, thereby providing insight into how pain may affect functional capacity.

During assessment, the person experiencing the covert behavior of experiencing pain is asked to communicate it to others but having collateral observable data aids in any assessment. The verbal reports of pain are under the control of environmental contingencies. A professional athlete will deny pain to the manager despite observable behaviors linked to pain because she knows that her career, financial well-being, praise from fans, and other sources of reinforcement may be at risk if she is placed on an injured list especially before a championship game. The self-reports of being angry and basic emotions are likewise under environmental conditions.

Emotions often designated as "problematic" within mental health contexts are not inherently problematic. Many behaviors categorized as "symptoms" by mental health professionals such as experiencing anger or sadness when disappointed or expressing happiness and excitement when pleasantly surprised are observed universally to varying degrees. These behaviors and emotional responses are considered "symptomatic" only when they lead to adverse outcomes for the individual or negatively affect others. Numerous actions exhibited by individuals living with SMI may not pose any danger but can cause discomfort, annoyance, or distress for those around them. Behaviors are classified as "abnormal" or problematic when they occur excessively, are overly intense, or manifest in inappropriate settings.

Problematic behaviors may not be governed by setting events; those demonstrated in inappropriate contexts often lack sufficient stimulus control. Behavior is considered under stimulus control when it occurs more frequently in the presence of specific stimuli—known as discriminative stimuli (S^D)—and less so when these stimuli are absent (Cooper et al., 2020). A deficit in stimulus control leads to behaviors manifesting in settings or contexts where they are inappropriate. For instance, individuals typically refrain from removing wet clothing in public areas following rainfall, opting instead to wait until they can do so privately. The act of "removing wet clothes" is deemed abnormal when performed in contexts that are not socially acceptable.

Behavior that lacks stimulus control is demonstrated in contexts where such actions or emotions are inappropriate, for example, laughing loudly during a funeral, raising one's voice at a judge or police officer during a traffic violation, or physically confronting a cashier over a pricing discrepancy. A person's behavior may be considered "abnormal" when it disrupts other adaptive responses or leads to negative outcomes for the individual. For instance, shouting at law enforcement during a traffic stop can result in additional legal charges and potential penalties, such as fines or incarceration. Behavior is further classified as "abnormal" if it occurs persistently, or if the individual expresses beliefs such as perceiving the police as malevolent supernatural entities that indicate significant departures from typical perceptions.

Definition of Anger

Anger is defined as a transient state with averse subjective experiences involving other private events, like cognition, beliefs, and somatic responses (Cassiello-Robbins & Barlow, 2016). The emotion of anger itself is not problematic or "abnormal"; it is a vital emotion for social functioning, motivating us to address individual, social, and systemic injustices. The function of anger is to facilitate goal attainment in situations involving challenges. Anger is theorized to be a coordinated response to the perception of obstacles to goals, prompting attention on obtaining the goal until it is either achieved or lost. This emotion organizes responses across cognitions, experiences, physiological responses, and behaviors to overcome obstacles and attain goals. Anger increases effort toward attaining a desired goal, frequently resulting in greater success, especially in challenging situations, promoting greater attention to goals, decision-making consistent with goals, and persistence in the face of difficulty (Lench et al., 2023).

Anger is normal and adaptative in response to perceived threat, powerlessness, injustice, betrayal, and other adverse conditions. However, for some individuals, anger can become problematic. Problematic anger is defined as anger that occurs with a level of frequency and intensity that causes significant distress and interferes with functioning. More than just an epiphenomenon or transdiagnostic feature of mental health problems, problematic anger—"dysfunctional anger"—has a unique contribution on the impacts of psychological trauma. These impacts include increased risk of harm to self and others, financial hardships, relationship difficulties, substance use, legal problems, and poor employment outcomes (American Psychological Association 2024; Fernandez & Johnson, 2016). Dysfunctional anger is linked to various adverse outcomes, including marital distress, long-term depression, and increased cardiovascular disease risk; suppression of anger is associated with experiencing higher intensity of pain and disability (Fernandez & Johnson, 2016).

Anger is a complex construct that includes antecedent conditions, motivational components, neurophysiological aspects, and a history of social and associative learning that result in behavioral chains of respondents and covert behaviors. Anger is characterized by unpleasant feelings and specific facial expressions, which can vary significantly among individuals due to social conditioning. Humans possess the capacity for emotional regulation, which enables a broader range of behavioral options compared to those available to lower animals.

Anger is viewed as a negative emotion; however, anger is conceptualized as a motivational state that enhances engagement in response to challenges and threats to a person's psychological and/or physical well-being (Harmon-Jones et al., 2013). It can function as a motivating operation (MO), specifically an establishing operation (EO) (i.e., increases the effectiveness of a reinforcer, making a behavior more likely to occur), or an abolishing operation (AO) (i.e., decreasing the effectiveness of a reinforcer) (Langthorne & McGill, 2009). Appropriate levels of anger can be an MO as it enhances performance in certain tasks like the righting of injustices and other perceived wrongs (e.g., the civil rights movements in the United States) (Fernandez & Johnson, 2016; Tamir et al., 2008). The display of anger by a person can be a MO/EO/AO for the observer as well. Observing the display of anger can result in behaviors on the part of the observer such as removing oneself from the situation, stopping the interaction, or emitting counter-control behaviors such as yelling, threatening, and other punitive responses (Delprato, 2002).

Anger is characterized as an approach emotion, triggered by perceived impediments to goal attainment, contrasting with avoidance emotions like fear (Fernandez & Johnson, 2016). It is characterized by tension and hostility arising from frustration, real or imagined injury by another, or perceived injustice or threat. The expression of anger is variable. It can manifest itself in behaviors designed to remove the object of the anger (e.g., determined action such as hitting) or behaviors designed merely to express emotion of anger (e.g., swearing). Anger is distinct from but a significant activator of aggression. Many individuals struggle with the appropriate expression of anger, particularly those with passive-aggressive tendencies. Factor analytic research indicates that affective and behavioral aspects of anger are separable, highlighting the complexity of anger and its management (Fernandez & Johnson, 2016). Despite their mutually influential relationship, anger is neither necessary nor sufficient for aggression to occur (American Psychological Association, n.d.-b; DiGiuseppe & Tafrate, 2007).

Anger is a core feature in five mental health problems in the Diagnostic and Statistical Manual of Mental Disorders (fifth ed., text rev.) (DSM-5-TR) (American Psychiatric Association, 2022) including the conditions of intermittent explosive (IED), borderline personality (BPD), bipolar (BP), disruptive mood dysregulation (DMDD), and oppositional defiant (ODD) mental health problems (Fernandez & Johnson, 2016). Presence of anger in the mental health problems mentioned in the DSM-5-TR finds that anger is elevated across these problems and is associated with negative consequences and treatment outcomes (Cassiello-Robbins & Barlow, 2016). Anger displayed by people living with these mental health problems is linked to poor outcomes, often due to difficulties in the regulation and expression of anger. The different mental health problems exhibit unique characteristics of anger, such as episodic high intensity of anger in IED and ODD, and chronicity in BD and BPD (Fernandez & Johnson, 2016).

Definition of Aggression

Aggression is a behavior aimed at harming others physically or psychologically. It can be distinguished from anger in that anger is oriented at overcoming the target but not necessarily through harm or destruction (American Psychological Association, n.d.-a). The aggressive behavior response class can be either physical, verbal, or both; the behaviors can be directed toward a living organism or an inanimate object. Aggressive behaviors correlate with the respondents (i.e., emotions) labeled as anger, annoyance, frustration, fear, boredom, and similar aversive emotional respondents although aggressive behavior can and does occur without the elicitation of anger (i.e., killing a store clerk during a robbery).

Violence is a form of extreme aggressive behavior that is explicitly directed against individuals or property; it is part of a longstanding repertoire of destructive or hurtful behavior or a sudden, paroxysmal reaction to a real or perceived provocation that at times results in the serious physical harm or death of the victim (Girasek et al., 2022). All violent acts are aggressive, but not all aggressive acts are violent. While aggressive behaviors and violence are often used interchangeably, they are not the same. Violence is a form of extreme aggression intended to cause serious physical harm, whereas aggression is a broader term encompassing any behavior intended to do harm to another person, either psychologically, socially, or physically. For this chapter, aggression will be used to define the broader verbal and physical topographies of aggressive behaviors.

Aggressive behaviors—verbal, physical, or responses of passivity—are serious behaviors that are associated with people living with SMI. The risk of being the victim of aggression by a person living with SMI is estimated at only 3–5%, much lower than that from a person living with a substance abuse mental health problem. However, people living with both SMI and co-occurring mental health problems are 73% more likely to exhibit aggression compared to non-substance abusers with mental health problems (Rueve & Welton, 2008). The use of substances and living with an SMI increases the risk of aggressive behaviors being emitted.

Threats and assaults on mental health staff are prevalent and are on the rise by people living with SMI (Anderson & West, 2011). The perception linking SMI to aggressive behavior results in significant stigma, with mental health service providers facing a 5–48% chance of physical assault during their careers with 40–50% of psychiatry residents experiencing attacks during training (Rueve & Welton, 2008). Nursing staff are at the greatest risk of an assault by a person living with SMI during an inpatient admission due to their frequent contact and close proximity (Anderson & West, 2011) as well as the types of interaction nursing staff have with a psychiatric inpatient population (Papadopoulos et al., 2012; Weltens et al., 2021).

The occurrence of aggressive behavior has considerable adverse consequences for individuals living with SMI and possibly contributes to the stigma attributed to individuals living with SMI. Studies show that individuals living with SMI are three times more likely to be arrested than the general population, often due to untreated symptoms and problem behaviors. Early offenders with mental health problems tend to commit more violent crimes and have higher recidivism rates, highlighting the complexity of mental health problems and criminal behavior (Rueve & Welton, 2008). It is conceivable that aggressive behaviors should be included in the list of positive symptoms associated with SMI; in the text, it will be treated as a positive symptom linked to SMI.

Certain mental health problems are associated with an increased risk of aggressive behaviors, influenced by factors of sex, age, and co-occurring mental health problems (Girasek et al., 2022; Gabbey & Raypole 2022; Liu et al., 2013; Van Dorn et al., 2011). In the DSM-5-TR (American Psychiatric Association, 2022), aggressive behaviors are specifically mentioned as associated features in schizophrenia spectrum mental health problems, a criterion for intermittent explosive condition (IED), and a functional consequence of substance-related mental health problems through the disinhibitory effect of the substance. IED is marked by repeated sudden outbursts of anger and aggression. About half of the people with IED also have another personality problem, with borderline personality (BPD) and antisocial personality mental health problems (ASPD) being the most common (Kolla et al., 2023).

Dimensions of Anger and Aggressive Behaviors

Anger, aggression, and related emotional states (e.g., hostility, annoyance, frustration) and the behavioral responses are multidimensional and are defined and differentiated in psychological/behavioral terms (Cassiello-Robbins & Barlow, 2016). Anger and aggression are conceptual domains that are broad areas of focus and research in people living with SMI. Each of these domains is composed of multiple dimensions that are operationally defined and assessed by various instruments (Hopwood et al., 2023).

Dimensions of Anger

Anger can be distinguished by various dimensions, including frequency, intensity, duration, antecedental and consequential factors, controllability, awareness, physiological responses, and the subjective distress experienced by individuals (Novaco, 2009). However, the dimensions in the published literature have considerably overlap with other dimensions as the operational definitions often lack specificity.

Cassiello-Robbins and Barlow (2016) differentiated domains of anger based on the dimensions of the experience of the respondent that is labeled as "anger" as follows:

- Hostility: characterized by persistent angry feelings and irritability, becoming angry over minor slights, insults, and frustrations. Results in mean and vengeful behaviors (i.e., insults, criticism). Considered a facet of the broader personality trait of antagonism.
- In the International Statistical Classification of Diseases and Related Health Problems (tenth ed., second rev.) (ICD-10) (World Health Organization [WHO], 2004), hostility is defined as a clinical characteristic that implies the recurring and enduring tendency to feel anger toward and a desire to inflict harm upon a person or group. It consists of cognitions associated with disapproval toward others, including thoughts and feelings of antagonism, resentment, and alienation.
- Irritability: described as being easily annoyed or provoked to anger.
- Anger attacks: sudden, intense experiences of anger with autonomic arousal symptoms, including tachycardia, sweating, and feelings of losing control. It occurs inappropriately in certain situations.
- Trait anger: refers to a person's increased probability of becoming angry based on history of experiencing angry across multiple antecedents.
- State anger: the intensity of an individual's angry feelings at a specific time and place.

The authors attempted to differentiate these subdomains, but there appear to be overlaps in the dimensions. For example, trait anger is defined as a history of becoming frequently angry, while hostility is defined as experiencing persistent feelings of anger and irritability (and their associated covert responses such as self-talk, and physiological respondents); irritability is defined as becoming angry over antecedent conditions that for others are not distressful and aversive but are otherwise for the individual experiencing "irritability." Skinner (1953) viewed anger as a grouping of responses that vary according to the environmental outcomes. The various subdomains of anger as stated by Cassiello-Robbins and Barlow (2016)) can be viewed as responses in the response class of "angry" behaviors that differentiate along dimensions of experiencing anger. The subdomains may serve as links in a behavioral chain that result in variability on the probability of engaging in a behavior in the aggressive response class, such as yelling, threatening, pushing, striking, and insulting that results in changes in the environment that reinforce the displayed behaviors. For example, the subdomain of irritability can be viewed as a link in the chain that is associated with the dimension of latency of responsiveness or reactivity during which a person's awareness of experiencing anger (onset of the stimulus) and the expression of the respondent or behavior is of shortened duration or known as inter-response time (IRT). This is defined as the amount of time that elapses between two consecutive instances of a response or a response class (Cooper et al., 2020).

In a review of assessment instruments of anger, Eckhardt et al. (2004) discussed the complexity and multifaceted construct of anger and the need for careful attention to various internal and external variables in its assessment. The authors concluded that assessment instruments and scales had weak psychometric characteristics, were only marginally related to each other, and were generally lacking in predictive or construct validity. Many scales were developed without explicit definitions for anger, hostility, or aggression, resulting in limited distinction between the internal experience and outward expression of anger. Additionally, most instruments lacked operational definitions, frequently measuring anger as a basic personality trait rather than as a clinically relevant, multidimensional affective domain that considers both experiential and behavioral components (Eckhardt et al., 2004).

The Multidimensional Anger Inventory (MAI) developed by Siegel (1986) did include scales on the following dimensions of anger: frequency, duration, magnitude/intensity, mode of expression, hostile outlook, and range of anger-eliciting situations. The mode of expression dimension was expected to contain measures indicating separate inward and outward expressions of anger, guilt, brooding, and discussing anger (during which the angry person would display assertive verbal behaviors seeking change from the target of the anger). Factor analyses of the MAI using college participants showed that the frequency, duration, and magnitude/intensity dimensions clustered together to form an anger-arousal factor that accounted for 64–71% of the variance. The range of anger-eliciting situations and hostile outlook emerged as separate dimensions and may be related to awareness of experiencing anger. Mode of anger expression was best described by two dimensions labeled as anger-in (repression of anger) and anger-out (externalizing/acting out).

Siegel (1986) identified a five-factor model of anger based on self-report measures, highlighting distinct dimensions of anger, comprising anger-arousal, anger-rumination, frustration-discomfort, anger-regulation, and socially constituted anger. The factors and their definitions are as follows:

- "Anger-arousal" dimension reflects frequent and intense anger experiences, indicating a stable dispositional characteristic (that may be similar to "trait anger").
- "Anger-rumination" involves covert cognitive-emotional processes and beliefs that can lead to emotional dysregulation. It is defined as having repetitive thinking about anger-inducing events, replaying of the anger-inducing event, thoughts of revenge, and thinking about the antecedents and consequences of the anger inducing event.
- "Frustration-discomfort" dimension focuses on cognitive self-statements (e.g., beliefs) related to entitlement, achievement, and discomfort.
- "Anger-regulation" identifies cognitive strategies for managing anger, distinguishing between control and regulation processes. This factor appears related to controllability of anger and the use of skills to control the intensity and expression of the emotion of anger.
- "Socially constituted" anger dimension examines anger within social variables and norms, emphasizing self-protection and identity. The person recognizes that anger can be a tool for expressing disagreement or protecting the self.

The study's findings show that gender, age, and ethnicity do not influence the five-factor model. Limitations include reliance on self-report measures, potential methodological artifacts, and constraints on generalizability due to predominantly Western college samples.

The Dimensions of Anger Reactions (DAR-5) is a 5-item self-report measure that assesses anger frequency, intensity, duration, aggression, and impact on a person's social functioning over the preceding four-week period. The responses to the items are on a five-point Likert scale (Forbes et al., 2004).

Maltby et al. (2023) attempted to consolidate over 50 years of research on the assessment of dimensions of anger using exploratory and confirmatory factor analyses of the 46 subscales in the 13 publicly available self-report measures assessing the domain of anger. Table 11.1 presents the instruments, along with the specific dimensions measured by each instrument.

Over 1000 participants responded via a public "crowd sourcing" website. The results from the items utilized from the 13 self-report instruments found five-dimensional factors of anger from the results that coincided with the dimensions measured by the Multidimensional Anger Inventory (MAI) developed by Siegel (1986). Presented below are the dimensions, the abbreviations of the self-report instruments as listed in Table 11.1, and sample items from the assessment instrument corresponding to each dimension:

1. Anger-arousal: focuses on the occurrence of expressions of anger and coping strategies such as avoidance, seeking distraction, and downplaying. It distinguishes between controlling and regulating anger. This dimension encompasses:

   a. Outward irritability (S): "I lose my temper and shout or snap at others."
   b. Anger traits (BPAQ): "I have trouble controlling my temper."

Table 11.1 Self-report instruments used to measure anger and dimensions measured in each instrument for factor analyses

Self-report measures of anger (and abbreviations)	Dimensions measured
Snaith irritability scale (SIS)	Outward and inward irritability.
Buss Perry aggression questionnaire (BPAQ)	Anger traits and hostility.
Anger-related reactions and goals inventory (ARGI)	Venting; downplaying; seeking distraction; giving feedback; submitting; humor; enforcing personal standards; enforcing social norms; protecting one's reputation; weighing costs; avoiding conflict; and downregulating affect.
Anger expression inventory (short form) (AEI-SF)	Anger-out and anger-in.
Multidimensional anger inventory (MAI)	Arousal, eliciting situations, and hostile outlook.
Anger rumination scale (AR)	Afterthoughts; thoughts of revenge; anger memories; and understanding causes.
Frustration discomfort scale (FDS)	Discomfort intolerance; entitlement; emotional intolerance; and achievement.
Behavioral anger response questionnaire (BARQ)	Avoidance; assertion; diffusion; and social support-seeking.
Irritability questionnaire (IQ)	Irritability; intensity; frequency.
Anger Reactions-5 scale (DAR-5)	Frequency; intensity; duration; antagonism; and social relationship impairment.
Self-expression and control scale (SCS)	Control; anger in and control anger out.
Metacognitive anger processing (MAP)	Positive and negative beliefs.
Anger discomfort scale (ADS)	Discomfort.

   c. Venting (ARGI): "I explode."
   d. Anger-out (AEI-SF): "I express my anger."

2. Anger-rumination: examines covert cognitive-emotional processes surrounding anger, including cognitive appraisals and cognition related to acting upon perceptions of wrongdoing. It includes repetitive thinking about past anger experiences and analyzing events that resulted in anger. It considers how beliefs about emotional stress influence behavioral and emotional dysregulation. The dimension encompasses:

   a. Rumination memories (ARS): "I ruminate about my past anger experiences."
   b. Afterthoughts (ARS): "Whenever I experience anger, I keep thinking about it for a while."

   c. Understanding of causes (ARS): "I analyze events that make me angry."
   d. Thoughts of revenge (ARS): "I have long living fantasies of revenge after the conflict is over."

3. Frustration-discomfort: focuses on cognitions/beliefs about entitlement, achievement, and alleviating discomfort. It explores how beliefs form expressions of anger. The dimension encompasses:

   a. Entitlement (FDS): "I can't stand it if other people act against my wishes."
   b. Discomfort intolerance (FDS): "I can't stand having to persist at unpleasant tasks."
   c. Achievement (FDS): "I can't bear the frustration of not achieving my goals."
   d. Emotional intolerance (FDS): "I can't bear disturbing feelings."

4. Anger-regulation: identifies cognitive strategies or processes that impact the expression and experience of anger, involving cognitive coping strategies like avoidance, seeking distraction, and downplaying. The dimension distinguishes between the abilities to control and regulate anger, highlighting that anger control measures that reflect the extent to which a person can manage her own anger, while anger regulation involves more complex cognitive processes and coping strategies. This distinction is crucial for understanding different approaches to handling anger and the underlying covert cognitive processes that mitigate the experience of anger. The dimension encompasses:

   a. Avoiding conflict (ARGI): "I want to avoid disagreements."
   b. Seeking distraction (ARGI): "I try to think of other things."
   c. Downplaying (ARGI): "I tell myself there are much worse things."
   d. Avoidance (BARQ): "I put the angering event out of my mind."

5. Socially constituted anger: considers anger within social dominance and conflict, recognizing anger in others and potential disagreements between individual values. It examines anger within the context of self-identity, social structures, and norms. This dimension is related to how anger functions within social dominance and conflict resolution, revealing motivations and potential disagreements between individuals. Social norms influence the protection and enhancement of the self, contribute to jointly constructed understandings of the world, and the values upheld by society. This dimension encompasses:

   a. Enforcing personal standards (ARGI): "I want to get the other person to do what I think is right."
   b. Enforcing social norms (ARGI): "I want to get the other person to act according to how one would expect."
   c. Protecting one's reputation (ARGI): "I want the other person to respect me."

While acknowledging the limitations of using self-report measures, Maltby et al. (2023) concluded that the five-factor model of anger that encompasses anger-arousal, anger-rumination, frustration-discomfort, anger-regulation, and socially constituted anger provides a meaningful assessment of the experience of anger. The items tend to focus on subjective self-statements that are associated with past experiences of anger but do not assess the awareness of antecedent and consequential conditions related to experiencing anger. The items on the frustration-discomfort and socially constituted anger dimensions attempt to identify antecedent conditions and MO/EOs but lack specificity as to the situations resulting in anger. For example, does the person become angry when she experiences violations of societal norms in general (e.g., seeing a driver tailgating) or only when the violations impact her personally (e.g., being tailgated)? Items on the dimension of anger-arousal and anger-rumination dimensions focus on the general topography and the perceptions of the anger-provoking event, respectively. There is no dimension that assesses the outcomes of the expression of anger and whether the expression has been reinforced. Analyzing an anger-eliciting event ought to result in the person becoming aware of events to avoid or mitigate by using behavioral self-management strategies. The anger-regulation dimension assesses general anger avoiding and reduction behaviors but does not assess the effectiveness of these overt and covert behavioral processes.

In a review of anger assessment scales, Eckhardt et al. (2004) proposed that there is a need for (a) an expansion of anger assessment methods beyond traditional approaches (e.g., self-reports), (b) scales to assess specific dimensions of the domain of the anger experience, (c) scales that assess unique content dimensions of the domain of the anger experience and expressions (i.e., context and situationally specific anger scales), and (d) scales that assess the clinical aspects of the anger construct in different populations.

Like any clinical behavior, the dimensions of anger ought to include the following relevant dimensions:

- Intensity: The strength or magnitude of the subjectively experienced anger.
- Frequency: How often is anger experienced and not experienced? Is anger experienced as phasic, tonic, or cyclic?
- Duration: How long does the anger last?
- Awareness: The degree that the person experiencing anger is aware of the respondents and covert responses.
- Expression: How anger is expressed, whether through physical actions, verbal outbursts, self-talk, sulking, or passivity?
- Latency of responsiveness or reactivity: What is the temporal duration of the person's awareness of experiencing anger (onset of the stimulus) and the expression of the respondent or behavior? Latency is the time elapsed between the presentation of an antecedent condition and the initiation of a behavior (Cooper et al., 2020). Reactivity can be operationally defined as inter-response time (IRT) or the amount of time that elapses between two consecutive instances of a response or a response class (Cooper et al., 2020).
- Antecedent conditions: What are the triggers or situations that are followed by the behavior of the anger response class.

- Self-control: How frequently does the person experiencing anger effectively control the display of anger? Self-control of the display of anger can be seen as related to impulsivity.
- Probability of the occurrence of aggressive behavior: How often does the experience of anger result in the display of an aggressive response by the person experiencing anger?
- Consequence: What are the environmental stimuli that follows the experience of anger?

These dimensions help in understanding and assessing the multifaceted nature of anger.

Dimensions of Aggressive Behavior

Aggressive behavior is defined as a behavior that is intended to harm another person who is motivated to avoid that harm (Allen & Anderson, 2017). Aggressive behavior is an observable operant although private events like thoughts and emotions may be in the chain of behavior that results in aggressive behaviors. The function of the behavior is to remove a target that is impeding the person who is emitting aggressive behavior from attaining a positive or negative reinforcing event (Ramiez, 2011). At times, aggressive behavior results in the intentional harming of the target of the aggressive behavior but at times unintentional harm also occurs (e.g., pushing a person that is in the way and the person falling and sustaining an injury) (Norton et al., 2006).

Aggression targets individuals and inanimate objects. Aggressive behavior differs in the topography of the response class of aggressive behaviors and can be classified as physical, verbal, or passive-aggressive behaviors. Physical aggression refers to both successful and unsuccessful attempts of overt physical acts directed at others that could cause harm. Examples include hitting, kicking, pushing, pinching, punching, biting, scratching, pulling hair, head-butting, or throwing objects at someone. Behaviors like hitting the wall or table with fists, stomping feet, glaring, clenching teeth, or making fists may be classified as threatening gestural behaviors but are not classified as aggression as these do not pose a direct threat of harm (Allen & Anderson, 2017). Verbal aggression involves verbal interactions with others whose function is again to remove the target who is perceived to be a threat or harmful to the aggressive individual or impeding the obtainment of a reinforcing event. Examples include swearing at someone, making overt threats of doing harm, using derogatory statements or name-calling, yelling at someone, teasing, or bullying (Allen & Anderson, 2017. Non-examples consist of interrupting, talking back, or telling vulgar jokes (Allen & Anderson, 2017) unless the function is to intimidate so the target removes himself from interacting with the aggressive individual in the immediate and future situations. Passive-aggressive behaviors typically involve avoidance of displaying overt aggressive behaviors, but the function is to harm the individual by setting up conditions for the target to experience frustration, distress, and adverse respondents through the absence of expected behaviors. Passive-aggressive behaviors include procrastination, stubbornness, unresponsiveness to requests/questions, or other subtle behaviors that result in frustration by the target of passive-aggressive behaviors.

The Buss-Warren Aggression Questionnaire (AQ) (Buss & Warren, 2000) is a self-report measure of aggressive behaviors. Participants respond to the items on 5-point Likert-type scale ranging from 1 ("not at all like me") to 5 ("completely like me") to 34 examples of five types of aggression (eight examples of "physical aggression," five examples of "verbal aggression." six examples of "indirect aggression," seven examples of "anger," and eight examples of "hostility"). Factor analyses yielded four scales or dimensions of aggression: physical aggression, verbal aggression, anger, and hostility. Further analysis revealed that the experience of anger is the bridge between both physical and verbal aggression and hostility (Buss & Perry, 1992).

Krahé (2013) and Parrott and Giancola (2007) have developed taxonomies of aggressive behavior that identify and define the dimensions in the behavioral domain of aggression. Both taxonomies highlight the diverse forms and dimensions of aggression. Krahé's (2013) taxonomy offers a multidimensional approach to aggression, examining its nature, visibility, intent, and impact.

- Response modality: verbal (e.g., shouting), physical (e.g., hitting), postural (e.g., threatening gestures), relational (e.g., spreading false rumors, online bullying).
- Immediacy: direct (e.g., punching someone) vs. indirect (e.g., spreading rumors).
- Response quality: action (e.g., forcing unwanted acts) vs. failure to act (e.g., withholding information).
- Visibility: overt (e.g., public humiliation) vs. covert (e.g., anonymous threats).
- Instigation: proactive/unprovoked (e.g., grabbing a toy) vs. reactive/retaliative (e.g., yelling after being attacked).
- Goal direction: hostile (e.g., hitting out of anger) vs. instrumental (e.g., taking a hostage for ransom).
- Type of harm: physical (e.g., broken bones) vs. psychological (e.g., inducing fear).
- Duration of effects: transient (e.g., minor bruises) vs. lasting (e.g., long-term relationship issues). Social units involved: individuals (e.g., intimate partner violence) vs. groups (e.g., riots).

The taxonomy by Parrott and Giancola (2007) identifies and defines two dimensions of aggressive behavior that are based on expression (active/passive) and immediacy (direct/indirect) resulting in four possible dimensions of aggressive behavior in a 2X2 dimensional taxonomy:

1. Active Expression:

   a. Direct: physical (e.g., hitting), verbal (e.g., insults), postural (e.g., threatening gestures), damage to property, theft.

   b. Indirect: same types of aggression but targeting the victim indirectly (e.g., spreading rumors, stealing anonymously, having others engage in aggressive behaviors toward the targeted individual).

2. Passive expression:

   a. Direct: failing to act in a way that helps the victim (e.g., withholding assistance).
   b. Indirect: subtle inaction that harms indirectly (e.g., neglecting responsibilities to harm someone).

The dimension of the relational response modality in the taxonomy of Krahé (2013) appears related to the context of the occurrence of aggressive behaviors than the topography of the behavior. Physical, verbal, postural, and passive responses (such as not responding after a request) can occur in the context of a relational interaction. The taxonomies that are cited above do overlap in certain dimensions both within and between the taxonomies. For example, the topography of aggressive behavior is defined in the dimension of "expression" in aggression taxonomy of Parrott and Giancola (2007), while it is defined in the "response modalities" by Krahé (2013). A comparison of the taxonomies by Krahé (2013) and Parrott and Giancola (2007) is presented in Table 11.2.

Table 11.2 Comparison of taxonomies of Krahé and Parrot and Giancola

Dimension	Krahé (2013) Taxonomy	Parrott & Giancola (2007) Taxonomy
Response modality	Verbal, physical, postural, relational	Physical, verbal, postural, damage to property, theft (direct); relational, anonymous (indirect)
Immediacy	Direct (e.g., punching) vs. indirect (e.g., spreading rumors)	Direct (e.g., hitting, insults, gestures) vs. indirect (e.g., rumors, stealing anonymously, using others to harm)
Response quality	Action (e.g., forcing unwanted acts) vs. failure to act (e.g., withholding information)	Active (doing harm) vs. passive (failing to help, neglecting responsibilities)
Visibility	Overt (e.g., public humiliation) vs. covert (e.g., anonymous threats)	Overt (observable) vs. covert (hidden, anonymous)
Instigation	Proactive/unprovoked vs. reactive/ retaliative	Not explicitly defined, but can be inferred in active/passive distinctions
Goal direction	Hostile (anger-driven) vs. instrumental (goal-driven, e.g., ransom)	Not explicitly defined in the taxonomy
Type of harm	Physical (e.g., broken bones) vs. psychological (e.g., inducing fear)	Physical, psychological, property, relational
Duration of effects	Transient (short-term) vs. lasting (long-term)	Not explicitly defined
Social units involved	Individuals (e.g., intimate partner violence) vs. groups (e.g., riots)	Not explicitly defined
Expression/ activity level	Not explicitly defined	Active expression (direct/indirect), passive expression (direct/indirect)

Allen and Anderson (2017)) have proposed a taxonomy of dichotomous dimensions of aggressive behaviors using the ones available in the mental health literature. For example, the dimension of "physical aggression" can be considered hostile or instrumental, direct or indirect, and active or passive. The same is true for verbal and relational aggression. Their classification of the dimensions of aggressive behaviors includes:

1) Hostile vs. instrumental:
    a. Hostile aggression: motivated by anger and the desire to harm (e.g., hitting someone out of frustration).
    b. Instrumental aggression: goal-oriented and calculated, where harm is a means to achieve another objective (e.g., harming someone to steal money). The experience of anger is not a part of the chain of behaviors resulting in aggression.
2) Direct vs. indirect:
    a. Direct aggression: The victim is physically present (e.g., punching someone).
    b. Indirect aggression: The victim is absent, and harm is caused indirectly (e.g., spreading rumors).
3) Active vs. passive:
    a. Active aggression: engaging in harmful actions (e.g., kicking someone).
    b. Passive aggression: failing to act in a way that helps, causing harm through inaction (e.g., withholding help intentionally).
4) Overt vs. covert:
    a. Overt aggression: highly visible actions (e.g., public insults).
    b. Covert aggression: low-visibility actions (e.g., anonymous threats).
5) Displaced vs. triggered:
    a. Displaced aggression: targeting an innocent substitute instead of the provocateur (e.g., yelling at a family member after a bad day at work).
    b. Triggered aggression: intentional targeting.
    c. Triggered displaced aggression: aggression toward a substitute target who has committed a minor offense (e.g., overreacting to a small mistake by someone else).
6) Legitimate vs. illegitimate:
    a. Legitimate aggression: considered acceptable or lawful in certain contexts (e.g., capital punishment).
    b. Illegitimate aggression: unlawful or socially unacceptable (e.g., murder).

7) Personological vs. situational:

   a. Personological aggression: driven by individual traits or personality (e.g., narcissism, hostile attitudes). An example would be an act of aggression based on the race or ethnicity of the target.
   b. Situational aggression: triggered by external factors (e.g., provocation, frustration, or environmental stressors).

These dimensions provide a nuanced framework for understanding the complexity of aggressive behaviors.

In assessing the construct and domains of aggressive behaviors in individuals living with SMI, it is imperative to be precise and thorough in ascertaining the dimensions so effective interventions can be developed and implemented. As in the dimension of anger, the dimensions of aggression ought to include the following relevant dimensions during assessment:

- Topography: What is the physical shape of the observable behavior? What does aggressive behavior look like?
- Expression: How is aggression expressed, whether through physical actions, verbal outbursts, self-talk, sulking, or passivity? This considers both overt and covert displays.
- Intensity: The strength or magnitude of aggressive behavior.
- Frequency: How often does aggression occur? Is the occurrence of aggression phasic, tonic, or cyclic?
- Duration: How long does the occurrence of aggression last? What is the duration between the display of aggressive behaviors.
- Awareness: The degree that the person engaging in aggressive behaviors is aware of the respondents and covert responses associated with aggression.
- Latency of responsiveness or reactivity: What is the temporal duration of the person's awareness of experiencing the onset of stimulus and the expression of the aggression (e.g., latency and IRT)?
- Antecedent conditions: What are the triggers or situations that lead to anger? Do the antecedents vary or is there a pattern?
- Self-control: How frequently does the person expressing aggressive behavior effectively control the occurrence? Self-control of aggression can be related to impulsivity and measured by IRTs.
- Consequence: What are the environmental stimuli that follow the experience of aggression?

Origins of Anger and Aggression

Neurological Substrates

Neurobiological factors—genetic, metabolic, neurochemical, and structural—and their corresponding mechanisms collectively contribute to the behavioral problem observed in people living with SMI, highlighting the complexity of the various problems displayed by people living with SMI (Pompili et al., 2017). Heightened anger and associated aggressive behaviors that occur in people living with SMI have serious consequences including more frequent and longer stays in psychiatric facilities, loss of relationships and employment opportunities, and increase of stigmatization of living with SMI.

The behavioral domains of anger and aggressive behaviors are complex in functioning and their relationships to various neuroanatomical areas of the brain. Many findings suggest that heightened anger and aggression in people living with SMI are associated with structural abnormalities in various brain regions, particularly those involved in emotion regulation, impulse control, and socio-emotional processing. Studies have implicated dysfunctional frontotemporal circuitry in impulsiveness and aggression in people living with SMI, particularly in the frontal cortical and subcortical areas. Using both fMRI and structural MRIs, studies have found problems with white matter integrity and volume of cortical structures.

The neural circuits implicated in anger and hostility in people living with SMI include the amygdala (Amyg), striatum, prefrontal cortex (PFC), anterior cingulate cortex (ACC), insula, and hippocampus (HC). These brain regions are involved in modulating hostile thoughts and behaviors, particularly in patients with schizophrenia who exhibit high levels of urgency, impulsivity, and aggressiveness. Imaging studies suggest that malfunctioning of these neural circuits contributes to the anger-related dimensions observed in SMI (Perlini et al., 2018). The brain regions that have been postulated to be involved in aggression regulation (Perlini et al., 2018) include:

- Amyg: Involved in the generation of aggressive responses and emotional processing. fMRI studies show increased amygdala activity in response to threats and frustrating stimuli (Blair, 2016). A significant correlation was found between self-report measures of aggressive behaviors and amyg reactivity to fearful faces in incarcerated violent offenders (Kolla et al., 2023).
- Striatum: Plays a role in the modulation of aggressive behaviors.
- PFC: The dorsolateral prefrontal cortex (dlPFC) and ventrolateral prefrontal cortex (vlPFC) are involved in impulse control and decision-making (Shahsavarani & Noohi, 2015). The ventromedial prefrontal cortex (vmPFC) and dorsomedial frontal cortex (dmFC) are involved in reinforcement-based decision-making related to aggression (Blair, 2016). vmPFC is believed to inhibit aggressive responses mediated by the amygdala, hypothalamus, and periaqueductal gray (PAG) regions. Lesions in the vmPFC have been shown to increase aggression in

both animals and humans. Some studies indicate vmPFC lesions lead to increased amygdala responses to threats, while others show typical emotional reactions. The vmPFC may not solely act as a brake on aggression but also represents potential rewards and costs of actions. vmPFC dysfunction can reduce amygdala responsiveness during decision-making, affecting optimal response choices. Increased impulsive aggression following vmPFC/OFC lesions may reflect poorer behavioral choices rather than disinhibition of aggression (Blair, 2016).

Neurofeedback studies show that manipulating PFC asymmetry affects emotional responses, with increased left activity linked to greater positive affect. Experiments indicate that anger can evoke both increased left and decreased right frontal activity, particularly when action is possible. Research using repetitive transcranial magnetic stimulation (rTMS), a noninvasive procedure that uses magnetic pulses to stimulate specific areas of the brain (American Psychological Association, n.d.-c), demonstrates that increased activity in the left PFC leads to attention toward angry faces, while increased activity in the right PFC leads to avoidance (Harmon-Jones et al., 2013).

- ACC: involved in emotion regulation and impulse control.
- Orbito-frontal Cortex (OFC): plays a role in decision-making and socio-emotional information processing.
- Insula: involved in socio-emotional information processing.
- Hippocampus (HC): associated with memory and emotional regulation.

Structural and fMRI scans on people living with SMI who display aggressive behaviors have revealed several key findings:

1. Frontal white matter: Disruption in the inferior frontal white matter is associated with impulsivity and aggression. Impairments in white matter integrity result in impaired connectivity between regions of the brain (Perlini et al., 2018). Impulsive aggression was associated with lower white matter integrity in the superior longitudinal fasciculus (Kolla et al., 2023).
2. Orbital frontal cortex (OFC): Higher assessed scores of aggressive behaviors correlate with larger grey and white matter volumes in the left OFC and bilateral OFC (Perlini et al., 2018). Amyg and OFC activation correlated with aggression, with some participants showing less differentiation in responses to angry versus neutral faces (Kolla et al., 2023).
3. Caudate: Increases in the frequency of aggressive behaviors are linked to larger grey and white matter volumes in the caudate (Perlini et al., 2018)..
4. Prefrontal Cortex (PFC): Violence is associated with cortical thinning in this area, particularly in the left medial inferior frontal and right lateral sensory motor cortex (Perlini et al., 2018). fMRIs have shown hyperactivation in medial PFC (mPFC) compared to individuals not living with SMI and displaying aggressive behaviors (Widmayer et al., 2019). Ventromedial PFC (vmPFC) influences decision-making related to aggression. Compromised vmPFC functioning disrupts reinforcement-based decision-making, potentially leading to impulsive behaviors, including aggression (Blair, 2016). Kolla et al. (2023)

reported results of reduced ventrolateral prefrontal cortex (vlPFC) activation and a tendency to approach angry faces, indicating dysfunction in emotional action control in individuals with SMI and reactive aggression.

5. Amyg, vPFC, and vmPFC: Structural MRIs have found reduced functional connectivity between the amyg and vPFC regions is inversely related to aggression levels. Higher scores on impulsivity/urgency predict lower cortical thickness and reduced connectivity between vPFC and limbic/executive brain regions (Perlini et al., 2018). fMRIs found hyperactivation in the right amyg. Increased amygdala reactivity to provocation was linked to higher aggression levels, showing reduced connectivity between the vmPFC and amyg (Kolla et al., 2023).
6. Medial OFC, dlPFC, ACC, and fronto-polar regions: Increased impulsivity in people living with co-occurring substance use mental health problems is related to grey matter volume losses in these regions (Chester & DeWall, 2016; Perlini et al., 2018).
7. Hypothalamus, putamen, cuneus/precuneus, and inferior frontal region: Individuals living with SMI and problem behaviors related to impulse control show increased grey matter volumes in these areas and decreased volumes in the inferior frontal region (Perlini et al., 2018).
8. Anterior cingulate cortex (ACC): People living with SMI who display aggressive behavior and those with conditions related to antisocial personality have significantly lower ACC volumes compared to individuals with no mental health issues (Perlini et al., 2018). fMRI has found this area to be significantly more reactive to negative stimuli in people living with SMI who display aggressive behaviors suggesting its role in aggression (Widmayer et al., 2019).
9. Inferior temporal area, middle temporal gyrus, temporal pole, and insular area: People living with SMI who display aggressive behavior show smaller volumes in these regions compared to nonviolent people living with SMI (Perlini et al., 2018). Using fMRIs, hyperactivations were noted in the frontal lobe and middle temporal gyrus in aggressive individuals living with SMI compared to healthy controls (Widmayer et al., 2019).
10. Right inferior parietal area. Hypoactivation in this region indicating possible working memory (WM) impairments (Widmayer et al., 2019).

These findings suggest that aggression in individuals living with SMI appears related to structural abnormalities in various brain regions, particularly those involved in emotion regulation, impulse control, and socio-emotional processing. .

Instrumental aggression is goal-directed behavior aimed at achieving desirable outcomes, such as financial gain. Key brain structures involved in reinforcement-based decision-making include the amygdala, ventromedial (vmPFC), and dorsomedical (dmPFC) prefrontal cortices, anterior insula cortices (AIC), and striatum. Instrumental aggression is more likely to be displayed by individuals due to a diminished perception and processing of the distress of others.

Increased impulsiveness reflects weaker striatal responsiveness to future rewards (Blair, 2016). Impulsivity in decision-making is assessed by using tasks in choosing between immediate and delayed rewards. Impulsive aggression linked to anger involves the acute threat response system that includes amygdala, hypothalamus, and periaqueductal gray (AG). This is modulated by the vmPFC, affecting response choices and impulsivity. Compromised neural structures, especially the ventromedial prefrontal cortex (vmPFC), the dorsomedial frontal cortex (dmFC), and the anterior insula cortex (AIC), may lead to increased impulsive aggression (Blair, 2016). Studies indicate that frustration and social provocation activate the dmFC, AIC, and vmPFC, which are linked to representations of outcomes and affect response choice; impairments in this neural circuit impact behavioral inhibition tasks that are correlated to increased impulsive aggression risk (Blair, 2016).

Neurotransmitter functions, particularly serotonin, have been linked to aggressive behavior. Other neurotransmitter systems involved include the dopaminergic, vasopressinergic, and glutamate systems (Pompili et al., 2017).

Evidence suggests that altered interactions between prefrontal and subcortical regions, particularly the amygdala, contribute to aggressive behaviors. Neuroimaging studies show frontal and temporal lobe abnormalities in people living with schizophrenia spectrum mental health problems who engage in aggressive behaviors (Pompili et al., 2017). A lack of clarity exists regarding the neural links between impulsiveness and aggression, with most studies relying on self-report measures. There is an identified need for more specific measures of aggression and a clearer distinction between the dimensions of aggressive behaviors. Future neuroimaging studies should address concerns about characteristics of samples used, methodological inconsistencies, and the use of a dimensional model to explore the interplay of multiple dimensions related to aggression and neurological substrates of the phenomenon (Kolla et al., 2023).

Psychological and Behavioral Substrates of Anger and Aggressive Behaviors

Anger and aggression are the result of a multifactorial interplay between biological and environmental influences. While genetic factors may provide a baseline propensity for anger and aggression, environmental factors such as associative and social learning, role modeling, interactions with the environment, and cultural norms shape how these behaviors are displayed by the individual. Skinner (1953) defines anger as:

> ...an emotional pattern that includes responses of glands and smooth muscles and a well-marked effect upon operant behavior which includes a heightened disposition to act aggressively toward the controlling agent and a weakening of other behavior. The emotion may be displaced from the controlling agent to other people or to things in general. (p. 262).

Anger is an innate emotional response; it is defined as a transient state with averse subjective experiences (e.g., physiological arousal) involving other private events, like cognition, beliefs, and somatic responses (Cassiello-Robbins & Barlow, 2016). The emotion of anger is a state of tension that is adaptative in response to perceived threat, powerlessness, injustice, betrayal, and other adverse conditions, arising from frustration and real or imagined injury by another. It is characterized as an approach emotion, triggered by perceived impediments to goal attainment, motivating people to address individual, social, and systemic injustices (Fernandez & Johnson, 2016).

Anger acts as a motivating operation (MO), which can either be an establishing operation (EO) that makes a reinforcer more effective and increases the likelihood of certain behaviors, or an abolishing operation (AO) that reduces the impact of a reinforcer (Langthorne & McGill, 2009). Moderate anger can serve as a motivating operation (MO), boosting performance in situations that involve addressing injustices or wrongdoings, such as the United States civil rights movements (Fernandez & Johnson, 2016; Tamir et al., 2008). When someone shows anger, it can act as an MO, EO, or AO for those observing. Witnessing anger may prompt observers to take actions like leaving the area, ending the interaction, or engaging in retaliatory behaviors such as shouting, making threats, or responding with punitive measures.

The expression of anger is subject to variation. It may be demonstrated through actions intended to eliminate the source of anger, such as purposeful intervention, or through behaviors that serve primarily to convey the emotion itself, for instance, verbal expressions like swearing. Anger is distinct from, but a significant activator of aggression (Novaco, 2017). Many individuals struggle with the appropriate expression of anger, particularly those with impulsive and passive-aggressive tendencies (Helfritz & Stanford, 2006; Hoptman, 2015). Factor analytic research indicates that affective and behavioral aspects of anger are separable, highlighting the complexity of anger and its management (Fernandez & Johnson, 2016; Novaco, 2017). Despite their mutually influential relationship, anger is neither necessary nor sufficient for aggression to occur (American Psychological Association, n.d.-a; Novaco, 2017).

The aggressive behavior response class can be either physical, verbal, or both; the behaviors can be directed toward a living organism or an inanimate object. Aggressive behaviors correlate with the respondents (i.e., emotion) of anger, annoyance, frustration, fear, boredom, and similar aversive emotional respondents.

In conclusion, anger and aggression are both innate and learned. Biological factors provide a foundation for anger and aggressive behavior, while social learning and cognitive processes significantly shape and regulate how anger is experienced and aggression is manifested (Novaco, 2017).

Anger dysregulation is associated with a wide range of mental health problems and affects the occurrence of aggressive behaviors in people living with SMI. Covert private events and processes such as perception of threat, hostile attribution bias, and rumination play significant roles in the activation and maintenance of anger and aggression. Anger is dysregulated when an individual experiences the emotion with greater frequency, intensity, and in situations and contexts when the anger is inappropriate (i.e., becoming angry when a baby is crying).

Anger is an emotional respondent marked by physiological and covert responses; it is behavior that is caused by a stimulus in the environment. The behavior is unlearned and reflexive (Skinner, 1953). Anger is closely linked to threat perception and is under the control of neurological structures such as the amygdala and the prefrontal cortex, which influence perceptions of threat. When individuals perceive a threat and hostility—real, imagined, or exaggerated—anger is experienced by the person, focusing attention on stimuli in the environment with survival significance (i.e., the source of the threat) (Novaco, 2017). Anger functions as the MO for behaviors to remove the agent of the threat and perceived hostile intent.

Nevertheless, anger can be conditioned and modified through interactions with the environment in which the individual learns how to mediate and modulate the experiences of anger and in so doing alters the dimensions of experiencing anger; that is altering the frequency, intensity, and the conditions in which the anger is experienced (Goldiamond, 2022).

The modulation of the experience of anger by an individual develops through associative learning, which is a process by which a person learns to associate two stimuli or a behavior and a stimulus (Enquist et al., 2016; Lind, 2018). This type of learning involves forming connections between different elements of the environment, leading to changes in behavior based on these associations. Associative learning is fundamental in understanding how animals and humans adapt their behaviors based on experiences and environmental cues.

There are two main types of associative learning:

1. Classical (Pavlovian)(respondent) conditioning: This occurs when a neutral stimulus becomes associated with a meaningful stimulus, resulting in the neutral stimulus eliciting a response similar to the meaningful stimulus. For example, a child is playing with a knife, and a parent responds by yelling resulting in a fear-generated response, and the child stops crying. If this is repeated by the parent, the child is conditioned to respond to knives with fear and avoidance. However, the child can also be conditioned to respond with anger to situations in which she is frustrated and controlled by an adult agent. It is possible that as an adult, she will experience anger when blocked in moving toward her goal (i.e., frustrated) by others in positions of authority (as a parent is to the child).

Prolonged anger that does not subside (e.g., trait anger, suppressed anger, unresolved anger) increases the chances that anger will be conditioned to other situations that are out of context and inappropriate to the situation (anger reactivity). An example may be a person who was admonished by his supervisor at work. While driving after work, he continues to engage in subvocal speech about this perceived injustice or implied threats to his job (Tourinho, 2006). The result is that he experiences anger that is related to the driving of others and at the slightest provocation engages in honking the horn and cursing other drivers. Excitation transfer is when residual arousal from unresolved anger events can transfer to future conflicts, further intensifying anger reactivity and increasing the probability of aggression (Novaco, 2017).

2. Instrumental (operant) conditioning: This involves learning to associate behavior with a consequence, such as being reinforced or punished. If the child in the previous example is physically punished by the parent (e.g., smacking her hand), the child will learn to avoid knives to avoid the hurt associated with the punish-

ment and may inhibit expressing anger in similar situations to avoid being punished. This can lead to a conditioned response where the child learns to suppress her anger and frustration to avoid the anticipated punishment.

People also learn about the dimensions of anger through social learning processes. Individuals observe the behavior of others in their social environments, particularly those individuals who are agents of control in their lives, are perceived as having domination of a situation, and are praised and reinforced by others. A person sees a professional athlete respond with anger when a play does not go as he desires; the person's friends and sports announcers praise his "passion and desire to win." The athlete is expressing anger and frustration in a maladaptive manner, but others may learn to imitate those behaviors because of the athlete's status and reinforcement that is observed.

The dimensions of the experience of anger are subject to environmental influences. The regulation of the experience of anger involves influencing the dimension of the emotion for instrumental benefits (i.e., positive reinforcement) or reducing the unpleasantness of the angry experience (i.e., negative reinforcement). Individuals may regulate unpleasant emotions to alleviate distressful reactions; alternatively, they may amplify such emotions when deemed beneficial for long-term outcomes, particularly within contexts that demand specific affective states such as anger. Research indicates that anger, while generally aversive, can enhance performance in tasks requiring confrontation, though it does not yield similar benefits in nonconfrontational situations. Consequently, individuals may intentionally increase feelings of anger prior to confrontational activities to leverage their functional advantages. The effectiveness of anger in facilitating goal attainment is notably context-dependent (Tamir et al., 2008).

Tamir et al. (2008) found that participants preferred anger-inducing activities over exciting or neutral ones when anticipating confrontational games. In contrast, preferences reversed for nonconfrontational games, indicating context-dependent emotional engagement and modulation. Overall, engaging in anger-inducing activities improved performance in confrontational games, highlighting the use of anger as a MO to increase the effectiveness of certain behaviors. Tamir et al. (2008) concluded that individuals may intentionally increase their experience of anger to enhance performance in confrontational tasks. The findings support a functional approach to emotional regulation, suggesting emotional preferences depending on contextual goals (Tamir et al., 2008).

The experience of anger and the display of aggressive behaviors are intertwined in complex manners, involving biological innate responses, perception, covert responses, and learning, resulting in a complex behavioral chain with multiple determinants. Anger significantly influences the display of aggressive behaviors through various mechanisms. Biological factors provide a foundation for aggressive behavior, while associative and social learning and shape and regulate how aggression is manifested (Novaco, 2017).

The display of aggressive behaviors is impacted by the environmental consequences of the behavior. An individual behaves aggressively toward another either verbally or physically and is punished by an agent of control (e.g., parents, police, teachers, supervisors). This happens repeatedly. Eventually, any situation in which aggressive behavior toward another person is likely to take place or any early stage of such action will generate the conditioned aversive stimulation associated with anxiety or guilt, leading to "self-control" (i.e., the display of behaviors that inhibit the aggressive responses). This is effective from the point of view of the victim and the controlling agent. The individual who is punished is more likely to engage in behaviors that compete with and inhibit aggressive behaviors, such as avoiding situations that elicit anger, generating incompatible respondents (i.e., relaxation), and subvocal covert verbal responses that mitigate against anger and aggressive behaviors (e.g., dismissing an affront by another as a "mistake"). By these responses, he "represses" his anger and aggression (Skinner, 1953).

The repression of anger and aggressive responses can be maladaptive if the person engages in substance use to become sedated and attenuate the aversive respondents (e.g., "numbing"), engages in aggressive behaviors toward other organisms that cannot respond protectively (e.g., animals, children), or displays self-harm to replace the emotional respondents associated with anger.

When aggressive behavior is reinforced and results in the avoidance or removal of a perceived threat, then the chances of aggressive behaviors being displayed in the near future increases. Aggressive behavior is reinforced if the consequences of aggression results in any desired outcome such as the acquisition of an item or relationship, verbal praise from others, and forcing someone into submission or control using aggressive responses (i.e., instrumental aggression).

Consequences also act to inhibit the display and intensity of aggressive responses. Aggressive behavior is regulated by inhibitory control mechanisms that are influenced by internal and external cues. These include physical constraints, expectations of punishment or retaliation, empathy, consideration of consequences, and conditioned prosocial values. When individuals consider the potential negative outcomes of their aggressive behaviors, such as punishment or harm to their social relationships, they are more likely to inhibit aggressive impulses. However, inhibition of aggressive behaviors can be impaired if the arousal of anger is intense and impairs covert cognitive and metacognitive processes, thinking about one's thinking (e.g., theory of mind [ToM]), consideration of the other person (i.e., empathy) and prosocial values, making it difficult to consider aggression-mitigating information (Novaco, 2017), resulting in the display of impulsive and reactive aggression.

The question remains as to why people living with SMI display anger and aggressive behaviors. Most violent acts (over 90%) are not attributed to mental health problems, and most individuals living with mental health problems are nonviolent. When aggression does occur, it is often linked to contextual factors like childhood abuse, substance use, and poorly resourced and punitive environments. Risk factors for the display of aggressive behaviors are relevant for those living with SMI including the use of psychoactive substances, adverse childhood experiences (e.g., abuse and other trauma), problems behaviors and symptoms of living with SMI such as high energy levels and impulsivity, beliefs of persecution and grandiosity, command auditory hallucinations, environmental factors (e.g., poor living conditions in high crime neighborhoods, homelessness), long-standing behaviors of acting aggressively, and financial and relationship stressors (DeAngelis, 2021). Furthermore, research indicates that approximately 39% of violent or aggressive incidents in psychiatric hospitals are preceded by staff–patient interactions, making this the most common antecedent overall. Analysis of these interaction themes demonstrates that limiting patients' freedoms, either through restrictions or denial of requests, constitutes the most frequent precursor to such incidents, representing an estimated 25% of all antecedents. This pattern suggests a response characterized by punitive and controlling measures (Ilkiw-Lavalle & Grenyer, 2003; Li et al., 2019).

Counter-control behavior is a functional class of human operant behavior that occurs in response to socially mediated aversive control. Counter-control behaviors on the part of the person who perceives being controlled by punitive consequences may manifest aggressive behaviors. When individuals are subjected to aversive conditions by others, they may respond by escaping or avoiding these conditions in ways that do not reinforce, and may even punish, the controlling behaviors of others. This can include actions such as moving out of range, attacking, or passively resisting. Counter-control highlights the principle that human behavior is both controlled and controlling, emphasizing that individuals are not passive and can actively oppose attempts at social control (Delprato, 2002). In a comprehensive review of prospectively recorded antecedents to aggressive and violent episodes in inpatient psychiatric environments, Papadopoulos et al. (2012) identified "behavioral cues"—such as changes in pacing, vocal tone, and volume, and facial expressions—and instances of "no clear cause" as predominant themes. These factors accounted for 38% and 33% of all documented aggressive incidents, respectively.

There is a fair large degree of variability in the prevalence of aggression behaviors in the research literature owing to lack of standardization, reliability of mental health problems, well defined and standardized operational definition of the domain of anger and aggression, and their respective behavioral dimensions.

Epidemiological Considerations

Anger and its related dimensions (including aggression) are present as a key criterion in five mental health problems cited in the DSM-5-TR (American Psychiatric Association, 2022) that include the following: intermittent explosive, oppositional defiant, disruptive mood dysregulation, borderline personality, and bipolar mental health problems (Cassiello-Robbins & Barlow, 2016; Fernandez & Johnson, 2016). There is no diagnostic category for problematic anger as a sole criterion in the DSM-5-TR or ICD-11 (WHO, 2022). Problematic anger is manifested in a wide variety of mental health problems although not considered essential for a determination of mental health conditions. Anger is often characterized by dysfunctionality and can be presented alongside delusions and command hallucinations in individuals experiencing psychotic mental health conditions. It may also be associated with emotional lability in personality conditions, irritability and episodic attacks in mood problems, as well as difficulties with impulse control and culturally specific mental health issues (Novaco, 2017). Anger is often a result of trauma, significantly affecting the severity and course of PTSD symptoms. The central characteristic of problematic anger in the clinical context is its dysregulation in which its activation, expression, and experience occur resulting in deleterious consequences and outcomes for the person and others.

The dysregulation of anger is characterized by frequency, reactivity, intensity, duration, and mode of expression, varying across mental health problems (Novaco, 2017). Despite its clinical relevance, no studies have been found that assess the point, period, or lifetime prevalence (National Mental Health Institute [NIMH], 2025) of problematic anger in people living with SMI.

Anger is a significant issue among hospitalized people living with SMI, linked to assaultive behavior both in facilities and post-discharge (Caruso et al., 2021; Li et al., 2019). Studies indicate that self-reported anger is a strong predictor of violence prior to hospitalization, during institutionalization, and in the community after discharge. Individuals reporting high levels of anger often have traumatic backgrounds, leading to possibility of anger as a coping mechanism to avoid or decrease adverse covert respondents associated with the trauma.

Given problematic anger's clinical relevance and adverse impact on functioning, there is a need to examine individuals transdiagnostically at different levels of anger severity and to provide a basis for considering anger severity in clinical research and practice. Using a five-item self-report rating measure of the experience of anger, Levin-Aspenson et al. (2023) found that increasing anger severity was associated with elevated ratings by service providers of psychosocial problems and poorer self-rated functioning and life satisfaction. The rating scale did not assess the occurrence of aggressive behaviors, but the experience of anger as problematic for the assessed person. Assessing anger yields crucial information about psychosocial functioning and the identification of mental health-related problems. Further research ought to be considered to assess the prevalence of problematic anger—without the display of aggressive behaviors—in people living with SMI (Joyal et al., 2011; Kurian et al., 2023).

Aggression can manifest as verbal or physical behavior, with verbal aggression being more common. Aggressive behaviors appear to occur along a continuum with behaviors with verbal aggression at one end and physical violence at the other (Morrison, 1992). Reports indicate that 2% to 3.7% of the general population in the United States commit violent acts annually, with a lifetime prevalence of 24% for aggressive behaviors (Girasek et al., 2022; Novaco, 2017).

The prevalence of aggressive behaviors in people living with SMI varies significantly based on the type of mental health issue and other contributing factors (Gopika et al., 2024). Studies indicate that people living with SMI are two to three times more likely to engage in aggressive behaviors than those without. The attributable risk of violence associated with serious mental illness is estimated to be between 3% and 5%, which is substantially lower than the risk linked to substance abuse (Anderson & West, 2011). Additionally, the prevalence of aggressive behavior among individuals living with SMI is reported at 14% during the month preceding admission to a psychiatric facility. In a survey, 72% of people who were labeled as assaultive were living with a type of schizophrenia spectrum disorder. Individuals diagnosed with multiple mental health conditions have an elevated risk of engaging in violent behavior, with those reporting more than three mental health conditions found to be 2 to 4.5 times more likely to exhibit such actions (Anderson & West, 2011; Joyal et al., 2011).

Females living with SMI exhibited aggressive behaviors violence at rates similar to male persons living with SMI, with the aggressive behaviors often directed at family members. People living with SMI under 30 years of age account for 68% of assaults. Risk factors for aggressive behaviors include a history of aggression with the probability of the occurrence of future aggressive behavior increasing linearly with the number of past violent events (Anderson & West, 2011).

Girasek et al. (2022) found that 28% of individuals who live with SMI and a history of childhood conduct problems exhibited significant aggressive behavior, compared to 14% of those without such a history. These findings underscore the influence of persistent aggressive behaviors as an established risk factor for future aggression. Only 12% had experienced psychotic-like problem behaviors and symptoms before the occurrence of violent acts. Rates of violence among individuals discharged from a psychiatric facility peak shortly after discharge, with an average of 2.12 violent acts per patient over 50 weeks (Rueve & Welton, 2008).

Ten percent of individuals living with schizophrenia spectrum mental health problems display aggressive behaviors living in the community post-discharge from the hospital. Individuals living with bipolar mood mental health problems showed a 12.2% lifetime prevalence of aggression, while individuals living with personality mental health problems (specifically borderline personality) have a 73% period prevalence rate of aggressive behavior within 1 year (Gopika et al., 2024).

People living with SMI and a co-occurring substance use problem show significant increase in frequency of aggressive behaviors, with alcohol being the most common substance associated with aggressive behavior. Girasek et al. (2022) reported that 28% of people living with SMI with previous offenses and residing in a forensic setting committed the offense under the influence of a psychoactive substance. Regular cannabis users are 2.4 times more likely to be involved in aggressive behavior, while heroin users have a 43% rate of suicide attempts in which aggressive behavior is directed to themselves (Novaco, 2017).

Aggressive behavior occurs at any stage of drug use including acute intoxication, drug-seeking behavior, withdrawal, or during episodes of drug-induced psychotic problem behaviors. Drugs and aggressive behaviors are related directly when the psychoactive substance induces instrumental aggressive behaviors as a method of obtaining the drug. Overall, the relationship between drugs and aggressive behaviors is complex and is multifactorial related to both transient and permanent physiological, psychological, environmental, and individual differences.

Aggressive behavior in inpatient psychiatric facilities was observed at rates ranging from 8–76%. Nursing staff, due to their frequent and close interactions with hospitalized individuals, were most often the victims of these aggressive incidents.

Explanatory factors of aggressive behavior were subdivided into patient, staff, and ward factors (Weltens et al., 2021).

Aggressive behavior has been observed in between 8 and 44% of individuals receiving acute psychiatric inpatient treatment. Research demonstrates that 2.5–7% of people experiencing delusions of jealousy may exhibit aggression linked to these erroneous beliefs (Novaco, 2017). Individual factors such as substance abuse, untreated mental health problems, young age, being male, history of aggressive behaviors, and poor living conditions increase the risk of the occurrence of aggressive behaviors (Girasek et al., 2022; Weltens et al., 2021). Environmental risk factors include untrained staff, job dissatisfaction and burnout, lack of high-quality interactions between staff and the people on the ward, overcrowding, and inadequate clinical leadership (Caruso et al., 2021; Ilkiw-Lavalle & Grenyer, 2003; Weltens et al., 2021). The results from Weltens et al. (2021) support the contention that the occurrence of aggressive behaviors displayed by people living with SMI is under the stimulus control of combination of environmental and interpersonal variables and not solely due to random neurological activity.

Cultural Considerations

Culture significantly influences various aspects of SMI, including the presentation of symptoms, coping strategies, family and community support networks, and individuals' likelihood of seeking treatment. Additionally, the cultural backgrounds of both clinicians and service systems affect the assessment, treatment, and delivery of mental health care. While cultural and social factors are not the sole determinants of mental health issues and service utilization among racial and ethnic minorities, they play critical roles in shaping these outcomes.

Mental health problems are highly prevalent across all populations, regardless of race or ethnicity. Cultural and social factors contribute to the causation of mental health problems, the problem behaviors displayed by the individuals with mental health problems, and the treatment received. The culture and social contributions vary by the mental health problem. Living with SMI is considered the product of complex interactions among biological, psychological, social, and cultural factors (Department of Health and Human Services [DHHS], 2001). The challenges in cross-cultural research on the prevalence of problem behaviors are the challenges of language across cultures and countries, standardization of operationalized definitions and assessments of the problem behaviors, and challenges of limited resources for research in mental health.

The studies on the occurrence of aggressive behaviors occurring in people living with SMI vary across different studies, locations, and settings. The prevalences are from people living with SMI exhibiting aggressive behaviors who have been admitted to inpatient psychiatric facilities:

1. In China, the study found that 35.4–53.0% of individuals living with schizophrenia spectrum mental health problems exhibit aggressive behaviors during hospitalization (Li et al.).
2. In Ethiopia, the study reported a 26.6% prevalence of aggressive behavior among individuals living with schizophrenia spectrum mental health problems. The prevalence of aggression in this study is higher than in studies from Canada (14.8%) and Nigeria (21.9%). The most common type of aggression reported was against property (15.89%) (Araya et al., 2020).
3. A study conducted in Nigeria found that 13.8% of individuals living with SMI demonstrated aggressive behaviors. Of these incidents, 69.8% occurred during the evening or nighttime hours, and 90.7% were directed toward living objects, with staff members comprising 57.5% of the targets (Amoo & Fatoye, 2010).
4. Caqueo-Urízar et al., 2016 studied the prevalence and risk factors of violent behavior in individuals living with SMI in community settings across three Latin American countries—Bolivia, Chile, and Peru. The overall prevalence of violent behavior was 24.4%, with significant differences between countries: 3.5% in Chile, 14.6% in Peru, and 55.4% in Bolivia. Younger age, severe symptoms/problem behavior corresponding to psychoses, lower family income, and unemployment were associated with violent behavior with more frequent occurrences of aggression occurring by individuals who experienced the onset of the SMI at a young age and frequent hospitalizations in the last 3 years. The authors concluded that the higher prevalence of aggressive behaviors in Bolivia and Peru compared to Chile was potentially due to economic disparities with more frequent occurrences of aggressive behavior related to countries with high unemployment and low incomes (Caqueo-Urízar et al. (2016)).

Types of Anger and Aggression

The domains of anger and aggression are composed of covert and overt behaviors. Within each of the domains are subdomains that vary along dimensions of behaviors. Domains and subdomains in mental health are composed of behavioral dimensions that are specific characteristics, behaviors, or measurements of that dimension. A domain is defined as a specific construct, activity, or scope (Gordon et al., 2022); within the domain of the construct of anger are types of anger that differ along behavioral dimensions.

The domain and subdomains of anger encompass covert events associated with the experience of anger including cognitions (subvocal speech that includes perceptions, appraisals and interpretations of antecedent conditions), emotional respondents (the dimensions of the respondents associated with anger including awareness of the experience), the behavioral display of anger (outward verbal and/or physical expressions of anger), the overt and covert consequences of the display that make up the types of anger experienced (perceptions, interpretations, and associated emotional respondents, of the consequences), and the function of the expression of aggressive response class (escape/avoidance of a aversive stimulus, acquisition of a desired stimulus). The subdomains of the expression of the experience of anger that is aggressive behaviors are composed of behavioral dimensions including frequencies, duration, intensities, latencies, and functional outcomes. Some behaviors labeled as aggressive are not associated with the experience of anger as an antecedent condition but vary along the same behavioral dimensions as other types of aggressive behaviors.

Types of Anger

All individuals experience anger at some point in their lives. Anger can be an adaptive response to antecedent environmental situations; anger is experienced along varying dimensions of frequencies, duration, intensities, latencies, and consequences. In certain instances, the environmental conditions preceding anger are recognized and accepted by the broader community. Conversely, individuals may sometimes encounter anger in contexts that are unique to their own perspective, where aspects of their emotional response extend beyond commonly accepted or "normal" boundaries.

The types of anger can be categorized according to salient dimensions. The types of anger categorized according to behavioral dimensions include:

- Chronicity: the temporal duration of the experience of anger.
- Latency: the time elapsed between a presented stimulus and the initiation of the emotional respondent of anger.
- Intensity: the magnitude of the angry experience.
- Expression: dimensions pertaining to the outward and inward expression of anger. Outward expression is labeled as blaming others; outward expression may involve display of aggressive response class that varies along types of aggression—verbal, physical, and both—and the targeted environmental stimulus of the displayed behaviors whether person, items, animals, or self. Inward expression involves self-blame, shame, and distressing respondents for the individual.
- Motivating operations (MOs) (establishing and abolishing operations (EOs/AOs)): MOs of anger change the reinforcing value of behaviors that lead to the removal of the aversive stimulus or the attainment of a desired outcome.
- Awareness of the experience: self-knowledge of the perception and associated covert of behaviors when angry (an aspect of the Theory of Mind [ToM]) and metacognitive abilities).
- Controllability: the degree of being able to control the dimensions of angry experience such as expression, intensity, and duration. This dimension involves resisting the situation or retaliating against it.
- Antecedent conditions: the environmental stimuli associated with the experience of anger. A sub-type of this type of anger is situational anger: This type arises in

response to specific events or situations, such as frustration at work or conflicts in personal relationships. It is typically temporary and situation-specific.

- Consequential conditions: the reinforcing and/or punitive consequences; the distress experienced by having the emotion of anger.
- Function of anger: The function of anger is theorized to facilitate goal attainment in situations involving challenges (Ramirez, 2011). Anger is theorized to be a coordinated response to the perception of obstacles to goals, prompting a focus on achieving the goal until it is either achieved or irrevocably lost. Subtypes of anger along the dimension of function include:
  - supportive anger, which is a mild form of anger that focuses on the need to find a resolution to the problem experienced. It includes feelings of mild anger, annoyance, frustration, and disappointment (Antonetti et al., 2020).
  - restorative vs. punitive anger. The function of this subtype is whether the anger functions to resolve a problem or inflict harm. Punitive or vindictive anger is an intense, high-arousal form of anger that focuses on seeking revenge against another entity for perceived wrongdoing, threat, or harm. It includes feelings of intense anger, rage, and outrage (Antonetti et al., 2020).
- Hostile anger: This is the situational expression of hostility that arises from interpersonal interaction that is characterized by challenge, evasion, and easily aroused irritation. Hostility involves the covert self-statements that others are motivated primarily by selfish concerns, and/or that people are likely to be hurtful and sources of mistreatment. Hostile anger may be expressed by a response in the domain of aggressive behaviors.

Mental health service providers have become increasingly aware of problematic anger and its negative impact on individuals. A recent poll reports that 42% of respondents to a poll said they were angrier in the past year than they had been at prior times (Hensley, 2019). More than a dozen different types of anger that people may experience have been identified by mental health professionals and organizations.

Various classifications and definitions of anger are frequently referenced within the mental health discipline. Smith (2022) and Kapur (2021) have identified several prevalent forms of anger. Table 11.3 presents these categories alongside their respective definitions as proposed by each author and indicates whether each type and definition is distinct.

The various types of anger listed by Kapur (2021) and Smith (2022) as seen in Table 11.3 have several commonalities and unique features that appear to be determined by various dimensions of the construct of anger such as: (a) the type of aggressive behavior displayed that is associated with the experience of anger (i.e., passive aggressive, verbal, silent); (b) the function of the displayed aggressive behavior (i.e., to obtain/acquire or avoid/escape stimuli); (c) the MO associated with the anger (i.e., judgmental and retaliatory anger); (d) the temporal duration of the experience of anger (i.e., chronic); (e) latency, the time elapsed between a presented stimulus and the initiation of the emotional respondent of anger (i.e., volatile,

Table 11.3 Comparison of anger types defined by Smith (2022) and Kapur (2021)

Type of Anger	Smith (2022) Definition	Kapur (2021) Definition	Features
Assertive anger	Constructive, aims for positive change, expressed respectfully, seeks resolution	Constructive, spurs positive change, clear respectful communication	Overlapping; both emphasize constructive use
Behavioral anger	Recognized by others, often from mistreatment/discrimination	Crosses from emotional to physical and include aggressive acts (e.g., hitting)	Kapur focuses on physical actions
Chronic anger	Long-lasting, affects mental health/social interactions, similar to "trait anger"	Low-level, continuous, manifests as frustration/resentment/irritability	Overlapping; both describe persistent anger
Destructive anger	Not listed	Intense, dangerous, can lead to violence/hatred	Unique to Kapur
Moral/judgmental anger	Arises from judgments and leads to negative outcomes	Righteous anger, stems from perceived injustices/moral flaws	Kapur adds moral/righteous aspect
Overwhelmed anger	From stressors, causes frustration	Builds up over time, leads to explosive outbursts	Kapur emphasizes buildup and explosion
Passive--aggressive anger	Indirect, subtle actions, avoids confrontation	Indirect, includes sarcasm, lack of response, "forgetting" requests	Overlapping; Kapur gives more examples
Retaliatory anger	Response to perceived wrongs, can escalate to aggression/violence	Vengeful, aggressive response to perceived threats	Overlapping; both focus on revenge
Self-abusive anger	Directed at oneself, linked to shame, self-harm	Associated with shame, negative thoughts, and leads to self-injury/substance abuse	Overlapping; Kapur adds substance abuse
Silent anger	Not listed	Expressed via facial expressions (e.g., scowling, "side eye"), subtype of passive-aggressive	Unique to Kapur
Verbal anger	Expressed through harsh words/yelling, impacts relationships	Displayed via yelling, cursing, sarcasm, criticism	Overlapping; Kapur expands behaviors
Volatile anger	Sudden, intense outbursts, severe consequences/aggression	Triggered by annoyances/frustrations, leads to rage, short latency	Overlapping; Kapur notes triggers
Deliberate anger	Not listed	Designed to hurt and be destructive	Unique to Kapur
Addictive/habitual anger	Not listed	Related to adrenaline/dopamine "high," cycle of seeking anger	Unique to Kapur

deliberate, overwhelmed); and (f) the intensity/magnitude of the experience of anger (i.e., destructive).

Anger becomes dysfunctional and problematic when it causes harm to the person experiencing anger and others who interact with that person. The types of anger that have been proposed have attempted to provide an operational definition of disturbed and problematic anger based on dimensions of the experience of anger and not just the outcome of the experience (DiGiuseppe & Tafrate, 2007).

Hecker and Lunde (1985) described six types of anger that are derived from the model of Spielberger et al. (1985), conceptualizing anger as a multifaceted construct. The theory distinguishes between "state anger" (i.e., temporary emotional responses to specific situations) and "trait anger" (i.e., a stable personality characteristic reflecting a predisposition to experience anger). Additionally, the theory identifies different styles of anger expression, including anger-in (internalized anger), anger-out (externalized anger), and anger control (the ability to regulate anger). It attempts to provide a framework for understanding how anger is experienced and expressed (Pease & Lewis, 2015). Hecker and Lunde (1985) divided anger into dimensions of inward-expression, outward-expression, and suppressed types. The first factor in their description distinguished between anger problems that were "under-controlled," "over-controlled," or "suppressed." The second factor had two levels of expression of anger, labeled as an impulsive-disorganized subtype contrasted with a deliberate-organized subtype.

From these dimensions, six types were derived (Hecker & Lunde, 1985):

1. Under-controlled impulsive: individuals experience high levels of anger and the impulsive expression of anger that is displayed by angry outbursts involving little deliberation or planning.
2. Under-controlled deliberate: individuals experience high levels of anger; having better impulse control, the expression of anger is planned for later retaliation.
3. Overcontrolled inward expression of anger: These people are over-controlled and stable individuals who maintain strong inhibitions about expressing anger. Anger is experienced frequently with high anger arousal, but it is not expressed. Physical or verbal aggressive behaviors rarely occur as these people take a passive stance and harbor resentment; nonetheless, anger interferes with daily functioning.
4. Overcontrolled unstable individuals: these individuals possess strong inhibitions about the outward expression of anger and occasionally lose control, displaying both physical and verbal aggressive behaviors.
5. Suppressed normal type: individuals suppress many emotions including anger. Reality testing is intact, but they do not consciously experience their anger, denying their experience of anger, but a hostile attitude often emerges.
6. Suppressed psychotic type: Individuals suppress anger, but their affect is inappropriate because of distortions of reality, lack of awareness of their anger, having disorganized thinking and speech, ideas of reference including paranoia and suspicions often having perceptions of others as critical of them.

Eckhardt and Deffenbacher (1995) offered two subtypes of the experience of dysfunctional anger:

- Situational anger: existence of problematic anger across a range of situations; specific stimuli or discrete situational antecedent domains trigger a dysfunctional level of anger.
- Generalized anger: dysfunctional anger is triggered across many situations.

The occurrence of aggression is an independent variable and can be present in both types of dysfunctional experiences of anger (Eckhardt & Deffenbacher, 1995).

DiGiuseppe and Tafrate (2007) conducted cluster analyses on data from a large sample (N > 1600) of people with and without mental health problems and dysfunctional anger using the Anger Disorders Scale (ADS). The ADS is a 74-item self-rated inventory designed to identify dysfunctional anger (DiGiuseppe & Tafrate, 2004). The analyses resulted in three subdomains being identified in the domain of dysfunctional anger composed of 13 subtypes or clusters of anger. The three subdomains and dimensional types/clusters in each subdomain were identified as follows:

- High expression and aggression without anger. Individuals express anger verbally and behave aggressively yet do not experience strong intense or frequent anger. This subdomain would include individuals living with an intermittent explosive mental health problem (IED).
  - Type 1: average anger and passive aggression: People in this group do not appear to get angry often nor stay angry for a long time, and do not self-identify as having an anger problem. However, when angry these individuals become noncooperative with the target of their anger. The sample was composed mostly of women.
  - Type 2: vengeful and indirect aggression: People who experience this type of anger have average trait anger but have a strong motive for revenge that they tend to accomplish through nonconfrontational, indirect yet aggressive means. Indirect aggression includes behaviors such as the secret destruction of property or hidden attempts to destroy the target of one's anger socially, emotionally, or professionally. These individuals do not see their anger as a problem; they do not display hostile attitudes typically associated with anger but have problems when experiencing anger having a strong desire for retaliation through indirect aggressive means.
  - Type 3: poly-aggressive, impulsive, with average anger: These people experience high levels of aggressive behavior but average levels on other dimensions of anger. The displayed aggression is more physical and occurs in interpersonal relationships. Individuals experiencing this type of anger have an average frequency of experiencing anger and little of the resentment and suspicion associated with anger; however, when they become angry, they impulsively act aggressively toward others by social disparagement and alienation, secretly trying to hurt the target of the anger. A moderate desire for revenge is felt, but these people cannot control their desire to attack the target of anger. Mostly men were found in this cluster.

  - Type 4: enduring, controlling, and nagging anger: The duration of anger is experienced for at least 6 months or more. Individuals in this cluster primarily express their anger through yelling, screaming, sarcasm, and banging objects. Anger is used to coerce or intimidate others into compliance.

- Higher anger with lower levels of expression and aggression (e.g., anger-in): includes people who experience frequent and intense dysfunctional anger but either hold their anger-in or express their anger less frequently than impulsive aggressive conditions.

  - Type 5: subclinical enduring anger with behavioral control: These individuals have longstanding experience of anger problems, yet they do not have frequent episodes that lead to aggression. They experience a low level of consistent subclinical anger characterized by rumination, resentment, suspicion, and a desire for retribution yet they do not display aggression. They do perceive that their anger impairs their life functioning.
  - Type 6: ruminating, high arousal, enduring anger: People in this cluster most likely have their anger triggered by social rejection, social disappointments, or failure to receive attention from others. They experience moderate levels of resentment and suspiciousness. The anger appears to be fueled by excessive rumination, holding their anger in, and failing to express it.
  - Type 7: low intensity, hostile attitudes, and anger-in: People in this cluster are characterized by rumination, physiological arousal, and the duration of anger as a problem. They experience less intense occurrences of anger than others with anger and outward expressive problems. Females comprised most of this group.

- High anger with expressive-aggressive behavior: individuals in this group experience both high levels of anger and expressive or aggressive.

  - Type 8: nonconfrontational vengeance: These individuals express their anger indirectly, secretly damaging the property of those with whom they are angry. Covert and subtle behaviors are displayed usually by not complying with activities or responsibilities. They have a strong desire for revenge, are suspicious of the motives of others, and expect hostility. These people experience resentment about circumstances of their life when they get angry and stay aroused for several days.
  - Type 9: social vengeance: People in this group are likely to alienate others socially with whom they are angry by making disparaging comments and forcing people to take sides. People in this cluster will fail to cooperate with the target of their anger and have strong desires for revenge, ruminating considerably about perceived transgressions against them and will be suspicious of others.
  - Type 10: impulsive, high-arousal, confrontational aggression: People in this cluster typically experience uncontrollable desires to confront others either verbally and physically; they are unlikely to hold their anger-in and will act on their anger when they experience it. They are unlikely to express anger covertly or indirectly and have no apparent motive for their expressions of

anger or aggressive behaviors. They also experience ruminative thoughts and high physiological arousal, although angry episodes are relatively short, lasting at most a few hours.

- Type 11: verbal or expressive, passive (not relational) aggression. Individuals in this group feel intense anger and often cannot control the urge to lash out at those they are upset with, frequently yelling, cursing, arguing, and insulting their targets. This verbal aggression can escalate into physical acts such as pushing or shoving, while subtle or indirect aggression is rare. These individuals tend to lose both behavioral and cognitive control, often dwelling on past wrongs and developing strong urges for revenge or to force others to comply, which disrupts their daily lives.
- Type 12: "total war": high-arousal, low anger-in: Individuals in this group are very likely to react with physical aggression when angry, feeling a powerful and uncontrollable urge to lash out combined with intense physiological excitement. They tend to dwell heavily on their anger, which seriously disrupts their daily lives, and they strongly desire revenge against those who wrong them. Additionally, they seek to force others to comply with their wishes, often using various forms of aggressive behavior to achieve control or retaliation.
- Type 13: extreme anger and aggression: People in this cluster were significantly more likely to display violent behaviors resulting in severe harm to others.

Types of Aggressive Behaviors

Variability exists in the cause and expression of aggressive behaviors. Multiple methods have been used to categorize and define aggressive behaviors. One major method has classified aggressive behaviors based on the typologies of aggressive behaviors: physical, verbal, and passive responses.

- Physical aggressive behavior is defined as behavior causing or threatening physical harm toward others. It includes hitting, kicking, biting, using weapons, and breaking items, objects, and the possessions of others (Kaye & Erdley, 2011).
- Verbal aggression is defined as the act of using language directed at a target. Verbal aggression topographies included insults, teasing, or hostile communication. It is considered a significant factor in interpersonal and social conflict and has antecedents and social consequences (Hamilton, 2012). Verbal aggression is operationally defined as any verbally statement or comment directed toward others that indicates intent to do physical or psychological harm to another person (e.g., "I am going to kick you in the leg!" or "You are a worthless and stupid person!") (Studco, 2021).
- Passive-aggressive behaviors are behaviors that indirectly express angry feelings by resistance to cooperation, procrastination, and intentional mistakes in response

to others' demands and requests. Rather than complying with the request, the person might express anger or resentment by failing to follow through or missing deadlines and passive opposition to the demands of others (Hall-Flavin, 2024).

Another method defines types of aggressive behaviors based on characteristics of the displayed aggressive behaviors and the aggressor's covert cognitive processes associated with the aggression (Babcock et al., 2014; Wrangham, 2018). The first type denotes a spontaneous lack of control that occurs with little if any thought or intention and has been called reactive, impulsive, affective, or hostile aggression. The second type denotes a planned intentional violent response and has been referred to as proactive, premeditated, predatory, or instrumental aggression. These two types of aggressive behaviors are supported by different physiological mechanisms and have distinct expressions, eliciting factors, and functions. The two types of aggressive behaviors following this framework are:

- Proactive aggression: defined as purposeful, planned attacks with the intent or goal of achieving a desired covert or overt reinforcer. It lacks an intention to harm others. The function is to coerce others into giving resources to the aggressor. It involves attention to a consistent target and often lacks emotional arousal. The topologies of this type of aggressive behavior include bullying, stalking, ambushes, premeditated homicides, robberies, and thefts (Babcock et al., 2014).
- Reactive aggression: defined as a response to a perceived threat or frustrating event whose function is the immediate removal of the provoking antecedent stimulus. It is associated with anger, and corresponding sudden sympathetic activation, failure of cortical regulation, easy switching among targets, and corresponding to an intent to cause harm to others. It is characterized by impulsivity, lack of planning, and short latency between the occurrence of the antecedent stimulus and the aggressive behavior being displayed. The typologies of this type of behavior included bar fights arising from mutual insults, crimes of passion immediately after discovering infidelity, and attacking a supervisor after being fired (Babcock et al., 2014).
- The types of aggressive behaviors can occur in conjunction with each other as physical and verbal aggressive behaviors can occur if the aggression is reactive or proactive (instrumental). Passive-aggressive behavior is considered as instrumental as the behavior is an intentional way of expressing negative feelings or achieving a goal, often through indirect actions, like silence (e.g., "silent treatment"), passive opposition (e.g., "forgetting" a birthday), or manipulation. The display of passive-aggressive behaviors is correlated with the experience of anger but is not overtly expressed.

Aggression is a behavioral domain composed of a response class of behaviors that consist of complex components, including subdomains, response classes within each subdomain, and dimensions of the specific behavioral response within the response class. The behavioral domain of aggression is composed of verbal, physical, and passive-aggressive subdomains. Within the subdomains are behavioral response classes that are group of responses that serve the same function, even if they differ in their specific form (Cooper et al., 2020). The behaviors in the response class are multidimensional in nature such as frequency, duration, latency, function, awareness, controllability, antecedent, and consequential conditions.

Why Do Anger and Aggressive Behaviors Occur?

Serious aggressive behaviors (i.e., violence) are rare events as is the prevalence of SMI, making it difficult to accurately assess societal risk. Most violent incidents involving individuals living with SMI occur within their social networks, often targeting family, friends, and sometimes service providers. The MacArthur Study indicated that 87% of violent incidents occurred at home (Stuart, 2003), with approximately 20% of family members of individuals living with SMI experiencing violence from the family member living with SMI annually (DeAngelis, 2021), while only 10.7% of incidents target strangers (Stuart, 2003). Research suggests that family variables, such as financial reliance and hostility, contribute to violence toward family members (DeAngelis, 2021). Population attributable risk (PAR: a measure in epidemiology that estimates the proportion of cases in a population that can be attributed to a specific exposure (Askari & Namayandeh, 2020)) for violence among those living with SMI is only 4.3%, suggesting limited impact on overall community violence although public fears about violence from the people living with SMI are often exaggerated, with individuals living with SMI to be victims than to victimize (Stuart, 2003).

Research indicates that while some individuals living with SMI may exhibit violent behavior, it is often linked to other factors (Stuart, 2003). Mental health problems do not directly cause violence, but socio-economic factors have been shown to play a crucial role (Powell & Williams, 2007). Contextual elements such as poverty, neighborhood crime rates, and substance use significantly influence violence, rather than mental illness alone. Adverse childhood experiences and unemployment are critical risk factors for violent behavior (DeAngelis, 2021; Stuart, 2003).

Part of the Reason May be Biochemical or Physical

- Anger and other problems of emotional self-control may be a direct result of the physical or chemical changes in the brain that are part of SMI. These differences may affect the areas of the brain that control emotions and the expression of emotions and make it more difficult for that person to control their emotions and the associated behaviors.
- The biochemical differences in brain functioning linked to living with SMI may disrupt sleep patterns or cause other problems (e.g., being up all night, sleeping during the day). This can result in impaired ability to cope with frustrating situations which, in turn, can result in anger and/or aggression.

- Irritability, anger, and agitation, as well as an inability to cope with them, can be unintended side effects of psychiatric or other medications rather than a result of living with SMI. These medications cause profound biochemical changes in brain functioning. Some medications may make the person living with SMI complain of feeling "jittery," "jumpy," or "not being able to sit still." These complaints may be a side-effect of some medications called "akathisia" that has been found to be related to agitation and impulsive aggressive behaviors (Lohr et al., 2015).

Part of the Reason May be Psychosocial

- People living with SMI often have more difficulty filtering out distractions in the environment. Excessive noise, activity, or crowding can lead to frustration, agitation, and anger. Individuals living with SMI may have a lower threshold for tolerating distractions compared to what others might anticipate. Consequently, an environment that seems tolerable to us may be very challenging for them. An example of this is being expected to respond to many questions and statements when too many people are talking at the same time.
- Working with a person living with SMI can be very frustrating. When others become critical or impatient with the person living with SMI, he may, in turn, become angry or agitated. Using the example above, it was observed by others that Charles has a problem paying attention. He can only do one thing at a time. The staff sometimes reminds him of things while he is already doing something else. He then forgets what they reminded him about. Later, many staff become upset and say "Charles, you'll never get better if you can't even remember simple things we ask you to do." When they said this, he often became angry, yelling that the service providers are picking on him, and saying "you'd better stop hassling me or else." In Charles' view, his anger is caused by their impatience with him. In certain situations, anger or agitation may arise as a result of unrealistic expectations imposed by others. A considerable number of individuals may lack awareness regarding the functional limitations associated with serious mental illness SMI and the increased patience required when interacting with those affected by SMI.
- Anger and aggression sometimes happen when people are unable to get something that they want. Such a problem is more likely to happen if a person has difficulty communicating and doesn't know how to properly go about asking for something. Sometimes, Charles wants a new video game but can't get to the store to buy it. When told that he'll have to wait several days before he can go, he starts to complain that he's being treated unfairly and that no one cares about him.
- Sometimes anger or aggression may accidentally be encouraged by other people. At times, a person living with SMI will become loud or unreasonable, and others may give in to the demands simply to quiet him down. If a person often gets something they want by threatening to get loud or hurt someone else, that person

is more likely to continue that behavior in the future as that behavior "works for them." For example, Charles often demands money from his parents. When he doesn't get what he wants, he gets louder, clenches his fists, and talks about feeling like he wants to start throwing furniture. His parents give in to calm him down. As a result, Charles is likely to act this way again when he wants money.
- For many adults living with SMI, anger and agitation may also be a natural reaction to the realization that many tasks which were once simple now require additional effort to perform, if they can be done at all. For example, if the person living with SMI began experiencing the mental health problem in early adulthood, they have memories of the friends they used to have and the good times that they had together. Many people will become angry about what they have lost.
- A history of childhood abuse has been found to be linked to anger and aggressive behaviors. Certain situations may "trigger" emotions and memories associated with the abuse, and these in turn make the person more likely to experience anger and display aggressive behaviors toward others or themselves.

Behavioral Support Strategies for Problems of Anger and Aggressive Behaviors Displayed by Individuals Living with SMI

To effectively prevent issues related to anger, one may consider implementing strategies in one or more of the following domains:

- Clearly define the problematic behaviors by specifying what the individual living with serious mental illness (SMI) does or says during episodes of anger or aggression. Examples of such behaviors may include yelling, pacing, throwing objects, or other similar actions. Recognize the early indicators that person living with SMI may be beginning to lose control. Warning signs of potential aggression, such as pacing, irritability, and reduced frustration tolerance, can often be managed through environmental interventions. Maintaining consistency in setting behavioral boundaries, offering positive reinforcement for self-control, and employing simple diversions are effective strategies for preventing the escalation of aggressive behaviors (Rueve & Welton, 2008).
- Be able to describe what is said and done and how frequently this happens. Anger and aggression can take many forms, and improvement is more likely if everyone is clear about what needs to be changed.
- Consider seeking a review of current medications. Increased irritability can be an unintended effect of medications being taken for other problem behaviors, symptoms, and physical problems. If anger and agitation seemed to increase after medication was started, seek a review of current medications with an experienced psychiatric prescriber. Another type of mediation may be more helpful in minimizing the anger/agitation and in preventing aggression.

- Change the problems that are making the person living with SMI angry. Engage and work with the person living with SMI to directly change the problems that result in anger. In some cases, support the person living with SMI to react differently to a problem situation and take steps to change it. In other cases, the person living with SMI may not be able to take the initiative to change a situation that is causing problems and needs more support. Simple interventions, such as maintaining a calm demeanor, can significantly impact violent outcomes. Aggressive behaviors are more likely to occur during transitional times when a person is changing from one state to another, such as waking up, eating meals, going to bed, and leaving the house (Randel, 2020; Rueve & Welton, 2008). If the person living with SMI complains about having to get up early on weekends to take medication, consult with the psychiatric service provider to change the times at which it needs to be taken. This is a common practice to make medication compliance.
- Change the way the person living with SMI reacts to these situations. Support the person living with SMI be less upset by the problems that they encounter. If the person living with SMI has seen a therapist, it is likely that they have talked about possible ways to lessen anger when it starts. These may include relaxation skills or a variety of other things to do (take a walk, go sit in a quiet room, count to 10 backward) when the angry feelings begin to build. Service providers know that Charles likes to shoot the basketball and suggest this (and, if possible, go with him) when they see that he's starting to get angry. In this example, the problem that caused anger hasn't changed, but the way that Charles responds to it has changed.
- Identify and avoid or change the situations that trigger anger.
- Determine the circumstances that trigger anger in individuals living with SMI and seek to mitigate or modify them. By proactively addressing these situations, it may be possible to prevent the onset of anger. Although this approach may not be feasible in every instance, it often represents an effective strategy for reducing the occurrence of anger and aggression.
- Watch for circumstances that provoke angry/agitated behavior. Try to become aware of the ways that the environment affects this behavior. Use the monitoring form in the Appendix to identify situations that contribute to anger. For example, certain people may often be the focus of the anger, or the problem may happen at certain times of the day, such as at mealtimes or when getting up in the morning (Randel, 2020; Rueve & Welton, 2008). This information is important for developing strategies to manage angry/agitated behaviors. Sometimes, the simplest and most realistic alternative is to try to avoid situations that provoke the problem.
- Simplify the environment. A person living with SMI is likely to have more difficulty in coping with a "busy" or chaotic environment. Consider simplifying the surroundings by minimizing noise, the number of people around, or other possible sources of frustration. It is often helpful to keep the daily routine consistent and predictable. For example, try to plan the daily activities so that lunch is

consistent at a certain time, and shopping is done on a certain day. Avoid sudden changes in routine as much as possible.

- Allow breaks during the day. Consider alternating specific break times with more active periods during the day. Encourage the person living with SMI to engage in a relaxing activity during these periods. For example, if the person living with SMI often becomes agitated during the late afternoon, allow for a rest period in the middle of the afternoon. This will make it less likely that the agitation will start to build later in the day.
- Distracting the person by using other activities when anger starts to build. It is important to identify the early indicators of escalating anger. For instance, Charles may exhibit warning signs such as staring at others and making threats in a low voice. Other individuals might display behaviors like pacing or raising their voice. When these signs are observed, it is advisable to calmly support the individual with SMI by removing them from the triggering situation or person. Offer gentle but firm guidance while maintaining a composed and reassuring tone or redirect their attention to a preferred activity. Avoid forcing the person to change activities abruptly.
- Establish a reminder or cue to use when signs of anger begin to appear. Prior to encountering challenging situations, have a discussion with the individual living with SMI regarding appropriate actions when they notice their anger increasing. Agree on a signal—such as raising a hand—that discreetly communicates escalating emotions. Ensure both parties understand and consent to the response plan; for instance, upon seeing the signal, the individual may count to ten, take a walk, or implement another strategy to manage their anger. This proactive approach fosters effective communication and supports emotional regulation.
- Watch for success. Watch for situations where the person living with SMI tolerates or successfully copes with frustrating situations or angry feelings. Provide compliments or praise for any success that you see (Randel, 2020; Rueve & Welton, 2008). This encourages the use of anger management skills. It's also important to pay attention to the person living with SMI at times when they aren't angry. For example, when Charles is calm, staff are instructed to play basketball with him, joke around (which he enjoys), or otherwise try to spend time with him.
- It is advisable to refrain from engaging in arguments, as doing so often exacerbates hostile behavior. If maintaining personal composure becomes challenging, consider taking a break and directing attention to an alternative activity. For instance, attempting to argue with Charles or match the volume of his speech tends to provoke additional threats and escalate tensions. Conversely, addressing him in a calm and neutral manner can help regulate his tone and prevent the situation from deteriorating.
- Let the anger subside before trying to discuss the situation. Consider the guidelines for communicating effectively as outlined in Chap. 4. These are even more important in situations where anger is getting out of control. Wait until after the anger or agitation has diminished before trying to talk about the problem. The person living with SMI will be much more likely to listen once the anger has

diminished. When addressing an individual living with SMI regarding a situation, it is advisable to use "I" statements to clearly communicate your perspective. Express disapproval of specific behaviors in a constructive manner (e.g., "I feel concerned when you raise your voice; I encourage you to try your best to refrain from this."), and avoid remarks that criticize or question the person's abilities or motivation (e.g., "Are you not aware of this?"; "Do you realize you are causing additional difficulties?"), as such comments may result in heightened frustration. When requesting that the individual cease certain actions, also suggest alternative approaches (e.g., "If you become upset, please avoid shouting; instead, consider discussing your feelings with me."). Following these recommendations can increase the likelihood that the individual will listen and retain guidance for handling similar situations in the future.

- Consider developing a behavioral contract to encourage better ways of dealing with anger and aggression. Such a contract makes it more likely that the person living with SMI will follow the steps to clarify the problem behavior and engage in adaptive alternative behaviors when getting angry as recognition for successful self-control is specified in the contract. With contracts, expectations are clearer, and it is less likely that problems will continue to happen. The contract can also have fines or other consequences for failing to meet expectations. These "negative consequences" (such as losing a trip to the mall or not going out to eat on Friday) should be agreed upon by all stakeholders and the person living with SMI and should be applied consistently (see the section on contracting for desired behaviors in Chap. 4). The contract should include both "positive" and "negative" consequences but should emphasize the positive. In the example of Charles, the staff worked with him to develop a contract. By doing certain things when he started to become angry—such as taking a walk or shooting baskets on the basketball court to control his anger and aggression—he could earn the opportunity to do certain things that he told the staff he liked (like being able to go to the mall on Friday night).
- Encourage the coping skills being taught by the others working with the person living with SMI. If the person living with SMI sees a service provider who is a therapist, that person has probably worked with him to develop a variety of coping skills to help reduce and manage anger and agitation. These may include several alternative activities to try as the anger builds (e.g., count to 10, go for a walk, shoot baskets, lie down and relax). Learn what these strategies are and encourage their use when you recognize that the person living with SMI's anger is increasing. In the example of Charles, the staff used problem-solving techniques (see section on problem solving in Chap. 4) after he calmed down. This helped him identify what it was that made him angry and what he could do next time to keep the situation from getting out of control.
- Be an advocate for the person living with SMI when it is appropriate. Sometimes the person living with SMI confronts situations that result in anger that simply shouldn't happen and can be changed. If the anger is brought on by such problems as long waits at the community mental health center or difficulty in explaining side effects to the physician, contact the source of frustration and help to

resolve the problem. While self-reliance should be encouraged, there will be times when the person living with SMI needs support to change a challenging situation.

- Be mindful of personal limitations regarding self-control. It is important to recognize that the anger or agitation exhibited by individuals living with SMI may cause discomfort and distress. In such situations, one's ability to communicate calmly can be reduced. Demonstrating impatience or irritability may escalate the situation further. If necessary, consider temporarily removing oneself from the environment to regain composure before determining the safest course of action.
- Recognize when the situation is getting out of control and have a plan. While the goal is to help the person living with SMI, there's no reason that one should have to tolerate aggressive behavior. If physical safety is threatened, stay out of reach of the person living with SMI and, if necessary, leave the situation. If the person living with SMI demands to leave the room, avoid blocking the exit or doing anything that might make the situation worse. Don't hesitate to call for help from neighbors, family members, friends, 911, the police, or staff members of the local community mental health center. It is best to have these telephone numbers handy and to have a clear and established plan as to who will be called. Setting clear and consistent limits is helpful.
- Consider seeking outside help for planning. It is very difficult to work with someone who has difficulty managing anger. Consult with a mental health service provider, usually a behavioral psychologist, to obtain a realistic assessment of self-management potential in consideration of the symptoms with a person living with SMI. When consulting the psychologist, be prepared to describe what the person living with SMI does when angry, the kinds of situations that seem to provoke such behavior, and this is currently handled.

Conclusion for Behavioral Support Strategies for Problems of Anger and Aggressive Behaviors Displayed by Individuals Living with SMI

When attempting to manage episodes of anger and agitation, consider the following steps:

1. Work with the psychiatric service provider of the person living with SMI to try to find the most effective medication(s) for the problem.
2. Make sure that the person living with SMI is taking the medication as prescribed. If there are concerns about the medications and side effects, consult with the prescriber and be specific about your concerns.
3. Take steps to identify circumstances that frequently bring on episodes of anger or agitation. For monitoring forms and examples see the forms in the Appendix.
4. Take steps to identify activities that the person living with SMI enjoys and which are calming such as taking walks, listening to music, playing checkers, or others.

These may include "self-control skills" that the person living with SMI has learned with a therapist.

5. Learn to recognize and watch for the early signs of increasing anger and agitation.
6. Be prepared to suggest alternative things to do as the anger builds. Practice giving this information in a clear, firm, but nonthreatening manner. Have the person living with SMI practice as to what to do when they experience anger/agitation.
7. Make sure that acknowledgment is given for self-control efforts and willingness to follow advice by the person living with SMI when agitation and anger increase.
8. Have a plan of what to do if the situation starts to get out of control. Know what help is available and don't be afraid to call for it.

What About Charles?

Several hospital staff quickly realized that trying to reason with Charles when he started becoming agitated only made things worse. Instead of trying to reason with him, they decided to try to get him involved in doing things that they knew he enjoyed. Sometimes they begin asking about the football game over the weekend and try to keep a conversation going on that topic. They sometimes offered to walk with him while talking about his last home visit or other topics that they knew he was interested in. Sometimes they offered to play a computer game against him. Later, after Charles had calmed down for several hours, they often tried to seek him out to talk about the situation that made him angry in the first place. When talking about this, they took special care to make sure that they let him know how impressed they were that he could put his anger aside and go and do things with them. In various ways, they tried to give him the message that being a "real man" means staying in control rather than losing control. They tried to let him know that they were impressed when he asked to be allowed to do certain things (sit in his room, ask to talk to certain staff) to calm himself down.

The staff who followed this plan became more influential with Charles and helped him to do better in the hospital. Several staff did not try these strategies. Some of these people felt that Charles should be able to calm himself and would continue to yell at him that he needed to calm down or he'd be punished. Other staff simply avoided interacting with him unless they had to. These people were much less influential with him.

In this example, the staff members who were effective with Charles followed several of the steps in this chapter:

1. They recognized that his complaining was an early sign that he was becoming agitated.
2. The team recognized that if they tried to reason with him, his agitation simply got worse.
3. They identified several alternative activities that Charles enjoyed doing.

4. The staff members learned how to calmly help him to engage in these alternative activities when they saw his agitation start to build.
5. They congratulated him (and allowed him to have certain reinforcers) whenever he was able to calm himself down with or without their help.

By approaching the anger problem this way, along with encouraging him to regularly take his medication, the number of anger episodes, and their severity, decreased.

Summary

Anger is a basic emotion that can lead to aggressive behavior, impacting mental health and social interactions. Anger is one of four basic emotions, alongside happiness, sadness, and fear, that are essential for adaptive functioning in human behavior. However, emotions are covert, private events that are often only known to the individual experiencing them and are assessed through self-reports that may be unreliable due to exaggeration or denial. Collateral sources, such as observable behaviors, can aid in assessing private events. Observable behaviors, like facial expressions and tone of voice, provide additional context for understanding emotions.

Emotions can become "problematic" in mental health when the experience and/or expression of emotions lead to unfavorable outcomes. "Symptomatic" behaviors occur when emotions result in distress for oneself or others. Problematic or "abnormal" behaviors are those behaviors displayed too frequently, intensely, or in inappropriate settings, lacking adequate stimulus control.

Anger is a complex and transient state involving subjective experiences, cognition, beliefs, and physiological responses. It is vital for social functioning and motivates addressing injustices. Anger facilitates goal attainment by organizing cognitive, emotional, and behavioral responses but may also lead to problematic outcomes when it results in harmful and deleterious results for the individual living with SMI and others in society.

Problematic anger occurs when the frequency and intensity of emotion cause distress and interfere with functioning. Problematic anger is linked to psychological trauma, increasing risks of harm, financial hardships, and relationship difficulties. Dysfunctional anger is associated with marital distress, long-term depression, and cardiovascular disease risk.

Anger is a complex multidimensional construct that includes antecedent conditions, social learning, and behavioral responses. It is characterized by unpleasant feelings and specific facial expressions, which vary among individuals. However, humans can regulate the experience and the expression of emotions, leading to more behavioral choices.

Anger is an "approach emotion" triggered by perceived impediments to goal attainment. It is expressed by behaviors aimed at removing the impeding stimulus or expressing the experienced emotional respondent and decreasing the adverse physiological responses correlated with the experience of anger. Anger is a motivational state that enhances engagement in response to challenges. It can function as a motivating operation, increasing the effectiveness of reinforcers. Appropriate levels of anger can enhance performance in tasks related to perceived injustices.

Many individuals struggle with appropriate expression, particularly those with passive-aggressive tendencies. Anger is a core feature in five DSM-5 conditions: Intermittent explosive (IED), borderline personality (BPD), bipolar (BP), disruptive mood dysregulation (DMDD), and oppositional defiant (ODD) mental health issues. Elevated anger is associated with negative treatment outcomes in these mental health challenges. Different mental health problems exhibit unique characteristics of anger, such as episodic intensity in IED and chronicity in BPD.

Aggression is behavior aimed at harming others, either physically or psychologically. It differs from anger, which is a covert event and may not be involved with any intention of inflicting harm. Violence is an extreme form of aggression intended to cause serious harm. Aggressive behaviors can be physical, verbal, or both, directed at living beings or objects; aggressive behaviors can also be expressed indirectly by facial expressions, delaying or not responding after a request, and subtle nonverbal responses such as sighing to express hostility and frustration (i.e., passive-aggressive behaviors).

Aggressive behaviors may be considered a positive symptom of SMI. Individuals living with SMI display less aggression than those without any mental health issue, accounting for less than 10% of violent crimes. Higher incidence of violence in individuals with SMI is linked to positive symptoms, history of aggression, and adverse environmental factors. Co-occurring mental health problems increase the risk of aggression in individuals with SMI. Fourteen percent of individuals admitted to mental health facilities had experienced violence in the preceding month. Among those living with SMI, 72% exhibited aggressive behaviors, while 68% of individuals under 30 with SMI demonstrated similar tendencies. The prevalence of aggressive behavior in psychiatric settings during acute treatment ranges from 8 to 44%. Mental health professionals are at considerable risk of experiencing physical assault during their careers, with estimates ranging from 5 to 48%. Among them, nursing staff are most vulnerable because they interact with hospitalized individuals more often. People who have multiple mental health conditions are 2 to 4.5 times more likely to display aggressive behavior. Those living with SMI face a somewhat lower likelihood—about 3–5%—of being aggressive compared to individuals struggling with substance abuse.

Certain mental health problems increase the risk of aggressive behaviors, influenced by sex, age, and co-occurring issues. DSM-5-TR mentions aggressive behaviors in relation to schizophrenia spectrum mental health problems and IED, which is characterized by repeated outbursts of anger and aggression, often co-occurring with personality disorders.

Incarcerated early offenders with mental health issues often commit more violent crimes and have higher recidivism rates. Individuals with SMI are three times more likely to be arrested than the general population.

Anger is a complex and multidimensional construct that involves behavioral dimensions such as frequency, intensity, duration, and controllability. Hostility, irritability, anger attacks, trait anger, and state anger are subdomains of the major construct of anger. Hostility is defined by sustained anger and retaliatory actions, whereas irritability pertains to a heightened sensitivity leading to frequent displays of anger. Trait anger represents an individual's overall predisposition toward experiencing anger, while state anger denotes the magnitude of anger felt during a particular moment.

Existing assessment instruments have weak psychometric characteristics and lack clear definitions of anger and aggression. The Multidimensional Anger Inventory (MAI) identifies dimensions like frequency, duration, and mode of expression. Factor analyses of MAI revealed that anger dimensions cluster into anger-arousal and anger-expression categories. A five-factor model of anger includes dimensions of anger-arousal, anger-rumination, frustration-discomfort, anger-regulation, and socially constituted anger. Anger-arousal reflects frequent intense anger experiences, while anger-rumination involves repetitive thoughts about anger-inducing events. Frustration-discomfort focuses on beliefs about entitlement and achievement, and anger-regulation identifies cognitive strategies for managing anger. Socially constituted anger examines anger within social contexts and norms.

The experience of anger is covert and private events and is assessed by self-reports. Limitations of self-report measures include a lack of specificity regarding antecedent conditions and outcomes of anger expression. There is a need for expanded assessment methods that include context-specific anger scales and clinical aspects of anger. Key dimensions for clinical assessment include intensity, frequency, duration, awareness, expression, and antecedent conditions related to the experience of anger.

Aggressive behaviors vary in topography and intent, complicating classification. Types of aggression include hostile, direct, displaced, instrumental, affective, and impulsive aggression. Hostile aggression aims to cause harm, while instrumental aggression seeks to achieve a goal.

Physical aggression includes hitting, kicking, and other harmful actions, regardless of intent. Verbal aggression involves insults and threats that cause emotional distress. Passive aggression is an indirect expression of anger, such as sarcasm or neglect. Revenge is a subjective intention to cause harm based on perceived injury.

Neurobiological factors, including genetic, metabolic, and neurochemical elements, contribute to problem behaviors in SMI like anger and aggressive behaviors. Heightened anger and aggression lead to longer psychiatric stays, relationship loss, employment issues, and increased stigma.

Recent research has shed light on how structural abnormalities in certain brain regions may play a role in aggression among individuals with SMI. Scientists have pinpointed key areas of the brain that are influential in shaping emotions like anger, as well as aggressive behaviors in this population.

The amygdala, for example, is known for its role in generating aggressive responses. Studies have shown that when activity in the amygdala is heightened, instances of aggression tend to increase. Meanwhile, the prefrontal cortex (PFC) is crucial for impulse control and decision-making. If lesions occur in this region, levels of aggression can rise—a finding that highlights the delicate balance required for regulation of behavior.

Another important area, the anterior cingulate cortex (ACC), contributes both to emotion regulation and impulse control. Researchers have observed that reduced volumes in the ACC are linked to higher rates of aggression. The insula and hippocampus also play significant roles: the insula participates in socio-emotional processing, while the hippocampus is vital for emotional regulation.

These observations are supported by functional MRI studies. Disruptions in frontal cortical white matter have been associated with impulsivity and aggressive tendencies. In fact, elevated aggression scores often coincide with increased grey and white matter volumes in the orbitofrontal cortex (OFC) and caudate. Further investigation has revealed that cortical thinning in the PFC is related to violent behavior, and hyperactivation of the medial PFC seems to be present in those who are more aggressive. Impaired function of the ventromedial PFC (vmPFC) can also contribute to impulsive aggression, influencing decision-making and behavioral choices. Increased impulsivity, researchers note, often corresponds with grey matter volume reduction in regions such as the medial OFC and ACC.

The display of aggressive behaviors is related to neurotransmitter systems including serotonin, dopaminergic, vasopressinergic, and glutamate systems. Altered interactions between prefrontal and subcortical regions, particularly the amygdala, contribute to the occurrence of aggression.

Future directions for research in the understanding of the neurobiological foundations of anger and aggressive behaviors in people living with SMI include the need for specific measures of aggression and clearer distinctions among the dimensions of aggressive behaviors. Future studies should address methodological inconsistencies and explore the interplay of dimensions of aggressive behaviors and neurological substrates.

Anger and aggression result from biological as well as environmental influences. Genetic factors may provide a baseline propensity for anger and aggression as anger is an innate emotional response linked to perceived threats and injustices that sometimes precede occurrences of aggressive behaviors. The respondent (emotion) of anger functions as a motivating operation (MO) that can enhance performance in confrontational tasks. Appropriate levels of anger can motivate actions against injustices, as seen in civil rights movements. Anger expression varies and can manifest as determined actions or mere emotional expressions. However, the expression and regulation of anger can be problematic for some individuals particularly individuals living with SMI. Anger dysregulation is linked to mental health issues and can lead to problematic aggressive behaviors resulting in negative outcomes for the individual living with SMI and society.

Anger can be conditioned through classical and instrumental learning. Prolonged unresolved anger can lead to inappropriate anger reactivity in unrelated situations. Environmental context influences the display of aggressive behaviors as aggressive behaviors are impacted by environmental consequences and social learning. Some individuals may suppress anger to avoid punishment, leading to maladaptive coping mechanisms.

Aggressive behaviors among individuals with SMI are multifaceted and extend across diagnostic categories. The majority of violent incidents are not solely attributable to mental health conditions; instead, contextual influences are often significant. Notably, 39% of violent episodes in psychiatric environments are associated with staff–patient interactions, frequently arising from perceived efforts to manage or control the individual exhibiting aggression.

Research in aggressive behavior displayed by people living with SMI has resulted in variability and a lack of generalizability of findings. The significant variability prevalent in research on aggression is due to lack of standardization in definitions and measures, small sample size, and other methodological limitations. .

Anger is a key criterion in five mental health disorders in DSM-5-TR. Problematic anger is not a standalone diagnostic category but is prevalent in various mental health issues. High levels of anger are linked to traumatic backgrounds and can predict violence. Dysregulation of anger is characterized by frequency, intensity, and mode of expression that is extreme and has negative outcomes for the person displaying the anger and the target of the anger.

At present, research that assesses the prevalence of the types of problematic anger in individuals with SMI is not available. Individuals living with SMI are two to three times more likely to engage in aggressive behaviors than those without. Fourteen percent of individuals living with SMI display aggressive behavior 1 month prior to psychiatric admission. Females with SMI exhibit aggressive behaviors similar to males, often directed at family members and close acquaintances. Young adults under 30 who are living with SMI account for 68% of physical assaults. History of aggression increases the likelihood of future violent behavior.

Co-occurring substance use significantly increases aggressive behavior frequency. Twenty-eight percent of individuals living with SMI committed offenses under the influence of psychoactive substances. Regular cannabis users are 2.4 times more likely to engage in aggression, and aggressive behaviors can occur at any stage of drug use, but at a higher risk during withdrawal and intoxication.

Aggressive behaviors among individuals with SMI residing in psychiatric facilities present significant challenges, with reported rates of aggression ranging from 8% to 76%. Nursing staff are frequently exposed to aggressive conduct from individuals who are admitted. Contributing individual factors include substance use, younger age, and a prior history of aggression. Additionally, environmental variables such as staff training and ward conditions play a role in influencing the prevalence of aggressive behaviors.

Social factors and culture are determinants of mental health issues and service utilization. Culture affects the expression of problem behaviors/symptoms, coping styles, and treatment willingness and engagement. Clinician and service system cultures also influence the identification and determination of mental health problems and treatment.

Aggressive behaviors in individuals with SMI vary by location and study. In a study from China, 35.4–53.0% of individuals living with a with schizophrenia spectrum mental health problem exhibit aggression during hospitalization. Researchers in Ethiopia report a 26.6% prevalence of aggressive behavior among individuals living with a schizophrenia spectrum mental health problem, while studies from Nigeria found 13.8% of individuals with SMI show aggressive behaviors, primarily targeting staff.

In addition, there are regional variations in the prevalence and rates of aggressive behaviors. A study in Latin America found 24.4% overall prevalence of violent behavior in community settings. Studies from countries in South America found the following prevalence by country: Bolivia: 55.4%; Peru: 14.6%; and Chile: 3.5%. Factors associated with violence include younger age, severe symptoms, low income, and unemployment. Economic disparities also may explain higher rates of aggression in Bolivia and Peru compared to Chile.

The experience of anger can be categorized by chronicity, latency, intensity, expression, antecedent, and consequential conditions. Situational anger arises from specific events, while chronic anger is low-level, persistent, and generalizes across antecedent conditions. Types of anger have been defined and include assertive, behavioral, chronic, moral, overwhelmed, passive-aggressive, retaliatory, self-abusive, silent, verbal, volatile, deliberate, and addictive/habitual anger.

Experiences of anger have several common dimensions including (a) anger being expressed outwardly (aggression) or inwardly (self-blame); (b) controllability that refers to the ability to manage anger's expression and intensity; and (c) awareness that involves understanding one's experience of anger and its triggers. Anger can facilitate goal attainment by focusing on overcoming obstacles. Supportive anger seeks resolution, while punitive anger aims for revenge. Hostile anger arises from interpersonal interactions and can lead to aggressive behaviors.

Anger has a significant impact on mental health. Forty-two percent of surveyed individuals reported increased anger in the past year. Problematic anger can harm individuals and their relationships. Mental health professionals identify over a dozen types of anger affecting well-being, especially dysfunctional anger.

Dysfunctional anger can be situational or generalized, leading to aggression. Different types of dysfunctional anger have been identified through cluster analyses. Types include high expression without anger, passive aggression, vengeful indirect aggression, and impulsive confrontational aggression.

In addition, the style of expressing the experience of anger varies dimensionally. Anger has been categorized into under-controlled, over-controlled, and suppressed types. Under-controlled individuals may express anger impulsively or deliberately. Overcontrolled individuals may harbor resentment without outward expression.

Research findings show various types of experiences of anger and their implications for mental health. Anger can lead to significant interpersonal consequences and affect daily functioning. Understanding anger's dimensions and expressions is crucial for effective management and resolution.

Aggressive behaviors are categorized into physical, verbal, and passive responses. Physical aggression involves causing or threatening physical harm. Verbal aggression includes insults, demeaning comments, sarcasm, and hostile communication, impacting social conflict. Passive-aggressive behaviors express anger indirectly through procrastination or intentional mistakes. Aggression can be reactive (impulsive) or proactive (planned), each with distinct physiological mechanisms. Proactive aggression aims to achieve a goal without intent to harm, while reactive aggression responds to perceived threats.

The causes of anger are likewise complex and multidimensional. Serious aggressive behaviors are rare, with most incidents occurring within the social networks of the person who aggresses. Eighty-seven percent of violent incidents involving individuals living with SMI occur at home with 20% of family members of individuals living with SMI experience violence annually. Mental health issues do not directly cause violence; adverse childhood experiences and unemployment are critical risk factors. Socio-economic factors, such as poverty and substance use, significantly influence the occurrence of violent behaviors. Individuals living with SMI are more often victims than perpetrators of violence.

The causes of anger and aggression are both biological and environmental. Anger and aggressive behaviors may have neurological underpinnings that result in physical or chemical changes in the brain due to living with SMI. Sleep disruptions can impair coping abilities, leading to anger and aggression. Medications can cause side effects like irritability and agitation, contributing to aggressive behaviors.

Part of the reason for the display of dysfunctional anger and aggression may be psychosocial. Individuals with SMI struggle to filter distractions, leading to frustration and anger. Frustration can arise from critical comments or impatient responses from others. Anger may stem from unmet desires or difficulties in communication. Childhood abuse history can trigger aggressive behaviors in certain situations.

When dealing with anger and aggression displayed by a person living with SMI, have the current medications reviewed by a psychiatric prescriber if irritability increases. The service provider needs to first clearly and precisely define the problem behaviors and identify early warning signs of aggression. If able, change situations that provoke anger and help the individual react differently. Simplify the environment to reduce distractions and maintain a consistent routine. Encourage coping skills and provide positive reinforcement for managing anger. Develop a behavioral contract to clarify expectations and consequences. Finally, seek outside help for planning and managing aggressive behaviors effectively.

References

Allen, J. J., & Anderson, C. A. (2017). Aggression and violence: Definitions and distinctions. In P. Sturmey (Ed.), *The Wiley handbook of violence and aggression* (pp. 1–14). John Wiley & Sons. https://doi.org/10.1002/9781119057574.whbva001

American Psychiatric Association. (2022). *Diagnostic and statistical manual of mental disorders* (5th ed., text rev.). doi:https://doi.org/10.1176/appi.books.9780890425787

American Psychological Association. (n.d.-a). Aggression. In *APA dictionary of psychology*. https://dictionary.apa.org/aggression

American Psychological Association. (n.d.-b). Anger. In *APA dictionary of psychology*. https://dictionary.apa.org/anger

American Psychological Association. (n.d.-c). Transcranial magnetic stimulation. In *APA Dictionary of Psychology*. https://dictionary.apa.org/transcranial-magnetic-stimulation

American Psychological Association. (2024). *Anger*. https://www.apa.org/topics/anger

Amoo, G., & Fatoye, F. O. (2010). Aggressive behaviour and mental illness: A study of in-patients at Aro neuropsychiatric hospital, Abeokuta. *Nigerian Journal of Clinical Practice, 13*(3), 351–355. https://www.ajol.info/index.php/njcp/article/download/59810/48086

Anderson, A., & West, S. G. (2011). Violence against mental health professionals: When the treater becomes the victim. *Innovations in Clinical Neuroscience, 8*(3), 34–39. https://innovationscns.com/violence-against-mental-health-professionals-when-the-treater-becomes-the-victim/

Antonetti, P., Crisafulli, B., & Katsikeas, C. S. (2020). Does it really hurt? Making sense of varieties of anger. *Psychology and Marketing, 37*(11), 1465–1483. https://doi.org/10.1002/mar.21392

Araya, T., Ebnemelek, E., & Getachew, R. (2020). Prevalence and associated factors of aggressive behavior among patients with schizophrenia at Ayder comprehensive specialized hospital, Ethiopia. *BioMed Research International, 2020*(1), 7571939. https://doi.org/10.1155/2020/7571939

Askari, M., & Namayandeh, S. M. (2020). The difference between the population attributable risk (PAR) and the potential impact fraction (PIF). *Iran Journal of Public Health, 49*(10), 2018–2019. https://doi.org/10.18502/ijph.v49i10.4713

Babcock, J. C., Tharp, A. L., Sharp, C., Heppner, W., & Stanford, M. S. (2014). Similarities and differences in impulsive/premeditated and reactive/proactive bimodal classifications of aggression. *Aggression and Violent Behavior, 19*(3), 251–262. https://doi.org/10.1016/j.avb.2014.04.002

Blair, R. J. (2016). The neurobiology of impulsive aggression. *Journal of Child and Adolescent Psychopharmacology, 26*(1), 4–9. https://doi.org/10.1089/cap.2015.0088

Buss, A. H., & Perry, M. (1992). The Aggression Questionnaire. *Journal of Personality and Social Psychology, 63*(3), 452–459. https://doi.org/10.1037/0022-3514.63.3.452

Buss, A. H., & Warren, W. L. (2000). *Aggression Questionnaire: Manual*. Western Psychological Services.

Caqueo-Urízar, A., Fond, G., Urzúa, A., Boyer, L., & Williams, D. R. (2016). Violent behavior and aggression in schizophrenia: Prevalence and risk factors. A multicentric study from three Latin-America countries. *Schizophrenia Research, 178*(1–3), 23–28. https://doi.org/10.1016/j.schres.2016.09.005

Caruso, R., Antenora, F., Riba, M., Belvederi Murri, M., Biancosino, B., Zerbinati, L., & Grassi, L. (2021). Aggressive behavior and psychiatric inpatients: A narrative review of the literature with a focus on the European experience. *Current Psychiatry Reports, 23*, 1–12. https://doi.org/10.1007/s11920-021-01233-z

Cassiello-Robbins, C., & Barlow, D. H. (2016). Anger: The unrecognized emotion in emotional disorders. *Clinical Psychology: Science and Practice, 23*(1), 66–85. https://doi.org/10.1111/cpsp.12139

Chester, D. S., & DeWall, C. N. (2016). The pleasure of revenge: Retaliatory aggression arises from a neural imbalance toward reward. *Social Cognitive and Affective Neuroscience, 11*(7), 1173–1182. https://doi.org/10.1093/scan/nsv082

Cooper, J. O., Heron, T. E., & Heward, T. E. (2020). *Applied behavior analysis* (3rd ed.). Pearson.

DeAngelis, T. (2021). Mental illness and violence: Debunking myths, addressing realities. *Monitor on Psychology, 52*(3), 31. Retrieved from https://www.apa.org/monitor/2021/04/ce-mental-illness

Delprato, D. J. (2002). Countercontrol in behavior analysis. *The Behavior Analyst, 25*(2), 191–200. https://www.ncbi.nlm.nih.gov/pmc/articles/PMC2733624/

DiGiuseppe, R., & Tafrate, R. C. (2004). *Anger disorders scale (ADS)*. Multi-Health Systems. https://doi.org/10.1037/t04936-000

DiGiuseppe, R., & Tafrate, R. C. (2007). *Understanding anger disorders*. Oxford University Press. https://academic.oup.com/book/1066

Eckhardt, C., & Deffenbacher, J. (1995). Diagnosis of anger disorders. In H. Kassinove (Ed.), *Anger disorders: Definition, diagnosis and treatment* (pp. 27–47). Taylor & Francis. https://doi.org/10.4324/9781315820361

Eckhardt, C., Norlander, B., & Deffenbacher, J. (2004). The assessment of anger and hostility: A critical review. *Aggression and Violent Behavior, 9*(1), 17–43. https://doi.org/10.1016/S1359-1789(02)00116-7

Enquist, M., Lind, J., & Ghirlanda, S. (2016). The power of associative learning and the ontogeny of optimal behaviour. *Royal Society Open Science, 3*, 160734. https://doi.org/10.1098/rsos.160734

Fernandez, E., & Johnson, S. L. (2016). Anger in psychological disorders: Prevalence, presentation, etiology and prognostic implications. *Clinical Psychology Review, 46*, 124–135. https://doi.org/10.1016/j.cpr.2016.04.012

Forbes, D., Hawthorne, G., Elliott, P., McHugh, T., Biddle, D., Creamer, M., & Novaco, R. W. (2004). A concise measure of anger in combat-related posttraumatic stress disorder. *Journal of Traumatic Stress, 17*(3), 249–256. https://doi.org/10.1023/B:JOTS.0000029266.74317.e3

Gabbey, A. E. & Raypole, C. (2022, March 3). *Aggressive behavior: Signs, causes, and treatment.* Healthline. https://www.healthline.com/health/aggressive-behavior

Girasek, H., Nagy, V. A., Fekete, S., Ungvari, G. S., & Gazdag, G. (2022). Prevalence and correlates of aggressive behavior in psychiatric inpatient populations. *World Journal of Psychiatry, 12*(1), 1. https://doi.org/10.5498/wjp.v12.i1.1

Goldiamond, I. (2022). *A programing contingency analysis of mental health.* Routledge. https://doi.org/10.4324/9781003260103

Gopika, G. G., Antony, S., Jayakumar, C., Moirangthem, S., Joseph, E., Gowda, G. S., & Reddi, V. S. K. (2024). Person-in-situation framework of aggression among persons with severe mental illness: A case series. *Indian Journal of Psychological Medicine, 46*(4), 358–362. https://doi.org/10.1177/02537176241251961

Gordon, J. A., Morris, S. E., & Avenevoli, S. (2022). A framework for integration of dimensional and diagnostic approaches to the diagnosis of schizophrenia. *Schizophrenia Research, 242*, 98. https://doi.org/10.1016/j.schres.2022.01.056

Gu, S., Wang, F., Patel, N. P., Bourgeois, J. A., & Huang, J. H. (2019). A model for basic emotions using observations of behavior in *drosophila*. *Frontiers in Psychology, 10*, 781. https://doi.org/10.3389/fpsyg.2019.00781

Hall-Flavin, D. K. (2024). What is passive-aggressive behavior? What are some of the signs? *Mayo Clinic.* https://www.mayoclinic.org/healthy-lifestyle/adult-health/expert-answers/passive-aggressive-behavior/faq-20057901#:~:text=Resentment%20and%20opposition%20to%20the,is%20%E2%80%94%20consider%20consulting%20a%20therapist

Hamilton, M. A. (2012). Verbal aggression: Understanding the psychological antecedents and social consequences. *Journal of Language and Social Psychology, 31*(1), 5–12. https://doi.org/10.1177/0261927X11425032

Harmon-Jones, E., Peterson, C., Gable, P. A., & Harmon-Jones, C. (2013). Anger. In A. Elliot (Ed.), *Handbook of approach and avoidance motivation* (pp. 399–413). Psychology Press. https://www.routledge.com/Handbook-of-Approach-and-Avoidance-Motivation/Elliot/p/book/9781848726753

Hecker, M. H. L., & Lunde, D. T. (1985). On the diagnosis and treatment of chronically hostile individuals. In M. A. Chesney & R. H. Rosenman (Eds.), *Anger and hostility in cardiovascular and behavioral disorders* (pp. 227–240). Hemisphere.

Helfritz, L. E., & Stanford, M. S. (2006). Personality and psychopathology in an impulsive aggressive college sample. *Aggressive Behavior, 32*(1), 28–37. https://doi.org/10.1002/ab.20103

Hensley, S. (2019, June 26). *Anger poll: 84% say we're madder than a generation ago.* NPR. Retrieved April 1, 2025, from https://www.npr.org/sections/health-shots/2019/06/26/735757156/poll-americans-say-were-angrier-than-a-generation-ago

Hoptman, M. J. (2015). Impulsivity and aggression in schizophrenia: A neural circuitry perspective with implications for treatment. *CNS Spectrums, 20*(3), 280–286. https://doi.org/10.1017/S1092852915000206

Hopwood, C. J., Morey, L. C., & Markon, K. E. (2023). What is a psychopathology dimension? *Clinical Psychology Review, 106*, 102356. https://doi.org/10.1016/j.cpr.2023.102356

Ilkiw-Lavalle, O., & Grenyer, B. F. (2003). Differences between patient and staff perceptions of aggression in mental health units. *Psychiatric Services, 54*(3), 389–393. https://doi.org/10.1176/appi.ps.54.3.389

Joyal, C., Côté, G., Meloche, J., & Hodgins, S. (2011). Severe mental illness and aggressive behavior: On the importance of considering subgroups. *International Journal of Forensic Mental Health, 10*(2), 107–117. https://doi.org/10.1080/14999013.2011.577136

Kapur, R. (2021). *Understanding the types of anger.* ResearchGate. https://www.researchgate.net/publication/350235712_Understanding_the_Types_of_Anger.

Kaye, A. J., & Erdley, C. A. (2011). Physical aggression. In S. Goldstein & J. A. Naglieri (Eds.), *Encyclopedia of child behavior and development*. Springer. https://doi.org/10.1007/978-0-387-79061-9_2156

Kolla, N. J., Tully, J., & Bertsch, K. (2023). Neural correlates of aggression in personality disorders from the perspective of DSM-5 maladaptive traits: A systematic review. *Translational Psychiatry, 13*(1), 330. https://doi.org/10.1038/s41398-023-02629-4

Krahé, B. (2013). *The social psychology of aggression* (2nd ed.). Psychology Press. https://doi.org/10.4324/9780203082171

Kurian, L. P., Rentala, S., Belsiyal, C. X., Srinivasan, P., & Thimmajja, S. G. (2023). Aggressive behavior and its associated factors among persons with mental illness: An observational study. *Journal of Education and Health Promotion, 12*(1), 249. https://doi.org/10.4103/jehp.jehp_195_23

Langthorne, P., & McGill, P. (2009). A tutorial on the concept of the motivating operation and its importance to application. *Behavior Analysis in Practice, 2*, 22–31. https://doi.org/10.1007/BF03391745

Lench, H. C., Reed, N. T., George, T., Kaiser, K. A., & North, S. G. (2023). Anger has benefits for attaining goals. *Journal of Personality and Social Psychology.* https://doi.org/10.1037/pspa0000350

Levin-Aspenson, H. F., Diehl, J. M., Boyd, S. I., & Zimmerman, M. (2023). Levels of anger severity in psychiatric patients. *The Journal of Nervous and Mental Disease, 211*(1), 29–34. https://doi.org/10.1097/nmd.0000000000001566

Li, Q., Zhong, S., Zhou, J., & Wang, X. (2019). Delusion, excitement, violence, and suicide history are risk factors for aggressive behavior in general inpatients with serious mental illnesses: A multicenter study in China. *Psychiatry Research, 272*, 130–134. https://doi.org/10.1016/j.psychres.2018.12.071

Lind, J. (2018). What can associative learning do for planning? *Royal Society Open Science, 5*(11), 180778. https://doi.org/10.1098/rsos.180778

Liu, J., Lewis, G., & Evans, L. (2013). Understanding aggressive behaviour across the lifespan. *Journal of Psychiatric and Mental Health Nursing, 20*(2), 156–168. https://doi.org/10.1111/j.1365-2850.2012.01902.x

Lohr, J. B., Eidt, C. A., Abdulrazzaq Alfaraj, A., & Soliman, M. A. (2015). The clinical challenges of akathisia. *CNS Spectrums, 20*(S1), 1–16. https://doi.org/10.1017/S1092852915000838

Maltby, J., Norton, W. H., McElroy, E., Cromby, J., Halliwell, M., & Hall, S. S. (2023). Refining anger: Summarizing the self-report measurement of anger. *Journal of Personality Assessment, 105*(6), 752–762. https://doi.org/10.1080/00223891.2022.2152345

Morrison, E. F. (1992). A hierarchy of aggressive and violent behaviors among psychiatric inpatients. *Hospital & Community Psychiatry, 43*(5), 505–506. https://doi.org/10.1176/ps.43.5.505

National Institute of Mental Health. (2025). *What is prevalence?* https://www.nimh.nih.gov/health/statistics/what-is-prevalence

Norton, R., Hyder, A. A., Bishai, D., & Peden, M. (2006). Unintentional injuries. In D. T. Jamison, J. G. Breman, A. R. Measham, G. Alleyne, M. Claeson, D. B. Evans, P. Jha, A. Mills, & P. Musgrove (Eds.), *Disease control priorities in developing countries* (2nd ed.). The International Bank for Reconstruction and Development/The World Bank. https://www.ncbi.nlm.nih.gov/books/NBK11779/

Novaco, R. W. (2009). Anger and psychopathology. In M. Potegal, G. Stemmler, & C. Spielberger (Eds.), *International handbook of anger: Constituent and concomitant biological, psychological, and social processes* (pp. 465–497). Springer. https://doi.org/10.1007/978-0-387-89676-2_27

Novaco, R. W. (2017). Cognitive–behavioral factors and anger in the occurrence of aggression and violence. In P. Sturmey (Ed.), *The Wiley handbook of violence and aggression* (pp. 1–13). John Wiley & Sons. https://doi.org/10.1002/9781119057574.whbva026

Papadopoulos, C., Ross, J., Stewart, D., Dack, C., James, K., & Bowers, L. (2012). The antecedents of violence and aggression within psychiatric in-patient settings. *Acta Psychiatrica Scandinavica, 125*(6), 425–439. https://doi.org/10.1111/j.1600-0447.2012.01827.x

Parrott, D. J., & Giancola, P. R. (2007). Addressing "the criterion problem" in the assessment of aggressive behavior: Development of a new taxonomic system. *Aggression and Violent Behavior, 12*(3), 280–299. https://doi.org/10.1016/j.avb.2006.08.002

Pease, C. R., & Lewis, G. J. (2015). Personality links to anger: Evidence for trait interaction and differentiation across expression style. *Personality and Individual Differences, 74*, 159–164. https://doi.org/10.1016/j.paid.2014.10.018

Perlini, C., Bellani, M., Besteher, B., Nenadić, I., & Brambilla, P. (2018). The neural basis of hostility-related dimensions in schizophrenia. *Epidemiology and Psychiatric Sciences, 27*(6), 546–551. https://doi.org/10.1017/S2045796018000525

Pompili, E., Carlone, C., Silvestrini, C., & Nicolò, G. (2017). Focus on aggressive behaviour in mental illness. *Rivista di Psichiatria, 52*(5), 175–179. https://doi.org/10.1708/2801.28344

Powell, L. H., & Williams, K. (2007). Hostility. In G. Fink (Ed.), *Encyclopedia of stress* (2nd ed., pp. 354–358). Academic Press. https://doi.org/10.1016/B978-012373947-6.00202-6

Ramırez, J. M. (2011). The usefulness of distinguishing types of aggression by function. *International Social Science Journal, 61*(200–201), 263–272. https://doi.org/10.1111/j.1468-2451.2011.01762.x

Randel, J. L. (2020). *The psychometric properties of an anger management routine outcome monitoring measure*. (Doctoral dissertation, St. John's University). St. John's Scholar. https://scholar.stjohns.edu/theses_dissertations/129

Rueve, M. E., & Welton, R. S. (2008). Violence and mental illness. *Psychiatry (Edgmont), 5*(5), 34–48. https://psycnet.apa.org/record/2008-07944-004

Shahsavarani, A. M., & Noohi, S. (2015). Explaining the bases and fundamentals of anger: A literature review. *International Journal of Medical Reviews, 1*(4), 143–149. https://www.ijmedrev.com/article_68914_c33f05764a1482053b57a85cecb38747.pdf

Siegel, J. M. (1986). The multidimensional anger inventory. *Journal of Personality and Social Psychology, 51*(1), 191–200. https://doi.org/10.1037/0022-3514.51.1.191

Smith, K. (2022, September 2). 14 types of Anger & how to manage them — Talkspace. Talkspace. https://www.talkspace.com/blog/types-of-anger/#:~:text=6.%20Overwhelmed%20Anger%20This%20type%20of%20anger,anger%20when%20the%20burden%20becomes%20too%20great

Spielberger, C. D. (1985). Anxiety, cognition and affect: A state–trait perspective. In A. H. Tuma & J. D. Maser (Eds.), Anxiety and the anxiety disorders (pp. 171–182). Lawrence Erlbaum Associates.

Spielberger, C. D., Johnson, E. H., Russell, S. F., Crane, R. J., Jacobs, G. A., & Worden, T. J. (1985). The experience and expression of anger: Construction and validation of an anger expression scale. In M. A. Chesney & R. H. Rosenman (Eds.), Anger and hostility in cardiovascular and behavioral disorders (pp. 5–30). Hemisphere/McGraw-Hill.

Stuart, H. (2003). Violence and mental illness: An overview. *World Psychiatry, 2*(2), 121–124. https://europepmc.org/articles/PMC1525086

Studocu. *(2021). 9 operational definitions of commonly occurring behaviors.* Edinboro University ofPennsylvania.https://www.studocu.com/en-us/document/edinboro-university-of-pennsylvania/psy-counselinginterviewing/9-operational-definitions-of-commonly-occurring-behaviors/22188684

Tamir, M., Mitchell, C., & Gross, J. J. (2008). Hedonic and instrumental motives in anger regulation. *Psychological Science, 19*(4), 324–328. https://doi.org/10.1111/j.1467-9280.2008.02088.x

Tourinho, E. Z. (2006). Private stimuli, covert responses, and private events: Conceptual remarks. *The BehaviorAnalyst, 29*(1), 13–31. https://www.ncbi.nlm.nih.gov/pmc/articles/PMC2223134/

U.S. Department of Health and Human Services. (2001). Mental health: Culture, race, ethnicity. *A supplement to mental health: A report of the surgeon general.* U.S. Public Health Service. https://www.ncbi.nlm.nih.gov/books/NBK44243/pdf/Bookshelf_NBK44243.pdf

Van Dorn, R., Volavka, J., & Johnson, N. (2011). Mental disorder and violence: Is there a relationship beyond substance use? *Social Psychiatry and Psychiatric Epidemiology, 47*, 487–503. https://doi.org/10.1007/s00127-011-0356-x

Weltens, I., Bak, M., Verhagen, S., Vandenberk, E., Domen, P., van Amelsvoort, T., & Sabbe, B. (2021). Aggression on the psychiatric ward: Prevalence and risk factors. A systematic review of the literature. *PLoS One, 16*(10), e0258346. https://doi.org/10.1371/journal.pone.0258346

Widmayer, S., Borgwardt, S., Lang, U. E., Stieglitz, R. D., & Huber, C. G. (2019). Functional neuroimaging correlates of aggression in psychosis: A systematic review with recommendations for future research. *Frontiers in Psychiatry, 9*, 777. https://doi.org/10.3389/fpsyt.2018.00777

World Health Organization (WHO). (2004). *ICD-10: International statistical classification of diseases and related health problems* (10 rev, 2nd ed). World Health Organization. https://iris.who.int/handle/10665/42980

World Health Organization (WHO). (2022). *ICD-11: International classification of diseases (11th rev.).* World Health Organization. https://icd.who.int/

Wrangham, R. W. (2018). Two types of aggression in human evolution. *Proceedings of the National Academy of Sciences, 115*(2), 245–253. https://doi.org/10.1073/pnas.1713611115

Chapter 12
Problems with the Use of Substances in Individuals Living with Serious Mental Illness (Co-occurring Disorders)

Introduction

The intersection of serious mental illness (SMI) and substance use disorders (SUD) represents one of the most complex and clinically significant challenges in contemporary mental health practice. Individuals living with SMI as defined by persistent, functionally impairing psychiatric conditions such as schizophrenia spectrum disorders, bipolar disorder, and severe major depression are disproportionately affected by substance-related problems. Epidemiological data consistently demonstrate elevated rates of alcohol, tobacco, cannabis, and stimulant use among this population, with co-occurring disorders (COD) contributing to poorer treatment outcomes, increased hospitalizations, and heightened risk for trauma, suicide, and social marginalization. Understanding the mechanisms that sustain this comorbidity is essential for developing effective, evidence-informed interventions.

This chapter examines the multifaceted relationship between substance use and SMI through a dimensional, biopsychosocial framework. It begins by outlining the DSM-5-TR criteria for substance use disorders, emphasizing the domains of impaired control, social impairment, risky use, and pharmacological effects such as tolerance and withdrawal. These criteria are contextualized within the lived experience of SMI, where substance use may serve as a maladaptive coping strategy, a neurobiological vulnerability, or a socially reinforced behavior. This chapter explores the types of substances most commonly used in this population, including legal substances such as caffeine and nicotine, and their reinforcing properties, metabolic interactions, and impact on psychiatric symptomatology.

Beyond diagnostic classification, this chapter delves into the behavioral dimensions of substance use, including craving, relapse, intoxication, and withdrawal through the lens of operant conditioning and motivating operations. Environmental contingencies, social learning, and trauma exposure are examined as antecedents and reinforcers of substance-related behaviors, while genetic predispositions and

G. F. McKeegan, *Behavior Change Interventions for Serious Mental Illness*, Evidence-Based Practices in Behavioral Health,
https://doi.org/10.1007/978-3-032-18372-9_12

neurological substrates are discussed as underlying contributors to vulnerability and chronicity. The limitations of categorical models are discussed and advocate for an integrated dimensional assessment that captures severity, frequency, and functional impact across both SMI and SUD domains.

By synthesizing clinical, behavioral, and neurobiological perspectives, a comprehensive understanding of co-occurring disorders in the context of serious mental illness is developed to enhance the critical evaluation of the functional relationships between substance use and psychiatric symptoms, and to apply dimensional, context-sensitive approaches to assessment and intervention. This foundation is essential for fostering competent, compassionate care and advancing integrated treatment models in diverse mental health settings.

> My relative gets worse when he drinks and uses weed. He becomes very depressed and says he wants to die. He has tried at times by trying to jump off a bridge or hanging himself. He has been to rehab a couple of times, but nothing seems to stick.

The Case of Jordan

Jordan is a 27-year-old man living with schizophrenia spectrum mental health problems and struggling with excessive substance use, including cannabis, alcohol, cigarettes, and caffeinated drinks. He presently lives in an adult care residence for people living with Co-occurring mental health problems (COD). First hospitalized at 19, Jordan had been staying away from friends and family, heard voices, and was prone to aggressive outbursts. While medication helped stabilize him, his daily habits—chain-smoking, drinking multiple energy drinks and coffee, and refusing structured activities—caused serious concern for his family and staff at the residence.

Jordan's behaviors included stealing cigarettes, spilling coffee throughout the house, and refusing to attend his work assignment, clubhouse, and recovery meetings. Staff reported that he sometimes smoked in his bedroom, creating a fire hazard. The other problems included frequent unscheduled visits to his sister's house (who was married and had two small children), refusing to attend a supervised work assignment at the clubhouse, stealing money and cigarettes, being inconsistent in taking his prescribed medications, and frequently complaining that family and staff were always telling him what to do and "into my business." Jordan also struggled with depression and social anxiety, using alcohol to help with anxiety and avoiding uncomfortable social situations. Recently, staff at the recovery center reported that he had been talking about committing suicide. Six months ago, the staff at the residence found him unconscious in his room with a loaded gun surrounded by empty beer cans and vodka bottles. He was admitted to a psychiatric hospital on an emergency basis.

Definition and Characteristics of the Use of Substances in Individuals Living with Serious Mental Illness (Co-occurring Disorders)

People living with SMI have higher rates of alcohol, tobacco, and drug use than the general population with around one out of four individuals who live with a mental health issue also living with a substance use disorder (SUD) (National Institute of Drug Abuse [NIDA], 2020). Recent national surveys have found that the use of substances has been increasing in people aged 12 years and older in the United States (National Center for Drug Abuse Statistics [NCDAS], 2025) with 13.5% having used substances in the past month with a 3.8% increase year-over-year prevalence. The prevalence of using illegal or misusing prescription substances within the last year was 21.4% with 50.0% of people having used illicit substances in their lifetime (Substance Abuse and Mental Health Services Administration [SAMHSA], 2020).

The use of legal and illegal drug use by people aged 12 years and older living in the United States in the past month in 2019 is reported to be as follows: 60.1 percent (or 165.4 million people) used a substance (i.e., tobacco, alcohol, kratom, or an illicit drug); 50.8 percent (or 139.7 million people) drank alcohol; 21.1 percent (or 58.1 million people) used a tobacco product; and 13.0 percent (or 35.8 million people) used an illicit drug. Nearly one-third of the population of the United States consumes alcohol and over 17% use tobacco or nicotine products (i.e., vaping). Twenty-two percent of males and 17% of females used illegal substances or misused prescription substances within the last year. Five percent of people in nonmetropolitan, rural counties used illegal drugs compared to 20.2% of people in larger metropolitan counties. Drug use is highest among people between the ages of 18–25 (39%) compared to persons aged 26–29 (34%). Forty-seven percent of young people use an illegal drug by the time they graduate from high school; 70 percent of users who try an illegal drug before age 13 develop a substance abuse problem (SUD) within the next 7 years compared to 27% of those who try an illegal drug after age 17 (NCDAS, 2025).

Individuals living with SMI smoke at rates two to three times higher than the general population (Rosen et al., 2023). Studies of dietary intake in individuals living with SMI find nearly double the consumption of caffeine compared to individuals without mental health problems (Strassnig et al., 2006). Caffeine and nicotine have reinforcing and sometimes beneficial consequences for their use. Individuals using caffeine experience cognitive benefits, boosting alertness, attention, and memory. It can impact mood, but high doses induce anxiety, restlessness, and insomnia. Moderate doses might address adenosine dysfunction and help neural system balance, especially in people living with SMI (Rosen et al., 2023). Dysregulation of adenosine homeostasis can result in various pathophysiological issues, such as memory loss, sleep disorders, and neuroinflammation (Jang & Song, 2024). Excessive caffeine use can increase risk for people living with a bipolar type of mental health problem as it may cause hyperactivity and irritability. Caffeine can also alter the metabolism of certain psychiatric medications by reducing their effectiveness (Rosen et al., 2023). Smoking accelerates caffeine metabolism, prompting higher caffeine consumption in smokers. High nicotine uses in individuals living with SMI may stem from its mood-regulating effects. Both substances are often used by those with mental illnesses to manage negative emotions or withdrawal, but their combined influence on mental health problems is not well-understood.

Behavioral research demonstrates evidence for concurrent caffeine and tobacco use, underscoring the metabolic interactions and significance of habitual patterns in the consumption of both substances. Habits are formed when behaviors are consistently repeated in the same contexts and antecedent conditions. Automaticity develops as the behavior is repeated in a similar context to strengthen the association between the antecedent stimuli and the behavior (Cooper et al., 2020; Gardner et al., 2012). Caffeine use may influence the desire to smoke and vice versa; the use of caffeinated beverages and nicotine sequentially is frequently associated as a behavioral "routine." A routine is defined as repeated behaviors involving a task associated in a moment of time that requires little awareness of the occurrence of the behaviors (e.g., brushing teeth) (Arlinghaus & Johnston, 2019).

Less is known about additional factors that may explain the relationship between caffeine use and SMI; the excessive use of caffeine may compensate for the sedative effects of psychiatric medications, coping with sleep deprivation, and pharmacokinetic interactions with other medications (Rosen et al., 2023).

Substance abuse refers to the use of a drugs in a way that is detrimental to self, society, or both (American Psychiatric Association, 2022). It includes both physical and psychological dependence. Physical dependence caused by prolonged use of a drug refers to an altered state in which withdrawal problems/symptoms develop when the drug is discontinued; psychological dependence refers to a state of intense need to continue taking a drug in the absence of physical dependence (Griffin, 1990). The psychological need to use the drug is known as "craving" which is an unrelenting desire, urge, or yearning to access and use the drug despite awareness of the drug's harmful and life-threatening consequences (American Psychiatric Association, 2025; American Psychological Association, n.d.-b).

Substance-use-related mental health problems (SUD) are a complex mental health condition in which there is uncontrolled use of a substance despite harmful consequences to the user and others. People with SUD have an intense focus on using substance(s) such as alcohol, tobacco, opioids, or other psychoactive substances, to the point where their ability to function in day-to-day life becomes impaired. People keep using the substance despite being aware of problems caused by its use.

The Diagnostic and Statistical Manual of Mental Disorders (5th ed., text rev.) (2022) (DSM-5-TR) (American Psychiatric Association, 2022) has established that the following substances can be misused: alcohol, caffeine, cannabis, hallucinogens, inhalants, opioids, sedatives, hypnotics, anxiolytics, stimulants, tobacco, and other or unknown substances. These substances are classified based on the type used, with distinct criteria for intoxication and withdrawal for each type. All the substances are in the substance intoxication category; tobacco and caffeine have no criteria for substance use disorder, and hallucinogens and inhalants are absent in the substance withdrawal category.

The DSM-5-TR has established 11criteria for SUD that can be grouped into four categories of problematic behavioral domains that are associated with the use of the substance(s) (American Psychiatric Association, 2022):

- Impaired control: Despite desires or efforts to reduce the use of the substance, the individual takes the substance more frequently, in larger amounts, and spends longer durations in acquiring the substance. The person may experience "cravings" or a strong urge to use the substance (American Psychological Association, n.d.-b).
- Social problems: Substance use causes failure to complete major tasks at work, school, or home; social, work, or leisure activities may be reduced or given up entirely, and interpersonal relationships suffer.
- Dangerous use: The substance is used in unsafe settings; the individual continues to use the substance and takes risks despite knowing or experiencing psychological, physical or both (e.g., overdoses).
- Drug effects: Tolerance (need for larger amounts to get the same effect) and withdrawal problem behaviors/symptoms are experienced and are different for each substance.

The severity of the problems can range from mild (two to three problem behaviors), moderate (four to five) to severe (five or more) with addiction being the most severe form of substance-related use problem. Although the term addiction is commonly used, it is not a mental health issue. Addiction is defined as state of psychological and/or physical dependence on the use of drugs or other substances or on activities or behaviors. Physical dependence is defined as a physical and/or psychological need for the substance and the appearance of withdrawal problem behaviors/symptoms when the substance is either stopped or reduced from an amount previously used (American Psychological Association, n.d.-c; Grant & Chamberlain, 2016; Hasin et al., 2013; Shahrokh & Hales, 2003).

The International Statistical Classification of Diseases and Related Health Problems (11th ed.) (ICD-11) (World Health Organization [WHO], 2019) classifies problems in the use of substances as to the extent of harmful consequences and outcomes (Hasin et al., 2013; Poznyak et al., 2018), ranging from the following:

- Harmful use refers to substance use that significantly harms physical or mental health, either of the user or others, due to intoxication, organ toxicity, or harmful administration methods.
- Hazardous use is a pattern of substance use that appreciably increases the risk of harmful physical or mental health consequences to the user or others, even if harm has not yet occurred. It is considered a behavior requiring health actions rather than a significant identified problem (e.g., disorder).
- Substance dependence is characterized by a strong internal drive to use the substance, impaired control over use, and prioritization of substance use over other activities. It includes physiological correlations with tolerance and withdrawal.

Substance-related use problems (SUD) affect over 20 million Americans aged 12 and over; the most common problematic conditions are related to marijuana and prescription pain relievers (NCDAS, 2025). People can develop an SUD to many substances including alcohol; cannabis; PCP; LSD and other hallucinogens; inhalants, such as paint thinners and glue; opioids, including pain killers and heroin; sedatives, hypnotics, and anxiolytics; stimulants (including cocaine, amphetamine-type substances, and other stimulants); nicotine (tobacco, vaping); and caffeine (coffee, tea, chocolate, energy drinks, OTC analgesics and cold remedies and weight lose aides) (American Psychiatric Association, 2022). Given that SUDs frequently persist as chronic conditions over many years, it is not unexpected that individuals require an average of three to four admissions to treatment facilities within a nine-year period to achieve a sustainable duration of recovery (Dennis & Scott, 2008).

In a recent study, Mojtabai (2022) found that the prevalence estimates for alcohol, cannabis, opioid, and stimulant use-related problems were significantly higher for the population of the United States than those reported by National Survey on Drug Use and Health (NSDUH) (Substance Abuse and Mental Health Services Administration [SAMHSA], 2024). Key findings from the combined 2018 to 2019 data indicate that the prevalence of alcohol use-related condition was 20.27% compared to 5.34%; cannabis use disorder was 7.57% versus 1.68%; opioid use disorder was 3.46% compared to 0.68%; and stimulant use disorder was 1.91% versus 0.85%. These results suggest that excessive substance use was nearly four to five times higher than previous estimates for the general population.

SMI is defined as complex behavioral, emotional, and mental health problems resulting in functional impairment that substantially interferes with or limits one or more major life activities (National Institute of Mental Health [NIMH], 2022). The burden of mental health problems is concentrated among those who experience disability due to SMI. Although SMI is a commonly used term in mental health, the definitions of SMI vary in policy and determine who is eligible for services and participation in research (Gonzales et al., 2022). The principal criterion for the term SMI is a significant, persistent, and chronic impairment in social, occupational, and educational functioning due to a mental health problem that results in a lower quality of life for the individual living with SMI (American Psychiatric Association, 2018; Gonzales et al., 2022). The analysis of the term SMI indicated that the presence of any DSM-5-TR mental health issue could be considered as living with SMI (Gonzales et al., 2022) as long as there is impairment in daily functioning in several domains.

Co-occurring mental health conditions (COD) refer to health issues that occur simultaneously, impacting problem behaviors/symptoms, treatment, and outcomes, especially in individuals living with substance use related problem (SUD) and SMI. In 2017, approximately 3.3 percent of the US adult population in the United States, or 7.7 million adults, were living with COD during the 12 months before interviewing for a national survey (Han et al., 2017). About 35% of US adults with mental health issues also experience SUD simultaneously, commonly linked to anxiety and depression (National Institute on Drug Abuse [NIDA], 2020).

The simultaneous occurrences of a SUD and a mental health problem do not mean that one problem caused the other. Research suggests possibilities that could explain why SUDs and other mental health problems may occur together (National Institute of Mental Health [NIMH], 2024) as follows:

- There are shared risk factors that contribute to both SUDs and other mental health problems. Both SUDs and other mental health problems can arise in families; certain biological variables (e.g., genetics) and environment may be factors in the genesis of COD. Environmental factors, such as stress, trauma, and social learning, can cause genetic changes that are to generations and may contribute to the development of mental health, substance use problems, or both.
- Mental health problems can contribute to SUDs. Studies found that people with a mental health problem may use drugs or alcohol as a form of self-medication to alleviate the distress of living with a mental health problem. Although some substances may temporarily reduce some aversive emotional respondents related to mental health problems, the problem behaviors/symptoms may worsen over time with the use of substances.
- The use of substances may place the person at risk for serious and harmful environmental events such as assaults, repeated trauma, becoming unhoused and unemployed, and life-threatening physical infections and injuries. Changes in people with mental health problems may increase the reinforcing effects of using substances by decreasing the aversive emotions associated with mental health problems making it more likely that substance use will continue.
- Substance use and SUDs can contribute to the development of other mental health problems. Substance use may trigger changes in brain structure, function, and cognitive capabilities that make a person more likely to develop a mental health problem (NIMH, 2024).
- Individuals living with SMI may have multiple SUDs that contribute to problematic use across different substances and increased risk of harm for the individual; this may set up a vicious cycle of continued use of multiple substances that increase the probabilities of trauma, physical harm, and possible neurological changes that result in further risk of using substances (NIDA, 2020).

COD involves both a substance-use-related condition (SUD) and another serious mental health problem (SMI). These concurrent mental health issues complicate assessment and treatment, as SUD can worsen the mental health problem, reduce treatment compliance, worsen prognosis, and increase the use of acute services (WHO, 1999).

SUD is the most common co-occurring condition among people living with SMI and is associated with poorer treatment outcomes (Siegfried, 1998). Using drugs, alcohol, or both range between a quarter to a third of samples in surveys conducted with people living with SMI (RachBeisel et al., 1999; Virgo et al., 2001). Research on the use of substances with persons living with SMI has many inconclusive results because of limitations due to small sample size, treatment drift and dropout, lack of an experimental design, short follow-up periods, and inadequate assessment of use (Siegfried, 1998).

It is well established that the use of drugs and alcohol by persons living with SMI is associated with many adverse impacts including increases in the severity of the problem behaviors/symptoms associated with SMI (i.e., increase in frequency and intensity of problems, reduced self-control), psychosocial functioning, decreased adherence to treatment recommendations, disruptive and aggressive behaviors, and higher rates of admissions to psychiatric facilities (SAMHSA, 2015; Van Dorn et al., 2011). The use of substances puts the individual living with SMI at greater risk for being traumatized by experiencing physical and sexual violence (RachBeisel et al., 1999) and the associated physical health risks associated with using drugs. However, the "occasional" use of substances by individuals living with SMI—not meeting the criteria for a COD—has not been thoroughly investigated. The question remains if "occasional" use negatively impacts the quality of life and recovery efforts. Given that most people living with SMI are prescribed medications, using alcohol and/or drugs can impact the body's metabolism of the prescribed medications and result in an increase in problem behaviors/symptoms and side effects from the medications (Levin, n.d.).

Both SMI and SUD are measurable patterns of thinking, feeling, and acting that deviate from the norm and are linked to underlying psychological, biological, and social-interpersonal problems, causing distress and/or impairment in the individual's life (Di Pierro et al., 2014). The difference between the two behavioral constructs of SMI and SUD is that SUD is composed of behavioral response classes that are intentional as the individual chooses to perform the behavior, rather than it being automatically emitted by a stimulus. The response class of behaviors displayed by people living with SUD are groups of behaviors that share a common function or purpose, even if they differ in their physical appearance (topography) (Cooper et al., 2020). The response class is aimed at achieving a specific outcome or goal—acquiring and using the substances and experiencing its effects. The consequences (reinforcement or punishment) following a behavior influence whether it is repeated in the future, like the behaviors of drug seeking and use.

The common definition of a co-occurring mental health problem (COD) is based on the temporal focus of problem behaviors related to living with a SMI and SUD that occur simultaneously in the same individual. Explanations of the interactions of SMI and SUD center on the effects that the behavioral constructs of SMI and SUD have on each other but do not expound on the possible functions of COD. Research supports the proposition that living with either SMI or SUD increases the probability that COD will develop; that is, living with SMI puts the person at risk for developing SUD and vice versa. A person living with either SUD or a SMI is at risk for developing a co-occurring mental health problem because of biological liabilities due to genetic inheritance, adverse developmental events, and the impact of substances on neurological substrates that may or may not be "primed" for impairments that result in SMI/SUD.

The mental health research literature lacks functional behavioral hypotheses and the impact that the environment has on the genesis of living with COD; the research focus is on the biological correlations of COD and pharmacological interventions. Correlational studies have shown that experiencing trauma, chronic stress, and adverse childhood experiences are associated with increased risk of developing both SMI and SUD; living in areas in which drug use and trauma occur also increases risk (NIDA, 2020). Young people exposed to multiple traumatic experiences face three to five times higher odds of developing SUD compared to those with a single event. Adolescents with PTSD are four times more likely to have alcohol use disorder (AUD) and nine times more likely to have SUD for other illicit drugs (Hinckley et al., 2024). A study by Poudel and Gautam (2017) indicated that early onset substance users—17 years and younger—compared to people living with late onset SUD are at higher risk for psychosocial problems in various areas of life including problematic behavior patterns (e.g., aggressive behaviors, impulsivity), mental health problems, impaired peer relationships, leisure/recreational activities, and work adjustment. Studies have shown that social acceptance among peers, availability of substances, and problematic behavior patterns contribute to onset of substance use at an early age (Luthar & D'Avanzo, 1999; Volkow et al., 2021). Pathways to developing a SUD include a history of engaging in deviant behaviors, stress/negative effects, and the reinforcing pharmacological effects of the substance. Developmental factors for developing SUD are early and high-frequency use, emotional dysregulation, and impulsivity. Racial and ethnic minority groups experience lower rates of substance use until adolescence, then face higher SUD risks and more drinking-related problems. Protective factors against SUD include positive parental influence and prosocial and community relationships (Boness et al., 2024) further support the influence that the environment has on both the onset and continuation of living with COD.

People living with substance-use-related conditions (SUD) are aware of the behaviors of seeking and taking the substances and the effects of the substances on their behaviors, including covert behaviors like thinking and feelings. The problem behaviors associated with SMI (e.g., symptoms) lack intentionality in that a person living with SMI does not voluntarily choose to experience hallucinations, disorganized thinking and speech, and false beliefs/delusions. The problem behaviors seen in people living with SMI are a complex interaction between bio-neurological conditions and the environment, including trauma, deprived conditions, and adverse, unfavorable social learning conditions. These conditions arise when individuals lack adequate opportunities or experience challenges in developing necessary behavioral skills, leading to difficulties in communication, social interaction, relationship building, and adaptive living skills which are behavioral impairments displayed by people living with SMI; these behaviors are in the response class of problematic behavioral symptoms either because of excessive frequencies of occurrence, inadequate stimulus control, or the absence of expected responses to presented stimuli (negative symptoms like social interactions, responding to a request, daily living skills). These problematic behaviors are considered operant in nature, and the consequences—whether reinforcement or punishment—that follow their occurrence significantly affect the likelihood of these behaviors being repeated in the future.

Co-occurring related conditions (COD) may be the result of using substances based on the impact of subjective experiences caused by the substances. The use of various substances has been shown to result in various alterations in subjective experiences ranging from increased relaxation and alertness, euphoria, altered sensations and perceptions, loss of inhibitions, and decreases in pain (Suncoast Practice Research Collaborative at the University of South Florida, 2002). Living with SMI has been identified as a source of significant psychological distress, which is distinct from anxiety and depression (Andrade et al., 2016). According to Andrade et al. (2016), psychological distress encompasses an individual's holistic emotional or psychological reaction to a persistent and severe mental health condition, such as SMI. This response is perceived as a traumatic event that disrupts daily functioning and requires adaptive strategies. The onset of SUD in conjunction with living with SMI may be a function of attempting to reduce the aversiveness of this distress by using substances that result in sedation, relaxation, or euphoria; in effect, substance use "numbs" the person living with SMI to the negative experiences of living with SMI (Di Pierro et al., 2014). The result is that COD is negatively reinforced by the immediate and temporary reduction of the unpleasant feelings of living with SMI.

The definition of COD is that a substance-use-related condition (SUD) and SMI occur concurrently. The assessment of the dimensions of COD is that the dimensions of both SUD and SMI are assessed by separate assessments and not integrated into dimensions that interact and function together. At present, there is no assessment instrument that identifies and examines the dimensions of COD. Possible dimensions of COD would be the function of SUD as an antecedent or consequential stimuli for the experience of a problem behavior related to SMI. For example, the individual experiences an increase in the loudness and frequency of auditory verbal hallucinations (AVH). Consequently, the individual experiences adverse respondents; he is unable to control the dimensions of loudness and frequency of the AVH. The individual uses an opioid that results in sedation, sleepiness, and the temporary cessation of the AVH; therefore, the use of the opioid is negatively reinforced. The assessment would entail measuring the frequency of this chain of responses and dimensions surrounding it such as when AVH occurs and the substance is not used and other behaviors are emitted, the antecedent stimuli associated with the onset of the AVH and substance use.

Dimensions of Co-occurring Conditions (COD)

A dimensional method to evaluate behaviors and symptoms linked to mental health issues has been suggested by researchers in the field. This approach not only identifies problem behaviors but also measures their intensity, frequency, and other aspects of the problem behaviors (Flynn & Brown, 2008). Dimensional measures that capture varying degrees of problem severity have been shown to be better predictors of outcomes. Marlowe et al. (1997) examined the impact of personality-based mental health problems on treatment outcomes among a sample of individuals with cocaine-related use issues. Researchers used both categorical and dimensional methods to assess mental health problems associated with personality problems.

Categorical assessment did not significantly affect treatment outcomes nor strongly correlate with drug use severity, depression, or anxiety. However, dimensional analyses of problems linked to personality problems revealed substantial influences on treatment success suggesting that dimensional assessments are more useful than categorical in planning effective treatment strategies.

Dimensional models and assessments provide more nuanced and precise information about the presentations of problem behaviors and the corresponding dimensional variables compared to categorical models, which often fail to capture the complexity of COD. Using a dimensional approach, Kircanski et al. (2017) found distinct dimensions of problem behaviors for anxiety and biological substrates, showing that dimensions of anxious arousal and apprehension resulted in fluctuations in cortisol levels in individuals living with co-occurring mental health problems (COD).

Assessment instruments for SMI and substance-use-related conditions (SUD) vary in statistical properties, length, and type of administration. Assessment tools for problem behaviors in individuals living with SMI include self-report questionnaires, clinical interview rating scales, and combined ratings by others familiar with the individual. Assessment of SUD is primarily self-report questionnaires and limited to the use and type of substances used (Moreira et al., 2022). Assessment tools emphasize various dimensions of substance use, including age of onset, duration and frequency of use, quantity consumed per occasion, length and frequency of abstinence periods, relapse rates, and related factors. They also address the substance's effects, adverse outcomes, cessation attempts, efforts to reduce usage, and both physiological and psychosocial consequences associated with substance use. However, functional outcomes—specifically, whether the substance's effects increase the likelihood of future use—are not typically assessed in the context of SUD evaluation. Additionally, these assessments consider whether substance use is influenced by overt antecedent stimuli (such as observing others using or proximity to substances) and covert antecedents (including thoughts and personal associations), or a combination of both. Assessment of SUD evaluates the social and interpersonal consequences of SUD, like the loss of employment, marriage, family relationships, and legal involvement. They overlook how substance-related use functions to avoid or escape unpleasant experiences, is reinforced by social outcomes like increased sociability, or prevents adverse physiological effects such as withdrawal.

The Addiction Severity Index (ASI) uses subscale composite scores to quantitatively evaluate the severity of substance-use-related problems on seven dimensions: medical, employment and support, drug use, alcohol use, legal issues (SAMHSA, 2024), family history, family and social relationships, and psychiatric status over the past 30 days (Cacciola et al., 2011; Public Health Management Corporation [PMHC], 2024). The medical dimension assesses the physical sequelae of substance use, while the severity of negative impacts on family and social relationships, employment status, and legal issues is rated. The psychiatric scale assesses the person's psychological and emotional status, including experiences of having problem behaviors, treatment history, and treatment needs. Key items include (a) treatment history including the number of treatments for psychological issues (hospital or outpatient); (b) mental health disability status; (c) recent and past experiences of depression, anxiety, hallucinations, concentration issues, violent behavior, or suicidal thoughts; (d) frequency and severity of mental health issues; (e) medications for mental health problems and perception of treatment. In addition, the interviewer rates any signs of depression and its severity, in addition to hostility, anxiety, reality testing issues, thought disorder, or neurocognitive problems. The ASI does evaluate the possibility of COD by asking if the experienced mental health problems are a result of the use of substances or occurred independent of substance use (PMHC, 2024).

The Alcohol and Addiction Research Domain Criteria (AARDoC) recently reconceptualized SUD, integrating behavioral, neurobiological, and genetic domains. The AARDoC developed the Addictions Neuroclinical Assessment (ANA) (Boness et al., 2024; Kwako et al., 2016) to assess these domains to increase the understanding and treatment of SUD. The ANA identified three domains that were included in the assessment guidelines: (1) reward/incentive salience that is linked to the mesocorticolimbic dopamine system that influences craving and relapse risk in individuals living with SUD; (2) negative emotionality which is characterized by increased dysphoria and "hypohedonia" (i.e., decreased ability to experience pleasure) that are driven by stress related biological systems; and (3) impairments in cognitive control/executive functions that are documented in various SUDs, affecting neurocognitive capabilities like attention, response inhibition, planning, working memory, and behavioral flexibility (Kwako et al., 2016).

The three domains identified in the ANA assessment focus on neurobiological correlates and substrates and not on observable and operationally defined behaviors. The reward/incentive salience domain entails craving and the renewed use of the substance. Craving in SUD is defined as an unrelenting desire or urge to use a substance despite awareness of the harmful and life-threatening consequences (American Psychological Association, n.d.-b; May et al., 2014). Craving can be viewed as a motivating operation (MO); that is, the desire to use the drug to obtain its pleasant effect (e.g., euphoria) or to decrease unpleasant effects (i.e., anxiety, dysphoria, fear) associated with the absence of the drug-induced experience. The MO can be elicited by overt and/or covert antecedent conditions (Montan & Banaco, 2021). MOs influence the likelihood of drug-seeking and self-administration behaviors by altering the reinforcing value of the substance. In classical conditioning, drug-related conditioned stimuli (CSs) can function as MOs because they increase the probability of substance-seeking behaviors when present. For example, stimuli associated with drug use, such as paraphernalia or specific locations and people, can evoke strong cravings and drug-seeking behaviors. These stimuli gain their MO function through a history of operant conditioning, where substance use alleviates aversive bodily states (negative reinforcement) or produces pleasurable effects (positive reinforcement) (Montan & Banaco, 2021).

The domain of "negative emotionality" can be behaviorally operationalized as the MO for the use of the substance by the consequences of alleviating the negative and aversive effects of dysphoria and a "hypohedonia." Impairments of cognitive control, including memory, flexibility, problem-solving, and response inhibition, affect a person's perception of controlling substance use when living with SUD.

Other dimensional assessments of COD/SUD include the PhenX toolkit for substance use (Hamilton et al., 2011). The PhenX project was to establish consensus measurement of dimensions in 21 research domains in health-related constructs (Hamilton et al., 2011). One of the identified domains is substance abuse. The dimensions assessed by the PhenX "toolkit" correspond to the following dimensions in the domain of substance use:

- Type of substance used: including alcohol, nicotine, sedatives/tranquilizers, painkillers, marijuana, cocaine/crack, stimulants, club drugs (Ecstasy, Rohypnol, GHB, Ketamine), hallucinogens, and inhalants.
- Duration: length of use from the age of the initiation of using the substance.
- Amount and frequency of use: assesses both point (past 30 days) and life-time prevalence.
- Perceived experience of using substances: euphoria, relaxation, and other pleasurable effects.
- Motives to use substances: include boredom, experimentation, craving, decrease tension, anger and/or frustration, and social.
- Abstinence: the duration and frequency of relapses.
- Controllability: perception of the ability to not use or perceived as beyond the control of the individual (i.e., need to have).
- Distress about using substances: impacting areas of functioning including family social relationships, negative outcomes (arrests, legal charges, incarceration).
- Presence of problem behaviors associated with mental health problems includes hallucinations, delusions, and neurocognitive problems.

Stewart et al. (2023) conducted a systematic review to identify and evaluate brief, free, readily accessible, and psychometrically valid self-report measures for substance-related use conditions (SUD) and treatment. Aims were to provide a list of psychometrically sound measures.

The results highlight gaps in existing measures and provide recommendations for future development and validation or measures that are related to dimensions of the use of specific substances and constructs of SUD. Stewart et al. (2023) categorized the assessments by the dimensions assessed by the self-report measures reviewed. The following are the labels and definitions of the specific dimensions of SUD:

1. Use: assesses the type of substance used including alcohol, stimulants, opioids, nicotine, benzodiazepines, cannabinoids, and general use across a broad range of substances.
2. Severity: measures the degree of SUD on a continuous scale related to amount, frequency, and duration of use and periods of abstinence.
3. Consequences: evaluate negative life outcomes (e.g., social, emotional, physical) related to substance use.
4. Withdrawal: assesses physical withdrawal symptoms from substance cessation.

5. Cravings/urges: measure psychological withdrawal symptoms or inclinations to use in the absence of physical withdrawal.
6. Expectancies: assesses beliefs about the positive and negative effects of substance use.
7. Motives: explores reasons for substance use to achieve desired outcomes. Related to the function of SUD and reinforcing consequences of use.
8. Self-efficacy: assesses confidence in one's ability to implement behaviors for desired effects and to control the use of the substance
9. Recovery: evaluates readiness for change, treatment engagement, and attitudes toward recovery.

The authors identified 73 instruments that satisfied the specified criteria. Assessment dimensions and corresponding measure counts were as follows: 25 evaluated use, 14 assessed severity, 8 examined consequences, 7 focused on withdrawal, 5 measured cravings or urges, 5 addressed expectancies, 3 explored motives, 6 considered self-efficacy, and 9 determined recovery readiness. Notably, six instruments encompassed multiple dimensions, including combinations such as recovery, self-efficacy, severity, urges, and expectancies (Stewart et al., 2023).

The authors recommended that future research needs to focus on creating measures for synthetic opioids and cannabinoids, stimulants (alone or concurrently), inhalants, caffeine, anti-Parkinsonian drugs, sedatives, and polysubstance use to address evolving public health crises (Stewart et al., 2023; Suncoast Practice Research Collaborative at the University of South Florida, 2002). There needs to be a priority on implementing measurement-based care in treatment settings using measures of dimensions of substance use related (SUD) and co-occurring mental health conditions (COD) instead of categorical and discrete measures (e.g., presence or absence) that would enhance the tailoring of treatment options. Broader psychometric properties, including clinical utility and "sensitivity to change" in specific dimensions would impact significantly the construct of SUD during treatment.

SUD and COD are complex concepts that are transdiagnostic and heterogeneous. Both concepts have covert and overt behavioral and physical response domains. All clinical behaviors are composed of domains, specific and defined constructs within the domains, and measurable dimensions of the domains (NIMH, n.d.).

An example of a complex concept composed of multiple domains and dimensions is pain. Like SUD and COD, pain is a complex transdiagnostic, idiosyncratic, and heterogeneous concept. Pain involves three domains: physical, psychological, and behavioral. These domains influence each other in intricate and dynamic ways. The subjective experience of the sensation of physical pain can lead to emotional distress, which then affects how someone behaves. The domains of pain include measurable dimensions that can be assessed. To illustrate, the physical domain of pain includes the results of scans, x-rays, and laboratory tests. The psychological domain refers to the awareness, perception, and experience of pain; the subjective intensity of the pain (sharp or dull ache); the perceived duration of the pain; and the emotions and private events associated with awareness of pain. The behavioral domain involves how the person responds to pain, such as avoiding or decreasing certain activities, taking substances to decrease the perception (e.g., sedation, euphoria) and the intensity of pain (e.g., analgesic, opioids), or participating in alternative behaviors to reduce the perception of pain (e.g., mindfulness meditation) (Zeidan & Vago, 2016).

The concept of COD involves the domains that encompass physical/biological dimensions, psychological/subjective response dimensions, and measurable behavioral dimensions. As with pain, these domains interact intricately with each other. It is not sufficient in an assessment to assess the presence or absence of a behavioral dimension, but detailed and operationally defined aspects of the dimension being assessed.

Based on the dimensions that are assessed in available self-report measures of SUD (Stewart et al., 2023) and the need for more comprehensive assessment measures, future instruments assessing COD should include the following relevant dimensions and subdimensions of the behavioral domain:

- Topography: the type of substances used alone, sequentially or simultaneously, dosage, and route of administration (e.g., smoking, injection).
- Intensity: the strength or magnitude of the subjectively experienced effect of the substance.
- Frequency and rate: the number of occurrences of use and abstinence of substances within a specified period. Is use and abstinence phasic, tonic, or cyclic? SUD can be continuous, episodic, or recurrent. Patterns of use are critical in determining the level of harm and the type of intervention required (Poznyak et al., 2018).
- Duration: length of time experiencing the effect of substance.
- Awareness: understanding the consequences of SUD-related behaviors, such as social, occupational, legal, and physical outcomes (e.g., overdose or withdrawal frequency).
- Respondents and covert responses: the perception of emotional respondents and covert responses (e.g., thoughts) that are linked to the use and abstinence of substances.
- Craving: consists of measures of intensity, intrusiveness, and frequency of covert responses related to using substances (May et al., 2014).
- Latency of responsiveness or reactivity: the duration of the person's awareness of experiencing craving after the onset of the stimulus associated with use of substances and the occurrence of drug-seeking and using behaviors. Latency is the time elapsed between the presentation of an antecedent condition and the initiation of behaviors (Cooper et al., 2020).
- Antecedent conditions: environmental triggers and overt and covert stimuli and events that lead to the use of drugs.
- Self-control: the frequency that the person experiencing craving effectively controls the use of drugs. Self-control is likely related to reactivity and shortened latency between onset of stimuli that is the MO and the use of drugs.

- Probability of the occurrence of drug use behavior: the frequency that the experience of craving will result in the display of drug seeking and responses of use by the person living with COD.
- Consequential conditions: the function of the environmental stimuli that follows the experience of using drugs. Does the use of a drug result in cessation/avoidance of physical and psychological distress associated with problems behaviors linked to SMI and/or results in euphoria and desired subjective experiences (e.g., alertness, sedation) that decrease the psychological distress of living with SMI?

These dimensions could assist in understanding and assessing the multifaceted nature of COD.

Origins and Maintenance of Co-occurring Mental Health Conditions (COD)

COD is a chronic and recurrent mental health condition that impacts the regulation of reward processing, motivational systems, memory function, and decision-making capabilities. COD leads to significant social, academic, and occupational impairments due to excessive consumption of various substances (i.e., substance-use-related condition (SUD)) and problem behaviors related to living with SMI. Factors influencing SUD include psychological, biological, sociocultural, and environmental elements, with COD increasing risk for occurrence. People living with COD use more types of substances and experience more negative outcomes than individuals with SUD alone. Compared to a single SUD condition, living with COD is associated with compulsive substance use behaviors, severity, and treatment resistance (Najt et al., 2011).

Polysubstance use among people living with COD complicates the assessment and treatment of these conditions (NIDA, 2020). Polysubstance use is common with people living with COD with many people developing multiple co-occurring SUDs. Among individuals with heroin use disorder, over 66% are dependent on nicotine, nearly 25% have an alcohol use-related condition, and over 20% have a cocaine use-related condition (NIDA, 2020). Among individuals with cocaine use-related condition, nearly 60% have an alcohol use problematic condition, 48% are dependent on nicotine, and over 21% have a marijuana use-related problem.

Neurological Substrates

The ontogenesis of COD is a complex interaction between neurobiological substrates that may have genetic influences and environmental factors. Studies of the brain using both structural and functional measures (Murnane et al., 2023; Paulus, 2022) have found several key areas that are impacted by drug use.

- Prefrontal Cortex (PFC): Impaired decision-making and impulse control are linked to reduced activation.
- Nucleus Accumbens (NAc): This area is central to reward processing; the use of substances increases dopamine (DA) levels, enhancing reinforcing effects and decreasing the related hypohedonia.
- Amygdala (amyg): Alterations in functioning are associated with emotional regulation and drug craving.
- Hippocampus (HC): Functional and structural changes impact memory and learning.
- Ventral tegmental area (VTA): Dysregulated systems of DA release/reuptake enhance drug responses (Murnane et al., 2023). Impaired release of DA may account for people living with alcohol use-related condition (AUD) and experiencing hypohedonia.
- Anterior cingulate cortex (ACC): This area is linked to behavioral control; studies have found reduced activation in stimulant users.
- Insula: This area is associated with craving and substance misuse risk.
- Striatum: The area is involved in reward and motor functions; cocaine craving increases available DA.
- Extended amyg (including the bed nucleus of the stria terminalis, the central nucleus of the amyg, and parts of the NAc): This structure plays a role in stress and emotional dysregulation during withdrawal.
- Thalamus: Reduced activity is correlated with SUD severity.

Several neurotransmitters are implicated in SUD with increases or decreases during activation of a specific area of the brain (Cadet et al., 2014):

- DA: It is central to the reward system and increased release contributes to SUD and relapse.
- Serotonin (5-HT): It affects mood regulation and is influenced by drugs like methylenedioxymethamphetamine (MDMA) (ecstasy or molly) and alcohol.
- GABA: It is enhanced by alcohol and benzodiazepines, leading to calming effects.
- Glutamate (Glu): This is disrupted by alcohol, affecting learning and memory.
- Endorphins: Opioids mimic natural painkillers that result in euphoria.
- Norepinephrine (NE): It is increased by stimulants, leading to heightened alertness.
- Acetylcholine (ACh): This is affected by nicotine, influencing attention and addiction.

Each drug type causes significant neurological impairments, including cognitive impairments, structural brain changes, and cerebrovascular complications, mediated by oxidative stress, receptor alterations, and neurological vascular damage. The following are substances used, and biological and functional changes brought about by their excessive use (Cadet et al., 2014):

- Marijuana cannabis: Cognitive effects include impairments in memory, attention, decision-making, and psychomotor speed, with increased risk of developing a psychotic-type of mental health problem. Structural changes involve reduced gray matter in HC, amyg, and PFC, and altered white matter integrity, especially in adolescent users. Cerebrovascular effects include increased blood pressure, cardiac ischemia, stroke risk, and decreased vascular resistance and oxygen uptake (Cadet et al., 2014).

- Cocaine: Cognitive impairments affect executive function, decision-making, memory, and psychomotor speed, with movement disorders mimicking Tourette-like symptoms. Structural changes show reduced volume in the PFC and gray matter density and altered DA transporter receptor levels. Cerebrovascular effects include vasoconstriction, endothelial damage, and risks of ischemic and hemorrhagic strokes (Cadet et al., 2014).
- Methamphetamine: Cognitive effects include impairments in episodic memory, executive function, and psychomotor abilities, with an increased risk of Parkinson's disease. Structural changes involve reduced DA levels, cortical gray matter loss, and enlarged striatum with HC volume loss. Cerebrovascular effects present stroke risk due to elevated blood pressure and vascular stenosis (Cadet et al., 2014).
- MDMA (methylenedioxymethamphetamine) (ecstasy, molly): Cognitive impairments include verbal memory, executive function, and prospective memory issues, along with paranoia and anxiety. Structural changes show reduced 5-HT transporter binding and gray matter loss in the orbitofrontal cortex (OFC) and thalamus. Cerebrovascular effects include hypertension, arrhythmias, intracranial hemorrhages, and cerebral edema (Cadet et al., 2014).
- Heroin: Cognitive effects include problems in visual memory, working memory, and processing speed, associated with hypoxic brain damage. Structural changes involve enlarged ventricles, reduced gray matter density, and white matter hyperintensities, with spongiform leukoencephalopathy in people who administer the drug by inhalation.Cerebrovascular effects include cerebral edema, ischemic strokes, and embolic phenomena due to foreign substances in heroin mixtures (Cadet et al., 2014).
- Synthetic cathinones (bath salts): Cognitive effects lead to long-term impairments in memory and executive function. Structural changes show limited evidence of direct neurotoxicity but potentiate effects of other neurotoxic drugs. Cerebrovascular effects include hyperthermia and potential vessel damage, though findings are nonspecific (Cadet et al., 2014).

Psychological/Behavioral Substrates

The mental health literature on co-occurring mental health problems (COD) suggests that biological factors such as heredity, impulsivity, and the reinforcing properties of drugs in relation to neurological mechanisms are significant determinants of substance-use-related conditions (SUD) and SMI. However, environmental and psychological aspects, such as interpersonal networks, expectations of drug effects, boredom, dysphoria, unemployment, poverty, lack of educational opportunities, and trauma, are also critical. The substances used by people living with SMI are a biopsychosocial phenomenon, with multiple contributing risk factors (Drake et al., 2002). Many researchers postulate that people living with SMI initiate using substances as a form of self-medication to manage or reduce behavior problems associated with the SMI, side-effects, and that certain substances are used to hinder the occurrence or reduce the severity of symptoms/behavior problems associated with specific mental health problems (Del Rio et al., 2021). It is important to consider that people living with SMI use the same psychoactive substances (e.g., alcohol, nicotine, cannabis, hallucinogens, and opioids) as persons living with SUD alone; the drugs used vary by availability rather than in relation to specific mental health problems or symptoms. People living with schizophrenia spectrum mental health problems who use substances begin doing so before the development of associated problem behaviors/symptoms (Drake et al., 2002). Biological research and risk factors remain important; however, they are predominantly the same as those that predict the risk of SUD in individuals without mental health problems, such as family history, childhood conduct issues and use of drugs, trauma, and other psychosocial problems (Mueser et al., 1998). There is no evidence that substances that are used are a function of the biologics of specific mental health problems, like delusions, hallucinations, and neurocognitive impairments. If the biology of SMI confers a special vulnerability to developing an SUD, it may be in the form of increased sensitivity to the effects of drugs. People living with SMI tend to experience adverse consequences in relation to small amounts of substances used, with minimal exposures causing serious relapses, lack of control, and exacerbations of problem behaviors with difficulty in returning to abstinence (Drake et al., 2002; Levin, n.d.). People living with SMI encounter many of the known environmental and psychological risk factors for SUD, such as poverty, living in high-risk neighborhoods, having deviant peer groups, social isolation, lack of education, unemployment, boredom, dysphoria, lack of family responsibilities, more frequent adverse encounters with law enforcement, and experiencing the stigma of living with a mental health problem (Drake et al., 2002). Important contributing factors in the development of SUD in people living with SMI are the role of social learning, respondent conditioning, and operant learning processes in the genesis and maintenance of SUD by an individual living with SMI.

Psychosocial and socio-environmental factors significantly contribute to the onset of a substance-use-related condition (SUD) for people living with SMI. Socio-environmental factors encompass peer influence, availability of drugs in neighborhoods where people living with SMI reside, financial and housing instability, and community and cultural norms. People living with co-occurring use mental health problems (COD) use substances at an early age, have easy access to drugs, and frequently are socially reinforced by peers during use (e.g., drinking beers at a party) (Drake et al., 2002). Psychosocial risk factors that are prevalent in individuals living with SMI include repeated occurrences of trauma, chronic stress, social isolation, co-occurring mental health issues, and maladaptive coping mechanisms (Drake et al., 2002). These elements collectively increase vulnerability to COD.

Classical conditioning (Pavlovian conditioning) explains how environmental cues associated with substance use can elicit conditioned responses (CRs) even in the absence of the substance itself. For example, cocaine is an unconditioned stimulus (US) that naturally produces unconditioned responses (URs) physiological responses and the subjective experience of euphoria. Neutral stimuli become conditioned stimuli (CSs) with the repeated pairing of stimuli associated with cocaine use (e.g., the observation of cocaine or a person or location associated with its use). Upon exposure to the CSs, the individual experiences the physical and subjective CRs that are like the actual effects of the drug (Montan & Banaco, 2021).

Drug-related CSs can increase the likelihood of craving, drug-seeking, and self-administration behaviors due to their eliciting and evoking properties. This occurs because the CRs involve aversive bodily changes that are alleviated by substance use, creating a history of operant conditioning where drug-seeking is reinforced by the removal of discomfort (negative reinforcement) or the pleasurable effects of the drug (positive reinforcement) (Montan & Banaco, 2021). The short latency of the administration and the effect of the drug results in the substance using behaviors becoming "habitual" despite experiencing adverse outcomes in the future. Substance abusers often prefer fast-acting drugs, which makes their behavior habitual despite future adverse outcomes. Drug delivery methods are crucial, with users favoring efficient ways to experience the effects quickly, like inhalation or injection (Sujatha et al., 2013). Drugs such as nicotine, fentanyl, and methamphetamine provide rapid effects, reinforcing drug dependence through repeated exposure and reinforcement (Ajit et al., 2013). This repeated exposure to CRs and the reinforcement by using substances strengthens the cycle of drug-seeking and dependence (Montan & Banaco, 2021).

Tolerance is defined as decreased responsiveness to a previous amount of drug (Siegel et al., 2000). This occurs as the body develops compensatory CRs. A compensatory CR (CCR) refers to a conditioned reaction that counteracts the effect of a stimulus (such as drugs) by producing an opposite effect; the CCR is the result of physiological responses to the ingestion of the drug. A CCR attenuates the drug's effects, requiring larger doses to achieve the same effect. Tolerance to drugs often develops in specific environments where the drug is repeatedly administered and not solely related to the pharmacological impact of the drug on the central nervous system (CNS). Drug-paired environmental cues can elicit conditional compensatory responses (CCRs) that counteract the drug's effects, making tolerance more pronounced in familiar drug-associated contexts than in novel ones. However, altering the situational cues and context of the usual use of a drug can disrupt tolerance, decreasing the CRR and increasing the risk of overdose (Siegel et al., 2000).

Withdrawal symptoms occur when CSs elicit aversive CRs in the absence of the drug, motivating the use of substances to alleviate discomfort. Relapses are often triggered by re-exposure to drug-related CSs after periods of abstinence, as these stimuli retain their ability to elicit CRs unless extinguished through repeated exposure without the drug (Siegel et al., 2000). Environmental cues associated with substance use can elicit withdrawal symptoms when the drug is absent. Similarly, pharmacological cues (e.g., small doses of the drug) can trigger withdrawal symptoms in individuals with prior drug experience (Siegel et al., 2000).

Motivating operations (MOs) in SUD refer to environmental or internal factors that influence the likelihood of drug-seeking and self-administration behaviors by altering the reinforcing value of the substance. Through classical conditioning, drug-related CSs can function as MOs because they increase the probability of substance-seeking behaviors when present. For example, stimuli associated with drug use, such as paraphernalia or specific locations, can evoke strong cravings and drug-seeking behaviors. These stimuli gain their MO function through a history of operant conditioning, where substance use alleviates aversive bodily states (negative reinforcement), produces pleasurable effects (positive reinforcement), and social reinforcement from peers (Montan & Banaco, 2021).

MOs play a role in withdrawal and relapses. When exposed to drug-related CSs, individuals may experience aversive CRs, such as discomfort or craving, which motivate substance use to remove these unpleasant states. Additionally, the reinforcing effects of the substance itself can act as an MO, further driving repeated use and dependence (Montan & Banaco, 2021).

Another factor in the genesis of SUD is social learning, which is learning that comes about through social interactions with other individuals. Social learning includes imitation, emulation, and mimicry. It is based on the individual observing the behaviors of others in the environment. People who are regarded as having "high social status" and being seen as receiving social and/or financial reinforcement from others are perceived as role models. This group of role models includes people in authority, having influence, and seen as successful according to the normative group. Repeatedly observing positive social reinforcement, such as peer acceptance, can encourage substance use behaviors in an individual (American Psychological Association, 2018).

When the role models of a person are observed using or under the influence of substances, the behavior of using substances and the stimuli related to the use of substances—including verbal behaviors—become part of the behavioral repertoire of the individual. By way of illustration, a child observes his father drinking alcohol frequently after work or with friends. His father is overheard saying that he needs a drink to relax or is seen laughing and socializing with friends. The child learns that a means to cope with stress and have fun is to drink alcohol. In conjunction, the child sees people having fun on commercials for alcoholic beverages and listens to songs with words pertaining to using alcohol to cope and have fun and enjoy life.

Individuals at risk for living with SMI may have a genetic liability to develop SMI but they also experience frequent maladaptive environmental situations including observing substance use, trauma, easily accessible drugs, and other stressors at an early age. By the principles of associative learning (in which stimuli paired with other environmental stimuli are learned (American Psychological Association, n.d.-a) and social learning, the outcome is that the use of alcohol is acceptable, adaptive, and rewarding despite awareness of possible negative consequences with the phenomenon of COD arising from the complicated interactions of both biological and environmental factors.

Epidemiological Consideration

Co-occurring mental health problems (COD) account for 26% of people living with SMI and 37% of substance-use-related conditions (SUD) cases among 76 million affected adults in the United States (Bahji, 2024). According to the 2023 NSDUH (SAMHSA, 2023), 35% of adults in the United States over 18 who have another mental health problem are also living with SUD. Mental health problems that commonly co-occur with SUD include anxiety, depression, post-traumatic stress disorder, problems related to psychosis, and borderline and antisocial personality-related mental health problems.

The risk of living with COD increases with early onset of substance use (Volkow et al., 2021). Knopf (2021) reported that the prevalence of developing SUD within a year after first use of a drug was about double for adolescents than for young adults. The lifetime prevalence for adolescents ages 12–17 years for a type of substance-related use condition is as follows: alcohol (26.3%); cannabis (5.4%); tobacco (13.4%); and prescription drugs (9.2%). For young adults ages 18–25, the lifetime prevalence rates for drug use are: alcohol (79.7%), cannabis (51.5%), tobacco (55.0%), cocaine (11.4%), methamphetamine (2.5%), heroin (1.3%), and prescription drugs (26.3%). Adolescents showed higher lifetime prevalence of SUDs within 12 months of initiation for cannabis and prescription drugs compared to young adults, while young adults had higher lifetime prevalence rates for most substances, including alcohol, cannabis, tobacco, and cocaine (Knopf, 2021).

Flynn and Brown (2008) reported the following from two national surveys:

- Lifetime prevalence rates for alcohol use-related condition (AUD) at 14.1%. to 16.5%
- Lifetime prevalence for drug use-related condition (DUD) was reported at 6.1% to 7.5%.
- Among individuals with DUD, 26% had co-occurring mood-related mental health problems and 28% had anxiety-related mental health problems.

Mojtabai (2022) re-analyzed the prevalence estimates for alcohol, cannabis, opioid, and stimulant use disorders using a "benchmark multiplier" that were reported by a recent 2018–2019 NSDUH survey. A benchmark multiplier is a method used in indirect prevalence estimations to calculate the total size of a target population (e.g., drug users) based on data from a subset of that population (United Nations Office on Drugs and Crime [UNODC], n.d.). Results showed that the rates of SUD were much higher than reported: AUD (20.27% vs. 5.34% (NSDUH)); Cannabis use-related condition (7.57% vs. 1.68%); opioid use-related condition (3.46% vs. 0.68%); and stimulant use-related condition: (1.91% vs. 0.85%).

In treatment populations, 50–70% of clients showed lifetime histories of COD, while 20–50% of mental health clients had SUD with 41% living with mood-related mental health problems. According to the 2018 NSDUH, approximately 1.6% of individuals aged 12 to 17 and 10.1% of individuals over age18 had a DSM-5 defined SUD in the past year (Boness et al., 2024; SAMHSA, 2019).

Williams et al. (2022) surveyed nearly 6000 veterans using the Mini International Neuropsychiatric Interview (MINI) to assess the prevalence of SUD. The results found that AUD prevalence is highest among younger patients (22.4%) and Hispanic/Latinx patients (17.7%); DUD prevalence is highest among younger patients (10.1%). Any SUD prevalence is highest among younger patients (27.7%) and Hispanic/Latinx patients (21.6%).

Using data from the Collaborative Psychiatric Epidemiology Studies, Mericle et al. (2012) cited a 53% prevalence of mental health problems co-occurring with an identified substance-use-related condition (SUD). Whites were found to have a higher lifetime prevalence of COD compared to other racial/ethnic groups except for Asians living with DUD (Mericle et al., 2012). Approximately 8.2% of Whites, 5.4% of Blacks, 5.8% of Latinos, and 2.1% of Asians met criteria for lifetime prevalence co-occurring mental health problem (COD). For Asian individuals, the prevalence of an anxiety type of mental health problem was 50.1%, while it was 46.4% for Latino individuals. Black individuals had a prevalence of 47.8% for any mental health problems (Mericle et al., 2012).

The overall lifetime prevalence of living with COD is 7.3%, with 8.2% of Whites affected compared to lower rates in Blacks (5.4%), Latinos (5.8%), and Asians (2.1%). Among individuals with alcohol-use-related conditions (AUD), Whites are more likely than Blacks to experience depressive and anxiety types of mental health problems. For drug use-related condition (DUD), Whites are also more likely to have depressive mental health problems compared to Blacks and Latinos. The average age of onset for SUD is younger for Whites than for Blacks. Whites living with COD are less likely to be unemployed compared to Blacks and Latinos, but more likely to have a history of psychiatric hospitalizations (Mericle et al., 2012), which may reflect better access to treatment. Most individuals with COD reported that mental health problem behaviors/symptoms preceded SUD symptoms, regardless of race/ethnicity. This finding by Mericle et al. (2012) is contrary to the finding reported by Drake et al. (2002) that substance use behaviors preceded problem behaviors/symptoms related to living with SMI. Further research is needed to clarify and help with the understanding of the complex relationship between SUD and COD.

The average age of onset for SUD is 20.4 years, with significant differences among racial/ethnic groups. Black individuals have a mean age of onset for SUD of 21.8 years, while onset for White individuals is 20.2 years. The percentage of SUD that is the primary mental health problem in people living with COD is similar for racial groups (Mericle et al., 2012).

Cross-Cultural Considerations of Co-occurring Mental Health Problems (COD)

The prevalence of co-occurring and substance-use-related issues varies across regions. It is a significant health problem with prevalence increasing in various populations. In Europe, Africa, and Asia, alcohol and opioid problems are escalating. Amphetamine and cannabis misuse are more prevalent in Asia, North America, and Europe, while cocaine is a significant substance use problem in North America and Europe. Indigenous psychoactive substances like "khat" are commonly misused in Africa and the Middle East and coca leaves in South America. Sub-Saharan Africa is predicted to have a 130% increase in alcohol and substance misuse by 2050 due to population growth and aging. Worldwide, substance-use-related conditions account for 5.4% of the total health-related problems, increasing to 9.1% when tobacco use is included (Baingana et al., 2015).

Co-occurring mental health problems (COD) occur in 25% to 74% of cases in developed countries (Temmingh, 2019). In South Africa, COD prevalence ranges from 50% to 68%. As in other countries, individuals living with COD experience shorter relapses but higher readmission rates and worse clinical outcomes compared to those without a substance-use-related condition. (SUD). Cannabis use problems are most prevalent among individuals with SMI, with a lifetime prevalence of 27.1%, followed by alcohol at 20.6%. The study found a lifetime prevalence of any SUD at 47.8% among individuals living with a schizophrenia spectrum mental health problem. The most prevalent substance use disorder was related to cannabis, affecting 39.6% of participants. Alcohol use-related problems (AUD) were identified in 20.5%, while methaqualone (Quaalude) use problems were reported in 6.2%. Methamphetamine use issues occurred in 4.8% of the sample. Only 0.6% of participants presented with other substance use conditions, which included cocaine and hallucinogens. Polysubstance use was notably frequent, as 40.1% of individuals with SUDs engaged in the use of two or more substances (Temmingh, 2019).

Significant associations were found between SUDs and younger age, male gender, inpatient status, and problematic behaviors related to living with PTSD in the sample from South Africa (Temmingh, 2019). Economic problems were reported in 41.9% of participants, and legal issues were noted in 7.6%. Many individuals had less than 12 years of education and were unemployed (93.9%) (Temmingh, 2019).

The prevalence of substance-use-related issues (SUDs) among individuals living with SMI ranged from 10% to 74%. More than 55% of those living with SMI met the criteria for SUD according to the DSM-5-TR (American Psychiatric Association, 2022). Specifically, cannabis and alcohol use issues were observed at rates of 34.3% and 30.6%, respectively. Reported problems associated with methamphetamine and methaqualone usage were 27.4% and 10.4%, respectively. Lifetime major depressive episodes occurred in 20.6% of individuals living with co-occurring mental health problems, while depressive symptoms were present in 55.7%. Anxiety symptoms were reported in 25% of people living with COD who also have higher rates of suicide attempts (Temmingh, 2019).

Temmingh (2019) found that younger age was significantly associated with problems with methamphetamine use, while lower educational attainment correlated with cannabis use problems in South Africa. Among participants with SUDs, 26.1% had arrests for "other crimes," while serious and major crimes were less common. Legal involvement was significantly elevated among participants with SUDs, particularly for cannabis and methaqualone users, while 67.3% had no history of arrests. Significant associations were found between male gender, substance-induced psychosis, and various SUDs (Temmingh, 2019).

A study from Norway (Stallvik & Nordahl, 2014) found that over 57% of individuals seeking treatment for substance-use-related conditions (SUD) had mental health problems; the percentages were in line with similar findings in previous research of 39% to 65%. Over 39% of the individuals who live with SMI reported a lifetime history of suicide attempts. Significant differences in age and work history were found among the three groups, with the individuals living with COD being younger and reporting higher rates of problem behaviors due to psychotic (17%) and PTSD (18%) related mental health problems.

Carra and Johnson (2009) conducted a systematic review of the literature on the prevalence of COD and SUD in the United Kingdom. The prevalence of COD varies significantly across different settings and populations. Rates of SUD among individuals living with SMI range from 20% to 37% with higher rates observed in inpatient, crisis resolution team, and forensic settings (38–50%). The prevalence of living with an SMI among SUD service users is reported to be between 6% and 15%. Rates are highest in urban areas, particularly inner cities, compared to rural and mixed areas. For example, alcohol use-related problems (AUD) in urban areas range from 22% to 32%, while rural areas report much lower rates (i.e., 12%). Black individuals are disproportionately represented among those living with co-occurring mental health problems (COD) relative to their percentage in the general population, with observed rates ranging from 1.8 to 5.8 times higher according to certain studies. The overall prevalence of COD within general medical practices has been estimated at 15%. Reported lifetime prevalence of alcohol use-related condition (AUD) varies between 22% and 47%, whereas current prevalence ranges from 15% to 49%. For drug-use-related issues (DUD), lifetime prevalence is reported between 16% and 68%, with current prevalence spanning from 17% to 48% (Carra & Johnson, 2009).

Using data from a nationwide survey in Canada, Rush et al. (2008a, 2008b) reported that the 12-month prevalence of COD in the population was 1.7%. Prevalence rates were higher among males (2.1%) compared to females (1.4%) and decreased with age, from 3.8% in individuals aged 15–24 years to 0.2% in those aged 55 years and over. The prevalence of COD is higher among individuals with DUD compared to SUD, and higher among those with substance dependence compared to less severe substance use problems. The exclusion of high-risk groups, such as Aboriginal people living on reserves and homeless individuals, may have underestimated the true prevalence of COD in Canada at the time of the survey.

Types of Co-occurring Use Mental Health Problems (COD)

COD is defined as the simultaneous presence of mental health and substance-use-related problems. Approximately 50% of individuals living with a type of SMI develop a type of substance-use-related conditions (SUD) during their lifetime. Higher prevalence of SUD is confirmed among people living with SMI as compared to the general population (RachBeisel et al., 1999). Approximately 35% of adults living in the United States are living with COD with the most common mental health problems being anxiety (including PTSD) and depression. A comprehensive survey of a mental health system conducted by Rush and Koegl (2008) identified that the overall prevalence of co-occurring mental health problems was 18.5%. The rate was highest among individuals receiving specialty tertiary inpatient care (28%), as well as within specific subpopulations, including younger adults (55%) and those diagnosed with personality disorders (34%).

Types of COD can be differentiated on the type of mental health problems the person is experiencing and the type of substances that are being used that are contributing to problems with living with an SMI. The use of more than one substance—polysubstance use—intensifies the overall effects of substance use and the negative outcomes in social, educational, and occupational domains. Both the mental health and substance use problems with which the person is living can be subtypes as to the levels of severity as defined by the DSM-5-TR (American Psychiatric Association, 2022). The result of "typing" co-occurring mental health problems is composed of categorizing the category of serious mental health problems (SMI), the type of substance-use-related conditions (SUD), and the dimensions related to SMI and SUD.

The mental health problems that a person experiences living with COD are the categories specified in the DSM-5-TR. SMI commonly refers to a person experiencing mental health problems involving psychosis, bipolar, and major depression. SMI can also include anxiety-related, eating-related, and personality-related mental health problems, if the degree of functional impairment is severe. SMIs are long-term conditions involving substantial functional impairment over multiple behavioral and symptom domains. These impairments often lead to an inability to maintain employment, poor social support, repeated psychiatric hospitalizations, homelessness, incarceration, and the increased risk of a coexisting SUD (Evans et al., 2016).

The DSM-5-TR (American Psychiatric Association, 2022) lists that following substances that can be misused: alcohol, caffeine, cannabis, hallucinogens, inhalants, opioids, sedatives, hypnotics, anxiolytics, stimulants, tobacco, and other or unknown substances. The substances are differentiated as to use, intoxication, and withdrawal with varying criteria for each. All these substances are listed in the substance intoxication category; tobacco and caffeine have no identifying criteria for substance-use-related condition (SUD) but have criteria for intoxication and withdrawal. Hallucinogens and inhalants have no criteria for the substance withdrawal category.

The DSM-5 (American Psychiatric Association, 2013) approach toward defining severity varies across disorders (Zimmerman et al., 2018). Severity across mental health problems is determined by the number of problem behaviors/symptoms, intensity, frequency, persistence, and functional impairment. For personality disorders, functional impairment is central, while for mental health problems of depression and anxiety, symptom-based measures are predominant (Zimmerman et al., 2018). The ratings of severity for most mental health problems are as follows:

- Number of problem behaviors that are displayed and present: "few" for mild, "substantially in excess" for severe.
- Dimension of intensity of problem behaviors: defined as "manageable" for mild, "seriously distressing and unmanageable" for severe.
- Functional impairment: "minor" for mild, "marked interference" in social and occupational functioning for severe.

There are no operational definitions for the degree of severity for the above criteria such as differentiating between "mild" and "marked interference" in functioning, "manageable to unmanageable" for intensity of problem behaviors, and "few" to "substantially in excess" for frequency of occurrence of problem behaviors. These are based on the subjective judgment of the treating service provider and feedback from the person living with SMI.

Personality mental health problems have a more detailed definition of severity (Zimmerman et al., 2018) but again involves the judgment of the treating service provider. Severity is often linked to:

- Functional impairment: maladaptive functioning in areas like identity formation, self-control, and interpersonal relationships. Concepts like identity formation need operationalized definitions for identification and measurement.
- The dimension of frequency and intensity of problem behavior: For example, the severity of a borderline personality mental health problem (BPD) can be measured by the frequency of self-injury or other behaviors.
- Comorbidity: Higher severity is associated with multiple co-occurring personality mental health problems or behaviors that occur across contexts and situations.

The severity of a substance-use-related condition (SUD) is determined by the number of problems encountered in the following behavioral domains and the dimensions that are listed in Table 12.1. Severity of SUD is determined by the number of DSM-5 criteria met (2–3 for mild, 4–5 for moderate, and 6 or more for severe).

To determine the types of co-occurring mental health problems (COD), it is imperative to assess the dimensional indicators of SMI and SUD that are simultaneously present. Assessing the dimensions of both SMI and SUD and the functions of SUD in service of the problems related to SMI will provide comprehensive understanding of the presenting behavior problems since it has been shown that severities of SUD and SMI impact treatment responsivity (Rush & Koegl, 2008). Types of COD can be differentiated on the type of mental health problems the person is experiencing and the type of substances that are being used that are contributing to

Table 12.1 DSM-5-TR domain criteria, dimensions and definitions for severity of SUD

Domain	Dimensions	Definition
Impaired control	Repeated attempts to quit/control use Craving (added to DSM-5) Larger/longer Amount of time spent using	Persistent desire or unsuccessful efforts to cut down or control substance use. A strong desire or urge to use the substance Using the substance in larger amounts or for longer than intended Spending more time obtaining, using, or recovering from the substance.
Social problems	Social/interpersonal problems related to use Neglect of major roles to use substance Activities given up to use	Continued use despite causing or exacerbating social or interpersonal issues (e.g., losing employment). Failing to fulfill major obligations at work, school, or home due to substance use. Reducing or abandoning important social, occupational, or recreational activities due to substance use.
Dangerous use	Physical/psychological problems related to use Hazardous use	Continued use despite knowing it causes or worsens physical or psychological problems (e.g., experiencing overdosing). Using the substance in situations where it is physically dangerous (e.g., using "dirty" needles to inject substances).
Drug effects	Withdrawal Tolerance	Experiencing withdrawal symptoms or using the substance to avoid withdrawal (cannabis withdrawal added in DSM-5). Needing more of the substance to achieve the desired effect or experiencing reduced effect with the same amount.

problems with living and exacerbating the mental health problems. Polysubstance use, which refers to the consumption of multiple substances simultaneously, can exacerbate the overall impact of substance use as well as increase adverse effects in social, educational, and occupational contexts. Mental health and substance use issues can be classified by severity levels defined in the DSM-5-TR (American Psychiatric Association, 2022), and classifying COD involves interactions of behavior problems and dimensions related to SMI and SUD. For instance, an individual living with COD can be classified as living with a schizophrenia spectrum mental health problem and an opioid use disorder. The mental health problems include the frequent experience of auditory-verbal hallucinations (AVH) during which he hears derogatory statements that cause psychological distress and anxiety. He perceives that he has no control over the intensity or frequency of the occurrence of the hallucinatory experiences. He also is living with an opioid use-related condition (SUD); the MO for the use of the drug is that the experience of sedation and euphoria from the drug temporarily decreases the AVH so its use is negatively reinforced. This example of a description of a person living with COD is dimensional and functional, leading to a more robust assessment and focus of treatment of the COD.

Understanding Co-occurring Mental Health Problems (COD): Substance Use Among Individuals with Living with SMI

Problems with substance use are common among people who are living with SMI. About half of all people who are hospitalized for SMI also have a problem with alcohol, cigarettes, coffee, and illicit drug use. Alcohol is the most common drug that is used followed by cannabis and amphetamines and is used with greater frequency than in the general population (RachBeisel et al., 1999).

Substances like caffeine (in coffee, tea, energy, and soft drinks) and nicotine (in cigarettes and vaping) are legal, widely available, and often used excessively by people living with SMI. Other drugs which may be misused include cocaine, heroin, "PCP," marijuana, "spice" (synthetic marijuana), and a variety of other drugs which are illegal; in the case of "spice," it is sold legally as jurisdictions have had difficulty defining "spice" as the chemicals used in its manufacture changes. Psychiatric medications, especially drugs that are prescribed for anxiety (e.g., "tranquilizers," benzodiazepines), depression, and sleeping aides (e.g., "sedatives," "barbiturates," and hypnotics) also can be misused. These drugs can be life-threatening when combined with alcohol. The abuse of legal "over the counter" (OTC) substances (e.g., cold and cough medicines), which bring on drowsiness, hallucinations, and other altered subjective experiences are common. Many people will use several of these drugs, sometimes simultaneously or sequentially, making evaluation and treatment more difficult. The OTC substances also interfere with the metabolism of psychiatric medication that may be prescribed for a person living with SMI, altering their effectiveness.

Excessive cigarette and/or caffeinated drink use are common problems among people living with SMI. For example, some individuals will consume a jar of regular instant coffee daily or drink the highly caffeinated "energy drinks." Excessive use of caffeinated drinks and cigarettes will affect a person's health and ability to think clearly. For people living with SMI, cigarette and caffeine use can interfere with necessary medications. Quitting or reducing these habits is challenging, especially when co-occurring mental health condition (COD) is a factor.

Problems with substances can appear in several forms. Physical dependence develops gradually as repeated administration of the drug leads the body—including neurological systems—to adapt to the presence of a consistent level of the substance. The body then needs more of the drug to have the same effect on mood and behavior (e.g., tolerance). If enough time passes without receiving the drug, the body begins a process of withdrawal during which the body and brain adapt to being without the drug. Withdrawal has uncomfortable physical and psychological effects and results in increases in craving and drug-seeking behaviors to obtain the drug to remove the adverse experiences of withdrawal and not experiencing the effects of the drug. The person in withdrawal may experience a wide variety of symptoms including being irritable, seeing things (e.g., visual hallucinations), feeling things on their skin (e.g., tactile hallucinations), and having difficulty thinking clearly (e.g., confusion, disorientation). In most cases, the symptoms are quickly relieved by taking the drug. When withdrawal symptoms happen, and the person uses the substance to relieve them, the person has a physical dependency; dependency on a substance is a DSM-5-TR criteria for a severe substance-use-related condition (SUD) (American Psychiatric Association, 2022).

Because of this physical process, it becomes very difficult to avoid drug use for a long period of time. The person living with COD develops a physical and psychological craving. Upon waking in the morning, individuals who consume coffee often anticipate their first cup with urgency. Some may assert that they are unable to begin their daily activities effectively until they have had one or two cups of coffee. Coffee drinkers who stop using coffee for a few days have withdrawal effects from the caffeine in the coffee (or tea, energy drinks), like decreased energy and alertness, drowsiness, decreased contentedness, depressed mood, difficulty concentrating, irritability, feeling foggy/not clearheaded, and headache. The severity of symptoms varies from mild to extreme. The incidence or severity of symptoms increases with increases in the daily amount consumed. Still, abstinence from low doses, such as one cup of coffee daily, can produce symptoms of withdrawal (Sajadi-Ernazarova & Hamilton, 2023). It is the same response but more severe with other drug use.

Living with SUD refers to where problems are caused by using a substance, with or without signs of physical dependency when the substances are stopped. Even though there is no physical dependency, substance use may cause or maintain many problems such as not doing well in school or on the job, arguing or fighting with other people, and being arrested for intoxication (SAMHSA, 2015; Volkow et al., 2021). While other people may see that SUD is contributing to these problems, the user does not, perceiving that the use of substances is under their control, and continues to use. While physical withdrawal may be absent, there are often many other factors (such as friends who use drugs, boredom, nervousness, depression) that strongly influence SUD. The use, therefore, becomes "habitual" and problems associated with drug use are repeated.

"Co-occurring" mental health problems refer to situations where the person is living with SMI and SUD (COD) at the same time. For example, a person who may be living with SMI, such as schizophrenia spectrum mental health problem, uses opioids. In this case, there are two mental health problems to treat. Unless both conditions are assessed and recognized that mental health problems interact with substance use problems and vice versa, treatment of either condition is likely to be ineffective. This makes the treatment of a person living with COD complex and challenging.

A complication for people living with co-occurring mental health problems (CODs) is that several different drugs may be used. This usually includes using alcohol and a wide variety of other drugs including cannabis, methamphetamines, opioids, inhaling fumes from gasoline, glue or solvents, and misuse of OTC medicines. This is called "polysubstance use"; it can be difficult for the service provider to identify the substances that are being used and complicates treatment.

Why Should a Person Living with SMI Avoid Substances

- Drugs and other substances can cause or worsen problems in a person living with SMI. COD can have different forms. Many problem behaviors/symptoms can be a direct result of severe SUD. Symptoms and problem behaviors that are related to living with SMI worsen by using a substance. For example, regular alcohol use over a long period of time can contribute to the development of depressive mental health problems. If the person is already depressed, alcohol use can increase the severity and frequency of the problem behaviors associated with living with depressive mental health problems. The use of stimulant drugs such as cocaine and amphetamines generates suspiciousness and delusional thinking that may not resolve when the drug use stops. This makes the assessment and treatment of mental health problems more difficult.
- Long-term substance use can cause physical alterations to the structures and neuronal connections in the brain. It may result in damage to the brain, which will then result in difficulty with paying attention, concentrating, remembering, and confusion. These symptoms may get better if substances use stops but some can be permanent. Such problems interfere with the person living with COD actively participating and benefiting from the help that is available.
- Substances interfere with many psychiatric medications. Even if the person living with COD uses substances in moderation, these chemicals can cause problems with the effectiveness of medications being prescribed for the problem behaviors/symptoms associated with SMI. For example, psychiatric medications prescribed for severe anxiety may strengthen the effects of alcohol and make its use physically risky. Alcohol interferes with the effect of many antipsychotic medications and, therefore, should be avoided by most people who take such medications. The biological effects of nicotine and caffeine impact the effectiveness of psychiatric medications but at the same time mitigate the uncomfortable side effects that happen with these medications, influencing the person to continue smoking and using caffeine.

Why Do Problems with Substance Use Occur with Individuals Living with Serious Mental Illness?

There is no simple answer as to why substance use becomes a problem when used by an individual living with SMI. Usually, there are several reasons that work together to bring on the problem and keep it from improving. The following are some of the most important of these possible reasons.

Part of the Reason May Involve Genetics and Biology

- Just as genetic factors are influential in the development of problem behaviors related to living with a SMI, genes are also important in whether substance-use-related conditions (SUD) develop (Zhang et al., 2022). While this isn't true for all drugs, many studies have shown that alcohol use-related issues (AUD) occur in biological families. If a relative has AUD, then other members of the family have an increased liability to develop the problem. In Jordan's case, his grandfather and an uncle lived with AUD. Despite the genetic influence, SUD can be prevented.
- Use of substances may make the user feel good (e.g., euphoria) or may help "numb" or decrease the distressing emotions about traumatic life events like abuse, loss of a loved one, and horrific experiences as in war. Because of their effect on the brain, substances influence the part of the brain that controls feelings and moods. Some substances result in pleasurable experiences for the user (commonly called a "high"). For example, a person who has few friends and challenges in finding a job may use substances to experience "good feelings" that hardly ever happen without the substance. As a result, substance use is more likely to happen.
- Cigarettes, "energy drinks," and coffee use are difficult to control because many factors are working together to keep the problem going. When several factors work together to cause a behavior, it is usually very hard to change that behavior by just focusing on one of those factors.
- Excessive substance use is more likely to happen if the substance relieves some of the distress associated with symptoms of living with a SMI. When using the substance, the person living with SMI may be less distressed about the symptoms that she experiences. The effects of some substances, however, can result in problematic behaviors/symptoms related to SMI. Some researchers believe that using substances may "mask" or cover up problem behaviors/symptoms of living with SMI; this has been labeled as "self-medicating." If a person is living with COD, it may take months before a mental health service provider determines that the problem behaviors shown by the person are due to living with SMI or SUD.
- Both cigarettes, "energy drinks," and coffee (or, more accurately, the substances—nicotine and caffeine—that they contain) can contribute to the development of a physical dependence. As a result, someone trying to quit cigarettes or caffeinated drinks temporarily will feel uncomfortable and/or irritable. This uncomfortable feeling can be quickly relieved by using caffeinated drinks or tobacco. Because of this, it is very difficult to stop using them. The nicotine in cigarettes and the caffeine in coffee and "energy drinks" are both stimulant substances, enhancing arousal, alertness, attention, and vigilance. Nicotine affects the central nervous system. It increases the release of neurotransmitters like dopamine, which can enhance mood and focus. For example, coffee helps to "wake you up" in the morning. This will make the person living with SMI reluctant to decrease the frequency of using coffee and cigarettes.

Part of the Reason May Involve Psychosocial Factors

- Environmental stress can affect whether a person uses substances. Many people believe that substance use helps to relieve stress or to be more effective in stressful situations. In most cases, substance use serves to worsen the situation. However, many people continue to believe that substance use can relieve stress. Thus, when a person living with SMI is experiencing stress, substance use is more likely to happen. For example, Jordan felt very nervous when he had to be around strangers. As a result of this, he avoided many social situations. At first, he felt more comfortable when he stayed away from these social situations. Later, however, he felt like a failure for avoiding them and became discouraged. He reported that drinking helped him to not think about how he was avoiding these situations. However, drinking also kept him from doing anything about his nervousness so it did not improve.
- The behavior of other people can be a very important influence on whether a person living with SMI uses substances. If other family members or friends use substances around the person living with SMI, then she will be more likely to use substances. If substances are kept in the home, it is likely that the person living with SMI may use them. Reducing the availability and making it more difficult to get the substances will result in a decreased likelihood that the individual will use the substances.
- It is important to remember that boredom can also be a stressor for some people living with SMI. A person living with SMI becomes involved in fewer activities than most other people. This doesn't mean that they don't want to do anything. A person living with SMI who doesn't talk very much and spends a lot of time sitting in the house can still get bored. The challenge is to encourage appropriate activities that will be beneficial for the person living with COD. The kinds of activities that are appropriate for a person living with SMI may be difficult to judge. Some activities may be so simple that they are not recognized as not interesting to the person. If the person has used substances in the past and has very little to do, substance use is more likely to happen as the best predictor of behaviors is past behaviors. It is important to get the person living with COD engaged and involved and engaged in any treatment decisions.
- Cigarette and caffeinated drink users frequently develop regular routines of use that are difficult to change. Cigarette and caffeinated drink use is more likely to happen at certain times of day, in certain situations (such as while watching TV), with certain other people and during emotional situations (e.g., stress, boredom, contentment). For example, many smokers like to smoke after a meal. When they eat and can't have a cigarette afterward, they feel that something is missing. As a result, the use of cigarettes and caffeinated drinks has become strong habits. This is particularly true if there are no alternative activities available for the person living with COD in which to engage. Many people use cigarettes and caffeinated drinks as a "break" during the day. This is their time to relax. Even though the physical effects of nicotine and caffeine work against physical relaxation, these

may be considered by the user to be "relaxing activities" if they have often been used during these breaks. The users have expectations that having a cigarette or drinking caffeinated drinks will help them to relax. Smoking cigarettes and caffeinated drinks can be "something to do" in a setting where there seems to be little else to do. For many people who have been hospitalized for SMI, caffeinated drinks (if available) and cigarette use increase during inpatient stays because there is a lack of meaningful and interesting activities. The same is true for home or community settings where the person living with COD may spend a lot of time with little to do. After the higher level of use has become habitual, it is difficult to reduce it even when other activities are made available. The person has become accustomed to consuming more caffeinated drinks and smoking more cigarettes, she will prefer to do these instead of other things.

In almost all cases, both psychosocial and biological influences should be assessed in trying to help the person stay refrain from substances. The challenge to mental health professional service providers is to identify what the influences are and pursue effective strategies.

Behavioral Support Strategies with Individuals Living with Co-occurring Mental Health Problems (COD)

The following suggestions represent steps that a service provider should consider when attempting to reduce the use of substances by a person living with SMI. Not all these suggestions will apply in all cases. It is likely that several of these can be helpful when used together.

- Conduct a comprehensive assessment of the issue. If there is suspicion that an individual who lives with an SMI is using substances, this factor must be incorporated into any treatment plan. Most mental health facilities have professionals specializing in co-occurring mental health conditions (COD), who should participate in developing the treatment strategy. Effective intervention requires the provider to address both substance-use-related conditions (SUD) and SMI.
- Specify which substances are being used and the timing of their use, including caffeine and nicotine. When substance use is identified as problematic, describe clearly the nature and patterns of usage. Document instances of use, including the context, location, people present, time of day, and associated emotional states. Determining these variables is critical in formulating an approach to reduce substance use. For example, if consumption tends to occur with specific individuals or in specific locations and times, avoidance strategies may be beneficial. If use frequently happens during certain times, such as before bed, alternative activities can be scheduled to provide distraction.
- For instance, alcohol consumption may be more prevalent during evening hours while watching television. Attempts to quit may coincide with periods of isolation

or low mood. Staff concerns regarding behaviors such as smoking in bed or consuming coffee outside designated areas—particularly if they result in safety or cleanliness issues—should be noted. Additionally, the timing of consumption is important; drinking coffee late in the day may adversely affect sleep quality. Precise identification of these factors enhances the development of effective treatment plans for individuals living with COD.

- Cigarette/caffeinated drinks use may be a problem for several reasons. For some, the unhealthy physical effects of using cigarettes and caffeine might be considered a problem. Some use of caffeinated drinks and smoking may be acceptable, but it becomes a problem when the amount is excessive or the context in which the substance is used by the person living with COD is not acceptable (e.g., on public transportation).
- Monitor medications carefully for individuals with COD. Substance use can alter the intended effects of psychiatric medicines, sometimes increasing them to dangerous levels or decreasing their benefits. If drug use cannot be stopped, seek advice from a psychiatric service provider who is familiar with the interaction between psychiatric medications and substances of use.
- Be clear about expectations. Substance use is something that should be avoided for anyone living with SMI. Be clear that substance use should not occur. State this goal in a clear but matter of fact and nonjudgmental manner (e.g., "I think that drinking alcohol can be dangerous with the medication that you take. I do not want you to drink alcohol as it is more important for you to continue taking the medication. Doing this will help you stay out of the hospital and make you feel better, so it is best for you not to drink."). The clearer that this behavior is to be avoided, the more likely it is that the person living with SMI will understand. This task may present significant challenges for many individuals. Those who have concerns about their capacity to manage this effectively are encouraged to consult with a mental health service provider. For additional guidance on discussing these matters with individuals living with SMI, refer to Chap. 4
- Identify activities that the person living with COD likes and can keep the person active in reinforcing and pleasurable activities. The MOs to use substances by individuals living with COD are to experience pleasure (e.g., release of dopamine) and decrease aversive respondents and private events (e.g., thoughts). The activities can help take the place of the effects of a substance, especially if boredom is an antecedent when the person living with COD has cravings. Make access to these activities easy for the person living with COD to engage in.
- Use access to certain activities that the person clearly enjoys as a reward for success in meeting the goals that have been set. Consider developing a contract for behavior to clarify the expectations and the rewards for progress.

What Are Reasonable Expectations for Change in a Person Living with Co-occurring Mental Health Problems (COD)?

COD can be difficult to treat. Substances that are used can interfere with the beneficial effect of the medications that treat many problem behaviors/symptoms of SMI. Abstinence (e.g., no use at all) is the safest goal but not easily attained. Even if abstinence is clearly identified as the preferred goal, it is usually very hard to achieve. Some people with SMI may stop using substances due to advice from providers or family, but others may not grasp the goal's importance and continue using them. Cravings often occur in familiar settings or moods, especially for those with past substance-use-related conditions (SUD). Abstinence can still be the goal that caregivers should communicate.

- Set realistic goals. Complete elimination of substances, especially cigarette and caffeinated drink use, may be unrealistic. Quitting substances is hard for anyone, but recovery can be more challenging for someone with COD (Dennis & Scott, 2008). If quitting completely is unrealistic, consider "harm reduction." Harm reduction refers to interventions aimed at reducing the negative effects of health behaviors without having the expectation that the problematic health behaviors will be completely or permanently eradicated (Hawk et al., 2017). The principles of harm reduction are defined and specified as follows (Hawk et al., 2017):
  - **Humanism**: Services are user-friendly, responsive to the needs of the individual, and free of moral judgments. Recognizes that harmful health behaviors provide some benefit to the individual, and understanding these benefits is empowering for service providers and users.
  - **Pragmatism**: Perfect health behaviors and abstinence may be both unrealistic. The goals need to focus on actual harm rather than moral or societal standards; service providers recognize the influence of social and community norms on health-related behaviors.
  - **Individualism**: Service providers recognize and assess individual strengths and needs without assumptions and maximize treatment options.
  - **Autonomy**: Service provider-user partnerships emphasize shared decision-making and reciprocal learning about treatment.
  - **Incrementalism**: Positive change is improvement; plateaus or setbacks are seen as part of the process; progress is slow and nonlinear.
  - **Accountability without Termination**: Individuals are responsible for their health choices; relapse is seen as part of the process; and individuals are supported in understanding the consequences of their decisions.
- Using harm reduction, the service provider and user work together to determine what is acceptable in terms of the dimension of substance use. Be cautious about setting goals that are too ambitious. For example, attempting to try to eliminate use of cigarette/caffeinated drink may create a variety of other problems such as stealing or "bumming" the desired items. Cutting off the use of some substances

may cause withdrawal symptoms and overdose. If the person living with COD becomes secretive about the SUD, the task will be much more difficult. It is usually best to seek small but more easily achievable changes in behavior and slowly increase expectations. It is often helpful to establish goals and specify rewards for success in a formal contract for the behaviors.

Be clear about your goals and expectations. Clarifying your goals can be best achieved by establishing a contract that specifies the dimension of the substance use targeted for change as well as the times and places where it is allowed. The contract should also state rewards for success and consequences if goals are not met. For example, Jordan and the service providers at the residence agreed that he would only smoke outside. The contract helped everyone understand what was expected and allowed Jordan to get a variety of things that he wanted for successfully meeting those expectations.

- In most cases, the goals should initially be set at the current level of use so they can be easily reached. Afterward, the goals can be changed gradually. Regardless of any rewards that are designated for progress, remember to compliment or praise the person living with COD for success in achieving any success.
- The use and possession of illicit substances in many countries have severe legal consequences. Harm reduction would be difficult with many substances as the principles accept the use of substances as part of the process of reducing health-related harmful outcomes. The possibility of legal consequences needs to be considered in harm reduction.
- Expectations should apply to all individuals interacting with someone living with COD. All stakeholders and mental health service providers should adhere to consistent expectations and goals. If the goal is abstinence or controlled use, service providers must act accordingly. Inconsistent goals can hinder progress toward achieving them.
- Individuals living with COD may resume substance use, leading to potential difficulties. This should not be perceived as a failure but as a reflection of the challenge in maintaining long-term abstinence. If substance use recurs, actions can be taken to address it (such as reminders, brief hospitalization, or more frequent recovery meetings) and initiate a new phase of recovery. It is important to persist with recovery efforts as progress is nonlinear. Many individuals who avoid substance use successfully have experienced multiple setbacks. Mental health service professionals can assist in identifying appropriate goals for individuals living with COD.
- Avoid having substances in the home. If you want to eliminate alcohol and other drug use in the living situation for the person living with SMI, whether home, group home, adult care residence, or an apartment, avoid having alcohol or other substances readily available. Some caregivers may be frustrated that they can't drink in their own home, but substance use is much less likely to occur if substances are not easily available and other members of the home avoid using them. It is the same for use of prescribed medications that can be abused, such as opioids ("pain killers"), benzodiazepines (antianxiety, hypnotics, "sleep

medications"), and stimulants ("ADHD medications," "weight loss"). OTC cold and cough medications can be abused. If the person living with COD has a problem with taking pills and OTC medications, keep these medications away from the person living with COD. Be sure that all medications are taken properly and stored away after they are used. Be aware that all medications, including commonly taken ones (e.g., Tylenol, Motrin, Pepcid, Robitussin DM), have side effects.

- Having access to cigarettes, caffeinated drinks, and alcohol is one important factor in whether use continues to happen. If other members of the family also smoke and drink coffee/energy drinks and/or alcohol, it is more likely that these will be accessible in the house. If friends of the person living with COD continue to smoke, they will probably "light up" in front of him. This makes it easier for the person living with SMI to use them; if it is harder for the person living with COD to get cigarettes and caffeinated drinks, the less likely it is that they will use them.
- Acknowledge successes; don't take them for granted. If substance use has been a problem in the past, don't ignore the effort to avoid use by the person living with COD. It is difficult to be certain if someone with COD is using substances, but one can observe if past substance-related behaviors persist. If the person living with COD is doing the activities suggested by their recovery team to help avoid using, such as going to the clubhouse and attending recovery meetings as scheduled, tell the person living with COD these efforts are appreciated. For example, one relevant challenge for most people living with COD is attending support group meetings. Most prefer not to go. Supportive comments from others are helpful in maintaining the person's willingness to attend support group meetings. If improvement in the behavior of the person living with COD is observed and the results are because of successfully staying away from substances (e.g., more agreeable, better mood, improvements in self-care), point out the improvement. For example, one can say: "I have noticed how you are getting up and taking a shower every morning since you stopped drinking. I also have seen your room is clean. Great job!"
- Don't expect immediate success. Stay aware of the potent incentives that serve to maintain SUD. The person living with COD becomes accustomed to using substances and may not be aware of the triggers—certain places, times, people linked to using substances. These are usually well-established habits that are resistant to change, like smoking and drinking coffee in the morning. Some initial failures should be expected in trying to manage the SUD. Early failures happen, and persistence is needed; progress is nonlinear.
- Although difficult, try to develop available alternatives to using substances. For example, using nicotine replacement gum, spray, or lozenges can help to lessen the uncomfortable feelings that may result when a person smokes less. Nonalcoholic beer has the same taste as alcoholic beer.
- If the person living with COD uses the nicotine replacement item and continues to smoke the same amount, the nicotine in his body can reach dangerous levels. Because of this, these items should be used only under close supervision. There

are a variety of techniques used by psychologists and other mental health service professionals to help people reduce the uncomfortable respondents correlated with cravings. Using mindfulness-based interventions can assist an individual living with COD to reduce the impact of cravings and reinforce not using substances (Tapper, 2018).

- Be prepared to assert oneself in a firm but nonjudgmental fashion. If you suspect substance use, communicate this in a brief, clear, and nonjudgmental fashion. Be prepared to speak up whenever there is evidence that there is a problem. However, don't expect that the person living with COD to suddenly change. Be prepared to encounter frustration in the efforts. It may be necessary to have a mental health service provider be a "coach" in this.

How to Determine If a Person Living with a Co-occurring Mental Health Problem (COD) Is Using Substances

By being familiar with the person living with COD, one is more likely to be aware of changes in behavior that appear suddenly. Alcohol has a lingering smell, and there are signs of abuse such as empty containers, bottles, and material that is associated with the use of other substances (e.g., plastic "baggies" with residue, pipes, bongs, needles); cigarettes leave a smell and ashes; there are used cigarettes and packages. If one becomes aware of the person's use of substances, observe the person to see what problems happen relapse.

- The person living with COD may attempt to hide the use of substances if they become aware of others knowing of their use. In some cases, observed behaviors may be related to drug use (sleeping late, talking louder and faster, yelling angrily, threatening, experiencing hallucinations, delusional speech) although there is no evidence of use of substances. In almost all cases, problems that can be caused by drug use possibly can be caused by other reasons as well, such as a worsening of the problem behaviors/symptoms of living with a SMI. In the end, focus primarily on the observables and what is known from past behaviors. If the person living with COD is "irritable" and substance use is suspected, one can briefly and clearly state concerns that substance use may be a part of the problem (but avoid accusing the person if unsure). However, continuing to talk and accusing them of using substances will only lead to an argument, especially if the person living with COD denies using any substance and there is no evidence of relapse. Focus on the problems that are observed but be more observant for substance use. Also check for involvement in activities (going to clubhouse, going to support and recovery groups, "hanging out" with others who use substances) that help the person living with COD stay in recovery. Compliment involvement in those recovery activities.
- Avoid pushing too hard; stay patient; success may take time. When encouraging an individual with a co-occurring mental health problem (COD) to discontinue

substance use, seek assistance from a mental health professional, or attend support group meetings, it is important to maintain a respectful approach and refrain from applying excessive pressure or engaging in confrontations. Often, the harder one tries, the less persuasive one becomes and is perceived as harassing. Instead, choose a time when the person living with COD seems to be doing well and is more willing to talk about the problem. Be patient. Usually, change occurs very slowly. Assistance from a professional mental health service provider may be necessary in understanding the challenges of staying in recovery.

- Consider developing a behavioral contract. If the person living with SMI shows willingness to attend therapy or support/recovery group meetings, include this in the contract. With the engagement and involvement of the person living with COD, the contract should specify certain preferred activities or other possible rewards that can be made available for progress in recovery. One can reward success at staying away from substances. Reinforce the behaviors that are important for continuing in recovery. For example, going to the mall and buying a desired item may be made contingent upon going to support group meetings every day during the week. Provide positive recognition for any progress that is observed (e.g., "I see that you went to the recovery clubhouse three days in a row. I am proud of you for taking your recovery seriously.")
- Seek support groups that are familiar with problems with people living with COD; be cautious about involvement in traditional substance treatments. Sometimes, meetings of traditional drug treatment programs and support groups (such as Alcoholics Anonymous (AA) or Narcotics Anonymous (NA)) may not be appropriate for someone who is living with COD. While these programs and support groups can be valuable sources of help, members in these groups who are not living with COD may not understand—or be accepting—the additional difficulties that are caused by COD. These programs are more likely to set expectations that are too high and can worsen the condition of the person living with COD. Plan attendance for these groups with the assistance of a professional mental health service provider who is familiar with support group meetings in the area. The COD service professional can suggest the most appropriate meetings to attend.
- Get support for oneself if caring for a person living with COD. Just as meetings of such organizations as the National Alliance on Mental Illness (NAMI) can be helpful in coping with having SMI in a family member, other groups, such as Al-Anon, which focuses on the challenges faced by family members of someone with substance-use-related issues (SUD), can clarify how substance use affects other members in the family. Members of these groups usually have appreciation for the challenges and problems faced by family members and caregivers. They can sometimes give practical information and support that even the most experienced professional mental health service provider cannot provide.

Conclusion for Behavioral Support Strategies with Individuals Living with Co-occurring Mental Health Problems (COD)

When faced with problems related to co-occurring mental health problems (COD), consider the following steps:

1. Take the use of substances seriously. Don't assume that problems related to COD will go away if the problem of living with SMI improves. Both problems—substance use and SMI—must be taken seriously.
2. Identify local "specialists" in treating COD who are familiar with how to intervene in cases where there is COD. Involve these people in treatment planning.
3. Try to be aware of the types and timing of the substances used. This information is the first step in planning strategies to minimize drug use.
4. Identify local programs and support groups that are available for people living with COD. The help of a local "specialist" may be helpful in identifying these programs.
5. "Model" the behaviors that are expected of the person living with COD. If expectations are that the person is to avoid substances, minimize use of, and access to substances around the person living with COD.
6. Try developing a contract to clarify expectations and reinforce any success. Specify the incentives to meet those expectations. This can help keep motivation as high as possible.
7. Seek support. Support groups such as Al-Anon or NAMI can provide practical advice and support in managing the level of stress. Staying calm, understanding COD, realistic expectations, or progress, and what to do is the best path to success.

What About Jordan?

During the hospitalization, the mental health service providers recognized that they needed to treat both Jordan's depression and alcohol use. When Jordan stopped drinking, he became very nervous, irritable, depressed, drank large amounts of caffeinated drinks, and smoked 2–3 packs of cigarettes daily. While Jordan's depression had responded well to medication, the treatment team knew that this improvement would not continue after discharge unless Jordan had help in learning to control dimensions of his use of alcohol. He was fortunate that his alcohol use had not resulted in serious neurological damage and physical problems. They also understood that while Jordan became friendly and cooperative after stabilizing, this did not mean that he would follow through with the recommendations that were given, particularly about the use of substances.

The residential staff had concerns about Jordan's smoking and using caffeinated drinks, stealing them from a nearby convenience store, and using cigarettes in unsafe places, especially his bedroom. Jordan was careless when he drank coffee and smoked, spilling ashes and drink on his clothes and furniture and burning holes in his clothes.

A behavioral oriented service provider met with Jordan to assess the smoking and caffeine use. Jordan did state it was better for him not to smoke and admitted not paying attention when he drinks coffee. Jordan was smoking more than a 2 packs of cigarettes a day, and he agreed that it would be more realistic to cut smoking down to a pack; everyone drank coffee at the residence (including staff), and there was always a pot brewing so eliminating it would be unrealistic. Because the cigarettes were very important to Jordan, the consultant worked with Jordan where and when he could drink coffee and smoke safely. Jordan was able to give his opinion and change the goals to be more realistic. This helped Jordan to feel more enthusiastic about the plan and in control of his treatment.

Service providers at the residence developed a contract with him to attend all group meetings that were intended for individuals living with COD, take his medication as prescribed, go to his clubhouse work assignment each day, smoke only outside of the house (in a designated area), and drink coffee in the kitchen at the table or outside.

Residential staff gave him a pack of cigarettes after breakfast each day when he got out of bed by 7 am and took his morning medications. If he was observed smoking inside the house, he would be allocated half a pack in the morning, and staff would allow him one cigarette per hour after he came back from meetings and activities. All agreed to stop complaining about how much he smoked if he was meeting expectations of the contract. A "reminder sign" was placed next to the coffee maker prompting Jordon where to smoke and drink as specified. If Jordan succeeded in meeting these expectations, Jordan would get $30 spending money on each Saturday morning (e.g., $5 for each weekday that he succeeded in meeting them and $5 extra for meeting them all week).

At the meetings for COD, he was introduced to a person who could be his sponsor in the community at these meetings. When Jordan returned from a meeting, he met with staff who showed positive interest in what he thought about the meeting and his recovery.

As with most behavioral contracts, there were problems getting everyone to work together during the first few weeks. For example, Jordan missed several meetings during the first few days; a pack of cigarettes to give him after breakfast was not always available. The residential staff, service providers, and Jordan persevered, resolved the problems, and became more consistent. After a couple of months, following the expectations of the contract had become "automatic" and the challenges subsided. While Jordan never quit smoking, he did reduce his smoking to one pack per day. He stopped smoking in the house and was much more consistent about taking his medications and going to the clubhouse and meetings for COD. By following this approach, Jordan maintained his interest in activities that helped him to remember the importance of avoiding substances. He worked with community mental health service providers who spent time with him to show interest in and encourage participation in the recovery groups and activities.

Summary

Co-occurring mental health problems (COD) involve the simultaneous presence of mental health and substance use problems. Approximately half of individuals living with SMI develop a substance use condition (SUD) in their lifetime. Higher prevalence of SUD is found in individuals with SMI compared to the general population. Common mental health issues in COD include anxiety, PTSD, and depression. SMI includes mental health problems like psychosis, bipolar, and major depression mental health conditions. Functional impairments from COD can lead to unemployment, poor social support, and homelessness.

Individuals with SMI have higher rates of substance use, with one in four also having an SUD. National surveys indicate a 3.8% year-over-year increase in substance use among those aged 12 and older. In 2019, 60.1% of US adults used substances, with 50.8% consuming alcohol and 21.1% using tobacco. Drug use was highest among ages 18–25, with 39% reporting illicit drug use. Individuals living with SMI use tobacco in cigarettes at rates 2–3 times higher than the general population. People living with SMI consume almost twice as much caffeine compared to the general population. Caffeine may provide cognitive benefits but can also induce anxiety and insomnia at high doses. Smoking accelerates caffeine metabolism, leading to higher consumption among smokers.

COD complicates the determination and treatment of mental health issues. Approximately 35% of adults with mental health issues living in the United States experience SUD. SUD is characterized by uncontrolled substance use despite harmful consequences, affecting over 20 million Americans. The DSM-5-TR outlines 11 criteria for SUD, including impaired control and social problems. Prevalence estimates of the problematic use of alcohol, cannabis, and opioid are significantly higher than previously reported. Shared risk factors for COD include genetics, environmental stressors, and self-medication behaviors.

Substance use can exacerbate symptoms of SMI, leading to increased severity and frequency of problem behaviors. Substance use can alter the metabolism of psychiatric medications, affecting treatment outcomes. Occasional substance use by individuals with SMI has not been thoroughly investigated for its impact on quality of life and exacerbation of problem behaviors.

Trauma and chronic stress are associated with increased risk of developing both SMI and SUD. Young people exposed to multiple traumatic experiences have a higher likelihood of developing an SUD. Protective factors against SUD include positive parental influence and community relationships.

Understanding the dimensions of co-occurring mental health problems (COD) is crucial for effective assessment and intervention strategies. A dimensional approach assesses behaviors and symptoms related to all mental health problems, focusing on severity and complexity. Research has shown that using dimensional measures predicts treatment outcomes better than categorical assessments.

Assessment tools for SMI and SUD vary in properties and types of administration. The Addiction Severity Index (ASI) evaluates addiction-related problems across seven dimensions, including medical, employment, and psychiatric status. ASI assesses the possibility of COD by determining if mental health issues are substance-related or independent. Alcohol Addiction Research Domain Criteria (AARDoC) integrates behavioral, neurobiological, and genetic domains to enhance understanding and treatment of SUD. The Addictions Neuroclinical Assessment (ANA) identifies three domains: reward/incentive salience, negative emotionality, and cognitive control impairments.

The PhenX toolkit establishes consensus measurements for various health-related constructs, including substance misuse. PhenX Toolkit assesses dimensions such as type of substance used, duration, frequency, motives for use, and perceived consequences.

Studies have identified 73 valid self-report measures for SUD treatment. The measures assess dimensions like use, severity, consequences, recovery readiness, and cravings; craving is defined as an unrelenting desire to use substances despite harmful consequences, influenced by both overt and covert stimuli. The studies concluded that future research should focus on developing measures for emerging substances and implementing measurement-based care in treatment settings.

Substance use (SUD) and co-occurring conditions (COD) are complex, transdiagnostic phenomenological concepts with multiple interacting domains including physical, psychological, and behavioral. An example of the complexity of COD is using the concept of pain. The assessment and treatment of pain involve physical, psychological (emotional), and behavioral aspects and their complex interactions. Similarly, a thorough evaluation of COD should encompass topography of the problematic behaviors, awareness, craving for the substance, and environmental triggers to gain a better understanding of the condition.

COD involves mental health issues affecting reward, motivation, memory, and decision-making. It leads to significant social, academic, and occupational impairments due to substance misuse. Factors influencing substance use conditions (SUD) include psychological, biological, sociocultural, and environmental elements. Individuals with COD use more substances and experience more negative outcomes than those with SUD alone. COD is associated with compulsive substance use, severity, and treatment resistance. In addition, people living with COD live with a greater incidence of polysubstance use that complicates the assessment and treatment of COD. Over 66% of individuals with heroin use problems are dependent on nicotine. Nearly 25% of individuals with heroin use problems also have problems with alcohol use. Among cocaine users, nearly 60% misuse alcohol, and 48% are nicotine dependent.

COD involves complex interactions between neurobiological substrates influenced by genetic and environmental factors. Key brain areas affected include the prefrontal cortex, nucleus accumbens, amygdala, hippocampus, and ventral tegmental area. Impaired dopamine release may lead to hypohedonia in individuals with alcohol use disorder. Neurotransmitters in SUD include dopamine (DA), which is central to the reward system; increased release contributes to relapse. Serotonin (5-HT) affects mood regulation and is influenced by substances like methylenedioxymethamphetamine (MDMA) and alcohol. GABA is enhanced by alcohol and benzodiazepines, leading to calming effects. Glutamate disruption affects learning and memory, while endorphins and norepinephrine are influenced by opioids and stimulants, respectively.

The substances used have substance-specific effects on the structures and functioning of the central nervous system. Marijuana impairs memory, attention, and decision-making, impacting structural changes in the hippocampus and prefrontal cortex. Cocaine affects executive function and memory with structural changes in the prefrontal cortex and risks of ischemic strokes. Methamphetamine impairs episodic memory and executive function and is associated with Parkinson's disease and stroke risk. Methylenedioxymethamphetamine (MDMA) causes verbal memory deficits and anxiety with structural changes in the orbitofrontal cortex and risks of cerebral edema. Heroin leads to visual memory deficits and hypoxic brain damage, and structural changes include enlarged ventricles and risks of ischemic strokes. Synthetic cathinones impair long-term memory and may cause vessel damage, although evidence of neurotoxicity is limited.

COD arises from the interaction of biological, psychological, and environmental factors affecting those with SMI. Substance use is often seen as self-medication to reduce psychological distress and problematic behaviors linked to SMI.

Environmental factors like trauma, poverty, and social isolation increase susceptibility to SUD. The environment affects the development and persistence of COD. Classical conditioning illustrates how environmental cues can elicit cravings and drug-seeking behaviors. Conditioned stimuli (CSs) can prompt cravings even when the drug is not present. Drug-related cues may lead to withdrawal symptoms, encouraging substance use to relieve discomfort. Tolerance occurs as the body adjusts to drug effects, necessitating larger doses for the same impact. Compensatory conditioned responses (CCRs) counteract drug effects, making tolerance more evident in familiar environments. Withdrawal symptoms can provoke relapses, particularly when exposed to drug-related cues.

Motivating operations (MOs) influence the likelihood of drug-seeking behaviors through environmental or internal factors. Social learning through observation of role models can encourage substance use behaviors. Individuals may view substance use as acceptable or rewarding due to social reinforcement from peers and media influences.

The prevalence and implications of co-occurring mental health problems (COD) among individuals with substance use conditions (SUD) and SMI varies according to age, sex, race, and other factors. Significant associations have been found between SUDs and younger age, male sex, and inpatient status. Individuals with COD experience shorter relapses but higher readmission rates. Economic problems are reported in 41.9% of individuals living with SUD.

Co-occurring mental health problems (COD) constitute 26% of individuals who live with SMI and 37% of those with substance use issues (SUD) in the United States. Approximately 35% of adults experiencing mental health challenges also have a SUD. It is further estimated that 50–70% of individuals in treatment for SUD present with COD, while 20–50% of those with mental health conditions are affected by SUD.

Early substance use increases the risk of COD; adolescents have double the prevalence of SUD after first use compared to young adults over 18 years of age. Lifetime prevalence of SUD after first use in adolescence is 26.3% for alcohol, 5.4% for cannabis use, and 13.4% for tobacco. Lifetime prevalence of SUD after initiation in young adulthood is 79.7% for alcohol, 51.5% for cannabis, and 55.0% for tobacco.

Racial and ethnic disparities have been found in studies with individuals living with COD. There is a higher lifetime prevalence of COD among Whites (8.2%) compared to Blacks (5.4%), Latinos (5.8%), and Asians (2.1%). Among individuals with alcohol use problems, Whites are more likely to experience mood-related issues than Blacks. Average age of onset for SUD is younger for Whites (20.2 years) than for Blacks (21.8 years).

The prevalence of COD varies globally; significant increases in alcohol and opioid problems are noted in Europe, Africa, and Asia. In South Africa, COD prevalence ranges from 50 to 68%. Cannabis use problems are most prevalent among individuals with SMI, with a lifetime prevalence of 27.1%. In Canada, 12-month prevalence of COD is 1.7%, and it is higher in males (2.1%) than females (1.4%). In the United Kingdom, COD prevalence ranges from 20–37%, with higher rates in urban areas. People of color living in the United Kingdom are overrepresented in COD cases compared to their proportion in the general population.

COD can be classified based on the mental health issue, substance type, and dimensions like onset age, severity, duration, use frequency, controllability, and negative outcomes. DSM-5-TR lists substances that can be misused, including alcohol, cannabis, opioids, and stimulants. The severity of substance use condition (SUD) is classified according to the number of DSM-5 criteria met, meeting 2–3 criteria indicate a mild case, 4–5 criteria signify a moderate case, and meeting six or more criteria constitutes severe SUD.

The assessment of behavioral dimensions in individuals living with both SMI and SUD is crucial for understanding the presenting behavior problems corresponding to COD. Severity of SUD and SMI impacts treatment responsivity. Types of COD can be classified based on the mental health problems and type of substances used. An example would be an individual living with schizophrenia spectrum disorder and opioid use who experiences auditory hallucinations (AH). The use of an opioid is functional in that the effect of the drug temporarily decreases AH, leading to the negative reinforcement of using the drug.

The presence of co-occurring mental health problems (COD) complicates treatment, requiring integrated approaches for both mental health and substance use issues. Approximately 50% of individuals hospitalized for problems associated with SMI also struggle with substance use issues. Alcohol, cannabis, and amphetamines are the most frequently used substances. Legal substances like caffeine and nicotine are excessively used by individuals living with SMI and can interfere with psychiatric medications.

Substance use issues arise from a combination of genetic, biological, psychosocial, and environmental factors. These factors can create a cycle of use that is difficult to break, especially for individuals with SMI. Genetic predisposition can increase the likelihood of developing SUD. Substances may provide temporary relief from distressing emotions or symptoms of SMI. Environmental stressors, history of trauma experiences, social influences, boredom, and the lack of reinforcing activities can contribute to substance use by individuals living with SMI.

Substance use can exacerbate symptoms of SMI, leading to a cycle of worsening mental health. Substances use can entail physical dependence, withdrawal symptoms, and habitual use, leading to various health and psychological issues. Withdrawal symptoms can include irritability, hallucinations, and cognitive difficulties, making it challenging for individuals to abstain from substance use. Physical dependence develops over time, requiring increased amounts of a drug for the same effect.

Effective treatment for individuals living with COD requires a comprehensive approach that includes thorough evaluation, clear communication by service providers, and the development of supportive activities. Strategies should focus on minimizing substance use while promoting engagement in healthier behaviors. A thorough evaluation of the dimensions of the substance use and problem behaviors linked to living with SMI is a priority. Service providers need to establish dimensions of substance use by tracking patterns of use to identify triggers and contexts of use and to establish clear expectations regarding substance use and its impact on health. Reinforcing activities and behaviors need to be identified and promoted to replace behaviors related to substance use.

Setting realistic goals for individuals with a co-occurring mental health problem (COD) involves establishing achievable objectives and gradually increasing expectations for behavior change. Achievements should be acknowledged, and positive reinforcement should be used to encourage progress. While abstinence is the safest goal, it may be challenging to attain. Harm reduction strategies can be utilized to reduce negative outcomes while progressively working toward reducing substance use. Harm reduction aims to lessen adverse effects rather than achieving complete cessation, recognizing that recovery is not linear and emphasizing progress toward this objective.

Support from mental health professionals, family, and community resources is essential for individuals living with COD. Engaging in support groups and developing contracts for behavior can help maintain motivation and accountability. Specialists familiar with COD should be involved in treatment planning. Identification of local support groups and programs tailored for individuals with COD needs to be part of any treatment plan. Behavioral contracts can be developed to clarify expectations and reinforce positive behaviors, encouraging participation in recovery activities and acknowledging progress.

References

Ajit, J., Abhishek, P., & Asheesh, K. (2013). Illicit drugs and their assessment: A brief review. *Research Journal of Forensic Sciences, 1*(1), 8–14. https://www.researchgate.net/publication/236165951_Illicit_Drugs_and_their_Assessment_A_Brief_Review

American Psychiatric Association. (2013). *Diagnostic and statistical manual of mental disorders* (5th ed.). https://doi.org/10.1176/appi.books.9780890425596

American Psychiatric Association. (2018). *What is mental illness?* American Psychiatric Association https://www.psychiatry.org/patients-families/what-ismental-illness

American Psychiatric Association. (2022). *Diagnostic and statistical manual of mental disorders* (5th ed., rev.). https://doi.org/10.1176/appi.books.9780890425787

American Psychiatric Association. (2025). *What is a substance use disorder?* Psychiatry.org. https://www.psychiatry.org/patients-families/addiction-substance-use-disorders/what-is-a-substance-use-disorder

American Psychological Association. (2018). Social learning theory. In *APA Dictionary of Psychology*. https://dictionary.apa.org/social-learning-theory

American Psychological Association. (n.d.-a). Associative learning. In *APA dictionary of psychology* https://dictionary.apa.org/associative-learning

American Psychological Association. (n.d.-b). Craving. In *APA dictionary of psychology*. https://dictionary.apa.org/craving

American Psychological Association. (n.d.-c). Substance dependence. In *APA dictionary of psychology*. https://dictionary.apa.org/substance-dependence

Andrade, M. C. R., Slade, M., Bandeira, M., Evans-Lacko, S., Komaroff, J., Martin, D., Gonçalves, D. A., Gouveia, M. C., Mari, J. J., Bressan, R. A., Wang, Y.-P., Fortes, S., & Andreoli, S. B. (2016). Subjective distress in a representative sample of outpatients with psychotic disorders. *Journal of Affective Disorders, 189*, 220–223. https://doi.org/10.1016/j.jad.2015.08.075

Arlinghaus, K. R., & Johnston, C. A. (2019). The importance of creating habits and routine. *American Journal of Lifestyle Medicine, 13*(2), 142–144. https://doi.org/10.1177/1559827618818044

Bahji, A. (2024). Navigating the complex intersection of substance use and psychiatric disorders: A comprehensive review. *Journal of Clinical Medicine, 13*, 999. https://doi.org/10.3390/jcm13040999

Baingana, F., Becker, A. E., & Pringle, B. (2015). Global research challenges and opportunities for mental health and substance-use disorders. *Nature, 527*(7578), S172–S177. https://doi.org/10.1038/nature16032

Boness, C. L., Carlos Gonzalez, J., Sleep, C., Venner, K. L., & Witkiewitz, K. (2024). Evidence-based assessment of substance use disorder. *Assessment, 31*(1), 168–190. https://doi.org/10.1177/10731911231177252

Cacciola, J. S., Alterman, A. I., Habing, B., & McLellan, A. T. (2011). Recent status scores for version 6 of the addiction severity index (ASI-6). *Addiction, 106*(9), 1588–1602. https://doi.org/10.1111/j.1360-0443.2011.03482.x

Cadet, J. L., Bisagno, V., & Milroy, C. M. (2014). Neuropathology of substance use disorders. *Acta Neuropathologica, 127*, 91–107. https://doi.org/10.1007/s00401-013-1221-7

Carra, G., & Johnson, S. (2009). Variations in rates of comorbid substance use in psychosis between mental health settings and geographical areas in the UK: A systematic review. *Social Psychiatry and Psychiatric Epidemiology, 44*, 429–447. https://doi.org/10.1007/s00127-008-0458-2

Cooper, J. O., Heron, T. E., & Heward, W. L. (2020). *Applied behavior analysis* (3rd ed.). Pearson. https://www.pearson.com/en-us/pearsonplus/p/9780137477210

Del Rio Szupszynski, K. P., & de Ávila, A. C. (2021). The transtheoretical model of behavior change: Prochaska and Diclemente's model. In A. L. M. Andrade, D. De Micheli, E. A. da Silva, F. M. Lopes, B. de Oliveira Pinheiro, & R. A. Reichert (Eds.), *Psychology of substance abuse: Psychotherapy, clinical management and social intervention* (pp. 205–216). Springer Nature Switzerland AG. https://doi.org/10.1007/978-3-030-62106-3_7

Dennis, M., & Scott, C. K. (2008). Managing addiction as a chronic condition. *Addiction Science & Clinical Practice, 4*(1), 45. https://doi.org/10.1151/ascp074145

Di Pierro, R., Preti, E., Vurro, N., & Madeddu, F. (2014). Dimensions of personality structure among patients with substance use disorders and co-occurring personality disorders: A comparison with psychiatric outpatients and healthy controls. *Comprehensive Psychiatry, 55*(6), 1398–1404. https://doi.org/10.1016/j.comppsych.2014.04.005

Drake, R. E., Wallach, M. A., Alverson, H. S., & Mueser, K. T. (2002). Psychosocial aspects of substance abuse by clients with severe mental illness. *The Journal of Nervous and Mental Disease, 190*(2), 100–106. https://doi.org/10.1097/00005053-200202000-00006

Evans, T. S., Berkman, N., Brown, C., Gaynes, B., & Weber, R. P. (2016). *Disparities within serious mental illness*. Agency for Healthcare Research and Quality (US). (Technical Briefs, No. 25.). https://www.ncbi.nlm.nih.gov/books/NBK368430/

Flynn, P. M., & Brown, B. S. (2008). Co-occurring disorders in substance abuse treatment: Issues and prospects. *Journal of Substance Abuse Treatment, 34*(1), 36–47. https://doi.org/10.1016/j.jsat.2006.11.005

Gardner, B., Lally, P., & Wardle, J. (2012). Making health habitual: The psychology of 'habit-formation' and general practice. *British Journal of General Practice, 62*(605), 664–666. https://doi.org/10.3399/bjgp12X659466

Gonzales, L., Kois, L. E., Chen, C., López-Aybar, L., McCullough, B., & McLaughlin, K. J. (2022). Reliability of the term "serious mental illness": A systematic review. *Psychiatric Services, 73*(11), 1255–1262. https://doi.org/10.1176/appi.ps.202100661

Grant, J. E., & Chamberlain, S. R. (2016). Expanding the definition of addiction: DSM-5 vs. ICD-11. *CNS Spectrums, 21*(4), 300–303. https://doi.org/10.1017/s1092852916000183

Griffin, J. B., Jr. (1990). Substance abuse. In H. K. Walker, W. D. Hall, & J. W. Hurst (Eds.), *Clinical methods: The history, physical, and laboratory examinations* (3rd ed.). Butterworths. https://www.ncbi.nlm.nih.gov/books/NBK709

Hamilton, C. M., Strader, L. C., Pratt, J. G., Maiese, D., Hendershot, T., Kwok, R. K., Hammond, J. A., Huggins, W., Jackman, D., Pan, H., Nettles, D. S., Beaty, T. H., Farrer, L. A., Kraft, P., Marazita, M. L., Ordovas, J. M., Pato, C. N., Spitz, M. R., Wagener, D., & Haines, J. (2011). The PhenX toolkit: Get the most from your measures. *American Journal of Epidemiology, 174*(3), 253–260. https://doi.org/10.1093/aje/kwr193

Han, B., Compton, W. M., Blanco, C., & Colpe, L. J. (2017). Prevalence, treatment, and unmet treatment needs of US adults with mental health and substance use disorders. *Health Affairs, 36*(10), 1739–1747. https://doi.org/10.1377/hlthaff.2017.0584

Hasin, D. S., O'Brien, C. P., Auriacombe, M., Borges, G., Bucholz, K., Budney, A., Compton, W. M., Crowley, T., Ling, W., Petry, N. M., Schuckit, M., & Grant, B. F. (2013). DSM-5 criteria for substance use disorders: Recommendations and rationale. *American Journal of Psychiatry, 170*(8), 834–851. https://doi.org/10.1176/appi.ajp.2013.12060782

Hawk, M., Coulter, R. W., Egan, J. E., Fisk, S., Reuel Friedman, M., Tula, M., & Kinsky, S. (2017). Harm reduction principles for healthcare settings. *Harm Reduction Journal, 14*, 1–9. https://doi.org/10.1186/s12954-017-0196-4

Hinckley, J. D., Adams, Z. W., Dellucci, T. V., & Berkowitz, S. (2024). Co-occurring trauma- and stressor-related and substance-related disorders in youth: A narrative review. *Medical Research Archives, 12*(8), 10–18103. https://doi.org/10.18103/mra.v12i8.5688

Jang, M. H., & Song, J. (2024). Adenosine and adenosine receptors in metabolic imbalance-related neurological issues. *Biomedicine & Pharmacotherapy, 177*, 116996. https://doi.org/10.1016/j.biopha.2024.116996

Kircanski, K., LeMoult, J., Ordaz, S., & Gotlib, I. H. (2017). Investigating the nature of co-occurring depression and anxiety: Comparing diagnostic and dimensional research approaches. *Journal of Affective Disorders, 216*, 123–135. https://doi.org/10.1016/j.jad.2016.08.006

Knopf, A. (2021). Teens more likely than young adults to develop SUD after first cannabis use. *The Brown University Child & Adolescent Psychopharmacology Update, 23*(5), 1–4. https://doi.org/10.1002/cpu.30572

Kwako, L. E., Momenan, R., Litten, R. Z., Koob, G. F., & Goldman, D. (2016). Addictions neuroclinical assessment: A neuroscience-based framework for addictive disorders. *Biological Psychiatry, 80*(3), 179–189. https://doi.org/10.1016/j.biopsych.2015.10.024

Levin, H. (n.d.). *Can I drink alcohol while taking schizophrenia medications?* WebMD. https://www.webmd.com/schizophrenia/features/alcohol-schizophrenia-meds

Luthar, S. S., & D'Avanzo, K. (1999). Contextual factors in substance use: A study of suburban and inner-city adolescents. *Development and Psychopathology, 11*(4), 845–867. https://doi.org/10.1017/S0954579499002346

Marlowe, D. B., Kirby, K. C., Festinger, D. S., Husband, S. D., & Platt, J. J. (1997). Impact of comorbid personality disorders and personality disorder symptoms on outcomes of behavioral treatment for cocaine dependence. *The Journal of Nervous and Mental Disease, 185*(8), 483–490. https://doi.org/10.1097/00005053-199708000-00006

May, J., Andrade, J., Kavanagh, D. J., Feeney, G. F. X., Gullo, M. J., Statham, D. J., Skorka-Brown, J., Connolly, J. M., Cassimatis, M., Young, R. M., & Connor, J. P. (2014). The craving experience questionnaire: A brief, theory-based measure of consummatory desire and craving. *Addiction, 109*(5), 728–735. https://doi.org/10.1111/add.12472

Mericle, A. A., Park, V. M. T., Holck, P., & Arria, A. M. (2012). Prevalence, patterns, and correlates of co-occurring substance use and mental disorders in the United States: Variations by race/ethnicity. *Comprehensive Psychiatry, 53*(6), 657–665. https://doi.org/10.1016/j.comppsych.2011.10.002

Mojtabai, R. (2022). Estimating the prevalence of substance use disorders in the US using the benchmark multiplier method. *JAMA Psychiatry, 79*(11), 1074–1080. https://doi.org/10.1001/jamapsychiatry.2022.2756

Montan, R. N. M., & Banaco, R. A. (2021). Cue exposure therapy for substance use: A complement to functional analysis. In S. M. Oliani, R. A. Reichert, & R. A. Banaco (Eds.), *Behavior analysis and substance dependence: Theory, research and intervention* (pp. 89–108). Springer Nature. https://doi.org/10.1007/978-3-030-75961-2_8

Moreira, D., Azeredo, A., & Dias, P. (2022). Instruments used for evaluation in substance use disorder: A systematic review. *Journal of Substance Use, 28*(5), 651–660. https://doi.org/10.1080/14659891.2022.2082334

Mueser, K. T., Drake, R. E., & Wallach, M. A. (1998). Dual diagnosis: A review of etiological theories. *Addictive Behaviors, 23*(6), 717–734. https://doi.org/10.1016/S0306-4603(98)00073-2

Murnane, K. S., Edinoff, A. N., Cornett, E. M., & Kaye, A. D. (2023). Updated perspectives on the neurobiology of substance use disorders using neuroimaging. *Substance Abuse and Rehabilitation*, 99–111. https://doi.org/10.2147/SAR.S362861

Najt, P., Fusar-Poli, P., & Brambilla, P. (2011). Co-occurring mental and substance abuse disorders: A review on the potential predictors and clinical outcomes. *Psychiatry Research, 186*(2–3), 159–164. https://doi.org/10.1016/j.psychres.2010.07.042

National Center for Drug Abuse Statistics (NCDAS). (2025). *Drug abuse statistics*. Retrieved April 12, 2025, from https://drugabusestatistics.org/

National Institute of Mental Health (NIMH). (2022). *Mental illness*. U.S. Department of Health and Human Services (DHHS), National Institutes of Health (NIH). Retrieved April, 2025, from https://www.nimh.nih.gov/health/statistics/mental-illness#:~:text=Serious%20mental%20illness%20(SMI)%20is,experience%20disability%20due%20to%20SMI

National Institute of Mental Health (NIMH). (2024). *Substance use and co-occurring mental disorders*. https://www.nimh.nih.gov/health/topics/substance-use-and-mental-health

National Institute of Mental Health (NIMH). (n.d.). *Development and definitions of the RDoC domains and constructs*. https://www.nimh.nih.gov/research/research-funded-by-nimh/rdoc/development-and-definitions-of-the-rdoc-domains-and-constructs

National Institute on Drug Abuse (NIDA). (2020, April). *Common comorbidities with substance use disorders: Research report*. National Institutes of Health. https://www.ncbi.nlm.nih.gov/books/NBK571451/

National Institute on Drug Abuse (NIDA). (2024, October). *Co-occurring disorders and health conditions*. U.S. Department of Health and Human Services, National Institutes of Health. https://nida.nih.gov/research-topics/co-occurring-disorders-health-conditions

Paulus, M. P. (2022). Neural substrates of substance use disorders. *Current Opinion in Neurology, 35*(4), 460–466. https://doi.org/10.1097/WCO.0000000000001077

Poudel, A., & Gautam, S. (2017). Age of onset of substance use and psychosocial problems among individuals with substance use disorders. *BMC Psychiatry, 17*, 10. https://doi.org/10.1186/s12888-016-1191-0

Poznyak, V., Reed, G. M., & Medina-Mora, M. E. (2018). Aligning the ICD-11 classification of disorders due to substance use with global service needs. *Epidemiology and Psychiatric Sciences, 27*(3), 212–218. https://doi.org/10.1017/S2045796017000622

Public Health Management Corporation. (2024). *Addiction severity index* (5th ed.). https://research.phmc.org/products/addiction-severity-index

RachBeisel, J., Scott, J., & Dixon, L. (1999). Co-occurring severe mental illness and substance use disorders: A review of recent research. *Psychiatric Services, 50*(11), 1427–1434. https://doi.org/10.1176/ps.50.11.1427

Rosen, R. L., Ramasubramani, R. S., Benowitz, N. L., Gandhi, K. K., & Williams, J. M. (2023). Caffeine levels and dietary intake in smokers with schizophrenia and bipolar disorder. *Psychiatry Research, 319*, 114989. https://doi.org/10.1016/j.psychres.2022.114989

Rush, B., & Koegl, C. J. (2008). Prevalence and profile of people with co-occurring mental and substance use disorders within a comprehensive mental health system. *Canadian Journal of Psychiatry, 53*(12), 810–821. https://doi.org/10.1177/070674370805301207

Rush, B., Urbanoski, K., Bassani, D., Castel, S., Wild, T. C., Strike, C., Kimberley, D., & Somers, J. (2008a). Prevalence of co-occurring substance use and other mental disorders in the Canadian population. *The Canadian Journal of Psychiatry, 53*(12), 800–809. https://doi.org/10.1177/070674370805301206

Rush, B. R., Dennis, M. L., Scott, C. K., Castel, S., & Funk, R. R. (2008b). The interaction of co-occurring mental disorders and recovery management checkups on substance abuse treatment participation and recovery. *Evaluation Review, 32*(1), 7–38. https://doi.org/10.1177/0193841X07307532

Sajadi-Ernazarova, K. R., & Hamilton, R. J. (2023). Caffeine withdrawal. In *StatPearls [Internet]*. StatPearls Publishing. https://www.ncbi.nlm.nih.gov/books/NBK430790/

Shahrokh, N. C., & Hales, R. E. (Eds.). (2003). *American psychiatric glossary* (8th ed.). American Psychiatric Publishing. https://doi.org/10.1176/appi.books.9780890425596

Siegel, S., Baptista, M. A., Kim, J. A., McDonald, R. V., & Weise-Kelly, L. (2000). Pavlovian psychopharmacology: The associative basis of tolerance. *Experimental and Clinical Psychopharmacology, 8*(3), 276–293. https://doi.org/10.1037/1064-1297.8.3.276

Siegfried, N. (1998). A review of comorbidity: Major mental illness and problematic substance use. *Australian and New Zealand Journal of Psychiatry, 32*(5), 707–717. https://doi.org/10.3109/00048679809113127

Stallvik, M., & Nordahl, H. M. (2014). Convergent validity of the ASAM criteria in co-occurring disorders. *Journal of Dual Diagnosis, 10*(2), 68–78. https://doi.org/10.1080/15504263.2014.906812

Stewart, R. E., Cardamone, N. C., Schachter, A., Becker, C., McKay, J. R., & Becker-Haimes, E. M. (2023). A systematic review of brief, freely accessible, and valid self-report measures for substance use disorders and treatment. *Drug and Alcohol Dependence, 243*, 109729. https://doi.org/10.1016/j.drugalcdep.2022.109729

Strassnig, M., Brar, J. S., & Ganguli, R. (2006). Increased caffeine and nicotine consumption in community-dwelling patients with schizophrenia. *Schizophrenia Research, 86*(1–3), 269–275. https://doi.org/10.1016/j.schres.2006.05.013

Substance Abuse and Mental Health Services Administration (SAMHSA). (2015). *Screening and assessment of co-occurring disorders in the justice system* (HHS Publication No. PEP19-SCREEN-CODJS). https://library.samhsa.gov/sites/default/files/pep19-screen-codjs.pdf

Substance Abuse and Mental Health Services Administration (SAMHSA). (2019). *Key substance use and mental health indicators in the United States: Results from the 2018 National Survey on Drug Use and Health* (HHS Publication No. PEP19–5068, NSDUH Series H-54). https://www.samhsa.gov/data/

Substance Abuse and Mental Health Services Administration (SAMHSA). (2020). *Key substance use and mental health indicators in the United States: Results from the 2019 National Survey on Drug Use and Health* (HHS Publication No. PEP20-07-01-001, NSDUH Series H-55). https://www.samhsa.gov/data/

Substance Abuse and Mental Health Services Administration (SAMHSA). (2023). *2023 National Survey on Drug Use and Health: Detailed tables*. https://www.samhsa.gov/data/report/2023-nsduh-detailed-tables

Substance Abuse and Mental Health Services Administration (SAMHSA). (2024). *2024 National Survey on drug use and health (NSDUH) releases*. U.S. Department of Health and Human Services. https://www.samhsa.gov/data/data-we-collect/nsduh-national-survey-drug-use-and-health/national-releases/2024

Sujatha, K., Arundathi, T., Rubina, S., Ramana, B. V., & Nagarajan, G. (2013). Drug delivery methods ranking addiction potential. *International Journal of Pharmaceutical Sciences and Research, 4*(4), 1287–1293. https://ijpsr.com/?action=download_pdf&postid=6881

Suncoast Practice Research Collaborative at the University of South Florida. (2002) *Co-occurring disorders treatment workbook*. Department of Mental Health Law & Policy, Louis de la Parte Florida Mental Health Institute, University of South Florida. https://www.usf.edu/cbcs/mhlp/documents/cdt_workbook.pdf

Tapper, K. (2018). Mindfulness and craving: Effects and mechanisms. *Clinical Psychology Review, 59*, 101–117. https://doi.org/10.1016/j.cpr.2017.11.003

Temmingh, H. (2019). *Epidemiology, diagnosis and aspects of treatment in persons with serious mental illness and co-occurring substance use disorders* (Doctoral dissertation, University of Cape Town, Department of Psychiatry and Mental Health, Faculty of Health Sciences). https://open.uct.ac.za/bitstream/11427/30422/1/thesis_hsf_2019_temmingh_hendrik.pdf

United Nations Office on Drugs and Crime (UNODC). (n.d.). *GAP Toolkit Module 2: Final English*. https://www.unodc.org/documents/GAP/GAP%20Toolkit%20Module%202%20Final%20ENGLISH%2002-60052.pdf

Van Dorn, R., Volavka, J., & Johnson, N. (2011). Mental disorder and violence: Is there a relationship beyond substance use? *Social Psychiatry and Psychiatric Epidemiology, 47*, 487–503. https://doi.org/10.1007/s00127-011-0356-x

Virgo, N., Bennett, G., Higgins, D., Bennett, L., & Thomas, P. (2001). The prevalence and characteristics of cooccurring serious mental illness (SMI) and substance abuse or dependence in the patients of Adult Mental Health and Addictions Services in eastern Dorset. *Journal of Mental Health, 10*(2), 175–188. https://doi.org/10.1080/09638230125422

Volkow, N. D., Han, B., Einstein, E. B., & Compton, W. M. (2021). Prevalence of substance use disorders by time since first substance use among young people in the US. *JAMA Pediatrics, 175*(6), 640–643. https://doi.org/10.1001/jamapediatrics.2020.6981

Williams, E. C., Fletcher, O. V., Frost, M. C., Harris, A. H., Washington, D. L., & Hoggatt, K. J. (2022). Comparison of substance use disorder diagnosis rates from electronic health record data with substance use disorder prevalence rates reported in surveys across sociodemographic groups in the veterans health administration. *JAMA Network Open, 5*(6), e2219651. https://doi.org/10.1001/jamanetworkopen.2022.19651

World Health Organization. (1992). *The ICD-10 classification of mental and behavioural disorders: Clinical descriptions and diagnostic guidelines*. World Health Organization.

World Health Organization (WHO). (2004). *ICD-10: International statistical classification of diseases and related health problems* (10 rev, 2nd ed.). World Health Organization. https://iris.who.int/handle/10665/42980

World Health Organization. (2019). *International classification of diseases for mortality and morbidity statistics* (11th rev.). World Health Organization. https://icd.who.int/

Zeidan, F., & Vago, D. R. (2016). Mindfulness meditation–based pain relief: A mechanistic account. *Annals of the New York Academy of Sciences, 1373*(1), 114–127.

Zhang, H., Grant, B. F., Hodgkinson, C. A., Ruan, W. J., Kerridge, B. T., Huang, B., Saha, T. D., Fan, A. Z., Wilson, V., Jung, J., Parsian, A., Goldman, D., & Chou, S. P. (2022). Strong and weak cross-inheritance of substance use disorders in a nationally representative sample. *Molecular Psychiatry, 27*(3), 1742–1753. https://doi.org/10.1038/s41380-021-01370-0

Zimmerman, M., Morgan, T. A., & Stanton, K. (2018). The severity of psychiatric disorders. *World Psychiatry, 17*(3), 258–275. https://doi.org/10.1002/wps.20569

Chapter 13
Problems with Social Functioning and Skills in Serious Mental Illness

Introduction

Social functioning is a cornerstone of human interaction and psychological well-being, yet it is profoundly disrupted in individuals living with serious mental illness (SMI). These disruptions extend beyond overt psychiatric symptoms, manifesting as impairments in social skills, pragmatic communication, and the neurocognitive substrates that support interpersonal engagement. While previous chapters have outlined the diagnostic features and symptomatic expressions of SMI, this chapter shifts focus to the behavioral, cognitive, and communicative dimensions that underlie social dysfunction—domains that are often overlooked yet critically influence quality of life, treatment outcomes, and community integration.

This chapter delineates the construct of social functioning, emphasizing its multidimensional nature. It explores how deficits in verbal and nonverbal communication, social cognition, and Theory of Mind contribute to maladaptive interpersonal behaviors. These impairments are not merely ancillary features of SMI but are central to its functional impact. The discussion integrates dimensional models of social behavior, which offer greater clinical utility than categorical approaches by capturing the variability and context dependence of social impairments. Particular attention is given to the role of negative symptoms such as avolition, anhedonia, and asociality, which are strongly predictive of poor social outcomes and resistant to pharmacological intervention.

Subsequent sections examine the neurological and environmental substrates of social dysfunction, including deficits in executive function, attention, and emotional processing, as well as the impact of institutionalization, social deprivation, and stigma. This chapter then transitions to assessment strategies, contrasting self-report measures with performance-based tools and highlighting the limitations and strengths of each. Pragmatic communication is addressed in depth, with reference to standardized tools and diagnostic criteria, including those outlined in the

G. F. McKeegan, *Behavior Change Interventions for Serious Mental Illness*, Evidence-Based Practices in Behavioral Health,
https://doi.org/10.1007/978-3-032-18372-9_13

DSM-5-TR. The behavioral dimensions of social competence are operationalized through frameworks such as Grice's Maxims and social reinforcement theory, providing students with concrete analytic tools for clinical observation and intervention planning.

Finally, the chapter concludes with a review of evidence-based behavioral support strategies and social skills training programs. These interventions are contextualized within broader rehabilitation efforts, emphasizing the need for individualized, culturally sensitive, and ecologically valid approaches. By integrating neurocognitive, behavioral, and environmental perspectives, comprehensive understanding of social functioning in SMI is presented to facilitate the assessment and interpretation of social functioning and skill impairment and intervene to promote meaningful social engagement and recovery.

> I take care of my aunt who is in her 40s. Recently, she was discharged from a state hospital after living there since she was 18. She has a hard time talking with others. She stays in her room, seldom talks to anyone in the family, and speaks only to ask for a cigarette. We have to remind her to shower and change clothes. Her room is a mess with trash and clothes on the floor. We cannot take her to a restaurant as she would embarrass us by asking others for money or a cigarette. She says rude things to other people when we go anywhere with her; we are afraid she is going to be arrested or assaulted if she says the wrong thing to someone.

The Case of Becky

Becky is a 40-year-old woman living with schizoaffective mental health problem. In the past, it was determined by service providers that she was living with a variety of other mental health problems including schizophrenia spectrum, bipolar, depression, personality-related mental health issues and "multiple personality disorder," and others. Since adolescence, she has attended special schools and been hospitalized many times in both private and public psychiatric hospitals. In the past, she has been prescribed a variety of medications. She is currently prescribed an antipsychotic medication and a medication to help stabilize mood as well as an antianxiety medication. Despite the professional attention she has received, she continues to do many things that make it difficult to get along with her at home.

Becky does not experience delusions or hallucinations. Her current problems involve the way that she interacts with other people. When she is with other people, she frequently cries and complains about the treatment she gets, saying that "my parents and doctors treat me unfairly and hate my guts." She typically continues to express these complaints despite the attempts of other people to help. She demands cigarettes, coffee, and other items from parents, service providers, and other people. When at home, she knocks on the doors of neighbors to complain that her parents don't feed her and ask for cigarettes and coffee. When they refuse, she curses at them and tries another house. When friends come to visit, she cuts into conversations that others are having and begins complaining that her medication causes her to have diarrhea or that she hasn't been able to go to the bathroom for several days.

Understandably, these behaviors have been very frustrating for her family and other people. Strangers typically show interest and sympathy when they first hear about her problems, but they tend to avoid her when they realize that she doesn't take steps to resolve the problems that she talks about. People who can't avoid her generally become very frustrated when she persists in complaining. Because of their frustration, many will eventually curse back at her, tell her to "get lost," tell her that she'll never get any better, or threaten to call the police.

Definitions and Characteristics of Problems Associated with Social Functioning in Individuals Who Live with Serious Mental Illness?

Social functioning refers to an array of behaviors that individuals use to get along with other people. These include such skills as listening to what others say, expressing what the person thinks and feels, starting and maintaining conversations, and asking for help from others when needed. Social functioning is a construct that is composed of domains of related behaviors. Social functioning behaviors are defined as a topographically broad class of responses; the responses are normative and socially sanctioned and that individuals use to interact effectively with other people. The responses include such things as dress and behavior codes, what to say and not to say, stylistic guidelines about the expression of affect, social reinforcement, interpersonal distance, and other dimensions of socially appropriate interpersonal behaviors (Kinnaman & Bellack, 2012).

Problems in social functioning are important dimensions in the assessment and treatment in people living with SMI. Social skills are crucial for adapting to social situations and maintaining interpersonal relationships, succeeding in assuming social roles including educational, occupational, vocational, and the development of mutually satisfying relationships. Individuals with competent social skills can navigate social environments more effectively, leading to better personal and social outcomes and increased quality of life. Limited social skills can result in dependency on others, hinder successful socialization, and decreased quality of life (Jurevičienė et al., 2012).

Problems in social functioning displayed by people living with SMI are heterogeneous, idiosyncratic, and transdiagnostic. Individuals living with SMI may display competent social skills in certain situations but not others. Social dysfunction in people living with SMI is particularly common, remains persistent when other symptoms (e.g., positive symptoms like hallucinations and delusions) improve, and does not beneficially respond to pharmacological treatment. It manifests as difficulties in initiating and maintaining conversations, meeting social goals, and fulfilling social roles, often leading to isolation and impaired social support.

Measures of social functioning frequently rely on self-reports by the individual living with SMI. Measures that directly assess social functioning through observations of social behaviors in analog (e.g., role play) or actual situations are time-consuming (Patterson et al., 2001). Bellack et al. (1990) employed the observation of performances in 12 role-plays of social encounters that were rated on various behavioral dimensions including gaze, speech duration, smoothness of conversation, verbal components (e.g., praise/appreciation, request/compliance), and overall performance of social skills.

Social functioning impairments are considered a "negative symptom" of living with SMI. Negative symptoms are defined as the absence of adaptive normative behaviors usually observed in adults including lack of interest and motivation to engage in behaviors such as personal hygiene, impaired social functioning and social isolation, and impaired awareness of problematic behaviors. They are broadly defined as a reduction of normal functions either related to motivation and interest (e.g., avolition, anhedonia, and asociality) or to expressive functions (e.g., blunted affect and alogia); they represent a loss or diminution in everyday experiences and abilities (Correll & Schooler, 2020). Although negative symptoms are a focus of research and treatment in the rehabilitation of people living with SMI, there is a lack of agreement as to the specificity of what are negative symptoms (Correll & Schooler, 2020). Studies have shown that 50%–60% of people living with SMI experience at least one negative symptom, and between 10% and 30% have two or more negative symptoms (Galderisi et al., 2021; Mosolov & Yaltonskaya, 2022). In a multicenter study, 57.6% of patients with schizophrenia spectrum mental health problems had negative symptoms.

According to the American Psychiatric Association (2022), negative symptoms comprise dimensions of social functioning, including:

(a) Diminished emotional expressions include both verbal and nonverbal aspects of emotional expression (i.e., facial expression and gestures) and verbal inflection and tone (i.e., prosody).
(b) Avolition is defined as a decrease or absence of self-initiated goal-directed activity.
(c) Alogia is defined as a lack of or decrease in expressed verbal behaviors.
(d) Anhedonia is defined as an inability to experience and express pleasure from an activity.
(e) Asociality is defined as a lack of interest to engage in social interactions with others (American Psychiatric Association, 2022, p. 88).

Individuals living with SMI experience challenges in social functioning, including both verbal and nonverbal communication skills (Francis & Penn, 2001). These difficulties may not be recognized as part of living with SMI. A lack of initiating social interactions with others and not wanting to go to clubhouse programs and groups is sometimes seen as "shyness," which is viewed as a character trait. Talking loudly, enthusiastically, and excessively about a unique and uncommon interest to strangers may be viewed as a tendency to overshare or being loquacious even when the other person leaves; it becomes a social problem when others avoid interacting with the person because the verbal behavior of the individual is annoying. Avoiding social interactions may be viewed by others as an indication that the individual is being unfriendly or lazy. These may be related to motivational impairments, which are an aspect of living with SMI that has not responded to treatment.

Social functioning impairment is not merely a consequence of positive or negative symptoms in individuals living with SMI. Negative symptoms significantly affect assessed social performance during role-plays (Bellack et al., 1990). Specific diminished behaviors typical of functioning, such as social withdrawal, psychomotor slowing, and blunted affect, are consistently linked to impairments across all domains of daily functioning, including social interactions. Impairments in neurocognitive skills—such as attention, executive function, working memory, verbal memory, and psychomotor speed—are strong predictors of functional difficulties. High correlations exist between measures of social functioning and negative symptoms, while positive symptoms show little to no relationship with social skills performance (Kurtz, 2006).

Negative symptoms are behaviorally characterized by a reduction in typical functioning, leading to diminished or absent expressions of behavior and emotional responses (Correll & Schooler, 2020). Certain diminished behaviors significantly impact social functioning. The behaviors that reflect reduced motivation for social engagement are the strongest predictors of everyday social functioning in individuals living with SMI. In contrast, active social avoidance and passive-apathetic social withdrawal account for the most variance in real-world social outcomes (Kalin et al., 2015). Impairments in neuropsychological performance, particularly in sustained attention and letter fluency, serve as significant predictors of social skill performance (Mahmood et al., 2018). Diminished behaviors exert both direct and indirect effects on social outcomes, with expression-related responses (e.g., impairments in emotional and verbal expressions) linked to social competence, while motivation-related responses (e.g., social withdrawal and avoidance) are directly correlated with social functioning. There appear to be distinct pathways to social functioning, highlighting the necessity for interventions to be tailored to individual differences in impairment (Tran et al., 2019).

To develop a comprehensive understanding of factors related to the social functioning of people living with SMI, it is essential to address negative symptoms and specific aspects of social behaviors. It may be critical to focus on impairments related to the initiation and maintenance of social interactions, specifically issues involving withdrawal and avoidance of social exchanges. Furthermore, it is important to examine how these impairments interact with verbal and emotional expressiveness and whether impairments in expressive skills impact the motivating operation (MO) of engaging in social exchanges. MOs for social functioning refer to environmental or situational factors that affect the value of a social interaction and the propensity to engage in it (Cooper et al., 2020). MOs can either enhance or diminish the efficacy of social reinforcers, such as attention, approval, acquisition, or reciprocity. The absence of social exchanges can result in a deficient history of being reinforced for engaging in such behaviors and the lack of opportunities to have effective social skills shaped and reinforced by the environment.

Social functional capacity involves completing social tasks in controlled environments (e.g., role-plays), while functional performance refers to doing them in real-world settings. Social functioning outcomes depend on both (Bromley & Brekke, 2010) as the individual needs to have the social behaviors in their repertoire that are needed for a successful exchange and to engage in the adaptive social behaviors in the correct context. Individuals with SMI might manage social tasks in artificial settings but struggle in everyday situations requiring adaptability and problem-solving.

Dysfunction in social functioning is a hallmark of living with SMI and leads to social isolation, impairments in major roles in life, and reduced sense of well-being and happiness in various areas of life (Bellack et al., 1990; Zhaoyang et al., 2019). Primary negative symptoms like anhedonia, avolition, and alogia are linked to social impairments. Secondary negative symptoms may result from positive symptoms (e.g., social withdrawal based on suspicion from persecutory delusions), co-occurring depression, side effects of medications, use of psychoactive substances (e.g., cannabis) or caused by social deprivation resulting from long-term hospitalizations and loss of significant relationships (Mosolov & Yaltonskaya, 2022). The distinction between primary and secondary symptoms has implications for treatment and understanding of problem behaviors related to living with SMI. Secondary negative symptoms can stem from social impairments and positive symptoms—hallucinations, delusions, and disorganized speech—rather than being their cause (Bellack et al., 1990; Mosolov & Yaltonskaya, 2022).

The DSM-5-TR (American Psychiatric Association, 2022) does not explicitly state that impairments in social functioning are a core criterion for the determination of an SMI; they are a significant aspect of many conditions and can be indicators of impairments in daily functional capabilities, which are part of the criteria for certain mental health problems linked to SMI.

Dimensions of Social Functioning Problems

Social functioning is a complex construct that presents challenges to define and operationalize. The domain of social functioning comprises social skills that are specific overt and covert behavioral responses that enable a person to competently perform particular social tasks. Social functioning is composed of domains of related behaviors that are defined as broad classes of learned responses or skills that are normative and socially sanctioned that individuals use to interact effectively with other people. The social skills used in interactions include dimensions of social pragmatic communication (Kinnaman & Bellack, 2012).

Social pragmatic communication is the ability to use language appropriately in social contexts, including understanding and responding to social cues, adapting communication styles to different situations, and following rules of conversations. Pragmatic communication in social situations requires an individual to have verbal and nonverbal expressive behaviors that mesh with the intent and goal of the interactions between people. For a competent social exchange, the individuals that are interacting need to be able to generate and comprehend each other's communication; they are required to have a degree of social understanding in which they acquire knowledge about the others' covert states—cognitive and emotional—and using it to guide social interactions (American Speech-Language-Hearing Association [ASHA], n.d.; Ihnen et al., 1998).

The DSM-5-TR (American Psychiatric Association, 2022) lists impairment in certain subdomains of communication to determine if an individual is living with social pragmatic communication problems. The domain of pragmatic communication involves the following subdomains:

- contextual understanding of the interaction and recognizing and adapting language and behavior to match the setting, listener, and the purpose of the communication.
- conversational management: using conversational rules including taking turns and conversational pauses, staying on topic, and being aware and rephrasing when misunderstood (Bellack et al., 1990).
- nonliteral language: understanding idioms, humor, metaphors, and other forms of nonliteral language.
- inferential reasoning: making inferences and drawing conclusions based on what is not explicitly stated but is communicated nonverbally.
- social etiquette: adhering to social norms and rules of etiquette in communication.

The DSM-5-TR (American Psychiatric Association, 2022) specifies that impairments in all subdomains need to be displayed for the presence of a social pragmatic communication problem (Yuan & Dollaghan, 2018).

Social pragmatics include both nonverbal and verbal communication. Nonverbal communication involves the behavioral dimensions of body language, gestures, facial expressions, and eye contact (ASHA, n.d.; Feldman et al., 1991). Competent verbal communication includes verbal behaviors that adhere to certain guidelines known as Grice's Maxims, which are measurable and observable dimensions of verbal behaviors (Feldman et al., 1991; Haroldfs, n.d.). There are four dimensions that entail Grice's Maxims (AHSA, n.d.):

1. Quantity: where one tries to be as informative as possible, gives information that is needed and no more. The individuals need to adjust the amount of information according to the context of the social situation. Discussing personal information with an Uber driver is dysfunctional.
2. Quality: where one tries to be truthful and does not give information that is false or that is not supported by evidence. Exaggeration and false beliefs brought up in communication would impair effective communication and mutual goal attainment.
3. Relation: where one tries to be relevant and says things that are pertinent to the discussion. Communicating off topic and engaging in loose association or flight of ideas would be a negative example of this dimension and contribute to dysfunctional pragmatic communication.

4. Manner: when one tries to be clear, brief, and orderly in what one says, and obscurity and ambiguity are avoided. Engaging in rapid, loud, rambling, and excessive verbal behaviors results in flawed pragmatic communication.

Social functioning can be categorized based on their expression (verbal, nonverbal) and function (intrapersonal/interpersonal; acquire/avoid). The complexity of social skills ranges from basic abilities (e.g., eye contact, verbal communication) to more advanced skills, such as decision-making and leadership (e.g., persuasion) (Jurevičienė et al., 2012).

The construct of social functioning can be categorized into three general domains. Effective social functioning requires the integration of all three functions to navigate social interactions successfully (Kinnaman & Bellack, 2012; Perez et al., 2007; Tenhula & Bellack, 2008). The three general domains of social functioning are:

1. The accurate reception or comprehension of relevant verbal and nonverbal interpersonal stimuli in different situations. The ability to accurately perceive social cues such as facial expressions, tone of voice, body posture, and speech content.
2. Processing these stimuli, generating response options, and choosing an appropriate response. It is the ability to analyze social situations by integrating current and historical information to identify an appropriate response.
3. Sending the chosen response (Perez et al., 2007). This is the ability to implement appropriate behavioral responses effectively, including using verbal and nonverbal communication skills like eye contact, body posture, gestures, facial expression, tone, and volume of voice.

Jurevičienė et al. (2012) developed a model of social skills comprising five behavioral domains of response classes that include interaction, communication, participation, and emotional and social cognitive skills. Each domain, which is made up of specific behavioral abilities and response classes, consists of specific behavioral class of responses that contribute to social functioning. The components are interrelated and interconnected. Performance in one domain can impact performance in another domain.

The various domains, characterized by distinct behavioral abilities and response classes, encompass specific behavioral response classes that play a crucial role in social functioning. These components are interrelated, interconnected, and multidirectional meaning that performance in one domain can significantly influence performance in another. Social competence is a general evaluative term referring to the quality or adequacy of an individual's overall performance on a particular task (Jurevičienė et al., 2012). It involves the ability to assess social situations and determine what is expected or required, to recognize the feelings and intentions of others, and to select behaviors that are most appropriate for that given context and the ability to vary responses given the unique stimuli in each social setting (American Psychological Association, n.d.-b). It is the effectiveness or skill in interpersonal relations and social situations requiring appropriate responses and certain cognitive-perceptual abilities (Bellack et al., 1990).

Behavioral competence in social functioning involves generating an appropriate response to a social situation, including the use of suitable verbal and nonverbal communication. This encompasses effective behaviors such as eye contact, posture, facial expression, interpersonal space, body movement, and gestures, which are collectively referred to as kinetics (Kinnaman & Bellack, 2012).

Social competence involves having competencies in behavioral skills that help individuals know when and how to respond in various situations. It relies on understanding what are the appropriate skills and the awareness of stimuli in a social context. Without recognizing these stimuli, a person may not exhibit necessary social skills. Social impairments can be rectified by skills training including being aware of social situations, stimuli associated with these situations, and behavioral responses linked to the situations. By virtue of the term social skills, these behaviors are both learnable and modifiable (Kinnaman & Bellack, 2012).

The effectiveness of social behaviors is determined if the behaviors that are displayed in a social exchange result in access to a desired outcome for the individuals in the exchange. If the outcome is reinforcing for them, then the covert and overt social behaviors displayed in that exchange are reinforced and have an increased probability of being displayed again in similar contexts and antecedent conditions (Skinner, 1953).

Competency in social functioning necessitates specific neurocognitive processes known as social cognition. This encompasses a range of neurocognitive functions associated with the recognition, understanding, processing, and appropriate application of social stimuli within one's environment (Ochsner, 2008; Penn et al., 2008). Social cognition pertains to how individuals perceive themselves and others in various social contexts. It incorporates mental representations, metacognitive experiences, and decision-making processes (Penn et al., 2008).

Social dysfunction (e.g., ineffective social functioning) occurs when individuals fail to learn, apply, or appropriately use effective social behaviors. It is linked to skills deficits, meaning that individuals either lack necessary social skills or lack adequate discriminative stimulus control (S^D) of the skills (e.g., fail to apply the skill when needed or display inappropriate and incorrect behaviors (S^{delta}). Neurocognitive impairments further hinder social perception and problem-solving, while environmental factors—such as isolation during critical developmental periods—limit opportunities to acquire necessary social skills. Impairments in the display of social skills by people living with SMI have been postulated to arise from inadequate learning experiences, anxiety, cognitive disturbances, and motivational problems. It may be the result of the individual living with SMI not having the appropriate behavioral response in their repertoire of social responses or having learned deficient responses due to lack of opportunity, social environmental influences, and faulty role models to learn and practice the responses in a particular context. Social dysfunction may stem from neurocognitive impairments affecting cognitive flexibility, attribution, perception of nonverbal emotional cues, and awareness of covert responses such as thoughts, beliefs, and emotions in oneself and others (Tenhula & Bellack, 2008), which are all aspects of the Theory of Mind (ToM) (i.e., the capability of thinking about oneself and others and predicting behaviors).

Individuals living with SMI consistently show impairments in aspects of social cognition across the following neurocognitive domains: attributional style, ToM, perception of emotion, and associated underlying processes (Healey et al., 2015; Penn et al., 2008). Disturbances in social functioning and impairments in aspects of social cognition have been shown to be independent of cognitive intelligence (i.e., IQ) (Tranel et al., 2003). The construct of social cognition includes expected verbal and nonverbal social behaviors and awareness of these behaviors in oneself and the exchange partner. It involves perceiving responses in a social interaction and the ability to be flexible and modify responses during the interactions (Penn et al., 2008).

Social cognition interfaces with neurocognition and negative symptoms, involving emotional and cognitive processing. Diminished salience of social rewards may link negative symptoms to social cognitive dysfunction. Studies indicate that social cognition is distinct from neurocognition and negative symptoms, with independent neural activation.

Key domains in social cognition encompass the perception of emotion, ToM, and attributional style. Attributional style pertains to how individuals interpret the causes of events, particularly their successes and failures (Janssen et al., 2006). It involves the reasoning patterns people employ to attribute outcomes to internal or external factors, stable or unstable causes, and global or specific influences. For instance, an individual with a negative attributional style may attribute failures to unchangeable personal flaws (e.g., lack of ability), whereas someone with a positive attributional style might ascribe failures to changeable factors such as effort or strategy. This attributional style can profoundly influence a person's motivation, expectations, performance, and emotional well-being (Anderson et al., 1983). ToM refers to the capacity to comprehend and infer the mental states of others, including their intentions, beliefs, desires, and emotions. It entails recognizing that others possess thoughts, feelings, beliefs, and knowledge distinct from one's own and utilizing this understanding to predict and interpret behaviors during both verbal and nonverbal social interactions (Hardy-Baylé et al., 2003). Furthermore, individuals living with SMI often exhibit significant impairments in perception of emotions, particularly negative emotions. These covert neurocognitive abilities are vital for effective social interactions and communication, enabling individuals to empathize with others, interpret social cues, and navigate complex social situations. Social cognition involves recognizing and interpreting facial expressions, body language, and vocal tones. ToM leverages this information to deduce what others may be thinking or feeling, allowing a person to grasp another's perspective and recognize emotional states essential for empathetic interactions (Cotter et al., 2017).

For instance, social cognitive deficits can lead to dysfunctional social behavior in individuals with SMI, especially when paranoia and negative perceptions are involved. Those living with paranoia may often blame others for negative events, known as "personalizing bias" (Janssen et al., 2006). Problems with ToM and attributional style can hinder realistic integration of contextual information, resulting in social dysfunction and impaired social behaviors.

Social functioning encompasses both verbal and nonverbal behaviors exhibited during social interactions. Verbal behavior refers to the use of spoken, sign, and written language in communication, including common disfluencies such as "you know" or "uh-uh." Nonverbal behaviors encompass facial expressions, gestures, and motor actions displayed during social exchanges.

Dimensions of domains of social functioning can be approached through topographical, functional, and information-processing perspectives (Liberman, 1982). Topographical dimensions of social functioning behaviors include the descriptions of the verbal and nonverbal behaviors that compose competent social responses in a particular social context; in essence, what verbal and nonverbal behaviors look like during a social exchange. Functional dimension is the consequence of the social exchange and whether the social behaviors result in access to overt and covert stimuli that are reinforcing or aversive. The dimensions of information processing in social functioning is the attending to, encoding, and interpretation of the meaning of social cues from the environment, such as actions or expressions of others, the identification of goals for the social situation (e.g., obtaining or avoiding/escaping a certain consequence), the generation and evaluation of possible responses based on goals and past learning experiences, enacting a response, and the adjustment of future responses based on feedback and attention to environmental cues during the exchange (Lemerise & Arsenio, 2000). Emotional awareness, regulation, and processing also play a critical role in shaping each step during the social exchange. These steps are influenced by past experiences, biologically determined capabilities, and covert feedback loops (perceptual, attributional) allowing for dynamic and adaptive social functioning (Lemerise & Arsenio, 2000).

Social pragmatic communication is defined as effective and appropriate use of language to comprehend ideas or to interact in social situations (Everyday Speech, n.d.). Pragmatic competence comprises several interrelated skills that are manifested in a range of adaptive behaviors. Rad (2014) summarized the assessment tools for adult pragmatic communication. Table 13.1 presents the instruments, dimensions assessed, the testing components (how assessed), and rating scales.

The tools in Table 13.1 assess various dimensions of social functioning that encompass the construct of social pragmatic communication. Dimensions are measurable aspects of behaviors, like scores on reliable assessments. Table 13.2 lists the dimensions that can be assessed by multimodal assessments of pragmatic communication.

Liberman (1982) rated the competency of social functioning by using over 200 different interpersonal role-plays covering contextual areas such as interactions in the hospital and community, friendship, and family relations. Each situation was role-played to assess and train the individual's "receiving," "processing," and "sending" social functioning. The dimensions that were assessed were (a) nonverbal components, including gaze, appropriateness of eye contact, duration of speaking, length of verbal responses, meshing and smoothness of turn-taking and conversational pauses; (b) affective dimensions including emotional expressiveness during interactions; (c) verbal components including request/compliance (defined as the ability to make requests or comply appropriately) and praise/appreciation, which

Table 13.1 Social pragmatic assessment: tools, dimensions, components, and rating scale

Instrument	Assessed dimensions	Components of assessment	Rating scale
Discourse Comprehension Test (DCT) (Brookshire & Nicholas, 1997)	Narrative processing	Two sets of five stories	Two-point scale (yes/no)
Pragmatic Protocol (PP) (Prutting & Kirchner, 1987)	Verbal, paralinguistic, and nonverbal aspects		Two-point scale (appropriate/inappropriate)
Profile of Communicative Appropriateness (PCA) (Penn, 1985)	Response to interlocutor, semantic content, cohesion, fluency, sociolinguistic sensitivity, nonverbal communication		Five-point scale (inappropriate to appropriate)
Communicative Abilities in Daily Living (CADL) (Holland, 1980)	Functional communication	Role-playing, social interactions	Three-point scale (correct/adequate/wrong)
Functional Communication Profile (FCP) (Kleiman, 2003)	Movement, speaking, understanding, reading, other activities		Nine-point scale (Normal to poor)
Functional Assessment of Communication Skills (FACS) (Frattali et al., 1995)	Social communication, basic needs, reading/writing/number concepts, daily planning		Five-point scale (qualitative), seven-point scale (communication independence)

entails the expression of gratitude or acknowledgment of what is said by the participant in the social exchange; and (d) overall social functioning, which is general rating of social competence based on the combination of verbal and nonverbal behaviors.

The limitations of Liberman's assessment approach are that social situations are nearly limitless, especially when assessing subtle features of social behaviors. Liberman used nearly 200 role-play situations in the assessment of social functioning. Certain critical and common domains of social situations could be used to evaluate the functioning of a person living with SMI but that does not predict the individual's general functioning. Measures of behaviors associated with living with SMI are not predictive of actual "real life" functioning (Harvey & Strassnig, 2012). Social situations (e.g., dating, job interviews) are sometimes unpredictable despite preparations made to display socially competent behaviors; being flexible, having a repertoire of social behaviors that could be used in these circumstances, and adequate social cognitions could assist in whether the social exchange is free of problems.

Bhola et al. (2016) developed an assessment tool (Social Skills Assessment Screening Scale [SSASS]), which measures dimensions of social functioning across three domains of social functioning: nonverbal behavior and communication, verbal

Table 13.2 Dimensions assessed using various tools assessing social pragmatic communication

Category	Behaviors
Verbal behaviors	Speech acts, message specificity, cohesion of message, topic selection, initiation, and maintenance of interaction (pausing, turn taking)
Paralinguistic behaviors	Fluency, prosody, volume and tone of speech, and speech intelligibility
Nonverbal behaviors	Facial expressions, eye gaze, and gestures (including touch)
Response to participant in conversation	Interaction and responsiveness during communication; asking for clarification and information, responding to verbal prompts and nonverbal cues; sequencing of verbal content to match the participant
Control of semantic content	Managing the meaning and relevance of communication; staying on message
Cohesion and fluency	Maintaining smooth and coherent communication; effort and consistency in topical transitions
Sociolinguistic sensitivity	Adapting communication to social norms and contexts; being aware of emotional cues
Functional communication	Ability to communicate effectively in real-life situations, including role-playing and social conventions
Daily communication skills	Reading, writing, number concepts, and daily planning

communication, and social behavior. The measure of each dimension is a combination of information from self-report responses by the individual living with SMI, people familiar with the person (e.g., family, caregivers), and members of the rehabilitation team who observed the person in the treatment setting. The domains of social functioning and the corresponding dimensions that are assessed by the SSASS are:

1. Nonverbal behavior and communication: grooming and appearance; establishing and maintaining eye contact; use of gestures and facial expressions; and maintaining interpersonal distance.
2. Verbal communication: appropriate greeting of other people; initiating a conversation; listening to a conversation; taking turns in conversation; communicating a meaningful message; and paralinguistic speech (e.g., clarity, tone, volume).
3. Social behavior: understanding social situations; changing behavior according to situation flexibility, awareness, inferential communications based on cues); knowledge and use of appropriate manners; engaging in activities with others; using appropriate language; sustaining a conversation/interaction; expressing/sharing day-to-day experiences; expressing/sharing emotions; helping others voluntarily; and able to empathize with others.

Bhola et al. (2016) used the SSASS with 380 individuals living with SMI who were admitted to a psychiatric facility in India. The findings were that dimensions assessed in the domain of social behavior showed that the most prominent impairments were in helping others voluntarily (26.3%) and empathizing with others (25.8%). In the domain of verbal communication, impairments were notable in the dimension of initiating conversations (24.3%) and taking turns (19.5%). In the domain of nonverbal behavior and communication, the dimensions were relatively less impaired, with the most common difficulty noted in the dimension of using gestures and facial expressions (16%). The dimensions of social functioning most frequently rated as impaired were mostly in the social domain, specifically helping others voluntarily (26.3%); empathizing with others/understanding their perspective (25.8%); expressing and sharing emotions (23%); and engaging in activities with others (23.3%). In the verbal communication domain, the dimension of initiating a conversation showed the most impairment (24.3%).

Another assessment tool measuring the dimensions of social functioning in people living with SMI is the Social Skills Performance Assessment (SSPA) (Patterson et al., 2001). The method of assessment is the examiner rating the performance of role-plays in two social situations evaluating dimensions of social functioning on the two domains of social competence and social appropriateness (Patterson et al., 2001). Miller et al. (2021) assessed nearly 1000 individuals living with SMI and people with no mental health problems using the SSPA. Each domain in the SSPA encompasses specific dimensions of social functioning including:

1. Interest: This refers to the participant's ability to show engagement and enthusiasm during social interactions.
2. Fluency: This measures smoothness and ease of communication, including the ability to express thoughts without significant pauses or disruptions.
3. Negotiation skills: The dimension assesses the participant's ability to effectively advocate for their needs or resolve conflicts, particularly in instrumental tasks like requesting a landlord to fix a leak.
4. Clarity: The person's ability to communicate ideas clearly and understandably is evaluated.
5. Persistence: This refers to the participant's ability to maintain effort and determination in achieving a goal during a social interaction, such as continuing to request action from a landlord.
6. Focus: It measures the participant's ability to stay on topic and maintain attention during a conversation.
7. Acting in accordance with norms: This refers to the individual's ability to conform to social norms, predict the impact of their behavior on others, and exhibit self-control to ensure that actions are socially acceptable. This dimension assesses the domain of "social appropriateness."

The results from the Miller et al. (2021) study found that individuals with SMI scored lower on measures of social competence compared to those without mental health issues, while differences in social appropriateness were less pronounced. Social competence correlated significantly with cognitive performance, functional capacity, and real-world outcomes like financial and residential independence, but social appropriateness had no impact (Miller et al., 2021). Miller et al. (2021) concluded that social competence and social appropriateness are distinct dimensions of social skills, as they were generally not correlated with each other but were within their domains.

The results from the Miller et al. (2021) study showed the importance of refining performance-based assessments. In addition, the identified dimensions in the SSPA could have overlap with other dimensions of social functioning. For instance, "interest," which is defined as showing enthusiasm and engagement in the social exchange, probably involves dimensions in the nonverbal domain of social functioning like posture, gaze, gestures, and emotional expressiveness. The dimension of "focus" likewise involves nonverbal behaviors as well as "clarity" and "persistence." A person who is paying attention to the content during a social exchange will ask questions and ask for clarification if their goal is not being supported by the interlocuter (an interlocuter is a person who participates in a social exchange with the speaker); if the person terminates a social exchange and is not reinforced by attaining his conversational goal, then "persistence" is not exhibited.

Another assessment instrument for social functioning is the Social Skills Inventory-2 Del-Prette (SSI-2-Del-Prette) (Del Prette et al., 2021), a self-report tool where individuals respond to 38 items depicting social interaction situations and potential reactions. The respondent estimates the frequency of responses on a 4-point Likert-type scale ranging from "never or rarely" to "always or almost always." The SSI-2-Del-Prette assesses five dimensions of social skills:

1. Assertive conversation: skills related to initiating and maintaining conversations, speaking in public, expressing displeasure, and requesting behavior changes.
2. Affective-sexual approach: skills involving affective and sexual expression, such as introducing oneself, declaring romantic feelings, and approaching sexual intercourse.
3. Expression of positive feeling: skills for expressing positive affection, including giving and receiving compliments, expressing love, and dealing with criticism.
4. Self-control/coping: skills for managing situations requiring self-control and assertive coping, such as reacting to criticism, expressing displeasure, and disagreeing in groups.
5. Social resourcefulness: general social skills for interacting with acquaintances, strangers, and authority figures, reflecting disinhibition and adaptability in various social contexts.

Google Scholar, PsycINFO, and PubMed databases were searched with the title of the instruments and the author. No study was found using this instrument with individuals living with SMI although a sample of over 4000 people living in Brazil was used in the update of its psychometric properties (Del Prette et al., 2021). This instrument is unique for dimensions pertaining to romanticized and intimate social interactions.

The Vellore Assessment of Social Performance (VASP) is a tool that was developed to evaluate social functioning in people living with SMI in India (Thamaraiselvi et al., 2020). VASP rates social behaviors on a seven-point incremental scoring system with higher scores in real-life and unfamiliar social situations that are culturally relevant. VASP uses either real-life observation or role-play situations assessing performance consisting of 20 items across five domains that contain:

- Nonverbal social skills: including eye contact, facial expressions, gestures, and proximity.
- Verbal social skills: including coherence, volume/tone of speech, initiation, termination of conversation, and asking for needs.
- Receptive social competence skills: including following directions, understanding questions, and taking turns.
- Processing social competence skills: including understanding others' behavior, impact of own behavior, and social norms.
- Expressive social competence skills: including answering questions, using social routines, offering help, modifying behavior, and participating in social situations.

VASP was used in the study on the effectiveness of social skills training with individuals living with SMI residing in India (Aruldass et al., 2022).

In a review of the multidimensional nature of social functioning, Perez et al. (2007) determined that functional social skills included the ability to receive, send, and control both verbal and nonverbal behaviors. Moreover, the nonverbal domain is dominated by skill in emotional communication because it primarily involves the sending, interpreting, and regulation of emotional messages. Focusing on the multidimensionality and heterogeneity of social functioning in individuals living with SMI, they postulated that global measures of competent social behaviors and social skill imbalances would be associated with severity of social dysfunction.

Perez et al. (2007) stated that social pragmatic communication involves the following aspects:

- Contextual understanding: awareness and comprehension of the environmental stimuli of the interaction and recognizing and adapting language and behavior to match the setting, listener, and the purpose of the communication.
- Conversation management: entails turn-taking and conversational rules, staying on topic, and being aware and rephrasing when misunderstood. (Bellack et al., 1990).
- Nonliteral language: understanding idioms, humor, metaphors, and other forms of nonliteral language.
- Inferential reasoning: making inferences and drawing conclusions based on what is not explicitly stated.
- Social etiquette: adhering to social norms and rules of etiquette in communication (like the domain of "social appropriateness" on the SSPA) (Patterson et al., 2001).

To summarize, social functioning is multidimensional and heterogenous. Studies on social functioning in people living with SMI have focused on different dimensions to assess. Currently, no assessment tool captures all the dimensions that have been identified in the studies.

Below is a summary of the dimensions that have been identified in the mental health literature on social functioning in people living with SMI:

1. Nonverbal Behavior and Communication (as defined in the SSASS) (Bhola et al., 2016): include grooming and appearance, eye contact; gestures and facial expressions; and interpersonal distance.
2. Verbal Communication (as defined in the SSASS) (Bhola et al., 2016): greeting others, initiating and sustaining conversations, listening and taking turns, communicating meaningfully, and using paralinguistic speech (tone, clarity, volume) are all essential aspects of social functioning. These elements contribute to effective communication and help individuals interact harmoniously within various social settings.
3. Social behavior (as defined in the SSASS) (Bhola et al., 2016): understanding social situations, being flexible and adapting behavior, using appropriate manners, engaging in activities with others, expressing emotions and experiences, and helping others by empathizing.
4. Social competence (as operationalized on the SSPA) (Patterson et al., 2001): interest and engagement in social interactions including (a) fluency in communication ensures that messages are conveyed accurately and understood by others; (b) negotiation skills that are crucial in resolving conflicts and reaching agreements; (c) clarity and persistence that help individuals convey their thoughts and ideas assertively; and (d) focusing during interactions enables individuals to stay on topic and respond appropriately to conversational cues.
5. Social appropriateness (as operationalized on the SSPA) (Patterson et al., 2001): acting in accordance with norms, predicting impact on others, and exhibiting self-control. These skills help individuals navigate social interactions effectively, ensuring that their behavior aligns with societal expectations and fosters positive relationships.
6. Assertive conversation (as operationalized in the SSI-2-Del-Prette) (Del Prette et al., 2021): ability to initiate and maintain discussions; able to express disapproval and displeasure; engage in requests to change interlocutor's behaviors.
7. Affective-sexual approach (as operationalized in the SSI-2-Del-Prette) (Del Prette et al., 2021): romantic and intimate interactions, expressing affection.
8. Expression of positive feelings (as operationalized in the SSI-2-Del-Prette) (Del Prette et al., 2021): giving and receiving compliments; able to express verbal messages of affection and attraction.
9. Self-control/coping (as operationalized in the SSI-2-Del-Prette) (Del Prette et al., 2021): able to manage critical comments, control emotional expressiveness, and respond assertively, requesting clarification.
10. Social resourcefulness (as operationalized in the SSI-2-Del-Prette) (Del Prette et al., 2021): display behaviors that show adaptation to social exchange with different individuals in various contexts.
11. Social pragmatic communication (Perez et al., 2007): contextual understanding, conversation management (e.g., pauses, conversational turn-taking), nonliteral language comprehension, inferential reasoning (e.g., showing understanding of interlocutor's goal for social exchange), and social etiquette (e.g., cultural manners).

These dimensions provide a unique perspective on social functioning, highlighting different aspects and heterogeneity of communication, behavior, and adaptability in social contexts and exchanges.

Social functioning is a complex concept involving multiple domains and behaviors. No single trait, response class of behaviors, or display of social behaviors in a single situation fully represents social functioning. There are no comprehensive assessment tools that measure the complexity of what makes up social functioning given the variety and possible permutations of situations in the domain of social exchanges. The behavioral domain of social functioning contains two major subdomains, verbal and nonverbal behaviors. Each subdomain encompasses specific response classes and dimensions that define the construct of social functioning.

A summary of the components of social functioning from the reviewed research of social functioning in the field of mental health and other related health sciences (e.g., speech and language pathology) is presented below.

- Verbal behaviors: include the following dimensions: the content of speech; message specificity; organization, intelligibility and coherence; topic selection; initiation and maintenance of interaction; awareness of verbal behaviors of the interlocutor and meshing with changes (meshing is the process of individuals smoothly integrating and interacting with others, creating a sense of mutual understanding and connection).
- Paralinguistic behaviors: defined as how things are said including dimensions of fluency, prosody, vocal quality, volume, rate, duration, and amount of speech; use of pauses.
- Responsive to interlocutor: includes the interaction and responsiveness during communication and meshing to verbal and nonverbal changes of speaker.
- Control of semantic content: defined as the responses that selectively access and manipulate meaningful information based on context or task demands; part of the management of the meaning and relevance of communication.
- Cohesion and fluency: maintenance of smooth and coherent communication; awareness of changes in the context of social exchange and altering the verbal behavior to match the change (e.g., changing from personal to humorous).
- Sociolinguistic sensitivity: adapting communication to social norms and contexts.
- Functional communication: behaviors related to communicating effectively in real-life situations, including role-playing and social conventions. Dimensions include staying on topic and behaviors in the response class of assertiveness (e.g., asking for clarification, answering questions).
- Nonverbal behaviors: including facial expressions; eye contact; maintaining gaze; gestures; touching.
- Appearance: dress and grooming.
- Posture and distance (e.g., proxemics): stance and distance during the exchange.
- Self-control: defined as expression of affect and emotion that meshes with verbal and nonverbal behaviors of the interlocutor. Self-control also includes dimensions of being socially appropriate in behavior such as using contextually appropriate language. Basic research in emotion regulation examines how individuals

influence which emotions they have, when they have them, and how they experience and express them (Perez et al., 2007).

- Self-monitoring: a dimension of self-awareness in which a person keeps a covert representation of identified behaviors in connection with efforts to change or control the behavior (American Psychological Association, n.d.-a). Furnham and Capon (1983) found that there was a significant difference in the ability to self-monitor between groups of socially skilled and unskilled adults.

The various dimensions used in studies highlight significant challenges in evaluating impairments in interpersonal interactions and social functioning displayed by individuals living with SMI. The use of dimensional assessment tools for social functioning shows specific behavioral dimensions that could be targeted for intervention. However, it needs to be noted that the dimensional impairments in the social behavior domain are linked to dimensions of social cognitions involving executive functioning, self-awareness, emotional awareness, and theory of mind (ToM) (i.e., the ability to understand that others have their own thoughts, feelings, and beliefs, different from one's own). Interventions for the impairments would need to ascertain the specific behaviors for each dimension of impaired social functioning that need to be instructed, modeled, prompted, reinforced, practiced, and generalized. Assessment of behavioral dimensions for social functioning should be multimodal and include self-report, information from others familiar with behaviors displayed by the individual living with SMI, role-plays, real-life observations, and neuropsychological assessment for identified neurocognitive capabilities linked to the dimension.

Origins of Problems in Social Skills

Social functioning encompasses a wide array of abilities, such as social skills, communication, empathy, awareness of how others perceive social interactions, emotional recognition, behavioral and cognitive flexibility, problem-solving, and various social-cognitive capabilities. These elements contribute to an individual's interactions and adaptations within social contexts. Key components include social perception, the knowledge and execution of behavioral responses in social settings, emotional regulation, and the capacity to adopt different roles in social situations. The interplay between abilities, components of social cognition, and the environment significantly influences and shapes behavioral responses. The behavioral responses exhibited in social situations originate from the interactions between the environment and neurological substrates.

Neurobiological Substrates

Social functioning is a construct that encompasses behavioral skills influenced by environmental factors, social-cognitive abilities, and neurological structures that operate as a network phenomenon. The concept of a network phenomenon highlights the intricate interactions and behaviors that arise within interconnected systems rather than concentrating on individual brain regions. No single brain region serves as the exclusive site for specific social response behaviors. Neurological structures operate in networks, facilitating social cognition, communication, and interaction. These neurological substrates reveal a complex, indirect relationship between neurocognition and social functioning.

Social functioning is multifaceted. The neurological substrates demonstrate a complex and indirect relationship between neurocognition and social functioning. Neurological impairments provide insights into how neural networks influence social functioning, as seen in conditions such as Williams syndrome, ASD, and other neurological events (i.e., strokes, tumors, traumatic brain injury). (Kennedy & Adolphs, 2012). Below are listed the brain structures involved in the associated functions that comprise social exchanges (Pinkham et al., 2003):

- The amygdala processes emotions, especially fear and social saliency. It is instrumental in recognizing emotional expressions and plays a significant role in social decision-making (Flechsenhar et al., 2022; Tranel et al., 2003).
- The ventromedial prefrontal cortex (vmPFC) regulates social emotions such as empathy and moral reasoning. It integrates emotional and social information to guide behavior. Lesions in this area result in disadvantageous personal choices (Tranel et al., 2003). Damage to this region leads to social behavior impairments. Individuals lose the ability to observe social conventions, and personal decisions prove to be problematic. Emotional expression and appropriate feelings in social situations are compromised. This area links memory, emotional responses, and feelings during judgment and decision-making. It integrates event categories from high-order association cortices with structures that manage emotional responses (Bechara, 2002).
- The fusiform face area (FFA) specializes in facial recognition. This area enables the identification of individuals and the interpretation of facial expressions. It is involved in social perception, the recognition of social cues (especially dealing with emotions), gaze direction, and communicative gestures (Flechsenhar et al., 2022).
- The insula plays a crucial role in empathy and emotional awareness, as it evaluates social contexts and accurately interprets the emotions of others. Neural representations of feelings are linked to the insula, the surrounding parietal cortices, and the cingulate regions, which are essential areas for emotional sharing and empathy (Bechara, 2002; Flechsenhar et al., 2022).
- The temporoparietal junction (TPJ) supports perspective-taking and theory of mind (ToM). It facilitates the comprehension of others' beliefs and intentions, thereby enhancing one's capacity to consider alternative perspectives.

- The superior temporal sulcus (STS) aids in interpreting social interactions, processing dynamic social cues like eye gaze direction and emotional expressions.
- The orbitofrontal cortex (OFC) plays a role in evaluating social rewards and decision-making. Damage to this area can result in inappropriate social behavior.
- The medial prefrontal cortex (mPFC) is involved in self-referential thinking and ToM. It is essential in forming social judgments and understanding the mental states of others.
- The anterior cingulate cortex (ACC) regulates social conflict resolution and emotional responses. It plays a role in monitoring social interactions.
- The corpus callosum (CC) facilitates communication between brain hemispheres. Proper connectivity in this region is crucial for integrating social information.

Social behavior, social cognition, and social functioning are intricately interconnected. These variables represent observable behaviors that yield consequences, covert events, and long-term interactional patterns, all stemming from the interplay of cognitive and environmental factors (Kennedy & Adolphs, 2012). Social cognition is dependent on extensive neural networks in the brain, which are essential for comprehending social dysfunction. Functional compensation and recovery enable individuals with damage to the central nervous system (CNS) to adapt and enhance their residual or alternative skills through behavioral, cognitive, or physical strategies. This approach underscores a behavioral model (Duca & Rose, 2011) that supports the notion that social behaviors are influenced by environmental factors and can be supported in individuals with impairments (Kinnaman & Bellack, 2012; Liberman, 1982).

Psychological and Behavioral Substrates

Social interactions play a vital role in mental health, significantly influencing overall well-being, as humans are inherently social creatures. These interactions can serve as a transformative experience for individuals facing mental health challenges. Numerous media reports highlight how positive social experiences have positively changed individuals' lifestyles. Furthermore, social connectedness is essential for mental health and can facilitate recovery from mental health issues while combating the stigma associated with SMI (Saeri et al., 2018).

Successful social interactions require ongoing moment-to-moment adaptations that enhance social competencies and feelings of connectedness. A critical dimension of social functioning is for an individual to possess the skills of attending to and being aware of the verbal and nonverbal behaviors of others during a social exchange and change their verbal and nonverbal behaviors to "mesh" with the other.

Social functioning skills encompass a range of learned behaviors that enable individuals to engage effectively and appropriately in social situations, resulting in positive outcomes. These skills include both verbal and nonverbal behaviors, shaped by the social environment, and are vital for establishing and nurturing relationships. Learning models such as operant conditioning, classical conditioning, and social learning theory can be effectively applied within social contexts (Flechsenhar et al., 2022).

Skinner (1953) defined social behavior "as the behavior of two or more people with respect to one another or in concert to a common environment" (p. 297). The presence and the behavior of the other person that is occurring in a particular environment are the stimuli available in a social interaction. These stimuli are the source of the MOs and the antecedent and contingent consequential stimuli in an exchange. Consider a simple example of Person A holding a door open for Person B who is carrying a child into a store. Person A is opening the door to leave the store; he sees Person B approaching with a child in her arms. He perceives that she is coming to the door where he is standing; he looks at her and the child. Based on previous learning experiences, Person A perceives respondents and covert feelings of empathy toward Person B. Person A engages in covert verbal behaviors that are in the response class of volunteering and self-statements of helping others that are in alignment with his empathic respondents. Person A delays his leaving after opening the door, steps aside, and makes eye contact with Person B while holding the door as Person B enters. Person B makes eye contact and verbally responds with "thank you" and a smile. Person A responds with saying "Welcome" and a smile. He allows the door to close as Person B clears the doorway.

Although a simple exchange, there are several dimensions of social functioning that are occurring. Person A displays awareness of an antecedent situation that he has experienced or observed. He has observed role models that have engaged in behaviors that he has in his repertoire. Person A has had reinforcing consequences for engaging in the response class of helping and volunteering behaviors. He likewise has experienced these behaviors from others in similar contexts like when he was carrying luggage, grocery bags, or carrying his own child. The nonverbal behaviors of eye gazing and smiling were a part of this specific chain of behaviors. Person A has the capability of perceiving empathetic respondents that may be the MO of engaging in the response class of helping and volunteering behaviors. Person A was positively reinforced by the social reinforcing stimuli of Person B's eye contact, smile, and verbal response as he held the door open. The outcome is that the chances of this response class of behaviors occurring in the future have increased for Person A.

This simple exchange could be a skill that a person living with SMI does not have in her repertoire. The individual living with SMI in the same context may not be aware of the person coming to the door carrying a small child as her attentional abilities are impaired. She may be aware of the contextual stimuli but does not experience empathetic respondents as an MO to engage in the response class of helping behaviors. She may have experienced aversive consequences because of being perceived and stigmatized as a person living with mental health problems. She may also lack control over competing verbal and nonverbal responses that would result in a negative social outcome (e.g., talking to herself, asking for money).

The relationship between social functioning and mental health is reciprocal, with social abilities not merely a consequence of mental health problems. Individual differences and contextual factors play a significant role in how social competencies are developed and adapted (Flechsenhar et al., 2022). People living with SMI frequently fail to become integrated into a natural social network that can assist them in coping with social demands and other life stressors. People living with SMI frequently reside in impoverished and under-stimulating environments with few available opportunities to engage in prosocial and reinforcing behaviors. The lack of a naturally occurring reinforcing social network often results in the family of the individual living with SMI as the only network to which they belong. However, the interactional patterns of families of individuals living with SMI are frequently deviant, punitive, and aversive, providing additional stress, where the individual lacks the appropriate interpersonal skills to resolve (Morrison & Wixted, 1989). In fact, studies have consistently found that people living with SMI whose family relationships are characterized by hostile and aversive interactions are particularly likely to be hospitalized within 9 months of discharge (Vaughn & Leff, 1976).

People living with SMI display impairments in social functioning for a variety of reasons. One reason may be that they may have never learned the skills as children or young adults due to deficient social learning environments and/or subtle cognitive impairments in childhood, which can interfere with later development of relationships and the acquisition of social skills (Tenhula & Bellack, 2008). Many individuals who live with SMI develop problem behaviors in young adulthood, which is a critical time for the development of more sophisticated interpersonal relationships and social functioning like work and serious romantic sexual relationships. Young people living with SMI have a greater risk of developing co-occurring mental health problems that interfere with normative interactional patterns. People living with SMI are repeatedly traumatized. Any semblance of a natural reinforcing environment is disrupted by repeated hospitalizations and events of being removed from the community (e.g., incarceration). Many individuals with SMI can develop isolated lifestyles with few opportunities to engage in high-quality age-appropriate interactions that prompt and reinforce competent social skills (Abel et al., 2021). Finally, neurocognitive impairments that many individuals living with SMI experience can interfere with both social perception and social problem-solving (Kinnaman & Bellack, 2012).

Individual differences and contextual factors significantly influence the development, adaptation, and exhibition of social competencies. A transdiagnostic, dimensional perspective is proposed for creating targeted support strategies for individuals living with SMI. The complexities of language and social functioning reflect our ability to respond both verbally and nonverbally to the subtle and intricate variables inherent in human experiences and interactions (Flechsenhar et al., 2022).

Various support strategies are designed to enhance the social functional capacities of individuals living with SMI. These strategies can lead to substantial improvements in social functioning. Social skills training has demonstrated effective benefits in acquiring skills essential for competent social functioning (Flechsenhar et al., 2022).

Social skills represent a complex construct that has proven challenging to quantify with precision. Characteristically, it is defined operationally by performance on an analog test of social interaction (e.g. role-plays or structured conversation) or by the self-report of the individual or others who are familiar with the person's social functioning. Adequate performances on the instruments imply that the individual has the requisite behaviors in their repertoire, although other factors may interfere with performance in real-life interactions. An individual who does not perform adequately may not possess the requisite skills or may fail to manifest them due to confounding factors (e.g. anxiety about being evaluated, structure of the role-play) (Bellack et al., 1990).

A meta-analysis of studies that evaluated the effectiveness of skills training for social functioning for individuals living with SMI has been conducted. In an analysis of 22 studies involving over 1500 people living with SMI, Kurtz and Mueser (2008) found positive effects for social skills training on content and performance measures for social and daily living skills, community functioning, beneficial impact on behaviors of diminished functioning, other problem behavioral excesses, and relapses. The results support the efficacy of social skills training for improving psychosocial functioning in people living with SMI. Dilk and Bond (1996) reported that social skills training was found to be moderately to strongly effective in increasing skill acquisition and reducing problem behaviors linked to SMI. However, effect size varied by type of outcome measure, with situationally specific measures yielding larger effects than measures of skill usage and role functioning. Majority of studies did not explore if acquired skills were used outside the training setting and generalized to real-life context (Dilk & Bond, 1996).

The basic format of a session in social skills training (SST) (U.S. Department of Veterans Affairs, n.d.) contains the following elements:

1. Review outside practice—attempts at practicing the skill are reinforced with acknowledgement of cultural/language adaptations.
2. Establish rationale—discussion of the importance of the skill, considering sociocultural and community factors.
3. Share relevant experiences—group members contribute personal insights while the facilitator summarizes rationale.
4. Explain the skill steps—trainees read and analyze each step, exploring modifications based on personal and cultural backgrounds.
5. Model the skill—facilitator demonstrates the skill, and members review the process.
6. Role-play—trainees engage in structured role plays tailored to their personal goals.
7. Elicit and provide corrective feedback—constructive feedback is given after an initial role play, with emphasis on positive reinforcement.
8. Repeat role-play and corrective feedback—members refine the skill through additional role-plays with continued feedback.
9. Develop outside practice assignments—personalized goal-driven exercises considering social, cultural, and linguistic factors.

This structured learning approach ensures effective skill building for people living with SMI, with a focus on personalization and adaptability emphasizing cultural, linguistic, and contextual adaptations (U. S. Department of Veterans Affairs, n.d.).

Although social and coping skills training can reduce problem behaviors, boost functioning, and improve quality of life for individuals living with SMI, these positive effects often do not carry over to different settings or responses. This lack of generalization is a challenge in skills training. Most behavioral skills fail to generalize across settings without explicit programming (Cooper et al., 2020). The generalization of social skills in which social behavior is displayed in natural occurring contexts does not happen automatically and must be deliberately embedded into the training programs.

To achieve better outcomes in social skills being used in real-life situations, Corrigan and Basit (1997) have outlined five strategies to increase generalization of social skills that have been trained:

1. Fading reinforcers: gradually reducing external rewards to encourage independent skill use.
2. Self-management strategies: teaching individuals to increase self-awareness and monitor and regulate their own behavior.
3. Judicious use of homework: incorporating tasks outside of training sessions to reinforce skills.
4. Recruiting significant others: involving family or mental health service providers to support skill application in everyday contexts.
5. Cognitive rehabilitation: enhancing cognitive functions that underpin effective skill transfer such as self-awareness, attention, cognitive flexibility, and response speed.
6. Independent practice: participants try out the skills learned in real-life situations, supervised by caregivers, with the next session starting with a review of this practice.

Additional strategies involve training skills across a variety of social contexts, ensuring that the stimuli in the training environment correspond with real-life situations. It is essential to promote flexibility by encouraging trainees to consider alternative stimuli that may arise in social contexts and to identify appropriate behaviors to employ. Furthermore, training should address scenarios where certain skills should not be exhibited, such as negative exemplars (Cooper et al., 2020). Aruldass et al. (2022) enhanced the SST format by involving the caregivers of individuals with SMI in the sessions, allowing participants to practice the skills learned during SST in real-life situations under the guidance and supervision of their caregivers. Each subsequent session commenced with a review of the supervised practice in real-life contexts, followed by feedback and problem-solving discussions.

Epidemiological Considerations

Impairment in social functioning is a critical aspect of ascertaining the presence of living with SMI (Roeling, 2010). Research on individuals who live with SMI indicates that impairments in social functioning are widespread. Social impairment is a criterion for the presence of only two mental health problems in the DSM-V-TR (American Psychiatric Association, 2022): autism spectrum disorder (ASD) and antisocial personality disorder (ASPD); it is a defining feature for ASD, whereas it is a contributing problem for ASPD where it is defined as the intentional disregard and violation of normative social behaviors.

As stated previously, social functioning is a construct that presents challenges to define and operationalize (Bellack et al., 1990). Multiple definitions of social functioning and social skills exist in the mental health literature. Publications and books were searched using the Google Scholar, PsycINFO, and PubMed database with the following key words in various combinations: prevalence, deficits, impairments, social skills, social functioning, chronic mental illness, serious mental illness, severe mental illness, schizophrenia, and bipolar disorder in various combinations. No studies were found that focused on the prevalence of and cultural influences on social functioning impairments among individuals living with SMI.

Mueser et al. (1991) investigated the prevalence and temporal stability of social skill deficits in 36 individuals diagnosed with schizophrenia spectrum mental health problems by comparing them to individuals without mental health issues. The study examined the stability of social skills over 6 months and 1 year following hospitalization. The findings indicated that approximately 50% of individuals living with SMI consistently exhibited social skill impairments over a 1-year period, while 11% consistently demonstrated skilled social interactions. Impairments in specific social skills were uncommon, with 14% of patients consistently displaying difficulties in conversational turn-taking. Overall, social skill impairments were prevalent but not universal among people living with SMI, with global social skill performance being more impaired than specific skill components.

In a related study, Druss et al. (2009) explored the prevalence of social role impairment, as assessed by the Sheehan Disability Scale (SDS). The SDS is a self-report scale that assesses disability in work/school activities, family relationships, and social functioning and evaluates the functional impact of mental health problems (Arbuckle et al., 2009). Results found that individuals living with SMI report severe social role impairment in 29.7% of cases. The mental health problems that resulted in the greatest impairment in the social domain were the mental health problems of bipolar (50.0%), major depression (49.1%), and PTSD (48.2%). Mental health problems were significantly more likely to cause severe social-role impairment compared to chronic medical conditions.

Types of Problems with Social Skills

The types of social skill impairments can be categorized according to domains and dimensions of social functioning, such as verbal and nonverbal behaviors that are impaired in social exchanges or along behavioral dimensions of functional social behaviors, such as meshing, eye gaze, and emotional expressiveness. The types of social functioning impairments also can be classified according to the behavioral response classes of social behaviors that are the basis of SST.

The following is a list of behavioral response classes that are trained in SST. The types of response classes are from research by the U. S. Department of Veterans Affairs (n.d.) (Kopelowicz et al., 2006; Koujalgi et al., 2014):

- Communication skills: involve expressing emotions, making and refusing requests, starting and ending conversations, exchanging compliments.
- Interpersonal skills: include active listening, empathy, respect, and cooperation.
- Responding or sending skills: effective use of verbal and nonverbal communication.
- Affiliative skills: expressing affection to family and friends and using self-disclosure judiciously.
- Problem-solving and conflict resolution; focus on understanding social situations, developing responses, negotiating, and compromising.
- Emotional regulation: recognizing and managing emotions and expressing them appropriately.
- Social perception: involves interpreting social cues, recognizing social rules, responding effectively, and accurate evaluation and appropriate interpretation of emotional expressions from others.
- Affiliative and interactional skills: include expressing affection, self-disclosure, starting and maintaining conversations, dating, and friendship.
- Instrumental role and norm-governed behavior: encompass practical tasks (e.g., renting an apartment) community living, and appropriate behavior in social settings.
- Vocational: employment interviews and work relationships.
- Health maintenance: communicating effectively with providers.
- Instrumental role skills: practical tasks such as purchasing food, renting an apartment.
- Behavior governed by social norms: examples include speaking politely to authority figures, such as a policeman.
- Other important skills: include refusing substances, asking for help, and handling unwanted advice.

Why Do Problems with Social Functioning Occur?

Part of the Reason May Be Problems with Neurocognitive Capabilities

- Sometimes, impaired social functioning will be due primarily to the neurocognitive impairments that affect many people living with SMIs (such as difficulty paying attention and concentrating). The person living with SMI may not have the ability to attend, learn, and remember acceptable ways to behave in many situations.

Part of the Reason May Be Biological

- Impaired social functioning may be a result of the imbalance of neurotransmitters that are associated with SMI. This imbalance can cause several other problems, such as having difficulty thinking clearly that contributes to the social functioning problems. The chemical imbalances can sometimes be caused by medications or other drugs. Medications that help to decrease such problems as delusions or hallucinations may make the person living with SMI drowsy, sluggish, sitting with eyes closed, and having problems with attention and concentration. The person living with SMI may be less able to use social skills that have been learned.

Part of the Reason May Be Psychosocial

- Living with SMI can result in the development of interpersonal relationships that fail to encourage the development and use of good social functioning. For example, a person who shows signs of SMI early in life may not be exposed to many friends and other interpersonal situations and not have the opportunities to learn and engage in adaptive and normative social behaviors. For instance, Becky began to experience symptoms of living with a SMI at age 14, a time when adolescents begin to develop skills in social functioning needed to deal with other people in an adult-like manner. Even if many social skills have been learned, the person living with SMI may have become dependent on a parent, siblings, or caretakers for most basic needs. This can influence the other family members to treat the person living with SMI as a child and enable the person living with SMI to be dependent on them and impair independent functioning. They may forget to encourage the person to independently do whatever they can. The frustration that others experience when the person living with SMI fails to use good social skills can result in critical interactions—such as blaming, arguing, and belittling—which often make matters worse. This will impair the ability of the person living with SMI to develop new social skills or use whatever skills that have been learned.

Part of the Reason May Be Motivational

- Impaired social skills may also result from apathy and avolition (i.e., low level of motivation) that is frequently a problem displayed by people living with SMI. Even if the person living with SMI learned adequate social skills when younger, a common and unfortunate effect of SMI is to have diminished motivation to use them. Diminished motivation is usually considered to be caused by the biochemical imbalance that causes the symptoms seen in persons living with SMI but is often not impacted by psychiatric medications (Correll & Schooler, 2020).
- Another possible reason is that there are not enough rewards—reinforcers—in their environment to display competent functional social skills. People living with SMI have been found to be isolated and have impoverished interpersonal interactions (Abel et al., 2021). Most people who display competent social functioning receive positive responses from other people. For people living with SMI, however, the common responses of other people, even when positive, may not be reasons to use good social skills. Occasional compliments from others often serve as motivators for many individuals to dress neatly. However, for someone living with SMI, such compliments may have little effect, as they might struggle to derive pleasure from experiences, a condition known as anhedonia. Typically, individuals who demonstrate competent social functioning receive positive responses from their peers. In contrast, those living with SMI may find that even affirmative feedback fails to motivate them to utilize appropriate social skills. For example, while compliments can inspire most people to maintain a tidy appearance, their impact on someone with SMI is often minimal. Using the example of Becky above, she seldom wears her shoes correctly. She doesn't tie them and frequently slips as she walks. She ties them when asked and seems to enjoy any compliments that she gets about dressing neatly, but these don't have a lasting impact. In her case, and many others, something more may be necessary, such as more frequent compliments or compliments that more clearly provide important and specific information (e.g., "I like the way you put on a warm shirt and button it all the way" instead of "You look nice today."). Without these extra features, some people living with SMI will not respond. Over time, other people may stop trying, making it even more unlikely that the person living with SMI will use the social skills.

It is improbable that any single reason among these is sufficiently significant to be evaluated in isolation from others. More likely, each of these factors contributes to the emergence of issues in social functioning. Therefore, all must be considered when determining appropriate interventions for such challenges. It is unlikely that any individual factor among these is sufficiently significant to be assessed in isolation from others. Rather, it is probable that each of these elements plays a role in the development of issues related to social functioning. Consequently, all must be considered when determining suitable support strategies for these challenges.

Behavioral Support Strategies for Social Skills Problems in a Person Living with SMI

Social skills encompass a range of behaviors essential for effective interpersonal interactions. Individuals living with SMI may exhibit proficiency in certain social skills while struggling with others. Consequently, a critical initial step is to clearly identify the specific social skills that require enhancement for the individual with SMI.

Before making any changes, it is essential to evaluate the necessity of such efforts. The presence of social skill challenges in an individual does not inherently imply that intervention is needed. These issues may occur infrequently or may not be perceived as significant by others. If the social skill difficulties of the individual do not disrupt critical activities such as medication adherence, participation in community programs, or employment, it is prudent to assess the value of attempting to modify these behaviors. For instance, if the individual does not initiate many social exchanges yet can attend community programs and engage with staff and peers, it may not be critical to promote additional interactions. A more pragmatic approach may involve accepting and accommodating existing abilities. Seeking guidance from a mental health service professional can be beneficial in establishing realistic and achievable goals.

Problematic Social Skills that Occur in Individuals Living with Serious Mental Illness

Problems with Interrupting Others

- It is essential to clearly identify the timing and context of interruptions. Utilize the form provided in the Appendix to document any variations in the observed behavior that may correlate with factors such as the time of day, the identity of the other individual, the subject matter being discussed, or other potential influences. This analysis will help ascertain the frequency of the issue. For instance, it may be observed that interruptions are more prevalent during phone conversations or when visitors are present. Such insights are crucial for formulating effective strategies to address the issue. In Becky's case, caregivers reported that she tended to engage in conversation with others while they were on the phone or talking with another person.
- Some medications may cause restlessness in the individual receiving care or hinder their capacity to regulate their own behavior. If these interruptions appear to stem from restlessness, it may be beneficial to consult a prescribing mental health service professional regarding the current medications being administered. Adjustments or changes to the medication regimen may be feasible to alleviate restlessness, sedation, or other issues induced by the medications.

- Establishing clear communication guidelines is essential for fostering effective interactions. It is advisable to develop straightforward rules that all service providers and caretakers can adhere to consistently. These guidelines may encompass taking turns during conversations, maintaining eye contact with the speaker, and using a moderate tone of voice, among others that are deemed primary. It is also important to acknowledge and commend individuals for adhering to these rules. For instance, in the case of Becky, who struggles with waiting her turn to speak with certain individuals, staff were instructed to observe instances when she successfully waited her turn. Upon such occasions, they were to affirm her behavior by stating, "Becky, you waited your turn to talk. Good job. What would you like to discuss with me?" This approach reinforces positive communication habits.
- Allocate dedicated time each day for the individual. It is advisable to establish a reasonable duration during which undivided attention is given to the person living with SMI. This time can often be integrated into regular daily routines. Optimal moments for this engagement may include morning coffee or shortly after dinner. Encourage the individual to select the discussion topics, ensuring that the topic of conversation is based on reality and not a false belief (i.e., delusion). Challenges, such as a lack of conversational topics, may arise when attempting to implement this schedule. Typically, persistence is essential for achieving success.
- Avoid placing expectations on the individual that exceed their capacity. Consider contracting for the behavior that is expected. It may be helpful to write a contract with a person living with SMI. The contract should specify a choice of various rewards for success in being patient and not interrupting. Involve the person living with SMI in the development of the behavioral contract like choosing the replacement behaviors and the reinforcers. In the beginning of such a plan, compliment and provide the reward for any improvement that is observed. Increase expectations as progress is made.
- It is imperative to ensure that conversational turns are taken appropriately. When interacting with an individual who is living with SMI, it is crucial to alternate speaking turns. Comments should be kept concise, allowing ample opportunity for the individual to respond. This method exemplifies the fundamental skills necessary for effective communication. Employing nonverbal signals, such as raising a hand, can facilitate the indication of a shift in the conversation and denote when it is one's turn to speak.
- Assist the individual living with SMI to learn appropriate methods to gain attention. They may not be aware of how to attract someone's attention without causing disruption. Demonstrate techniques for interjecting into a conversation respectfully, such as saying, "Excuse me, may I ask you something?" Additionally, acknowledge and commend any successful attempts that are made.
- Be prepared to correct mistakes. When the person living with SMI fails to follow a rule, provide correction in a composed and objective approach, characterized by neutrality and professionalism. This may require practice to do well. If unsure about how this is done, seek the advice of a mental health service professional.

Be prepared to provide the same corrective feedback to others that give care to the person living with SMI if they also have difficulty following the rules. When giving corrective feedback, be prepared to clearly explain what is being done wrong and what behaviors should be done instead. For example: "You're talking when it's my turn. If you can wait patiently for a few more minutes, I'll come see what you want." This increases the likelihood that guidance will be understood and followed. Using the example above, Becky has difficulty waiting her turn in conversations. She often continues to talk even when the other person is saying something. Rather than continuing to listen to her (and becoming impatient and angry with her), the staff hold up their hand and say, "It's my turn to talk." If she stops and listens, they thank her.

- When rules aren't followed, be prepared to stop the conversation. If the person living with SMI continues to interrupt after being corrected, do not continue the conversation. Attend to other matters and leave the conversation (e.g., "I won't continue to talk to you unless you can take turns."). In the example with Beckey, if she does not stop interrupting and talking after the staff has prompted her to take turns, the staff walked away.
- Coaching effective communication techniques with individuals living with SMI is essential. It is important to assist friends, relatives, and others in understanding the challenges the person faces during conversations. Furthermore, providing support to help others develop the techniques outlined in this section is crucial for fostering better interactions.
- It is advisable to seek assistance when necessary. Many recommendations in this section may present challenges in implementation. If difficulties are encountered in making progress, consider consulting a mental health service professional with expertise in behavioral support methods. Typically, this would be a clinical psychologist experienced in working with individuals living with SMI.

Problems with Rude Comments

- Clearly articulate your intentions. "Rudeness" can manifest in various ways. Specify the behaviors exhibited by individuals living with SMI that are perceived as rude. Is the issue the use of profanity in public settings, inquiring about sensitive topics such as personal hygiene, or making disparaging remarks like "You have a big nose." A precise definition of these behaviors increases the likelihood of effectively addressing the situation.
- Note when the problem occurs. Use the form in the Appendix to keep data and look for possible differences in behavior according to the people who are the target of the rude comments, where the behavior happens, or other issues that may be important. For example, a male may make rude comments when around females, such as "I'd like to take a shower with you." In the example, Becky tells certain males that they have a "nice butt" and sometimes adds that "I'd like to have sex with you." Being aware of who she makes these comments to will likely

be very important in creating more effective ways to minimize the problem. It is possible that if such situations can be predicted, these can be avoided in the future, and this may be the simplest method to minimize the problem.

- Consider seeking a review of medications. Some medications sometimes make a person more irritable and may contribute to rudeness or impatience. If the medications of the person living with SMI have not recently been reviewed, seek the advice of a mental health service prescriber regarding whether a change in medication will be helpful.
- Clearly define realistic expectations and establish straightforward, consistent rules for addressing situations involving rude comments. An example would be: "there is no cursing or yelling in the house." These conversational rules should apply to everyone. If others around the person living with SMI make rude comments, correct them also.
- Watch for examples of the desired behavior. Stay alert for circumstances in which the person living with SMI interacts competently. If he says something nice to a friend who comes to visit, compliment such success (e.g., "I liked what you said to Mary about her dress."). It is important to acknowledge any progress that is observed.
- Provide corrections in a calm and matter-of-fact manner. Avoid displaying shock, surprise, or disgust when interacting with individuals living with SMI who may make rude comments or gestures. Such comments are sometimes intended to provoke a reaction, which may inadvertently encourage further inappropriate behavior. Address this conduct in a composed, deliberate, and professional manner. If feeling upset, it may hinder any ability to respond effectively. In such instances, it is advisable to take a break, remove oneself from the situation, and return once composure is regained. Refrain from making statements that could exacerbate the situation. This approach may necessitate practice with a mental health service professional.
- When providing corrections, it is essential to articulate expectations clearly. When addressing inappropriate remarks from individuals with SMI, it is important to specify what was inappropriate and suggest preferred alternatives. For instance, one might say, "I've asked that you do not curse or swear; you can express the same sentiment without using to such language." Additionally, acknowledge and commend any positive changes that are observed following corrective feedback.
- If necessary, be prepared to stop the conversation. If the person living with SMI continues to make rude comments after being corrected, do not continue the interaction. Excuse yourself to other matters (e.g., "I don't like the language you're using. I'm leaving. When you think you can use better language, come see me."). Don't allow the interaction to continue unless more acceptable behavior occurs.
- Consider developing a behavior contract. Consider developing a contract like the example in Chap. 4. This contract should clearly specify what behaviors are expected to be manifested by the person living with SMI when talking to other people and identifies specific positive consequences for meeting the expectations

(e.g., agreeing to take the person living with SMI to a favorite restaurant if he succeeds at refraining from using curse words during a family visit). With Becky, the staff developed a contract that allowed her to earn money to buy her own cigarettes and sodas if she did not ask for the items from other people. It may be necessary to seek the advice of a mental health service professional to do this well.

- Provide guidance to others. Help others understand that the rude comments may occur and help them learn how to deal with them. This will help to reduce their uncertainty and frustration. Most people will appreciate the assistance about what to expect and what they should do about it.

Problems with Social Withdrawal, Isolation, and Not Initiating Conversations

- Be clear about what the person living with SMI does. Withdrawal, isolation, and lack of motivation to initiate conversations will mean different things to different people. Be clear about what the person living with SMI does that defines the problem (e.g., "He just sits in the family room and watches soap operas for several hours every afternoon.").
- Note when the problem is likely to happen. Use the form in the Appendix to become aware of any variation in the situations when, with whom, and what the person living with SMI does when he "withdraws" or "isolates." Watch to see if and how this varies according to time of day, the setting, who else is present, or other factors. Be cognizant of any behavioral patterns that emerge. Be particularly aware of times when the person living with SMI may be overstimulated such as during groups, social gatherings, parties, or visits by neighbors. At the same time, watch for situations in which the person living with SMI seems more motivated or willing to talk to others. This information is often important in planning more effective ways to deal with the problem.
- Consider having medications reviewed. Some medications contribute to lethargy or confusion, which makes social interactions or other activities difficult to initiate and maintain. If there are concerns that social withdrawal has intensified following a modification or increase in medication, it is advisable to consult a mental health service prescriber for a comprehensive evaluation of currently prescribed medications.
- Establish daily routines for important activities. Life can often become very chaotic and unstructured. This is a poor environment for a person living with SMI who is inclined to be socially withdrawn. The person living with SMI is more likely to become involved in social activities if they are routine, familiar, and predictable (e.g., having dinner at approximately the same time each day with a brief conversation time afterward).

- Consider developing a behavioral contract to encourage more activity. This contract should identify specific activities that the person living with SMI could do and identify rewards that will be made available to the person living with SMI for following through and doing specified activities or behaviors. An example would be taking the person to a preferred movie if he goes to the community mental health center as scheduled. Remember expectations when beginning a contract must be modest. Provide an opportunity for the person living with SMI to succeed before setting higher expectations.
- Encourage preferred activities to prompt conversations with someone living with SMI. Pair these activities, like going to the store or eating out, with social opportunities, such as inviting a friend. Use these activities as rewards in a behavior contract, setting easy-to-achieve expectations to ensure success and interest.
- Determine which individuals are preferred conversational partners for the person. Identify those with whom the individual living with SMI feels most comfortable and maintains regular interaction. Encourage these selected individuals to increase their engagement with the person. These preferred individuals can help the person gradually get used to new situations and meet new people. Just like with preferred activities, you can use access to these individuals as a reward in a behavior contract.
- Strive to facilitate progress while exercising caution against excessive pressure. In efforts to promote social interaction, it is crucial to refrain from overwhelming individuals living with SMI. Such pressure may induce anxiety and potentially result in adverse effects. Instead, motivate individuals living with SMI to participate in uncomplicated interactions with others. It is important to refrain from forcing these interactions; for instance, if an individual living with SMI spends 30 minutes watching television with family members or caregivers—when they typically prefer solitude in their room—this should be recognized as progress, even if verbal communication is minimal. Additionally, refrain from making light-hearted remarks, teasing, or displaying impatience when the individual opts out of engaging in available activities, as they may misconstrue such comments as criticism. If gentle encouragement does not yield immediate results, it is advisable to withdraw and revisit the approach later or with more manageable expectations.
- For instance, Becky had a hard time staying in groups of people but then would complain that she was bored because there was nothing to do. The staff involved her in a needlepoint project for a sewing group. They set a timer for 5 minutes. If Becky worked on the needlepoint project until the timer expired, she earned points that she could trade in for something she wanted. As she succeeded, the time slowly increased over several months until she was working for 20 minutes without leaving the group; as she spent more time in the room with other people, her conversations with them increased and improved.
- Acknowledge and appreciate the individual living with SMI for their interactions, even if they appear trivial. Gradually raise expectations as progress is made.

- Avoid perceiving the problem as insurmountable. It is important to recognize that changes may not occur rapidly, even if there is a belief that individuals living with SMI possess the capacity for greater achievements.
- Be mindful of reactions toward the individual. In some instances, others may have resigned themselves to the situation, ceasing to take any proactive measures. Conversely, certain behaviors from others may inadvertently exacerbate social withdrawal by expressing frustration or criticism.
- Provide guidance to others. Help other people to be aware that the person living with SMI tends to stay alone. Help them to understand how to behave (e.g., avoid appearing impatient or pushing too hard) as they will likely appreciate the guidance that is offered regarding how to handle such situations.
- If efforts are unsuccessful, seek help. Social withdrawal and lack of motivation are often identified as the most frustrating problems faced by family and mental health service providers (Provencher & Mueser, 1997). Medications have not been found to be very helpful in reducing these problems (Correll & Schooler, 2020). Many of the suggestions that have been made are much more difficult to carry out than people expect them to be. Do not hesitate to seek guidance from a mental health service professional.

Problems with Inappropriate Behaviors in the Homes of Other People and Public Places

- Be clear about what the problem is. "Inappropriate" means different things to different people. Be clear and specific about what the person living with SMI does that is inappropriate (e.g., "She helps herself to whatever is in the refrigerator without asking"). This helps to reduce confusion among those who are working to improve the behavior of the person living with SMI.
- Plan for any visit. Anticipate potential behavioral challenges that may arise. Establish clear and realistic expectations with the individual living with SMI prior to the visit; confirm their understanding by having them rehearse the expectations. Avoid setting expectations that may be difficult for the individual to meet. If the individual frequently requests cigarettes from those around them, inform them that cigarettes will be available, upon asking, refraining from asking others, and it must be smoked outside.
- It may be beneficial to agree on a discreet signal to indicate when a behavior change is necessary (e.g., raising the hand as a signal for the individual to cease asking others for cigarettes). Remember to acknowledge and commend the individual whenever they respond positively to the agreed upon signal. When setting expectations, include guidance for what to do as well as what not to do. Just before a visit, remind the person living with SMI of the expectations for what they should do during the visit. Remember that these expectations should be

realistic. Consider making a list of the expected behaviors to go over just before leaving.

- Acknowledge and celebrate successes. Consider the potential challenges that may arise when the individual visits a friend's home or goes to a public space. Clearly define expected behaviors for the person living with SMI. Establish consistent "rules of conduct" and offer praise or rewards when these rules are adhered to. These guidelines should be uniform for expectations both at the residence of the person living with SMI and in public settings. If the rules are consistently followed, it is likely that they will be observed in other settings. After outings, commend the individual with SMI for their adherence to the rules (e.g., "I appreciate how you waited your turn to speak.").
- When providing corrections, it is essential to consider the most effective approach. In certain situations, it may be beneficial to promptly inform the individual living with SMI about their behavior and suggest appropriate alternatives. For instance, if the individual is speaking loudly and disrupting others, it is advisable to request that he steps aside and say, "Please lower your voice," or "There is no need to speak so loudly." In a specific scenario, when Becky spoke loudly and interrupted others, caregivers were instructed to communicate the following: "Becky, I am currently talking with someone; please wait for your turn. I will speak with you as soon as I am finished." Conversely, there are instances where immediate feedback may cause embarrassment, leading to a negative reaction from the individual.
- Be prepared to terminate a visit if corrective attempts are not working. Despite attempts to set realistic expectations, some situations will be encountered in which the person living with SMI cannot achieve an acceptable level of success. If the person living with SMI is not responding to attempts and prompts to encourage more acceptable behavior, be prepared to leave the place that is being visited. For example, if the person living with SMI asks others for cigarettes in a restaurant and won't stop when requested, be prepared to leave. Experience is the best guide as to when it is necessary to leave.
- Include visits to places that the person living with SMI prefers. Be aware of places to which the person living with SMI likes to go and plan occasional visits to these places, such as a preferred restaurant or a friend's home. The person living with SMI will be more motivated to follow guidelines when visiting such places. This will provide an opportunity for success that can be reinforced. With such success, the person living with SMI is more likely to succeed in other situations. Also, having to leave preferred places because of them may have more impact.
- Guide family and friends on what to expect and how to act when interacting with someone living with SMI. Encourage open communication at places frequented by the individual, helping them understand potential behaviors and set realistic expectations. This can reduce concerns and make them appreciate the advice. Help align their expectations with those at the person's residence and provide tips on effective interaction.

Problems with Not Listening to What Is Said

- Consider seeking a hearing examination. Difficulty listening may simply be due to a hearing problem.
- Observe when the issue occurs by using the form in the Appendix. This will help identify variations based on topics, time of day, speakers, or other factors, which are crucial for understanding and addressing the issue. For example, patterns may indicate that an individual with SMI listens more attentively when discussing a movie compared to discussing cleaning the bedroom.
- Identify potential distractions in the environment that may hinder the ability of individuals living with SMI to focus. These distractions can include noise, television, radio, the presence of other people, and various environmental factors. It is advisable to initiate conversations when there are minimal distractions present.
- Simplify requests. When giving multiple instructions, break them down into clear, manageable steps. For instance, instead of saying, "go downstairs, get clean sheets and make your bed," provide the information in smaller parts, one step at a time. This approach can enhance understanding. Additionally, it may be beneficial for the person living with SMI to repeat the instructions to ensure comprehension. If they accurately repeat the steps, offer praise for their attentiveness, such as, "That is exactly what I said and want you to do. Thank you for listening." If the message is complex (containing several steps), consider putting the information down on paper. For many situations, it may be helpful to provide a written set of instructions that breaks down expectations to several smaller and simple steps, as in the bed-making example above. This will assist individuals living with SMI in recalling instructions.
- Be patient. Improvement will take time. Remain patient in attempts to communicate with the person living with SMI. Do not become easily frustrated or give up. Be willing and able to invest time to minimize the likelihood that the message is ignored. Seek support from others if needed.
- Demonstrate to the individual living with SMI that effective communication is a priority. To enhance the individual's attention, employ strategies such as using their name, maintaining an appropriate distance, establishing eye contact (while avoiding prolonged staring), utilizing a warm tone of voice, and encouraging them to paraphrase statements periodically. Prior to conveying important information, preface remarks with a phrase like, "It is important that you listen to what I am about to say." In the case of Becky, staff members were advised to utilize concise sentences and prompt her to repeat key points. By addressing the behavioral challenges exhibited by Becky, caregivers demonstrated their commitment to ensuring her comprehension of the information presented. These communication guidelines should be consistently applied by all individuals within the residential and recovery environments. Look for success. Watch when and where the person living with SMI listens well. Remember to compliment this success. When complimenting, be clear about what the person living with SMI is

doing is competent and adaptive (e.g., "I like the way you were able to keep looking at me while I talked with you.").

- Monitor stress levels. It is essential to be cognizant of frustration levels while implementing these recommendations. Engage with the individual living with SMI in a supportive manner, avoiding a critical tone. Maintain objectivity and treat the individual respectfully. It is important to recognize that a person living with SMI may experience difficulties in processing information, and this should not be interpreted personally, nor should it be assumed that the person lacks the desire to improve.

Conclusion for Behavioral Support Strategies for Social Skills Problems in a Person Living with SMI

When you want to try to improve the social functioning of the person living with SMI, consider the following steps:

1. Identify the specific changes that should be implemented. Rather than solely concentrating on eliminating issues, think about the positive outcomes that are desired for the individual living with SMI.
2. Evaluate the severity of the problem to determine if it justifies effort to change it.
3. Ensure that the medications prescribed to the individual living with SMI are appropriate and being administered as directed.
4. Clearly articulate objectives regarding the desired improvements in the person's behavior. It is generally advisable to initiate with straightforward, achievable behaviors that are already in the individual's behavioral repertoire but may not be exhibited frequently or of sufficient magnitude and duration.
5. Observe and acknowledge the positive behaviors exhibited by the individual living with SMI; provide positive reinforcement for these actions. For monitoring forms and examples, refer to the Appendix.
6. Raise expectations as progress is observed.
7. Consider developing a contract to delineate the goals and objectives agreed upon by the individual living with SMI and the support that is needed for success.
8. Educate friends and others who interact with the individual on the most effective support strategies to be used.
9. If efforts do not yield satisfactory results, do not hesitate to seek professional assistance.

What About Becky?

At the hospital, the staff decided to develop a contract with her. First, they had all her physical complaints evaluated by a physician and confirmed that she required no additional treatment. They were very aware that she liked cigarettes, coffee, sodas, time with certain other people, and a variety of possible reinforcers. They set up a schedule for her to get access to these if she was able to successfully go an identified short amount of time without cursing, yelling, threatening, or hitting other people. When she began complaining of physical problems, they were instructed to ignore that topic and bring up another topic. They agreed to use a signal (e.g., putting their hands up) if she continued to complain. If this didn't work, they were instructed to turn their backs and say, "When you're ready to talk with me, I'll be ready to listen." If this didn't work after 10 seconds, they walked away and did something else. They helped her to identify staff members who would meet with her for a specified time-period (e.g., 15 minutes) if she was able to refrain from the problem behaviors for a period of 3 hours.

To help Becky, the staff members did the following:

1. They clarified the problems that they hoped to reduce (i.e., cutting in on conversations; complaining about her treatment; complaining about her bowel habits; demanding cigarettes and sodas; frequent cursing).
2. They clarified the behaviors that they wanted to see Becky do instead (take turns in conversations; talking to others without cursing, complaining about her treatment or bowel habits; refraining from demands for cigarettes or other items).
3. They identified several things that Becky liked (cigarettes, sodas, time with certain other people) and could be used to reinforce adaptive behaviors.
4. They made an agreement to give Becky certain of these reinforcers when she was able to successfully do what was specified.
5. They knew that the expectations were realistic when the plan began (refrain from asking for sodas and cigarettes for 1 hour). Higher expectations were planned as they saw success. They also accepted that Becky may not ever act in a completely "normal" manner.
6. They watched when Becky did well and complimented her at those times. In doing so, they were providing compliments to her that they may not give to most other people who had better control of problem behaviors.

Summary

Individuals living with SMI often experience significant impairments in social functioning, which can greatly affect their daily lives. Impairments in functional social skills may result in dependency, isolation, and strained relationships. These challenges arise from a combination of neurocognitive, biological, psychosocial, and motivational factors. Effective social functioning encompasses behaviors essential for successful interpersonal interactions, including communication and social skills. Notably, social dysfunction is prevalent in SMI and can persist even when other problematic behaviors and symptoms show improvement.

Negative symptoms, which are defined as diminished or absent expression of expected and normative behaviors and emotions, significantly impact social functioning and are linked to social withdrawal and avoidance. Negative symptoms include diminished emotional expressiveness, impairments in motivation (avolition), diminished verbal and nonverbal communication (alogia) and experiencing pleasure (anhedonia), and lack of social interactions (asociality). Fifty-to-sixty percent of individuals with SMI experience at least one negative symptom, and people living with a schizophrenia spectrum mental health problems experience more than two diminished behaviors. Understanding the distinction between primary and secondary negative symptoms is crucial for effective treatment. Secondary negative symptoms may arise from social impairments or positive symptoms rather than being their cause.

Addressing the initiation and maintenance of social interactions is crucial for enhancing social functioning in individuals with SMI. There is a notable distinction between social functional capacity and real-world performance, as many individuals face challenges in everyday situations. Assessments of social functioning frequently depend on self-reports, which can be subjective, while observational measures tend to be labor-intensive. Impairments in neurocognitive skills are significant predictors of difficulties in social functioning. This domain encompasses a complex array of behaviors, including the skills and cognitive processes necessary for effective social interactions. Social functioning is a multifaceted construct that includes various social skills and behaviors essential for successful interpersonal interactions. It involves both verbal and nonverbal communication, social cognition, and the ability to adapt to diverse social contexts. Individuals living with SMI encounter numerous challenges and impairments in social functioning, largely due to issues with social pragmatic communication.

Social functioning encompasses learned responses and skills that are both normative and socially accepted. It includes the appropriate use of language in social contexts, known as social pragmatic communication. Effective social functioning necessitates the integration of three key domains of pragmatic communication: the reception of social stimuli, the processing and generation of responses, and the delivery of appropriate replies. The DSM-5-TR identifies impairments in specific subdomains of communication to determine the presence of social pragmatic communication issues.

Social pragmatic communication consists of several subdomains that contribute to effective social interactions. These subdomains are essential for understanding and managing social exchanges. Contextual understanding involves adapting language and behavior to match the social setting and purpose. Conversational management includes turn-taking, staying on topic, and rephrasing when misunderstood. Nonliteral language comprehension is necessary for understanding idioms, humor, and metaphors. Inferential reasoning allows individuals to make inferences based on implicit information. Social etiquette involves adhering to social norms and rules during communication. Pragmatic social communication behaviors include verbal behaviors such as speech acts and message cohesion, paralinguistic aspects like fluency and tone, nonverbal cues including facial expressions and gestures, and the significance of responsive interaction. It also highlights the management of semantic content, the need for cohesion and fluency in communication, sociolinguistic sensitivity to social norms, and functional communication skills necessary for effective real-life interactions.

Social competence refers to the overall quality of an individual's performance in social tasks, requiring the ability to be aware of and assess situations and respond appropriately. It is crucial for successful interpersonal relations. Social competence includes recognizing the feelings and intentions of others and selecting appropriate behaviors. Socially competent behaviors involve generating appropriate responses using verbal and nonverbal communication and are influenced by cognitive perceptual abilities and the effectiveness of interpersonal exchanges. Social impairments can be addressed through skills training and awareness of social situations and contexts.

Social functioning relies on specific neurocognitive processes known as social cognitions, which are essential for recognizing and processing social stimuli. These processes are critical for effective social interactions. Social cognition includes understanding oneself and others in social contexts, involving mental representations and decision-making. Impairments in social cognition can lead to social dysfunction, particularly in individuals living with SMI. Key domains of social cognition include attributional style, theory of mind (ToM), and perceptions of emotions. Individuals with SMI often show impairments in social cognition independent of their cognitive intelligence.

Various assessment tools have been developed to measure the dimensions of social functioning in individuals, particularly those living with SMI. These tools evaluate different aspects of social skills and behaviors. The Social Skills Assessment Screening Scale (SSASS) measures nonverbal behavior, verbal communication, and social behavior. Findings from SSASS indicate significant impairments in social behavior in people living with SMI, particularly in the response classes of helping others voluntarily (26.3%) and empathizing (25.8%). The Social Skills Performance Assessment (SSPA) evaluates social competence and appropriateness through role-plays. The Social Skills Inventory-2 Del-Prette assesses assertive conversation, affective-sexual approach behaviors, and self-control through self-report measures.

Assessment tools of social pragmatic communication include various instruments like the Discourse Comprehension Test (DCT) focusing on narrative processing, the Pragmatic Protocol (PP) assessing verbal and nonverbal aspects, and the Profile of Communicative Appropriateness (PCA) evaluating multiple dimensions of communication. Other tools include the Communicative Abilities in Daily Living (CADL) for functional communication, the Functional Communication Profile (FCP) assessing various communication activities, and the Functional Assessment of Communication Skills (FACS) covering social communication and daily planning with qualitative and quantitative scales.

Social functioning is inherently multidimensional, encompassing various behaviors and skills that are dependent on context. Understanding this complexity is essential for effective assessment and intervention. Comprehensive assessments should utilize multimodal approaches, including self-reports, observations, and role-plays to capture the complexity of social interactions.

Deficits in social cognition, executive functioning (EF), and emotional awareness can lead to significant impairments in social functioning. The key domains of social functioning encompass both verbal and nonverbal behaviors, emotional communication, and sociolinguistic sensitivity. Additionally, dimensions of social functioning include grooming, maintaining eye contact, initiating conversations, and effectively expressing emotions. All behaviors exhibited by individuals are influenced by neurobiological, psychological, and behavioral factors. Environmental and neurological elements interact to shape social behavior. Social functioning encompasses communication, empathy, emotional recognition, and cognitive flexibility. The essential components involve social perception, emotional regulation, and behavioral responses.

The neurobiological substrates linked to the manifestation of impairment of social functioning in individuals living with SMI rely on interconnected neurological networks rather than isolated brain regions. Key brain structures in this complex network include the following: (a) amygdala: processes emotions and social decision-making; (b) ventromedial prefrontal cortex (vmPFC): regulates empathy and moral reasoning; (c) fusiform face area (FFA): specialized for facial recognition; (d) insula: important for empathy and emotional awareness; (e) temporoparietal junction (TPJ): supports perspective-taking; (f) superior temporal sulcus (STS): processes dynamic social cues; (g) orbitofrontal cortex (OFC): evaluates social rewards; (h) medial prefrontal cortex (mPFC): involved in self-referential thinking; (i) anterior cingulate cortex (ACC): regulates social conflict resolution; and (j) corpus callosum: facilitates communication between brain hemispheres.

Social interactions are crucial for mental health and recovery from mental health problems. Social skills are learned behaviors essential for building relationships. Successful social interactions require awareness of and attention to verbal and nonverbal behaviors. Individuals with SMI may have diminished social skills due to various factors, including cognitive impairment and negative social environments. The family and social environments can significantly impact social functioning in individuals living with SMI through the absence or infrequent occurrence of role modeling of adaptive social functioning by significant and influential people in the individual's environment. Social skills training (SST) has shown effectiveness in improving social functioning. Meta-analysis of 22 studies indicated positive effects on social skills and community functioning. Basic SST format includes identifying the skill, reviewing practice, establishing rationale, modeling skills, role-playing, and providing feedback. Generalization of skills to real-life contexts is a challenge; strategies include fading reinforcers and involving significant others in training.

Social functioning impairments are critical in the evaluation of people living with SMI. The assessment of the presence of impairments in social functioning manifested by individuals living with SMI is challenging as the definitions of social functioning and skills vary in the mental health literature. There is a lack of prevalence data on impairment in social functioning in people living with SMI although it is agreed upon that it is a major challenge in recovery in living with SMI and does contribute to decreased quality of life, stigmatization, and disability. No studies were found that focused on cultural influences on social functioning impairments in SMI.

Mueser et al. (1991) studied 36 individuals with schizophrenia spectrum mental health problems. Approximately 50% exhibited consistent social skill deficits over 1 year. Only 11% demonstrated skilled social interactions consistently. Specific deficits, like conversational turn-taking, were uncommon (14%). Global social skill performance was more impaired than specific skills. Druss et al. (2009) assessed social role impairment using the Sheehan Disability Scale (SDS). Severe social role impairment was reported in 29.7% of individuals with SMI. Mental health conditions including bipolar (50.0%), major depression (49.1%), and PTSD (48.2%) caused the greatest social impairment. Mental health problems are significantly more likely to cause severe social-role impairments compared to chronic medical and physical conditions.

Social skill impairments can be classified into verbal and nonverbal behaviors, as well as functional social behaviors, along with specific response classes of behavioral skills that target various aspects of social functioning. The areas of social functioning addressed through Social Skills Training (SST) encompass communication, interpersonal skills, emotional regulation, and problem-solving. Additionally, other essential skills include health maintenance, vocational skills, and behaviors that adhere to social norms.

The improvement of social skills in individuals living with SMI focuses on addressing specific challenges such as interrupting others, fostering effective communication, and controlling oneself in public settings. Social skills are crucial for effective interpersonal interactions. Individuals with SMI may have mixed proficiency in social skills exceling in some areas while struggling in others. Social skills encompass various behaviors necessary for interaction. Identifying specific skills that need improvement is essential for targeted intervention. Clear identification of skills needing enhancement is a critical first step.

Before implementing changes, it is vital to assess whether impairment in a specific response class of social skill warrants intervention. Assess the necessity of changing social skills before acting. Problems may not interfere with critical activities like medication adherence or employment. If this specific impairment does not significantly disrupt essential activities, it may be more beneficial to accept the individual's current capabilities. Acceptance of current capabilities may be more realistic in some cases.

To enhance social functioning in individuals with SMI, a structured approach is necessary. Evaluate the severity of social skill issues to determine the necessity for intervention. Identify specific changes needed for improvement in social skills. This includes identifying specific changes and providing positive reinforcement for desired behaviors. Provide positive reinforcement for observed improvements and gradually raise expectations.

Interrupting others while they are speaking can be problematic in social interactions, and understanding the context is key to addressing this behavior. Strategies include establishing rules, reviewing medications, and providing positive reinforcement for appropriate behavior. Identify when and where interruptions occur to develop effective strategies. Review medications that may contribute to restlessness or impulsivity. Establish clear communication rules and provide positive reinforcement for adherence.

Rude comments can be manifested in various ways, and it is essential to define and address these behaviors clearly. Consistent expectations, monitoring the occurrence of positive behaviors, and providing corrections calmly are crucial for improvement. Clearly articulate what constitutes rude behavior to reduce confusion. Establish consistent rules regarding acceptable language and behavior.

Social withdrawal and lack of motivation can hinder interactions, necessitating clear definitions and strategies to encourage social engagement. Establishing routines, using preferred activities, and gradually increasing expectations can help motivate individuals. Define what social withdrawal looks like for the individual. Establishing daily routines helps to create a structured environment. Use preferred activities to encourage social interactions and gradually increase expectations.

Inappropriate behaviors in public settings require clear definitions and proactive planning. Setting realistic expectations, monitoring behavior, and providing immediate corrections can help to manage these situations effectively. Clearly define what inappropriate behavior entails to reduce confusion. Plan ahead for visits and establish realistic expectations. Monitor behavior during visits and provide immediate corrections when necessary.

Listening difficulties may stem from various factors, including hearing issues and environmental distractions. Simplifying communication, being patient, prompting rehearsal, and demonstrating effective communication techniques can enhance listening skills. Consider a hearing examination if listening issues persist. Identify distractions that may interfere with attention during conversations. Use simple language and be patient while communicating expectations, making requests, and asking questions.

References

Abel, D. B., Salyers, M. P., Wu, W., Monette, M. A., & Minor, K. S. (2021). Quality versus quantity: Determining real-world social functioning deficits in schizophrenia. *Psychiatry Research, 301*, 113980. https://doi.org/10.1016/j.psychres.2021.113980

American Psychiatric Association. (2022). *Diagnostic and statistical manual of mental disorders* (5th ed., text rev.). https://doi.org/10.1176/appi.books.9780890425787

American Psychological Association. (n.d.-a). Self-monitoring. In *APA dictionary of psychology*. https://dictionary.apa.org/self-monitoring

American Psychological Association. (n.d.-b). Social competence. In *APA dictionary of psychology*. https://dictionary.apa.org/social-competence

American Speech-Language-Hearing Association (ASHA). (n.d.). *Components of social communication*. ASHA Practice Portal. https://www.asha.org/Practice-Portal/Clinical-Topics/Social-Communication-Disorder/

Anderson, C. A., Horowitz, L. M., & French, R. D. (1983). Attributional style of lonely and depressed people. *Journal of Personality and Social Psychology, 45*(1), 127–136. https://doi.org/10.1037/0022-3514.45.1.127

Arbuckle, R., Frye, M. A., Brecher, M., Paulsson, B., Rajagopalan, K., Palmer, S., & Degl'Innocenti, A. (2009). The psychometric validation of the Sheehan Disability Scale (SDS) in patients with bipolar disorder. *Psychiatry Research, 165*(1–2), 163–174. https://doi.org/10.1016/j.psychres.2007.11.018

Aruldass, P., Sekar, T. S., Saravanan, S., Samuel, R., & Jacob, K. S. (2022). Effectiveness of social skills training groups in persons with severe mental illness: A pre–post intervention study. *Indian Journal of Psychological Medicine, 44*(2), 114–119. https://doi.org/10.1177/02537176211024146

Bechara, A. (2002). The neurology of social cognition. *Brain, 125*(8), 1673–1675. https://doi.org/10.1093/brain/awf169

Bellack, A. S., Morrison, R. L., Wixted, J. T., & Mueser, K. T. (1990). An analysis of social competence in schizophrenia. *British Journal of Psychiatry, 156*(6), 809–818. https://doi.org/10.1192/bjp.156.6.809

Bhola, P., Basavarajappa, C., Guruprasad, D., Hegde, G., Khanam, F., Thirthalli, J., & Chaturvedi, S. K. (2016). Development of a social skills assessment screening scale for psychiatric rehabilitation settings: A pilot study. *Indian Journal of Psychological Medicine, 38*(5), 395–403. https://doi.org/10.4103/0253-7176.191392

Bromley, E., & Brekke, J. S. (2010). Assessing function and functional outcome in schizophrenia. In N. Swerdlow (Ed.), *Behavioral neurobiology of schizophrenia and its treatment* (Current topics in behavioral neurosciences) (Vol. 4, pp. 3–31). Springer. https://doi.org/10.1007/7854_2010_40

Brookshire, R. H., & Nicholas, L. E. (1997). *Discourse comprehension test* (2nd ed.). Psychological Corporation. https://discoursecomptest.com

Cooper, J. O., Heron, T. E., & Heward, W. L. (2020). *Applied behavior analysis* (3rd ed.). Pearson Education. https://www.pearson.com/en-us/subject-catalog/p/applied-behavior-analysis/P200000003531000053

Correll, C. U., & Schooler, N. R. (2020). Negative symptoms in schizophrenia: A review and clinical guide for recognition, assessment, and treatment. *Neuropsychiatric Disease and Treatment, 16*, 519–534. https://doi.org/10.2147/NDT.S225643

Corrigan, P. W., & Basit, A. (1997). Generalization of social skills training for persons with severe mental illness. *Cognitive and Behavioral Practice, 4*(1), 191–206. https://doi.org/10.1016/S1077-7229(97)80018-1

Cotter, J., Granger, K., Backx, R., Hobbs, M., Looi, C. Y., & Barnett, J. H. (2017). Social cognitive dysfunction as a clinical marker: A systematic review of meta-analyses across 30 clinical conditions. *Neuroscience and Biobehavioral Reviews, 80*, 365–371. https://doi.org/10.1016/j.neubiorev.2017.11.014

Del Prette, Z. A. P., Del Prette, A., & Peixoto, E. M. (2021). Social skill inventory-2 Del-Prette: Expanding and updating psychometric properties. *Estudos de Psicologia (Campinas), 38*, e190124. https://doi.org/10.1590/1982-0275202138e190124

Dilk, M. N., & Bond, G. R. (1996). Meta-analytic evaluation of skills training research for individuals with severe mental illness. *Journal of Consulting and Clinical Psychology, 64*(6), 1337–1346. https://doi.org/10.1037/0022-006X.64.6.1337

Druss, B. G., Hwang, I., Petukhova, M., Sampson, N. A., Wang, P. S., & Kessler, R. C. (2009). Impairment in role functioning in mental and chronic medical disorders in the United States: Results from the National Comorbidity Survey Replication. *Molecular Psychiatry, 14*(7), 728–737. https://doi.org/10.1038/mp.2008.13

Duca, L., & Rose, J. (2011). Functional compensation. In J. S. Kreutzer, J. DeLuca, & B. Caplan (Eds.), *Encyclopedia of clinical neuropsychology* (pp. 1110–1111). Springer. https://doi.org/10.1007/978-0-387-79948-3_400

Everyday Speech. (n.d.). *Understanding pragmatic skills: A comprehensive guide to assessment tools*. https://everydayspeech.com/sel-implementation/understanding-pragmatic-skills-a-comprehensive-guide-to-assessment-tools/

Feldman, R. S., Philippot, P., & Custrini, R. J. (1991). Social competence and nonverbal behavior. In R. S. Feldman & B. Rimé (Eds.), *Fundamentals of nonverbal behavior* (pp. 329–350). Editions de la Maison des Sciences de l'Homme; Cambridge University Press. https://psycnet.apa.org/record/1991-98576-009

Flechsenhar, A., Kanske, P., Krach, S., Korn, C., & Bertsch, K. (2022). The (un)learning of social functions and its significance for mental health. *Clinical Psychology Review, 98*, 102204. https://doi.org/10.1016/j.cpr.2022.102204

Francis, J. L., & Penn, D. L. (2001). The relationship between insight and social skill in persons with severe mental illness. *The Journal of Nervous and Mental Disease, 189*(12), 822–829. https://doi.org/10.1097/00005053-200112000-00002

Frattali, C. M., Thompson, C. K., Holland, A. L., Wohl, C. B., & Ferketic, M. M. (1995). *Functional assessment of communication skills for adults (ASHA FACS)*. American Speech-Language-Hearing Association. https://apps.asha.org/eweb/OLSDynamicPage.aspx?Webcode=olsdetails&title=American+Speech-Language-Hearing+Association+Functional+Assessment+of+Communication+Skills+for+Adults+%28ASHA+FACS%29

Furnham, A., & Capon, M. (1983). Social skills and self-monitoring processes. *Personality and Individual Differences, 4*(2), 171–178. https://doi.org/10.1016/0191-8869(83)90017-X

Galderisi, S., Mucci, A., Dollfus, S., Nordentoft, M., Falkai, P., Kaiser, S., Bitter, I., Giordano, G. M., Nibbio, G., Vignapiano, A., Rocca, P., Rossi, A., Samochowiec, J., & Gaebel, W. (2021). EPA guidance on assessment of negative symptoms in schizophrenia. *European Psychiatry, 64*(1), e23. https://doi.org/10.1192/j.eurpsy.2021.11

Hardy-Baylé, M. C., Sarfati, Y., & Passerieux, C. (2003). The cognitive basis of disorganization symptomatology in schizophrenia and its clinical correlates: Toward a pathogenetic approach to disorganization. *Schizophrenia Bulletin, 29*(3), 459–471. https://doi.org/10.1093/oxfordjournals.schbul.a007019

Haroldfs. (n.d.). *Grice's maxims*. University of Pennsylvania. Retrieved May 5, 2025, from https://www.sas.upenn.edu/~haroldfs/dravling/grice.html

Harvey, P. D., & Strassnig, M. (2012). Predicting the severity of everyday functional disability in people with schizophrenia: Cognitive deficits, functional capacity, symptoms, and health status. *World Psychiatry, 11*(2), 73–79. https://doi.org/10.1016/j.wpsyc.2012.05.004

Healey, K. M., Combs, D. R., Gibson, C. M., Keefe, R. S., Roberts, D. L., & Penn, D. L. (2015). Observable social cognition – A rating scale: An interview-based assessment for schizophrenia. *Cognitive Neuropsychiatry, 20*(3), 198–221. https://doi.org/10.1080/13546805.2014.999915

Holland, A. L. (1980). *Communicative abilities in daily living*. Pro-Ed. https://www.proedinc.com/Products/14650/cadl3-communication-activities-of-daily-livingthird-edition.aspx

Ihnen, G. H., Penn, D. L., Corrigan, P. W., & Martin, J. (1998). Social perception and social skill in schizophrenia. *Psychiatry Research, 80*(3), 275–286. https://doi.org/10.1016/S0165-1781(98)00079-1

Janssen, I., Versmissen, D., Campo, J. A., Myin-Germeys, I., Van Os, J., & Krabbendam, L. J. P. M. (2006). Attribution style and psychosis: Evidence for an externalizing bias in patients but not in individuals at high risk. *Psychological Medicine, 36*(6), 771–778. https://doi.org/10.1017/S0033291706007422

Jurevičienė, M., Kaffemanienė, I., & Ruškus, J. (2012). Concept and structural components of social skills. *Baltic Journal of Sport and Health Sciences, 3*(86), 42–52. https://doi.org/10.33607/bjshs.v3i86.266

Kalin, M., Kaplan, S., Gould, F., Pinkham, A. E., Penn, D. L., & Harvey, P. D. (2015). Social cognition, social competence, negative symptoms and social outcomes: Inter-relationships in people with schizophrenia. *Journal of Psychiatric Research, 68*, 254–260. https://doi.org/10.1016/j.jpsychires.2015.07.008

Kennedy, D. P., & Adolphs, R. (2012). The social brain in psychiatric and neurological disorders. *Trends in Cognitive Sciences, 16*(11), 559–572. https://doi.org/10.1016/j.tics.2012.09.006
Kinnaman, J. E. S., & Bellack, A. S. (2012). Social skills. In W. T. O'Donohue & J. E. Fisher (Eds.), *Cognitive behavior therapy: Core principles for practice* (pp. 251–272). Wiley. https://doi.org/10.1002/9781118470886.ch10
Kleiman, L. I. (2003). *Functional communication profile—Revised (FCP-R)*. Western Psychological Services. https://www.wpspublish.com/fcp-r-functional-communication-profile-revised
Kopelowicz, A., Liberman, R. P., & Zarate, R. (2006). Recent advances in social skills training for schizophrenia. *Schizophrenia Bulletin, 32*(Supplement 1), S12–S23. https://doi.org/10.1093/schbul/sbl023
Koujalgi, S. R., Patil, S. R., Nayak, R. B., Chate, S. S., & Patil, N. M. (2014). Efficacy of social skill training in patient with chronic schizophrenia: An interventional study. *Journal of the Scientific Society, 41*(3), 156–161. https://doi.org/10.4103/0974-5009.141201
Kurtz, M. M. (2006). Symptoms versus neurocognitive skills as correlates of everyday functioning in severe mental illness. *Expert Review of Neurotherapeutics, 6*(1), 47–56. https://doi.org/10.1586/14737175.6.1.47
Kurtz, M. M., & Mueser, K. T. (2008). A meta-analysis of controlled research on social skills training for schizophrenia. *Journal of Consulting and Clinical Psychology, 76*(3), 491–504. https://doi.org/10.1037/0022-006X.76.3.491
Lemerise, E. A., & Arsenio, W. F. (2000). An integrated model of emotion processes and cognition in social information processing. *Child Development, 71*(1), 107–118. https://doi.org/10.1111/1467-8624.00124
Liberman, R. P. (1982). Assessment of social skills. *Schizophrenia Bulletin, 8*(1), 62–94. https://doi.org/10.1093/schbul/8.1.62
Mahmood, Z., Burton, C. Z., Vella, L., & Twamley, E. W. (2018). Neuropsychological predictors of performance-based measures of functional capacity and social skills in individuals with severe mental illness. *Journal of Psychiatric Research, 102*, 201–206. https://doi.org/10.1016/j.jpsychires.2018.04.011
Miller, M. L., Strassnig, M. T., Bromet, E., Depp, C. A., Jonas, K., Lin, W., McCarrick, P., McCormack, J., McIntosh, E., McLaughlin, D., Moore, R. C., Moran, M., Morra, L., Mueser, K. T., Neuchterlein, K. H., Nuechterlein, K. H., Reichenberg, A., Ventura, J., & Harvey, P. D. (2021). Performance-based assessment of social skills in a large sample of participants with schizophrenia, bipolar disorder and healthy controls: Correlates of social competence and social appropriateness. *Schizophrenia Research, 236*, 80–86. https://doi.org/10.1016/j.schres.2021.08.012
Morrison, R. L., & Wixted, J. T. (1989). Social skills training. In A. S. Bellack (Ed.), *A clinical guide for the treatment of schizophrenia*. Springer. https://doi.org/10.1007/978-1-4757-8979-9_10
Mosolov, S. N., & Yaltonskaya, P. A. (2022). Primary and secondary negative symptoms in schizophrenia. *Frontiers in Psychiatry, 12*, 766692. https://doi.org/10.3389/fpsyt.2021.766692
Mueser, K. T., Bellack, A. S., Douglas, M. S., & Morrison, R. L. (1991). Prevalence and stability of social skill deficits in schizophrenia. *Schizophrenia Research, 5*(2), 167–176. https://doi.org/10.1016/0920-9964(91)90044-5
Ochsner, K. N. (2008). The social-emotional processing stream: Five core constructs and their translational potential for schizophrenia and beyond. *Biological Psychiatry, 64*(1), 48–61. https://doi.org/10.1016/j.biopsych.2008.04.024
Patterson, T. L., Moscona, S., McKibbin, C. L., Davidson, K., & Jeste, D. V. (2001). Social skills performance assessment among older patients with schizophrenia. *Schizophrenia Research, 48*(2–3), 351–360. https://doi.org/10.1016/S0920-9964(00)00109-2
Penn, C. (1985). *The profile of communicative appropriateness: A clinical tool for the assessment of pragmatics*. University of the Witwatersrand, Department of Speech Pathology and Audiology. https://1library.net/document/y9319pdy-profile-communicative-appropriateness-clinical-tool-assessment-pragmatics.html

Penn, D. L., Sanna, L. J., & Roberts, D. L. (2008). Social cognition in schizophrenia: An overview. *Schizophrenia Bulletin, 34*(3), 408–411. https://doi.org/10.1093/schbul/sbn014

Perez, J. E., Riggio, R. E., & Kopelowicz, A. (2007). Social skill imbalances in mood disorders and schizophrenia. *Personality and Individual Differences, 42*(1), 27–36. https://doi.org/10.1016/j.paid.2006.05.011

Pinkham, A. E., Penn, D. L., Perkins, D. O., & Lieberman, J. (2003). Implications for the neural basis of social cognition for the study of schizophrenia. *American Journal of Psychiatry, 160*(5), 815–824. https://doi.org/10.1176/appi.ajp.160.5.815

Provencher, H. L., & Mueser, K. T. (1997). Positive and negative symptom behaviors and caregiver burden in the relatives of persons with schizophrenia. *Schizophrenia Research, 26*(1), 71–80. https://doi.org/10.1016/s0920-9964(97)00043-1

Prutting, C. A., & Kirchner, D. M. (1987). A clinical appraisal of the pragmatic aspects of language. *Journal of Speech and Hearing Disorders, 52*(2), 105–119. https://doi.org/10.1044/jshd.5202.105

Rad, D. S. (2014). A review on adult pragmatic assessments. *Iranian Journal of Neurology, 13*(3), 113–118. https://pdfs.semanticscholar.org/c792/82e41106002a16534fac8d873e0554bcb2f9.pdf

Roeling, M. P. (2010). Functioning is the cornerstone of life: Assessing chronic impairment in social functioning. *Journal of European Psychology Students, 2*, 1–14. https://doi.org/10.5334/jeps.aj

Saeri, A. K., Cruwys, T., Barlow, F. K., Stronge, S., & Sibley, C. G. (2018). Social connectedness improves public mental health: Investigating bidirectional relationships in the New Zealand attitudes and values survey. *Australian & New Zealand Journal of Psychiatry, 52*(4), 365–374. https://doi.org/10.1177/0004867417723990

Skinner, B. F. (1953). *Science and human behavior.* Macmillan. https://doi.org/10.1037/11149-000

Tenhula, W. N., & Bellack, A. S. (2008). Social skills training. In K. T. Mueser & D. V. Jeste (Eds.), *Clinical handbook of schizophrenia* (pp. 240–248). The Guilford Press. https://psycnet.apa.org/record/2008-01373-016

Thamaraiselvi, S., Priyadarshini, A., Arisalya, N., Samuel, R., & Jacob, K. S. (2020). Development and validation of Vellore assessment of social performance among clients with chronic mental illness. *Indian Journal of Psychiatry, 62*(2), 121–130. https://doi.org/10.4103/psychiatry.IndianJPsychiatry_510_19

Tran, T., DeRosse, P., Burdick, K., Malhotra, A., Welikala, T., & Bowie, C. (2019). Real-world functioning in schizophrenia: Negative symptoms as a bridge in pathways from neurocognition, social cognition, and functional competence. *Schizophrenia Bulletin, 45*(Supplement_2), S352–S353. https://doi.org/10.1093/schbul/sbz020.666

Tranel, D., Denburg, N. L., & Bechara, A. (2003). Exploring the neurological substrate of emotional and social intelligence. *Brain, 126*(8), 1790–1800. https://doi.org/10.1093/brain/awg177

U.S. Department of Veterans Affairs. (n.d.). *Brief overview of SST and the VA SST training program.* https://www.mirecc.va.gov/visn5/training/sst/Brief-Overview-of-SST-and-the-VA-SST-Training-Program.asp#presentation-citations

Vaughn, C. E., & Leff, J. P. (1976). The influence of family and social factors on the course of psychiatric illness: A comparison of schizophrenic and depressed neurotic patients. *British Journal of Psychiatry, 129*(2), 125–137. https://doi.org/10.1192/bjp.129.2.125

Yuan, H., & Dollaghan, C. (2018). Measuring the diagnostic features of social (pragmatic) communication disorder: An exploratory study. *American Journal of Speech-Language Pathology, 27*(2), 647–656. https://doi.org/10.1044/2018_AJSLP-16-0219

Zhaoyang, R., Sliwinski, M. J., Martire, L. M., & Smyth, J. M. (2019). Social interactions and physical symptoms in daily life: Quality matters for older adults, quantity matters for younger adults. *Psychology & Health, 34*(7), 867–885. https://doi.org/10.1080/08870446.2019.1579908

Chapter 14
Problems with Functional Impairments in Daily Living Skills in Individuals Living with Serious Mental Illness

Introduction

Functional impairments represent some of the most enduring and complex challenges faced by individuals living with serious mental illness (SMI). Beyond the hallmark symptoms of psychosis, mood disturbance, or cognitive disorganization, SMI often disrupts the ability to perform essential daily tasks that sustain independence and social participation. These impairments manifest across multiple dimensions of functioning, ranging from basic activities of daily living (ADLs), such as hygiene and nutrition, to more complex instrumental activities of daily living (IADLs), including financial management, transportation, and social engagement. The persistence of these difficulties, even in the presence of symptom reduction through pharmacological treatment, underscores the importance of understanding functional impairment as a distinct and clinically significant domain of SMI.

This chapter examines the multidirectional and multidimensional nature of functional impairments, situating them within idiographic and nomothetic frameworks that highlight both individual variability and broader patterns across populations. Central to this discussion are the roles of executive functions, social cognition, and neurocognitive processes, which interact with negative symptoms such as avolition to shape the trajectory of daily functioning. Neurological substrates and environmental influences further complicate this picture, as impairments are not only rooted in brain-based dysfunctions but also shaped by contextual factors such as stigma, resource availability, and cultural expectations. By integrating these perspectives, the need for comprehensive models is emphasized that capture the heterogeneity of functional capacities in SMI.

The structure of this chapter proceeds in three parts. First, it delineates the dimensions of functional activities, distinguishing between ADLs and IADLs, and explores their relevance to quality of life and disability. Second, it critically reviews existing assessment tools, highlighting their limitations and the necessity for

G. F. McKeegan, *Behavior Change Interventions for Serious Mental Illness*, Evidence-Based Practices in Behavioral Health,
https://doi.org/10.1007/978-3-032-18372-9_14

updated, psychometrically sound measures that reflect contemporary contexts and diverse populations. Finally, the chapter considers intervention strategies, including functional skills training and behavioral approaches, that aim to enhance independence and social role performance. Together, a framework is presented for understanding functional impairment not merely as a secondary consequence of SMI but as a central construct requiring targeted assessment and intervention in clinical practice and research.

The Case of Michael

Michael lives in a group home where I work as a staff. He has problems with taking care of himself—he refuses to take a shower, and it has been as long as 3 weeks before he does take one. When he does shower, he must be told to use soap and wash his hair, or he would just stand under the water. He does not wash his clothes and must be told to wear clean ones, or he will wear dirty ones after he showers. He wears a winter coat all the time even in the summer; for his safety, it is taken from him when it gets too hot. When he does change his clothes, he leaves them on the floor with other trash. He just ignores me; then I tell him that he has a horrible odor and needs a shower. Some of the other residents have told staff that he smells so bad that they do not want to be around him. He does not brush his teeth, but he sometimes says his mouth hurts but refuses to go to the dentist. When Michael receives some money from his family, he spends all of it quickly on sodas and snacks. When he has no money, he asks other residents and strangers, leading to people avoiding him. His "bumming" money has resulted in several "run-ins" with the police.

Definition and Characteristics of Problems with Daily Functioning and Living Skills

SMI negatively impacts many areas of functioning, including daily hygiene, toileting, dressing, nutrition, washing clothes, cooking, shopping, managing finances, using transportation, work, academics, completing goals, social and family relationships, leisure activities, taking care of possessions, and behaviors related to wellness and healthcare (Brown & Velligan, 2016; Harvey & Strassnig, 2012; Tanner et al., 2019). Functional impairment refers to significant limitations in performing these activities in fulfilling the expected social roles. It is the inability to perform necessary behaviors for a specific purpose, not entirely due to other problems (Spaulding et al., 2003).

Functional impairment serves as a key criterion for identifying the presence of certain mental health issues. Individuals living with SMI often experience clinically significant impairment or distress in social, occupational, or other vital areas of functioning (McIntyre et al., 2013). Impairments can be used to determine the presence of a mental health issue or an associated feature as described in the Diagnostic and Statistical Manual of Mental Disorders, fifth edition, text revision (DSM-5-TR) (American Psychiatric Association, 2022). The inclusion of the criterion highlights that the occurrence of expected behaviors is significantly disrupted by a mental health condition, hindering the individual's ability to function effectively in daily life.

Although functional impairment is a necessary criterion for several mental health conditions, the impairments vary widely in topography, intensity, and frequency across different behavioral dimensions, even for levels of severity that are identical (Verboom et al., 2011). Clinical observations have noted that some people experience significant incapacitation from relatively mild mental health problems, while others manage daily activities despite moderate-to-severe problem behaviors; this results in a disassociation between mental health problems and the inability to fulfill daily tasks. The dimensions of the impairments associated with living with SMI (e.g., severity, lack of control) have a more significant impact on everyday functioning than environmental factors (Verboom et al., 2011).

Functional impairment must be considered "clinically significant" to indicate a mental health issue, causing considerable distress or disrupting daily activities. Individuals with SMI may have difficulty performing daily tasks (Njenga, 2009; Ustün & Kennedy, 2009). The DSM-5-TR (American Psychiatric Association, 2022) includes "clinical significance" as a criterion for identifying mental health problems linked to SMI. It consists of subjective distress and observable impairment in expected functioning. Distress may be shown by the individual or their loved ones through worry, concern, or suffering, even if it is sometimes denied.

Functional impairment is one of the most enduring, intractable problem behaviors linked to living with SMI. The term "functional impairment" refers to the persistent interference in daily life activities and role performance because of mental health problems (McGrath et al., 2013). Even when certain problem behaviors abate through intervention, quality of life (QoL) does not always improve (Harvey et al., 2011). Effective and beneficial effects of psychiatric medication on functional impairment are meager.

Functional impairment and disability are interconnected. Disability involves limitations in performing activities or participating in life due to mental health issues (American Psychological Association, n.d.-a). Functional impairment refers to dysfunction in social and occupational areas, often signaling a mental health problem that contributes significantly to disability. It specifically describes the loss or reduction of performing certain functions of the body and/or mind, leading to daily activity limitations (Ustün & Kennedy, 2009). SMI is common among individuals with disability and is the primary cause of disability in the United States (Strassnig et al., 2018; Xie et al., 2022).

Individuals with SMI often experience functional and behavioral impairments. Rubin and Panzano (2002) conducted a comprehensive evaluation in a large catchment area in a mid-Western state of the United States. This assessment utilized a rating scale completed by case managers for more than 3600 clients undergoing mental healthcare services. The results showed that the range of individuals living with SMI needing daily supervision in functional behaviors ranged from 15% to 29% of the sample. Functional areas assessed included basic living skills, use of community resources, taking medications independently, and leisure and vocational pursuits. The authors found that the most disabled persons—those with the greatest impairment needing daily supervision—resided with family or in residential facilities.

The non-performance of expected life skills is persistent and not amenable to change with medications. Although problem behaviors like hallucinations and delusions may decrease along behavioral dimensions (i.e., frequency, intensity, control), the functional capacities of the individuals living with SMI remain unaltered (Harvey et al., 2011). In addition, the functional problems that are displayed in certain contexts have consequences in the real world. Individuals living with SMI have reduced opportunities to engage in mutually reinforcing social interactions. Meaningful academic and vocational opportunities are likewise diminished given the stigma associated with living with SMI. As an outcome of the lessened financial opportunities in job settings, many individuals living with SMI are dependent on disability payments; keeping those payments requires the person to continue to display functional impairments to qualify. Community resources have limited availability for individuals living with SMI resulting in fewer than 40% of individuals receiving ongoing treatment and rehabilitation (Kessler et al., 2001).

Negative symptoms substantially impair the development and manifestations of functional life skills, leading to reduced social-role performance in individuals living with SMI (Fulford et al., 2013; Marder & Galderisi, 2017). Findings suggests that "negative symptoms" are correlated with functional impairments, whereas disorganized and positive symptoms, such as hallucinations and delusions, have limited predictive value. Behaviors related to anxiety and depressive disorders exert the most substantial impact on functional impairment, with fatigue and concentration difficulties being particularly noteworthy (Tanner et al., 2019).

It has been postulated that avolition (i.e., amotivation) represents the critical component that influences the manifestations of functional impairments (Foussias & Remington, 2010). Avolition is defined as a reduced initiation and persistence of goal-directed activities (Shahrokh & Hales, 2003) and is considered a primary negative symptom (Mosolov & Yaltonskaya, 2022); negative symptoms are defined as the diminished or absent expression of typical and expected behaviors and emotions (Correll & Schooler, 2020). It is often interchangeable with terms like decreased drive, amotivation, and apathy. It is assessed based on both observed behavior and the individuals self-reported interest or desire to engage in activities (Marder & Galderisi, 2017). It is important to distinguish avolition from secondary causes like paranoia, depression, or lack of opportunities, which may also lead to reduced initiation and persistence of behaviors.

Avolition is linked to motivation, involving pursuit of experiences, reward prediction, valuation of effort, and decision-making (Marder & Galderisi, 2017). Studies indicate that individuals with SMI enjoy activities but struggle to anticipate future rewards, leading to decreased effort valuation and goal-directed behavior. It is hypothesized that those with SMI experience pleasure less intensely (i.e., hypohedonia) than those without mental health issues (Kayton & Koh, 1975).

Neurocognitive impairments (Green et al., 2000) include issues in memory, attention, executive functioning, and verbal fluency. In individuals with SMI, these impairments are often linked to avolition. Problems in planning and decision-making can lead to difficulties in starting and maintaining goal-directed activities, worsening functional impairments (Marder & Galderisi, 2017).

Problems in the functional domains of neurocognition must be considered for a complete picture of the individual's problems in independent functioning. Negative symptoms and neurocognitive impairments in people living with SMI share many features and are correlated in their severity on a cross-sectional basis (Harvey et al., 2006). Studies have shown that individuals living with SMI demonstrate problems in composite scores on assessments of neurocognitive functioning. Long-term and short-term memories, executive functioning (EF) and planning, vigilance, and psychomotor speed appear to be correlated with higher levels of functional capacities in certain domains (Green, 1996; Heinrichs & Zakzanis, 1998). EF is composed of cognitive skills, such as task initiation, organization, flexibility, setting priorities, problem solving, working memory, and control of impulsivity and emotions (Baggetta & Alexander, 2016).

The negative symptoms of avolition and neurocognitive impairments interact in a complex manner, although research has been inconsistent. It is believed that people living with SMI have limited neurocognitive resources, which include abilities for performing tasks such as executive functions (EFs). These tasks demand elevated resources and capacity, impacting performance in other cognitive areas. Neurocognitive resources link an individual's capability and motivation during training or when engaging in cognitive tasks. The theory suggests that goal-directed activities heavily tax cognitive processes, and limited resources may reduce activity and observable functional behaviors (American Psychological Association, n.d.-b).

Dimensions of Functional Impairments

Assessing the problems in functioning with people living with SMI confronts many challenges (Bellack et al., 2007; Harvey & Strassnig, 2012). A major limiting factor in the development of reliable and valid assessment instruments is the failure to develop a model of functional abilities and its primary mediators and moderators (Bellack et al., 2007). The assessment tools should be efficient, accurate, demonstrate sensitivity to change and be comprehensive in the identification and measurement of the response classes in the domains and dimensions that comprise functional life skill behaviors. The challenges in developing reliable and valid measures of functioning are compounded by the multiple dimensions of the behavioral response classes in each of the functional capacities and the heterogeneity of functioning in individuals living with SMI (Barker et al., 1994; Endicott & Spitzer, 1972).

Normative functioning in the multiple domains and dimensions of functioning is also culturally relevant. Culture is a set of beliefs and values within a particular group about what is considered normal and acceptable behavior. They can vary across different cultures and subgroups. These are the specific actions and attitudes that are deemed appropriate, expected, and acceptable within a given context, based on cultural norms (American Psychological Association, n.d.-c). For example, in a professional setting, there might be expectations about how an individual dresses, communicates, and interacts with colleagues, which are influenced by business etiquette and cultural norms but may be different in a social setting. At present, there is no norm-based scale of adaptive daily functioning.

It is difficult to capture "a snapshot" of the problems in daily functioning in an individual living with SMI given the dimensions of the behavioral response classes involved. The domains of functional capacities in a person living with SMI are heterogenous, complex and multidimensional, and multidirectional in the behavioral response classes that constitute each functional impairment. The domains of functional behavioral capacities and impairments are composed of several response classes each made up of more than one behavior and vary on several behavioral dimensions (e.g., frequency, duration, antecedent condition, and context). For instance, the construct of independent functioning covers several contextual domains including work/vocational, residence/household, personal care, community/social, health/wellness, and mobility. In each of these domains are dimensions related to the topographies of expected behaviors, the complexity of the behavior that is expected (e.g., steps involved), the observable and measurable criterion defining completion of task within a specified amount of time, or the amount of support/prompting/supervision needed to complete the task.

There are several instruments that are presently utilized. Bellack et al. (2007) concluded that every instrument has strengths and weaknesses and recommends that a multimodal and multimethod approach be used in assessing the functional problems of persons living with SMI; that is, combinations of self-reports from the person living with SMI, surrogates and caretakers on multiple instruments, and real-time observations of the functioning of the person. As the domains of functional capacities are heterogeneous and multidimensional, then the assessment needs to be individual and based on the needs of the person living with SMI. Multimethod and multimodal individual assessment can ascertain the dimensions of the behaviors in each functional capacity on the amount of supervision needed for a person living with SMI to successfully complete the targeted task, self-initiation, the type and immediacy of reinforcement for the completion of the task to be maintained, and the need for shaping of the expected behaviors to be manifested.

Impairments in functioning can be classified into two broad domains: activities of daily living (ADLs) and instrumental activities of daily living (IADLs). These are domains of functional abilities that enable a person to manifest behaviors that allow successful completion of tasks that are expected in certain contexts (Edemekong et al., 2019). They are components of a person's functional status. ADLs refer to fundamental skills required for individuals to independently care for themselves. These include basic tasks such as eating, bathing, dressing, toileting, mobility, and maintaining personal hygiene. The inability to perform them can lead to dependence on others, unsafe conditions, and a reduced quality of life (QoL) (Edemekong et al., 2019). IADLs are those activities that allow an individual to live independently in a community (Guo & Sapra, 2022). Although it is not necessary for functional living, the ability to perform IADLs can significantly improve the quality of life (QoL) by expanding the situations in which the person can function without supervision and oversight. The major domains of IADLs include cooking, cleaning, transportation, laundry, and managing finances. The assessment of IADLs can determine the level of an individual's need for assistance and neurocognitive functioning (Guo & Sapra, 2022).

IADLs are commonly confused with ADLs. The major dimensions of ADLs are feeding, dressing, bathing, and walking. In contrast with IADLs, ADLs are necessary for basic functional living. Severe impairments in performing ADLs may indicate the need for home healthcare or placement in a supervised facility. IADLs involve more complex tasks that are essential for independent living in the community (Guo & Sapra, 2022). Specific dimensions of IADLs include:

1. Transportation and shopping: ability to procure groceries, attend events, and manage transportation (e.g., driving or organizing other means of transport).
2. Managing finances: paying bills and managing financial assets.
3. Meal preparation: shopping for food and preparing meals.
4. Housecleaning and home maintenance: cleaning living areas, maintaining tidiness, and performing home maintenance tasks.
5. Laundry: washing and maintaining clothing.
6. Managing communication: handling telephone calls and mail.
7. Managing medications: obtaining and taking medications as directed.

These tasks require organizational and neurocognitive skills. Individuals impaired in these dimensions of functioning often require assistance to perform the tasks associated within the domain of IADLs.

Multiple scales exist for the evaluation of IADLs. The Pfeffer Functional Activities Questionnaire (Pfeffer, 1982; Fuentes-García, 2023) evaluates the following domains and dimensions of IADLs:

1. Financial management: writing checks, paying bills, balancing checkbook.
2. Organizational tasks: assembling personal records, business affairs, or papers.
3. Shopping: shopping alone for clothes, household necessities, or groceries.
4. Leisure activities: playing a game of skill or working on a hobby.
5. Basic kitchen tasks: heating water, making coffee, turning off the stove.
6. Meal preparation: preparing a balanced meal.
7. Awareness of current events: keeping track of current events.
8. Media engagement: paying attention to and discussing current events.
9. Memory: remembering appointments, family occasions, holidays, medications.
10. Transportation: traveling out of the neighborhood, driving, or arranging transportation.

Each dimension is rated by the individual using the following scale: "dependent = 3"; "requires assistance = 2"; "has difficulty but does by self=1"; "normal = 0"; "never did but could do now=0"; and "never did and would have difficulty now=1." The total score gives the degree of functional and neurocognitive impairments (Pfeffer, 1982; Fuentes-García, 2023).

The Lawton–Brody Instrumental Activities of Daily Living Scale (Lawton–Brody IADL Scale) assesses eight domains of functioning related to independent living skills (Graf, 2008; Lawton & Brody, 1969). These domains and their dimensions include:

1. Ability to use a telephone: operating a telephone.
2. Shopping: shopping for needed items.
3. Food preparation: covers planning and preparing meals.
4. Housekeeping: maintaining a residence.
5. Laundry: doing personal laundry.
6. Mode of transportation: assesses ability to travel.
7. Responsibility for own medications: managing and dispensing medications.
8. Ability to handle finances: managing financial matters and handling money.

Each domain is scored based on the individual's highest level of functioning, with scores ranging from 0 (low function, dependent) to 8 (high function, independent) for women, and 0 to 5 for men (excluding food preparation, housekeeping, and laundry). The scoring needs updating to reflect current normative behaviors as IADL performance is not determined by gender roles.

There are significant limitations in using these instruments in assessing functional status of people living with SMI (Barker et al., 1994). These instruments were developed and psychometrically evaluated with a population of older adults living in the community (Lawton & Brody, 1969; Pfeffer, 1982). The instruments are dated; for instance, males are excluded from the response classes of functioning in laundry, food preparations, and housekeeping. On the Lawton–Brady IADL Scale, a dimension assesses the use of a telephone, whereas a large percentage of people—if not a majority—now use a cellular phone (that is in essence a handheld computer) and text to communicate instead of talking (over 70%) (CallHub, n.d.). These instruments are also self-reported. Most individuals are biased toward their abilities to perform specific tasks, and thus, they may overestimate or underestimate their abilities. In addition, individuals living with SMI may be unreliable in any self-reports of behaviors because of impairments in verbal comprehension of what is being asked and recall of performances. Gathering data from collateral sources who are acquainted with the individuals being evaluated, as well as from real-life behavioral observations, would significantly enhance the external validity of the assessment instruments. The instruments need to be updated and psychometrically evaluated on a representative sample of people living with SMI.

The domains of functional behaviors cover many behavioral response classes, some of which are interdependent and multidirectional; that is, an impairment in one area may impact the person's ability in one or several additional areas. An example could be seen in a person's demonstrated impairment in recall of information that is verbally given to the person—that is, someone telling her what needs to be done. The individual's problem in recalling what she has been instructed to do may interfere with her ability to function without reminders or follow-up requests in daily hygiene activities, getting to a vocational activity on time, and remembering tasks associated with the vocational activity. The assessment of a behavioral outcome being done "competently," "independently," and "completely" would be challenging unless the assessment measure was precise and the raters were applying consistently the criteria for each of the concepts of "competent," "independent," or "successful."

Assessment questions about functional capacities often lack specific details. For instance, instead of asking "How do you get along with others in leisure activities?" a more detailed approach would be helpful. Examples of vague questions include: "How often do you engage in activities with others?"; "How well do you perform hygiene skills?"; "How is the quality of your work?"; and "To what extent do attention, memory, or planning issues affect your daily activities?" These challenges are similar when assessments rely on reports from surrogates or caretakers.

Detailed assessments focus on measurable aspects of behaviors, such as time taken to complete tasks, task frequency, and the need for prompts. These assessments take longer and require clear understanding of questions from the respondents. For example, in the social domain: "How often do you ask others to play cards or go to the movies?"; "What would you do before going to the movies?"; and "How would you get to the movies?" In the personal hygiene domain, items might include observing or role-playing teeth brushing.

Assessing a specific behavioral response class by self-report from the person living with SMI may be unreliable given impairments in intelligible and coherent speech as well as neurocognitive factors (e.g., memory, comprehension) (Harvey & Strassnig, 2012; Green, 1996). Using surrogates/caretakers may be limited in the validity and reliability of the data given limitations in the opportunities to observe the person doing the targeted task or behavior across several contexts (Bellack et al., 2007).

Self-monitoring and self-control skills are necessary skills to have and use in daily life. These are the tasks and strategies that individuals living with SMI use to successfully live with and manage the physical, social, and emotional impact of living with SMI (Lean et al., 2019). Problems in self-monitoring and self-control may be related to impairments in self-awareness (e.g., "insight"); the lack of self-awareness has similarities with the neurocognitive impairment of "anosognosia" that can be present in persons with neurogenerative disease and averse neurological events, such as CVAs and head trauma (Shahrokh & Hales, 2003). If a person living with SMI is not aware of what they are doing, then the person is unable to monitor their behaviors; with a lack of self-monitoring, a person would have difficulty with refraining from doing a maladaptive problematic behavior and display the adaptive alternative behaviors. For example, when an individual is hungry, people having self-monitoring and self-control skills can determine when and how to reduce the impact of hunger and not act impulsively; poor self-control can result in maladaptively responses to reduce the aversive state of hunger (e.g., stealing food; eating out of trash) and have worse aversive consequences for the individual (e.g., being arrested).

Self-management and self-control skills are associated with better overall adjustment on a wide range of personal and interpersonal measures, including less substance use, binge eating, academic success, better emotional responses, and better interpersonal relationships (Tangney et al., 2004). Individuals that who impairments in self-awareness and self-control skills may not display response classes of functional behaviors like daily hygiene, taking medications, paying bills, buying groceries, getting to appointments, or work on time.

Lack of self-control and self-management may stem from functional skill impairment. People learn behaviors by observing others and seeing what works. Effective behaviors, including associated self-talk, are reinforced and become part of their skill set, while ineffective ones are not, leading to their elimination.

The World Health Organization Disability Assessment Schedule (WHODAS-2.0) (World Health Organization (WHO), 2010) is a standardized tool designed to measure limitations in activity and social restrictions experienced by individuals over the past 30 days. It is a generic, non-health-condition-specific, cross-cultural measure that can be used across various health conditions. WHODAS is available in 12-item and 36-item versions and can be self-administered or interviewer-administered. Responses can be provided by the individual, a caregiver, or a clinician. The instrument assesses impairments across six domains (American Psychiatric Association, n.d.):

1. Understanding and communicating: include activities like concentrating, remembering, problem-solving, learning new tasks, understanding speech, and maintaining conversations (American Psychiatric Association, n.d.).
2. Getting around: covers mobility-related activities such as standing, moving inside the home, getting out of the home, and walking longer distances (American Psychiatric Association, n.d.).
3. Self-care: focuses on personal care tasks like washing, dressing, eating, and staying alone (American Psychiatric Association, n.d.).
4. Getting along with people: assesses interpersonal interactions, including dealing with strangers, maintaining friendships, getting along with close people, making new friends, and sexual activities (American Psychiatric Association, n.d.).
5. Life activities include: (a) household tasks such as responsibilities, completing tasks, and efficiency; (b) work or school tasks including daily activities, task performance, and efficiency; and (c) participation in society involving community activities, barriers, dignity, emotional impact, financial strain, family issues, and ability to relax or enjoy leisure activities (American Psychiatric Association, n.d.).

The Multidimensional Scale of Independent Functioning (MSIF) is a semi-structured interview designed to measure functional impairment in individuals living with SMI (Jaeger et al., 2003). It assesses an individual's ability to perform daily activities across multiple domains of functioning, concentrating on their level of independence and functionality. The MSIF examines various aspects of daily life, including work, education, social interactions, and self-care. The MSIF covers the domains of:

- Work/education: evaluates the ability to maintain employment or participate in educational activities.
- Social functioning: assesses interpersonal relationships and social engagement.

- Self-care: measures the ability to manage personal hygiene, health, and daily living tasks.

The MSIF scoring system quantifies functional impairment by rating performance in each domain. Higher scores indicate better functioning and greater independence. MSIF ratings are determined through a detailed interview with the individual living with SMI, supplemented by collateral sources such as family members, employers, residential staff, and mental health service providers (Jaeger et al., 2003).

The MSIF evaluates the daily activities of the person in work, education, and residential environments. For example, when a rating is made for the work environment, the MSIF would consider not only the job title but also what tasks the job involves, when and at what pace tasks are completed, with what level of supervision or self-initiation tasks are performed, what assistance is received, and to what performance standard the work is held. Ratings consider factors like job responsibilities, tasks, supervision, assistance, and performance standards. Information for each environment is coded on three dimensions: role responsibility, support presence and level, and performance quality. The interviewer also provides global ratings for each environment and overall independent functioning, based on their subjective judgment (Jaeger et al., 2003).

McGrath et al. (2013) (used a version of the RAND 36-Item Health Survey (SF-36) (RAND Corporation, n.d.) to assess functional impairment in a sample of individuals living with SMI. SF-36 (RAND Corporation, n.d.) is a comprehensive questionnaire designed to evaluate perceived health-related functioning. This instrument encompasses various items that assess physical functioning, role limitations due to physical health, bodily pain, general health perceptions, vitality, social functioning, and role limitations due to general emotional and mental health issues over the preceding 4 weeks. It is divided into two assessment domains:

- Health perceptions: based on respondents' overall health status and comparisons to the previous year, including any limitations in daily activities.
- Impact of physical and emotional health on daily life: evaluates the extent to which physical and emotional problems have influenced daily activities and social interactions.

Although used as an assessment of functional impairment in people living with SMI, it relies on the person's subjective perception of their activity level. It does not assess the extent to which lack of motivation, incentives, and/or opportunities to engage in the activities influences the perceptions of functional impairment by the person responding. The SF-36 is commonly utilized as a tool in medical settings with groups that report different levels of ill-health (Jenkinson et al., 1994).

The Butajira Functioning Scale (BFS) is a culturally competent measure that assesses functioning across three main domains in people living in rural areas in Ethiopia (Habtamu et al., 2018). It is composed of 41 items with 33 common to both men and women and 8 items specifically for women.

The BFS has domains that include ADLs and IADLs: self-care, work, and social functioning. Items on the domain of "**self-care" i**nclude tasks related to personal hygiene and eating, such as washing the body, cutting nails, using the toilet properly, and preparing and eating food. The domain of work is divided into shared work items for men and women (e.g., farming, kitchen gardening, attending livestock) and gender-specific work items for women (e.g., domestic tasks like cooking, cleaning, and fetching water). "Social functioning" domain covers family and community participation, such as maintaining social contact with relatives, advising children, participating in local self-help groups, attending community meetings, and engaging in religious activities (Habtamu et al., 2018).

These domains highlight the sociocultural context of rural Ethiopia, focusing on essential survival tasks. Factor analysis identified subdomains such as hygiene and eating, farming and domestic tasks within work, and family/children and community participation within social functioning. Self-care factors include eating and hygiene (e.g., dimensions include "washing own body," "washing hands," "cutting nails"); work factors involve fieldwork, kitchen gardening, and livestock care. Women-specific work domains include items focusing on dimensions about farming tasks (e.g., "cutting grass," "splitting firewood") and domestic tasks (e.g., "preparing food," "cleaning the house"). Social functioning factors cover family/children (e.g., "following up children's health," "helping elders") and community participation (e.g., "participating in self-help groups," "attending community meetings") (Habtamu et al., 2018).

Wallace (1986) reviewed various assessment instruments for evaluating functional living skills in people living with SMI. The assessment tools ranged from global to specific measurable dimensions of functional living skills including problem behaviors, social behaviors, role performance, perceptions of distress, and instrumental skills. The tools varied in coverage, reliability, and ease of use. Instruments such as the Katz Adjustment Scale (KAS) (Katz & Lyerly, 1963) and Personal Adjustment and Role Skills Scale (PARS) (Ellsworth et al., 1979) are straightforward to administer and commonly utilized in treatment studies; however, they lack detailed planning for comprehensive rehabilitative interventions. Conversely, scales like the Social Behavior and Adjustment Scale (SBAS) (Platt et al., 1980) and Social Adjustment Scale (SAS) (Weissman et al., 1981) provide extensive evaluations of household burdens and social roles, though they necessitate long and expansive interviews.

The Denver Community Mental Health Questionnaire (DCMHQ) (Ciarlo & Reihman, 1977) and Social Stress and Functioning Inventory for Psychotic Disorders (SSFIPD) (Serban, 1978) are instruments used to assess antisocial behaviors, stress, and community adaptation. These tools have limited psychometric properties. The Independent Living Skills Survey (ILSS) (Wallace et al., 1985) offers a thorough analysis of daily living skills but demonstrates restricted variance in certain areas. Meanwhile, tools such as the Psychiatric Status Schedule (PSS) (Spitzer et al., 1970), Psychiatric Evaluation Form (PEF) (American Psychiatric Association, 2006), and Current and Past Psychopathology Scale (CAPPS) (Spitzer et al., 1968) are highly reliable for evaluating problem behaviors and social adjustment, although their administration is costly.

Other assessments, including the Community Adaptation Schedule (CAS) (Burnes & Roen, 1967) and Rehabilitation Evaluation (REHAB) (Baker & Hall (1988), primarily focus on specific aspects of social function and may require additional evaluations to support rehabilitation planning.

Overall, the reviewed instruments differ significantly in their ability to provide comprehensive and reliable assessments of functional behavior. No single instrument is wholly adequate for assessing impairments functional living skills given the heterogeneity of dimensional skills in each domain of functioning. Global instruments are useful for broad evaluations, while specific instruments are better for pinpointing behaviors for rehabilitation efforts. Combining instruments tailored to the assessment purpose is recommended for comprehensive evaluations. Many assessment instruments lack criterion validity, meaning their items do not align with real-world functional behaviors. Additionally, tools for assessing functional living behaviors evaluate other behaviors associated with SMI, such as social interactions, speech clarity, and response to auditory hallucinations.

The Rehabilitation Evaluation (REHAB) by Baker and Hall (1988) uses ratings from two independent observers on behaviors like table manners, hygiene, dressing, care of possessions, care of personal items including money, social interactions, and how much prompting is needed. The ratings are based on a scale that measures competent performance in tasks such as washing and cleaning oneself. However, functional life skills involve multiple behaviors, such as brushing teeth, which include steps like finding the toothbrush, turning on the water, wetting the head of the brush, opening and then applying toothpaste. Impairments can occur at any step, like using too much paste, not locating the toothbrush, and eating the toothpaste.

The Assessment of Lifespan Functioning Attainment (ALFA) (Joseph et al., 2015) is a novel brief self-report scale designed to evaluate functional outcomes across various functional domains in individuals living with SMI. The ALFA evaluates functioning across different decades of life before and after the onset of living with SMI. It assesses present status and historical engagement in functional domains, providing a measure of functioning. The ALFA evaluates five functional domains, which are defined as follows (Joseph et al., 2015):

- Paid employment: Individuals are asked about their engagement in being paid for work activities during specific periods of their life including defining full-time childcare or full-time student status as equivalent to working.
- Living independently: defined as residing in an unsupervised private or cooperative house, apartment, or boarding house where no staff or meals are provided.
- Close friendships: defined as having contact with someone at least once a month.
- Romantic relationships: defined as having a significant other.
- Recreational engagement: defined as engaging in activities with people who are not part of the participant's family.

The results from interviews with over 60 men and women living with SMI in the community revealed significant declines in multiple areas of life in sociability (friendship and recreational engagement) and independence (paid employment, living independently, romantic partnerships) since the beginning of the individual living with SMI. Significant correlations were found between ALFA and items on a measure of quality of life (QoL) related to employment, living situation, and romantic partnerships (Joseph et al., 2015). It should be noted that the domains of close and romantic relationships and recreational engagement are social in nature and are assessed on some scales of social functioning.

The Independent Living Skills Survey (ILSS) and the Independent Living Skills Inventory (ILSI) for assessing the community functioning of individuals living with SMI have been used to assess functional skills necessary for competency living in the community (Menditto et al., 1999). Two versions were developed: (1) informant (ILSS-I) and (2) self-report (ILSS-SR). Data from over 300 participants were analyzed for internal consistency, stability, interrater reliability, and validity. Results suggested that both versions are reliable and valid for treatment planning and program evaluation.

The ILSS covers various life skills necessary for self-sufficiency and successful adjustment to living in community settings. The response class domains and some of the dimensions measured by the ILSS include:

- Money management: assesses knowledge of coins, currency, and transaction skills; evaluates understanding of budgeting and saving concepts; includes ability to manage a checking account and read bank statements.
- Food management: covers hygiene practices like handwashing before food preparation; assesses knowledge of cooking utensils and appliances; evaluates ability to prepare meals and create grocery lists.
- Personal appearance: assesses self-care skills including dressing, bathing, and dental hygiene; evaluates ability to maintain clean clothing and perform laundry tasks.
- Health: evaluates knowledge of medication management and health symptoms; assesses ability to seek medical help and understand first aid.
- Housekeeping: covers skills related to cleaning, laundry, and general home maintenance; assesses ability to manage waste disposal and managing repairs.
- Transportation: evaluates knowledge of safe transportation methods including biking and public transport; assesses ability to read maps and understands seat belt usage.
- Emergency and safety skills: assess knowledge of emergency services and evacuation procedures; evaluate ability to use safety equipment like smoke alarms and fire extinguishers.
- Knowledge of community resources: covers ability to access local services like grocery stores and pharmacies; assesses knowledge of emergency contacts and public facilities.
- Interpersonal skills: evaluate social skills including communication and conflict resolution; assess ability to maintain friendships and seek help when needed.
- Legal issues: cover understanding of legal rights and responsibilities; assess knowledge of legal resources and voting registration.

The ILSS covers many areas of functioning that are expected in society except for occupational or academic roles. The ILSS scoring on the dimensions is a discrete response of "yes" or "no" as to the questions asked (e.g., "Do you know how to write a check?") without any observed performance of the skill being asked. Self-reports either by the person living with SMI or by a familiar informant can be influenced by contextual and neurocognitive factors like memory, comprehension, and social desirability that call into question the validity and reliability of the responses.

The Schizophrenia Outcomes Functioning Interview (SOFI) (Kleinman et al., 2009) was developed to provide an assessment of functional outcomes in people living with SMI; it was reported by the authors to address limitations of existing measures and emphasized observable behaviors and multiple relevant domains. SOFI relies on discrete responses based on interviews of the person living with SMI and informants who live with the person or is a paid caretaker. The questions asked are closed-ended and pertaining to the person performing behaviors and activities contained in the questions. For instance, a question related to independent functioning asks if the person can leave the residence without permission. The SOFI-P version is administered directly to the person living with SMI; the SOFI-I version is administered to a caregiver informant, who can be either a formal paid caregiver (e.g., case manager, group home staff) or an informal caregiver (e.g., family member or friend). Informants must have observed the person for at least 1 month and directly interacted with them at least twice per month.

Both versions aim to gather comprehensive information about the individual's functioning across various domains (Kleinman et al., 2009). The contextual domains and dimensions of response classes of behaviors include:

- Living situation: current residence, ability to access residence without supervision, autonomy in scheduling. Sample items include: (a) does the person have unsupervised access to their home or room, (b) does the person decide when to wake or eat, and (c) can the individual come and go as they wish?
- Instrumental activities of daily living (IALs): self-care, psychiatric treatment adherence, money management, planning skills, transportation, and leisure activities. Sample behavior response classes examined were: (a) whether the individual requires assistance with shopping, (b) whether the individual independently seeks medical care, (c) the extent to which the individual can travel independently, and (d) whether the individual organizes their daily activities autonomously.
- Productive activities: working, volunteering, parenting, vocational training, education, or attendance at a day treatment program. Response classes evaluated included: (a) does the individual have a job coach at work, (b) does the individual need help staying on-task, and (c) what other productive activities does the individual engage in?
- Social functioning: social interactions and initiation of activities. Response classes examined include: (a) can the individual depend on their family, (b) does the individual maintain appropriate social distance, and (c) what kind of social network does the individual have?

The SOFI reportedly was designed to be sensitive to changes in functional impairment and is based on observable behaviors rather than self-report, with the intent to capture the real-world functioning of individuals (Kleinman et al., 2009). Although agreement between individual and informant ratings on the SOFI had general good concordance ratings, the SOFI still relied on data from interview-based assessments. Interview data can be biased and subject to recall issues, social desirability, and subjective impressions. SOFI's convergent validity was computed using interview-based instruments and not on performance- or observation-based measures. The domain of social functioning is linked to behaviors evaluated by assessments of competent social functioning although it could be considered an aspect of adaptive daily functioning that is needed for independent living in the community. In addition, the interviewer was the same for both the individual and informant; the lack of independent interviewers could affect the reliability and validity of the ratings by introducing biases and inflating the correlations (Kleinman et al., 2009).

The University of California San Diego Performance-Based Skills Assessment (UPSA) (Becattini-Oliveira et al., 2018; Patterson et al., 2001) directly assesses functional capabilities among community dwelling individuals living with SMI. This test measures everyday functional skills using standard role-plays to evaluate skills in five different domains. A more recent version of the instrument, the UPSA-2 (Henry et al., 2013), quantifies functional abilities across six domains, including (1) household management and chores (e.g., planning grocery shopping); (2) communication (e.g., using the telephone for an appointment); (3) financial skills (e.g., paying bills); (4) transportation (e.g., public transportation); and (5); comprehension/planning (e.g., organizing trips). The assessment takes about 30 minutes to be completed.

The domains, assessed dimensions, and the corresponding role-plays are listed below:

- Household management—developing a comprehensive shopping list: In this simulation, participants are provided with a recipe and are tasked with compiling a shopping list for essential items at a grocery store, while omitting items already available in a simulated pantry (University of California, San Diego Performance-Based Skills Assessment (UPSA), 2025).
- Communication—conducting telephone calls: Participants are given a non-functional push-button phone and instructed to make telephone calls, such as requesting assistance in an emergency, seeking directory information, or reading and responding to a medical appointment letter. Points are awarded for executing accurate actions, including accessing a dial tone, dialing correctly, and successfully completing the call (UPSA, 2025).
- Financial skills—(1) counting change: Participants receive "play money" in the form of bills and coins and are required to count specific amounts and calculate the correct change for a transaction; (2) paying bills: Individuals must comprehend a utility bill and write a check to pay the bill, ensuring that the correct due date, amount, and description are included (UPSA, 2025).

- Transportation—navigating public transit: Participants are provided with a bus schedule and must identify the appropriate bus for traveling between specified locations. Accurate determination of departure and arrival times, as well as the cost of a ticket, is essential (UPSA, 2025).
- Comprehension and planning—organizing recreational activities: Individuals read a scenario regarding participation in a recreational activity and are tasked with planning their transportation to the activity, determining what items to bring, and outlining the actions to take upon arrival at the destination (UPSA, 2025).
- Medication management—demonstrating proficiency in following a mock medication regimen: Participants are tasked with managing a medication schedule, utilizing four different medications to be taken at various times throughout the day (UPSA, 2025).

The predictive utility for assessing independent living status in older adults living with SMI was conducted by Fortuna et al. (2018) using both the ILSS and the UPSA. The ILSS and UPSA predicted independent living status at baseline and 1-year follow-up. The ILSS was associated with self-efficacy and employment status, while neither the ILSS nor UPSA correlated with hospitalizations or health status.

The Test of Adaptive Behavior in Schizophrenia (TABS) (Velligan et al., 2007) is an instrument developed to assess functional capacity in two domains important to functioning: (1) initiation of tasks in the real world and (2) identifying problems that occur during functional activities. It is a performance-based measure that addresses limitations of existing measures by focusing on initiation and problem identification. Individuals living with SMI are observed and assessed while performing tasks rather than relying solely on self-report from either the person or an informant.

Six domains are assessed by observing dimensional response classes of behaviors that pertain to the domains, including awareness of problems, problem solving, and initiation of responses required to solve problems. The individuals are scored by a "percent correct" score for each of the six domains.

The domains, dimensional response class of behaviors, and specific scoring details for each dimension assessed are as follows:

1. Medication management skills: taking medications as directed, identifying when pills will run out, and generating solutions. Points are awarded for correct placement of medication, identifying problems (e.g., running out of medication), and generating solutions. More points are given for spontaneously identifying and solving problems compared to responding after prompts.
2. Daily hygiene: identifying items needed for daily use in an empty bathroom. Points are given for naming necessary items, categorizing responses, and generating appropriate items that are needed.
3. Shopping skills: navigating a store, shopping for items, and identifying incorrect change. Points are earned for navigating a map, remembering items, purchasing correctly, and noticing errors (e.g., missing items, being short-changed). Spontaneous identification of problems earns more points.

4. Dressing: selecting appropriate clothing. Points are given for selecting appropriate outfits for specific events like a doctor's appointment, trip to the park, and weather conditions. A mannequin is used, and the individual selects the clothes, some of which are dirty and/or torn. Additional points are awarded for asking relevant questions (e.g., about the weather).
5. Work and productivity: completing tasks like collating flyers. Points are awarded for organizational strategies, correctly assembling packets, and persistence in completing tasks.
6. Social skills: evaluating eye contact, speech, and other social behaviors during the test. Rated on a 3-point scale (0–2) for dimensions like eye contact, speech volume, and initiating conversation.

The TABS scores are significantly correlated with other measures of functional outcomes and to "negative symptoms" but not the presence of problem behaviors associated with living with SMI (i.e., "positive symptoms"). Further research is needed to establish its utility in predicting real-world outcomes (e.g., employment and independent community living) and its responsiveness to interventions (Velligan et al., 2007).

Independent Living Scales (ILS) (Loeb, 1996) is a self-report instrument used to assess a person's ability to care for themselves and their property. It is a standardized, reliable, and valid measure for identifying areas of competence in five domains and two factor-analyzed subscales:

1. Memory and orientation: include items that measure dimensions of orientation to time and place, recall of a brief shopping list, and recognition of a missing object (Loeb, 1996; Revheim and Medalia, 2004).
2. Managing money: focuses on dimensions related to monetary calculations and budgetary precautions (e.g., not having enough money to pay bills) (Loeb, 1996; Revheim & Medalia, 2004).
3. Managing home and transportation: measures performances of response classes of use of the telephone, public transportation, and home management skills (Loeb, 1996; Revheim & Medalia, 2004).
4. Health and safety: assesses dimensions of awareness of health problems, medical emergencies, and potential hazards around the home (Loeb, 1996; Revheim & Medalia, 2004).
5. Social adjustment: measures self-reported perceptions about interpersonal relationships (Loeb, 1996; Revheim & Medalia, 2004).

The factor-analyzed subscales include:

- Performance–information factor: reflects actual knowledge or dimensional skills used to perform tasks, such as using a telephone book or making change (Loeb, 1996; Revheim & Medalia, 2004).
- Problem-solving factor subscale (ILS-PB): comprises 33 items across all subscales that evaluate dimensions of abstract reasoning, judgment, cognitive flexibility required for daily living, with items like "What would you do if your lights

and television went out simultaneously?" and "What would you do if you unintentionally lost ten pounds in a month?" (Loeb, 1996; Revheim & Medalia, 2004).

The ILS has not been widely utilized for individuals living with SMI. Revheim and Medalia (2004) evaluated over 160 individuals living with SMI who resided in the community. The key finding is that ILS-PB effectively distinguishes between all three levels of functional outcomes, from maximum to minimal supervision. This indicates that ILS scores are sensitive to varying levels of supervision needs. ILS-PB problem-solving skills are significant predictors of living status. Individuals requiring maximum supervision scored lower on the ILS-PB, while those requiring minimal supervision approached the recommended cutoff score of 50 for independent living. The authors concluded that the ILS -PB is an appropriate tool for aftercare follow-up among individuals who live with SMI transitioning from institutional settings to community living, as it specifically addresses daily problem-solving skills linked to functional outcomes.

No "gold standard" tool exists that assesses functional behaviors in people living with SMI (Bellack et al., 2007); research has shown that performance-based measures show the most evidence for predicting abilities to care for oneself and exhibit behaviors that are expected to live independently (Mausbach et al., 2009). The reviews that have been conducted on these assessment tools focus on ease of administration (e.g., length of time needed for administration, required training, ease of scoring), psychometric properties, relationship to real-world behaviors and outcomes, and sensitivity to change when used in clinical trials (Mausbach et al., 2009).

Measuring daily functional behaviors of people living with SMI presents several challenges. Functional outcomes encompass various domains, including daily living skills, social skills, and vocational performance. These include the need to measure multiple domains and dimensions, conflicting interests among care stakeholders, limitations of self-report and informant reporting data, and other methodological issues. Self-reports of functional abilities by the individual living with SMI are popular, but their relevance to different stakeholders must be carefully considered (Brown & Velligan, 2016).

The selection of functional outcome measures is complicated by the heterogeneity in the presentations of functional impairments in individuals living with SMI. Recent studies identified 59 potential functional assessments, highlighting the need for consensus on relevant measures (Brown & Velligan, 2016). Many assessment tools focus on self-care and social relationships while not consistently addressing quality of life, health status, and work skills. Individual instruments have limitations such as lacking behavioral anchors for scale items (i.e., specific behaviors related to various levels of performance (Murphy & Constans, 1987)), insufficient specificity for individuals with SMI, and scoring that inaccurately represents their impairments, like needing prompts or rarely displaying certain behaviors (Dickerson, 1997).

Performance-based measures have demonstrated strong external and predictive validity for assessing the functional behaviors of individuals living with SMI (Mausbach et al., 2009). However, there are no instruments that comprehensively measure the various domains that comprise functional behaviors. The deficit may be attributable to the impracticality of such an instrument in clinical and research settings, due to the extensive number of domains and dimensions that would require evaluation. Instead, the research on assessing functional behaviors investigates a few functional domains and searches for correlations on other factors, such as degree of supervision needed, duration of living in the community post discharge, scores obtained on neuropsychological performance measures, and other measures of functional behaviors (Brown & Velligan, 2016).

Impairments in functional living skills are an important focus with individuals who have had adverse neurological events; these events often result in impairment in many of the same domains that have shown impairments in individuals living with SMI. The most frequently impaired skills included residential independence, money management, and leisure activities. Neurocognitive deficits were highly correlated with disruptions in everyday functioning. However, improvements were noted even for participants more than 1-year post-injury (Lewis & Horn, 2013), whereas the functional impairments observed in people living with SMI are persistent and do not respond to pharmacological intervention (McGrath et al., 2013).

An example of functional assessment with people who have had adverse neurological events is the Neuro Skills Independent Living Skills Assessment (NSILS). It is an observational tool used by staff members assigned to a specific individual to collect observational data over 1-week periods (Centre for Neuro Skills Independent Living Scale, n.d.). The NSILS was shown to have good construct validity, inter-rater reliability, internal consistency, instrument stability, and convergent validity (Ashley et al., 2001).

The domains assessed in the independent living skills assessment (Centre for Neuro Skills Independent Living Scale, n.d.) include: (1) money management; (2) food management; (3) personal appearance; (4) health; (5) housekeeping; (6) transportation; (7) emergency and safety skills; (8) knowledge of community resources; (9) interpersonal skills; and (10) legal issues. In each of the domains are behavioral dimensions that are observed and rated according to degree of independence, need for prompting and/or assistance, not currently manifesting, not applicable, and desire to learn the skill. Each domain has several specific dimensions in the response classes that are rated. For instance, the domain of food management is assessed by evaluating the individual's ability to perform the following tasks:

1. Wash hands before eating and preparing food.
2. Know the name and use of most cooking utensils.
3. Use cooking utensils effectively and safely.
4. Use kitchen appliances effectively and safely.
5. Understand how to use dates on food packages to prevent spoilage.
6. Store perishable items in the refrigerator.
7. Recognize signs of spoilage in food.
8. Follow instructions for preparing canned or frozen foods.
9. Prepare recipes from a cookbook.
10. Fix lunch for one.

11. Fix dinner for one.
12. Make a grocery shopping list.
13. Shop for a week's menu and stay within a budget.
14. Set the table properly.

Each dimension is assessed based on the individual's observed level of functioning (Centre for Neuro Skills Independent Living Scale, n.d.).

The NSILS (Centre for Neuro Skills Independent Living Scale, n.d.) is relatively comprehensive in evaluating the domains of independent functioning. It has been reported to be a psychometrically sound instrument. The dimensions are ones that are measured in other validated and reliable instruments. For instance, the dimensions of making a grocery list, shopping for items by using a menu, and staying within budget are dimensions on several performance instruments, such as USPA-2 (Henry et al., 2013). Preparing a meal is a dimension assessed on the Pfeffer Functional Activities Questionnaire (Pfeffer, 1982; Fuentes-García, 2023).

Although the domains and dimensions are similar to those that are impaired and need support and intervention in people living with SMI, the NSILS was developed and tested on samples of individuals living with different types of averse neurological events. It is a lengthy and time-consuming assessment, needing dedicated staff to conduct the observations. Additionally, scoring on this instrument could be expanded to include IADLs to account for the diverse range of impairments experienced by individuals with SMI. Individuals with SMI may not show functional behavior due to limited resources, lack of incentives, or may have previously had functional ability but can no longer independently demonstrate these skills due to neurocognitive impairments such as memory retrieval difficulties or lack of stimulus control.

Domains and response classes of the corresponding dimensions have been assessed using various methods, including self-reports, informant reports, role-playing, and direct observation, with scoring systems tailored to measure independence, assistance required, and performance quality. Below is a summary of the response classes of the dimensions that have been assessed by the various tools measuring the functional competence and abilities of individuals living with SMI across multiple domains including activities of daily living (ADLs) and instrumental activities of daily living (IADLs):

ADLs:

- Feeding: ability to eat independently.
- Dressing: selecting and wearing appropriate clothing.
- Bathing: personal hygiene and cleanliness.
- Toileting: managing bathroom needs.
- Mobility: walking and moving around.
- Maintaining personal hygiene: grooming and cleanliness.

IADLs:

- Transportation: navigating public transit, reading schedules, attending events, managing transportation (e.g., driving or organizing other means of transport).

- Managing finances: paying bills, balancing checkbooks, and handling financial assets.
- Meal preparation: shopping for food, preparing meals, and following recipes.
- Housecleaning and home maintenance: cleaning living areas, maintaining tidiness, and performing home maintenance tasks.
- Laundry: washing and maintaining clothing.
- Managing communication: handling telephone calls, mail, responding to appointment letters, texts and calls, and other forms of communication.
- Financial skills: counting change, paying bills, budgeting.
- Comprehension and planning: organizing recreational activities, planning trips. Planning grocery shopping, organizing chores.
- Managing medications: obtaining and taking medications as directed.
- Maintaining friendships: engaging in social activities and resolving conflicts.
- Maintaining a romantic relationship: having a significant other.
- Community participation: attending meetings, participating in self-help groups.
- Awareness of health problems: recognizing symptoms and seeking medical help.
- Emergency preparedness: using safety equipment, evacuation procedures.
- Task completion: organizing and completing work-related tasks; persistence: maintaining focus and effort in tasks.
- Understanding legal rights: knowledge of voting registration and legal resources.
- Accessing community resources: navigating local services like grocery stores, restaurants, and pharmacies.

The problem with conducting observations and training skills in functional abilities is that it is time-consuming, complex, and challenging. The behaviors that comprise independent functioning have many steps for the person to perform with or without prompting and assistance. For instance, below is an outline of the steps required to competently perform tooth brushing (excluding the movements of the brush head on various parts of the teeth):

1. Pick up your toothbrush.
2. Open the water tap.
3. Wash and rinse toothbrush.
4. Pick up your toothpaste.
5. Open the lid of the paste.
6. Squeeze out some paste on the brush head.
7. Close the lid of the paste.
8. Put down the toothpaste tube.
9. Brush the teeth.
10. Spit out any paste and saliva in mouth.
11. Open the tap.
12. Rinse the toothbrush.
13. Place the toothbrush back in its holder.
14. Take a rinsing cup.
15. Fill it with water.
16. Rinse the mouth with water.

17. Spit out the water.

Functional impairment in people living with SMI is multifaceted and varies among individuals (Bechi et al., 2017; Harvey & Strassnig, 2012). Research on functional impairments in various aspects of daily life for individuals who live with SMI has typically used nomothetic methods, which involve aggregating data from groups (Barlow & Nock, 2009). The nomothetic approach (i.e., the study of interindividual variation) dominates analyses of research data on different observed and noted impairments, even though its assumption of homogeneity across people and time is often violated. The idiographic approach (i.e., the study of intraindividual variation) is best suited for analyses of heterogeneous data (Beltz et al., 2016); it focuses on the intraindividual variations in results on performance measures in people living with SMI. The reliance on the nomothetic approach has resulted in limitations in flexibility and generalizability of the findings of the research and use in clinical practice (Barlow & Nock, 2009). In addition, functional impairment studies often compare self-reports and performance measures between individuals with SMI and those without. Some assessment tools use small samples or lack robust validity and reliability data.

Assessing functional behaviors of people with SMI, such as age of onset, duration, behavior frequency, severity, and context (e.g., residence), provides detailed information for creating effective, individualized interventions. Normative data may not capture the nuances and complexities of impairments in people living with SMI, potentially leading to inaccurate or misleading conclusions about an individual's mental health and ability to function without oversight. Using clinical norms based on clinical clusters allows for personalized statistical inferences about deviations from typical patterns allowing for individual-level statistical inferences about deviations from normative patterns, accommodating diverse outcome pathways (Marquand et al., 2019; Pratt et al., 2017). Research and assessment in SMI need to shift focus to understanding the specific experiences, strengths, and challenges for each person rather than comparing them to a "norm." As noted by researchers, there is a lack of "real world data" that support the external validity of the assessment (Abel et al., 2021; Harvey & Strassnig, 2012).

Measurement of impairments should include whether the expected behaviors are part of the person's behavioral repertoire. The non-occurrence of the expected behaviors could be a result of other variables like deficits in reinforcing consequences, lack of opportunities to engage in the expected behaviors, and impairments in neurocognitive abilities such as comprehension and recall. A determination can be made as to whether the diminished or absent manifestations of the expected behaviors are a skill deficit or a problem in the density of reinforcement (i.e., the frequency and magnitude of reinforcement).

Individualized rehabilitation and skills training in specific functional behaviors could be achieved by using instruments that use data from informants as to a person's ability to frequently engage in certain functional behaviors and supplemented by self-reports from the individual living with SMI and existing performance-based measures such as REHAB (Velligan et al., 2007), TABS (Baker & Hall, 1988), and

UPSA-2 (Henry et al., 2013). Based on data from these tools, observations on the domains and dimensions that the data indicate are impaired can be tailored for the person displaying the impairments.

Origins of Functional Impairments

Neurological Substrates

Impairments in daily functioning represent a major treatment issue with people living with SMI. A more in-depth knowledge of underlying constructs is crucial for interventions to translate into better outcomes. Studies that aim to investigate variables influencing both functional capacity and real-life behavior in individuals living with SMI have found no significant correlation between functional capacity and real-life behavior (Bechi et al., 2017; Harvey & Strassnig, 2012). The assessment of functional capacity was significantly predicted by IQ (i.e., neurocognition), while real-life behavior was significantly predicted by social-cognitive variables such as empathy and emotional recognition. Functional capacity seems to be related to neurocognition, whereas real-life behavior appears more complex, requiring the integration of different factors and interventions (Bechi et al., 2017; Schretlen et al., 2000).

Goodkind et al. (2015) conducted a meta-analysis of structural neuroimaging studies across multiple mental health problems. The study found a transdiagnostic pattern of gray matter loss in the anterior insula and dorsal anterior cingulate cortex (dACC) among individuals with mental health problems corresponding to SMI. The decrease in gray matter in these regions correlates with impaired functioning in the domain of executive functions (EFs) in participants with no known mental health problems. The neurocognitive domain of EF is composed of neurocognitive dimensions, such as task initiation, organization, flexibility, setting priorities, problem-solving, working memory, and control of impulsivity and emotions (Baggetta & Alexander, 2016). EF is crucial for self-regulation and goal-directed behavior that is needed for performance of behaviors related to daily functioning. Impairments in EF are prevalent across various mental health problems linked to living with SMI, with the largest deficits observed in individuals living with schizophrenia spectrum mental health problems followed by bipolar and major depressive mental health problems (Baggetta & Alexander, 2016).

The findings suggest that cortical thinning and gray matter loss in the anterior insula, frontotemporal regions, and dACC may contribute to functional impairments in EF and working memory (WM) rather than specific symptoms (Goodkind et al., 2015; Huang et al., 2025). Effects related to specific mental health problems were observed only in participants with schizophrenia spectrum and major depressive mental health problems. No significant effects of medications or co-occurring health problems were found on gray matter volume.

Goodkind et al. (2015) concluded that there are neurological commonalities across mental health problems contrasting with previous studies related to specific mental health problems; future research should explore how gray matter loss relates to the severity, chronicity, and dimensions of symptoms and behavior problems linked to specific mental health problems as the findings suggest shared neural substrates and structural brain changes for mental health problems, particularly those corresponding to SMI.

Gray matter loss indicates a common neural idiosyncrasy in individuals with SMI, regardless of different causes. Results from structural MRIs have found the loss of gray matter in the following brain structures and possible impact of associated functions (Goodkind et al., 2015):

- Dorsolateral prefrontal context (dlPFC): This region is crucial for executive functions like WM, planning, and decision-making. Reduced activity and gray matter volume in the dlPFC are often observed in individuals living with SMI, contributing to difficulties with these neurocognitive processes.
- Ventromedial prefrontal cortex (vmPFC): This area plays a vital role in emotional regulation and social cognition. Abnormalities in the vmPFC are associated with difficulties processing emotions, understanding social cues, and avolition (impairments with experiencing motivation) in people living with SMI.
- Anterior cingulate cortex (ACC): The ACC is important for error detection, conflict monitoring, and attention. Dysfunction in the ACC is linked to impaired cognitive control, difficulty focusing, and problems with emotional processing in SMI.
- Hippocampus (HC): This structure is essential for memory formation and spatial navigation. Reduced hippocampal volume and activity are frequently found in individuals living with SMI, particularly those with depression, impacting memory and potentially contributing to difficulties in daily life and learning.
- Amygdala (amyg): The amygdala is the brain's primary center for processing emotions, particularly fear and anxiety. Altered amygdala activity, either increased or decreased, is observed in individuals living with SMI, influencing emotional responses and potentially contributing to symptoms like anxiety, fear, and social withdrawal.
- Striatum (STR): This structure is part of the brain's reward system and is involved in motivation and habit formation and is essential for learning which actions lead to reward and for implementing those actions in the future (Cox & Witten, 2019). Changes in the striatum, including altered activity and gray matter volume, are associated with difficulties experiencing pleasure (anhedonia) and impaired motivation, particularly in individuals with depressive and schizophrenia spectrum mental health problems. Structural changes in the area may be associated with decreasing the effectiveness of reinforcement in people living with SMI.

Studies on neurological substrates of functional impairments in people living with SMI need to consider that it is not just about individual brain structures but also about the communication and coordination between them. Altered functional connectivity patterns between these structures are observed in individuals living with

SMI, disrupting the coordinated activity necessary for adaptive cognitive, emotional, and daily functioning. Individuals with SMI show varying patterns of brain structure and function, highlighting the complexity of the construct of SMI contributing to the diverse range of problem behaviors and functional impairments seen in people living with SMI. Antipsychotic medications, commonly used to treat schizophrenia spectrum conditions, can impact brain structure, particularly in the basal ganglia (BG). The influence of medication on observed brain changes needs to be considered when interpreting research findings (Goodkind et al., 2015).

Progress has been made, but the precise mechanisms by which alterations in brain structures and neural connections lead to specific functional impairments are elusive. Continued research using advanced neuroimaging techniques and longitudinal studies is crucial for a deeper understanding of the neurobiological basis of SMI and its associated symptoms and problematic behaviors and for developing targeted interventions for specific impairments.

Psychological and Behavioral Substrates

An individual living with SMI may not have had opportunities to learn functional adaptive skills (i.e., life skills). Many skills that are expected from functional adults are learned in mid-to-late adolescence. If the onset of living with SMI occurs during this developmental period, the person living with SMI may not have had chances to learn necessary skills. The young person living with SMI may have disruptions in his life due to being admitted to psychiatric facilities, entanglements with legal authorities, placements outside of the home and family, and problems with school attendance. The young person living with SMI may be experiencing neurocognitive problems in memory, attention, and planning; they will have fewer opportunities to engage in meaningful and practical skill acquisitions to improve quality of life (QoL). The results are the persistent and pervasive functional problems that are common across many contexts for the person living with SMI, including skills in self-control.

Adaptive skills in daily functioning encompass a range of learned behaviors that enable individuals to engage effectively and appropriately in everyday tasks that are expected in adult living; successfully performing these tasks result in positive outcomes, such as receiving verbal praise for appearance, hygiene, and self-care, enabling close personal friendships, participating in enjoyable activities, independence in traveling, preparing and eating appetizing meals, and paid employment. Life skills, also known as adaptive skills or daily living skills, are the behaviors that people need to effectively maneuver through their daily lives. Learning models such as operant conditioning, classical conditioning, and social learning theory can be effectively applied in the contexts in which these functional skills do and should occur.

Functional skill impairments are characterized by the absence of behaviors required for independent functioning and successful interaction with the environment to handle daily tasks and demands. Environments that are not conducive to learning and practicing new skills can contribute to impairments. With functional impairments, the expected behaviors do not occur either because the behaviors were not learned as the person had limited exposure to the response class of behaviors that encompass living skills or that the individual has not been taught or given sufficient opportunities to practice essential life skills, whether due to a lack of formal education, supportive environment, or underlying developmental challenges. The opportunities to learn may have been deficient in reinforcing the behavior in situations when the behavior should and should not occur (i.e., stimulus control). Lack of or ineffective use of positive reinforcement results in the absence of motivating operations (MOs) to engage in the skills in the appropriate context or situation. MOs refer to environmental or situational factors that affect the value of engaging in certain behaviors and the propensity to engage in them (Cooper et al., 2020). MOs can either enhance or diminish the efficacy of reinforcers, such as attention, approval, acquisition, or reciprocity. The absence of engaging in life skill behaviors could result in a deficient history of being reinforced for engaging in such behaviors, the lack of opportunities to have effective skills shaped and reinforced by the environment, and the lack of motivating stimuli to engage in the behaviors. Learning also occurs through observing and imitating others. If appropriate life skills are not effectively modeled, individuals would not acquire these behaviors. Insufficient modeling of the desired behaviors or modeling of behaviors results in ineffective daily functioning. Living skills like hygiene, cooking, and dressing may lack enough opportunities to occur and be reinforced, preventing them from becoming habitual responses. Habits are "automatic behaviors triggered by environmental cues, developed through consistent repetition in stable contexts" (Lally & Gardner, 2011, p. 484). Strong habits diminish the influence of deliberate intentions on behavior, making them crucial for both promoting healthy actions and disrupting unhealthy ones. Habits are essential for achieving long-term goals, as they promote consistent behavior over time. Interventions that focus on habit formation enhance the sustainability of adaptive behaviors beyond the active intervention period (Lally & Gardner, 2011).

Additional environmental factors can influence the acquisition of functional living skills. Sensory sensitivities and difficulties expressing needs and understanding others' communication can limit the ability to learn and interact. Challenges with organization, time management, and transitions can make it difficult to initiate, plan, and carry out everyday tasks, impacting life skills like managing personal hygiene or completing chores.

Trauma or negative interactions can lead to emotional and behavioral responses that hinder skill development. The person might lack the skills to handle disappointment and frustration, especially if he has faced inconsistent or frequent punishment. Repeated punishment, failures, or perceived lack of control often leads to a sense of helplessness, making it difficult to try and learn new skills as the individual avoids any situation if he perceives decreased control over negative outcomes, even when having the opportunity to change the situation (American Psychological Association, n.d.-d).

People living with SMI often struggle with daily functioning due to various factors. They may not have learned essential skills during childhood or young adulthood due to deficient learning environments or neurocognitive impairments. This lack of skill development can lead to problem behaviors during a crucial time for acquiring advanced functions such as working, driving, cooking, and paying bills. Additionally, they are at higher risk for developing co-occurring conditions that disrupt typical behavior patterns. Repeated trauma and isolated lifestyles further hamper their access to positive reinforcement. Frequent hospitalizations and removal from the community exacerbate these issues. The absence of competent role models and neurocognitive impairments like attention and memory deficits contribute to the difficulty in learning necessary life skills. Functional impairment in people with SMI is influenced by a combination of lack of knowledge, motivation, proper stimulus control, or all the above.

People living with SMI frequently fail to become integrated into a natural social network that can assist them in coping with life demands and other life stressors. They frequently reside in impoverished and under-stimulating environments with few available opportunities to engage in prosocial and reinforcing behaviors. The lack of a naturally occurring reinforcing network often results in the family of the individual living with SMI as the only network to which they belong. The response patterns of families of individuals living with SMI often include deviant, punitive, and aversive behaviors, adding stress that the individual who lives with SMI lacks the skills to manage (Morrison & Wixted, 1989). Studies have repeatedly found that people with SMI who have family relationships characterized by hostile and aversive interactions are more likely to be hospitalized within 9 months of discharge (Vaughn & Leff, 1976).

Individual differences and contextual factors play a significant role in how functional competencies are developed and adapted. A transdiagnostic, dimensional perspective is necessary for creating targeted behavioral supports for individuals living with SMI. The variety and complexities of domains of adaptive functioning reflect the challenges in the assessment and effective treatment of these impairments.

Interventions have been developed to enhance the functional capacities and abilities of individuals living with SMI. These interventions can result in improvements in life functioning. Life skills training has demonstrated some effective benefits in acquiring skills essential for competent adaptive functioning (Patterson et al., 2003, 2006).

Functional living skills are a construct that has defied operationalized definitions and measurement. It is typically measured by performance on functional behavior tests or by self-report or observations from those familiar with the person. Adequate test results suggest that the individual has the necessary behaviors, though real-life factors may affect performance. An individual who does not perform adequately might not possess the requisite skills or fail to manifest them due to confounding factors (e.g. anxiety about being evaluated, structure of the role-play, history of trauma, problems with neurocognitive abilities) (Bellack et al., 1990).

The Functional Adaptation of Skills Training (FAST) was developed to enhance functional independence and quality of life in a sample of middle-aged and older adults residing in community board and care home. The FAST targeted six key domains of daily life functioning for training in living skills: medication management, social skills, communication skills, organization and planning, transportation, and financial management (Patterson et al., 2003, 2006). Specifically, the behavioral dimensions that were trained for each domain were:

- Medication management: tracking medication, monitoring symptoms, communicating with healthcare providers, and problem-solving.
- Social skills: engaging in appropriate conversations, including initiation, maintenance, and termination of conversations.
- Communication skills: recognizing communication styles (passive, assertive, aggressive).
- Organization and planning: scheduling events, healthcare appointments, and preparing for outings.
- Transportation: reading maps, transportation schedules, and seeking help when needed.
- Financial management: counting money, writing checks, and reading account statements.

The structure of the sessions included a review of previous concepts, reinforcement (e.g., verbal praise) of skills learned during the session, and praise for homework completion and attempts at completing assignments.

The format of the sessions was like other behavioral skills training (e.g., Social Skills Training (SST) (U.S. Department of Veterans Affairs, n.d.)). Sessions included in-class practice through behavioral modeling and role-playing, reinforcing skills through repetition and review. Participants discussed generalizing these skills to other life domains and were encouraged to apply them outside the sessions. Homework assignments, such as medication tracking or using pillboxes, helped reinforce the application of skills in real-life scenarios. Problem-solving support was given to those who struggled with homework or had difficulty completing tasks using behavioral modeling, prompting, and role-playing.

The intervention consisted of 24 semiweekly, 120-minute group. The results showed that FAST significantly improved everyday functioning (measured by the UCSD Performance-Based Skills Assessment [UPSA]) immediately post-intervention and at a 3-month follow-up. However, it did not significantly affect the occurrence of problem behaviors (e.g., depression, hearing voices) or health-related quality of life issues (Patterson et al., 2003, 2006).

Although Patterson et al., (2003, 2006) reported positive findings, a review comparing seven randomized controlled life skills training programs for over 460 individuals living with SMI with outcomes for standard "treatment as usual" (TAU) found no significant differences in life skills performance or retention rates between the groups. Quality of life (QoL) scores were comparable, with no notable differences in measures of problematic behaviors associated with living with SMI (Tungpunkom et al., 2012).

Learning IADLs is essential for achieving independence and well-being; community-based interventions have been found to be more effective than institutional approaches. Patmisari et al. (2025) reviewed 30 studies focusing on interventions to enhance IADLs. Interventions were categorized into simple, complex, and recreational IADLs, each crucial for independent living. The studies show significant improvements in daily engagement and social interactions through individualized tailored support plans. Variables that enhanced the acquisition of daily living skills included individualized approaches, structured programs, and technology integration (e.g., use of smart phones to prompt occurrence of behaviors). The authors noted variability in study designs and the need for long-term follow-up with future research recommended to focus on diverse IADL interventions.

The life skills programs reviewed by Tungpunkom et al. (2012) failed to provide details on key aspects of the training. Most of the studies used verbal praise for completion of homework assignments and compliance with the requirements of the training program (e.g., attending session, participation). Only one study used a token economy but did not provide details as to the frequency and schedule of reinforcement and type of backup reinforcers available in the token economy. One study reported the use of criticizing participants for non-completion of homework, which could negatively impact the perceptions and behaviors of people living with SMI (Vaughn & Leff, 1976).

The skills training programs reviewed by Tungpunkom et al. (2012) did not assess specific skill impairments or the function of the impaired skill. Training occurred in hospital and community settings but lacked details on the specific environments and whether training was conducted where the skills would be applied. The training was done by professional staff, but the studies did not mention if staff who interacted daily with the individuals living with SMI were excluded from training. The studies did not show whether skills were encouraged outside the training setting or if generalization was considered. Without repetitive prompting and reinforcement in appropriate settings, these skills likely would not develop into daily life habits (Lally & Gardner, 2011).

When training desired behaviors that are not in a person's behavioral repertoire, it is important to provide continuous immediate reinforcement for behavior that closely approximates the targeted behavior and gradually shape the topography to the final targeted behavior by breaking down complex life skills into smaller steps, providing targeted instruction, modeling, prompting, and reinforcement; once this is occurring, then the schedule of reinforcement can be gradually "thinned" depending on outcome data (Cooper et al., 2020).

In summary, impairments in life skills, from a behavioral perspective, stem from a complex interaction of factors related to learning history, underlying abilities, environmental influences, and challenges in acquiring and performing the necessary behaviors. Interventions that utilize behavioral principles, such as ABA therapy, can be beneficial in addressing these impairments and helping individuals develop greater independence. Understanding how behaviors are learned and how to use positive reinforcement and other behavioral support strategies to promote desired behaviors can be effective in breaking down complex life skills into smaller steps and providing targeted instruction and support.

Epidemiological Considerations

Living with SMI significantly impacts everyday functioning across multiple domains, including social, vocational, and self-care activities. Individuals living with SMI often fail to achieve traditional milestones such as marriage, stable relationships, competitive employment, and independent living. These impairments appear early in living with mental health issues and are stable and persistent even when other problem behaviors decrease, continuing to affect functionality (McGrath et al., 2013; Schretlen et al., 2000; Tanner et al., 2019). Neurocognitive impairments, such as poor memory, attention, and processing speed, are the most consistent determinants of functional impairments and are minimally affected by current psychopharmacological interventions. Diminished and absent expressions of expected behaviors and emotions like motivation (avolition) and experiencing pleasure (anhedonia) further contribute to functional impairments.

Important areas of impairment in everyday functioning impact individuals living with SMI with a substantial proportion not being able to live without support and supervision. Harvey et al. (2012) report the following areas that are negatively impacted by living with SMI:

- Independent living: Approximately 25%–40% of individuals can live independently, frequently receiving support through disability compensation or assistance from family members. Of these, 75% depend on disability compensation for their financial needs.
- Health and medication management: Managing medications and co-occurring medical conditions can be challenging, potentially leading to adverse health outcomes and reduced life expectancy.
- Self-care activities: Tasks like personal hygiene, cooking, shopping, and transportation are often impaired, with only a minority capable (20%) effectively performing these activities.
- Driving: A small percentage hold valid driver's licenses or drive regularly, with impairments linked to neurocognitive impairments and diminished frequency of expected behavior and emotions. Approximately 50% of individuals have a valid driver's license, but only 40% actively drive, compared to 96% of healthy controls.
- Social functioning: Individuals often have reduced social networks, impaired social skills, and difficulty maintaining relationships, which can lead to job terminations and social isolation. Marriage and stable relationships are rare, and social networks are significantly reduced.
- Neurocognitive functioning: Especially relevant is the prevalence of neurocognitive impairment or the low prevalence of "neuropsychological normality" in people living with SMI. If "neuropsychological normality" is defined as performance on a neuropsychological assessment battery greater than one standard deviation below the "healthy" mean, the number of cases across studies is about 20%–30%. This contrasts with 83% of the population with no mental health problems scoring at this level.

These impairments are persistent, minimally responsive to treatment, and intrinsic to living with SMI, underscoring the need for disability support to improve functioning and recovery.

Rubin and Panzano (2002) conducted a comprehensive evaluation in a large catchment area in a mid-Western state of the United States. This assessment utilized a rating scale completed by case managers for more than 3600 clients undergoing mental healthcare services. The results showed that the range of individuals living with SMI needing daily supervision in functional behaviors ranged from 15% to 29% of the sample. Estimates of the prevalence data of the impairments in the domains of life skills in people living with SMI in the United States are lacking although reports have the prevalence as high as 48% (Mahmood et al., 2021). No prevalence data were found using searches for "functional impairments," "serious mental illness," "SMI," "schizophrenia," "bipolar disorder," "life skills," and "independent skills" in PubMed, Google Scholar, and PsycINFO.

Cultural Considerations

Functional skills and impairments in these skills are contextually dependent in that the situation influences the behavior that is emitted. Culture, which is defined as the values, beliefs, language, rituals, traditions, and other behaviors that are passed from one generation to another within any social group (American Psychological Association, n.d.-c), plays an encompassing and significant role in how the functional skills are learned, practiced, and displayed. Cultural norms, values, and beliefs influence how people communicate, interact, and determine what behaviors are expected by people living in that culture and society.

Assessing prevalence and types of impairments in functional behaviors in people living with SMI begins with the culturally relevant domains and dimensions of living skills that are displayed by individuals living in that culture (McIntosh et al., 2011). For instance, Habtamu et al. (2018) developed an instrument that measured functional impairment among individuals living with SMI in rural Ethiopia. The items on the instrument reflected the impact of sociodemographic, economic, and clinical characteristics of the functioning of these individuals. The domains and dimensions measured covered the tasks and expected roles for adult men and woman living in a rural agricultural community such as getting water from the community well, cooking, tending livestock, and child care.

Velligan et al. (2012) reviewed available scales of functional abilities and impairments in people living with SMI. Problems were identified for specific subscales on all the performance-based assessments across multiple countries. Problems were identified for specific subscales on all the performance-based assessments across multiple countries. India, China (McIntosh et al., 2011), and Mexico presented the greatest challenges in adaptation. There is a lack of data on the prevalence and types of impairments in life skills among individuals with SMI across different cultures.

Types of Functional Impairments

Functional and life skill impairments can be broadly categorized into activities of daily living (ADLs) and instrumental activities of daily living (IADLs). These are domains of functional abilities that enable a person to manifest behaviors that allow successful completion of tasks that are expected in certain contexts (Edemekong et al., 2019). ADLs refer to fundamental skills required for individuals to independently care for themselves. These include basic tasks such as eating, bathing, dressing, toileting, mobility, and maintaining personal hygiene. The inability to perform them can lead to dependence on others, unsafe conditions, and a reduced quality of life (Edemekong et al., 2019). IADLs are those activities that allow an individual to live independently in a community (Guo & Sapra, 2022). Although these skills are not necessary for living with minimal support and supervision from others, the ability to perform IADLs can significantly improve the quality of life (QoL) by expanding the context in which the person can function without oversight and supervision. The major domains of IADLs include cooking, cleaning, transportation, laundry, and managing finances. The assessment of IADLs can determine the level of an individual's need for assistance and neurocognitive functioning (Guo & Sapra, 2022).

IADLs are commonly confused with ADLs. The major dimensions of ADLs are feeding, dressing, bathing, and physical mobility. In contrast with IADLs, ADLs are necessary for basic functional living. Severe impairments in performing ADLs may indicate the need for home healthcare or placement in a supervised facility. IADLs involve more complex tasks that are essential for independent living in the community (Guo & Sapra, 2022). Specific dimensions of IADLs include:

1. Transportation and shopping: ability to procure groceries, attend events, and manage transportation (e.g., driving or organizing other means of transport).
2. Managing finances: paying bills and managing financial assets; budgeting, interacting with banks; assembling tax records or papers; performing competently during financial problems.
3. Shopping: shopping alone for clothes, household necessities.
4. Meal preparation: planning, shopping, and preparing food; heating water, making coffee, turning off the stove.
5. Housecleaning and home maintenance: cleaning living areas, maintaining tidiness, and performing home maintenance tasks; competently handling household emergencies.
6. Laundry: washing and maintaining clothing on a regular basis.
7. Managing communication: handling telephone calls, messages, and mail.
8. Managing medications: obtaining and taking medications as directed.
9. Awareness of current events: keeping track of current events.
10. Media engagement: paying attention to and discussing TV, books, or magazines.
11. Memory: remembering appointments, family occasions, holidays, medications.

12. Transportation: traveling outside of the neighborhood, knowing directions and how to use public transportation, driving, or arranging other means of transportation.
13. Health maintenance: scheduling medical appointments both routine and when necessary; engaging in healthful behaviors; awareness of physical health indices.
14. Leisure activities: accessing and participating in individual and/or group pleasurable activities.

Functional Challenges in Self-Care Skills that Occur in Individuals Living with Serious Mental Illness

Functional impairments in individuals living with severe mental illness often manifest in everyday tasks, including problems with self-care skills and financial management. Self-care skills refer to a variety of behaviors that are important for personal hygiene (bathing, tooth brushing, washing clothes) and care of living areas, such as making the bed or cleaning the room. Some problem behaviors that occur are functional living skills in people living with SMI including poor hygiene (e.g., infrequent showering, not brushing teeth); wearing inappropriate or dirty clothing; living in unhygienic environments and not taking care of personal possessions (e.g., room cluttered with trash); refusal or apathy toward improving appearance or cleanliness; spending money impulsively and on non-essential items; and inability to budget and pay bills.

These difficulties may stem from neurocognitive challenges, medication side effects, psychosocial factors, or environmental influences. These skills are key to assessing the independence of someone with SMI. It's not unusual for some individuals to excel in some self-care areas while struggling with others.

Why Do Problems with Self-Care Skills Happen?

Self-care skills can be affected by various factors. Multiple elements may contribute to the difficulties faced by the individual living with SMI who is in need of supervision and enhanced support.

Part of the Reason May Be Biological

Poor self-care skills may be a result of the imbalance of neurotransmitters that are believed to be the cause of the problem behaviors that are seen in people living with SMI. This imbalance can bring on a variety of problems, such as having difficulty thinking clearly, remembering, and experiencing pleasure. People with SMI may hear voices telling them not to wash or that water is harmful, believe they must wear the same clothes, or lack motivation to shower and change. These imbalances can hinder learning and performing self-care skills, resulting in problems in accomplishing basic tasks. Delusions and hallucinations are called "positive symptoms" that may be distressful to the person who experiences them. It is often the "negative symptoms," such as lack of interest or motivation to engage in self-care and other activities, that many service providers find most frustrating. This is complicated by the fact that it is often difficult to tell whether the lack of involvement in an activity is a "negative symptom" linked to living with an SMI or due to psychosocial issues. Negative symptoms of SMI should not be mistaken for laziness. Caregivers might wrongly believe that the person can perform self-care behaviors if they truly want to, viewing them as defiant and oppositional, instead of perceiving the impairments as a need for support.

Sometimes the psychiatric medications that are used to help with delusions, hallucinations, and other problematic behaviors and symptoms of SMI may cause drowsiness or interfere with thinking, concentration, and attention. In such cases, the treatment of some symptoms can cause other problems. This has been a problem with many of the medications that have been used to treat SMI, particularly schizophrenia spectrum mental health problems. Second-generation antipsychotic medications may help to improve negative symptoms and enhance self-care skills, unlike older medications. Switching medication could better manage positive symptoms while controlling side effects that affect self-care.

Part of the Reason May Be Psychosocial

People living with SMI may struggle to learn self-care skills due to positive symptoms like delusions and hallucinations that impair the ability to learn, pay attention, and concentrate. Medication can help control these symptoms, providing a better chance to learn functional and self-care skills. However, poorly managed problem behaviors or emotional and motivational issues may still hinder their ability or willingness to use self-care skills.

Environmental factors may impede the development of self-care skills. Over time, service providers might underestimate the potential for individuals with SMI to perform self-care activities independently, which can result in a lack of appropriate incentives and corrective experiences necessary to foster or support these skills.

Behavioral Strategies for Problems with Self-Care Skills and Functioning

Self-care skills can refer to many different responses in many self-care response classes. People with SMI may excel in some self-care skills while struggling with others. Before attempting to implement strategies to improve these skills, assess if it's worth the effort. Inadequate self-care does not always require intervention from service providers, especially if it doesn't frequently disrupt daily life or social interactions.

- Setting realistic goals is an important first step. Evaluate whether addressing the issue justifies time and effort. It may be more realistic to accept the level at which the person is able to function. For example, Michael would leave his clothes on the floor next to his bed when he goes to bed. Some staff members felt that he should be required to put them in the laundry basket; it was decided by the clinical team that it wasn't important enough to spend time on changing this as he was improving by taking a shower, brushing his teeth, and changing his clothes. As he improved in other areas, the staff stopped being concerned about it and decided to focus on what was more important.
- Consider seeking a review of medications. Most medications for SMIs are more successful in reducing positive symptoms such as delusions and hallucinations than at helping the person do more independently. Some medications may cause side effects like drowsiness, which can hinder self-care activities such as showering. If prescribed these medications, request a review and specify concerns.
- Identify behaviors to address and set clear goals. For instance, rather than "wasting money," set a goal to limit daily spending to three dollars. Be specific in defining the goal. If Michael does not use soap when showering or wears dirty clothes afterward, the objective is for him to use soap every time and wear clean clothes. Specify self-care and functional skills that need improvement, like wearing clean and weather-appropriate clothes, buttoning shirts, and budgeting money.
- Clear, specific instructions are more effective than vague phrases. For instance, staff wanted Michael to wash his favorite clothes weekly and wear a jacket when it is cold outside. A vague request might be, "Michael, you need to wear clean clothes and dress appropriately," it is better to say "Michael, your favorite shirt and pants are dirty; you will need to wash them first." When Michael was going outside, it is best to be explicit about the weather and wearing a coat: "Michael, it is very cold; you need to wear the coat that keeps you warm."
- Ensure that the individual living with SMI has the necessary items to complete the task. Provide sufficient materials to assist them in improving. If showering is an issue, provide towels, soap, shampoo, and clean clothes before the shower time. If dressing is challenging, supply a pair of shoes and other comfortable clothing.
- Consider the preferences of the individual with SMI when aiming to encourage specific behaviors. When shopping for clothes, or other self-care items, engage

with the person living with challenges with self-care behaviors and allow the person to be involved in picking out the items (clothing, toothpaste, style of haircut, deodorant, and shaving cream). Ask the person what time he would like to shower. He is more likely to utilize these items and take a shower at the time he indicates. In the hospital, Michael could use the washer and dryer only at certain times. To improve his laundry skills, Michael and the staff agreed on a suitable time for him to use the washer and dryer.

- Identify when/where problem behaviors occur and if any people or setting variables affect behavior such as seeing other people having money or items that they desire. Identify patterns of behavior that occur and do not occur and what variables may be influencing the behaviors.
- Set examples for the skills being encouraged, as everyone in the environment is a role model. Avoid saying "do what I say, not what I do." Ensure that others practice good habits like wearing clean clothes, maintaining hygiene, and budgeting money. If staff smoke outside without jackets but expect residents to wear them, it undermines their message. People respond better to those who practice what is preached.
- Support the person living with SMI by suggesting appropriate clothing, ensuring that shoes are tied, and providing laundry detergent. Do not force assistance. Praise any cooperation. The group home staff initially assisted Michael with his laundry to ensure that he learned to use the washer/dryer and the correct amount of detergent.
- Develop memory aids like lists of expectations, reminders, and schedules. Post clear expectations for tasks such as cleaning a bedroom, taking a shower, and using money. Make "rules" consistent and followed by others; list them visibly as reminders. For example, staff created a simple list for Michael's housekeeping of his bedroom—bed made, dirty clothes in laundry bag, clean clothes in drawers, no food—and he was occasionally reminded of his scheduled tasks like laundry or cleaning. If remembering expectations is challenging, establish a checklist for regular tasks (clothes match, pants zipped, shirt buttoned, showering schedule, money requests). Regularly check the list to ensure that tasks are done. Verbally praise the person on aspects of dressing, personal hygiene, and self-management that are done correctly.
- Consider formal ways of monitoring and rewarding success, such as a "contract." If attempts to change the behaviors don't seem to be enough, consider writing a "contract." Contracting for behavior change is outlined in Chap. 4. Whenever possible, the contract should be written with the engagement of the person living with SMI including the behaviors to change, the goals, and the reinforcing outcomes; it should specify the self-care and self-management functions that are expected and the specific rewards that are available when the person succeeds. Adjust expectations over time as success increases. For Michael, the staff contracted for him to wash his clothes at least once per week, wear a jacket when the outside temperature is less than 60 degrees, get out of bed and get shaved by 7 a.m., wear pajamas or underwear in bed at night, and take a shower every 2 days. By meeting these expectations, Michael was able to get several items that

he told the staff he wanted. These included such items as music CDs, sweat bands, batteries for a CD player, and sports videos.

- Be as clear as possible about what needs to be corrected and give directions on how to change it. When giving corrective feedback to the person living with SMI, explain clearly what was done, how it should be corrected, and why. Do not assume that the person living with SMI "knows better." For example, if the shoes of the person living with SMI are untied, the feedback might be "Michael, your shoes are untied. I want you to tie them so that you won't trip and fall. Please tie them now." Say this in a calm and matter-of-fact manner. Avoid making indirect criticism when this is done (e.g., "Don't you understand that you need to wear a coat in weather like this?"). If the person does what is requested, be sure to compliment and verbally praise.
- Recognize successes. Observe achievements in meeting expectations, self-care, and functional behaviors. Praise and reward these accomplishments, emphasizing the effort made. Compliments can have varying effects; although they may initially cause embarrassment for some, they typically contribute to positive feelings overall. Michael particularly responded well to compliments from certain staff members, even when receiving other reinforcers like batteries or CDs.
- Prioritize the problem behaviors that have been identified, focusing on one or two at a time. Initially, it is probably best to focus on improving the behaviors that are important but also relatively easy to change so the person living with SMI can experience success. Do not overlook those tasks that are currently done well. Remember to give the person living with SMI credit for what is currently being done well.
- Establishing a consistent routine for providing feedback can be beneficial. Even without a formal contract, regularly checking the progress of individuals living with SMI may help ensure that expectations are met. It is advisable to specify times for various activities such as room cleaning, showering, laundry, and money access. For instance, staff checked Michal's room between 8:15 and 8:30 every morning. This routine helped Michael plan his time.
- Utilize the natural consequences associated with engaging in targeted desired behaviors to promote specific skills. Even in the absence of a behavioral contract, there are various scenarios where natural consequences can be applied effectively. For instance, an individual living with SMI may enjoy visiting the mall or a preferred restaurant, which typically has standard expectations for appearance. Clear expectations should be established that stipulate such outings are contingent upon the individual's adherence to personal hygiene, wearing clean attire, and financial preparedness. It is crucial to consistently enforce these expectations through both positive and negative outcomes. Should the individual fail to meet the expected standards of appearance or lack money, the planned activity should be scheduled for a time when the expectations are met. Implementing this consequence may be challenging due to feelings of guilt or self-perception of not being compassionate when denying an anticipated activity. However, if defined expectations are not upheld, the person living with SMI will begin to disregard

them. Consistently applied clear expectations and consequences are essential for effective behavioral conditioning.
- It is crucial that individuals living with SMI have access to essential resources required to perform daily life and functional skills. Ensure that all necessary materials, such as soap, towels, washcloths, shampoo, clean clothing, and available funds, are provided to meet expectations for personal hygiene and financial management. Adequate availability of resources is fundamental; for instance, effective money management is not feasible without having funds to manage.

What About Michael?

At the group home residence, Michael had to live with others and had to share a bedroom. He did not shower or change his clothes, and this resulted in his roommate complaining about the odor in the room. He would spend money quickly on sodas and snacks, leading to episodes of requesting money from others; he littered the floor with soda cans, partially eaten food, and wrappers. There was concern that this would result in roaches and mice. The staff were faced with the challenge of helping Michael do the self-care behaviors that most people take for granted. The first step was to see if there were times that he did take a shower on his own or when asked by staff; the staff observed him and recorded this as well as if there was any difference in the time of day that he did shower (with or without asking) and who asked him to take a shower. The staff recorded the observations for 8 weeks. The results showed that Michael took a shower about once every 3 weeks; he showered in the evening when others were not around. He ignored staff requests. The staff did the same data collection for the behavior of Michael changing and washing his clothes.

After the observations were gathered, the staff met with Michael and developed a plan. Michael agreed to take a shower every other day after 7 p.m. He stated that he would like to be reminded to take a shower after dinner by a male staff member since he stated, "I feel like a kid being asked to do this by someone like my mom." The team and Michael also came up with a time that Michael would wash his clothes weekly. They agreed to place this schedule with signs to remind him. Michael agreed to a contract that if he took a shower and washed his clothes, a staff member would take him to a store to buy a music CD. Michael only took two showers the first week and did not access the trip; he took his scheduled showers and washed his clothes as scheduled for the following weeks. After this success, the staff next focused on his room and took the same steps to obtain Michael's engagement. A schedule was negotiated with Michael as to when his room was to be cleaned (e.g., twice weekly with no trash on floor and clothes in basket). Room cleaning became part of the contract. Staff also began spending time with Michael as they found out what kind of music he liked. He began speaking to staff about his music and would offer to play his favorites for them.

In offering support for Michael, the group home staff engaged with him and completed the following actions:

1. Clarified behaviors for improvement: Michael and staff came up with specific, realistic, and observable behaviors that hindered his recovery.
2. Decided whether change was necessary: Both prioritized what functional behaviors were important to Michael in his recovery.
3. Use of positive reinforcement: With Michael's engagement, reinforcers were found for defined success and efforts.
4. Employed natural consequences: The support by the staff allowed real-world outcomes to help with generalization and further progress.
5. Clear expectations were established: Visual cues, prompting, routines, and modeling were used to establish when and where the adaptive behavior was to occur.
6. Behavior contracts were created: The contract included input from Michael and adjusted over time and progress.
7. Staff gave support: The staff engaged Michael socially and meaningfully and not just telling him what to do.
8. Professional guidance was sought when needed: Behavioral specialists can assist with complex cases.

After a few months, Michael made sufficient progress, and he was able to move out of the group home and into a supervised apartment.

Summary

Living with SMI impacts the manifestation of functional behaviors, significantly impairing daily living activities, including hygiene, nutrition, and social relationships. Functional impairment is a key criterion for identifying mental health issues, indicating distress in social and occupational areas. Individuals with SMI may experience varying levels of incapacity, with some managing daily tasks despite severe symptoms. Negative symptoms—defined as the diminished or absent expression of expected behaviors and emotions—particularly affects motivation (i.e., avolition), experiencing pleasures (i.e., anhedonia), and expressing emotions and interest (i.e., apathy). Neurocognitive deficits are critical factors influencing functional impairments.

Functional impairments in living skills that indicate limitations in daily activities due to mental health issues are linked to disability. Living with SMI is a primary cause of disability in the United States, affecting individuals' ability to perform essential tasks. A significant percentage (15%–29%) of individuals living with SMI require daily supervision for basic living skills.

Avolition, or reduced motivation, is a key component affecting functional impairments in individuals living with SMI. It is associated with difficulties in initiating and persisting in goal-directed activities, impacting overall functioning. Individuals living with SMI may experience hypohedonia (i.e., a decrease in experiencing pleasure), leading to decreased effort in pursuing activities that result in natural occurring reinforcers, such as verbal praise for personal hygiene and appearance. In addition, neurocognitive impairments in memory, attention, and executive functioning are prevalent in individuals with SMI, are often correlated with avolition, and contribute to challenges in independent functioning. Limitations in neurocognitive resources can exacerbate functional impairments, affecting the ability to engage in daily activities.

The assessment of impairment in daily functional behaviors presents challenges and complexities, focusing on the dimensions of activities of daily living (ADLs) and instrumental activities of daily living (IADLs). Assessing the domains and dimensions of functional impairments in individuals living with SMI is difficult due to the complex and heterogeneous presentation of functional behaviors and skills, resulting in multiple operational definitions of functional impairments and the lack of reliable and valid assessment tools, particularly in measuring real-life functional behaviors. The development of valid instruments is hindered by the absence of a comprehensive model of functional capacity, its mediators, and operationalized definitions. The complexity and multidimensionality of functional capacities complicate assessments. In addition, cultural relevance is crucial in defining normative functioning. Currently, a norm-based scale for adaptive daily functioning does not exist.

Functional impairments can be categorized into activities of daily living (ADLs) and instrumental activities of daily living (IADLs), each with distinct domains and dimensions. ADLs are essential for basic self-care, while IADLs enhance independent living in the community. ADLs include basic tasks like eating, bathing, and personal hygiene. IADLs involve more complex tasks such as cooking, managing finances, and transportation. Severe impairments in ADLs may necessitate home healthcare or supervised placement. IADLs significantly improve quality of life by allowing greater independence.

There are several instruments available to evaluate functional capacities, each with its own advantages and limitations. A multimodal and multimethod approach is suggested for thorough assessment. Instruments like the Pfeffer Functional Activities Questionnaire (PFAQ) and Lawton–Brody IADL Scale assess different domains of IADLs. These tools have limitations such as outdated norms, reliance on self-reports, and potential biases. They are in need of updated norms and validation for use with individuals living with SMI.

Self-monitoring and self-control are critical living and functional skills for individuals living with SMI to manage daily life effectively. Impairments in these areas can lead to maladaptive behaviors and reduced quality of life. Lack of self-awareness can hinder self-monitoring and self-control. Poor self-control may result in impulsive behaviors, negatively impacting daily functioning. Individuals with better self-management skills show improved emotional responses and interpersonal relationships.

Performance-based measures are essential for accurately assessing functional capabilities in individuals with SMI. These types of measures have strong predictive validity for independent living and focus on observable behaviors rather than self-reports. The University of California San Diego Performance-Based Skills Assessment (UPSA) evaluates skills across multiple domains. The Test of Adaptive

Behavior in Schizophrenia (TABS) assesses initiation and problem identification in real-world tasks.

Individualized assessment approaches are necessary to address the unique functional impairments of individuals with SMI. A focus on intraindividual variations can lead to more effective interventions. Current assessments rely on nomothetic methods, which may overlook individual differences. Personalized assessments can provide insights into specific experiences and challenges faced by individuals. A shift toward understanding individual pathways rather than comparing to normative data is essential for effective rehabilitation.

Daily functioning impairments are major treatment concerns for individuals living with SMI. The impairments involve neurological and environmental factors. Studies show no significant correlation between the assessment of functional capacities and the manifestation of functional real-life behaviors. Functional capacity is predicted by neurocognitive factors like IQ, while real-life behavior is influenced by social cognitive variables such as empathy. Gray matter loss in specific brain regions correlates with impaired executive functions (EF) in individuals living with SMI.

Common structural changes in individuals living with SMI include gray matter loss in certain regions of the brain including areas in the dorsolateral prefrontal (dlPFC) and ventral medial prefrontal cortices (vmPFC); the anterior cingulate cortex (ACC); hippocampus; amygdala; and striatum. The dlPFC is crucial for executive functions; reduced volume affects planning and decision-making. The vmPFC is vital for emotional regulation; abnormalities lead to difficulties in processing emotions and social cues. ACC dysfunction is linked to impaired cognitive control and emotional processing. Hippocampal volume loss impacts memory formation, particularly in depression. Altered amygdaloid activity influences emotional responses, contributing to anxiety and social withdrawal. Changes in the striatum are associated with a lessened ability to experience pleasure (i.e., anhedonia) and impaired motivation (avolition and apathy).

Studies have emphasized the importance of communication and coordination between brain structures for the display of functional behaviors and skills. Altered functional connectivity patterns disrupt adaptive cognitive and emotional functioning in individuals with SMI. Variability in brain structure and function highlights the complexity of SMI and its associated behavioral impairments. Antipsychotic medications can impact brain structure, particularly in the basal ganglia. The influence of medication on brain changes must be considered in research findings.

Continued research using advanced neuroimaging and longitudinal studies is essential for understanding the neurobiological basis of impairment in people living with SMI. Targeted interventions for specific impairments can be developed based on deeper insights into brain structure and function.

Individuals with SMI often lack opportunities to learn essential life skills during adolescence resulting in challenges in life skills development. Disruptions such as psychiatric admissions and legal issues hinder skill acquisition. Neurocognitive problems like memory and attention deficits further impede learning. Functional impairments result from insufficient exposure to adaptive behaviors, deficits in reinforcement, and the lack of adaptive role models from which to observe and learn functional living skills.

Adaptive skills are necessary for effective engagement in daily tasks and achieving positive outcomes. Life skills training can enhance functional capacities and improve quality of life. Learning models like operant conditioning and social learning theory can be applied to teach these skills.

Impairments arise from a lack of knowledge, motivation, and proper stimulus control. Environmental factors, sensory sensitivities, and trauma can limit skill development. Individuals may struggle with daily functioning due to co-occurring conditions and isolated lifestyles.

Life skills training has shown effectiveness in improving essential skills for adaptive functioning. The Functional Adaptation of Skills Training (FAST) program targets key domains like medication management and social skills. Studies indicated significant improvements in everyday functioning post-intervention, though not in problem behaviors.

Community-based approaches are more effective than institutional methods for enhancing independent living skills. Individualized interventions and technology integration have shown positive outcomes in skill acquisition. Long-term follow-up and diverse intervention strategies are recommended for future research.

Studies on life skills training programs lack detailed assessments of specific skill impairments and do not consider generalization of skills. The training programs did not specify schedules of reinforcement used. Continuous reinforcement and appropriate training environments are crucial for developing life skills into habits.

Behavioral principles can effectively address impairments and promote independence in individuals living with SMI. SMI significantly affects daily functioning in multiple aspects of life, requiring continual support for recovery.

Individuals living with SMI experience significant difficulties in social, vocational, and self-care activities, often failing to achieve typical developmental milestones. Neurocognitive impairments, such as poor memory and attention, are consistent predictors of functional limitations. Only 25%–40% of individuals with SMI live independently, typically relying on disability compensation. Approximately 20%–30% of individuals with SMI score within the range of "neuropsychological normality," in contrast to 83% of the general population.

The management of medications and co-occurring conditions presents considerable challenges, resulting in negative health outcomes. Only 20% effectively engage in self-care activities, and approximately 50% possess valid driver's licenses, with only 40% actively driving. Social networks for these individuals are notably diminished, with stable relationships being rare and job terminations frequently occurring due to impaired social skills.

Functional skills impairments are contextually dependent, influenced by cultural norms and values. Culturally relevant domains must be assessed to understand functional behaviors in individuals with SMI. An instrument developed in rural Ethiopia measured functional impairment based on sociodemographic and clinical characteristics.

Performance-based assessments face adaptation challenges in countries like India, China, and Mexico. There is a lack of data on the prevalence and types of impairments in life skills among individuals with SMI across different cultures.

Functional impairments can be categorized into ADLs and IADLs that are essential for independent living. ADLs include basic self-care tasks like eating, bathing, and dressing. Inability to perform ADLs can lead to dependence and reduced quality of life. ADLs are fundamental skills necessary for self-care and basic living. IADLs allow individuals to live independently in the community and include more complex tasks. Major domains of IADLs include transportation, managing finances, meal preparation, and housecleaning. IADLs significantly improve quality of life by expanding functional contexts without oversight.

Self-care skills in individuals living with SMI are influenced by biological and psychosocial factors, requiring individualized tailored behavioral support plans. Biological factors include neurotransmitter imbalances, which can lead to poor self-care skills and problem behaviors. Positive symptoms like delusions and hallucinations can hinder self-care, while negative symptoms may reflect lack of motivation and diminished experience in feeling pleasure. Psychiatric medications can cause side effects that impact self-care abilities, necessitating careful management of treatment options.

Environmental support is crucial for learning self-care skills; low expectations can hinder progress. Impairment in functional living skills may persist despite medication, requiring targeted interventions. Service providers should avoid misconceptions about attributing impairments in functioning due to characterological impediment (e.g., laziness) and focus on understanding the challenges faced by the individual living with SMI.

It is recommended that service providers assess the necessity of intervention based on the impact of inadequate self-care on daily life. Interventional support in improving impairment if self-care skills and functional behaviors include:

- Review medications to address side effects that may hinder self-care.
- Set specific, realistic goals for self-care improvement, focusing on detailed instructions and necessary resources.
- Involve the individual living with SMI in decision-making regarding aspects of the support plan including choosing self-care items and routines to enhance engagement.
- Use role modeling and consistent feedback to encourage positive behaviors and establish routines.
- Recognize and praise successes to motivate continued improvement in self-care skills.

References

Abel, D. B., Salyers, M. P., Wu, W., Monette, M. A., & Minor, K. S. (2021). Quality versus quantity: Determining real-world social functioning deficits in schizophrenia. *Psychiatry Research, 301*, 113980. https://doi.org/10.1016/j.psychres.2021.113980

American Psychiatric Association. (2006). *Practice guideline for the psychiatric evaluation of adults* (2nd ed.). https://psychiatryonline.org/pb/assets/raw/sitewide/practice_guidelines/guidelines/psychevaladults.pdf

American Psychiatric Association. (2022). *Diagnostic and statistical manual of mental disorders* (5th ed., text rev.). https://doi.org/10.1176/appi.books.9780890425787

American Psychiatric Association. (n.d.). *WHODAS 2.0 self-administered*. https://www.psychiatry.org/File%20Library/Psychiatrists/Practice/DSM/APA_DSM5_WHODAS-2-Self-Administered.pdf

American Psychological Association. (n.d.-a). Disability. In *APA Dictionary of Psychology*. https://dictionary.apa.org/disability

American Psychological Association. (n.d.-b). Cognitive resource theory. In *APA dictionary of psychology*. https://dictionary.apa.org/cognitive-resource-theory

American Psychological Association. (n.d.-c). Culture. In *APA dictionary of psychology*. https://dictionary.apa.org/culture

American Psychological Association. (n.d.-d). Learned helplessness. In *APA dictionary of psychology*. https://dictionary.apa.org/learned-helplessness

Ashley, M. J., Persel, C. S., & Clark, M. C. (2001). Validation of an independent living scale for post-acute rehabilitation applications. *Brain Injury, 15*(5), 435–442. https://doi.org/10.1080/02699050010005896

Baggetta, P., & Alexander, P. A. (2016). Conceptualization and operationalization of executive function. *Mind, Brain, and Education, 10*(1), 10–33. https://doi.org/10.1111/mbe.12100

Baker, R., & Hall, J. N. (1988). REHAB: A new assessment instrument for chronic psychiatric patients. *Schizophrenia Bulletin, 14*(1), 97–111. https://doi.org/10.1093/schbul/14.1.97

Barker, S., Barron, N., McFarland, B. H., & Bigelow, D. A. (1994). A community ability scale for chronically mentally ill consumers: Part I. Reliability and validity. *Community Mental Health Journal, 30*(4), 363–383. https://doi.org/10.1007/BF02207489

Barlow, D. H., & Nock, M. K. (2009). Why can't we be more idiographic in our research? *Perspectives on Psychological Science, 4*(1), 19–21. https://doi.org/10.1111/j.1745-6924.2009.01088.x

Becattini-Oliveira, A. C., de Farias Dutra, D., de Oliveira Campos, B. S., de Araujo, V. C., & Charchat-Fichman, H. (2018). A systematic review of a functional assessment tool: UCSD Performance-based skill assessment (UPSA). *Psychiatry Research, 267*, 12–18. https://doi.org/10.1016/j.psychres.2018.05.005

Bechi, M., Bosia, M., Spangaro, M., Buonocore, M., Cavedoni, S., Agostoni, G., Cocchi, F., Guglielmino, C., Smeraldi, E., & Cavallaro, R. (2017). Exploring functioning in schizophrenia: Predictors of functional capacity and real-world behaviour. *Psychiatry Research, 251*, 118–124. https://doi.org/10.1016/j.psychres.2017.02.019

Bellack, A. S., Morrison, R. L., Wixted, J. T., & Mueser, K. T. (1990). An analysis of social competence in schizophrenia. *The British Journal of Psychiatry, 156*(6), 809–818. https://doi.org/10.1192/bjp.156.6.809

Bellack, A. S., Green, M. F., Cook, J. A., Fenton, W., Harvey, P. D., Heaton, R. K., Laughren, T., Leon, A. C., Mayo, D. J., Patrick, D. L., Patterson, T. L., & Wykes, T. (2007). Assessment of community functioning in people with schizophrenia and other severe mental illnesses: A white paper based on a NIMH-sponsored workshop. *Schizophrenia Bulletin, 33*(3), 805–822. https://doi.org/10.1093/schbul/sbl035

Beltz, A. M., Wright, A. G., Sprague, B. N., & Molenaar, P. C. (2016). Bridging the nomothetic and idiographic approaches to the analysis of clinical data. *Assessment, 23*(4), 447–458. https://doi.org/10.1177/1073191116648209

Brown, M. A., & Velligan, D. I. (2016). Issues and developments related to assessing function in serious mental illness. *Dialogues in Clinical Neuroscience, 18*(2), 135–144. https://doi.org/10.31887/DCNS.2016.18.2/dvelligan

Burnes, A. J., & Roen, S. R. (1967). Social roles and adaptation to the community. *Community Mental Health Journal, 3*, 153–158. https://doi.org/10.1007/BF01421314

CallHub. (n.d.). *13 eye-opening text message statistics to boost customer engagement.* https://callhub.io/blog/text-messaging/text-message-statistics/#:~:text=social%20media,under%20the%20age%20of%2050.

Centre for Neuro Skills. (n.d.). *Independent living scale.* https://www.tbims.org/ils/ils2012b.pdf

Ciarlo, J. A., & Reihman, J. (1977). The Denver community mental health questionnaire: Development of a multidimensional program evaluation instrument. In J. A. Ciarlo (Ed.), *Program evaluation for mental health: Methods, strategies, and participants* (pp. 131–167). Academic Press. https://doi.org/10.1016/B978-0-12-172250-8.50012-3

Cooper, J. O., Heron, T. E., & Heward, W. L. (2020). *Applied behavior analysis* (3rd ed.). Pearson. https://www.pearson.com/en-us/subject-catalog/p/applied-behavior-analysis/P200000003465/9780134752556

Correll, C. U., & Schooler, N. R. (2020). Negative symptoms in schizophrenia: A review and clinical guide for recognition, assessment, and treatment. *Neuropsychiatric Disease and Treatment, 16*, 519–534. https://doi.org/10.2147/NDT.S225643

Cox, J., & Witten, I. B. (2019). Striatal circuits for reward learning and decision-making. *Nature Reviews Neuroscience, 20*, 482–494. https://doi.org/10.1038/s41583-019-0189-2

Dickerson, F. B. (1997). Assessing clinical outcomes: The community functioning of persons with serious mental illness. *Psychiatric Services, 48*(7), 897–902. https://doi.org/10.1176/ps.48.7.897

Edemekong, P. F., Bomgaars, D., Sukumaran, S., & Levy, S. B. (2019). Activities of daily living. *StatPearls*. https://digitalcollections.dordt.edu/faculty_work/1222

Ellsworth, R. B., Collins, J. F., Casey, N. A., Schoonover, R. A., Hickey, R. H., & Nesselroad, J. R. (1979). Some characteristics of effective psychiatric treatment programs. *Journal of Consulting and Clinical Psychology, 47*(5), 799–817. https://doi.org/10.1037/0022-006X.47.5.799

Endicott, J., & Spitzer, R. L. (1972). What! Another rating scale? The psychiatric evaluation form. *The Journal of Nervous and Mental Disease, 154*(2), 88–104. https://doi.org/10.1097/00005053-197202000-00005

Fortuna, K. L., Lohman, M. C., Bruce, M. L., & Bartels, S. J. (2018). Utility of functioning measures in the prediction of independent living status in older adults with serious mental illness. *International Journal of Geriatric Psychiatry, 33*(2), 423–431. https://doi.org/10.1002/gps.4764

Foussias, G., & Remington, G. (2010). Negative symptoms in schizophrenia: Avolition and Occam's razor. *Schizophrenia Bulletin, 36*(2), 359–369. https://doi.org/10.1093/schbul/sbn094

Fuentes-García, A. (2023). Pfeffer functional activities questionnaire. In F. Maggino (Ed.), *Encyclopedia of quality of life and well-being research*. Springer. https://doi.org/10.1007/978-3-031-17299-1_2158

Fulford, D., Niendam, T. A., Floyd, E. G., Carter, C. S., Mathalon, D. H., Vinogradov, S., Loewy, R. L., Stuart, B. K., Stuart, S. R., & Stuart, T. J. (2013). Symptom dimensions and functional impairment in early psychosis: More to the story than just negative symptoms. *Schizophrenia Research, 147*(1), 125–131. https://doi.org/10.1016/j.schres.2013.03.024

Goodkind, M., Eickhoff, S. B., Oathes, D. J., Jiang, Y., Chang, A., Jones-Hagata, L. B., Ortega, B. N., Zaiko, Y. V., Roach, E. L., Korgaonkar, M. S., Grieve, S. M., Galatzer-Levy, I., Fox, P. T., & Etkin, A. (2015). Identification of a common neurobiological substrate for mental illness. *JAMA Psychiatry, 72*(4), 305–315. https://doi.org/10.1001/jamapsychiatry.2014.2206

Graf, C. (2008). The Lawton instrumental activities of daily living scale. *American Journal of Nursing, 108*(4), 52–62. https://doi.org/10.1097/01.NAJ.0000314810.46029.74

Green, M. F. (1996). What are the functional consequences of neurocognitive deficits in schizophrenia? *The American Journal of Psychiatry, 153*(3), 321–330. https://doi.org/10.1176/ajp.153.3.321

Green, M. F., Kern, R. S., Braff, D. L., & Mintz, J. (2000). Neurocognitive deficits and functional outcome in schizophrenia: Are we measuring the "right stuff"? *Schizophrenia Bulletin, 26*(1), 119–136. https://doi.org/10.1093/oxfordjournals.schbul.a033430

Guo, H. J., & Sapra, A. (2022, November 14). Instrumental activity of daily living. In *StatPearls*. StatPearls Publishing. https://www.ncbi.nlm.nih.gov/books/NBK553126/

Habtamu, K., Alem, A., Medhin, G., Fekadu, A., Prince, M., & Hanlon, C. (2018). Development and validation of a contextual measure of functioning for people living with severe mental disorders in rural Africa. *BMC Psychiatry, 16*, 1–13. https://doi.org/10.1186/s12888-016-1022-3

Harvey, P. D., & Strassnig, M. (2012). Predicting the severity of everyday functional disability in people with schizophrenia: cognitive deficits, functional capacity, symptoms, and health status. *World Psychiatry, 11*(2), 73–79. https://doi.org/10.1016/j.wpsyc.2012.05.004

Harvey, P. D., Koren, D., Reichenberg, A., & Bowie, C. R. (2006). Negative symptoms and cognitive deficits: What is the nature of their relationship? *Schizophrenia Bulletin, 32*(2), 250–258. https://doi.org/10.1093/schbul/sbj011

Harvey, P. D., Raykov, T., Twamley, E. W., Vella, L., Heaton, R. K., & Patterson, T. L. (2011). Validating the measurement of real-world functional outcomes: Phase I results of the VALERO study. *American Journal of Psychiatry, 168*(11), 1195–1201. https://doi.org/10.1176/appi.ajp.2011.10121723

Harvey, P. D., Heaton, R. K., Carpenter, W. T., Jr., Green, M. F., Gold, J. M., & Schoenbaum, M. (2012). Functional impairment in people with schizophrenia: Focus on employability and eligibility for disability compensation. *Schizophrenia Research, 140*(1–3), 1–8. https://doi.org/10.1016/j.schres.2012.03.025

Heinrichs, R. W., & Zakzanis, K. K. (1998). Neurocognitive deficit in schizophrenia: A quantitative review of the evidence. *Neuropsychology, 12*(3), 426–445. https://doi.org/10.1037/0894-4105.12.3.426

Henry, B. L., Minassian, A., & Perry, W. (2013). Everyday functional ability across different phases of bipolar disorder. *Psychiatry Research, 210*(3), 850–856. https://doi.org/10.1016/j.psychres.2013.04.006

Huang, Y., Wang, W., Hei, G., Shao, T., Li, L., Yang, Y., Wang, X., Long, Y., Xiao, J., Peng, X., Song, C., Cai, J., Song, X., Xu, X., Gao, S., Huang, J., Kang, D., Wang, Y., Zhao, J., et al. (2025). Subgroups of cognitive impairments in schizophrenia characterized by executive function and their morphological features: a latent profile analysis study. *BMC Medicine, 23*(1), 13. https://doi.org/10.1186/s12916-024-03835-9

Jaeger, J., Berns, S. M., & Czobor, P. (2003). The multidimensional scale of independent functioning: A new instrument for measuring functional disability in psychiatric populations. *Schizophrenia Bulletin, 29*(1), 153–167. https://doi.org/10.1093/oxfordjournals.schbul.a006987

Jenkinson, C., Wright, L., & Coulter, A. (1994). Criterion validity and reliability of the SF-36 in a population sample. *Quality of Life Research, 3*, 7–12. https://doi.org/10.1007/BF00647843

Joseph, J., Kremen, W. S., Glatt, S. J., Franz, C. E., Chandler, S. D., Liu, X., Vuoksimaa, E., Lyons, M. J., & Twamley, E. W. (2015). Assessment of Lifespan Functioning Attainment (ALFA) scale: A quantitative interview for self-reported current and functional decline in schizophrenia. *Journal of Psychiatric Research, 65*, 102–107. https://doi.org/10.1016/j.jpsychires.2015.04.001

Katz, M. M., & Lyerly, S. B. (1963). *Katz adjustment scales*. Psychological Reports. https://psycnet.apa.org/doi/10.1037/t04041-000

Kayton, L., & Koh, S. D. (1975). Hypohedonia in schizophrenia. *Journal of Nervous and Mental Disease, 161*(6), 412–420. https://doi.org/10.1097/00005053-197512000-00005

Kessler, R. C., Berglund, P. A., Bruce, M. L., Koch, J. R., Laska, E. M., Leaf, P. J., Manderscheid, R. W., & Wang, P. S. (2001). The prevalence and correlates of untreated serious mental illness.

Health Services Research, 36(6 Pt 1), 987–1007. https://www.ncbi.nlm.nih.gov/pmc/articles/PMC1089279/

Kleinman, L., Lieberman, J., Dube, S., Mohs, R., Zhao, Y., Kinon, B., Marder, S., Carpenter, W., Loebel, A., Green, A. I., Mintz, J., Alphs, L., & Revicki, D. A. (2009). Development and psychometric performance of the schizophrenia objective functioning instrument: an interviewer administered measure of function. *Schizophrenia Research, 107*(2–3), 275–285. https://doi.org/10.1016/j.schres.2008.10.002

Lally, P., & Gardner, B. (2011). Promoting habit formation. *Health Psychology Review, 7*(sup1), S137–S158. https://doi.org/10.1080/17437199.2011.603640

Lawton, M. P., & Brody, E. M. (1969). Assessment of older people: Self-maintaining and instrumental activities of daily living. *The Gerontologist, 9*(3), 179–186. https://doi.org/10.1093/geront/9.3_Part_1.179

Lean, M., Fornells-Ambrojo, M., Milton, A., Lloyd-Evans, B., Harrison-Stewart, B., Yesufu-Udechuku, A., Kendall, T., & Johnson, S. (2019). Self-management interventions for people with severe mental illness: Systematic review and meta-analysis. *The British Journal of Psychiatry, 214*(5), 260–268. https://doi.org/10.1192/bjp.2019.54

Lewis, F. D., & Horn, G. J. (2013). Traumatic brain injury: Analysis of functional deficits and posthospital rehabilitation outcomes. *Journal of Special Operations Medicine, 13*(3), 56–61. https://doi.org/10.55460/ATYP-5WSB

Loeb, P. A. (1996). *ILS: Independent living scales manual*. Psychological Corporation, Harcourt Brace Jovanovich. https://www.worldcat.org/title/ils-independent-living-scales-manual/oclc/35662607

Mahmood, Z., Vella, L., Maye, J. E., Keller, A. V., Van Patten, R., Clark, J. M., & Twamley, E. W. (2021). Rates of cognitive and functional impairments among sheltered adults experiencing homelessness. *Psychiatric Services, 72*(3), 333–337. https://doi.org/10.1176/appi.ps.202000065

Marder, S. R., & Galderisi, S. (2017). The current conceptualization of negative symptoms in schizophrenia. *World Psychiatry, 16*(1), 14–24. https://doi.org/10.1002/wps.20385

Marquand, A. F., Kia, S. M., Zabihi, M., Wolfers, T., Buitelaar, J. K., & Beckmann, C. F. (2019). Conceptualizing mental disorders as deviations from normative functioning. *Molecular Psychiatry, 24*(10), 1415–1424. https://doi.org/10.1038/s41380-019-0441-1

Mausbach, B. T., Moore, R., Bowie, C., Cardenas, V., & Patterson, T. L. (2009). A review of instruments for measuring functional recovery in those diagnosed with psychosis. *Schizophrenia Bulletin, 35*(2), 307–318. https://doi.org/10.1093/schbul/sbn152

McGrath, L. M., Cornelis, M. C., Lee, P. H., Robinson, E. B., Duncan, L. E., Barnett, J. H., Huang, J., Gerber, G., Sklar, P., Sullivan, P., Perlis, R. H., & Smoller, J. W. (2013). Genetic predictors of risk and resilience in psychiatric disorders: A cross-disorder genome-wide association study of functional impairment in major depressive disorder, bipolar disorder, and schizophrenia. *American Journal of Medical Genetics Part B: Neuropsychiatric Genetics, 162B*(7), 530–548. https://doi.org/10.1002/ajmg.b.32190

McIntosh, B. J., Zhang, X. Y., Kosten, T., Tan, S. P., Xiu, M. H., Rakofsky, J., & Harvey, P. D. (2011). Performance-based assessment of functional skills in severe mental illness: Results of a large-scale study in China. *Journal of Psychiatric Research, 45*(8), 1089–1094. https://doi.org/10.1016/j.jpsychires.2011.01.012

McIntyre, R. S., Cha, D. S., Soczynska, J. K., Woldeyohannes, H. O., Gallaugher, L. A., Kudlow, P., Alsuwaidan, M., Law, C. W. Y., Carvalho, A. F., Mansur, R. B., & Baskaran, A. (2013). Cognitive deficits and functional outcomes in major depressive disorder: Determinants, substrates, and treatment interventions. *Depression and Anxiety, 30*(6), 515–527. https://doi.org/10.1002/da.22063

Menditto, A. A., Wallace, C. J., Liberman, R. P., Wal, J. V., Jones, N. T., & Stuve, P. (1999). Functional assessment of independent living skills. *Psychiatric Rehabilitation Skills, 3*(2), 200–219. https://doi.org/10.1080/10973439908408384

Morrison, R. L., & Wixted, J. T. (1989). Social skills training. In A. S. Bellack (Ed.), *A clinical guide for the treatment of schizophrenia*. Springer. https://doi.org/10.1007/978-1-4757-8979-9_10

Mosolov, S. N., & Yaltonskaya, P. A. (2022). Primary and secondary negative symptoms in schizophrenia. *Frontiers in Psychiatry, 12*, 766692. https://doi.org/10.3389/fpsyt.2021.766692

Murphy, K. R., & Constans, J. I. (1987). Behavioral anchors as a source of bias in rating. *Journal of Applied Psychology, 72*(4), 573–577. https://doi.org/10.1037/0021-9010.72.4.573

Njenga, F. (2009). Factors that influence functional impairment and outcome of mental illness. *World Psychiatry, 8*(2), 95–96. https://doi.org/10.1002/j.2051-5545.2009.tb00225.x

Patmisari, E., Huang, Y., McLaren, C., Bhatia, P., Orr, M., Govindasamy, S., Rathi, S., Alford, K., & McLaren, H. (2025). Review of community-based interventions for people with serious mental illness, focusing on learning instrumental activities of daily living and enhancing wellbeing. *Scandinavian Journal of Occupational Therapy, 32*(1), 2468421. https://doi.org/10.1080/11038128.2025.2468421

Patterson, T. L., Goldman, S., McKibbin, C. L., Hughs, T., & Jeste, D. V. (2001). UCSD performance-based skills assessment: development of a new measure of everyday functioning for severely mentally ill adults. *Schizophrenia Bulletin, 27*(2), 235–245. https://doi.org/10.1093/oxfordjournals.schbul.a006870

Patterson, T. L., McKibbin, C., Taylor, M., Goldman, S., Davila-Fraga, W., Bucardo, J., & Jeste, D. V. (2003). Functional adaptation skills training (FAST): A pilot psychosocial intervention study in middle-aged and older patients with chronic psychotic disorders. *The American Journal of Geriatric Psychiatry, 11*(1), 17–23. https://doi.org/10.1097/00019442-200301000-00004

Patterson, T. L., Mausbach, B. T., McKibbin, C., Goldman, S., Bucardo, J., & Jeste, D. V. (2006). Functional adaptation skills training (FAST): A randomized trial of a psychosocial intervention for middle-aged and older patients with chronic psychotic disorders. *Schizophrenia Research, 86*(1–3), 291–299. https://doi.org/10.1016/j.schres.2006.05.017

Pfeffer, R. I. (1982). Measurement of functional activities in older adults in the community. *Journal of Gerontology, 37*(3), 323–329. https://doi.org/10.1093/geronj/37.3.323

Platt, S., Weyman, A., Hirsch, S., & Hewett, S. (1980). The Social Behaviour Assessment Schedule (SBAS): Rationale, contents, scoring and reliability of a new interview schedule. *Social Psychiatry, 15*, 43–55. https://doi.org/10.1007/BF00577960

Pratt, S. I., Mueser, K. T., Wolfe, R., Santos, M. M., & Bartels, S. J. (2017). One size doesn't fit all: A trial of individually tailored skills training. *Psychiatric Rehabilitation Journal, 40*(4), 380. https://doi.org/10.1037/prj0000261

RAND Corporation. (n.d.). *36-item short form survey instrument*. RAND Health Care. https://www.rand.org/health-care/surveys_tools/mos/36-item-short-form/survey-instrument.html

Revheim, N., & Medalia, A. (2004). The independent living scales as a measure of functional outcome for schizophrenia. *Psychiatric Services, 55*(9), 1052–1054. https://doi.org/10.1176/appi.ps.55.9.1052

Rubin, W. V., & Panzano, P. C. (2002). Identifying meaningful subgroups of adults with severe mental illness. *Psychiatric Services, 53*(4), 452–457. https://doi.org/10.1176/appi.ps.53.4.452

Schretlen, D., Jayaram, G., Maki, P., Park, K., Abebe, S., & DiCarlo, M. (2000). Demographic, clinical, and neurocognitive correlates of everyday functional impairment in severe mental illness. *Journal of Abnormal Psychology, 109*(1), 134–138. https://doi.org/10.1037/0021-843X.109.1.134

Serban, G. (1978). Social Stress and Functioning Inventory for Psychotic Disorders (SSFIPD): Measurement and prediction of schizophrenics' community adjustment. *Comprehensive Psychiatry, 19*(4), 337–347. https://doi.org/10.1016/0010-440X(78)90016-0

Shahrokh, N. C., & Hales, R. E. (2003). *American psychiatric glossary* (8th ed.). American Psychiatric Publishing. https://www.worldcat.org/title/american-psychiatric-glossary/oclc/52874762

Spaulding, W. D., Sullivan, M. E., & Poland, J. S. (2003). *Treatment and rehabilitation of severe mental illness*. Guilford Press. https://www.guilford.com/books/Treatment-and-Rehabilitation-of-Severe-Mental-Illness/William-D-Spaulding/9781572308059

Spitzer, R. L., Endicott, J., Conti, L., Cassano, G. B., & Castrogiovanni, P. (1968). *Current and past psychopathology scales (CAPPS)*. Università di Pisa, Istituto di Psichiatria. https://www.worldcat.org/title/current-and-past-psychopathology-scales-capps/oclc/492593413

Spitzer, R. L., Endicott, J., Fleiss, J. L., & Cohen, J. (1970). The psychiatric status schedule: A technique for evaluating psychopathology and impairment in role functioning. *Archives of General Psychiatry, 23*(1), 41–55. https://doi.org/10.1001/archpsyc.1970.01750010043009

Strassnig, M., Bowie, C., Pinkham, A. E., Penn, D., Twamley, E. W., Patterson, T. L., & Harvey, P. D. (2018). Which levels of cognitive impairments and negative symptoms are related to functional deficits in schizophrenia? *Journal of Psychiatric Research, 104*, 124–129. https://doi.org/10.1016/j.jpsychires.2018.06.018

Tangney, J. P., Boone, A. L., & Baumeister, R. F. (2004). High self-control predicts good adjustment, less pathology, better grades, and interpersonal success. *Journal of Personality, 72*(2), 271–324. https://doi.org/10.4324/9781315175775-5

Tanner, J., Zeffiro, T., Wyss, D., Perron, N., Rufer, M., & Mueller-Pfeiffer, C. (2019). Psychiatric symptom profiles predict functional impairment. *Frontiers in Psychiatry, 10*, 37. https://doi.org/10.3389/fpsyt.2019.00037

Tungpunkom, P., Maayan, N., & Soares-Weiser, K. (2012). Life skills programmes for chronic mental illnesses. *Cochrane Database of Systematic Reviews, 2012*(1), CD000381. https://doi.org/10.1002/14651858.CD000381.pub3

U.S. Department of Veterans Affairs. (n.d.). *Brief overview of SST and the VA SST training program*. https://www.mirecc.va.gov/visn5/training/sst/Brief-Overview-of-SST-and-the-VA-SST-Training-Program.asp#presentation-citations

University of California, San Diego Performance-Based Skills Assessment (UPSA). (2025, May 27). In *Wikipedia*. https://en.wikipedia.org/wiki/University_of_California,_San_Diego_Performance-Based_Skills_Assessment#UPSA-21

Ustün, B., & Kennedy, C. (2009). What is "functional impairment"? Disentangling disability from clinical significance. *World Psychiatry, 8*(2), 82–85. https://doi.org/10.1002/j.2051-5545.2009.tb00219.x

Vaughn, C. E., & Leff, J. P. (1976). The influence of family and social factors on the course of psychiatric illness: A comparison of schizophrenic and depressed neurotic patients. *The British Journal of Psychiatry, 129*(2), 125–137. https://doi.org/10.1192/bjp.129.2.125

Velligan, D. I., Diamond, P., Glahn, D. C., Ritch, J., Maples, N., Castillo, D., & Miller, A. L. (2007). The reliability and validity of the Test of Adaptive Behavior in Schizophrenia (TABS). *Psychiatry Research, 151*(1–2), 55–66. https://doi.org/10.1016/j.psychres.2006.10.007

Velligan, D. I., Rubin, M., Fredrick, M. M., Mintz, J., Nuechterlein, K. H., Schooler, N. R., Marder, S. R., Liberman, R. P., Green, M. F., Kern, R. S., Bellack, A. S., Fenton, W. S., & Dube, S. (2012). The cultural adaptability of intermediate measures of functional outcome in schizophrenia. *Schizophrenia Bulletin, 38*(3), 630–641. https://doi.org/10.1093/schbul/sbq136

Verboom, C. E., Sentse, M., Sijtsema, J. J., Nolen, W. A., Ormel, J., & Penninx, B. W. (2011). Explaining heterogeneity in disability with major depressive disorder: Effects of personal and environmental characteristics. *Journal of Affective Disorders, 132*(1–2), 71–81. https://doi.org/10.1016/j.jad.2011.01.01

Wallace, C. J. (1986). Functional assessment in rehabilitation. *Schizophrenia Bulletin, 12*(4), 604–630. https://doi.org/10.1093/schbul/12.4.604

Wallace, C. J., Kochanowicz, N., & Wallace, J. (1985). *Independent living skills survey*. Unpublished manuscript, Mental Health Clinical Research Center for the Study of Schizophrenia, West Los Angeles VA Medical Center, Rehabilitation Medicine Service (Brentwood Division).

Weissman, M. M., Sholomskas, D., & John, K. (1981). The assessment of social adjustment: An update. *Archives of General Psychiatry, 38*(11), 1250–1258. https://doi.org/10.1001/archpsyc.1981.01780360066006

World Health Organization (WHO). (2010). *World Health Organization Disability Assessment Schedule (WHODAS-2.0)*. https://iris.who.int/bitstream/handle/10665/43974/9789241547598_eng.pdf?sequence=1

Xie, Z., Tanner, R., Striley, C. L., & Marlow, N. M. (2022). Association of functional disability with mental health services use and perceived unmet needs for mental health care among adults with serious mental illness. *Journal of Affective Disorders, 299*, 449–455. https://doi.org/10.1016/j.jad.2021.12.040

Chapter 15
Problems with Behaviors of Health and Wellness: Sleep, Dietary Habits, Physical Activity and Healthcare in Individuals Living with Serious Mental Illness

Introduction

Serious mental illness (SMI) is associated not only with profound psychiatric symptoms but also with pervasive disruptions in health and wellness behaviors that significantly compromise quality of life and longevity. Individuals living with SMI experience elevated rates of premature mortality, often 10–25 years earlier than the general population, largely due to preventable physical health conditions. Sleep disturbances, poor dietary habits, physical inactivity, and sedentary lifestyles emerge as critical domains of concern, each contributing to cardiometabolic disease, obesity, and diminished health-related quality of life. These behavioral health challenges are compounded by neurocognitive impairments, negative symptoms, and environmental influences, which collectively hinder motivation, self-regulation, and engagement in healthcare. Understanding these multidirectional pathways is essential for clinicians, educators, and researchers seeking to address the complex interplay between mental and physical health in this population.

In this chapter, the dimensions of wellness behaviors as functional living skills are examined, situating them within idiographic and nomothetic frameworks that highlight both individualized experiences and broader epidemiological patterns. Sleep hygiene, dietary regulation, and physical activity are explored not only as lifestyle factors but also as behaviors deeply embedded in executive functioning, social cognition, and neurocognitive processes. The role of neurological substrates and environmental contexts is emphasized, illustrating how biological vulnerabilities intersect with psychosocial stressors and systemic barriers to care. By framing wellness behaviors as integral to recovery and community participation, the necessity of integrating physical health promotion into mental health services is underscored.

A central focus is placed on behavioral support strategies and functional skills training, which offer pragmatic avenues for intervention. Approaches such as

G. F. McKeegan, *Behavior Change Interventions for Serious Mental Illness*, Evidence-Based Practices in Behavioral Health,
https://doi.org/10.1007/978-3-032-18372-9_15

reinforcement-based techniques, motivational operations, and structured skills training are discussed as mechanisms to counteract learned helplessness, apathy, and other negative symptoms that impede wellness. These strategies are considered within the broader context of integrated care, highlighting how coordinated interventions can reduce health disparities and improve both mental and physical outcomes. The importance of tailoring interventions to individual needs while maintaining fidelity to evidence-based practices is addressed, thereby balancing idiographic precision with nomothetic generalizability.

In sum, this chapter provides a comprehensive overview of the health and wellness challenges faced by individuals with SMI, linking behavioral risk factors to mortality, quality of life, and functional outcomes. By weaving together epidemiological evidence, neurocognitive insights, and behavioral strategies, a multidimensional framework for understanding and addressing these issues is offered. The discussion sets the stage for sections that detail specific problems in sleep, diet, and physical activity, while also presenting practical approaches to skills training and behavioral support that can foster resilience, autonomy, and improved health trajectories in this vulnerable population.

The Case of Marcus: Complex Challenges in Sleep, Dietary Habits, and Activity Levels

Marcus is a 24-year-old individual with a long history of neurodevelopmental and behavioral challenges. Diagnosed in early childhood with autism spectrum disorder (ASD), intellectual disability, and signs of early-onset psychosis, Marcus had received support through special education and day treatment programs. Though intervention efforts have reduced aggression and self-injury over time, several problematic behaviors related to sleep, diet, and activity remain prominent and interfere with his quality of life and community participation. He lives at home with his parents and attends a day support program. He is overweight. He does not exercise and has gained a lot of weight; he becomes irritated and screams when he is denied food. He is difficult to awaken, and he will lie in his bed for long periods of time just looking at his fingers or watching old movies. He coughs a lot but refuses to go see the doctor. His ankles are swollen, and his parents are afraid that his heart is being affected by his obesity, overeating, and sedentary behaviors.

Marcus faces challenges in three areas: dietary habits, sleep difficulties, and a sedentary lifestyle. He exhibits erratic eating behaviors, including rapid food consumption completing a meal in less than 2 minutes, which has caused choking, vomiting, and regurgitation. He drinks caffeinated and sugary drinks excessively. His sleep is disrupted by inconsistent routines and excessive screen time, contributing to daytime fatigue and irritability; day program staff have been concerned about his falling asleep in the middle of the day at the program; at times he will lie down in the middle of the floor in the lunchroom and sleep. Additionally, Marcus spends excessive time in sedentary activities, resisting physical prompts, which has led to weight gain and reduced mobility. These behaviors have led to social exclusion and health risks.

Definition and Characteristics of Problematic Behaviors of Health and Wellness in Individuals Living with SMI

Physical health issues frequently co-occur with severe mental health problems, leading to significant challenges in healthcare (Ostrow et al., 2014). Individuals living with SMI face a 10–25-year reduction in life expectancy due to chronic health issues. Chronic health problems are common among people living with SMI, often due to reduced exercise and physical activity, poor dietary habits, and adverse effects of medications (Spurrier et al., 2023).

Physical health is often overlooked in individuals presenting with SMI, leading to inadequate monitoring and assessment. Medical management is challenging, with difficulties in seeking treatment for physical symptoms while managing mental health conditions and poor coordination between mental and physical health services, complicating the experiences of people living with SMI with chronic physical conditions (Ostrow et al., 2014; Spurrier et al., 2023).

Living with SMI is a risk factor for developing serious life-threatening health problems (De Mooij et al., 2019). Unhealthy lifestyle behaviors undoubtedly play a role in the development of poor physical health and chronic disease; research indicates that low physical activity, poor diet, smoking, substance use, and risky sexual behavior are common in individuals with SMI and place the person at risk for serious physical health problems (De Mooij et al., 2019; Rush et al., 2008).

Individuals living with SMI experience higher rates of obesity, tobacco use, metabolic syndrome, diabetes mellitus, as well as cardiovascular and respiratory diseases. These elevated incidences of chronic health conditions contribute substantially to an increased mortality risk, leading to as many as 30 years of potential loss (Scott & Happell, 2011). Research indicates that people with SMI have a reduced life expectancy, living 10–25 years fewer than the general population (Hayes et al., 2017; John et al., 2018; De Mooij et al., 2019; Spurrier et al., 2023).

Recent evidence shows a growing gap in physical health and mortality rates between people with SMI and the general population. Those with SMI have higher rates of poor health and unhealthy behaviors, highlighting the need for mental health providers to address these issues (Scott & Happell, 2011).

Several prevalent physical health problems and unhealthy lifestyle behaviors have been identified among people living with SMI (Firth et al., 2019). Physical health problems include:

- Cardiometabolic diseases: The risk of obesity, diabetes, and cardiovascular diseases is nearly twice as high compared to the general population. Metabolic syndrome prevalence is significantly elevated in various mental health conditions (Firth et al., 2019).
- Noncommunicable diseases: There is a higher prevalence of hypertension, stroke, osteoporosis, and autoimmune disorders with mixed evidence for cancer risk (i.e., increased risk for lung and liver cancer but decreased risk for colorectal and prostate cancer) (Firth et al., 2019).

- Infectious diseases: There is an elevated and significant prevalence of hepatitis B, hepatitis C, HIV, and tuberculosis in people living with SMI (Firth et al., 2019).
- Premature mortality: Reduced life expectancy occurs due to poor physical health with cardiovascular diseases and metabolic disorders being significant factors (Firth et al., 2019).

In addition, people living with SMI engage in unhealthy lifestyle behaviors that crucially impact physical health and wellness. These unhealthy lifestyle behaviors include:

- Smoking: Higher rates of smoking and nicotine dependence are prevalent across all mental health diagnoses. Individuals living with SMI smoke at rates 2–3 times higher than that of the general population (Rosen et al., 2023).
- Poor diet: People living with SMI have increased caloric and sodium intake, lower diet quality, and dysregulated eating behaviors compared to those without mental health problems (Mueller-Stierlin et al., 2022; Teasdale et al., 2019). Studies of dietary intake in individuals living with SMI find nearly double the consumption of caffeine compared to individuals without mental health problems (Rosen et al., 2023; Strassnig et al., 2006). Caffeine use may influence the desire to smoke and vice versa (Rosen et al., 2023). The use of caffeinated beverages and nicotine sequentially is frequently associated as a behavioral "routine." A routine is defined as repeated behaviors involving a task associated in a moment of time that requires little awareness of the behaviors (e.g., brushing teeth) (Arlinghaus & Johnston, 2019), which probably contributes to the excessive use of both substances in individuals living with SMI.
- Physical inactivity and sedentary behavior: Around 60%–70% of individuals living with SMI do not meet minimal physical activity guidelines (Firth et al., 2016). People living with SMI have long periods of sedentary time ranging from 8 to 11 hours per day (Firth et al., 2016).
- Excessive alcohol and other substance use: Survey data indicate elevated rates of alcohol use disorders, particularly in bipolar mental health problems and post-traumatic stress disorder (PTSD) (Drake & Mueser, 1996). Using drugs, alcohol, or both ranges between a quarter to a third of samples in surveys conducted with people living with SMI (RachBeisel et al., 1999; Rush et al., 2008; Virgio et al., 2001).
- Sleep disturbance: Sleep disturbances are prevalent in people living with SMI with poor sleep quality and reduced sleep depth being most notable (Briguglio et al., 2020; Firth et al., 2016).

These physical health problems and lifestyle behaviors contribute to the increased burden of illness and premature mortality in people with mental illness. There is an urgent need to address these issues through integrated healthcare and lifestyle interventions.

Mental health issues affect almost 30% of individuals worldwide, contributing to economic burden and disability. Despite advancements in treatment, many people with mental health problems do not fully recover and exhibit residual behaviors.

Access to mental healthcare remains limited, particularly for those with low and middle incomes. There has been limited progress in preventing mental health issues, with rising rates of depression and anxiety among younger generations (Firth et al., 2020).

A strong link between mental and physical health has been established, but pathways are not well understood (Ohrnberger et al., 2017). Data from over 10,000 individuals aged 50 and over from the English Longitudinal Study Cross-sectional Evidence show that a range of mental health problems are associated with adverse health behaviors, such as poor dietary and sleeping patterns, low levels of physical activity, and higher rates of tobacco use, compared to healthy controls; this is especially evident in people living with mental health problems that are linked to living with SMI including schizophrenia spectrum, mood-related problems (e.g., bipolar and depression), and anxiety and stress-related mental health problems like post-traumatic stress disorder (e.g., PTSD) (Briguglio et al., 2020; Firth et al., 2020). Additionally, recent findings found that the relationships between many of these lifestyle risk factors are also evident in low- and middle-income countries (Firth et al., 2020).

Unhealthy sleep patterns, diet, and lack of physical activity are significant risk factors for mental health problems and contribute to the interplay of genetic, epigenetic, and environmental influences that underlie these problems. Saunders (2003) conducted a review of studies identifying various problematic behaviors in individuals living with SMI perceived as burdensome and negatively impacting caregivers. These behaviors encompass problem behaviors like delusions, hallucinations, bizarre and disorganized actions, as well as aggressive tendencies and substance use. Negative symptoms, like reduced or missing emotional responses and behaviors (Correll & Schooler, 2020)—including blunted affect, limited speech, apathy, lack of pleasure, poor social interactions, low drive (Foussias & Remington, 2010), and unhealthy eating and sleeping habits, were identified by caregivers of people living with SMI as particularly challenging and demanding (Provencher & Mueser, 1997). Problematic behaviors associated with low motivation and disrupted daily routines (e.g., sleep, dietary habits, physical activity) can pose significant challenges for caregivers. These issues often present greater difficulty than managing violence or substance abuse, potentially leading to heightened levels of psychological stress and depression among caregivers (Hatfield et al., 1994).

Poor sleep hygiene, including insufficient sleep duration and quality, is linked to worse mental health outcomes such as depression, anxiety, and cognitive decline. Sleep disturbances are common in many mental health problems, especially in schizophrenia spectrum and mood-related mental health problems. Circadian rhythm disruptions can exacerbate problem behaviors and even correlate to clinical responses to treatments (Briguglio et al., 2020). Poor dietary choices, such as high-sugar intake, are associated with neurocognitive impairments and worse mental health outcomes. Nutritional deficiencies are common in individuals living with SMI, further worsening their conditions as diet can lead to inflammation and altered brain functioning, impacting mental health (Briguglio et al., 2020). Physical inactivity and sedentary behavior are prevalent among individuals living with SMI contributing to longer illness duration and poorer outcomes, increasing the risk of anxiety, depression, and cognitive decline. Regular physical activity improves brain health, mood, and cognitive function through mechanisms like enhanced neurogenesis (e.g., forming new neurons and neural connections) (American Psychological Association, n.d.-i) and better circulation (Briguglio et al., 2020). Addressing these risk factors through lifestyle interventions focusing on wellness behaviors like healthy eating, regular physical activity, and sleep hygiene can reduce the burden of mental health problems and improve overall mental and physical health (Briguglio et al., 2020).

Wellness behaviors are related to states of physical, mental, and social well-being. These behaviors are part of the domain of functional living skills that individuals engage in to maintain daily life, resolve problems, live with minimal supervision, and have a satisfactory quality of life (QoL). Common elements of QoL include "personal health (physical, mental, and spiritual), relationships, education status, work environment, social status, wealth, a sense of security and safety, freedom, autonomy in decision-making, social belonging, and physical surroundings" (Teoli & Bhardwaj, 2023, p. 1). The concept of wellness is that healthcare should actively involve the promotion of good mental and physical health rather than being concerned merely with the prevention and treatment of identified physical and mental conditions (American Psychological Association, n.d.-n). Some researchers and clinicians have viewed wellness as the result of four key factors over which an individual has some control: biology (i.e., body condition and fitness), environment, lifestyle, and healthcare management (American Psychological Association, n.d.-l). The wellness behaviors that promote health are not smoking; getting regular physical activity (i.e., participating in aerobic physical for at least 150 minutes per week); limiting use of alcohol to less than two drinks daily; maintaining a normal body weight; and sleeping at least 7 hours per 24-hour period (Liu et al., 2016).

Problems with Sleep

Sleep is a naturally recurring and reversible biobehavioral state characterized by relative immobility, perceptual disengagement, and altered consciousness. As a predictable and easily reversible phenomenon, sleep is distinct from other states of consciousness such as coma, which typically involve the absence or suppression of neural activity (Tubbs et al., 2019). Proper sleep necessitates the interaction between voluntary decisions and involuntary biological activities. Actions such as turning off the lights, reducing noise, and lying down are voluntary behaviors that result in an involuntary increase in melatonin and a series of shifts in brain activity patterns throughout the night (Tubbs et al., 2019). Melatonin, a metabolic product of the neurotransmitter serotonin, regulates seasonal changes in physiology and plays a role in initiating sleep, regulating the sleep–wake cycle, and managing circadian rhythm sleep problems (American Psychological Association, n.d.-h;

Kennaway, D. J., & Wright, H. (2002). Ultimately, sleep depends on the collaboration between behavior and biology; and impairments in either can disrupt sleep (Tubbs et al., 2019).

Good sleep is essential for our health and emotional well-being. Getting enough good sleep quality is essential for wellness. The amount of sleep you need changes as you age; getting the recommended hours of sleep helps a person stay healthy with less illness, maintain a healthy weight, reduce stress and improve mood, improve heart health and metabolism, lower risk of chronic conditions, lessen risk for accidents, and improve neurocognitive behaviors like memory and concentration (Centers for Disease Control and Prevention [CDC], n.d.-a). It is not just a quantity of sleep but quality as well with less awakenings, ease of getting to sleep, and feeling rested when awakened. Adequate amount and quality of sleep are crucial for cognitive and emotional well-being, with poor quality of sleep linked to various mental health problems (Briguglio et al., 2020; Freeman et al., 2017).

There is an interconnection between sleep and mental health problems. Sleep disturbances are commonly seen in individuals living with SMI. Research indicates that sleep disorders, such as insomnia, occur in about 50% of individuals living with schizophrenia spectrum mental health conditions (Freeman et al., 2020). The Diagnostic and Statistical Manual of Mental Disorders (5th ed, rev.) (DSM-5-TR) (American Psychiatric Association, 2022a) list 10 problems that are related to disruptions to sleep with insomnia, circadian rhythm disorders, sleep-disordered breathing, narcolepsy, parasomnias, and restless legs syndrome/periodic limb movement disorders being most common (Huo et al., 2025). Sleep problems are associated with a range of health conditions, including heart disease, brain disorders, psychological changes, hypertension, diabetes, and obesity. Approximately 40%–50% of the global population suffers from a form of sleep deprivation (Huo et al., 2025).

Sleep disturbances can occur before the appearance of psychotic symptoms, such as persecutory delusions. Longitudinal studies show that insomnia doubles the risk of developing depression and is commonly reported by individuals with depressive mental health issues, with about 85% experiencing insomnia (Freeman et al., 2020). Sleep disturbances are linked to increased suicidal ideation and behaviors, often independent of depression. Nightmares show a unique association with suicidality, with frequent nightmares increasing suicide risk by 105%. Insomnia and poor sleep quality are also significant risk factors, with insomnia predicting a 34% increased risk for suicide (Bernert & Joiner, 2007).

Sleep apnea is a condition that occurs when a person's breathing stops and restarts many times while asleep, resulting in reduced quantity and quality of sleep (American Psychological Association, n.d.-l). This prevents the body—and especially the brain—from getting enough oxygen. The result of living with sleep apnea is snoring, gasping for air during sleep, frequent awakening, poor sleep quality, and excessive daytime sleepiness and drowsiness. Sleep apnea affects 3.3% of the U.S. adult population. Serious psychological distress is 2.88 times more prevalent among those with sleep apnea. Individuals with sleep apnea have 3.11 times higher odds of developing a depression-related mental health problem and 3.68 times higher odds of anxiety-related problems. People with sleep apnea are 2.75 times more likely to experience suicidal thoughts. Individuals with sleep apnea demonstrate higher rates of mental health service use but also report unmet needs for care (Kaufmann et al., 2017).

Sleep apnea has a bidirectional influence on physical health and well-being including obesity, COPD, cardiovascular problems, diabetes, kidney problems, vision and neurocognitive problems, and other chronic conditions (National Heart, Lung, and Blood Institute [NHLBI], n.d. -b). The prevalence of sleep apnea among individuals with SMI varies according to specific mental health conditions. PTSD exhibits the highest prevalence, with rates ranging from 1.3% to 83% in clinical settings and from 46.4% to 50% in general populations. Anxiety disorders show a clinic-based prevalence of 47.5%, with population prevalence ranging from 6.4% to 58.1%. Mood-related mental health issues display varying prevalence rates. The prevalence of sleep apnea among individuals with bipolar mental health problems ranges from 2.9% to 69% in clinical settings and is reported at 6.94% within general populations. For depression-related conditions, rates vary between 0% and 66% in clinics and from 7.4% to 44% in broader population studies. Among those with schizophrenia spectrum problems, sleep apnea occurrence is comparatively lower, ranging from 0.7% to 48% in clinical environments and 4.52% in population samples. Sleep apnea is notably more frequent in individuals living with major depressive mental health problems (MDD) and posttraumatic stress conditions (PTSDs), while the evidence concerning its association with other mental health conditions remains inconsistent (Gupta & Simpson, 2015).

Disrupted sleep is frequently regarded as a chronic behavioral concern, often interpreted as a consequence or a nonspecific outcome of mental health conditions; this perception can lead to sleep disturbances being given low treatment priority. Alternatively, some research suggests that disturbed sleep may play a contributory role in the development of various mental health issues associated with SMI. A worsening cycle can occur between mental health distress, impaired daytime functioning, and difficulty achieving restorative sleep. This may lead to the use of non-prescribed psychoactive substances to aid sleep, which can further aggravate behavioral problems associated with SMI and affect sleep quality (Freeman et al., 2017).

Problems with Dietary Habits

A healthy and balanced diet plays an important role in wellness and managing life in people living with SMI. Unhealthy eating patterns may affect mental health and result in adverse health consequences. It has been found that individuals living with SMI have higher caloric and sodium intakes, lower diet quality, and unbalanced eating behaviors compared to those without mental health problems (Mueller-Stierlin et al., 2022; Teasdale et al., 2019). Individuals with SMI had significantly higher dietary energy and sodium intake compared to controls. Qualitative synthesis indicated that higher energy and sodium intakes correlated with poorer diet quality and unhealthy eating patterns (Teasdale et al., 2019).

Individuals living with SMI described negative experiences related to their dietary habits, including feelings of burdensomeness and physiological discomfort. Living with SMI is linked to altered dietary behaviors and food addictions. Weight gain and medication side effects are associated with anxiety and depressive episodes. Eating is perceived as troublesome and a cause for worry and distress by some individuals living with SMI due to negative physiological effects like sleepiness, restlessness, and feeling heavy; this might lead to lessened motivation and energy to shop for and prepare healthy foods, thereby relying on prepared and fast-food high in sodium and fats. Increased perceptions of stigmatization and discrimination were reported to be related to weight gain (Caton et al., 2015; Mueller-Stierlin et al., 2022).

Individuals living with SMI often experience challenges and internal conflict regarding their dietary decisions. The process of selecting between healthy and unhealthy foods can result in feelings of guilt, distress, and overall dissatisfaction. Individuals reported perceiving that they were unable to maintain healthy eating habits despite being aware of benefits of a healthy diet (Mueller-Stierlin et al., 2022). Many people living with SMI are financially dependent on limited disability benefits and may not be able to afford healthy foods (Kessler et al., 2001). Unhealthy food choices are linked to neurocognitive deficits and a preference for inexpensive, ready-made meals and a low consumption of fruits and vegetables, with high intake of fats, sugars, and sodium (Kalinowska et al., 2021).

The convergence of multiple factors may result in "learned helplessness," wherein individuals experience repeated stressors, perceive a lack of control over environmental events (Caton et al., 2015), and cease attempts to alter their situation. This condition fosters vulnerability to depression (American Psychological Association, n.d.-g). Depression serves as a risk factor for emotional eating, where individuals consume food in response to stress and negative emotions, frequently leading to weight gain. Research demonstrates that emotional eating is predictive of weight gain in adults (Konttinen, 2020). High-sugar intake is correlated with depressive mental health conditions. Emotional eaters typically consume high-energy, palatable foods rich in sugar, which contribute to weight gain. The resultant overeating and weight gain exacerbate feelings of guilt and frustration, amplify stigmatization and discrimination, reduce social interactions, and deepen dysphoria, distress, hopelessness, and perpetuate poor dietary habits (Mueller-Stierlin et al., 2022; Teasdale et al., 2019).

Individuals living with SMI often exhibit poor nutritional habits due to various factors such as limited resources to purchase nutritious foods, medication side effects, weight gain, learned helplessness, dysphoria, and depression. These elements contribute to increased stigmatization and social isolation, emotional distress stemming from weight gain, lack of motivation to engage in physical exercise, and emotional eating, which further compounds weight gain. Additionally, there is a perception that service providers stigmatize weight gain; dietary concerns were often dismissed by healthcare providers and often failed to offer support to address dysfunctional eating habits and manage weight gain (Mueller-Stierlin et al., 2022; Teasdale et al., 2019).

Problems with Engaging in Physical Activity

Physical activity has been recognized as a key component of a wellness approach to recovery within mental health services with the potential benefits ranging from improved quality of life (QoL), reduction in distress and problem behaviors, and an improvement in service engagement and utilization (Rosenbaum et al., 2014). Direct and indirect effects were identified in self-assessed measures of mental and physical health, with indirect effects accounting for 10% of the influence of prior mental health on physical health and 8% in the reverse direction. Past physical activity and social interaction were significant mediators in the relationship between baseline mental and physical health. Specifically, indirect effects comprised 9.7% of this association, with physical activity contributing 77.27% and social interaction 13.63%. Regarding mental health outcomes, physical activity was identified as the sole mediator, representing 8% of the total effect (Ohrnberger et al., 2017).

Although being physically active contributes to perceptions of wellness and health, physical inactivity is prevalent among individuals living with SMI, contributing to longer duration and poorer outcomes of the mental health problems (Briguglio et al., 2020; Snethen et al., 2021; Soundy et al., 2014). Individuals living with SMI spend a large portion of their day in sedentary activities, which negatively impacts their physical and mental health (Bort-Roig et al., 2020). High amounts of sedentary behavior are associated with physical and mental health risks, including obesity, metabolic disorders, poor emotional well-being, and more severe psychiatric symptoms (Bort-Roig et al., 2020).

Only a minority of individuals living with SMI engage in physical activity and exercise at a level compatible with public health recommendations (Soundy et al., 2014). One explanation is that individuals living with SMI often lack the necessary motivation to adopt and maintain an active lifestyle (Soundy et al., 2014). Additionally, there is an absence of consistent and effective incentives to encourage engagement in physical activity. Negative symptoms (i.e., defined as the absence or reduction of normal emotional and behavioral functions) are associated with low physical activity, while positive symptoms show a negative correlation with physical activity levels (Kalinowska et al., 2021). Manifestations of problem behaviors such as avolition (amotivation) (Foussias & Remington, 2010), apathy, and impairments in neurocognitive functions can further hinder the development of wellness behaviors and habits.

The lack of motivation and incentives can be explained by several factors. The presence of mental health problems may result in people living with SMI being disinterested and not valuing the beneficial health outcomes to make physical activity a priority (Vancampfort et al., 2015). Individuals living with SMI have a decreased responsiveness to pleasurable and reinforcing events (Kayton & Koh,

1975) and do not engage in reinforcing self-statements after completing an activity or meeting a goal. Individuals living with SMI also experience a lack of motivation and apathy that are problem behaviors that do not respond to pharmacological interventions, are persistent, and occur after other problems behaviors remit (Li et al., 2023; Marder & Galderisi, 2017; Mosolov & Yaltonskaya, 2022).

Motivation is multidimensional, existing along a continuum from extrinsic motivation to intrinsic self-determination. In the context of physical activity engagement, amotivation lies at the low end of this continuum, where an individual lacks the motivation to participate in goal-directed behaviors such as walking around a track (Vancampfort et al., 2015).

Regulation of physical activity can be either overt or covert. Overt regulation refers to engaging in physical activity due to overt contingencies, such as avoiding negative consequences (e.g., criticism) or gaining access to rewards (Vancampfort et al., 2015). Overt regulation involves the imposition of stimuli contingent upon physical activity, such as praise and other forms of reinforcement and negative outcomes like criticism, shame, or fines if the activity does not occur. Physical activity is undertaken to obtain reinforcement or to avoid adverse consequences. The external stimuli may originate from sources such as teammates or coaches, with reinforcement potentially taking the form of social approval or monetary incentives for winning a race.

Covert regulation consists of private events, including self-talk (i.e., cognition), which act as motivating operations (MOs) and antecedent conditions (S^d and S^{delta}) for initiating physical activity. MOs represent the "motivations" that drive or inhibit certain behaviors. MOs are events or conditions that temporarily alter the value of a stimulus, such as a reinforcer or punisher, and the likelihood of behaviors associated with obtaining the stimulus or avoiding it (Cooper et al., 2020). The individual engages in an activity in anticipation of covert reinforcement (e.g., self-talk regarding mental health improvements, weight loss, prevention of somatic conditions, or to avoid critical self-talk (e.g., self-statements and feelings of inadequacy).

Intrinsic motivation is defined as the drive to engage in an activity for its inherent satisfaction or pleasure rather than for some separable consequence. This type of motivation arises from curiosity, the desire for novelty, or the pursuit of mastery, exemplified by activities such as running a marathon, painting a picture, biking a mountain trail, or building a doghouse. It stands in contrast to extrinsic motivation, where behaviors are performed to obtain external rewards or avoid punishments (Di Domenico & Ryan, 2017). Even when behaviors are motivated by the desire for novelty or mastery, other stimuli, both overt and covert, may influence the occurrence of these behaviors, such as attention from others or self-talk regarding personal accomplishment.

Individuals living with SMI experience anhedonia, which is the inability to enjoy experiences or activities that normally would be pleasurable (Amercian Psychologicl Association, n.d.-b; Shahrokh & Hales, 2003); individuals living with SMI may experience problems with the anticipation of reinforcing outcomes for engaging in behaviors (American Psychological Association, n.d.-a) like physical activity. Some individuals may experience "anticipatory anhedonia" in which experiencing pleasure from anticipating future rewards is diminished or "consummatory anhedonia" in which experiencing the reward itself does not result in feelings of pleasure or satisfaction (Sepúlveda et al., in press). The result is a diminished experience of pleasurable outcomes.

People living with SMI may have diminished capabilities to put intention into action and maintain engagement due to impairments in neurocognition (Green, 1996; Harvey et al., 2006; Heinrichs & Zakzanis, 1998), particularly aspects of executive functioning (EF). EFs are "higher-level" cognitive processes composed of neurocognitive dimensions, such as task initiation, organization, flexibility, setting priorities, problem-solving, working memory, and control of impulsivity and emotions (American Psychological Association, n.d.-e; Baggetta & Alexander, 2016); impairments in EFs are prevalent across various mental health problems corresponding to SMI (Baggetta & Alexander, 2016). Executive function (EF) is important for self-regulation and goal-directed behavior, which are necessary for daily activities such as physical activity and exercise. Challenges in self-regulation, task initiation, and setting priorities among individuals living with SMI can negatively affect the ability to engage in physical activity. This includes planning and initiating activities, determining the duration and location (e.g., gym, track, or park), and problem-solving (e.g., addressing poor weather conditions).

Firth et al. (2016) did a systematic review and meta-analysis of research examining the motivating factors and barriers to participation in physical activity among individuals living with SMI. "Improving health" was the primary reason for exercising (91%), followed by "losing weight" (83%), "improving mood" (81%), and "reducing stress" (78%). Despite the acknowledgment of the benefits of exercise, individuals who live with SMI face significant barriers that impede their participation and impact motivation to engage in physical activity. Low mood and stress were the most common barriers, reported by 61% of individuals followed by a lack of support affecting 50% of individuals. These barriers often counteract motivating factors, making it essential to provide professional support to help individuals manage and overcome them to engage in physical activity.

Individuals living with SMI may be suffering from health-related co-occurring physical challenges that present a real or perceived barrier (Stubbs et al., 2016; Vancampfort et al., 2014), especially given the prevalence of obesity and smoking in people living with SMI (Jo et al., 2002). It is estimated that as many as 70%–85% of people living with SMI smoke (National Institute on Drug Abuse (NIDA), 2023) while 70% of individuals with SMI were found to be overweight or obese, despite consuming fewer calories than the general population (Bradshaw & Mairs, 2014; Jo et al., 2002).

Nevertheless, a better understanding of the motivational limitations in people with SMI may be a critical component to increase physical activity in people living with SMI. There is a need for research investigating the motivational processes linked to the adoption and maintenance of physical activity in people living with SMI (Vancampfort & Faulkner, 2014). Exercise can significantly improve clinical outcomes for individuals living with SMI, yet many engage in low levels of physical activity. Understanding the motivating factors for exercise can enhance participation rates among this population.

Dimensions of Wellness Behaviors of Sleep, Dietary Habits, and Physical Activity

Having a healthy lifestyle is defined by engaging in several key behaviors: sufficient sleep, nondrinking or moderate drinking of alcohol, not smoking, meeting recommendations for aerobic physical activity, and maintaining a normal weight (Liu et al., 2016). Liu et al. (2016) found that a small proportion of respondents in the general population reported not engaging in any of the five health-related behaviors while 24% and 6% reported engaging in four or all five behaviors, respectively. Adults 65 and older had the highest rate (10.1%) of all five health-related behaviors among age groups.

As stated previously, individuals living with SMI do not consistently manifest behaviors associated with a healthy lifestyle (Briguglio et al., 2020; Firth et al., 2019). This factor contributes to the early mortality in people living with SMI (De Mooij et al., 2019; John et al., 2018). Between 50% and 70% of people living with SMI do not engage in any of the healthy behaviors due to various factors including environment, motivation, lack of support and resources, trauma-related behaviors, and neurocognitive impairments.

Health-related behaviors and the absence of healthy behaviors in individuals with SMI are multidimensional and heterogeneous, like other functional behavioral impairments (Bechi et al., 2017; Harvey & Strassnig, 2012). Research on behavioral impairments in various aspects of daily life for individuals living with SMI has typically utilized nomothetic methods, which involve aggregating data from groups (Barlow & Nock, 2009). The nomothetic approach, which focuses on interindividual variation, dominates analyses of research data on different observed and noted impairments and problem behaviors. However, its assumption of homogeneity across people and time is often violated. The idiographic approach, which focuses on intraindividual variation, is more suitable for analyzing heterogeneous data (Beltz et al., 2016); it examines intraindividual variations in measures of observable behaviors in individuals with SMI. The reliance on the nomothetic approach has resulted in limitations in the flexibility and generalizability of research findings and their application in clinical practice (Barlow & Nock, 2009).

The dimensions of the behaviors that comprise the behaviors related to health need to be operationally defined and measured for individuals living with SMI so individualized support plans can be developed with the person's engagement and collaboration. Research has been done that shows that these behaviors are modifiable when the person living with SMI is engaged and supported in the behaviors linked to their recovery (Freeman et al., 2017; Hassan et al., 2022; Vancampfort et al., 2015).

Use of alcohol and tobacco products is discussed in Chap. 12. The following are the dimensions of the health-related behaviors of sleep, dietary habits, and engaging in motoric activities to assist in the development of wellness behaviors that contribute to improved clinical outcomes and higher quality of life (QoL).

Dimensions of Sleep

Sleep results from both behavioral choices and biological processes. It is a reversible state characterized by stillness, reduced awareness, and neural changes. Sleep depends on voluntary actions (like turning off lights) and involuntary ones (such as melatonin production), with melatonin, derived from serotonin, regulating sleep and circadian rhythms (Kennaway & Wright, 2002; American Psychological Association, n.d.-h).

Sleep is a complex and essential physiological process affecting cognition, health, and overall well-being. Problems with sleep are common among people who live with SMI. The Diagnostic and Statistical Manual of Mental Disorders (5th ed. rev.) (DSM-5-TR) (American Psychiatric Association, 2022c) lists 10 psychiatric problems that are related to disruptions to sleep. Approximately 40%–50% of individuals who live with a sleep disorder also live with a mental health problem (American Psychiatric Association, 2022c). Freeman et al. (2020) report that 50% of individuals with schizophrenia spectrum disorders and 80% with depressive disorders experience sleep problems, including insomnia.

Sleep is a multidimensional construct. It is more than just closing your eyes; it is a complex phenomenon defined along three complementary dimensions: behavior, physiology, and phenomenology (Andrillon & Oudiette, 2023). Sleep is characterized behaviorally by a transient reduction in responsiveness to external stimuli, often interpreted as a form of disconnection from the external world. To the observer, a sleeping person has eyes closed, relatively motionless, and does not overtly respond to most external stimuli. However, sleepers can still process external stimuli covertly without waking up (Andrillon & Oudiette, 2023). Physiologically, sleep involves distinct changes in brain dynamics and physiological variables (e.g., muscle tone, heart rate). The neurological dimension of sleep is divided into two main phases measured by EEG: (a) non-rapid eye movement (NREM), characterized by slow waves, K-complexes, and sleep spindles; and (b) rapid eye movement (REM) features wake-like brain activity, muscular atonia, and rapid eye movements (Andrillon & Oudiette, 2023). Phenomenological definition includes subjective experiences such as dreaming and perceptual experiences while emerging from unconsciousness. Dreams can occur in both REM and NREM sleep, challenging the traditional association of REM with dreaming and NREM with unconsciousness. These dimensions are complementary and interact to characterize sleep, which is not a unitary experience but can vary across people and in brain regions of an individual (Andrillon & Oudiette, 2023).

The domain of sleep involves multiple dimensions that include quantity, timing, environment, and quality (Briguglio et al., 2020). Other dimensions include latency of onset and sleep disruptions (National Sleep Foundation [NSF], 2024; Ohayon et al., 2017).

- Quantity: "Sleep duration" refers to the total amount of sleep obtained, either during the nocturnal sleep episode or across a 24-hour period (Seow et al., 2020) with 7–8 hours of sleep recommended for wellness (NSF, 2024).
- Timing: Exact sleeping times will vary between people, but for the majority, the best quality of sleep is achieved at night, going to sleep between 10 P.M. and waking around 7 in the morning as these hours coincide with naturally occurring circadian rhythms (NHLBI, n.d.-a). Circadian rhythm is a biological system that synchronizes the body's activities to the 24-hour day cycle (NHLBI, n.d.-a). Having a regular sleep schedule can affect key areas in daily life including perceptions and performance in mental and physical aspects of health, like alertness, attention, and timely responding. Getting enough sleep from a regular sleep schedule can enhance the ability to cope with stress and is less likely to be impacted by minor negative events that develop (NSF, 2024).
- Sleep intrusions are sleeping outside of hours of wakefulness (Andrillon & Oudiette, 2023). Sleep-like slow EEG waves can intrude during wakefulness, particularly in fatigued or sleep-deprived individuals. These intrusions are associated with lapses in attention, impulsive errors, sluggish responses, and impaired neurocognitive performances. They are specific to a brain region, with frontal slow waves linked to impulsivity and posterior slow waves tied to sluggish responses (Andrillon & Oudiette, 2023).
- Sleep deprivation increases the risk of local sleep intrusions, causing attentional lapses and errors. Even without deprivation, extended mental effort can have similar effects (Andrillon & Oudiette, 2023). In individuals living with SMI, cognitive resources may be overtaxed by daily demands, particularly when executive functions are required (American Psychological Association, n.d.-c; Cohen et al., 2012). Disrupted sleep patterns in this group may worsen neurocognitive impairments. Notably, 50%–80% of people who live with SMI report sleep problems, which may contribute to cognitive and functional difficulties (Freeman et al., 2020).
- Latency of onset: Latency is an aspect of the subdomain of sleep continuity (Ohayon et al., 2017) with duration ranging from 20 to 30 minutes being problematic (NSF, 2024).
- Frequency of arousals during sleep: This is defined as the number of awakenings greater than 5 minutes after sleep onset (NSF, 2024).
- Duration of wakefulness after arousals: Another dimension is the duration of being awake after each arousal.
- Sleep efficiency: This is defined as the ratio of time asleep to time lying in bed (NSF, 2024).
- Sleep quality: This dimension is a composite of dimensions of sleep that comprise sleep continuity including sleep latency, number of awakenings, duration of

arousals greater than 5 minutes, duration of sleep before and after arousals, duration of latency returning to sleep after arousal, sleep efficiency, subjective indices of sleep (such as depth of sleep), how well-rested one feels upon awakening, and general satisfaction with sleep (NSF, 2024; Ohayon et al., 2017; Seow et al., 2020). Poor sleep quality is a stronger indicator for psychological and overall health compared to sleep duration. Sleep quality and quantity are crucial for cognitive and emotional well-being, with poor sleep linked to various mental health problems (Seow et al., 2020).

- Environment: Sleep problems take many different forms. One type of problem is with the time of day or where sleep occurs, such as falling asleep while driving a car or taking public transportation (and missing where to disembark). Many of these problems are similar to problems experienced by people not living with SMI. Environmental factors significantly influence sleep health, including physical and social surroundings. Aspects of the social environment (including neighborhood characteristics such as crime, safety, air pollution, and noise) could be salient for understanding differences in sleep (Knutson, 2013). Vulnerable populations, such as racial/ethnic minorities and low-socioeconomic-status (SES) individuals, experience higher rates of sleep problems. Better sleep health is related to access to green spaces. Urban density and recreational facilities impact sleep duration and quality. Natural environments promote physical activity, reduce stress, and improve sleep (Billings et al., 2020). Having a place—a bed and a bedroom—that is associated with sleep is part of developing healthy sleep habits. The bed should be reserved for sleep and quiet, non-active activities such as reading, conversing, or listening to calming music or sounds. It is advisable to avoid using the bed for eating, studying, engaging in arguments, or any other activities associated with physical activity or emotional and physiological arousal. It is essential to establish a clear association between sleep and the bed environment (Billings et al., 2020; Suni & Rosen, 2024). In addition, factors like light pollution, noise, and air quality significantly affect sleep. Artificial light exposure at night can delay sleep onset and disrupt circadian rhythms. Noise pollution is associated with insomnia and fragmented sleep (Billings et al., 2020; Suni & Rosen, 2024).

Methods of assessing sleep include sleep diaries and questionnaires that provide subjective reports about sleep behaviors but are susceptible to various problems with validity and reliability. Advances in technology like the use of smart phones may improve the psychometric properties of these types of measures (Gopalakrishnan et al., 2022). Polysomnography and actigraphy are objective methods for monitoring sleep patterns (Briguglio et al., 2020). Polysomnography is a recording of various physiological processes (e.g., eye movements, brain waves, heart rate, respiration) throughout the night for the presence of sleep-related problems (American Psychological Association, n.d.-m). Actigraphy is a watch-shaped device that is generally placed on the non-dominant wrist and contains motion detectors (accelerometers) to monitor and record movements (American Psychological Association, n.d.-a; Fekedulegn et al., 2020).

Dimensions of Dietary Habits and Eating Behaviors

Many kinds of problems with eating and dietary habits are prevalent in people living with SMI. Eating disorders (EDs) are severe mental health problems characterized by abnormal eating or weight-controlling behaviors (Huo et al., 2025). They can take many forms such as eating too much, eating too little, eating the wrong kinds of foods, eating at the wrong times, binge eating, or ritualized eating patterns (Huo et al., 2025). The eating behaviors may be tied to problem behaviors of living with SMI, improve as other symptoms improve, or persist even though the other symptoms improve.

Certain problematic eating conditions, like bulimia and anorexia nervosa, have been linked to SMI (Huo et al., 2025). The problematic eating conditions are marked by excessive concern with weight and body image. However, among individuals who live with SMI, bulimia, and anorexia are rare; more common issues involve poor diet and obesity.

The measurable dimensions of dietary habits include the amount, frequency, type of foods, and duration spent eating and rate of eating between meals. Various methods exist to evaluate dietary habits effectively. Dietary quality, quantity, meal timing, and environment are key features of eating patterns. Dietary history questionnaires and 7-day food diaries are common assessment tools (Briguglio et al., 2020).

Dietary habits are a multidimensional domain. The dimensions are aimed at identifying patterns related to dietary habits that lead to weigh gain, fat, starch and protein intake, and calories. The key dimensions in this domain are as follows (Greenwood et al., 2012; Mizia et al., 2021):

- Meal frequency: defined as the number of meals consumed within a 24-hour period. Most individuals eat between three and four meals daily, usually on a routine basis with consistent times.
- Rate of eating: This dimension is defined as the amount of food consumed per unit of time. Eating rates are contingent on an individual's drive to eat and the structure and nutritive properties of the food being consumed. Food texture can directly impact eating rate, where food textures that have shorter breakdown during chewing requiring less lubrication and taking less time to ingest. A growing body of research has shown that when meals are eaten at a faster rate, this leads to larger amounts that are ingested (Heuven et al., 2024), leading to overeating and weight gain.
- Snacking habits: the frequency, amount, and type of food that is consumed between meals. Research has shown that 83% of respondents snacked between meals with women preferring fruits while men preferred sweets and salty snacks (Heuven et al., 2024).
- Breakfast: Bread was common. Women leaned toward whole-wheat types of bread and produce while men preferred meat-based items (Heuven et al., 2024).

- Lunch and dinner: These are defined as the meals typically consumed and type of food like soup, meat, potatoes, and vegetables. Men more commonly ate meat while women chose more vegetables (Heuven et al., 2024).
- Fats used: the type of oils used in cooking (Heuven et al., 2024).
- Water intake: the frequency and amount of water with recommendation of up to 6 or more 8-ounce glasses daily (Heuven et al., 2024).
- Liquid consumed: type, frequency, and amount consumed in a specified duration, including water, diet and non-diet beverages, vegetable and fruit juices, and cold/hot teas and coffees (Heuven et al., 2024).
- Alcohol use: frequency, amount, and duration of using alcohol during a specified duration (Heuven et al., 2024).
- Fast food/restaurant: frequency and amount of food consumed over a specified duration (Heuven et al., 2024).

Dimensions of Physical Activity

Physical activity is defined as "any bodily movement produced by skeletal muscles that results in energy expenditure" (Caspersen et al., 1985, p. 129) and that can be measured in kilocalories (Caspersen et al., 1985). Sedentary behaviors are activities performed in sitting, reclining, or lying posture such as watching television, screen time, or doing nothing that does not increase energy expenditure. Sedentary behaviors are distinct from physical inactivity, which refers to not engaging in sufficient levels of moderate-to-vigorous physical activity (Bort-Roig et al., 2020).

Assessing physical activity involves understanding the quality, type (aerobic and anaerobic), quantity, timing, and the environment in which the activity occurs. Individuals living with SMI are significantly less active with 70%–75% of individuals who live with SMI not meeting the recommendations for daily physical activity (Lindamer et al., 2008; Scheewe et al., 2013). According to the current Physical Activity Guidelines for Americans (Office of Disease Prevention and Health Promotion [ODPHP], n.d.), it is recommended that adults participate in at least 150 minutes of moderate-intensity physical activity and 2 days of muscle-strengthening activity each week (ODPHP, n.d.). It should be noted that 25% of the general population does not meet these recommendations (Briguglio et al., 2020).

Individuals living with SMI accumulate less than 38 minutes of moderate-to-vigorous activity per day, compared with 47 minutes per day in individuals living without SMI (Hassan et al., 2022). Low activity levels are linked to increased risk for individuals living with SMI due to the occurrence of obesity, diabetes, and cardiovascular diseases with rates twice as high compared to the general population (Firth et al., 2019). Metabolic syndrome prevalence is significantly elevated across various mental health problems (Firth et al., 2020; Stubbs et al., 2018), which in turn elevates their risk of cardiovascular disease by 78% compared with the general population (Correll et al., 2017). A deficiency in physical activity has been shown as one of the main causes for the reduced life expectancy by up to 25 years in people living with SMI (Briguglio et al., 2020). It has also been reported that individuals living with SMI are more likely to participate in unhealthy behavior such as smoking, drinking alcohol, and excessive sedentary behavior compared to the general population (Firth et al., 2019).

Physical activity can be measured by the dimensions that comprise the domain of physical activity. The dimensions include the following:

- Type of activity: the topography of the behavior (e.g., running, walking, swimming).
- Intensity: Moderate-intensity aerobic physical activity is defined as resulting in increases in heart rate and breathing to the point that one can talk but not continuously. Vigorous-intensity aerobic activity is defined as breathing is hard and fast, heart rate is higher than with moderate activity, and talking becomes difficult to do (CDC, n.d.-b).
- Frequency: how often the activity occurs.
- Duration: the length of time in which the activity is engaged.
- Periods of inactivity: both during the activity (e.g., resting times) and the times between periods of activity.
- Amount and frequency of sedentary and physically inactive behaviors: sitting or lying in bed, reading, or sleeping.
- Timing: the time of day when the activity occurs and does not occur.
- Environmental stimuli: the place and the individual(s) with whom the activity occurs.
- Perception of activity: the individual's subjective experience before, during, and after the activity, especially regarding its enjoyment.
- Perceived difficulty in doing the activity: perceived impediments and adverse experiences when doing the activity.
- Covert events associated with the activity: the cognitions that the individual experienced before, during, and after the performance of the activity.
- Consequences: stimuli presented or available after the activity, such as self-reinforcing thoughts, external rewards (like a coffee treat), or verbal praise.

Actigraphy is a noninvasive method to monitor physical activity as it measures movement (American Psychological Association, n.d.-a). There are many types of commercially available "sport watches" that have functions that measure some of the dimensions of physical activity including subjective evaluation of the individual's performance. Subjective questionnaires can provide additional data but may vary in reliability as biases and social desirability occur (Fernandez-Ballesteros, 2004).

Origins of Problems in Wellness Behaviors

Neurological Substrates

Real-life behaviors are multifaceted. Impairments in fundamental functional capacities, like sleep, dietary behaviors, and physical activity, are common among individuals living with SMI and stem from a complex interplay of neurocognitive functions, neurological substrates and connections, as well as environmental and developmental factors. The occurrence or absence of daily behaviors is influenced by numerous variables, necessitating the integration of various factors and interventions (Bechi et al., 2017).

Goodkind et al. (2015) conducted a meta-analysis of structural neuroimaging studies, revealing gray matter loss in the anterior insula and dorsal anterior cingulate cortex (dACC) among individuals living with SMI. This reduction correlates with impaired executive functions (EFs), which include task initiation, organization, flexibility, prioritization, problem-solving, working memory, and impulse control (Baggetta & Alexander, 2016). EF is essential for self-regulation and goal-directed behavior required for daily tasks and behaviors. The study suggested that cortical thinning and gray matter loss in regions such as the anterior insula, frontotemporal areas, and dACC may impact EF and working memory (WM) rather than specific symptoms associated with a mental health problem (Goodkind et al., 2015; Huang et al., 2025). Goodkind et al. (2015) concluded that neurological similarities exist across different mental health problems, and these findings indicate shared neural substrates in individuals who live with SMI.

Sleep and neurological substrates: Sleep is an essential behavior for humans that serves many adaptive functions. It has been proposed that sleep and wakefulness are separate processes that serve a singular function on both a neurological and a behavioral level that, if dysregulated, can be detrimental to the organism (Van Someren, 2021).

There have been numerous studies that explore the underlying mechanisms in sleep-regulating systems of the brain. A collection of brain regions interacts to influence sleep regulation, emotional adaptation, and arousal. Dysfunction in these areas is central to sleep problems, like insomnia.

A summary of the brain regions and functions associated with sleep and its dysregulations (Van Someren, 2021) follows below:

- Locus coeruleus (LC): regulates noradrenaline activity during sleep, especially REM sleep. Insufficient silencing during REM sleep links to restless sleep and emotional dysregulation (Van Someren, 2021).
- Salience network: Comprising the anterior cingulate cortex (ACC), orbitofrontal cortex (OFC), and insular cortex (IC), this network manages emotional regulation, arousal, and consciousness. Alterations are associated with hyperarousal and insomnia (Van Someren, 2021).

- Anterior cingulate cortex (ACC): This area is active during REM sleep and involved in emotional distress regulation. Persistent activation may contribute to hyperarousal in insomnia (Van Someren, 2021).
- Orbital frontal cortex (OFC): Plays a role in evaluation of reinforcing stimuli and emotional regulation. Reduced gray matter density correlates with insomnia symptoms like early awakening and fragmented sleep (Van Someren, 2021).
- Insular cortex (IC): The area is involved in interoceptive awareness and emotional processing. Increased activation is linked to negative mood and heightened arousal in insomnia (Van Someren, 2021).
- Claustrum: It is connected to the ACC and is involved in consciousness and REM sleep activation.
- Caudate nucleus: It is associated with emotional processing and cortical excitability. Reduced connectivity with the OFC is observed in insomnia (Van Someren, 2021).
- Anterior limb of the internal capsule: The area is composed of white matter bundles connecting key regions such as the ACC, OFC, and caudate nucleus. Changes in this area are consistently found in insomnia (Van Someren, 2021).
- Amygdala (amyg): This brain area is involved in emotional memory processing. Insomnia relates to insufficient overnight adaptation of amyg responses to emotional stimuli (Van Someren, 2021).

Dietary behaviors and neurological substrates: Key brain regions and neurochemical factors regulate eating behaviors, with implications for eating problems and developmental influences. Key brain regions are involved in regulating eating behaviors, including the hypothalamus (HYP), hindbrain, insular cortex (IC), amygdala (amyg), prefrontal cortex (PFC), ventral tegmental area (VTA), and the mesolimbic reward system (Stover et al., 2023). In addition, the gut–brain axis has an important role in appetite regulation. Various serious eating problems such as obesity, anorexia nervosa, eating addiction, and binge eating problems are heavily influenced by developmental vulnerabilities and early life programming (Stover et al., 2023). The neurological areas and structures that are implicated in eating and dietary behaviors are:

- Hypothalamus (HYP): central regulator of energy homeostasis, integrating hunger and satiety signals through its nuclei. Certain neurons promote hunger and suppress appetite (Stover et al., 2023).
- Hindbrain: processes visceral signals via the nucleus tractus solitarius, regulating meal size and satiety through neurons in the parabrachial nucleus that is in the brain stem (Stover et al., 2023).
- Insular cortex (IC): serves as a hub for interoception, integrating visceral, gustatory, and perceptions of pleasurable sensations that signals to guide eating behavior (Stover et al., 2023).
- Amygdala: assigns emotional valence to taste stimuli, mediating responses to sweet and bitter tastes, influencing food preferences and aversions (Stover et al., 2023).

- Prefrontal cortex (PFC): enables EFs such as decision-making, impulse control, and goal-directed eating; area does not fully mature until age 25 (Stover et al., 2023).
- Ventral tegmental area (VTA): contains dopaminergic neurons involved in reward signaling related to food intake, overlapping with circuits for other motivated behaviors (Stover et al., 2023).
- Mesolimbic reward system: this includes the nucleus accumbens (NAc), driving pleasurable aspects of eating, such as liking and wanting food (Stover et al., 2023).
- Gut–brain axis: it facilitates communication between gut and brain via the vagus nerve, hormones, and microbiota, influencing appetite and satiety (Stover et al., 2023).
- Eating disorders and dysfunctions: obesity involves altered circuits and hormones, leading to overeating; anorexia nervosa may involve pathway dysfunctions; eating addiction relates to reward system activation; binge eating links to microbiota and neuroendocrine changes (Stover et al., 2023).
- Developmental influences: adolescents show increased reward sensitivity, and early life exposures can program eating behaviors (Stover et al., 2023). Obesity modifies energy homeostasis circuits and hormone profiles. Individuals living with obesity respond differently to food cues with heightened visual attention. Neuroimaging studies have shown altered brain responses to perceived food cues (Stover et al., 2023).

Physical activity and neurological substrates**:** A minority of individuals living with SMI engage in physical activity and exercise at levels compatible with public health recommendations (Soundy et al., 2014). A lack of motivation and effective incentives may explain the low engagement in an active lifestyle (Soundy et al., 2014). Negative symptoms like reduced emotional and behavioral functions correlate with low physical activity, while positive symptoms negatively correlate with activity levels (Kalinowska et al., 2021). Behaviors such as avolition, apathy, and neurocognitive impairments further hinder wellness habits.

Several factors contribute to low motivation in individuals with SMI. Mental health issues can result in disinterest and neglect of physical activity, despite its benefits (Vancampfort et al., 2015). Individuals living with SMI often have a diminished response to rewarding events (Kayton & Koh, 1975) and lack self-reinforcement after completing tasks or goals. Persistent amotivation and apathy that are resistant to pharmacological treatment may persist even after other symptoms improve (Marder & Galderisi, 2017; Mosolov & Yaltonskaya, 2022).

Apathy and avolition are linked to dysfunctions in several neurological areas and circuits (Giordano et al., 2018), primarily involving the frontostriatal network (Goodkind et al., 2015). Key regions and their functions include:

1. Ventromedial prefrontal cortex (vmPFC): associated with decision-making, reward valuation, and emotional regulation. Damage or dysfunction in this area can impair goal-directed behavior and volition (Goodkind et al., 2015).

2. Dorsal anterior cingulate cortex (dACC): plays a role in effort-based decision-making, integrating effort costs and reward benefits, and action initiation. Impairment in this region is strongly associated with apathy (Goodkind et al., 2015).
3. Basal ganglia: includes the nucleus accumbens (NAc) and ventral pallidum (VP), which are critical for motivation, reward processing, and effort exertion. Dopaminergic signaling in these areas is essential for initiating and sustaining motivated behavior (Goodkind et al., 2015; Stepien et al., 2018).
4. Ventral tegmentum area (VTA): a source of dopaminergic projections to the NAc and PFC, crucial for reward anticipation and reinforcement learning (Goodkind et al., 2015).
5. Orbital frontal cortex (PFC): involved in reward evaluation and responses linked to reinforcement. Atrophy in this region is linked to apathy in neurodegenerative diseases (Benoit et al., 2012; Goodkind et al., 2015; Kluge et al., 2018).
6. Anterior insula: area associated with interoception and physiological arousal during reward anticipation. Dysfunction may impair motivational states (Goodkind et al., 2015).
7. Amyg: plays a role in emotional processing and its connections with the ACC influence motivation (Goodkind et al., 2015).
8. Locus coeruleus (LC): produces noradrenaline, which is involved in effort allocation and anticipatory arousal. Degeneration in the LC is linked to apathy in Parkinson's and Alzheimer's diseases (Goodkind et al., 2015).
9. Right superior temporal gyrus (rSTG): Compared to healthy controls, individuals living with SMI who have problems with apathy and amotivation showed smaller gray matter in this region, which is linked to social and emotional processing (Benoit et al., 2012).

These regions collectively mediate processes such as option generation, cost–benefit decision-making, reward sensitivity, action initiation, and sustaining effort. Disruption in their connectivity or neurotransmitter systems (e.g., dopamine, noradrenaline, acetylcholine) contributes to apathy and avolition across various neurological and mental health conditions (Goodkind et al., 2015).

Psychological and Behavioral Substrates

Individuals living with SMI may demonstrate impairments in functional skills due to limited opportunities to develop these behaviors during their formative years. Many skills expected of functional adults are acquired throughout childhood and adolescence. However, if the onset of SMI occurs during early developmental stages, individuals may not have had sufficient opportunities to learn essential skills. Young individuals with SMI may face numerous disruptions, including admissions to psychiatric facilities, interactions with legal authorities, placements outside the home and family, and issues with school attendance. These disruptions can result in neurocognitive challenges affecting memory, attention, and planning, thereby reducing opportunities to acquire meaningful and practical skills that enhance quality of life. Consequently, individuals with SMI often experience persistent and widespread functional difficulties across various contexts, including wellness behaviors such as sleep, diet, and physical activity.

The response class of wellness behaviors encompasses a range of functional learned behaviors that enable individuals to manifest them, leading to a healthy lifestyle and minimizing the risk of developing preventable physical problems; successfully performing these tasks results in positive outcomes, such as receiving verbal praise and subjective experiences of wellness.

Wellness, quality of life (QoL), and well-being refer to the positive, subjective state that is opposite to illness. Wellness is not just the absence of disease and illness but is a unique positive state. QoL, well-being, and wellness are multidimensional, comprising physical, social, emotional/psychological, intellectual, and spiritual domains (Meiselman, 2016).

Wellness behaviors are crucial for individuals to effectively navigate their daily activities and achieve a satisfactory QoL. The application of learning models such as operant conditioning, classical conditioning, and social learning theory can be highly effective in understanding and promoting these behaviors within relevant contexts.

Impairments in wellness behaviors are characterized by the lack of engagement in actions that promote a healthy lifestyle and the presence of behaviors that negatively impact an individual's overall well-being. Environments that do not facilitate learning and practicing adaptive behaviors related to wellness can contribute to these impairments. Impairments refer to a persistent or temporary decline in functioning (American Psychological Association, n.d.-f). Expected behaviors may not be manifested because they were not learned, potentially due to limited exposure to wellness-related behaviors, or because the individual has not been adequately taught or provided with sufficient opportunities to practice essential wellness behaviors. This behavioral challenge may result from a lack of formal education, an unsupportive environment, or underlying developmental challenges. Insufficient opportunities to learn these behaviors may have led to inadequate reinforcement of the behavior in relevant contexts (i.e., stimulus control). The ineffective use of positive reinforcement reduces the presence of motivating operations (MOs) necessary to engage in these behaviors appropriately. MOs refer to environmental or situational factors that influence the value of certain behaviors and the likelihood of their occurrence (Cooper et al., 2020). MOs can either enhance or diminish the effectiveness of reinforcers, such as attention, approval, acquisition, or reciprocity. The failure to engage in wellness behaviors may arise from a deficient history of reinforcement for such behaviors, the absence of opportunities for environmental shaping and reinforcement, and the lack of motivating stimulus to encourage these behaviors.

Learning occurs through observation and imitation of others. If appropriate wellness behaviors are not demonstrated, individuals will not acquire these behaviors. Wellness behaviors associated with sleep, nutrition, and physical activity may be insufficiently present or rarely exhibited, limiting the reinforcement necessary for them to develop into habitual responses. Habits are defined as "automatic behaviors triggered by environmental cues and developed through consistent repetition in stable contexts" (Lally & Gardner, 2011, p. 484). Strong habits reduce the impact of deliberate intentions on behavior, making them vital for promoting healthy actions and disrupting unhealthy ones. Habits are crucial for achieving long-term goals, as they facilitate consistent behavior over time. Support plans that focus on habit formation enhance the sustainability of adaptive behaviors beyond the active intervention period (Lally & Gardner, 2011).

Additional environmental factors can influence the acquisition of wellness behaviors. Sensory sensitivities and difficulties expressing needs and understanding others' communication can limit the ability to learn and interact. Challenges with organization, time management, and transitions can make it difficult to initiate, plan, and carry out everyday tasks, like managing a healthy diet, sleep, or engaging in physical activity. Trauma or negative interactions can lead to emotional and behavioral responses that hinder the development of health-related behaviors. The person might lack the skills to manage himself, especially if he has faced inconsistent or frequent punishment. Repeated punishment, failures, or perceived lack of control often leads to a sense of "learned helplessness," making it difficult to engage in and learn novel behaviors as the individual avoids any situation if he perceives decreased control over negative outcomes, even when having the opportunity to change the situation (American Psychological Association, n.d.-g).

Individuals who live with SMI frequently encounter challenges in consistently engaging in health-promoting behaviors because of multiple contributing factors. They may not have learned skills linked to a healthy lifestyle during childhood or young adulthood due to deficient learning environments or neurocognitive impairments. This lack of skill development can lead to problems of poor sleep, diet, and activity that result in decreased quality of life (QoL) and physical problems. Additionally, they are at higher risk for developing co-occurring mental health problems that disrupt typical behavior patterns (e.g., substance use). Repeated trauma and isolated lifestyles further hamper their access to positive reinforcement. Frequent hospitalizations and removal from the community exacerbate these issues. The absence of competent role models and neurocognitive impairments like attention and memory impairments contribute to the difficulty in learning adaptive healthy behaviors. Challenges in engaging in wellness behaviors that are prevalent in people living with SMI are influenced by a combination of lack of knowledge, motivation, proper stimulus control, or all the above; these factors are complex and multidirectional in that impairment—and improvement—in one area can impact functioning in other areas.

Individuals living with SMI often encounter difficulties integrating into natural social networks that could support them in managing life demands and stressors. They frequently reside in impoverished and unstimulating environments with limited opportunities and resources for engaging in wellness behaviors such as maintaining healthy diets and participating in physical activity. When a naturally occurring reinforcing network is lacking, families often serve as the primary or exclusive social network for individuals living with SMI. Unfortunately, families of individuals with SMI often exhibit response patterns that include deviant, punitive, and aversive behaviors, exacerbating the stress that the individual may lack the skills to manage (Morrison & Wixted, 1989). Research has consistently demonstrated that individuals who live with SMI experience family relationships characterized by hostile and aversive interactions, which often result in increases in problematic behaviors and relapses that necessitate hospitalizations (Vaughn & Leff, 1976).

Individual differences and contextual factors influence the development and adaptation of behavioral competencies. A transdiagnostic, dimensional perspective is useful for creating targeted interventions for individuals living with SMI. The variety and complexity of wellness behavior domains present challenges in assessing and effectively treating these impairments.

Modifiable lifestyle behaviors are health-related actions that can be altered, and these changes may affect an individual's health. These include alcohol consumption, eating behavior, physical activity, sedentary behaviors, sleep pattern, and smoking (Siew et al., 2022). Wellness-related behaviors are modifiable using techniques of behavior change, like behavior skills training (BST) (Bellack, 2004; Chafetz et al., 2008). Programmatic interventions have been developed to enhance various adaptive abilities and skills in individuals living with SMI.

When training desired behaviors that are not part of an individual's behavioral repertoire, it is crucial to provide continuous and immediate reinforcement for behaviors that closely approximate the targeted behavior. This involves gradually shaping the topography toward the final targeted behavior by breaking down complex wellness behaviors into smaller steps, providing targeted instruction, modeling, prompting, and reinforcement. Once this process is established, the schedule of reinforcement can be gradually "thinned" based on data; "thinning of reinforcement" is the gradual decrease in the frequency of rewards or reinforcers for a specific behavior (Cooper et al., 2020). Without consistent prompting and reinforcement in appropriate settings, these skills are unlikely to develop into daily life habits (Lally & Gardner, 2011).

In summary, impairments in wellness behaviors result from a complex interaction of factors related to learning history, underlying abilities, environmental influences, and challenges in acquiring and performing the necessary behaviors. Interventions that apply behavioral principles, such as ABA therapy, can be effective in addressing these impairments and fostering greater independence in individuals. Understanding the mechanisms of behavior learning and employing positive reinforcement and other strategies to encourage desired behaviors can be instrumental in deconstructing complex behaviors into observable and measurable components, thus facilitating targeted instruction and support.

Epidemiological Considerations of Problems with Wellness Behaviors of Sleep, Dietary Habits and Eating, and Physical Activity in Individuals Living with Serious Mental Illness

Prevalence of Problems with Sleep

Understanding and addressing sleep problems in the SMI populations are critical for improving mental health outcomes. The prevalence and types of sleep problems in individuals living with SMI are significant and are common across various mental health problems linked to SMI (Heron et al., 2022; Stafford et al., 2024). The prevalent rates of sleep disturbances in individuals living with SMI are estimated to range between 26% and 80% of individuals living with SMI (Heron et al., 2022; Stafford et al., 2024). Besides experiencing decreased sleep efficiency, individuals living with SMI live with many types of sleep disorders that are listed in the DSM-5-TR (American Psychiatric Association, 2022d) including:

- Insomnia: difficulty falling or staying asleep; occurs across almost all the mental health problems linked to SMI (Heron et al., 2022; Stafford et al., 2024).
- Circadian rhythm disorders: disruption in the sleep–wake cycle, particularly in schizophrenia spectrum mental health problems (Heron et al., 2022; Stafford et al., 2024).
- Hypersomnia: excessive sleepiness, often seen in bipolar type of mental health problems (Heron et al., 2022; Stafford et al., 2024).
- Restless legs syndrome: frequent moving of the legs due to an effort to relieve uncomfortable and distressing sensations in the legs (Stafford et al., 2024); can occur in all hours of the day but are most severe at night (American Psychiatric Association, 2022c).
- Delayed sleep phase: difficulty in falling asleep at conventional times, observed in people living with schizophrenia spectrum mental health problems (Heron et al., 2022).
- Sleep-disordered breathing (SDB): increased prevalence in bipolar type of mental health problem, including obstructive sleep apnea syndrome (OSAS), partly due to psychiatric medications contributing to obesity and metabolic syndrome (Heron et al., 2022; Stafford et al., 2024).

Sleep disturbances in people living with SMI can exacerbate problem behaviors, including mood dysregulation and neurocognitive and functional impairments (Heron et al., 2022). Problems with sleep are elevated in the SMI populations compared to the general population (Stafford et al., 2024). Stafford et al. (2024) reported that only 12% of people living with SMI and supported by early intervention and community mental health teams were identified as having sleep problems, suggesting potential under-identification and undertreatment.

Prevalence of Problems with Eating and Dietary Habits

Living with mental health problems related to eating behaviors places one at risk for experiencing a co-occurring mental health problem during the person's lifetime (Hambleton et al., 2022). Obesity is a major problem in people living with SMI with the global prevalence of obesity among people living with SMI reported to be 25.9%; the combined prevalence of overweight and obesity is over 60% (Afzal et al., 2021). Research demonstrates that 55%–97% of people identified to be living with a challenging eating condition also are identified as living with at least one additional mental health problem (National Eating Disorders Collaboration [NEDC], n.d.). According to Momen et al. (2022), approximately 40% of individuals living with anorexia nervosa (AN) or other problematic eating problems (OED) also experience a comorbid mental health condition. The most common mental health problems that co-occur with conditions of problematic eating include mood and anxiety mental health problems, PTSD and trauma-related problems, substance use problems, personality-related mental health problems, sexual dysfunction, non-suicidal self-injury, and suicide ideation (NEDC, n.d.). The most prevalent mental health problems co-occurring with eating-related mental health problems include anxiety (62%), mood (54%), and substance use mental health problems (27%) (Hambleton et al., 2022).

A mental health problem related to dysfunctions in eating is a behavioral problem with persistent eating-related disturbances resulting in altered consumption of food and usually associated with distressing emotions and thoughts affecting physical, psychological, and social function (American Psychiatric Association, 2022b; American Psychological Association, n.d.-d). Eating-related mental health problems listed in the DSM-5-TR (American Psychiatric Association, 2022b) are as follows:

- Anorexia nervosa: characterized by restriction of food intake leading to significantly low body weight, intense fear of gaining weight, and a distorted perception of body shape or weight.
- Bulimia nervosa: involves recurrent binge eating episodes followed by inappropriate compensatory behaviors (e.g., vomiting, laxatives, fasting, excessive exercise) to prevent weight gain.
- Binge eating disorder: defined by recurrent rapid eating until uncomfortably full, or when not hungry, and often accompanied by the occurrence of private events of guilt or distress.
- Avoidant/restrictive food intake disorder: a disturbance in eating that leads to significant weight loss, nutritional deficiency, dependence on supplements, or interference with psychosocial functioning without body image concerns.
- Pica: persistent eating of non-nutritive, non-food substances (e.g., dirt, paper, cigarette butts).
- Rumination disorder: repeated regurgitation of food (which may be re-chewed, re-swallowed, or spit out).

- Other specified feeding or eating disorder (OSFED) and unspecified feeding or eating disorder (UFED): applies when eating behaviors either can cause significant distress or impairment but do not meet full criteria or fit into any specific disorder

The prevalence of co-occurring problems with eating among individuals living with SMI is notable high. Individuals living with SMI showed elevated risks of developing eating problems (Momen et al., 2022). The bidirectional nature of living with problematic eating conditions (ED) and SMI simultaneously is supported by the finding that the risk of developing either challenging condition is four to five times higher with the presence of either mental health problem related to SMI or ED (Momen et al., 2022).

Kouidrat et al. (2014) performed a qualitative review of the published literature on the co-occurrence of EDs and SMIs. According to the results, there is a high prevalence of comorbidity between living with SMI and EDs as follows:

- Anorexia nervosa: affects 1%–4% of individuals living with SMI with women (4%) more commonly affected than men (less than 1%) (Kouidrat et al., 2014).
- Bulimia nervosa: prevalence in people living with SMI is 0.73% for men and 1.57% for women (Kouidrat et al., 2014).
- Binge eating disorder: Prevalence ranges from 5.9% to 20% in individuals living with SMI, which is approximately five times higher than in the general population (Kouidrat et al., 2014).
- Night eating syndrome: an abnormal increase in food intake in the evening and nighttime, manifested by large consumption of food after the evening meal, and/or nocturnal awakenings followed by further consumption (Allison et al., 2010). Prevalence ranges from 8% to 25% in individuals living with SMI, significantly higher than the 1.5% prevalence in the general population (Kouidrat et al., 2014).

The physical complications associated with problematic eating conditions (EDs) impact severity, treatment outcomes, and overall functioning of the individual. Medical co-occurrences related to EDs can affect various systems, including neuroendocrine, skeletal, nutritional, gastrointestinal, dental, and reproductive health. Examples of common complications include cardiovascular issues, bone health problems such as osteoporosis, gastrointestinal conditions, and reproductive health concerns like infertility and menstrual irregularities. These co-occurrences can occur before, alongside, or as consequences of the ED (Hambleton et al., 2022).

Prevalence of Problems Engaging in Physical Activity

People living with SMI exhibit high levels of sedentary behaviors. On average, they spend nearly 8 hours a day in sedentary activities, significantly more than healthy controls of the same age and gender (Chapman et al., 2016; Vancampfort et al., 2017). Adults living with SMI are sedentary for about two-thirds of their waking time, with accelerometer data showing a median of 9.2 hours per day of being sedentary (Chapman et al., 2016). One-third of this behavior occurs in bouts lasting over 20 minutes. Self-reported sedentary behavior is slightly higher, with a median of 10.3 hours per day.

Chapman et al. (2016) identified the following common sedentary activities:

- Watching TV: contributed most to sedentary behaviors, with a median of 2.8 hours/day.
- Sitting for travel: reported by 96% of participants.
- Reclining (not including sleep): an important contributor to sedentary behavior, more so than sitting for work or computer use.

In addition, Chapman et al. (2016) reported that people living with SMI participated in the following types, frequencies, and durations of physical activity:

- Walking for transport: Reported more frequently and for longer durations than other activities, with a median of two hours/week.
- Moderate-to-vigorous physical activity (MVPA): Self-reported median was 4.5 hours/week, while accelerometer-derived was 26 minutes/day. Only 7% of MVPA time was accumulated in durations of 10 minutes or more.

A high proportion of participants reported activity levels consistent with physical activity guidelines (i.e., adults participate in at least 150 minutes of moderate-intensity physical activity weekly (Office of Disease Prevention and Health Promotion [ODPHP], n.d.); however, only a small portion of activity was accumulated in durations of 10 minutes or more. Participants also engaged in significant sedentary behaviors, with approximately one-third of these occurring in periods exceeding 20 minutes (Chapman et al., 2016). This resulted in prolonged inactivity interrupted by brief intervals of light-to-moderate physical activity. Chapman et al. (2016) concluded that interventions to increase physical activity could target increasing recreational walking and reducing television watching.

Cultural Considerations

Cultural, ethnic, and racial differences in mental health reveal significant disparities in the prevalence, severity, and persistence of mental health conditions (Yip & Cheon, 2020). Compared to White adults, ethnic and racial minority groups, including Black, Latinx, Asian, and Native American populations, experience higher rates of persistent and severe mental health problems and report a lower quality of life (QoL). Contributing factors to these disparities include discrimination, socioeconomic status, residential segregation, healthcare access, provider bias, and geographic differences (Yip & Cheon, 2020). Given the impact of cultural, ethnic, and racial influences on mental health issues, it can be inferred that wellness behaviors are similarly affected.

Culture and Sleep

There is a significant connection between sleep and mental health. Inadequate sleep hygiene, characterized by insufficient duration and poor quality of sleep, is associated with adverse mental health outcomes, including depression, anxiety, and cognitive decline. Sleep disturbances are frequently observed in various mental health conditions, particularly those related to schizophrenia spectrum and mood-related mental health problems. Disruptions in circadian rhythms can worsen problematic behaviors and may even be correlated with clinical responses to treatments (Briguglio et al., 2020).

Yip and Cheon (2020) have reported differences in dimensions of sleep across racial and ethnic groups. Black, Latinx, and Asian adults are more likely to sleep less than 6 hours per night compared to White adults. Black adults are 1.6 times more likely to exhibit poor sleep efficiency, to experience more light sleep and less slow wave deep sleep. and nearly twice as likely to report daytime sleepiness. Latinx adults are 1.4 times more likely to exhibit poor sleep efficiency and 1.2 times more likely to report daytime sleepiness. Chinese adults are nearly twice as likely to exhibit poor sleep efficiency compared to White adults. Black adults experience more light sleep and less deep (slow wave) sleep compared to White adults. These disparities are consistent across self-reported measures, actigraphy, and polysomnography and persist across all age groups.

Culture and Dietary Habits

Culturally, the shared values, beliefs, and attitudes that characterize any group of people are often influenced by their food choices, the context of their meals, and the people around them when eating. Dietary habits in cultures form a cornerstone of traditions. Cultural awareness of eating patterns is essential for understanding dietary habits and problems with eating behaviors in individuals living with SMI (Jayasinghe et al., 2025; Nemec, 2020).

Obesity is a global problem. Worldwide adult obesity has more than doubled since 1990, and adolescent obesity has quadrupled. In 2022, 2.5 billion adults (18 years and older) were overweight. Of these, 890 million were living with obesity. In 2022, 43% of adults aged 18 years and over were overweight and 16% were living with obesity (World Health Organization [WHO], 2024).

Obesity affects 25.9% of people with SMI globally, and over 60% are either overweight or obese (Afzal et al., 2021). One in eight people in the world is living with obesity. Afzal et al. (2021) reported regional differences in prevalence of obesity in people living with SMI as follows:

- Sub-Saharan Africa: 13.4% (lowest prevalence of obesity).
- South Asia: 17.7%.
- East Asia and Pacific: 22.5%.

- Europe and Central Asia: 27.5%.
- North America: 30%.
- Latin America and Caribbean: 31.7%.
- Middle East and North Africa: highest prevalence at 35.8%.

The prevalence of problematic eating conditions varies across cultures but shows notable similarities and differences. No ethnic differences were found in the prevalence of eating problems in a sample of different racial and ethnic groups living in the United States but more shared rates and risk factors than ethnic differences (Cheng et al., 2019).

Challenging eating behaviors appear widespread across cultures, influenced by diverse motivations including religious, cultural, and societal factors, with Westernization playing a significant role in the increasing prevalence of shape and weight-related conditions in non-Western region (Yassin, 2023). In Africa, studies indicate rates of bulimia nervosa around 0.87% and unspecified eating conditions about 4.45%, comparable to Western countries like the United States, where bulimia is approximately 1.5% and unspecified conditions about 4.78%. No cases of anorexia nervosa were identified, but some women exhibited problematic eating driven by religious fasting rather than body image concerns. In Asian countries such as Hong Kong and India, early studies also reported eating-related conditions without a focus on shape and weight, often linked to physical discomfort or cultural practices. However, with Western influence and media, there has been a shift toward problematic conditions related to eating characterized by body dissatisfaction and a desire for thinness, aligning prevalence rates more closely with Western patterns (Yassin, 2023).

Culture and Physical Activity

Geographical differences exist, with people in Europe being less sedentary compared to those in North America, South America, or Asia. Additionally, people with bipolar-related mental health problems are the most sedentary, spending 615 minutes per day, compared to those with schizophrenia spectrum mental health problems (493 minutes) and major depressive mental health problems (414 minutes) (Vancampfort et al., 2017).

Cultural differences in sedentary behaviors were observed in a study performed by Vancampfort et al. (2017). People living with SMI in Europe were significantly less sedentary (413 minutes per day) compared to those in North America (586 minutes), South America (555 minutes), and Asia (579 minutes). These differences may be influenced by variations in healthcare practices, lifestyle, and the integration of physical activity into mental health care settings. For example, in many European mental healthcare settings, physical activity is often an integral part of multidisciplinary treatment, which may contribute to lower sedentary behavior levels.

Beliefs and practices about physical activity are influenced by a complex variety of cultural and contextual factors. Providing culturally relevant contexts to the meaning of physical activity allows opportunities for improving programs that would engage individuals and communities in physical activity in culturally meaningful ways. Incorporating cultural and contextual factors is critical to promote physical activity, especially vulnerable communities like people living with SMI (Rio & Saligan, 2023).

The prevalence and amount of physical activity among individuals vary significantly across regions and cultures due to factors such as socioeconomic conditions, cultural norms, gender roles, and environmental contexts (Rio & Saligan, 2023):

- Africa: Research covering 22 African countries indicated that 79% of the population adhered to the physical activity recommendations of WHO (2022), which entail engaging in 150 minutes of moderate-intensity physical activity per week, or at least 75 minutes of vigorous-intensity activity, or an equivalent combination of both. Leisure-time physical activity was minimal (5.3%), whereas occupation-related physical activity constituted nearly half (48.6%) of the total physical activity (Rio & Saligan, 2023).
- Arab Countries: In Arab countries, cultural norms generally result in lower levels of physical activity among women compared to men, particularly due to restrictions on exercising in public areas without gender segregation or chaperones (Rio & Saligan, 2023).
- United States: Within the United States, Asian Americans who primarily spoke English at home were more likely to meet WHO physical activity guidelines. Similarly, English-speaking Hispanics exhibited higher physical activity levels than their Spanish-speaking counterparts, underscoring the influence of language and socioeconomic factors (Rio & Saligan, 2023).
- China: In China, parents, and especially fathers, play a crucial role in motivating children's physical activity. However, academic activities often take precedence over sports or other forms of physical exercise (Rio & Saligan, 2023).
- Global Trends: Income disparity emerges as a significant predictor of physical activity engagement. Countries with high income inequality typically have a higher percentage of physically inactive individuals, irrespective of overall national wealth (Rio & Saligan, 2023).

Impact of Problem Behaviors of Sleep, Eating, and Level of Activity with Overall Perceptions of Wellness

Health Related Quality of Life (HRQoL)

The concept of quality of life (QoL) has emerged as a critical outcome in both the research and treatment of SMI (Barnes et al., 2012). QoL of individuals living with SMI is generally low (de Medina-Moragas et al., 2024). This construct focuses on overall life satisfaction, physical HRQoL, and mental HRQoL (Barnes et al., 2012). Current efforts attempt to distinguish between objective QoL—encompassing aspects like employment and housing—and subjective QoL, which focuses on perceived life satisfaction that aligns with the recovery model (Barnes et al., 2012). Studies indicate that employment status, intensity and frequency of problem behaviors, support from service providers, and family relationships significantly impact overall QoL (de Medina-Moragas et al., 2024).

The absence of standardized definitions and measurements of QoL poses significant challenges. Research suggests that the determinants of overall QoL in individuals living with SMI are multidimensional. As stated above, key determinants affecting QoL in individuals who live with SMI emphasize the role of problem behaviors and social support. Mental health issues such as depression and negative symptoms exhibit variable connections with life satisfaction; symptom improvement alone does not necessarily lead to improved QoL. Certain studies associate life satisfaction with neurocognitive functioning (Barnes et al., 2012). The relationship between neurocognitive functioning and life satisfaction is complex, with studies reporting varying results with some indicating correlations while others finding no relationship or even inverse associations (Barnes et al., 2012).

Both QoL and HRQoL have been recognized as important measures of mental health–related problems that impact individuals living with SMI; it has been shown to be considerably impaired in this population (Barnes et al., 2012; Defar et al., 2023). Health-related quality of life (HRQoL) integrates the effects of physical and mental health (Barnes et al., 2012). It evaluates how health impacts quality of life, including overall well-being and the frequency of "unhealthy" days (Yin et al., 2016). HRQoL focuses on individual perceptions of the individual's physical and mental health.

Key dimensions assessed in HRQoL (Barnes et al., 2012) include:

- Physical health: evaluates the impact of physical conditions and problem behaviors on daily functioning (Barnes et al., 2012).
- Mental health: assesses emotional well-being, coping ability, and psychological resilience (Barnes et al., 2012).
- Social functioning: examines interpersonal relationships and social support (Barnes et al., 2012).
- Functional status: measures the ability to perform daily activities and maintain independence (Barnes et al., 2012).

HRQoL is increasingly utilized in healthcare research to assess subjective health status, condition-related burden, and coping mechanisms, complementing traditional population-level measures like mortality and morbidity rates. This multidimensional concept involves subjective evaluations of physical, psychological, emotional, social, functional, and environmental states (Anderson & Ozakinci, 2018). Its importance is underscored by the high rate of medical co-occurring conditions and early mortality among individuals living with SMI (De Mooij et al., 2019; Firth et al., 2020; Hayes et al., 2017; John et al., 2018). People living with SMI experience declining HRQoL, comparable to or worse than individuals living with medical conditions (Defar et al., 2023). Colillas-Malet et al. (2020) found significant gender disparities in HRQoL for those living with SMI, with women scoring lower in physical well-being and satisfaction.

Individuals living with SMI encounter numerous issues related to health behaviors, particularly regarding sleep, dietary habits, weight maintenance, and physical activity. These factors significantly contribute to chronic physical health problems (Briguglio et al., 2020; Firth et al., 2019) and consistently low HRQoL by individuals who live with SMI (Barnes et al., 2012). Wu et al. (2025) found that sleep difficulties mediate the impact of chronic diseases on HRQoL in middle-aged and older adults within the general population. The prevalence rates of sleep disturbances among individuals with SMI are estimated to range between 26% and 80% (Heron et al., 2022; Stafford et al., 2024). Given the high incidence of sleep disturbances in individuals living with SMI, it can be inferred that their HRQoL is significantly affected.

Individuals who live with SMI often experience challenging dietary habits, including feelings of burden and physiological discomfort. Living with SMI affects dietary behaviors and can lead to food addiction. Weight gain and medication side effects increase anxiety and depression. Eating is seen as burdensome due to effects like sleepiness and restlessness, reducing motivation to shop for and prepare healthy foods, leading to reliance on unhealthy fast foods. Stigmatization and discrimination linked to weight gain are also common (Mueller-Stierlin et al., 2022).

Up to 63% of individuals diagnosed with schizophrenia spectrum mental health problems and 68% of those identified with living bipolar-type mental health problems are classified as overweight or obese (Kolotkin et al., 2008). A study examining the impact of obesity on individuals living with SMI has demonstrated that obesity is associated with decreased HRQoL. Obese participants reported lower weight-related HRQoL compared to their non-obese counterparts. HRQoL scores for the obese sample of individuals with SMI were more impaired than those in outpatient weight-loss samples but less impaired than individuals undergoing gastric-bypass surgery (Kolotkin et al., 2008).

Cross-Cultural Considerations with Health-Related Quality of Life (HRQoL)

Deenik et al. (2017) examined the relationship between physical activity and quality of life (QoL) in long-term hospitalized people living with SMI (Deenik et al., 2017). Increasing physical activity among long-term hospitalized people living with SMI is correlated with enhanced QoL. Physical activity was notably associated with improved QoL across physical, psychological, and social domains but excluding the environmental domain. The largest improvements in QoL are observed when individuals shift from sedentary behavior to light physical activity (Deenik et al., 2017).

These findings indicate that even slight increases in physical activity can enhance QoL for long-term hospitalized individuals living with SMI.

Positive attitudes toward physical activity do not necessarily lead to increased physical activity. Perceptions about physical activity and self-efficacy (e.g., subjective perception of an individual's capability to perform in each setting or to attain a desired result (American Psychological Association, n.d.-k) related to physical activity were not found to be aligned with actual frequency of being physically active, suggesting a disparity between intention and behavior. The study underscores the complexity of QoL and the need for integrated, peer-supported interventions to promote physical activity among inpatients with SMI.

Defar et al. (2023) investigated HRQoL among people living with SMI in southern Ethiopia. The study aimed to identify predictors of HRQoL among individuals living with SMI and undergoing outpatient follow-up in the Sidama region of southern Ethiopia. Scores of HRQoL were positively associated with social support and being single. Functional disability, being a student, jobless status, and depression type of mental health problem negatively impacted HRQoL (Defar et al., 2023). HRQoL among individuals living with SMI in southern Ethiopia is significantly influenced by social support, marital status, occupation, type of mental health condition, and functional disability; these factors are similar to key determents in Western cultures as well.

Research on health-related quality of life (HRQoL) among individuals who live with SMI indicates the significance of addressing both physical and mental health needs. The results point to the potential benefit of educational interventions, individualized support plans for people with SMI and their caregivers, and collaborative care models to improve mental healthcare outcomes. It is also suggested that measures to support functioning, social support, and employment opportunities may be beneficial for individuals living with SMI.

Changing Behaviors Related to Sleep, Dietary Habits, and Sedentary Behaviors in Individuals Living with SMI

Problems with sleep, dietary habits, and sedentary behaviors are common among individuals living with SMI. In a survey of service providers of people with SMI, nearly three out of four service providers identified issues with eating and sleeping as problematic. These issues were rated as more concerning than problems such as poor self-care, arguing, hitting others, and drug/alcohol abuse (Hatfield et al., 1994; Saunders, 2003). Various sleep, dietary, and physical activity challenges may arise when providing mental health services to individuals with SMI. These issues have practical and emotional impacts, highlighting the need for comprehensive support strategies.

Why Do Problems with Sleep, Eating, and Physical Activity Occur?

Part of the Problem May Be Biological or Physical:

Medical conditions: There are varieties of medical conditions that can cause problems with sleep, dietary habits, and being physically active. For example, heart and lung problems can make it very hard for that person to sleep while lying down or walking up a flight of stairs. It is recommended that the person living with SMI have a comprehensive physical examination to rule out that she is not living with a physical illness or condition that can interfere with engaging in wellness behaviors.

- Biological and neurochemical influences:
  - Neurochemical disruptions: Many SMIs, such as depression or schizophrenia spectrum mental health problem, involve imbalances in neurotransmitters like serotonin and dopamine—key regulators of mood, appetite, and circadian rhythms. This can lead to irregular hunger cues and disrupted sleep cycles, often manifesting as insomnia, hypersomnia, overeating, or loss of appetite.
  - Biochemical imbalances: Imbalances in neurotransmitters are commonly associated with SMI and can impair areas responsible for alertness, appetite regulation, and circadian rhythms. These imbalances may lower motivation, which in turn disrupts structured mealtimes and sleep schedules. Medications prescribed for SMI or other medical conditions, such as antidepressants or antipsychotics, can cause side effects like drowsiness or appetite changes, compounding both eating and sleep disturbances. Use of substances like alcohol, nicotine, caffeine, and illicit drugs can further destabilize neurochemical regulation, affecting hunger signals, sleep–wake cycles, and levels of motivation.
- Psychosocial and environmental stressors: Lack of structured routines or meaningful daily activities can lead to daytime sleep, erratic eating patterns, and sedentary behaviors. Boredom and unoccupied time often prompt dysregulated sleeping, dysfunctional eating, and lack of being physically active. Stressors related to socioeconomic challenges—such as financial strain, housing instability, or unemployment—can lead to chronic stress, anxiety, and depression, all of which impair sleep quality, dietary habits, and motivational states. Cognitive impairments tied to SMI (e.g., attention deficits, memory issues) may hinder an individual's ability to maintain regular schedules for eating, sleeping, and exercise. Social isolation or inadequate support may reduce access to healthy meals and emotional regulation, making it harder to maintain both sleep hygiene and nutritional balance.

Interactions with Other Problem Behaviors

Besides the impact of neurological and environmental substrates, living with SMI often creates a compounding effect on eating, sleeping, and being physically active with each issue influencing the other through interconnected biological, behavioral, and psychosocial pathways. The observed problems in wellness-related behaviors tend to overlap by the following complex mechanisms:

- Medication side effects: Pharmacological treatments for SMI frequently involve medications (e.g., antipsychotics, mood stabilizers) that alter appetite, levels of sedation, and affect the environmental and social incentives to engage in physical activity. A person might sleep excessively due to drowsiness or experience restless nights while also dealing with increased appetite or weight gain—sometimes from the same medication. Being overweight may influence a person's mood, his overall perceptions of being physically healthy, and increase difficulty in doing physical activity like shortness of breath or joint pain.
- Disrupted daily routines: Living with SMI can erode the ability to maintain structured schedules. When a person lacks predictable mealtimes, sleep/wake patterns, and daily routines, the occurrence of certain behaviors becomes erratic. Sleeping during the day due to low motivation, for instance, often leads to skipping meals or late-night eating as well as missing scheduled and unscheduled available physical activities.
- Neurocognitive and motivational impairments: Conditions like schizophrenia spectrum or major mood mental health problems may reduce initiative, planning, and executive functioning. This can result in a lack of interest in preparing meals, following bedtime routines, planning on and the execution of participating in activities that are fundamental elements of healthy sleep, dietary habits, and being physically active.
- Psychosocial stress and environment: Individuals living with SMI frequently face greater financial stress, housing instability, lack of resources, live in poor and toxic environments, and are socially isolated. Environmental instability—such as lack of routines or stimulation—reduces contextual cues (e.g., S^D) that typically signal mealtime, bedtime, and other active behaviors leading to irregular behavioral patterns. These stressors increase depression, anxiety and dysregulated sleep, eating, and activity. A person preoccupied with safety or food access may struggle to fall asleep, maintain consistent nutrition, and have the energy, motivation, and forethought to engage in physically active routines.

Over time, the disturbance in one response class of wellness behaviors can influence and worsen other response classes. Poor nutrition affects energy, mood, and sleep quality; inadequate sleep increases food cravings, impairs judgment, and weakens appetite control mechanisms; being sedentary for long periods results in increases in anxiety, dysphoria, and helplessness and decreases in perceptions of wellness creating a self-perpetuating cycle. Sleep deprivation can function as an establishing operation (EO) for emotional dysregulation, increasing food-seeking and emotional eating as a coping behavior. An EO is a particular type of MO that increases the value of a stimulus and alters the chances of engaging in a behavior that will access the stimulus (Cooper et al., 2020). Poor diet and lack of physical activity can reduce sleep quality, which in turn further degrades behavior regulation—establishing a compounding, cyclical pattern.

Behavioral Support Strategies for Problems with Sleeping, Dietary Habits, and Sedentary Behaviors

- Define the behavior and understand its function: Identify and clearly define the problem behaviors related to eating (e.g., excessive intake, avoidance, poor diet), sleeping (e.g., insomnia, hypersomnia, poor sleep hygiene), and physical activity (e.g., lying in bed watching TV for more than 4 hours). Be clear as to what the behavior is and avoid the use of assumptions about the occurrence of the behaviors such as "Marcus never sleeps," "Marcus is always eating," or "Marcus does not walk with others as he wants to be alone."
- Describe the behavior: Describe the behavior as close as possible as to what can be observed by the senses (Molloy et al., 1997). Putting the description of the targeted behavior into words is often difficult but is a necessary first step before any assessment can occur. To accurately describe the behavior, it is imperative to put into words exactly what is seen, heard, or experienced when the behavior occurs. Labels and explanations of behavior need to be avoided. For example, lying in bed is described as "being in a supine horizontal position, with the body supported by a mattress." Someone lying in bed with their eyes closed is not necessarily asleep; additional methods are needed to confirm sleep.
- Seek a review of medications: The medications that are prescribed for people living with SMI have side effects. Some medications can contribute to restlessness, irritability, drowsiness, hunger, sedation, and other problems, which can interfere with behavioral patterns and routines. Consider having the current medications evaluated by a prescribing mental health service provider to determine whether changes in the medications may be helpful. For example, if the medications cause drowsiness, it may be possible to arrange a dosage that can be given once a day during the evening hours. The evaluation by the prescribing service provider may result in a referral of the person living with SMI to a medical specialist to make sure that the problem is not caused by a physical illness or condition.
- Decide whether the behavior needs to change: Developing and implementing an intervention for problem behaviors are complex and require considerable effort. One of the most important decisions that a service provider must make is whether to try to change a problem behavior. In almost every case, an attempt to change such a problem will require a lot of time, effort, and persistence by the members of the recovery team. The efforts of the service provider to change a problem

may cause new conflicts with the service user who is expected to change behaviors that probably have been happening for a long time. Because of this, the service provider must balance the time and effort that will be required and the risk and benefits of implementing a behavioral support plan and the likelihood that an acceptable level of success can be achieved. In some cases, the service provider may decide that the benefit of change is not worth the effort. For example, a person living with SMI may sleep during the afternoon hours because of drowsiness brought on by medications to treat the SMI; his sleeping in the afternoon results in him missing the afternoon scheduled activities. If the medication cannot be changed, dosage decreased, or given at a different time of day, it may be more realistic to accept the afternoon "nap" and plan other activities around it. The assistance of a mental health professional service provider should be helpful in determining whether it is realistic to go ahead with a plan.

- Engage the person living with SMI who is manifesting the behaviors: Members of the recovery team need to engage and collaborate with each other and the person living with SMI. Using a recovery orientation in everyday clinical work involves eliciting information on subjective life goals and working with people living with SMI to help them achieve their goals, including management of problem behavior that may be impeding her recovery (Whitley et al., 2015). The recovery service team begins by establishing rapport and trust with the person living with SMI. The use of active listening lays the foundation of a trusting relationship with members of the recovery team. The key points of active listening—eye contact, paraphrasing, reflective statements, empathy, using gestures and other nonverbal communication behaviors—need to be utilized during any discussion with the person living with SMI (Karnieli-Miller & Salyers, 2011). Using the principles and techniques of active listening communicates to the individual living with SMI that the team members are paying respectful attention to the content and feeling expressed in their communication. Meeting with the team becomes a safe place to discuss concerns and issues; disagreements are not the end point of the discussion, but the beginning as active listening and motivational interviewing facilitates further discussion, leading to the use of solution-focused techniques in resolving the differences and enabling progress toward recovery.
- Operationally define the problem that needs intervention: Use operational definitions by which the behavior can be observed and measured (American Psychological Association, n.d.-j). Define the behavior specifically in measurable terms such as frequency, magnitude/intensity, duration of the problem when it occurs, and the context in which the problems occur (e.g., where the problem behavior occurs, what was person doing before the behaviors occurs, who was in the vicinity of the person when the problem occurs, what was the outcome of the problem behavior, what was done about the problem) (Molloy et al., 1997).
- Observe and track the behavior that is defined: Watch for changes in the problem behavior. Observe the problematic behavior and assess the dimensions of the behavior like how frequently the behavior is manifested, the duration, intensity/magnitude of the manifested behavior, the conditions and contexts in which the behavior occurs and does not occur. The data should include any changes that

occur with the behavior according to such factors as day of the week, changes in the environment, (e.g., person, place, situation), activities that occurred (or did not occur), or other ways that the environmental context influences the behavior. Monitoring sheets are in the appendix to record what is observed according to the operational definition of the behavior. If there are times when the problematic behavior seems better or worse than at other times, consider what are the variables that might be contributing to this. This information is likely to be valuable in developing support plans to minimize the problem and to develop an understanding as to the function of the behavior and answer the question of "why" the behavior occurs. In Marcus's situation, observations indicated that he frequently slept during the day when he did not have scheduled activities; this pattern suggests that daytime sleeping might be maintained by relief from boredom, which can be considered an aversive stimulus (Molloy et al., 1997).
- Look for contextual patterns for the occurrence and non-occurrence of the targeted behavior: Patterns from the data can be used to ascertain environmental conditions that occur before and after the occurrence and non-occurrence of the problem behaviors. If using remote data from technology, it may be more difficult as the person living with SMI (or a person familiar with the person) would need to identify what the antecedental and consequential conditions of the behavior were. At times this may be difficult because of problems with memory, social desirability, and other problems associated with self-report (Shipman et al., 2023).
- Use self-monitoring and technology: Self-awareness of one's behavior can be encouraged, shaped, and reinforced. Food, sleep, and activity diaries can be utilized to help monitor specific aspects of the targeted behavior. Self-monitoring can be facilitated by prompting individuals to track and record the targeted behavior through calls, texts, or automatic prompts at designated times to log the occurrence or non-occurrence of the behavior on a tablet, smartphone, or watch. Positive reinforcement can be provided for successfully completing self-monitoring.

Interventions to Change the Wellness Behaviors of Sleep, Dietary Habits, and Levels of Activity

- Environmental structuring and establishment of routines: Individuals living with SMI may lack routines, habits, or behaviors that support the regular occurrence of behaviors like eating, sleep, and physical activity. Neurocognitive impairments, social isolation, and low motivation can hinder activities like food preparation or adhering to bedtime rituals and participation in physical activity. Existing habits like daytime sleeping and dysregulated eating patterns may be negatively reinforced by short-term avoidance of boredom or anxiety/distress. Social isolation reduces access to cues that help maintain healthy sleep, eating patterns, and exercise, thereby reinforcing maladaptive behaviors.

- Develop and reinforce consistent daily routines that structure wake times, meals, sleep, and activity with the collaboration of the person living with SMI: Anchoring routines to notable environmental events promote predictability and reduce environmental ambiguity. Examples of salient or notable environmental events would be (a) eating meals in the morning upon awakening and evening meal when the sun is rising and setting; (b) going to bed at night; and (c) going for walk after breakfast. A person cannot be "forced" to go to sleep, eat healthy food, and exercise, but routines can help by establishing consistent and specific times to sleep, eat, and exercise.
- Increase control of environmental stimuli as cues for the behavior to occur: Encouraging food intake, sleep, and physical activity to occur at certain times and in designated areas will assist in establishing stimulus control as to when and where the behaviors should occur. Changing cues in the environment can prompt and encourage changes in the targeted behaviors.

  Sleep: Sleeping should occur only in the bedroom and in bed; minimize computer and TV use, caffeine, and stimulating activities before bed; plan preferred "quiet time" activities into the daily routine before bedtime. If getting to sleep during the night has been a problem, the person living with SMI may be overly sensitive to stimulation in the environment. Encourage preferred "quiet" activities such as taking a shower, listening to soft music, or reading a book, for about 20–30 minutes before going to bed. Avoid video games and other electronic devices before bedtime.

  Dietary behaviors: Eating meals at certain times and in one location without excessive noise and distractions will assist the person to attend to the behaviors associated with eating. If overeating is the problem, use smaller plates to decrease the amount of food that is seen and place snacks and other food items out of sight of the person living with SMI. Collaborate with the person to develop a list of healthy snack items and food items and make these foods available.

  Physical activity: With the collaboration of the person living with SMI, decide on type of activity, time, place, frequency, intensity, and duration of activity in which to engage. Set realistic and obtainable goals together. Ensure that the person is physically capable of engaging in physical activity.

- Use verbal and visual prompts and reminders: Provide verbal and visual cues or assistance to enhance the chances of the targeted behavior to occur. Have the person living with SMI read the prompts periodically to help with memory about the details of the encouraged behavior.
- Set realistic and obtainable goals: Set small and obtainable behavior changes with the collaboration of the person living with SMI. If the person is sedentary more than 8 hours, then a goal may be to have the person walk around the residence every 3–4 hours or after meals. Objectives and goals can be set depending on the data that are collected.
- Use reinforcement strategies: Reinforce adaptive eating, sleeping, and engaging in physical activity (e.g., praise for preparing and eating a balanced meal, adher-

ing to a bedtime, or taking a walk around the block). Use positive reinforcement (verbal praise, access to preferred activities, snack, privileges.) for behavior indicating progress. Consider realistic incentives for manifesting the behavior that is encouraged. If getting out of bed has been a problem, think about the incentives to use when the person living with SMI follows the routine for sleep and awakening. For example, a preferred food can be made available at breakfast when the person living with SMI gets up on time. Sometimes, another reinforcing preferred activity can also be made available for progress, like using a tablet or computer for a defined period.

- Do not overlook successes: Praise individuals living with SMI for adaptive behaviors, such as sticking to three meals when managing obesity. Recognize and reinforce every success, no matter how small.
- Reinforce the behavior as soon as possible after the behavior occurs so that there is an association between the targeted behavior and reinforcement: This is especially important when attempting to change a behavior that has been occurring for a long time and has a been effective for the person living with SMI. People living with SMI have problems with neurocognitive capabilities (e.g., memory) and with experiencing pleasure (e.g., anhedonia, hypohedonia). Therefore, the consequence for engaging in adaptive alternative behaviors must be potent and salient to the person.
- Initiate behavioral contracts: With the collaboration of the person living with SMI, define the alternative behaviors (e.g., getting out of bed by 8 a.m., eating one vegetable per meal, walking to the bus stop) and determine the reinforcers for displaying the adaptive behaviors. Include reinforcers chosen by the individual to increase compliance, ownership, and individualization. Include incentives into an agreement to encourage adaptive behaviors. Make specific rewards available for success in meeting the objectives specified in the contract. Acknowledge and praise small improvements to foster momentum in adherence and shape lasting change.
- Promote maintenance by fading prompts and support while continuing intermittent reinforcement for success.

Skills Training and Activity Scheduling

- Incorporate activity scheduling to counter inactivity, boredom, and low motivation: Plan stimulating and preferred daytime activities that reduce daytime sleep, appetite dysregulation, and sedentary behaviors.
- Use task analyses to break down complex self-care routines (e.g., preparing meals, getting ready for bed, preparing for physical activity).
- Train self-monitoring and self-management skills, such as using timers or visual prompts to signal when and where the alternative behavior is to occur.

Conclusion for Behavioral Strategies with Problematic Behaviors of Wellness

1. Be clear about what the problem is.
2. Observe the problem behavior to determine exactly what is occurring.
3. Provide a clear and concise definition of the adaptive alternative behavior (such as "Getting out of bed by 7a.m." or "Sleeping on bed only in the bedroom with lights and screens turned off.").
4. Decide whether it is worth the effort to try to accomplish the goal.
5. Engage and collaborate with the person living with SMI before any attempt is made to change a behavior.
6. Make sure that medications are correct, are being taken as prescribed, and the side effects have little impact on the problem behavior. Understand the effect they have on sleep, appetite, and motivation. Some medications are likely to impact drowsiness; others can make it more difficult to relax. Adjust expectations accordingly.
7. Avoid stimulating activities and the use of foods containing caffeine during the hours before going to bed. These make it more difficult to sleep.
8. Develop a regular schedule of routine and behaviors during certain hours of the day and be as consistent as possible. This helps to minimize boredom during the day and provides consistency as to expectations.
9. Consider working incentives into the routines that are developed. As much as possible, use incentives that the person who lives with SMI identifies. Consider developing a formal behavioral contract.
10. Remember to acknowledge the effort that the person living with SMI is making. It probably will take time to reestablish a routine and constantly engage in adaptive alternative behaviors.

What About Marcus?

Due to the interconnected nature of Marcus's eating, sleep, and activity patterns, the care team has prioritized a coordinated intervention strategy. Initial steps focused on moderating mealtime behaviors using controlled food pacing and prompting and reinforcing slow, regulated eating. His parents held ongoing consultations with a nutritionist, and weekly meal plans were developed. Soft drinks and juices were no longer purchased and were not available to Marcus. Marcus's parents established consistent bedtime routines and limiting evening screen exposure to improve sleep hygiene. To address inactivity, the team at the support program introduced brief, scheduled movement breaks supported by preferred reinforcers (like limited tablet time) and gradual exposure to structured recreational activities that he can do (e.g., slowly walking around building, shooting a basketball for 10–15 minutes). Slow and steady progress has been made. After 3 months of no episodes of regurgitation,

Marcus and his parents ate lunch at a fast-food restaurant for the first time in 15 years.

Summary

People with SMI frequently have notable physical health issues, which can result in a life expectancy that is 10–20 years shorter than that of the general population. Individuals living with SMI present health and wellness behavior challenges, specifically in the domains of sleep, diet, and physical activity. The interplay between chronic health issues and mental health conditions complicates healthcare access and management for these individuals. Chronic health problems are common due to health compromising behaviors such as dysregulated sleep patterns, physical inactivity, poor diet, smoking, and substance use. These findings present serious challenges in the assessment and treatment of people living with SMI given the poor coordination between mental and physical health services, which complicates treatment. There is an urgent need for coordinated care models that incorporate wellness behavior interventions into mental health services.

Individuals who live with SMI are at elevated risk for chronic conditions such as obesity, smoking-related conditions, metabolic syndrome, diabetes, and cardiovascular diseases. This increased risk contributes to substantially higher mortality rates and may result in up to 30 years of potential loss of life. Unhealthy lifestyle behaviors are more common among those who live with SMI and play a significant role in adverse physical health outcomes. These behaviors encompass higher rates of tobacco use, inadequate dietary patterns, and insufficient physical activity. Smoking prevalence is two to three times greater among individuals with SMI compared to the general population. Approximately 60%–70% of individuals with SMI do not achieve recommended physical activity levels. Poor nutritional habits are characterized by elevated caloric consumption and reduced diet quality, including excessive intake of sugars and starches.

There is an urgent need for integrated healthcare approaches to address the physical health issues of individuals living with SMI. Integrated healthcare can reduce the burden of mental health problems. Lifestyle interventions focusing on wellness behaviors can significantly improve overall health outcomes. Lifestyle interventions should focus on healthy eating, regular physical activity, and sleep hygiene. Addressing physical health can improve mental health outcomes and quality of life.

Sleep disturbances are common in individuals with SMI and are linked to various mental health issues, including depression and anxiety. Poor sleep quality can exacerbate mental health conditions and lead to increased risk of suicidal ideation. Approximately 40%–50% of people worldwide experience sleep deprivation. Insomnia is associated with a twofold increase in risk for developing depression and is present in about 85% of individuals who have depressive mental health conditions. Sleep apnea is prevalent among individuals who live with SMI, increasing the risk of depression and anxiety.

Individuals with SMI often face nutritional challenges that adversely affect their mental and physical health. Factors such as medication side effects, financial limitations, and emotional distress contribute to unhealthy eating patterns. Higher caloric and sodium intakes are common among individuals with SMI. Emotional eating is predictive of weight gain and is linked to feelings of guilt and distress. Limited resources and stigma around weight gain hinder access to healthy food options.

Physical inactivity is prevalent among individuals living with SMI, with various barriers preventing them from engaging in regular exercise. Understanding these barriers is crucial for promoting physical activity within this population. Low mood and stress are the most common barriers to physical activity, affecting 61% of individuals. Only a minority engage in physical activity at levels compatible with public health recommendations.

Motivational factors and external support are essential for encouraging physical activity. Motivation is a key factor influencing the participation of individuals who live with SMI in physical activity. Understanding the motivational processes can enhance participation rates and improve health outcomes. Individuals with SMI often experience low motivation and apathy, hindering physical activity engagement. Anticipatory and consummatory anhedonia can diminish the pleasure derived from physical activity. External and covert regulation can influence motivation for physical activity, highlighting the need for supportive interventions.

A healthy lifestyle is characterized by five primary behaviors: obtaining adequate sleep, practicing moderate alcohol consumption, abstaining from smoking, engaging in regular aerobic exercise, and maintaining a normal body weight. Among respondents without mental health conditions, only 6% practice all five healthy behaviors, while 24% engage in four of these behaviors. Adults aged 65 and over demonstrate the highest compliance with all five behaviors, at 10.1%. Between 50% and 70% of individuals who live with SMI do not participate in any of the recommended healthy behaviors, often due to multiple barriers. This lack of engagement contributes to early mortality, as a substantial proportion of this population does not adopt the advised health-related practices.

Sleep is a critical aspect of health that is often disrupted in individuals with SMI, affecting their overall well-being and cognitive function. Sleep problems are prevalent among this population, with significant implications for mental health. Sleep is defined as a reversible biobehavioral state involving neural activity and physiological changes. Mental health issues co-occur in 40%–50% of individuals with dysregulated sleep. Sleep problems are prevalent with 50% of individuals living with schizophrenia spectrum mental health problems and 80% with depression-type mental health problems experiencing sleep problems.

Sleep is a multidimensional phenomenon, characterized by behavior, physiology, and subjective experiences. The quality of sleep is influenced by various dimensions, including quantity, timing, environment, and subjective impressions of quality. Understanding these dimensions is essential for improving sleep health in individuals living with SMI. The recommended sleep duration is 7–8 hours for perceptions of feeling well. The best sleep quality is achieved by sleeping at night, ideally from 10 p.m. to 7 a.m. Sleep intrusions can occur during wakefulness, leading to cognitive impairments and experiences of dysphoria and anxiety. Sleep quality is a stronger indicator of psychological health than sleep duration.

Dietary habits among individuals with SMI are often problematic, leading to various health issues. Poor dietary habits are linked to obesity and other health problems. Understanding these habits is crucial for developing effective interventions. Eating-related mental health conditions are prevalent, characterized by abnormal eating behaviors. Dietary habits include meal frequency, rate of eating, snacking habits, and types of food consumed. Common assessment tools include dietary history questionnaires and food diaries.

Physical activity is essential for health, yet individuals living with SMI are significantly less active than the general population. Physical activity is defined as any bodily movement resulting in energy expenditure. Low activity levels are associated with increased risks of obesity, diabetes, and cardiovascular diseases. Most people who live with SMI—about 70%–75%—do not achieve the recommended 150 minutes of moderate exercise per week, increasing their risk of physical illnesses.

Assessing health-related behaviors in individuals living with SMI involves various methods, both subjective and objective. These assessments are crucial for understanding and improving health outcomes. Subjective methods include sleep diaries and dietary questionnaires, which may have validity issues. Objective methods like polysomnography and actigraphy provide more reliable data on sleep and physical activity. Actigraphy measures movement and can help monitor physical activity levels effectively.

Individuals with SMI frequently exhibit impairments in essential functional domains such as sleep, dietary habits, and physical activity. These challenges result from a complex interaction among neurocognitive dysfunction, neurological factors, and environmental conditions. Disruptions in sleep, nutrition, and exercise are prevalent in this population. Given the multifactorial nature of these real-world behaviors, comprehensive and integrated interventions are required.

Research indicates that individuals living with SMI exhibit gray matter loss in specific brain regions, which correlates with impaired executive functions (EFs) essential for daily tasks. Gray matter loss was found in the anterior insula cortex (aIC) and dorsal anterior cingulate cortex (dACC). Impaired EF includes difficulties in task initiation, organization, flexibility, and impulse control. Cortical thinning in key areas may impact EF and working memory rather than specific mental health symptoms.

Sleep is crucial for adaptive functioning, and dysregulation in sleep processes can lead to significant health issues, particularly in individuals who live with SMI. Sleep and wakefulness are separate processes that, if dysregulated, can harm the individual. Key brain regions involved in sleep regulation include the locus coeruleus (LC), salience network, anterior cingulate cortex (ACC), and insula cortex (INS). Dysfunctions in these areas are linked to sleep-related mental health conditions like insomnia, characterized by hyperarousal and emotional dysregulation.

Various brain regions and neurochemical factors regulate eating behaviors, which can lead to serious eating disorders influenced by developmental vulnerabilities. The hypothalamus (HYP) is central to energy homeostasis, integrating hunger and satiety signals. The insula context (INS) and amygdala (amyg) play roles in interoception and emotional responses to food. Eating disorders such as obesity and anorexia nervosa are linked to altered brain circuits and early life programming.

Most individuals who live with SMI do not participate in physical activity at recommended levels, largely attributable to diminished motivation and negative symptoms. Contributing factors include avolition, apathy, and neurocognitive impairments. Mental health challenges may result in reduced interest in physical activity, despite the well-established benefits associated with regular exercise. Apathy and avolition are linked to dysfunctions in the frontostriatal network and key brain regions like the ventromedial prefrontal cortex (vmPFC) and dorsal anterior cingulate cortex (dACC).

Individuals with SMI may lack essential functional skills due to disruptions during formative years, impacting their ability to engage in wellness behaviors. Early onset of SMI can limit opportunities to learn critical skills expected of functional adults. Disruptions such as psychiatric admissions and legal issues hinder skill acquisition. Neurocognitive challenges affect memory, attention, and planning, leading to persistent functional difficulties.

Wellness behaviors are essential for navigating daily activities and achieving a satisfactory quality of life (QoL), encompassing physical, social, emotional, and spiritual domains. Impairments in wellness behaviors can lead to decreases in QoL and physical health problems. The absence of learned wellness behaviors can result from inadequate exposure, lack of reinforcement, and environmental factors. Learning models like operant conditioning can effectively promote wellness behaviors.

Environmental factors substantially influence the development of wellness behaviors, with sensory sensitivities and exposure to trauma affecting the learning process. Inadequate positive reinforcement and the absence of effective role models can further impede the acquisition of adaptive behaviors. Additionally, negative interactions and traumatic experiences may evoke emotional responses that hinder the formation of health-promoting behaviors. Difficulties in organization and time management also present significant barriers to maintaining healthy practices.

Behavior-change techniques, such as Behavior Skills Training (BST), have demonstrated efficacy in modifying lifestyle behaviors among individuals who live with SMI. Interventions that prioritize habit formation can promote the long-term maintenance of adaptive behaviors beyond the duration of active intervention. Continuous and immediate reinforcement remains essential for establishing desired behaviors. Furthermore, complex wellness behaviors are more effectively learned when they are systematically shaped into manageable, incremental steps.

Understanding and addressing the epidemiological and cultural considerations of wellness behaviors, specifically focusing on sleep, dietary habits, and physical activity in individuals living with SMI are essential for assessment and treatment. Treating and assessing sleep issues in individuals living with SMI are necessary to enhance mental health outcomes. Sleep disturbances are prevalent in the SMI population, affecting their overall well-being and functioning. Sleep disturbances affect 26%–80% of individuals living with SMI. Common sleep-related challenges include insomnia, circadian rhythm problems, hypersomnia, restless legs syndrome, delayed sleep phase, and sleep-related breathing problems. Sleep issues can exacerbate mood dysregulation and cognitive impairments. Only 12% of individuals with SMI in community mental health settings are identified as having sleep problems, indicating potential under-identification.

As observed with sleep disturbances, individuals who live with SMI face an elevated risk of developing eating-related conditions, which may further complicate their overall mental health. The prevalence of eating-related mental health problems in those with SMI is significantly higher than in the general population, presenting considerable challenges for treatment and recovery. Dietary challenges can include overeating, undereating, and unhealthy eating patterns, which may persist even when other behaviors improve. Research indicates that most individuals with eating and dietary problems have at least one additional mental health condition, with estimates suggesting that 55%–97% of those with SMI experience a co-occurring eating problem.

Approximately 25.9% of individuals with SMI are classified as obese, and over 60% fall into the overweight or obese categories. Individuals exhibiting dysregulated dietary patterns and behaviors often present with co-occurring mental health conditions, including anxiety (62%), mood (54%), and substance use–related mental health issues (27%). Research indicates that having either an eating or dietary problem, or living with SMI, is associated with a four- to fivefold increased likelihood of developing the other.

Individuals with SMI tend to have higher levels of sedentary behavior, which is associated with physical and mental health outcomes. Research on these behaviors is important for designing appropriate interventions. People with SMI spend around 8 hours a day sedentary, more than healthy controls. Typical sedentary activities include watching television (2.8 hours per day) and sitting during travel (reported by 96% of participants). Physical activity levels are generally low, with a median of 2 hours per week spent walking and 4.5 hours per week engaged in moderate-to-vigorous physical activity. Interventions need to aim to promote more recreational walking and reduce time spent watching television.

Cultural, ethnic, and racial differences significantly influence mental health outcomes, including the prevalence and severity of mental health conditions. These disparities highlight the need for culturally sensitive approaches in mental healthcare. Factors contributing to disparities include discrimination, socioeconomic status, and healthcare access. Ethnic and racial minority groups experience higher rates of severe mental health problems compared to White adults. Black, Latinx, and Asian adults report poorer sleep quality and efficiency compared to White adults.

Obesity represents an escalating global health issue, with individuals living with SMI exhibiting notably higher prevalence rates. Recognizing regional variations in obesity and eating-related problematic conditions is essential for developing targeted interventions. Since 1990, global adult obesity has more than doubled, with 2.5 billion adults classified as overweight and 890 million living with obesity as of 2022. Among those with SMI, the obesity prevalence stands at 25.9%, demonstrating significant disparities across regions. The presentation of eating-related conditions also varies cross-culturally, shaped by diverse societal influences. For example, the prevalence of bulimia nervosa is approximately 0.87% in Africa compared to around 1.5% in the United States.

Physical activity levels vary significantly across cultures and regions, influenced by socioeconomic conditions and cultural norms. Understanding these differences is crucial for promoting physical activity among individuals with SMI. In Africa, 79% of the population meets the World Health Organization's (WHO) physical activity recommendations, primarily through occupational activity. Cultural norms in Arab countries lead to lower physical activity levels among women. In the United States, English-speaking Asian Americans and Hispanics show higher physical activity levels than their non-English-speaking counterparts. Income disparity is a significant predictor of physical activity engagement globally.

Quality of life (QoL) is recognized as a crucial outcome in health-related research and mental health treatment. Individuals who live with SMI frequently report a reduced QoL. A distinction exists between objective QoL indicators—such as employment and housing—and subjective QoL, which refers to perceived life satisfaction. Key determinants impacting QoL include employment status, problematic behaviors, and social support.

The factors influencing QoL are multifaceted, with diverse elements contributing to the overall well-being of individuals with SMI. Notably, mental health conditions such as depression do not invariably correspond with decreased life satisfaction, and neurocognitive functioning demonstrates a complex association with life satisfaction.

Health-related quality of life (HRQoL) measures the impact of physical and mental health on overall well-being. It assesses individual perceptions of health and evaluates daily functioning and perceptions of being well. High rates of co-occurring medical challenges and early mortality are prevalent in individuals living with SMI. Significant gender disparities exist, with women scoring lower in physical well-being satisfaction.

Individuals living with SMI often experience challenges related to sleep, nutrition, and physical activity. Reported sleep disturbances among people with SMI range from 26% to 80%, which can impact health-related quality of life (HRQoL). Dietary habits and medication side effects are factors that may contribute to chronic health conditions affecting perceived wellness. Studies indicate that up to 63% of those identified with schizophrenia spectrum mental health problems and 68% of those with bipolar-type of mental health problems are classified as overweight or obese. Obesity has been associated with lower HRQoL, with individuals who are obese reporting reduced weight-related HRQoL compared to those who are not obese.

Studies have found a correlation between increased physical activity and enhanced QoL in long-term hospitalized individuals with SMI. Improvements in QoL were noted across physical, psychological, and social domains, with the most significant changes occurring when moving from sedentary to light activity. Positive attitudes toward physical activity do not always translate into actual engagement, highlighting the need for integrated peer-supported interventions.

Health-related quality of life (HRQoL) among individuals living with SMI in southern Ethiopia was evaluated. Significant predictors of HRQoL included social support, marital status, occupation, diagnosis, and level of functional disability. Detrimental effects on HRQoL were linked to unemployment, presence of functional disabilities, and symptoms of depression.

Common problems among individuals with SMI include sleep disturbances, dietary habits, and sedentary behaviors. A survey indicated that nearly 75% of service providers identified eating and sleeping issues as more concerning than self-care or substance abuse problems.

Individuals living with SMI often face biological and physical challenges that contribute to issues with sleep, eating, and physical activity. These challenges include medical conditions, neurochemical disruptions, and the side effects of medications. Medical conditions like heart and lung issues can hinder sleep and physical activity. Neurochemical imbalances in neurotransmitters such as serotonin and dopamine disrupt mood, appetite, and sleep cycles. Medications for problem behavior linked to SMI can cause side effects like drowsiness and appetite changes, exacerbating wellness issues. Substance use can further destabilize neurochemical regulation, affecting hunger signals and the sleep–wake cycles.

Psychosocial and environmental factors significantly impact the wellness behaviors of individuals living with SMI. Stressors such as lack of daily routines, socioeconomic challenges, and social isolation contribute to irregular eating and sleeping patterns. Lack of structured routines can lead to erratic eating and sleeping behaviors. Socioeconomic challenges, including financial strain and housing instability, increase chronic stress and anxiety. Cognitive impairments associated with SMI can hinder the ability to maintain regular schedules for eating and sleeping. Social isolation reduces access to healthy meals and emotional support, complicating wellness management.

Difficulties related to eating, sleeping, and physical activity behaviors are interconnected and contribute to wellness challenges among individuals living with SMI, with these factors influencing one another through biological, behavioral, and psychosocial mechanisms. Medication side effects can lead to increased appetite and disrupted sleep patterns. Disrupted daily routines contribute to irregular eating and sleeping behaviors. Neurocognitive impairments reduce motivation and initiative for healthy behaviors. Environmental stressors can exacerbate emotional dysregulation, leading to a cycle of poor wellness behaviors.

Implementing effective behavioral support strategies necessitates a thorough understanding of everyone's unique needs and circumstances. Actively involving individuals living with SMI in the process is fundamental to achieving successful outcomes. It is important to clearly identify and define problematic behaviors related to eating, sleeping, and physical activity.

Work collaboratively with the individual to establish goals that are both achievable and realistic, taking into account their unique preferences and circumstances. This joint process fosters a sense of ownership and ensures that objectives are meaningful and attainable.

Consistently monitor and record behaviors related to wellness, such as eating, sleeping, and physical activity patterns. Systematic tracking helps identify relevant trends, triggers, and barriers, informing future interventions and adjustments to routines.

Utilize reinforcement strategies to encourage the adoption of adaptive behaviors. Recognize and formally celebrate accomplishments, whether they are incremental improvements or significant milestones, to sustain motivation and reinforce ongoing progress.

Creating structured routines and effectively controlling environmental stimuli play a crucial role in enhancing wellness behaviors for individuals living with SMI. Establishing consistent schedules for key activities—including meals, sleep, and physical exercise—provides a reliable framework that supports healthy behavioral patterns. By developing daily routines anchor to notable environmental events, individuals can more easily integrate adaptive behaviors into their everyday lives.

It is important to encourage the use of specific times and designated locations for eating, sleeping, and engaging in physical activity. This consistency helps reinforce behavioral expectations and reduces confusion or uncertainty around daily activities. To further support adherence to these routines, both verbal and visual prompts can be utilized. These cues serve as helpful reminders, enhancing memory and supporting individuals in maintaining their routines.

Reinforcing adaptive behaviors through positive reinforcement and incentives is also essential. Recognizing and rewarding efforts—whether through verbal praise or tangible rewards—can motivate individuals to continue engaging in healthy behaviors, ultimately leading to sustained improvements in overall wellness.

Engaging individuals with SMI in their recovery process fosters a sense of ownership and increases the likelihood of successful behavior change. Building trust and rapport is essential for effective collaboration. Develop rapport by utilizing active listening skills and demonstrating empathetic communication. Collaborate with individuals to identify personal goals and preferences and employ motivational interviewing strategies to support open dialog regarding behavioral changes and wellness improvement. Recognize and praise incremental achievements to reinforce ongoing progress.

References

Afzal, M., Siddiqi, N., Ahmad, B., Afsheen, N., Aslam, F., Ali, A., Ayesha, R., Bryant, M., Holt, R., Khalid, H., Ishaq, K., Koly, K. N., Rajan, S., Saba, J., Tirbhowan, N., & Zavala, G. A. (2021). Prevalence of overweight and obesity in people with severe mental illness: Systematic review and meta-analysis. *Frontiers in Endocrinology, 12*, 769309. https://doi.org/10.3389/fendo.2021.769309

Allison, K. C., Lundgren, J. D., O'Reardon, J. P., Geliebter, A., Gluck, M. E., Vinai, P., Serafini, P., Cassone, S., Nasser, J. A., Grilo, C. M., & Stunkard, A. J. (2010). Proposed diagnostic criteria for night eating syndrome. *International Journal of Eating Disorders, 43*(3), 241–247. https://doi.org/10.1002/eat.20693

American Psychiatric Association. (2022a). *Diagnostic and statistical manual of mental disorders* (5th ed., text rev.). https://doi.org/10.1176/appi.books.9780890425787

American Psychiatric Association. (2022b). Feeding and eating disorders. In *Diagnostic and statistical manual of mental disorders* (5th ed., text rev.). https://doi.org/10.1176/appi.books.9780890425787.x10_Feeding_and_Eating_Disorders

American Psychiatric Association. (2022c). Restless legs syndrome. In *Diagnostic and statistical manual of mental disorders* (5th ed., text rev.). https://doi.org/10.1176/appi.books.9780890425787

American Psychiatric Association. (2022d). Sleep-wake disorders. In *Diagnostic and statistical manual of mental disorders* (5th ed., text rev., pp. 361–422). American Psychiatric Publishing. https://doi.org/10.1176/appi.books.9780890425787

American Psychological Association. (n.d.-a). Actigraphy. In *APA dictionary of psychology*. https://dictionary.apa.org/actigraphy

American Psychological Association. (n.d.-b). Anhedonia. In *APA dictionary of psychology*. https://dictionary.apa.org/anhedonia

American Psychological Association. (n.d.-c). Cognitive resource theory. In *APA dictionary of psychology*. https://dictionary.apa.org/cognitive-resource-theory

American Psychological Association. (n.d.-d). Eating disorders. In *APA dictionary of psychology*. https://www.apa.org/topics/eating-disorders

American Psychological Association. (n.d.-e). Executive functions. In *APA dictionary of psychology*. https://dictionary.apa.org/executive-function

American Psychological Association. (n.d.-f). Impairment. In *APA dictionary of psychology*. https://dictionary.apa.org/impairment

American Psychological Association. (n.d.-g). Learned helplessness. In *APA dictionary of psychology*. https://dictionary.apa.org/learned-helplessness

American Psychological Association. (n.d.-h). Melatonin. In *APA dictionary of psychology*. https://dictionary.apa.org/melatonin

American Psychological Association. (n.d.-i). Neurogenesis. In *APA dictionary of psychology*. https://dictionary.apa.org/neurogensis

American Psychological Association. (n.d.-j). Operational definition. In *APA dictionary of psychology*. https://dictionary.apa.org/operational-definition

American Psychological Association. (n.d.-k). Self-efficacy. In *APA dictionary of psychology*. https://dictionary.apa.org/self-efficacy

American Psychological Association. (n.d.-l). Sleep apnea. In *APA dictionary of psychology*. https://dictionary.apa.org/sleep-apnea

American Psychological Association. (n.d.-m). Polysomnography. In *APA dictionary of psychology*. https://dictionary.apa.org/polysomnography

American Psychological Association. (n.d.-n). Wellness. In *APA dictionary of psychology*. https://dictionary.apa.org/wellness

Anderson, N., & Ozakinci, G. (2018). Effectiveness of psychological interventions to improve quality of life in people with long-term conditions: Rapid systematic review of randomised controlled trials. *BMC Psychology, 6*, 1–17. https://doi.org/10.1186/s40359-018-0225-4

Andrillon, T., & Oudiette, D. (2023). What is sleep exactly? Global and local modulations of sleep oscillations all around the clock. *Neuroscience & Biobehavioral Reviews, 155*, 105465. https://doi.org/10.1016/j.neubiorev.2023.105465

Arlinghaus, K. R., & Johnston, C. A. (2019). The importance of creating habits and routine. *American Journal of Lifestyle Medicine, 13*(2), 142–144. https://doi.org/10.1177/1559827618818044

Baggetta, P., & Alexander, P. A. (2016). Conceptualization and operationalization of executive function. *Mind, Brain, and Education, 10*(1), 10–33. https://doi.org/10.1111/mbe.12100

Barlow, D. H., & Nock, M. K. (2009). Why can't we be more idiographic in our research? *Perspectives on Psychological Science, 4*(1), 19–21. https://doi.org/10.1111/j.1745-6924.2009.01088.x

Barnes, A. L., Murphy, M. E., Fowler, C. A., & Rempfer, M. V. (2012). Health-related quality of life and overall life satisfaction in people with serious mental illness. *Schizophrenia Research and Treatment, 2012*(1), 245103. https://doi.org/10.1155/2012/245103

Bechi, M., Bosia, M., Spangaro, M., Buonocore, M., Cavedoni, S., Agostoni, G., Cocchi, F., Guglielmino, C., Smeraldi, E., & Cavallaro, R. (2017). Exploring functioning in schizophrenia: Predictors of functional capacity and real-world behaviour. *Psychiatry Research, 251*, 118–124. https://doi.org/10.1016/j.psychres.2017.02.019

Bellack, A. S. (2004). Skills training for people with severe mental illness. *Psychiatric Rehabilitation Journal, 27*(4), 375–391. https://doi.org/10.2975/27.2004.375.391

Beltz, A. M., Wright, A. G., Sprague, B. N., & Molenaar, P. C. (2016). Bridging the nomothetic and idiographic approaches to the analysis of clinical data. *Assessment, 23*(4), 447–458. https://doi.org/10.1177/1073191116648209

Benoit, A., Bodnar, M., Malla, A. K., Joober, R., & Lepage, M. (2012). The structural neural substrates of persistent negative symptoms in first-episode of non-affective psychosis: A voxel-based morphometry study. *Frontiers in Psychiatry, 3*, 42. https://doi.org/10.3389/fpsyt.2012.00042

Bernert, R. A., & Joiner, T. E. (2007). Sleep disturbances and suicide risk: A review of the literature. *Neuropsychiatric Disease and Treatment, 3*(6), 735–743. https://doi.org/10.2147/ndt.s1248

Billings, M. E., Hale, L., & Johnson, D. A. (2020). Physical and social environment relationship with sleep health and disorders. *Chest, 157*(5), 1304–1312. https://doi.org/10.1016/j.chest.2019.12.002

Bort-Roig, J., Briones-Buixassa, L., Felez-Nobrega, M., Guàrdia-Sancho, A., Sitjà-Rabert, M., & Puig-Ribera, A. (2020). Sedentary behaviour associations with health outcomes in people with severe mental illness: A systematic review. *European Journal of Public Health, 30*(1), 150–157. https://doi.org/10.1093/eurpub/ckz016

Bradshaw, T., & Mairs, H. (2014). Obesity and serious mental ill health: A critical review of the literature. *Healthcare, 2*(2), 166–182. MDPI. https://doi.org/10.3390/healthcare2020166

Briguglio, M., Vitale, J. A., Galentino, R., Banfi, G., Zanaboni Dina, C., Bona, A., Panascì, S., Ricevuti, G., & Glick, I. D. (2020). Healthy eating, physical activity, and sleep hygiene (HEPAS) as the winning triad for sustaining physical and mental health in patients at risk for or with neuropsychiatric disorders: Considerations for clinical practice. *Neuropsychiatric Disease and Treatment, 16*, 55–70. https://doi.org/10.2147/NDT.S229206

Caspersen, C. J., Powell, K. E., & Christenson, G. M. (1985). Physical activity, exercise, and physical fitness: Definitions and distinctions for health-related research. *Public Health Reports, 100*(2), 126–131. https://doi.org/10.2307/20056429

Caton, S. J., Nolan, L. J., & Hetherington, M. M. (2015). Alcohol, appetite and loss of restraint. *Current Obesity Reports, 4*, 99–105. https://doi.org/10.1007/s13679-014-0130-y

Centers for Disease Control and Prevention (CDC). (n.d.-a). *About sleep*. U.S. Department of Health & Human Services. https://www.cdc.gov/sleep/about/index.html

Centers for Disease Control and Prevention (CDC). (n.d.-b). *What counts as aerobic activity?* U.S. Department of Health & Human Services. https://www.cdc.gov/physical-activity-basics/adding-adults/what-counts.html

Chafetz, L., White, M., Collins-Bride, G., Cooper, B. A., & Nickens, J. (2008). Clinical trial of wellness training: Health promotion for severely mentally ill adults. *The Journal of Nervous and Mental Disease, 196*(6), 475–483. https://doi.org/10.1097/NMD.0b013e31817738de

Chapman, J. J., Fraser, S. J., Brown, W. J., & Burton, N. W. (2016). Physical activity and sedentary behaviour of adults with mental illness. *Journal of Science and Medicine in Sport, 19*(7), 579–584. https://doi.org/10.1016/j.jsams.2015.07.017

Cheng, Z. H., Perko, V. L., Fuller-Marashi, L., Gau, J. M., & Stice, E. (2019). Ethnic differences in eating disorder prevalence, risk factors, and predictive effects of risk factors among young women. *Eating Behaviors, 32*, 23–30. https://doi.org/10.1016/j.eatbeh.2018.11.004

Cohen, A. S., Morrison, S. C., Brown, L. A., & Minor, K. S. (2012). Towards a cognitive resource limitations model of diminished expression in schizotypy. *Journal of Abnormal Psychology, 121*(1), 109–118. https://doi.org/10.1037/a0023599

Colillas-Malet, E., Prat, G., Espelt, A., & Juvinyà, D. (2020). Gender differences in health-related quality of life in people with severe mental illness. *PLoS One, 15*(2), e0229236. https://doi.org/10.1371/journal.pone.0229236

Cooper, J. O., Heron, T. E., & Heward, W. L. (2020). *Applied behavior analysis* (3rd ed.). Pearson Education. https://www.pearson.com/en-us/pearsonplus/p/9780137477210

Correll, C. U., & Schooler, N. R. (2020). Negative symptoms in schizophrenia: A review and clinical guide for recognition, assessment, and treatment. *Neuropsychiatric Disease and Treatment, 16*, 519–534. https://doi.org/10.2147/NDT.S225643

Correll, C. U., Solmi, M., Veronese, N., Bortolato, B., Rosson, S., Santonastaso, P., Pigato, G., Favaro, A., Monaco, F., Spinazzola, E., & Stubbs, B. (2017). Prevalence, incidence and mortality from cardiovascular disease in patients with pooled and specific severe mental illness: A large-scale meta-analysis of 3,211,768 patients and 113,383,368 controls. *World Psychiatry, 16*(2), 163–180. https://doi.org/10.1002/wps.20420

de Medina-Moragas, A. J., Lima-Serrano, M., Fernández-Fernández, M. J., & Lima-Rodríguez, J. S. (2024). Quality of life of individuals with serious mental illness and family caregivers. *Current Psychology, 43*(25), 21756–21767. https://doi.org/10.1007/s12144-024-05961-2

De Mooij, L. D., Kikkert, M., Theunissen, J., Beekman, A. T., De Haan, L., Duurkoop, P. W., Peen, J., & Dekker, J. J. M. (2019). Dying too soon: Excess mortality in severe mental illness. *Frontiers in Psychiatry, 10*, 855. https://doi.org/10.3389/fpsyt.2019.00855

Deenik, J., Kruisdijk, F., Tenback, D., Braakman-Jansen, A., Taal, E., Hopman-Rock, M., van Gool, A. R., & van Harten, P. (2017). Physical activity and quality of life in long-term hospitalized patients with severe mental illness: A cross-sectional study. *BMC Psychiatry, 17*, 298. https://doi.org/10.1186/s12888-017-1466-0

Defar, S., Abraham, Y., Reta, Y., Deribe, B., Jisso, M., Yeheyis, T., Tadesse, M., & Ayalew, M. (2023). Health related quality of life among people with mental illness: The role of socio-clinical characteristics and level of functional disability. *Frontiers in Public Health, 11*, 1134032. https://doi.org/10.3389/fpubh.2023.1134032

Di Domenico, S. I., & Ryan, R. M. (2017). The emerging neuroscience of intrinsic motivation: A new frontier in self-determination research. *Frontiers in Human Neuroscience, 11*, 145. https://doi.org/10.3389/fnhum.2017.00145

Drake, R. E., & Mueser, K. T. (1996). Alcohol-use disorder and severe mental illness. *Alcohol Health and Research World, 20*(2), 87–93. https://pubs.niaaa.nih.gov/publications/arh20-2/87.pdf

Fekedulegn, D., Andrew, M. E., Shi, M., Violanti, J. M., Knox, S., & Innes, K. E. (2020). Actigraphy-based assessment of sleep parameters. *Annals of Work Exposures and Health, 64*(4), 350–367. https://doi.org/10.1093/annweh/wxaa007

Fernandez-Ballesteros, R. (2004). Assessment and evaluation, overview. In C. D. Spielberger (Ed.), *Encyclopedia of applied psychology* (Vol. 1, pp. 163–176). Academic Press. https://doi.org/10.1016/B0-12-657410-3/00373-1

Firth, J., Rosenbaum, S., Stubbs, B., Gorczynski, P., Yung, A. R., & Vancampfort, D. (2016). Motivating factors and barriers towards exercise in severe mental illness: A systematic review and meta-analysis. *Psychological Medicine, 46*(14), 2869–2881. https://doi.org/10.1017/S0033291716001732

Firth, J., Siddiqi, N., Koyanagi, A. I., Siskind, D., Rosenbaum, S., Galletly, C., Allan, S., Alexis, D., Carney, R., Carvalho, A. F., Chatterton, M. L., Correll, C. U., Curtis, J., Gaughran, F., Heald, A., Hoare, E., Jackson, S. E., Kisely, S., Lovell, K., et al. (2019). The Lancet Psychiatry Commission: a blueprint for protecting physical health in people with mental illness. *The Lancet Psychiatry, 6*(8), 675–712. https://doi.org/10.1016/S2215-0366(19)30132-4

Firth, J., Solmi, M., Wootton, R. E., Vancampfort, D., Schuch, F. B., Hoare, E., Gilbody, S., Torous, J., Teasdale, S. B., Jackson, S. E., Smith, L., Eaton, M., Jacka, F. N., & Stubbs, B. (2020). A meta-review of "lifestyle psychiatry": The role of exercise, smoking, diet and sleep in the prevention and treatment of mental disorders. *World Psychiatry, 19*(3), 360–380. https://doi.org/10.1002/wps.20773

Foussias, G., & Remington, G. (2010). Negative symptoms in schizophrenia: Avolition and Occam's razor. *Schizophrenia Bulletin, 36*(2), 359–369. https://doi.org/10.1093/schbul/sbn094

Freeman, D., Sheaves, B., Goodwin, G. M., Yu, L. M., Nickless, A., Harrison, P. J., Emsley, R., Luik, A. I., Foster, R. G., & Espie, C. A. (2017). The effects of improving sleep on mental health (OASIS): A randomised controlled trial with mediation analysis. *The Lancet Psychiatry, 4*(10), 749–758. https://doi.org/10.1016/S2215-0366(17)30328-0

Freeman, D., Sheaves, B., Waite, F., Harvey, A. G., & Harrison, P. J. (2020). Sleep disturbance and psychiatric disorders. *The Lancet Psychiatry, 7*(7), 628–637. https://doi.org/10.1016/s2215-0366(20)30136-x

Giordano, G. M., Koenig, T., Mucci, A., Vignapiano, A., Amodio, A., Di Lorenzo, G., Siracusano, A., & Maj, M. (2018). Neurophysiological correlates of avolition-apathy in schizophrenia: A resting-EEG microstates study. *NeuroImage: Clinical, 20*, 627–636. https://doi.org/10.1016/j.nicl.2018.08.031

Goodkind, M., Eickhoff, S. B., Oathes, D. J., Jiang, Y., Chang, A., Jones-Hagata, L. B., Ortega, B. N., Zaiko, Y. V., Roach, B. J., Korgaonkar, M. S., Grieve, S. M., Galatzer-Levy, I., Fox, P. T., & Etkin, A. (2015). Identification of a common neurobiological substrate for mental illness. *JAMA Psychiatry, 72*(4), 305–315. https://doi.org/10.1001/jamapsychiatry.2014.2206

Gopalakrishnan, A., Venkataraman, R., Gururajan, R., Zhou, X., & Genrich, R. (2022). Mobile phone enabled mental health monitoring to enhance diagnosis for severity assessment of behaviours: A review. *PeerJ Computer Science, 8*, e1042. https://doi.org/10.7717/peerj-cs.1042

Green, M. F. (1996). What are the functional consequences of neurocognitive deficits in schizophrenia? *The American Journal of Psychiatry, 153*(3), 321–330. https://doi.org/10.1176/ajp.153.3.321

Greenwood, J. L., Lin, J., Arguello, D., Ball, T., & Shaw, J. M. (2012). Healthy eating vital sign: A new assessment tool for eating behaviors. *International Scholarly Research Notices, 2012*(1), 734682. https://doi.org/10.5402/2012/734682

Gupta, M. A., & Simpson, F. C. (2015). Obstructive sleep apnea and psychiatric disorders: A systematic review. *Journal of Clinical Sleep Medicine, 11*(2), 165–175. https://doi.org/10.5664/jcsm.4466

Hambleton, A., Pepin, G., Le, A., Maloney, D., National Eating Disorder Research Consortium, Touyz, S., & Maguire, S. (2022). Psychiatric and medical comorbidities of eating disorders: Findings from a rapid review of the literature. Journal of Eating Disorders, 10(1), 132. https://doi.org/10.1186/s40337-022-00654-2

Harvey, P. D., & Strassnig, M. (2012). Predicting the severity of everyday functional disability in people with schizophrenia: Cognitive deficits, functional capacity, symptoms, and health status. *World Psychiatry, 11*(2), 73–79. https://doi.org/10.1016/j.wpsyc.2012.05.004

Harvey, P. D., Koren, D., Reichenberg, A., & Bowie, C. R. (2006). Negative symptoms and cognitive deficits: What is the nature of their relationship? *Schizophrenia Bulletin, 32*(2), 250–258. https://doi.org/10.1093/schbul/sbj011

Hassan, J., Shannon, S., Tully, M. A., McCartan, C., Davidson, G., Bunn, R., & Breslin, G. (2022). Systematic review of physical activity interventions assessing physical and mental health outcomes on patients with severe mental illness (SMI) within secure forensic settings. *Journal of Psychiatric and Mental Health Nursing, 29*(5), 630–646. https://doi.org/10.1111/jpm.12832

Hatfield, A., Coursey, R., & Slaughter, J. (1994). Family responses to behaviors and illness. *Innovation and Research, 3*, 41–47. https://psycnet.apa.org/record/1995-28887-001

Hayes, J. F., Marston, L., Walters, K., King, M. B., & Osborn, D. P. (2017). Mortality gap for people with bipolar disorder and schizophrenia: UK-based cohort study 2000–2014. *The British Journal of Psychiatry, 211*(3), 175–181. https://doi.org/10.1192/bjp.bp.117.202606

Heinrichs, R. W., & Zakzanis, K. K. (1998). Neurocognitive deficit in schizophrenia: A quantitative review of the evidence. *Neuropsychology, 12*(3), 426–445. https://doi.org/10.1037/0894-4105.12.3.426

Heron, P. N., Henderson, L. M., Crosland, S., Gilbody, S. M., Johnston, G. A., Moriarty, A. S., Armitage, C. J., Hann, M., & Peckham, E. (2022). Sleep health among people with severe mental ill health during the COVID-19 pandemic: Results from a linked UK population cohort study. *Frontiers in Psychiatry, 13*, 975593. https://doi.org/10.3389/fpsyt.2022.975593

Heuven, L. A., van Bruinessen, M., Tang, C. S., Stieger, M., Lasschuijt, M. P., & Forde, C. G. (2024). Consistent effect of eating rate on food and energy intake across twenty-four ad libitum meals. *British Journal of Nutrition, 132*(4), 535–546. https://doi.org/10.1017/S0007114524001478

Huang, Y., Wang, W., Hei, G., Shao, T., Li, L., Yang, Y., Zhang, Y., Zhang, X., & Wu, R. (2025). Subgroups of cognitive impairments in schizophrenia characterized by executive function and their morphological features: A latent profile analysis study. *BMC Medicine, 23*(1), 13. https://doi.org/10.1186/s12916-024-03835-9

Huo, K., Shao, F., & Zhang, Z. (2025). Causal effects of schizophrenia on sleep and eating disorders: A Mendelian randomization study. *Medicine, 104*(18), e42334. https://doi.org/10.1097/MD.0000000000042334

Jayasinghe, S., Byrne, N. M., & Hills, A. P. (2025). Cultural influences on dietary choices. *Progress in Cardiovascular Diseases*. https://doi.org/10.1016/j.pcad.2025.02.003

Jo, Y. H., Talmage, D. A., & Role, L. W. (2002). Nicotinic receptor-mediated effects on appetite and food intake. *Journal of Neurobiology, 53*(4), 618–632. https://doi.org/10.1002/neu.10147

John, A., McGregor, J., Jones, I., Lee, S. C., Walters, J. T., Owen, M. J., O'Donovan, M. C., DelPozo-Banos, M., Hall, J., & Lloyd, K. (2018). Premature mortality among people with severe mental illness - New evidence from linked primary care data. *Schizophrenia Research, 199*, 154–162. https://doi.org/10.1016/j.schres.2018.04.009

Kalinowska, S., Trześniowska-Drukała, B., Kłoda, K., Safranow, K., Misiak, B., Cyran, A., & Samochowiec, J. (2021). The association between lifestyle choices and schizophrenia symptoms. *Journal of Clinical Medicine, 10*(165), 165. https://doi.org/10.3390/jcm10010165

Karnieli-Miller, O., & Salyers, M. P. (2011). Clinical communication with persons who have serious mental illness. In A. Rudnick & D. Roe (Eds.), *Serious mental illness: Person-centered approaches* (pp. 155–167). Radcliffe Publishing.

Kaufmann, C. N., Susukida, R., & Depp, C. A. (2017). Sleep apnea, psychopathology, and mental health care. *Sleep Health, 3*(4), 244–249. https://doi.org/10.1016/j.sleh.2017.04.003

Kayton, L., & Koh, S. D. (1975). Hypohedonia in schizophrenia. *Journal of Nervous and Mental Disease, 161*(6), 412–420. https://doi.org/10.1097/00005053-197512000-00005

Kennaway, D. J., & Wright, H. (2002). Melatonin and circadian rhythms. *Current Topics in Medicinal Chemistry, 2*(2), 199–209. https://doi.org/10.2174/1568026023394380

Kessler, R. C., Berglund, P. A., Bruce, M. L., Koch, J. R., Laska, E. M., Leaf, P. J., Manderscheid, R. W., & Wang, P. S. (2001). The prevalence and correlates of untreated serious mental illness. *Health Services Research, 36*(6 Pt 1), 987–1007. https://www.ncbi.nlm.nih.gov/pmc/articles/PMC1089240/

Kluge, A., Kirschner, M., Hager, O. M., Bischof, M., Habermeyer, B., Seifritz, E., Walther, S., & Kaiser, S. (2018). Combining actigraphy, ecological momentary assessment and neuroimaging to study apathy in patients with schizophrenia. *Schizophrenia Research, 195*, 176–182. https://doi.org/10.1016/j.schres.2017.09.034

Knutson, K. L. (2013). Sociodemographic and cultural determinants of sleep deficiency: Implications for cardiometabolic disease risk. *Social Science & Medicine, 79*, 7–15. https://doi.org/10.1016/j.socscimed.2012.05.002

Kolotkin, R. L., Corey-Lisle, P. K., Crosby, R. D., Swanson, J. M., Tuomari, A. V., L'Italien, G. J., & Mitchell, J. E. (2008). Impact of obesity on health-related quality of life in schizophrenia and bipolar disorder. *Obesity, 16*(4), 749–754. http://www.nature.com/doifinder/10.1038/oby.2007.133

Konttinen, H. (2020). Emotional eating and obesity in adults: The role of depression, sleep and genes. *Proceedings of the Nutrition Society, 79*(3), 283–289. https://doi.org/10.1017/S0029665120000166

Kouidrat, Y., Amad, A., Lalau, J. D., & Loas, G. (2014). Eating disorders in schizophrenia: Implications for research and management. *Schizophrenia Research and Treatment, 2014*(1), 791573. https://doi.org/10.1155/2014/791573

Lally, P., & Gardner, B. (2011). Promoting habit formation. *Health Psychology Review, 7*(Suppl. 1), S137–S158. https://doi.org/10.1080/17437199.2011.603640

Li, Y., Rekhi, G., Ang, M. S., & Lee, J. (2023). Impact of negative symptoms on health-related quality of life in schizophrenia. *Frontiers in Psychiatry, 14*, 1252354. https://doi.org/10.3389/fpsyt.2023.1252354

Lindamer, L. A., McKibbin, C., Norman, G. J., Jordan, L., Harrison, K., Abeyesinhe, S., & Patrick, K. (2008). Assessment of physical activity in middle-aged and older adults with schizophrenia. *Schizophrenia Research, 104*(1–3), 294–301. https://doi.org/10.1016/j.schres.2008.04.040

Liu, Y., Croft, J. B., Wheaton, A. G., Kanny, D., Cunningham, T. J., Lu, H., Greenlund, K. J., & Giles, W. H. (2016). Clustering of five health-related behaviors for chronic disease prevention among adults, United States, 2013. *Preventing Chronic Disease, 13*, E70. https://doi.org/10.5888/pcd13.160054

Marder, S. R., & Galderisi, S. (2017). The current conceptualization of negative symptoms in schizophrenia. *World Psychiatry, 16*(1), 14–24. https://doi.org/10.1002/wps.20385

Meiselman, H. L. (2016). Quality of life, well-being and wellness: Measuring subjective health for foods and other products. *Food Quality and Preference, 54*, 101–109. https://doi.org/10.1016/j.foodqual.2016.05.009

Mizia, S., Felińczak, A., Włodarek, D., & Syrkiewicz-Świtała, M. (2021). Evaluation of eating habits and their impact on health among adolescents and young adults: A cross-sectional study. *International Journal of Environmental Research and Public Health, 18*(8), 3996. https://doi.org/10.3390/ijerph18083996

Molloy, D. W., Bédard, M., Guyatt, G. H., & Lever, J. (1997). Dysfunctional behavior rating instrument. *International Psychogeriatrics, 8*(S3), 333–341. https://doi.org/10.1017/S104161029700358X

Momen, N. C., Plana-Ripoll, O., Yilmaz, Z., Thornton, L. M., McGrath, J. J., Bulik, C. M., & Petersen, L. V. (2022). Comorbidity between eating disorders and psychiatric disorders. *International Journal of Eating Disorders, 55*(4), 505–517. https://doi.org/10.1002/eat.23687

Morrison, R. L., & Wixted, J. T. (1989). Social skills training. In A. S. Bellack (Ed.), *A clinical guide for the treatment of schizophrenia*. Springer. https://doi.org/10.1007/978-1-4757-8979-9_10

Mosolov, S. N., & Yaltonskaya, P. A. (2022). Primary and secondary negative symptoms in schizophrenia. *Frontiers in Psychiatry, 12*, 766692. https://doi.org/10.3389/fpsyt.2021.766692

Mueller-Stierlin, A. S., Cornet, S., Peisser, A., Jaeckle, S., Lehle, J., Moerkl, S., & Teasdale, S. B. (2022). Implications of dietary intake and eating behaviors for people with serious mental illness: A qualitative study. *Nutrients, 14*(13), 2616. https://doi.org/10.3390/nu14132616

National Eating Disorders Collaboration (NEDC). (n.d.). *Co-occurring conditions*. https://nedc.com.au/eating-disorders/types/co-occurring-conditions

National Heart, Lung, and Blood Institute (NHLBI). (n.d.-a). *Circadian rhythms and the sleep-wake cycle*. U.S. Department of Health and Human Services, National Institutes of Health. https://www.nhlbi.nih.gov/health/sleep/sleep-wake-cycle

National Heart, Lung, and Blood Institute (NHLBI). (n.d.-b). *Sleep apnea*. U.S. Department of Health and Human Services, National Institutes of Health. https://www.nhlbi.nih.gov/health/sleep-apnea

National Institute on Drug Abuse (NIDA). (2023, February 24). *Do people with mental illness and substance use disorders use tobacco more often?* https://nida.nih.gov/publications/research-reports/tobacco-nicotine-e-cigarettes/do-people-mental-illness-substance-use-disorders-use-tobacco-more-often

National Sleep Foundation (NSF). (2024, April 12). *What is sleep quality?* https://www.thensf.org/what-is-sleep-quality

Nemec, K. (2020). Cultural awareness of eating patterns in the health care setting. *Clinical Liver Disease, 16*(5), 204–207. https://doi.org/10.1002/cld.1019

Office of Disease Prevention and Health Promotion (ODPHP). (n.d.). *Physical activity guidelines for Americans*. U.S. Department of Health and Human Services. https://odphp.health.gov/our-work/nutrition-physical-activity/physical-activity-guidelines/current-guidelines

Ohayon, M., Wickwire, E. M., Hirshkowitz, M., Albert, S. M., Avidan, A., Daly, F. J., Ferber, R., & Vitiello, M. V. (2017). National sleep foundation's sleep quality recommendations: First report. *Sleep Health, 3*(1), 6–19. https://doi.org/10.1016/j.sleh.2016.11.006

Ohrnberger, J., Fichera, E., & Sutton, M. (2017). The relationship between physical and mental health: A mediation analysis. *Social Science & Medicine, 195*, 42–49. https://doi.org/10.1016/j.socscimed.2017.11.008

Ostrow, L., Manderscheid, R., & Mojtabai, R. (2014). Stigma and difficulty accessing medical care in a sample of adults with serious mental illness. *Journal of Health Care for the Poor and Underserved, 25*(4), 1956–1965. https://doi.org/10.1353/hpu.2014.0185

Provencher, H. L., & Mueser, K. T. (1997). Positive and negative symptom behaviors and caregiver burden in the relatives of persons with schizophrenia. *Schizophrenia Research, 26*(1), 71–80. https://doi.org/10.1016/S0920-9964(97)00043-1

RachBeisel, J., Scott, J., & Dixon, L. (1999). Co-occurring severe mental illness and substance use disorders: A review of recent research. *Psychiatric Services, 50*(11), 1427–1434. https://doi.org/10.1176/ps.50.11.1427

Rio, C. J., & Saligan, L. N. (2023). Understanding physical activity from a cultural-contextual lens. *Frontiers in Public Health, 11*, 1223919. https://doi.org/10.3389/fpubh.2023.1223919

Rosen, R. L., Ramasubramani, R. S., Benowitz, N. L., Gandhi, K. K., & Williams, J. M. (2023). Caffeine levels and dietary intake in smokers with schizophrenia and bipolar disorder. *Psychiatry Research, 319*, 114989. https://doi.org/10.1016/j.psychres.2022.114989

Rosenbaum, S., Tiedemann, A., Sherrington, C., Curtis, J., & Ward, P. B. (2014). Physical activity interventions for people with mental illness: A systematic review and meta-analysis. *The Journal of Clinical Psychiatry, 75*(9), 14465. https://doi.org/10.1016/j.jsams.2014.11.161

Rush, B., Urbanoski, K., Bassani, D., Castel, S., Wild, T. C., Strike, C., Kimberley, D., & Somers, J. (2008). Prevalence of co-occurring substance use and other mental disorders in the Canadian population. *The Canadian Journal of Psychiatry, 53*(12), 800–809. https://doi.org/10.1177/070674370805301206

Saunders, J. C. (2003). Families living with severe mental illness: A literature review. *Issues in Mental Health Nursing, 24*(2), 175–198. https://doi.org/10.1080/01612840305301

Scheewe, T. W., Backx, F. J. G., Takken, T., Jörg, F., Van Strater, A. C. P., Kroes, A. G., Mulder, T., & Cahn, W. (2013). Exercise therapy improves mental and physical health in schizophrenia: A randomised controlled trial. *Acta Psychiatrica Scandinavica, 127*(6), 464–473. https://doi.org/10.1111/acps.12029

Scott, D., & Happell, B. (2011). The high prevalence of poor physical health and unhealthy lifestyle behaviours in individuals with severe mental illness. *Issues in Mental Health Nursing, 32*(9), 589–597. https://doi.org/10.3109/01612840.2011.569846

Seow, L. S. E., Tan, X. W., Chong, S. A., Vaingankar, J. A., Abdin, E., Shafie, S., Chua, B. Y., Ong, H. L., & Subramaniam, M. (2020). Independent and combined associations of sleep duration and sleep quality with common physical and mental disorders: Results from a multi-ethnic population-based study. *PLoS One, 15*(7), e0235816. https://doi.org/10.1371/journal.pone.0235816

Sepúlveda, P., Aitsahalia, I., Kumar, K., Atkin, T., & Iigaya, K. (in press). Addressing altered anticipation as a transdiagnostic target through computational psychiatry. *Biological Psychiatry: Cognitive Neuroscience and Neuroimaging*. https://doi.org/10.1016/j.bpsc.2025.02.014

Shahrokh, N. C., & Hales, R. E. (2003). *American psychiatric glossary* (8th ed.). American Psychiatric Publishing. https://psycnet.apa.org/record/2003-04362-000

Shipman, A., Dezecache, G., & Majumdar, A. (2023). A quantification of the reliability of self-reports following a simulated stressful event. *International Journal of Disaster Risk Reduction, 86*, 103502. https://doi.org/10.1016/j.ijdrr.2022.103502

Siew, R. V. K., Nabe-Nielsen, K., Turner, A. I., Bujtor, M., & Torres, S. J. (2022). The role of combined modifiable lifestyle behaviors in the association between exposure to stressors and allostatic load: A systematic review of observational studies. *Psychoneuroendocrinology, 138*, 105668. https://doi.org/10.1016/j.psyneuen.2022.105668

Snethen, G., Brusilovskiy, E., McCormick, B. P., Hiremath, S. V., & Salzer, M. S. (2021). The relationship between community participation and physical activity among individuals with serious mental illnesses. *Mental Health and Physical Activity, 20*, 100381. https://doi.org/10.1016/j.mhpa.2021.100381

Soundy, A., Wampers, M., Probst, M., De Hert, M., Stubbs, B., Vancampfort, D., & Ströhle, A. (2014). Physical activity and sedentary behaviour in outpatients with schizophrenia: a systematic review and meta-analysis. *International Journal of Therapy and Rehabilitation, 20*(12), 588–595. https://doi.org/10.12968/ijtr.2013.20.12.588

Spurrier, G. F., Shulman, K., Dibich, S., Benoit, L., Duckworth, K., & Martin, A. (2023). Physical symptoms as psychiatric manifestations in medical spaces: A qualitative study. *Frontiers in Psychiatry, 13*, 1074424. https://doi.org/10.3389/fpsyt.2022.1074424

Stafford, A., Oduola, S., & Reeve, S. (2024). How sleep in patients with serious mental illness is recorded and treated, and its impact on service engagement. *Sleep Medicine, 124*, 58–69. https://doi.org/10.1016/j.sleep.2024.09.002

Stepien, M., Manoliu, A., Kubli, R., Schneider, K., Tobler, P. N., Seifritz, E., Herdener, M., & Kirschner, M. (2018). Investigating the association of ventral and dorsal striatal dysfunction during reward anticipation with negative symptoms in patients with schizophrenia and healthy individuals. *PLoS One, 13*(6), e0198215. https://doi.org/10.1371/journal.pone.0198215

Stover, P. J., Field, M. S., Andermann, M. L., Bailey, R. L., Batterham, R. L., Cauffman, E., Frühbeck, G., Iversen, P. O., Starke-Reed, P., Sternson, S. M., Vinoy, S., Witte, A. V., Zuker, C. S., & Angelin, B. (2023). Neurobiology of eating behavior, nutrition, and health. *Journal of Internal Medicine, 294*(5), 582–604. https://doi.org/10.1111/joim.13699

Strassnig, M., Brar, J. S., & Ganguli, R. (2006). Increased caffeine and nicotine consumption in community-dwelling patients with schizophrenia. *Schizophrenia Research, 86*(1–3), 269–275. https://doi.org/10.1016/j.schres.2006.05.013

Stubbs, B., Firth, J., Berry, A., Schuch, F. B., Rosenbaum, S., Gaughran, F., Bannert, M. M., & Vancampfort, D. (2016). How much physical activity do people with schizophrenia engage in? A systematic review, comparative meta-analysis and meta-regression. *Schizophrenia Research, 176*(2–3), 431–440. https://doi.org/10.1016/j.schres.2016.05.017

Stubbs, B., Vancampfort, D., Hallgren, M., Firth, J., Veronese, N., Solmi, M., Gaughran, F., Kahl, K. G., & Schuch, F. B. (2018). EPA guidance on physical activity as a treatment for severe mental illness: A meta-review of the evidence and position statement from the European psychiatric association (EPA), supported by the International Organization of Physical Therapists in mental health (IOPTMH). *European Psychiatry, 54*, 124–144. https://doi.org/10.1016/j.eurpsy.2018.07.004

Suni, E., & Rosen, D. (2024). *Sleep hygiene*. National Sleep Foundation (NSF). Retrieved June 16, 2025, from https://www.sleepfoundation.org/sleep-hygiene

Teasdale, S. B., Ward, P. B., Samaras, K., Firth, J., Stubbs, B., Tripodi, E., & Burrows, T. L. (2019). Dietary intake of people with severe mental illness: Systematic review and meta-analysis. *The British Journal of Psychiatry, 214*(5), 251–259. https://doi.org/10.1192/bjp.2019.20

Teoli, D., & Bhardwaj, A. (2023). Quality of life. In *StatPearls [Internet]*. StatPearls Publishing. https://www.ncbi.nlm.nih.gov/books/NBK536962/

Tubbs, A. S., Dollish, H. K., Fernandez, F., & Grandner, M. A. (2019). The basics of sleep physiology and behavior. In M. A. Gardner (Ed.), *Sleep and health* (pp. 3–10). Academic Press. https://doi.org/10.1016/B978-0-12-815373-4.00001-0

Van Someren, E. J. (2021). Brain mechanisms of insomnia: New perspectives on causes and consequences. *Physiological Reviews, 101*. https://doi.org/10.1152/physrev.00046.2019

Vancampfort, D., & Faulkner, G. (2014). Physical activity and serious mental illness: A multidisciplinary call to action [Editorial]. *Mental Health and Physical Activity, 7*(3), 153–154. https://doi.org/10.1016/j.mhpa.2014.11.001

Vancampfort, D., Stubbs, B., Venigalla, S. K., & Probst, M. (2015). Adopting and maintaining physical activity behaviours in people with severe mental illness: The importance of autonomous motivation. *Preventive Medicine, 81*, 216–220. https://doi.org/10.1016/j.ypmed.2015.09.006

Vancampfort, D., Firth, J., Schuch, F. B., Rosenbaum, S., Mugisha, J., Hallgren, M., Probst, M., Mikkelsen, S., & Stubbs, B. (2017). Sedentary behavior and physical activity levels in people with schizophrenia, bipolar disorder and major depressive disorder: A global systematic review and meta-analysis. *World Psychiatry, 16*(3), 308–315. https://doi.org/10.1002/wps.20458

Vaughn, C. E., & Leff, J. P. (1976). The influence of family and social factors on the course of psychiatric illness: A comparison of schizophrenic and depressed neurotic patients. *British Journal of Psychiatry, 129*(2), 125–137. https://doi.org/10.1192/bjp.129.2.125

Virgio, G. B., Higgins, D., Bennett, L., & Thomas, P. (2001). The prevalence and characteristics of co-occurring serious mental illness (SMI) and substance abuse or dependence in the patients of adult mental health and addictions services in eastern Dorset. *Journal of Mental Health, 10*(2), 175–188. https://doi.org/10.1080/09638230020023732

Whitley, R., Palmer, V., & Gunn, J. (2015). Recovery from severe mental illness. *CMAJ, 187*(13), 951–952. https://doi.org/10.1503/cmaj.141558

World Health Organization (WHO). (2022, October 5). *Physical activity* [Fact sheet]. https://www.who.int/news-room/fact-sheets/detail/physical-activity

World Health Organization (WHO). (2024, June 9). *Obesity and overweight* [Fact sheet]. https://www.who.int/news-room/fact-sheets/detail/obesity-and-overweight

Wu, Y., Chen, Z., Cheng, Z., Yu, Z., Qin, K., Jiang, C., & Xu, J. (2025). Effects of chronic diseases on health related quality of life is mediated by sleep difficulty in middle aged and older adults. *Scientific Reports, 15*(1), 2987. https://doi.org/10.1038/s41598-025-86420-1

Yassin, F. (2023, October 24). *How do eating disorders change between cultures?* The Wave Clinic. https://thewaveclinic.com/blog/how-do-eating-disorders-change-between-cultures/

Yin, S., Njai, R., Barker, L., Siegel, P. Z., & Liao, Y. (2016). Summarizing health-related quality of life (HRQOL): Development and testing of a one-factor model. *Population Health Metrics, 14*, 1–9. https://doi.org/10.1186/s12963-016-0091-3

Yip, T., & Cheon, Y. M. (2020). Sleep, psychopathology and cultural diversity. *Current Opinion in Psychology, 34*, 123–127. https://doi.org/10.1016/j.copsyc.2020.02.006

Chapter 16
Problems with Adherence to Medications and Treatment by Individuals Living with Serious Mental Illness

Introduction

Treatment adherence remains one of the most critical challenges in the management of serious mental illness (SMI). Despite advances in pharmacological and psychosocial interventions, a substantial proportion of individuals living with schizophrenia-spectrum, bipolar, and major depressive disorders struggle to consistently follow prescribed treatment regimens. Nonadherence is not a singular phenomenon, but a multidimensional construct encompassing missed doses, irregular scheduling, partial compliance, outright refusal, and disengagement from therapeutic recommendations. Its prevalence across diagnostic categories underscores the complexity of sustaining long-term engagement with treatment, particularly in populations facing persistent symptoms, cognitive impairments, and systemic barriers to care.

Understanding nonadherence requires careful attention to its defined types and dimensions. Research has identified patterns ranging from intermittent lapses to persistent refusal, each associated with distinct clinical trajectories and outcomes. These behaviors are shaped by interacting biological, psychological, and social factors, including neurological substrates such as deficits in insight and executive functioning, as well as environmental influences like stigma, socioeconomic strain, and fragmented healthcare systems. The heterogeneity of nonadherence highlights the need for dimensional frameworks that move beyond categorical definitions, situating adherence within broader domains of functioning and lived experience.

The consequences of nonadherence are profound, extending beyond symptom relapse to encompass hospitalization, suicide risk, cognitive decline, social instability, and increased healthcare costs. Medication-related factors such as side effects, pill burden, and perceived ineffectiveness further complicate adherence, often reinforcing negative attitudes toward treatment. These outcomes not only compromise individual recovery but also place significant strain on families, communities, and health systems. Addressing nonadherence therefore requires a comprehensive

G. F. McKeegan, *Behavior Change Interventions for Serious Mental Illness*, Evidence-Based Practices in Behavioral Health,
https://doi.org/10.1007/978-3-032-18372-9_16

understanding of its multifactorial origins and its cascading impact on clinical, psychosocial, and economic domains.

This chapter examines the problem of treatment and medication nonadherence in individuals living with SMI through an integrative lens. It explores the defined types and dimensions of nonadherence, the role of neurological substrates and environmental influences, and the impact of medication side effects. Outcomes of nonadherence are analyzed in terms of relapses, hospitalization, functional decline, and systemic burden. Finally, the chapter considers behavioral support strategies and culturally sensitive interventions designed to enhance adherence, emphasizing the importance of personalized, multidimensional approaches. By situating nonadherence within its broader context, the discussion aims to present a nuanced understanding of this pervasive challenge and its implications for clinical practice and mental health systems.

> My brother doesn't do what his doctors and therapists tell him to do. He misses appointments and argues or ignores what his treatment team suggests would be good to keep him in recovery. He refuses to discuss taking long-acting medications and says he does not need medications and feels fine without them. He thinks if he misses a dose, he can take more to make up for it.

The Case of Fred

Fred is a 41-year-old man who presently is living in a supervised apartment. His last admission to a psychiatric hospital happened after he called the police and told them that he was going to "get a rifle and shoot up the McDonald's." Later, after the police took him into custody, he explained he began feeling "shaky" and that he needed to be hospitalized. He later said this was the only way that he could think to get attention and the help that he needed.

Since high school, Fred had often complained about feeling uncomfortable with other people and having difficulty "fitting in." In his early 20s, his thinking became increasingly confused and disorganized, and he had severe problems even with short conversations. He was first hospitalized at the age of 22. Over the years, psychiatric service providers identified a variety of possible mental health problems with which he was living, but eventually it was determined that he was living with a schizophrenia spectrum mental health problem. While his thinking improved with medications, he continued to have problems with daily functioning and required a supported living placement. He also complained about a variety of side effects brought on by his medications. Shortly after being discharged to a supported apartment, he stopped taking his medications and left. He lived in shelters while looking for a job. After a while, his mental health problems worsened, and he was readmitted to the hospital and placed back on medications.

This pattern was repeated several times over the next 20 years. Fred held a variety of jobs but quit shortly after starting. He would often hitchhike to places where he thought that he could find a job. He lived in shelters while in that area. Eventually, he would return home. Throughout these years, there were 12 brief hospitalizations during which Fred was "stabilized" and discharged to a suitable placement in the community. Soon after, he would leave the placement, stop taking his medications, and search for a job.

While Fred had frequently attracted the attention of mental health service organizations over the years, he had never consistently followed the treatment recommendations that were offered. When admitted to a hospital, he modestly improves with medications. However, he seldom participated in any of the therapy groups and activities that were available to him. When he did attend, he usually sat quietly and did not speak unless someone else asked him a question. He preferred to walk around the hospital grounds and would spend many hours each day alone during his walks. When this became evident by his history and the staff at the mental health center began asking him about it, he attributed his behavior to "wanderlust" that he had felt since his teen years. He explained that he felt a desire to go explore places that he had not seen before and get a job because he didn't want to be a burden on other people. Because he knew that other people would not understand, he would simply gather a few belongings and leave. At the supervised apartment, the staff was left with the challenge of helping him to be more consistent in following the treatment and support that was available to him.

Definition and Characteristics of Problems with Adhering to Medication and Treatment Recommendations by Individuals Living with Serious Mental Illness

Problems with taking prescribed medications and following treatment recommendations are common in individuals living with SMI. Nonadherence includes behaviors such as taking lower or higher doses than prescribed, following a different schedule, completely abandoning treatment, or refusing regular visits or hospital admissions. Nonadherence to medications refers to the failure to follow prescribed recommendations given to the individual by a prescribing psychiatric service provider.

People who live with SMI mental health problems often have high rates of nonadherence: 61% for those living with schizophrenia-spectrum; 57% for bipolar; and 52% for depressive problems (Malik et al., 2020). Injectable long-acting psychiatric (LAIs) medications still see significant nonadherence within one year (Malik et al., 2020). Understanding and addressing the reasons for nonadherence—such as poor insight and lack of awareness, negative attitudes toward medication, substance abuse, medication side effects, and neurocognitive impairments—are critical for improving adherence and optimizing outcomes. Interventions targeting these modifiable factors can help mitigate the risks associated with nonadherence (Acosta et al., 2012; Velligan et al., 2017).

Current criteria for defining nonadherence to medication regimens include taking less than 80% prescribed doses, experiencing gaps in medication intake of at least seven days, or not adhering to the prescribed regimen for at least 75% of the time (Acosta et al., 2012; Lincoln et al., 2016). Adherence, however, is a dynamic process that can vary over time and is not a discrete unitary phenomenon (Malik et al., 2020). Most nonadherent patients are only partially nonadherent. Approximately 20% of individuals diagnosed with schizophrenia spectrum disorders demonstrate medication refusal, either initially with eventual consent, or through intermittent or consistent refusal, regardless of an initial period of adherence (Lincoln et al., 2016). Lambert et al. (2010) found that 33.7% of first-episode individuals living with SMI were fully adherent to antipsychotic medications; 47.4% displayed at least one phase of nonadherence; and 18.8% were persistent medication refusers, never receiving adequate trials of psychiatric medications. "Persistent refusers" are persons living with SMI who do not take medication over a longer duration (Lambert et al., 2010). Present refusers disengaged from provider services at a rate of 50%, compared to 27.9% for intermittently nonadherent, and none for fully adherent patients (Lambert et al., 2010).

Approximately 49% of patients with major psychiatric disorders exhibit medication nonadherence. Nonadherence rates are higher in specific mental health problems linked to living with SMI: 56% for schizophrenia-spectrum mental health problems, 50% for major depressive type of problems, and 44% for bipolar mental health problems (Semahegn et al., 2020). Previous systematic reviews have reported medication adherence levels ranging from 24% to 90%, indicating a significant challenge in treatment compliance. Problems with adhering to treatment recommendations involve the discontinuation of psychiatric treatment (e.g., attending follow-up appointments with recovery team, following treatment plan, attending therapy appointments) or "dropping out." Dropping out is defined as termination of treatment despite therapeutic need and before completing the agreed-upon treatment plan or reaching therapeutic goals (Tehrani et al., 1996). Depending on the operationalized definition of dropping out, nonadherence of treatment also has included missed sessions, failure to complete treatment protocols, and therapists' judgments (Kullgard et al., 2022). Research conducted in Canada and the United States has identified dropout rates ranging from 17% to 22%. A World Health Organization (WHO) survey (Kessler et al., 2006) reported an overall dropout rate of 31.7%, with high-income countries experiencing rates of 26.3% (Wells et al., 2013). One study found that 26% of individuals living with SMI discontinued treatment within the first year (Tehrani et al., 1996). Recent studies have reported dropout rates ranging from 19.7% to 47%, underscoring variability that can be attributed to disparate definitions and research contexts (Kullgard et al., 2022). Notably, during follow-up visits after discharge from psychiatric admission, 30–50% of individuals with SMI miss appointments within 30 days, which may contribute to adverse outcomes (Ojo et al., 2024).

Nonadherence to psychiatric medication and treatment remains a widespread challenge, linked to notable clinical and social consequences and increased healthcare costs (Acosta et al., 2012; Buchman-Wildbaum et al., 2020; Dennis et al.,

2020; Grover et al., 2021; Guo et al., 2023; Kreyenbuhl et al., 2016; Laranjeira et al., 2023; Lincoln et al., 2016; Marcus et al., 2017; Velligan et al., 2017; Wells et al., 2013). Among individuals living with SMI, failure to comply with treatment recommendations can lead to severe clinical ramifications including the following:

- Relapses and symptom exacerbations: Nonadherence is linked to substantially higher relapse risk: 82% relapse rate over 5 years in individuals living with a schizophrenia spectrum mental health problem (Acosta et al., 2012; Emsley 2013). Interruptions of taking medications as short as 1–10 days increase the risk of hospitalization (Velligan et al., 2017).
- Hospitalization and psychiatric emergencies: Nonadherence increases use of emergency services and psychiatric crises (Kreyenbuhl et al., 2016). Hospitalizations occurred in 69% of people living with SMI after discontinuing medication (Acosta et al., 2012).
- Suicide risk and mortality: Nonadherence correlates with higher mortality and violent behavior (Velligan et al., 2017). After stopping treatment, 22% of people who live with SMI attempted suicide (Acosta et al., 2012).
- Cognitive and functional deterioration: Reduced treatment participation results in lower social and occupational functioning (Laranjeira et al., 2023). Impaired memory and executive dysfunction were observed in nonadherent persons who live with SMI (Guo et al., 2023).

Nonadherence with medications and treatment likewise resulted in adverse psychosocial and behavioral consequences:

- Social instability and isolation: Linked to housing instability, social withdrawal, and reduced family engagement (Grover et al., 2021).
- Legal system involvement: Associated with increased incarceration, arrests, and violence due to resurgence of problem behaviors (Velligan et al., 2017).
- Stigma and self-stigmatization: Individuals living with SMI may refrain from seeking care due to perceived stigma, which can further contribute to disengagement from ongoing treatment and support services (Buchman-Wildbaum et al., 2020; Docksey et al., 2022).

In addition, the economic burden for treatment nonadherence is considerable, with nonadherence accounting for approximately 40% of the total cost associated with treating individuals with SMI (Acosta et al., 2012). The outcomes for individuals who decline medication remain a significant concern, as over half demonstrate disengagement from services and/or ongoing substance use. Additionally, two-thirds do not achieve remission from problematic behaviors and symptoms, and only a minority are employed. Collectively, these factors suggest unfavorable long-term prognoses and limited prospects for recovery (Lambert et al., 2010). The economic and systemic outcomes linked to treatment nonadherence include the following:

- Excess healthcare costs: In the United States, individuals with serious mental illness (SMI) account for 40% of total mental health service expenditures. The economic burden attributable to SMI exceeds $10 billion annually (Acosta et al., 2012; Dennis et al., 2020).

- Disrupted continuity of care: Nonadherence increases the burden on emergency services and reduces coordinated long-term care (Marcus et al., 2017).
- High dropout rates from mental health services: The global treatment dropout rate is approximately 31.7%, leading to incomplete recovery and missed follow-ups (Wells et al., 2013).

Difficulties with medication adherence, attending follow-up appointments, participating in therapy, engaging in recovery and case management sessions, and following recommendations such as maintaining sobriety, are frequently observed among individuals who live with SMI, and represent several key dimensions contributing to treatment nonadherence. Adherence and nonadherence are multifactorial and dynamic, shaped by an array of complex, heterogenous, and transdiagnostic personal, relational, clinical, and systemic factors. While poor insight/lack of awareness and medication side effects remain significant predictors, variables like stigma, financial strain, lack of transportation, therapeutic misalignment, negative interactions with service providers, shortfalls in social support, and substance use consistently emerge as core drivers of nonadherent behaviors.

Factors related to the personal aspects of the individual such as the presence of a co-occurring disorder, problems in self-management and self-awareness, and covert self-statements about living with SMI highly impact the person's willingness to adhere to treatment recommendations including taking medications (Acosta et al., 2012; Grover et al., 2021; Guo et al., 2023; Lincoln et al., 2016; Magura et al., 2014; Malik et al., 2020; Velligan et al., 2017). The factors related to the person living with SMI include the following:

- Lack of insight (anosognosia): A diminished awareness of issues associated with SMI, commonly referred to as "insight" in mental health literature, has been identified by some researchers as a negative symptom (Brucato et al., 2017; Mader & Galderisi, 2017). Negative symptoms—defined as the absence or reduced expression of behaviors typically expected in healthy functioning (Correll & Schooler, 2020)—are often resistant to treatment and may persist even as other symptoms related to SMI respond to intervention. This challenge in recognizing mental or physical health problems closely parallels anosognosia, which is described as "the failure to recognize the existence of a deficit or disorder, such as cognitive impairment, hearing loss, poor vision, or paralysis" (American Psychological Association, n.d.-a).
- Impairments in self-awareness observed in individuals with SMI are analogous to neurocognitive deficits seen in conditions such as neurodegenerative diseases or following adverse neurological events, including cerebrovascular accidents (CVAs) and head trauma. When an individual living with SMI does not acknowledge their mental health challenges, they are unlikely to perceive a need for treatment and may subsequently refuse to adhere to recommended interventions. This phenomenon is particularly prevalent in populations experiencing mental health disorders associated with SMI (Acosta et al., 2012; Lincoln et al., 2016).

- Negative attitudes and perceptions toward medication: Beliefs that medication is unnecessary, ineffective, or harmful (Lincoln et al., 2016; Velligan et al., 2017). Negative beliefs about SMI and its treatments, including myths and misconceptions, significantly affect adherence (Alekhya et al., 2015).
- Socioeconomic status: Lower socioeconomic status is linked to nonadherence due to financial constraints and limited access to healthcare resources (Alekhya et al., 2015).
- Substance abuse: Linked to both intentional and unintentional nonadherence across various SMI populations as using some substances can mimic and/or worsen problem behaviors in persons living with SMI (Grover et al., 2021; Magura et al., 2014). Habits such as smoking or alcohol consumption are associated with higher rates of nonadherence (Alekhya et al., 2015).
- Forgetfulness and poor organization: Impacts adherence, especially in those with neurocognitive impairments, especially impairments in executive functioning and memory capabilities (Guo et al., 2023; Malik et al., 2020).
- Grief and internalized stigma: Emotional distress, shame, and identity loss from illness contribute to avoidance of stimuli associated with living with SMI and discourages individuals from seeking or continuing care (Buchman-Wildbaum et al., 2020; Deng et al., 2022). Internalized stigma has been recognized as a factor associated with delayed engagement with services, with some outpatient populations experiencing delays of up to two years. Among individuals living with SMI, higher levels of internalized stigma are linked to reduced social support and integration, increased hopelessness, lower self-esteem, and decreased sense of coherence. Lower self-esteem is a key associated factor and appears to mediate both quality of life and the likelihood of avoiding treatment. Research suggests that the risk of lowered self-esteem may be greater in those with higher insight, particularly when accompanied by loss of valued social identity (Vieira et al., 2023).

Medication-related factors are frequently cited as reasons for nonadherence, often associated with the effects, side effects, dosage, and scheduling of medications (Benjet et al., 2022; Dennis et al., 2020; Lucca et al., 2015; Mert et al., 2015; National Alliance on Mental Illness (NAMI), 2024; Velligan et al., 2017). The factors related to medications that contribute to nonadherence are as follows:

- Side effects: Common reasons for discontinuation include sedation, weight gain, cognitive dulling, and impairments in behavioral responsivity (e.g., diminished responsiveness to external stimuli) (Lucca et al., 2015; Velligan et al., 2017).
- Pill burden and complexity: Multiple medications or frequent and complicated dosing negatively impact adherence. (Dennis et al., 2020; Mert et al., 2015). On the average, research suggests that individuals living with SMI are often prescribed multiple medications daily, typically ranging from 2 to 5 psychotropic drugs, with some receiving even more due to co-occurring physical health conditions (Dennis et al., 2020; Mert et al., 2015). A study found that polypharmacy—the use of two or more psychiatric medications—was common among adults who live with schizophrenia-spectrum and bipolar mental health problems, with

over 50% of people with SMI receiving three or more psychotropic medications (Essock et al., 2009). An analysis of Medicaid data showed that individuals living with SMI were prescribed an average of 7–11 total medications daily, including both psychiatric and non-psychiatric drugs (Essock et al., 2009). This high medication burden reflects the complexity of treating individuals who live with SMI, which often involves managing intransigent problem behaviors like psychosis, mood instability, anxiety, and sleep disturbances, as well as addressing chronic physical health issues such as diabetes or cardiovascular disease.
- Perceived ineffectiveness: Individuals may discontinue medications when they feel better or if outcomes do not meet expectations (Benjet et al., 2022; NAMI, 2024).

The following factors highlight the complexity of managing illness-related variables that influence nonadherence to treatment of the problem behaviors linked to SMI (Guo et al., 2023; Lambert et al., 2010; Lincoln et al., 2016; Magura et al., 2014; Wells et al., 2013). Several factors related to dimensions of the mental health problem contribute to nonadherence including the following:

- Duration of illness: Studies indicate that patients with an illness duration exceeding one year exhibit higher rates of nonadherence, reaching over 51% (Alekhya et al., 2015; Lambert et al., 2010; Wells et al., 2013).
- Relapses and hospitalizations: Research indicates that individuals who experience relapses have higher rates of nonadherence (39.79%) compared to those without relapses (30.09%) (Alekhya et al., 2015; Lincoln et al., 2016; Wells et al., 2013). Furthermore, individuals living with SMI in community settings who have not required hospital admission for treatment demonstrate higher nonadherence rates (50.48%) (Alekhya et al., 2015).
- Comorbidities: Nonadherence is more common in individuals living with comorbid physical health problems conditions such as hypertension (7.76%), diabetes (6.79%), and endocrine disorders (1.94%). Co-occurring physical or mental health conditions make adherence more difficult (Alekhya et al., 2015; Guo et al., 2023; Magura et al., 2014).
- Untreated depression: Individuals who live with SMI and live with a co-occurring and untreated depressive mental health problem for extended periods exhibit higher nonadherence rates (36.89% for untreated depression) (Alekhya et al., 2015).
- Suicide ideation and attempts: Nonadherence is higher in patients with thoughts of suicide (35.92%) and those who have attempted suicide (17.47%) (Alekhya et al., 2015).

System-related and environmental factors also negatively affect adherence to treatment (Alekhya et al., 2015; Buchman-Wildbaum et al., 2020; Deng et al., 2022; De Soet et al., 2024; Ljungberg et al., 2016; Lincoln et al., 2016; Malik et al., 2020; Marcus et al., 2017; Ojo et al., 2024). These factors include the following:

- Limited access to services and care: Insufficient or absent reimbursement from health insurance plans and ineffective medication distribution systems impede treatment adherence. Interruptions in follow-up, restricted availability of services, or fragmented healthcare systems may disrupt ongoing care (Marcus et al., 2017; Ojo et al., 2024). Delays between referral and appointment scheduling reduce the likelihood of continued adherence (Alekhya et al., 2015). Disruptions during significant life transitions are associated with increased risk of treatment dropout (De Soet et al., 2024).

- Financial and logistical barriers: Cost of medication, denials and delays in insurance coverage for treatment, transportation, or limited community mental health resources impeded access to ongoing care and contribute to nonadherence (De Soet et al., 2024; Malik et al., 2020).
- Poor therapeutic alliance: Unsupportive, paternalistic, or disengaged relationships with service providers reduce trust and motivation (Lincoln et al., 2016; Ljungberg et al., 2016). Service providers may lack training in managing SMI and co-occurring mental health problems, which affects their ability to effectively support the individuals living with SMI. Lack of knowledge on adherence and effective interventions for improving it further contributes to nonadherence. Providers responsible for significant workloads frequently have constrained time for consultations with individuals who live with SMI, which may adversely affect the quantity, duration, and quality of care delivered. Consequently, this can lead to insufficient patient education and limited support for treatment adherence. The healthcare system's restricted capacity to inform patients and facilitate consistent follow-up has also been recognized as a barrier to adherence (Alekhya et al., 2015). In addition, difficulties in developing community support structures and self-management programs hinder adherence rates (Alekhya et al., 2015).

- The quality of relationships between individuals who live with SMI and mental health professionals, particularly prescribing service providers, plays a crucial role in treatment outcomes (Ljungberg et al., 2016). Non-helpful relationships, characterized by professionals who are pessimistic, uncaring, paternalistic, and disrespectful, can significantly hinder recovery and well-being and result in nonadherence to treatment recommendations, treatment dropout, or termination. These professionals often lack engagement, show emotional detachment, and display indifference toward the situations of the person living with SMI, leading to feelings of alienation and distrust among patients (Ljungberg et al., 2016). Additionally, professionals may operate in an impersonal, mechanical manner, prioritizing documentation over meaningful interactions, which further exacerbates the sense of being treated as mere cases rather than as individuals. The paternalistic approach, where professionals make decisions without considering the input and collaboration of the individual who lives with SMI, contributes to a perception of loss of control and active participation in their own care (Ljungberg et al., 2016). Furthermore, professionals' reliance on stereotypes and preconceptions, along with their pessimistic attitudes, fosters hopelessness and low expectations and furtherance of learned helplessness and stigmatization that negatively impacts the mental health of the individual living with SMI (Ljungberg et al., 2016). Negative emotional expressions from professionals, such as anger, irritation, and high expressed emotionality (American Psychological Association, n.d.-b) can also harm the therapeutic relationship, leaving lasting impressions on the service user living with SMI. Organizational factors, including discontinuity in care, lack of time, and insufficient communication, further contribute to non-helpful relationships, leading to repeated retelling of painful stories and feelings of betrayal when relationships end. These detrimental interactions result in increased suffering, loss of self-respect, and feelings of hopelessness among individuals with SMI, highlighting the need for organizations to create conditions that allow professionals to engage meaningfully with their respective service users who live with SMI (Ljungberg et al., 2016).

Several cultural, social, and contextual factors influence individuals living with SMI to nonadhere to treatment (Alekhya et al., 2015; Benjet et al., 2022; Deng et al., 2022; De Soet et al., 2024; Grover et al., 2021; Laranjeira et al., 2023). These include the following:

- Family and social support: Strong familial support is associated with better adherence (Grover et al., 2021; Laranjeira et al., 2023; Zimet et al., 1988). Negative attitudes by family members or lack of support from family members can impact adherence. Nonadherence was found to be high in patients with non-cooperative and critical family members. Limited family support and lack of community engagement can reduce adherence (Alekhya et al., 2015).
- Cultural perceptions regarding mental health problems and treatment: Misconceptions about mental health problems may decrease engagement (Benjet et al., 2022; Deng et al., 2022). The use of interpreters by therapists and cultural variations in the understanding of mental health issues and their interventions can impede adherence. Enhancing adherence rates and treatment outcomes can be supported by addressing cultural and social factors through education, community engagement, and family involvement (Alekhya et al., 2015).

Dimensions of Medication and Treatment Nonadherence

The National Institute of Mental Health (NIMH) proposed the Research Domain Criteria (RDoC) initiative to organize research of mental health problems, by looking at dimensions of functioning rather than being tied to categorical domains and constructs (NIMH, n.d.; Pacheco et al., 2022). The aim is to understand the dimensional aspects of mental health problems in terms of varying degrees of impairment in fundamental psychological, behavioral, and biological systems (NIMH, n.d.). A dimension is defined as a factor or component that is applied in measuring a set of variables (American Psychological Association, n.d.-c); dimensionality is the number of dimensions applied in measuring a construct or domain of a class of responses (American Psychological Association, n.d.-d). A dimension in the context of mental health is a measurable aspect or characteristic that contributes to understanding mental health or related phenomena (Korkeila, 2000). Dimensions include emotional, neurocognitive, behavioral, social, and physical aspects, such as anxiety, depression, hallucinations, delusions, coping strategies, social support, and quality of life. These dimensions are assessed using various scales and indicators to evaluate the dimension of the construct, variable or response class of behaviors in individual with mental health problem (Korkeila, 2000; Korkeila et al., 2003).

The concept of treatment nonadherence by individuals living with SMI is complex, multidimensional, multidirectional, and heterogeneous. An example of such a concept in a health-related field is pain. Pain is a complex transdiagnostic, idiosyncratic, and heterogenous concept. Pain involves three domains: physical, psychological, and behavioral. These domains influence each other in intricate and dynamic ways. The subjective experience of the sensation of physical pain can lead to emotional distress, which then affects how someone behaves, indicating multidirectionality. The domains of pain include measurable dimensions that can be assessed. To illustrate, the physical domain of pain includes the results of scans, x-rays, and laboratory tests. The psychological domain refers to the awareness, perception and experience of pain; the subjective intensity of the pain (sharp or dull ache); the perceived duration of the pain; and the emotions and private events associated with awareness or pain. The behavioral domain involves how the person responds to pain, such as avoiding or decreasing certain activities, taking substances to decrease the perception (e.g., sedation, euphoria) and the intensity of pain (e.g., analgesic, opioids), or participating in alternative behaviors to reduce the perception of pain, like mindfulness meditation.

Treatment nonadherence by individuals living with SMI involves domains that encompass physical/biological dimensions, psychological/subjective response dimensions, and behavioral dimensions. These domains interact with each other. It is not sufficient in an assessment to assess the presence or absence of a behavioral dimension but detailed and operationally defined aspects of the dimension being assessed.

The assessment of the problem with treatment and medication adherence by individuals living with SMI uses objective data and subjective measures (e.g., self-report, judgment by evaluator). Data on treatment adherence to medications can be obtained by self-reports from the individuals living with SMI and other informants familiar with the person. Adherence to certain medications can be obtained objectively using blood levels of the metabolites of the medications (Hiemke et al., 2018). Therapeutic drug monitoring (TDM) is commonly used in psychiatry to assess blood levels of certain medications that have narrow therapeutic windows, variable metabolism, or significant toxicity risks (Hiemke et al., 2018). The following are the classes and medications that can be monitored objectively by blood levels:

1. Mood Stabilizers (Hiemke et al., 2018)

   Lithium: Regular monitoring is essential due to its narrow therapeutic index.

   Valproic acid/divalproex sodium: Monitoring for therapeutic efficacy and potential hepatotoxicity is required.

   Carbamazepine: Requires monitoring because of autoinduction and the risk of toxicity.

Lamotrigine: Therapeutic drug monitoring is less common but may be warranted in certain clinical scenarios.

2. Antipsychotics (Hiemke et al., 2018)

   Clozapine: Plasma concentrations are monitored to assess efficacy and mitigate the risk of agranulocytosis.

   Olanzapine, Risperidone, Quetiapine, Haloperidol: Therapeutic drug monitoring may be considered in cases of suspected nonadherence or toxicity, though it is not standard practice.

   Paliperidone, Aripiprazole: Monitoring is occasionally indicated in complex clinical cases.

3. Antidepressants (Hiemke et al., 2018)

   Tricyclic Antidepressants (e.g., amitriptyline, nortriptyline): Blood-level assessment is frequently employed to guide dosing and minimize toxicity.

   SSRIs and SNRIs: Routine blood-level monitoring is generally not recommended except in research contexts or select patient populations.

4. Other Agents (Hiemke et al., 2018)

   Benzodiazepines: Monitoring is infrequent and typically reserved for situations involving suspected overdose or impaired metabolism.

   Stimulants (e.g., methylphenidate, amphetamines): Serum-level monitoring is not routinely performed but is available.

   Adherence to certain treatment recommendations can be obtained objectively. Abstaining from substance use can be monitored by urine and blood tests (Hadland & Levy, 2016).

Many of the dimensions of problems in treatment adherence involve covert and private events that can only be measured by self-report and other subjective modalities. One such dimension in treatment adherence is stigmatization and reports of negative interactions with service providers. Other dimensions can be measured by factual, quantifiable information, which can be measured and verified through objective methods like prescriptions that are filled by pharmacies. Some dimensions can include observations and reports from informants (e.g., staff at residences, family members); these dimensions include the frequency and severity of side effects as well as behavioral dimensions of the concept of stigmatization that include social withdrawal, isolation, and hesitancy to seek treatment (Corrigan & Watson, 2002).

Based on the dimensions that are assessed in available measures of the response classes of behaviors associated with problems with medications and treatment adherence, there is a need for comprehensive assessment measures; future instruments assessing factors associated with treatment adherence by individuals living with SMI need to include the following relevant dimensions:

- Topography: The categories of medications omitted, the nature of missed appointments, the therapies and recommendations not implemented, and a detailed account of observed nonadherent behaviors.
- Frequency and rate: The number of occurrences of adherence and nonadherence during a specified duration of time. Patterns of adherence and nonadherences are critical in determining the function of the behavior of nonadherence.

- Duration: Length of time that adherence and nonadherence occur.
- Awareness: Understanding the consequences of nonadherence like relapses, increase in mental health crises, and hospitalization.
- Respondents and covert responses: The perception of emotional respondents and covert responses (e.g., thoughts) that are linked to nonadherence. Dimensions or treatment adherence can be a motivating operation (MO) that increases covert self-statements and respondents linked to self-stigmatization. MO is an environmental stimulus that changes the value of a consequence and influences the likelihood of behaviors that have been previously associated with those consequences (Cooper et al., 2020). Nonadherence to medications and treatment may temporarily reduce the increased intensity of the distressing respondents connected to self-stigmatization and result in nonadherence being negatively reinforced.
- Antecedent conditions: Environmental triggers and overt and covert stimulus and events that lead to the occurrences of nonadherence. Individuals who live with SMI may stop taking medications due to a rapid increase in weight or having visible tremors in the arms and legs that result in shame and embarrassment.
- Consequential conditions: Environmental stimuli and events that occur after instances of nonadherence. Nonadherence may lead to the avoidance or reduction of physical and psychological effects, as well as stigmatization, which are sometimes associated with following treatment protocols, such as increased distress and other aversive respondents.
- Function of nonadherent behaviors with treatment: The function of a behavior is the purpose or reason for the occurrence of the behavior. The common functions are to obtain attention, escape or avoid an aversive event or stimulus, to obtain a desired item or stimulus, and to engage in behavior that is reinforcing, pleasurable or novel (Cooper et al., 2020). Behavior can have more than one function. Skydiving may be reinforcing because it is an exhilarating and novel experience but also can be reinforced by gaining the attention of a social group. Nonadherence can transpire to escape from the distress linked with aversive self-statements associated with stigmatization or to escape stigmatization from others. Nonadherence can be manifested if the person living with SMI has negative interactions with the prescribing service provider and drops out of treatment to avoid any further interactions. In a study by Mirhaj Mohammadabadi et al. (2022), a group of individuals living with a personality type of SMI (i.e., borderline personality) were assessed on a 16 item inventory asking their attitudes towards psychiatric medications, psychotherapy, and genaral treatment adherence. The two most common reasons for discontinuation of treatment were medication side effects (53.1%) and dissatisfaction with the service provider (40.3%) indicating that they did not have a good relationship with the prescribing service provider. Developing a functional hypothesis for the problem behavior of nonadherence to treatment can clarify the dimensions of nonadherence for the individual.

Medication and nonadherence to treatment in people who live with SMI are heterogenous, transdiagnostic, and multidirectional, meaning that one dimension influences another dimension. An example would be that negative interactions with mental health service provider can impact the severity and degree of hopelessness, helplessness, and stigmatization (all subjective experiences) that can then influence the adherence to treatment recommendations (that can be assessed objectively). The problems with nonadherence to medications and treatment recommendations are composed of multidimensional response classes of behaviors.

A multidimensional response class of the behaviors of adherence to medications is the frequency of taking and missing doses of prescribed medication. Lambert et al. (2010) defined various dimensions of medication adherence as follows:

- Full adherence: These individuals consistently took their medication as prescribed and had no lapses of adherence for seven days or longer during treatment (Lambert et al., 2010).
- Nonadherence: Defined as at least one phase where medication was not taken for a week or more, indicating issues beyond missed doses. Service discontinuation despite ongoing treatment need (e.g., dropout) also counts as nonadherence (Lambert et al., 2010).
- Medication refusal: Individuals were classified as having refused medication if they consistently declined to take prescribed drugs during treatment, with allowance for up to three weeks of nonadherence. Participants who discontinued treatment prior to completing three weeks were also categorized as refusers, given that shorter durations are insufficient to evaluate medication efficacy. Additionally, individuals who did not engage with the facility, refused contact, or became untraceable were similarly considered to have refused all prescribed medications (Lambert et al., 2010).

The following dimensions response classes of nonadherence to medications and treatment can be assessed using validated tools, clinical interviews, or observational data:

A. Person-Related Factors

  - Insight into illness: Poor insight (anosognosia) is a strong predictor of nonadherence, especially in people living with SMI (Velligan et al., 2017). This can be measured by the "Scale to Assess Unawareness of Mental Disorder," which assesses discrete and global aspects of awareness across a variety of manifestations of problem behaviors linked to SMI (Amador et al., 1993; Rozalski & McKeegan, 2019).
  - Attitudes toward medication: Negative beliefs, fear of dependency, or preference for alternative treatment modalities (e.g., homeopathic) (Lincoln et al., 2016) can be measured using the Drug Attitude Inventory (DAI) (Hogan et al., 1983). The Drug Attitude Inventory (DAI) is a 30-item scale designed to evaluate private self-statements about medication use in relation to compliance. It is commonly used to assess subjective responses to medication and to predict adherence among individuals who live with SMI. The items on the scale were chosen based on feedback from individuals about their medications. Respondents are asked to answer "true" or "false" to each of the 30 statements (Hogan et al., 1983). The Medication Adherence Rating Scale

(MARS) (Fialko et al., 2008; Velligan et al., 2017) is a ten-item self-report measure for medication adherence. It measures three dimensions of taking medications including the following:

(a) Medication adherence behavior: The first four items address behaviors associated with taking medication, including instances of forgetting or discontinuing medication due to changes in health status.
(b) Attitude toward taking medication: Items five to eight examine perspectives regarding medication, such as beliefs about its effectiveness and necessity.
(c) Negative side effects and attitudes to psychotropic medication: Items nine and 10 pertain to subjective experiences of side effects, including sensations of fatigue, sluggishness, or feeling significantly altered while on medication.

The Morisky Medication Adherence Scale-8 (MMAS-8) (Morisky et al., 1986) is an 8-item self-report tool; it is a widely used instrument that screens for intentional/unintentional nonadherence with medications. It was initially developed to screen for adherence to medications for physical ailments (Morisky et al., 1986).

- Neurocognitive impairment: Deficits in memory and executive function (EF) can negatively impact medication adherence and are typically evaluated using neuropsychological assessments (Velligan et al., 2017). Individuals with such impairments may have difficulty remembering medication schedules, risk taking incorrect dosages, or fail to plan for timely prescription refills.
- Problems with adherence to treatment recommendations are closely linked to functional impairments in a person living with SMI. An impairment is defined as an observable decrement in an individual's capabilities to function adaptively in basic self-care skills (American Psychological Association, n.d.-f; Harvey & Strassnig, 2012). Functional impairment refers to the inability or reduced ability to perform everyday activities necessary for independent living, productive work, and social interactions. Functional impairment in people living with SMI spans major domains such as residential independence, vocational activities, and social functioning. It is influenced by various factors, including neurocognitive impairments, functional capacity, symptoms (e.g., depression, negative symptoms), environmental factors (e.g., financial disadvantage, stigma), and health status (e.g., obesity, physical fitness). These impairments result in challenges in expected social roles and performing essential skills (Harvey & Strassnig, 2012).
- Functional impairment encompasses limitations in essential life activities, including self-care, employment, social relationships, and independent living (Harvey & Strassnig, 2012). Nonadherence to psychotropic medication among people living with SMI was associated with increased functional impairment and inability to manage illness in the community (Semahegn et al., 2020). Treatment nonadherence may further aggravate functional impairment by intensifying psychiatric symptoms and problem behaviors, elevating the risk of relapse, and diminishing the capacity to manage daily responsibilities (Semahegn et al., 2020).

- Research indicates that individuals who live with SMI who do not adhere to treatment protocols are at greater risk for increased hospitalization, compromised social and occupational functioning, elevated rates of homelessness and incarceration, and diminished quality of life (QoL). Although adherence itself is not categorized as a formal domain of functioning—such as neurocognition or social skills—it remains a critical behavioral factor impacting functional outcomes (Semahegn et al., 2020).
- Frameworks like the World Health Organization's (WHO) (2001) International Classification of Functioning, Disability and Health (ICF) include adherence behaviors within "personal factors" influencing overall functioning. Likewise, psychiatric rehabilitation models frequently incorporate adherence as an important consideration when assessing an individual's ability to participate in treatment and sustain stability (Semahegn et al., 2020).
- Substance use, including alcohol and drug misuse, has been consistently linked to unintentional nonadherence (Magura et al., 2014). Assessment tools such as Tobacco, Alcohol, Prescription Medication, and other Substance (TAPS) use screen (National Institute on Drug Abuse [NIDA], n.d.) are available for evaluating substance use. The TAPS tool comprises an initial combined screening component (TAPS-1), followed by a brief assessment (TAPS-2) for individuals who screen positively. This instrument provides both self-administered and clinician-administered formats, facilitating the evaluation of problematic substance use within the past three months. In addition to self-reported tools, objective monitoring through random urine and blood testing is also utilized to assess substance use (Hadland & Levy, 2016).
- Stigma and self-stigmatization (Buchman-Wildbaum et al., 2020). Internalized or self-stigma can be measured using validated scales and is linked to social withdrawal and treatment avoidance (Ritsher et al., 2003). It can be measured by collateral reports from informants that the individuals living with SMI engage in social avoidance and self-statements indicative of worthlessness and hopelessness. (Corrigan & Watson, 2002).
- Negative symptoms: Adhering to medications and treatment recommendations requires the voluntary and overt behaviors of swallowing the pills, attending therapies and other appointments with service providers. Studies have shown that individuals living with SMI who complied poorly with medications had significantly greater severity of negative symptoms, especially avolition, apathy, and alogia (Tattan & Creed, 2001). Duration of illness and duration of being prescribed medications were associated with compliance (Tattan & Creed, 2001). The findings suggest that the dimension of negative symptoms (i.e., the absences or decrements in behaviors coupled with typical functioning) are one of the important factors in determining whether a person who lives with SMI will adhere to treatment recommendations.

B. Medication-Related Factors

- Side effects: Sedation, weight gain, and "extrapyramidal symptoms" (EPS) are common reasons for discontinuation and can be tracked using side effect checklists (Lincoln et al., 2016). EPS refers to medication side effects that result in limb rigidity, tremors, Parkinson-like symptoms, dystonia (abnormal movements), and akathisia (restlessness) (American Psychological Association, n.d.-e). Psychiatric medications are sometimes discontinued due to "metabolic syndrome" (Vázquez-Bourgon et al., 2021), which raises the risk of cardiovascular disease, stroke, and Type 2 diabetes. Side effects include hypertension, elevated insulin, nonalcoholic fatty liver disease, and obesity (American Psychological Association, n.d.-g).

- Pill burden and regimen complexity: These factors are assessed by quantifying the number of daily medications and doses, as they have been shown to correlate with adherence rates (Acosta et al., 2012). Refill data from insurance providers and pharmacies can provide objective evidence of medication adherence. Additionally, collateral information from informants—such as staff at residential facilities or members of assertive community treatment teams (American Psychological Association, n.d.-d)—can be valuable when supporting individuals who live with serious SMI in maintaining adherence.
- Cost and access: Financial barriers are measurable via patient surveys, reports by informants, or insurance data (Lucca et al., 2015).

C. Illness-Related Factors

- Symptom severity: Higher symptom burden (e.g., psychosis, mania, disorganized speech and thinking) is associated with lower adherence. Tools like the Positive and Negative Symptom Syndrome (PANSS) scale (Kay et al., 1987) or the Brief Psychiatric Rating Scale (BPRS) (Andersen et al., 1989) can quantify (by subjective judgments of the professional interviewer) the intensity of problem behaviors connected to living with SMI (Guo et al., 2023).
- Duration of illness: The onset and length of time living with SMI can be determined by examining admission and treatment records, as well as reports from individuals with SMI and informants. Extended durations of living with SMI have been associated with lower adherence rates, potentially due to treatment fatigue (Mert et al., 2015).
- Comorbidities: Co-occurring physical or mental health conditions complicate treatment and can be tracked via diagnostic records (Dennis et al., 2020).

D. System-Related Factors

- Therapeutic alliance: The quality of the patient–provider relationship is a measurable predictor of adherence (Ljungberg et al., 2016). Instruments like the Working Alliance Inventory (WAI) have been used (Horvath & Greenberg, 1989). The WAI consists of 36 items, with 12 items for each of the three dimensions: (a) tasks: The specific in-therapy behaviors and cognitions that both the clinician and person perceive as relevant and effective for achieving therapeutic goals. Both parties must accept responsibility for performing these tasks; (b) goals: The mutually agreed-upon outcomes or objectives of

the therapeutic process that both the clinician and person value and endorse; and (c) bonds: The positive personal attachments between the clinician and person, including mutual trust, acceptance, and confidence (Horvath & Greenberg, 1989). The individual and clinician rate all items on a Likert scale.
- Continuity of care: Missed follow-ups and poor care transitions (e.g., post-discharge) are linked to dropout and can be tracked via appointment data (Marcus et al., 2017).
- Access to services: Geographic, financial, or logistical barriers (e.g., transportation) can be assessed through structured interviews or administrative data (Ojo et al., 2024).

E. Social and Environmental Factors

- Family and social support: Lack of support is a key predictor of nonadherence (Grover et al., 2021). This can be measured using tools like the Multidimensional Scale of Perceived Social Support (MSPSS). The MSPSS is a 12-item self-report inventory that assesses the magnitude of different sources of support from family, friends, and significant other. Respondents are asked to rate their perception of support from various subgroups on a 7-point Likert scale (i.e., "very strongly agree" = 7 to "very strongly disagree" = 1).
- Living situation and stability: Housing instability or social isolation are measurable risk factors (Benjet et al., 2022) and can be obtained from records, insurance and identification cards, self-report, and informants.
- Cultural beliefs and stigma: Cultural attitudes toward mental health problems and treatment influence adherence and can be assessed through qualitative or survey-based methods (Laranjeira et al., 2023).

Origins of Problems with Medications and Treatment Nonadherence

Treatment nonadherence by individuals living with SMI is complex, multidimensional, multidirectional, and heterogeneous. Treatment nonadherence is a problem behavior that occurs in people with other major health problems, like diabetes, cardiovascular disease, obesity, and kidney failure. There is a significant occurrence of medication nonadherence among individuals with multimorbidity, with a prevalence rate of 42.6% (Foley et al., 2021). Multimorbidity is the co-occurrence of at least two chronic conditions in the same individual and that has a substantial impact on the individual, their families, and on health systems and society (Skou et al., 2022). Multimorbidity is distinct from the concept of comorbidity as multimorbidity refers to the combined effects of additional conditions in relation to the original or first condition in an individual (Skou et al., 2022).

Nonadherence rates in general differ widely depending on the method used to measure adherence, with self-reported methods indicating the highest rates (76.5%) and electronic monitoring the lowest (44.1%) (Foley et al., 2021). Frequently cited predictors of medication nonadherence include a history of previous nonadherence and beliefs related to treatment. Other factors that have been assessed are the number of prescribed medications, an individual's health status, and beliefs about their physical conditions. No demographic predictors, such as age, sex, or marital status, were identified. Lower medication adherence was linked to reduced QoL and impaired performance on memory assessments (Foley et al., 2021).

The prevalence of nonadherence varies between physical conditions and mental health problems (Foley et al., 2021). In studies involving individuals with both physical conditions and depression or anxiety-related mental health problems, nonadherence was higher for antidepressants medications. Among those living with both mental health problems and physical conditions, nonadherence to psychiatric medications was higher in three out of seven studies, while nonadherence to medications for physical conditions was higher in four studies. These findings highlight the variability of medication nonadherence across different health conditions (Foley et al., 2021).

Treatment adherence is regarded not as a "symptom" of SMI, but rather because of living with SMI. The issue of adhering to treatment recommendations affects individuals with physical health conditions as well (Foley et al., 2021; Skou et al., 2022). Nonadherence is a complex phenomenon that involves beliefs (i.e., covert self-statements) about physical and/or mental health problems and health status, past occurrences of nonadherence, side effects of the medications and treatment, degree of social support, and quality of interactions with the prescribing and other service providers. Nonadherence also may involve certain problem behaviors that are reductions on typical functioning (i.e., negative symptoms (Correll & Schooler, 2020)) like apathy and impairments in motivation, and neurocognitive impairments in planning and memory (Mert et al., 2015; Semahegn et al., 2020; Velligan et al., 2017).

Behavioral challenges observed in individuals who live with SMI are associated with both neurological and environmental influences. Nonadherence to treatment recommendations is also present among the general population without mental health problems, particularly among those with impaired memory functioning (Foley et al., 2021). In people living with SMI, forgetfulness has been identified as the most common self-reported reason for nonadherence (Velligan et al., 2017). Impaired executive function (EF) predicted nonadherence by individuals living with SMI while other cognitive functions like long-term memory and attention did not. Individuals prescribed fewer medications showed better adherence, possibly due to reduced burden of planning and remembering dosing schedules (Velligan et al., 2017).

Neurological Substrates

Apathy, avolition, and other negative symptoms stem from disruptions in the integration of motivational, emotional, cognitive, and motor processes within complex neural circuits and associated neurotransmitter systems, particularly those regulating dopamine transmission in frontal and subcortical regions. These disturbances contribute to negative symptoms observed in various mental health and neurological health problems (Brown & Pluck, 2000; Goodkind et al., 2015; Hovington & Lepage, 2012). Gray and white matter loss in the frontal regions of the brain indicates a frequent neural idiosyncrasy in individuals with SMI, regardless of different causes. Results from structural MRIs have found the loss of gray and white matter in the following brain structures and possible impact on associated functions (Chuang et al., 2014; Goodkind et al., 2015; Hovington & Lepage, 2012):

Key structures include the following:

A. Frontal Cortex

- Dorsolateral prefrontal cortex (DLPFC): Linked to executive functions and cognitive processes. DLPFC is crucial for executive functions like working memory (WM), planning, and decision making. Reduced activity and gray matter volume in the DLPFC are often observed in individuals living with SMI, contributing to difficulties with these neurocognitive processes (Brown & Pluck, 2000; Chuang et al., 2014; Goodkind et al., 2015; Hovington & Lepage, 2012). Reduced gray matter density in DLPFC and regionally selective thinning are associated with negative symptoms (Hovington & Lepage, 2012).
- Medial and lateral PFC: Reduced gray matter density has been shown on MRIs with reduced connectivity in these areas and with the posterior cingulate cortex (PCC), impacting decision making and memory (Chuang et al., 2014; Hovington & Lepage, 2012).
- Ventromedial PFC (VMPFC): This area plays a vital role in emotional regulation and social cognition. Abnormalities in the VMPFC are associated with difficulties processing emotions, understanding social cues, and avolition (impairments with experiencing motivation) in people living with SMI (Goodkind et al., 2015).
- Medial orbitofrontal cortex (MOFC): Involved in emotional and motivational regulation (Brown & Pluck, 2000).
- Anterior cingulate cortex (ACC): Plays a role in decision making and emotional processing. The ACC is important for error detection, conflict monitoring, and attention. Dysfunction in the ACC is linked to impaired cognitive control, difficulty focusing, and problems with emotional processing in SMI (Brown & Pluck, 2000; Chuang et al., 2014; Goodkind et al., 2015).
- Superior temporal gyrus (STG): Reduced gray matter density has been shown to impact speech perception, auditory sensory memory, and language comprehension (Hovington & Lepage, 2012).

B. Subcortical Structures

- Basal ganglia: Includes the caudate nucleus, putamen, and globus pallidus, which are involved in motor and cognitive functions (Brown & Pluck, 2000; Chuang et al., 2014).
- Ventral striatum (VS) (e.g., Nucleus accumbens (NAc)): Central to motivation and reward processing. This structure is part of the brain's reward system and is involved in motivation and habit formation and is essential for learning which actions lead to reward and for implementing those actions in the future (Cox & Witten, 2019). Changes in the striatum, including altered activity and gray matter volume, are associated with difficulties experiencing pleasure (anhedonia) and impaired motivation, particularly in individuals with depressive and schizophrenia spectrum mental health problems. Structural changes in the area may be associated with decreasing the effectiveness of reinforcement in people living with SMI (Brown & Pluck, 2000; Chuang et al., 2014; Goodkind et al., 2015). Reduced activation during reward-related tasks correlates with anhedonia and negative symptoms (e.g., avolition) (Hovington & Lepage, 2012).
- Substantia nigra pars compacta (SNpc): Provides dopamine input to the striatum, crucial for regulating goal-directed behavior.
- Ventral tegmental area (VTA): Supplies dopamine to limbic and cortical areas, influencing motivation and reward.

C. Limbic System

- Amygdala (amyg): Processes emotional responses and motivation. The amyg is the brain's primary center for processing emotions, particularly fear and anxiety. Altered activity in the amyg, either increased or decreased, is observed in individuals living with SMI, influencing emotional responses and potentially contributing to symptoms like anxiety, fear, and social withdrawal (Brown & Pluck, 2000; Chuang et al., 2014; Goodkind et al., 2015).
- Hippocampus (HC): Contributes to memory and emotional regulation. This structure is essential for memory formation and spatial navigation. Reduced HC volume and activity are frequently found in individuals living with SMI, particularly those with depression, impacting memory and potentially contributing to difficulties in daily life and learning (Brown & Pluck, 2000; Chuang et al., 2014; Goodkind et al., 2015).
- Volume reductions in the amyg–HC complex (AHC), particularly the left anterior AHC, which is critical for memory function, has been shown with structural MRIs (sMRI) along with greater asymmetry in the shape and volume of the AHC and reduced volumes and connectivity. Correlations between reduced AHC volume and negative symptoms have been found (Chuang et al., 2014; Hovington & Lepage, 2012).
- Thalamus: Acts as a relay center, connecting limbic, striatal, and cortical structures; reduced thalamic volume correlates with negative symptoms (Brown & Pluck, 2000; Chuang et al., 2014; Hovington & Lepage, 2012).
- Lateral ventricles: Enlargement of the lateral ventricles has been linked to decreased volumes of cortical and subcortical gray matter, as well as an

association between ventricular enlargement and the presence of negative symptoms (Hovington & Lepage, 2012).

Goodkind et al. (2015) conducted a meta-analysis of studies using sMRIs across multiple mental health problems. The study found a transdiagnostic pattern of gray matter loss in the anterior insula (aINS) and dorsal ACC (dACC) among individuals with mental health problems corresponding to SMI. The decrease in gray matter in these regions correlates with impaired functioning in the domain of executive functions (EF) in participants with no known mental health problems. The neurocognitive domain of EF is composed of neurocognitive dimensions, such as task initiation, organization, flexibility, setting priorities, problem solving, working memory, and control of impulsivity and emotions (Baggetta & Alexander, 2016). Executive function (EF) plays a vital role in self-regulation and goal-directed behavior, both of which are essential for adhering to treatment recommendations. Impairments in EF are commonly observed across a range of mental health problems related to SMI, with the most significant impairments reported among individuals diagnosed with schizophrenia spectrum disorders, followed by those with bipolar and major depressive mental health problems (Baggetta & Alexander, 2016). This finding aligns with the high rates of nonadherence observed in these populations; for example, the prevalence of nonadherence among individuals with SMI in the referenced study was 54% (Khan et al., 2024).

The findings suggest that cortical thinning and gray matter loss in the aINS, fronto-temporal regions and dACC may contribute to impairments in EF and WM rather than specific symptoms (Goodkind et al., 2015; Huang et al., 2025). No significant effects of medications or comorbid health problems were found on gray matter volume.

Goodkind et al. (2015) concluded that there are neurological commonalities across mental health problems contrasting with previous studies related to specific mental health problems; future research should explore how gray matter loss relates to the severity, chronicity, and dimensions of symptoms and behavior problems linked to specific mental health problems as the findings suggest shared neural substrates and structural brain changes for mental health problems, particularly those corresponding to SMI.

Psychological and Behavioral Substrates

An individual living with SMI may not have had opportunities to learn functional adaptive skills, including health-related behaviors like treatment adherence. Many skills that are expected from functional adults are learned in mid-to-late adolescence. If the onset of living with SMI occurs during this developmental period, the person may not have chances to learn necessary skills. The young person living with SMI may have disruptions in his life due to being admitted to psychiatric facilities, entanglements with legal authorities, placements outside of the home and family, and problems with school attendance. The young person living with SMI may be experiencing neurocognitive problems in memory, attention, planning, and task initiation, having fewer opportunities to engage in meaningful and practical skill acquisitions. The results are the persistent and pervasive problems that are common across many contexts for the person living with SMI, including skills in self-control, self-monitoring, and self-regulation.

Adaptive skills in functioning encompass a range of learned behaviors that enable individuals to engage effectively and appropriately in everyday tasks that is expected in adult living; successfully performing these tasks results in positive outcomes, such as enabling close personal friendships, participating in enjoyable activities, independence in traveling, preparing and eating appetizing meals, and paid employment, including being able to maintain adequate mental health. Adaptive skills are the behaviors that people need to effectively manage their lives. Learning models such as operant conditioning, classical conditioning, and social learning theory can be effectively applied in the contexts in which these functional skills do and should occur.

Functional impairments are characterized by the absence of behaviors required for independent functioning and successful interaction with the environment to handle tasks and demands. Environments that are not conducive to learning and practicing new skills can contribute to behavioral skill impairments. With functional impairments, the expected behaviors do not occur either because the behaviors were not learned as the person had limited exposure to the response class of behaviors that encompass those skills or that the individual has not been taught or given sufficient opportunities to practice essential life skills, whether due to a lack of formal education, supportive environment, or underlying developmental challenges. The opportunities to learn may have been deficient in reinforcing the behavior in situations when the behavior should and should not occur (i.e., stimulus control). Lack of or ineffective use of positive reinforcement results in the absence of motivating operations (MOs) to engage in the skills in the appropriate context or situation. MOs refer to environmental or situational factors that affect the value of engaging in certain behaviors and the propensity to engage in them (Cooper et al., 2020). MOs can either enhance or diminish the efficacy of reinforcers, such as attention, approval, acquisition, or reciprocity. The absence of engaging in treatment adherent behaviors could result in a deficient history of being reinforced for engaging in adherent behaviors in similar contexts (e.g., following school schedules), the lack of opportunities to have effective skills shaped and reinforced by the environment and the lack of motivating stimuli to engage in the behaviors.

Learning can take place through observation and imitation. If life skills are not consistently demonstrated, individuals may not acquire these behaviors. Limited opportunities to observe modeled behaviors can affect daily functioning. Skills such as medication management, maintaining a healthy lifestyle, personal hygiene, and attending health-related appointments may not become routine if they are not regularly modeled and reinforced. Habits are "automatic behaviors triggered by environmental cues, developed through consistent repetition in stable contexts" (Lally & Gardner, 2011, p. 484). Strong habits diminish the influence of deliberate intentions on behavior, making them crucial for both promoting healthy actions and disrupting unhealthy ones, including nonadherence. Habits are essential for achieving long-term goals, promoting consistent behavior over time. Interventions that focus on habit formation enhance the sustainability of adaptive behaviors beyond the active intervention period (Lally & Gardner, 2011).

Additional environmental factors can influence the acquisition of adaptive skills. Sensory sensitivities and difficulties expressing needs and understanding others' communication can limit the ability to learn and interact. Challenges with capabilities to organize, time management, and transitions can make it difficult to initiate, plan, and carry out tasks, impacting skills like managing health-related behaviors.

Trauma or negative interactions can lead to emotional and behavioral responses that hinder skill development. The person might lack the skills to handle disappointment and frustration, especially if he has faced inconsistent or frequent punishment. Repeated exposure to punishment, failure, or a perceived lack of control can foster feelings of helplessness and hopelessness. This may inhibit individuals from attempting to learn new skills, as they tend to avoid situations where they believe their ability to influence negative outcomes is limited—even when opportunities for change exist. The presence of negative interactions with others because of living with SMI will result in increases in aversive self-statements and respondents related to self and other stigmatization. Adhering to treatment recommendations can function as a discriminative stimulus and an MO to experience adverse private events and an increase in distress; nonadherence and treatment discontinuation are negatively reinforced by the temporary reduction of the distress associated with being labeled as living with SMI and the stigma associated with it.

People living with SMI often struggle with adaptive functioning due to various factors. They may not have learned essential skills during childhood or young adulthood due to deficient learning environments or neurocognitive impairments. This lack of skill development can lead to problem behaviors during a crucial time for acquiring advanced functions such as taking care of one's health. Additionally, individuals living with SMI are at higher risk for developing co-occurring disorders (i.e., substance use) that disrupt typical behavior patterns such as adherence to treatment. Repeated trauma and isolated lifestyles further hamper access to positive reinforcement. Frequent hospitalizations and removal from the community exacerbate these issues. The absence of competent role models and neurocognitive impairments in attention, memory, planning, and task initiation contributes to the difficulty in learning necessary adaptive skills. Impairments in adaptive behaviors in people who live with SMI are influenced by a combination of lack of knowledge, motivation, proper stimulus control, or all the above.

People living with SMI frequently fail to become integrated into a natural social network that can assist them in coping with life demands and other life stressors. They frequently reside in impoverished and under-stimulating environments with few available opportunities to engage in prosocial and reinforcing behaviors. The lack of a naturally occurring reinforcing network often results in the family of the individual living with SMI as the only network to which they belong. The response patterns of families of individuals living with SMI often include deviant, punitive, and aversive behaviors, adding stress that the individual lacks the skills to manage (Morrison & Wixted, 1989). Studies have repeatedly found that people living with SMI who have family relationships characterized by hostile and aversive interactions are more likely to be hospitalized shortly discharge from a psychiatric facility (Vaughn & Leff, 1976) resulting in disruptions to the acquisition of adaptive habits and behaviors.

Individual differences and contextual factors play a significant role in how functional competencies are developed and adapted. A transdiagnostic, dimensional perspective is necessary for creating targeted interventions for individuals living with SMI. The variety and complexities of domains of adaptive functioning reflect the challenges in the assessment and effective treatment of these impairments.

Epidemiological Considerations

Nonadherence to treatment recommendations and medications is highly relevant because it significantly impacts the treatment outcomes for individuals living with SMI. Psychiatric medication like all medications, is effective only when taken as prescribed, and nonadherence undermines the potential benefits of treatment, such as reduction in distressing problem behaviors and possible improved functioning (Acosta et al., 2012; Velligan et al., 2017).

The consequences of nonadherence are deleterious and detrimental to ongoing recovery and improved QoL. Nonadherence to treatment results in increased use of emergency psychiatric services and increased risk of relapses and hospitalization. Interruptions in treatment, even as short as one to 10 days, are associated with a higher likelihood of hospitalization in people living with SMI (Acosta et al., 2012; Velligan et al., 2017). Nonadherence is linked to poor social and occupational functioning, increased risk of suicide attempts, violence, arrests, and overall diminished QoL.

Nonadherence rates vary depending on the assessment method. Self-reported nonadherence is the highest at 76.5%, followed by pharmacy data at 69.4%, and electronic monitoring at 44.1%. Overall, reported nonadherence rates range from 7.0% to 83.5%. Various demographic factors influence nonadherence and show differing prevalence rates of nonadherence. Age, gender, socioeconomic status, and illness severity are commonly cited as key factors associated with nonadherence to treatment regimens in individuals who live with SMI. Both younger (<34) and older adults (≥60) show elevated nonadherence (Grover et al., 2021). Lower educational attainment has been linked to higher rates of nonadherence (Lucca et al., 2015). Being unemployed is a predictor across several studies (Benjet et al., 2022; Semahegn et al., 2020). There is mixed evidence for gender being a crucial factor, but, in general, males tend to have higher rates of noncompliance; this may be linked to males having higher rates of co-occurring mental health problems (NIDA, 2020). Sociocultural variations exist (Benjet et al., 2022) with low income showing a positive correlation with cost-related nonadherence (Lucca et al., 2015; Magura et al., 2014). Socioeconomic status (SES) influences adherence: lower SES can hinder follow-up due to transportation and cost issues (Dennis et al., 2020), while higher SES is linked to better adherence rates (Ghosh et al., 2022).

Nonadherence to psychotropic medication varies among different mental health problems. Individuals living with schizophrenia spectrum mental health problems showed the highest nonadherence rate at 56% (Guo et al., 2023; Malik et al., 2020; Semahegn et al., 2020), followed by major depressive disorder (MDD) at 50% (Laranjeira et al., 2023; Semahegn et al., 2020), and bipolar disorder that ranged from 44% to 57% (Malik et al., 2020). Semahegn et al. (2020) reported a 49% pooled prevalence rate of nonadherence in individuals living with SMI.

The mental health problem of borderline personality has been classified as an SMI (U.S. Department of Health and Human Servcies [HHS], National Institute of Health [NIH], 2023). Nonadherence to treatment has been a challenge in people living with this mental health problem. Studies have reported rates of nonadherent behaviors ranging from 35% to 70%, depending on the population, setting, and how adherence is measured (Gunderson & Choi-Kain, 2018; Magura et al., 2014). Psychotherapy dropout rates for BPD are also high, with estimates between 20% and 50%, especially in early sessions (Kullgard et al., 2022; Wells et al., 2013). Long-term refusal of medication over 18 months is about 19% in individuals experiencing first-episode psychosis and living with BPD traits (Lambert et al., 2010).

Types of psychiatric medications have shown to have variable influence on nonadherence by individuals living with SMI. Nonadherence to oral antipsychotics is estimated to be 50%; LAIs may reduce nonadherence and dropout rates (Acosta et al., 2012) and nonadherence is notably lower than with oral antipsychotics (Velligan et al., 2025). However, studies have found that between 56% and 45% of individuals initially accept LAIs but between 20% and 40% later display nonadherent behaviors with the medications (Velligan et al., 2025).

Mood-stabilizing medications are reported to have a 45.5% nonadherence prevalence by individuals living with bipolar type of mental health problem (Mert et al., 2015). Antidepressant medications often show high prevalence of nonadherence in co-occurring and comorbid populations (Alekhya et al., 2015). Individuals living with multimorbidity have shown a 42.6% pooled nonadherence rate (Foley et al., 2021).

Cultural Considerations

Cultural and regional variations in the prevalence of nonadherent behaviors have been reported (Benjet et al., 2022; Deng et al., 2022; Semahegn et al., 2020). A prevalence rate for nonadherence of 57% has been reported for the Asian region (Semahegn et al., 2020). Deng reported that rates of medication nonadherence in the People's Republic of China (PRC) vary according to the type of mental health condition. Individuals diagnosed with schizophrenia spectrum mental health problems exhibited a nonadherence prevalence of 56%, those with bipolar type of mental health problem demonstrated a rate of 48%, and individuals experiencing major depressive problems had a prevalence of 51%. This lack of adherence has contributed to approximately 60% of people who live with SMI in the PRC experiencing significant disability, frequent rehospitalization, and elevated suicide rates.

Khan et al. (2024) found the following prevalence of nonadherence in a sample of individuals living with mental health problems in India. Nonadherence rates vary significantly among different mental health problems. Substance use disorders had the highest nonadherence rate, with 77% of individuals discontinuing treatment after the initial visit with only 16.2% adhering to regular follow-ups. Fifty percent of people living with common mental health problems discontinued treatment after the first visit. The rate of nonadherence in people living with SMI was that 36% discontinued treatment after the first visit (Khan et al., 2024).

The prevalence of nonadherence in other regions is as follows: Africa (48%); North America: (48%); and Europe (49%). Dropout rates also differ by country, with the United States at 9%, Mexico at 18.9%, and Peru at 22.6% (Benjet et al., 2022).

Cultural and regional factors affect how people follow treatment recommendations for SMI. Key cultural factors affecting treatment adherence by people living with SMI include the following:

- Medication acceptance: Beliefs about mental health problems shape adherence to treatment. Individuals may turn to traditional healing due to cultural faith, limited success with allopathic medicine, economic concerns, stigma, and accessibility (Viswanath & Chaturvedi, 2012).
- Family involvement: Families play a critical role in supporting treatment adherence (Viswanath & Chaturvedi, 2012).
- Sociocultural beliefs: A disregard for the beliefs of an individual living with SMI can reduce follow-up rates; integrating these beliefs into care improves adherence (Viswanath & Chaturvedi, 2012).
- Traditional healing: Use of traditional practices alongside modern medicine is common and may support adherence (Viswanath & Chaturvedi, 2012).
- Stigma: Stigma remains a major barrier, especially in rural areas where discrimination is more overt, hindering ongoing treatment (Viswanath & Chaturvedi, 2012).
- Coping strategies: Some traditional cultures rely on avoidance or meditation rather than medical intervention, unlike Western counterparts (Viswanath & Chaturvedi, 2012).

Despite the impact of culture on treatment aspect of SMI, it is notable that the prevalence of nonadherence is remarkably similar in the reported regions (Semahegn et al., 2020; Benjet et al., 2022).

Types of Problems with Adhering to Medication and Treatment Recommendations

Problems with adherence to treatment recommendations by people living with SMI are heterogeneous; types or patterns of nonadherence to treatment recommendations help service providers tailor interventions effectively. The heterogeneity of nonadherent behaviors presents challenges as to defining subtypes of nonadherence (Vega et al., 2020).

Researchers have identified several forms of treatment nonadherence among people living with SMI. Types of treatment nonadherence are as follows:

- Intentional and unintentional nonadherence (Hugtenburg et al., 2013; Lincoln et al., 2016; Magura et al., 2014; Vega et al., 2020): Intentional nonadherence is defined as the choosing not to follow treatments due to beliefs, attitudes, lack of insight, financial burden of following treatment recommendations, or perceived side effects of medications. Unintentional nonadherence occurs due to forgetfulness, neurocognitive impairments, or logistical barriers, like transportation or late delivery of medications (Lincoln et al., 2016; Vega et al., 2020).
- Voluntary vs. involuntary nonadherence (Velligan et al., 2017). Voluntary nonadherence refers to a conscious decision by the individuals to stop taking medication or to take less than prescribed. This is often influenced by factors such as poor insight, negative attitudes toward medication, distressing side effects, poor therapeutic alliance, or stigma. Involuntary nonadherence occurs when practical problems or impairments related to the individual's mental health problems interfere with their ability to take medication regularly. Examples include substance abuse, neurocognitive impairments, depression, lack of family/social support, limited access to mental health care, or social instability. Although similar to the type of intentional/unintentional nonadherence, Velligan et al. (2017) does emphasize that the person must have the "capacity" to intentionally interrupt or drop out of treatment. "Capacity" is defined as the ability of to receive or retain information and knowledge and to competently function in mental or physical tasks. The person demonstrating capacity must demonstrate an understanding of the information about their health condition, treatment options, and potential risks and benefits, and make a voluntary choice based on that understanding (Barstow et al., 2018).
- Primary and secondary nonadherence (Semahegn et al., 2020): Primary nonadherence is defined as the person does not initiate the prescribed treatment while secondary nonadherence is defined as the individual starts but does not continue with the recommended treatments (such as dropping out of therapy after a few sessions) (Semahegn et al., 2020).
- Partial and complete nonadherence (Vrijens et al., 2012): Partial nonadherence is defined when the person living with SMI follows some aspects of the treatment recommendations but not others. Examples would be taking medication inconsistently, taking only one class of medications or lowering the dose of medications,

or skipping therapy sessions. Complete nonadherence is when the person discontinues all forms of treatment (Vrijens et al., 2012).

- Persistent and intermittent nonadherence (Lambert et al., 2010): Persistent nonadherence is defined as the long-term refusal or avoidance of treatment. Intermittent nonadherence is when nonadherence fluctuates over time, often linked to exacerbations of mental health problems or life stressors (Lambert et al., 2010).
- Nonadherence can be subtyped by the duration or length of time of the occurrence of nonadherent behaviors. Long-term treatment nonadherence typically refers to a sustained failure to follow prescribed treatment over an extended period—often six months or more. This definition is especially relevant in chronic conditions and with SMI, where adherence is expected to be continuous. Lambert et al. (2010) defined persistent medication refusal as nonadherence lasting at least 18 months, despite clinical recommendations for continued treatment. This definition highlights a pattern of consistent disengagement, rather than intermittent lapses. Vrijens et al. (2012) introduced a taxonomy where "persistence" refers to the duration of time from treatment initiation to discontinuation. Long-term nonadherence reflects a premature end to treatment before the recommended course is completed.
- Full adherence and nonadherence: These individuals consistently took their medication as prescribed and had no lapses of seven days or longer during treatment (Lambert et al., 2010). Nonadherence is defined as at least one phase where medication was not taken for a week or more, indicating issues beyond missed doses. Service discontinuation despite ongoing treatment need (e.g., dropout) also was defined as nonadherence (Lambert et al., 2010).
- Medication refusal: Individuals were considered to have refused medication if they consistently declined to take prescribed drugs during treatment, with up to three weeks of nonadherence allowed. Those who left treatment three weeks after initiation of treatment also were classified as "refusers," as shorter trials are insufficient to assess medication effectiveness. Individuals not engaging with the service providers, refusing contact, or being untraceable were likewise deemed to have refused all medications (Lambert et al., 2010).

Nonadherent behaviors can be categorized according to the dimensions of the nonadherence. These dimensional types include the following:

- The types of medications, treatments, and therapies prescribed to which types of adherences/nonadherences occur.
- Length of adherence, nonadherence, and intervals of switching between them for each treatment type. Subtypes of adherence/nonadherence would include the amount and schedule of medications being taken, frequency of occurrences when dosing and schedule are altered by the person living with SMI, and the duration of the altered dosing and schedule.
- Magnitude of nonadherence: The amount of adherence/nonadherence that occurs in treatment recommendations. Does the person living with SMI discontinue all treatment recommendations? Some individuals living with SMI will continue

with certain therapies but discontinue or are nonadherent to medications (Mirhaj Mohammadabadi et al., 2022).

The assessment of the types of adherence/nonadherent can facilitate the determination of the effective treatment for an individual living with SMI. For example, LAIs may be a beneficial and effective treatment for the person who unintentionally is nonadherent to medication, but may not be effective in a person living with SMI who has a history of nonadherence and displays intentional and intermittent nonadherence.

Why is Nonadherence to Medications and Treatment Recommendations Problematic with Individuals Living with SMI?

People who live with SMI usually require a combination of medication and other forms of treatment, like group and individual therapies and case management. At times, medications are an important factor in minimizing problem behaviors such as delusions and hallucinations. SMI is a chronic condition and, if medications are not taken as prescribed, the problem behaviors may return. The return of problematic symptoms may be gradual, leading the person (and perhaps the family members) to think that the medications are not important. However, stopping medication has been demonstrated to be one of the major reasons that rehospitalizations and mental health crises occur.

While the medications help, they are usually not enough. Medications alone will not overcome unemployment, poverty, homelessness, stigmatization, and lack of basic social and self-care skills that are often a part of living with a SMI. To do this, rehabilitative therapies as well as guidance and support from other people are critical. Social support—defined as the assurance that individuals have reliable advocates—is frequently one of the most significant determinants in whether a person living with SMI utilizes available resources.

Seeking and following the advice of mental health service professionals may seem obvious to most people, and this is usually much easier said than done. There are a variety of possible reasons why it may be very difficult for the person living with SMI to seek or follow the advice and help that are available.

Part of the Problem May Be Biochemical or Physical

- Avoidance of side effects (American Medical Association [AMA], 2023): The medications that are prescribed for mental disorders are potent. While they may have a good effect on some symptomatic problem behaviors linked to living with SMI, they may also bring on a variety of uncomfortable side effects which the person wishes to avoid. Sometimes nonadherence occurs because of wanting to avoid a serious side effect of metabolic syndrome. Unfortunately, in the view of the person living with SMI, the benefits don't outweigh the side effects. Many will stop taking the medications to avoid the side effects (Aljofan et al., 2023).

- People take medications for certain symptoms of which they are aware (Grover et al., 2021): If one has a headache, usually people take something like acetaminophen or a NSAID. If the person does not have a headache, the importance of taking the medication fades. It is the same for any health problem. It takes time and effort to take medications daily; it is difficult to remember what and when to take the medications. "Pill boxes" are available that can be filled and help the person take the medication correctly and as scheduled. Pill boxes, however, need to be refilled and sometimes people forget. In addition, when a person feels better and has fewer distressing symptoms, the importance of taking the medications lessens.
- Impairments related to living with an SMI often interfere with a person's ability to think clearly (Lincoln et al., 2016; Smith et al., 2017): Because of this, the person who lives with SMI may have more difficulty remembering the schedule for taking medications or for times of appointments and meetings (Lincoln et al., 2016; Smith et al., 2017). SMI may also interfere with the ability to recognize and appreciate the improvements by the person living with SMI because of taking medication or seeing a therapist (Grover et al., 2021). As a result, the individual may perceive no compelling or valid reason to adhere to prescribed medications or attend scheduled appointments.
- The biochemical imbalance that is assumed to cause SMI may result in problem behaviors, such as delusions and lack of awareness (e.g., insight) that directly interferes with the willingness to follow treatment recommendations (Grover et al., 2021). For example, the person living with SMI may claim that "I don't have a mental illness" or say that "the doctors are against me. They never listen to what I say." He may claim that "the medications are destroying my insides." Beliefs about medications and the presence of living with SMI make it much more difficult to convince the person who lives with SMI to do what service providers are recommending.

Part of the Problem May Be Psychosocial

- Stigmatization: The person who lives with SMI may be reluctant to accept help and treatment because of misunderstandings that he and other people have about SMI. Some people believe that living with SMI is simply a lack of will power and if the person "just tries hard enough," things would be better. The person who lives with SMI and their support group may consider medications or counseling to be an unnecessary "crutch." Many people are unsure how to view SMI and may avoid those displaying unusual behaviors. Terms like "crazy" or "psycho" carry stigma, leading to discrimination, isolation, and hopelessness for those with SMI. This stigma can discourage individuals from recognizing their condition or seeking support (Benjet et al., 2022; Buchman-Wildbaum et al., 2020; Deng et al., 2022; Lincoln et al., 2016).

- People living with SMIs have a problem with developing trust in other people. Most people will be uncomfortable about meeting with someone with whom they are unfamiliar. This uncomfortable feeling will usually be greater when the other person is evaluating their behaviors and speech, asking them very personal questions about their experiences, thoughts and feelings, and giving recommendations about their experiences. If the interaction with a service provider is perceived as critical and dismissive, the individual may stop going to the appointments. In some cases, this is a part of living with an SMI. In other cases, it may be a result of how they have been treated by mental health service professionals in the past and may avoid further interactions. Dissatisfaction with prescribing service providers, feeling poorly informed about medication, experiencing emotional detachment, paternalism, and lack of empathy by service providers have been found to be barriers to adherence and a key factor in discontinuation of treatment (Grover et al. 2021; Lincoln et al. 2016; Ljungberg et al. 2016).
- The services required to treat SMI can often be complicated: For example, a person living with SMI may require several types of medications (Acosta et al., 2012; American Medical Association [AMA], 2023). These may include an antipsychotic drug for major symptoms, a second medication for side effects brought on by the antipsychotic medications, and a third medication to decrease physiological arousal and help the person sleep. These may need to be taken at various times throughout the day (such as four times daily, with meals, or at bedtime) and could include specific instructions for administration (for example, before or after meals, avoiding dairy products or salads, or taking with water). Pills can appear similar, making it challenging to distinguish between different types of medications. Different brands of the same medication may also vary in appearance, which can lead individuals to question whether they have received the correct medication. Such issues have been associated with some people living with SMI discontinuing their medications (Acosta et al., 2012; AMA, 2023).
- A reason that some people stop taking medications is that sometimes they work very well. A person with problematic psychiatric behavioral symptoms may improve with proper medications and feel and do much better. Because the symptoms have decreased, the person may no longer see any need to take the medicine (Benjet et al., 2022; NAMI, 2024). Living with SMI is a lifelong condition, and some problem behaviors may require long-term treatment. Any reduction or discontinuation with treatment needs to be done slowly and be supervised by a professional provider (Benjet et al., 2022; NAMI, 2024).

Behavioral Support Strategies to Increase Adherence to Follow Treatment Recommendations by Individuals Living with Serious Mental Illness

Steps can be taken to make it more likely that the person living with SMI will follow the treatment recommendations. Some or all the following suggestions may be useful depending on the situation:

- Seek a review of current medications: It may be helpful to obtain a review of current medications by a psychiatric service provider. This is particularly true if side effects appear to be a problem for the person who lives with SMI. The psychiatric service prescriber needs to be aware of the side effects that are bothersome and when they occur. The prescribing service provider may be able to change to other medications which have fewer or less severe side effects. In the example above, Fred reported experiencing drowsiness as a side effect of his medications. After discussing this with the prescribing healthcare provider, an adjustment to a different medication with a lower likelihood of causing drowsiness could have been considered. The prescriber might also have adjusted the dosage so that Fred would take the medication once daily before bedtime. For many side effects, there are additional medications that help to reduce how distressing and severe the side effects are. These are only a few of the possible changes that might help the person who lives with SMI to be more consistent in taking the medications.
- Watch for circumstances that affect the adherence to follow treatment recommendations by the person who lives with SMI: Usually, the primary problem with treatment adherence is that it is inconsistent and not that the person refuses outright. Watch for any variation in the willingness to take the medication as prescribed or attend scheduled therapy meetings by the person living with SMI. Note any issues that seem to be tied to refusals, such as time of day, mood, complaints of side effects, or other factors, like transportation and finances. These may be important in devising strategies to minimize the problem. For example, the person who lives with SMI may have difficulty getting out of bed in the morning. This may be due to sedation brought on by the medicine. If aware, the psychiatric provider can adjust the dosage, schedule, or medication to reduce morning sedation.
- Make meeting or medication times a clear daily priority: Since treatment adherence can't be assumed, integrate it into the routine for both individuals who live with SMI and their support teams. Set clear schedules for medications and appointments, post them visibly, and plan other activities around these times. Reviewing the day's schedule after breakfast each day can help reinforce this habit and ensure that these tasks are treated as essential.
- Use memory aids to help remember when medications are to be taken or appointments kept: Many people, including those living with SMI, may struggle to remember when to take their medications. A variety of methods to assist people

have been developed. One example is a pill box. This will hold a week's worth of medication in compartments that are marked by day of the week and time of the day. The compartments help the person remember when it is time to take the next dose. For appointments, a calendar, small appointment book or automatic reminders on smart phones can be helpful in remembering when appointments are scheduled.

- Establish familiarity with the community mental health service providers: If the person living with SMI is reluctant to go to appointments, it may be helpful to escort the individual to the first few meetings. This can help the person who lives with SMI become familiar with that setting and other people. Some "nervousness" is to be expected when meeting new people or going to an unfamiliar place. The "nervousness" will lessen as they become more familiar with the people and the expectations. Using the example above, Fred's family took him to visit his case manager before being discharged from his last admission. This was done to help Fred "connect" with the case manager before he left the hospital.
- Make sure that the person who lives with SMI is familiar with directions, transportation, and other factors necessary to attend appointments and meetings: Even if the person who lives with SMI has attended appointments or meetings in the past, don't assume that they remember where the building is located, the layout of the building, the location of the office of the case manager and other service providers, and what assistance is available to get there. Having a few "practice runs' 'before the next meeting is usually helpful. Using the example above, Fred said that he was very nervous about being able to find his way to the community clinic. He was also nervous about meeting with his case manager. His parents took him for brief visits to the clinic to become familiar with the setting. They arranged for a visit during a time that his case manager would be there. This way he became more familiar (and less nervous) about visiting the clinic.
- Establish a contract for taking medications or keeping appointments: A contract for desired behaviors can help to specify when the medications need to be taken as well as identifying what reinforcing activities are available for adherence. The contract outlines the expectations for individuals living with SMI and clarifies their responsibilities. It also serves as a framework for involving the individual in developing the terms of a behavior contract, specifying which activities, benefits, and reinforcing events are linked to adherence to treatment recommendations. The person who lives with SMI should be involved in specifying the rewards for following the contract. This helps to make sure that the rewards truly act as incentives for the behaviors that are being encouraged. Using the example above, it was important to Fred that he was able to spend time walking in a park by himself. The staff at the supervised apartment agreed to give him specific times for walking if he attended certain group meetings and took his medications as scheduled. Later, they developed an arrangement in which Fred could spend time at his father's house if he agreed to spend a specific amount of time at the community mental health center. Each of these agreements helped Fred to do things that he would have avoided. Remember that a contract is a temporary measure that helps to get the desired behavior started. If the medication and/or treatment

meetings truly benefit the person who lives with SMI, the behavior should become reinforcing itself as Fred has opportunities to meet friends and engage in other activities that are rewarding.

- Do not overlook examples of adherence in other areas: If the person who lives with SMI has been inconsistent about attending appointments or following the treatment recommendations, be aware of other behaviors that are being manifested that show adherence to requests, like doing the laundry when asked. When the person living with SMI takes medications or attends treatment meetings as scheduled, they need to be verbally praised for the willingness to do so.
- Inquire about a "long-acting" medication option: If consistent adherence to medication has been challenging, there may be psychiatric medications available that require less frequent dosing. These are often referred to as "LAs" or long-acting medications and may only have to be taken once each month. Some are available in an "injectable" form so the medication can be given at a monthly visit to the doctor. Not all psychiatric medications are available as LAs, so some prescribed drugs for people who live with SMI may not be offered in this form. This is a decision that can be made with the mutual engagement of the treating psychiatric provider and the person living with SMI.
- Do not overlook the value of basic education: The experience of coping with SMI can be very confusing and frustrating, for the person living with SMI and the support individuals. Getting familiar with what problems to expect from a specific mental health problem related to SMI and the common treatments for the problem can help reduce that confusion. Informative booklets on specific mental health problems and interventions are available at the local community mental health center and from advocacy groups, like NAMI and NIMH. These booklets can help people living with SMI and their support networks better understand the situation and possible actions. While they may not answer every question or solve all issues, they will enhance understanding of SMI.

Conclusion for Behavioral Support Strategies to Increase Adherence to Follow Treatment Recommendations by Individuals Living with Serious Mental Illness

When an individual living with SMI does not consistently adhere to treatment recommendations, such as by irregularly taking prescribed medications or missing scheduled appointments, the following strategies may be beneficial:

1. Seeking the opinion of a psychiatric provider about current medications to see if side effects can be minimized by an alternative medicine.
2. Discuss "long-acting" alternatives for the current medications.
3. Watch for factors (such as mood, type of meeting, who is in the meeting) that seem to make a difference in whether the person who lives with SMI adheres to recommendations.

4. Plan daily routine around the behaviors that are being encouraged. Develop a daily schedule and review the schedule with the person who lives with SMI at a convenient time, such as after breakfast.
5. Make sure that the person who lives with SMI knows what is expected of him and how to follow through. Spend time helping him get used to where he must go and what he is supposed to do.
6. If adherence is inconsistent, watch for success and verbally praise the person who lives with SMI when adherence is exhibited even in other areas of functioning, like daily hygiene.
7. Create a contract to clarify expectations for the person with SMI and outline incentives for desired behaviors.

What About Fred?

The staff was made aware of Fred's history of leaving treatment shortly after discharge. They also recognized that he preferred to stay away from other people and avoided becoming actively involved in any treatment program. They made efforts to encourage his participation in the treatment options available to him. They decided that pushing him too aggressively to be involved in activities and groups would only provoke him to run away. Thus, they were patient and accepted the level of participation that he was currently able to show. The case manager worked with him and suggested two groups at the community clinic that he could try that had fewer members attending. The staff at the apartment made a point to ensure that Fred took the medication as prescribed and attended the groups (they set no expectations beyond attending the groups); they arranged his schedule so that he would have plenty of time to leave the apartment, walk around the park and go to a fast food restaurant. While they showed interest in him by occasionally asking him how he was, they kept their interactions short unless he appeared interested in keeping the conversation going. They emphasized that their priority for him was to help him to be stable, decrease the distressing problem behaviors, and not be admitted to the hospital.

The staff at the clinic and apartment worked to help Fred increase his social engagement. In group therapy, the psychologist let Fred participate at his own pace, occasionally inviting his input but never pressuring him. Gradually, structured activities required Fred to be a bit more involved, always allowing others to go first so he could observe. As Fred grew more comfortable, the psychologist expressed interest in his contributions; over time, Fred took greater initiative both in group sessions and in other settings.

After several weeks, when he returned to the apartment after his stay at the clinic, the staff acknowledged him. Some staff members spent time outside with him and talked about his day. He was recognized for continuing his treatment rather than leaving the group or the clinic. At this point, Fred responded to these interactions, which led him to view his "wanderlust" as discomfort in unfamiliar social situations.

After a few months, he began to meet with a therapist to examine living independently. They discussed places to live that were near his parents' home. They found an apartment and arranged for Fred to have a series of brief overnight passes to become more familiar with the apartment. He continued attending activities at the local community clinic. Fred was eventually discharged to the independent living apartment and has successfully stayed there and became more involved in the programs at the mental health center.

In this example, the various service providers took several steps to help Fred become more willing and able to follow the treatment advice that he was being given:

1. They recognized that Fred was very nervous about participating in most of the treatment but that they could not allow him to avoid becoming involved in it.
2. They recognized that Fred spent much of his time "walking off" his nervousness. This also helped him to stay away from other people.
3. They identified a small number of groups that they felt he could tolerate better, and which would be beneficial for him.
4. They made sure to give him a brief reminder before each group was held. However, they left the decision to attend the group up to him. They made sure that he had plenty of time to do his walking.
5. The group leader developed structured exercises that involved all members of the group. He made sure that other group members went first so Fred could see how they did and minimized any perceptions of "being singled out."
6. The group leader and other staff made sure to compliment his efforts at participating in discussions in the group.
7. The staff at the supervised apartment helped Fred with his medication adherence. The staff got him a pill box and prompted and supervised him to fill it weekly; as he became more reliable, the staff allowed him to refill the pill box independently with only occasional checking to make sure that he was taking the medications and refilling it correctly.
8. The staff assisted him by organizing his medication schedule and clinic appointments on two large calendars, placing one in his bedroom and the other in the kitchen.
9. As Fred became more comfortable with others, he began visiting potential independent living apartments near his parents.

Fred was ultimately discharged to his own apartment. His engagement in his treatment increased significantly, which contributed to more consistent and lasting progress with this approach.

Summary

Nonadherence to medication and treatment is a prevalent issue among individuals living with SMI, leading to significant clinical and social consequences, including relapses, hospitalization, and increased suicide risk.

Approximately 49% of all individuals living with SMI exhibit medication nonadherence. Nonadherence rates remain substantial among individuals who live with certain types of mental health problems linked to SMI, with prevalence reported at 61% for schizophrenia-spectrum mental health problems, 57% for bipolar-type, and 52% for depressive-type of mental health problems. Additionally, long-acting injectable (LAI) medications are associated with significant nonadherence within the first year of treatment. Nonadherence behaviors include taking incorrect doses, altering schedules, abandoning treatment, and refusing visits.

Nonadherence to treatment can result in serious negative consequences for the person living with SMI. Failure to adhere to treatment recommendations can result in severe clinical ramifications and increased healthcare costs. Nonadherence is linked to an 82% relapse rate over five years in schizophrenia spectrum mental health problems. Interrupting medication for one to 10 days has been associated with an increased risk of hospitalization. Among individuals with SMI who discontinue treatment, 69% are hospitalized and 22% attempt suicide. Nonadherence is also linked to higher mortality rates. Additionally, societal impacts include an economic cost exceeding $10 billion annually in the United States.

Nonadherence to treatment among individuals with SMI is influenced by a range of personal, relational, clinical, and systemic factors. On the individual level, impaired insight—also known as anosognosia—plays a significant role in whether a person follows their treatment plan. Negative beliefs about medication and doubts about its effectiveness can further reduce adherence. Socioeconomic challenges and substance use are also associated with higher rates of nonadherence. Organizational difficulties, often stemming from neurocognitive impairments like forgetfulness, can make it harder to stick to medication schedules. Internalized stigma and feelings of grief may discourage individuals from seeking care or continuing with treatment.

Medication-related issues are common barriers to adherence. Side effects such as sedation and weight gain frequently lead individuals to stop taking their medication. The complexity of treatment regimens and the number of medications prescribed—often between two and five psychotropic drugs—can also lower adherence. If patients perceive medications as ineffective, they are more likely to discontinue treatment prematurely.

Certain characteristics of the mental health problem itself, including how long a person has been living with the mental health problem and the presence of additional health problems, can impact adherence rates. Nonadherence is especially common among those who have lived with the mental health issues for more than a year and among those with repeated relapses. Additional physical health conditions and untreated depression are also linked to worse adherence.

Environmental and systemic barriers have a substantial effect on treatment adherence. Poor access to mental health services, inadequate insurance reimbursement, financial difficulties, and transportation problems can all interfere with ongoing care. A weak therapeutic alliance with healthcare providers can erode trust and motivation, making it less likely individuals will follow treatment recommendations.

Culture and social support are key influences on whether individuals who live with SMI adhere to treatment. Misunderstandings and misconceptions about mental illness among family and social networks can undermine engagement in care. Conversely, strong family support improves adherence, while negative family attitudes make adherence more difficult. Addressing cultural beliefs and strengthening community support are important for improving adherence rates.

Medication nonadherence in SMI is complex and multifaceted, requiring comprehensive assessment tools that consider psychological, behavioral, and social factors. NIMH Research Domain Criteria (RDoC) framework encourages understanding mental health issues through various dimensions of functioning. Just as pain is understood as involving physical, psychological, and behavioral domains, treatment nonadherence should be viewed as multidimensional. Assessments should include objective measures (like blood levels) and subjective tools (such as self-report questionnaires), as well as factors like the specifics of nonadherent behavior, frequency, duration, awareness, antecedents, and the reasons behind nonadherence.

Other personal variables strongly influence whether someone with SMI adheres to treatment. Memory impairments can all affect adherence. Limited insight into one's illness and negative attitudes toward medication can be measured with tools like the Drug Attitude Inventory (DAI) and the Medication Adherence Rating Scale (MARS), Substance use and stigma also play a role. Adverse medication effects, complicated dosing schedules, and financial constraints further challenge adherence.

Clinical features, such as symptom severity and duration of illness, often influence engagement with treatment. Comorbid physical or psychiatric conditions may complicate care and hinder adherence even more. On the system level, the quality of the therapeutic relationship and continuity of care are critical; strong provider relationships help, while missed follow-up and poor care transitions hinder ongoing treatment.

Finally, social and environmental circumstances—such as family support, stable housing, and community resources—play a vital role in ensuring that individuals living with SMI can adhere to their treatment plans. Cultural beliefs and the stigma associated with mental illness can shape adherence behaviors in profound ways.

Treatment nonadherence in individuals who live with SMI is a multifaceted concern impacted by numerous factors, such as multimorbidity and neurocognitive impairments. The complexities and neurological foundations of medication nonadherence in this population are significant, with cognitive and emotional factors playing a substantial role in influencing treatment adherence.

Treatment nonadherence is prevalent in individuals with SMI and other chronic health conditions, with a 42.6% rate among those with multimorbidity. Nonadherence rates vary based on measurement methods: self-reported methods show 76.5% adherence, while electronic monitoring shows 44.1%. Predictors of nonadherence include previous nonadherence history, beliefs about treatment, number of prescribed medications, and health status. Lower medication adherence correlates with reduced QoL and impaired memory performance. Nonadherence rates differ between physical and mental health conditions, with higher rates for antidepressants in individuals with both physical and mental health issues. Nonadherence is influenced by cognitive impairments, particularly in executive function, and is often linked to forgetfulness, which is not uncommon in individuals living with a depressive type of mental health problem.

Alterations in brain structure and function observed in individuals who live with SMI are associated with negative symptoms and challenges in treatment adherence. Apathy and avolition stem from disruptions in neural circuits, particularly those regulating dopamine in frontal and subcortical regions. Structural MRIs reveal gray and white matter loss in key brain areas, including the dorsolateral prefrontal cortex (DLPFC) and anterior cingulate cortex (ACC). Impairments in executive functions, such as working memory (WM) and decision making, are linked to reduced gray matter in the anterior insula (aINS) and dorsal anterior cingulate cortex (dACC). The ventral striatum (VS) is crucial for motivation and reward processing, with structural changes associated with anhedonia and impaired motivation. Meta-analytic studies indicate shared neural substrates across various mental health problems, suggesting commonalities in gray matter loss.

Individuals who live with SMI often lack essential adaptive skills due to developmental disruptions, leading to difficulties in treatment adherence and daily functioning. Many people who live with SMI may not have the opportunity to acquire functional skills during adolescence because of psychiatric hospitalization or other significant life disruptions. Adaptive skills are necessary for effective daily functioning and include health-related behaviors like treatment adherence. Learning models, such as operant conditioning and social learning theory, can be applied to improve skill acquisition. Environmental factors, including sensory sensitivities and trauma, hinder the development of adaptive skills. The absence of positive reinforcement and competent role models contributes to difficulties in learning necessary life skills. Individuals with SMI often experience aversive family interactions, which can exacerbate functional impairments and lead to increased hospitalization rates.

Different types and patterns of medication nonadherence among individuals who live with SMI can be identified, which may inform the development of interventions tailored to specific nonadherence profiles. Nonadherent behaviors can be categorized as intentional–unintentional; voluntary–involuntary; primary–secondary; partial–complete; and persistent– intermittent.

Intentional and unintentional types of nonadherences are influenced by beliefs, insight, and logistical barriers. Intentional nonadherence involves conscious decisions to skip treatment due to side effects or financial burdens. Unintentional nonadherence results from forgetfulness or cognitive impairments.

Voluntary nonadherence is a conscious choice to stop medication, often due to negative attitudes or stigma. Involuntary nonadherence occurs when mental health issues hinder the ability to adhere to treatment.

Primary nonadherence refers to not starting prescribed treatment, while secondary nonadherence involves discontinuing after initiation. Partial nonadherence means following some treatment aspects, while complete nonadherence indicates total discontinuation of treatment.

Persistent nonadherence is long-term refusal of treatment, whereas intermittent nonadherence fluctuates with mental health status. Long-term nonadherence is sustained failure to follow treatment for six months or more, with persistent refusal lasting at least 18 months.

Full adherence is defined as consistent medication intake without lapses, while nonadherence includes any missed doses or service discontinuation. Medication refusal is defined when the individual living with SMI consistently declines prescribed drugs for up to three weeks. Dimensions of nonadherence also can be categorized by medication types, length of adherence intervals, and magnitude of nonadherence behaviors.

Nonadherence to treatment recommendation among individuals living with SMI present challenges to continuation, beneficial outcomes of treatment and recovery. Nonadherence to medications and treatment recommendations can lead to the return of symptoms and problem behaviors in individuals living with SMI and a substantial delay in recovery.

Medications are crucial for minimizing symptoms like delusions and hallucinations. Nonadherence is a major reason for rehospitalizations. Living with an SMI is chronic and requires ongoing treatment, including medication and therapy. Social support is vital for encouraging adherence to treatment. Strategies need to be developed to improve adherence to treatment recommendations.

Various factors contribute to the difficulty individuals with SMI face in adhering to treatment recommendations. Biochemical or physical issues can lead to avoidance of medications due to side effects and metabolic syndrome. Impairments in thinking and memory can hinder the ability to follow medication schedules. Psychosocial factors, such as stigma and mistrust of service providers, can discourage seeking help. Complicated medication regimens can be overwhelming and lead to discontinuation. Implementing specific strategies can enhance adherence to treatment recommendations for individuals living with SMI.

Current medications should be reviewed with a psychiatric provider to address side effects. Identify and prioritize medication and appointment times in daily routines. Memory aids, such as pill boxes and calendars, need to be employed to help remember medication schedules. Establish familiarity with service providers and treatment settings to reduce anxiety. Contracts that specify expectations and incentives for treatment adherence can be developed collaboratively with individuals who live with SMI and who exhibit nonadherent behaviors.

A comprehensive approach can help improve adherence to treatment recommendations for individuals with SMI including the following:

- Seek psychiatric review for medication adjustments to minimize side effects
- Monitor factors affecting adherence, such as mood and time of day
- Develop a structured daily routine that incorporates medication and appointments
- Praise and acknowledge any instances of adherence, even in other areas of functioning
- Consider long-acting medication options to reduce the frequency of doses required

References

Acosta, F. J., Hernández, J. L., Pereira, J., Herrera, J., & Rodríguez, C. J. (2012). Medication adherence in schizophrenia. *World Journal of Psychiatry, 2*(5), 74–82. https://doi.org/10.5498/wjp.v2.i5.74

Alekhya, P., Sriharsha, M., Priya Darsini, T., Reddy, S., Venkata Ramudu, R., Shivanandh, B., & Hrushikesh Reddy, Y. (2015). Treatment and disease related factors affecting non-adherence among patients on long term therapy of antidepressants. *Journal of Depression and Anxiety, 4*(2), 1000175. https://doi.org/10.4172/2167-1044.1000175

Aljofan, M., Oshibayeva, A., Moldaliyev, I., Saruarov, Y., Maulenkul, T., & Gaipov, A. (2023). The rate of medication nonadherence and influencing factors: A systematic review. *Electronic Journal of General Medicine, 20*(3), em471. https://doi.org/10.29333/ejgm/12946

Amador, X. F., Strauss, D. H., Yale, S. A., Flaum, M. M., Endicott, J., & Gorman, J. M. (1993). Assessment of insight in psychosis. *The American Journal of Psychiatry, 150*(6), 873–879. https://doi.org/10.1176/ajp.150.6.873

American Medical Association (AMA). (2023, February 22). *8 reasons patients don't take their medications*. https://www.ama-assn.org/delivering-care/physician-patient-relationship/8-reasons-patients-dont-take-their-medications

American Psychological Association. (n.d.-a). Anosognosia. In *APA Dictionary of Psychology*. https://dictionary.apa.org/anosognosia

American Psychological Association. (n.d.-b). Expressed emotion. In *APA Dictionary of Psychology*. https://dictionary.apa.org/expressed-emotion

American Psychological Association. (n.d.-c). Dimension. In *APA Dictionary of Psychology*. https://dictionary.apa.org/dimension

American Psychological Association. (n.d.-d). Assertive community treatment. In *APA Dictionary of Psychology*. https://dictionary.apa.org/assertive-community-treatment

American Psychological Association. (n.d.-e). Extrapyramidal symptoms. In *APA Dictionary of Psychology*. https://dictionary.apa.org/extrapyramidal-symptoms

American Psychological Association. (n.d.-f). Impairment. In *APA Dictionary of Psychology*. https://dictionary.apa.org/impairment

American Psychological Association. (n.d.-g). Metabolic syndrome. In *APA Dictionary of Psychology*. https://dictionary.apa.org/metabolic-syndrome

Andersen, J., Larsen, J. K., Schultz, V., Nielsen, B. M., Kørner, A., Behnke, K., Munk-Andersen, E., Butler, B., Allerup, P., & Bech, P. (1989). The brief psychiatric rating scale: Dimension of schizophrenia–reliability and construct validity. *Psychopathology, 22*(2–3), 168–176. https://doi.org/10.1159/000284591

Baggetta, P., & Alexander, P. A. (2016). Conceptualization and operationalization of executive function. *Mind, Brain, and Education, 10*(1), 10–33. https://doi.org/10.1111/mbe.12100

Barstow, C., Shahan, B., & Roberts, M. (2018). Evaluating medical decision-making capacity in practice. *American Family Physician, 98*(1), 40–46. https://www.aafp.org/pubs/afp/issues/2018/0701/p40.html

Benjet, C., Borges, G., Orozco, R., Aguilar-Gaxiola, S., Andrade, L. H., Cia, A., Hwang, I., Kessler, R. C., Piazza, M., Posada-Villa, J., Sampson, N., Stagnaro, J. C., Torres, Y., Viana, M. C., Vigo, D., & Medina-Mora, M. E. (2022). Dropout from treatment for mental disorders in six countries of the Americas: A regional report from the World Mental Health Surveys. *Journal of Affective Disorders, 303*, 168–179. https://doi.org/10.1016/j.jad.2022.02.019

Brown, R. G., & Pluck, G. (2000). Negative symptoms: The 'pathology' of motivation and goal-directed behaviour. *Trends in Neurosciences, 23*(9), 412–417. https://doi.org/10.1016/S0166-2236(00)01626-X

Brucato, G., Masucci, M. D., Arndt, L. Y., Ben-David, S., Colibazzi, T., Corcoran, C. M., Candan, K. A., Altschuler, R. H., Wall, M. M., Lehembre-Shiah, E., Nossan, D., Terrillion, C. E., Girgis, H., Kantrowitz, J. T., Lieberman, J. A., Malaspina, D., Goetz, R. R., Schobel, S. A., Small, S. A., et al. (2017). Baseline demographics, clinical features and predictors of conver-

sion among 200 individuals in a longitudinal prospective psychosis-risk cohort. *Psychological Medicine, 47*(11), 1923–1935. https://doi.org/10.1017/S0033291717000319
Buchman-Wildbaum, T., Váradi, E., Schmelowszky, Á., Griffiths, M. D., Demetrovics, Z., & Urbán, R. (2020). Targeting the problem of treatment non-adherence among mentally ill patients: The impact of loss, grief and stigma. *Psychiatry Research, 290*, 113140. https://doi.org/10.1016/j.psychres.2020.113140
Chuang, J.-Y., Murray, G. K., Metastasio, A., Segarra, N., Tait, R., Spencer, J., Ziauddeen, H., Dudas, R. B., Fletcher, P. C., & Suckling, J. (2014). Brain structural signatures of negative symptoms in depression and schizophrenia. *Frontiers in Psychiatry, 5*, 116. https://doi.org/10.3389/fpsyt.2014.00116
Cooper, J. O., Heron, T. E., & Heward, W. L. (2020). *Applied behavior analysis* (3rd ed.). Pearson. https://psycnet.apa.org/record/2020-62773-000
Correll, C. U., & Schooler, N. R. (2020). Negative symptoms in schizophrenia: A review and clinical guide for recognition, assessment, and treatment. *Neuropsychiatric Disease and Treatment, 16*, 519–534. https://doi.org/10.2147/NDT.S225643
Corrigan, P. W., & Watson, A. C. (2002). Understanding the impact of stigma on people with mental illness. *World Psychiatry, 1*(1), 16–20. https://www.ncbi.nlm.nih.gov/pmc/articles/PMC1489832/
Cox, J., & Witten, I. B. (2019). Striatal circuits for reward learning and decision-making. *Nature Reviews Neuroscience, 20*(8), 482–494. https://doi.org/10.1038/s41583-019-0189-2
De Soet, R., Vermeiren, R. R. J. M., Bansema, C. H., Van Ewijk, H., Nijland, L., & Nooteboom, L. A. (2024). Drop-out and ineffective treatment in youth with severe and enduring mental health problems: A systematic review. *European Child & Adolescent Psychiatry, 33*(10), 3305–3319. https://doi.org/10.1007/s00787-023-02182-z
Deng, M., Zhai, S., Ouyang, X., Liu, Z., & Ross, B. (2022). Factors influencing medication adherence among patients with severe mental disorders from the perspective of mental health professionals. *BMC Psychiatry, 22*(1), 22. https://doi.org/10.1186/s12888-021-03681-6
Dennis, J. A., Gittner, L. S., Payne, J. D., & Nugent, K. (2020). Characteristics of US adults taking prescription antipsychotic medications, National Health and Nutrition Examination Survey 2013–2018. *BMC Psychiatry, 20*, 1–6. https://doi.org/10.1186/s12888-020-02895-4
Docksey, A. E., Gray, N. S., Davies, H. B., Simkiss, N., & Snowden, R. J. (2022). The stigma and self-stigma scales for attitudes to mental health problems: Psychometric properties and its relationship to mental health problems and absenteeism. *Health Psychology Research, 10*(2), 35630. https://doi.org/10.52965/001c.35630
Emsley, R. (2013). Non-adherence and its consequences: Understanding the nature of relapse. *World Psychiatry, 12*(3), 234. https://doi.org/10.1002/wps.20067
Essock, S. M., Covell, N. H., Leckman-Westin, E., Lieberman, J. A., Sederer, L. I., & Kealey, E. (2009). Identifying clinically questionable psychotropic prescribing practices for Medicaid recipients in New York State. *Psychiatric Services, 60*(12), 1595–1602. https://doi.org/10.1176/appi.ps.60.12.1595
Fialko, L., Garety, P. A., Kuipers, E., Dunn, G., Bebbington, P. E., Fowler, D., & Freeman, D. (2008). A large-scale validation study of the Medication Adherence Rating Scale (MARS). *Schizophrenia Research, 100*(1–3), 53–59. https://doi.org/10.1016/j.schres.2007.10.029
Foley, L., Larkin, J., Lombard-Vance, R., Murphy, A. W., Hynes, L., Galvin, E., & Molloy, G. J. (2021). Prevalence and predictors of medication non-adherence among people living with multimorbidity: A systematic review and meta-analysis. *BMJ Open, 11*(9), e044987. https://doi.org/10.1136/bmjopen-2020-044987
Ghosh, P., Balasundaram, S., Sankaran, A., Chandrasekaran, V., Sarkar, S., & Choudhury, S. (2022). Factors associated with medication non-adherence among patients with severe mental disorder—A cross sectional study in a tertiary care Centre. *Exploratory Research in Clinical and Social Pharmacy, 7*, 100178. https://doi.org/10.1016/j.rcsop.2022.100178
Goodkind, M., Eickhoff, S. B., Oathes, D. J., Jiang, Y., Chang, A., Jones-Hagata, L. B., Ortega, B. N., Zaiko, Y. V., Roach, E. L., Korgaonkar, M. S., Grieve, S. M., Galatzer-Levy, I., Fox, P. T.,

& Etkin, A. (2015). Identification of a common neurobiological substrate for mental illness. *JAMA Psychiatry, 72*(4), 305–315. https://doi.org/10.1001/jamapsychiatry.2014.2206

Grover, S., Mallnaik, S., Chakrabarti, S., & Mehra, A. (2021). Factors associated with dropout from treatment: An exploratory study. *Indian Journal of Psychiatry, 63*(1), 41–51. https://doi.org/10.4103/psychiatry.IndianJPsychiatry_87_19

Gunderson, J. G., & Choi-Kain, L. W. (2018). Medication management for patients with borderline personality disorder. *American Journal of Psychiatry, 175*(7), 709–711. https://doi.org/10.1176/appi.ajp.2018.18050576

Guo, J., Lv, X., Liu, Y., Kong, L., Qu, H., & Yue, W. (2023). Influencing factors of medication adherence in schizophrenic patients: A meta-analysis. *Schizophrenia, 9*(1), 31. https://doi.org/10.1038/s41537-023-00356-x

Hadland, S. E., & Levy, S. (2016). Objective testing: Urine and other drug tests. *Child and Adolescent Psychiatric Clinics, 25*(3), 549–565. https://doi.org/10.1016/j.chc.2016.02.005

Harvey, P. D., & Strassnig, M. (2012). Predicting the severity of everyday functional disability in people with schizophrenia: Cognitive deficits, functional capacity, symptoms, and health status. *World Psychiatry, 11*(2), 73–79. https://doi.org/10.1016/j.wpsyc.2012.05.004

Hiemke, C., Bergemann, N., Clement, H. W., Conca, A., Deckert, J., Domschke, K., Eckermann, G., Egberts, K., Gerlach, M., Greiner, C., Gründer, G., Haen, E., Havemann-Reinecke, U., Hefner, G., Helmer, R., Janssen, G., Jaquenoud, E., Laux, G., Messer, T., Müller, M. J., et al. (2018). Consensus guidelines for therapeutic drug monitoring in neuropsychopharmacology: Update 2017. *Pharmacopsychiatry, 51*(1–2), 9–62. https://doi.org/10.1055/s-0043-116492

Hogan, T. P., Awad, A. G., & Eastwood, R. (1983). A self-report scale predictive of drug compliance in schizophrenics: Reliability and discriminative validity. *Psychological Medicine, 13*(1), 177–183. https://doi.org/10.1017/S0033291700050182

Horvath, A. O., & Greenberg, L. S. (1989). Development and validation of the Working Alliance Inventory. *Journal of Counseling Psychology, 36*(2), 223–233. https://doi.org/10.1037/0022-0167.36.2.223

Hovington, C. L., & Lepage, M. (2012). Neurocognition and neuroimaging of persistent negative symptoms of schizophrenia. *Expert Review of Neurotherapeutics, 12*(1), 53–69. https://doi.org/10.1586/ern.11.173

Huang, H., Wang, X., Qin, X., Xu, R., Xiong, Y., Chen, C., Li, Y., Zhang, L., Liu, S., Zhao, Q., Wang, Y., Zhou, H., Sun, J., & Palaniyappan, L. (2025). Distinct structural deficits in treatment-resistant schizophrenia and their putative neurotransmitter basis: A source-based morphometry analysis. *Neuropsychopharmacology, 50*(12), 1807–1816. https://doi.org/10.1038/s41386-025-02135-x.

Hugtenburg, J. G., Timmers, L., Elders, P. J., Vervloet, M., & van Dijk, L. (2013). Definitions, variants, and causes of nonadherence with medication: A challenge for tailored interventions. *Patient Preference and Adherence*, 675–682. https://doi.org/10.2147/PPA.S29549

Kay, S. R., Fiszbein, A., & Opler, L. A. (1987). The positive and negative syndrome scale (PANSS) for schizophrenia. *Schizophrenia Bulletin, 13*(2), 261–276. https://doi.org/10.1093/schbul/13.2.261

Kessler, R. C., Haro, J. M., Heeringa, S. G., Pennell, B. E., & Üstün, T. B. (2006). The World Health Organization world mental health survey initiative. *Epidemiology and Psychiatric Sciences, 15*(3), 161–166. https://doi.org/10.1017/S1121189X00004395

Khan, J., Khan, J. A., Kumari, S., & Charan, D. (2024). Treatment non-adherence patterns among patients with mental illness: A study from the district mental health care center in India. *Cureus, 16*(2), e54495. https://doi.org/10.7759/cureus.54495

Korkeila, J. (2000). *Measuring aspects of mental health (Themes 6/2000).* National Research and Development Centre for Welfare and Health (STAKES). https://urn.fi/URN:NBN:fi-fe201210169453

Korkeila, J., Lehtinen, V., Bijl, R., Dalgard, O. S., Kovess, V., Morgan, A., & Salize, H. J. (2003). Establishing a set of mental health indicators for Europe. *Scandinavian Journal of Public Health, 31*(6), 451–459. https://doi.org/10.1080/14034940210165208

Kreyenbuhl, J., Record, E. J., & Palmer-Bacon, J. (2016). A review of behavioral tailoring strategies for improving medication adherence in serious mental illness. *Dialogues in Clinical Neuroscience, 18*(2), 191–201. https://doi.org/10.31887/DCNS.2016.18.2/jkreyenbuhl

Kullgard, N., Holmqvist, R., & Andersson, G. (2022). Premature dropout from psychotherapy: Prevalence, perceived reasons and consequences as rated by clinicians. *Clinical Psychology in Europe, 4*(2), e6695. https://doi.org/10.32872/cpe.6695

Lally, P., & Gardner, B. (2011). Promoting habit formation. *Health Psychology Review, 5*(2), 137–155. https://doi.org/10.1080/17437199.2011.603640

Lambert, M., Conus, P., Cotton, S., Robinson, J., McGorry, P. D., & Schimmelmann, B. G. (2010). Prevalence, predictors, and consequences of long-term refusal of antipsychotic treatment in first-episode psychosis. *Journal of Clinical Psychopharmacology, 30*(5), 565–572. https://doi.org/10.1097/JCP.0b013e3181f058a0

Laranjeira, C., Carvalho, D., Valentim, O., Moutinho, L., Morgado, T., Tomás, C., Gomes, J., & Querido, A. (2023). Therapeutic adherence of people with mental disorders: An evolutionary concept analysis. *International Journal of Environmental Research and Public Health, 20*(5), 3869. https://doi.org/10.3390/ijerph20053869

Lincoln, T. M., Jung, E., Wiesjahn, M., Wendt, H., Bock, T., & Schlier, B. (2016). The impact of negative treatment experiences on persistent refusal of antipsychotics. *Comprehensive Psychiatry, 70*, 165–173. https://doi.org/10.1016/j.comppsych.2016.07.009

Ljungberg, A., Denhov, A., & Topor, A. (2016). Non-helpful relationships with professionals – A literature review of the perspective of persons with severe mental illness. *Journal of Mental Health, 25*(3), 267–277. https://doi.org/10.3109/09638237.2015.1101427

Lucca, J. M., Ramesh, M., Parthasarathi, G., & Ram, D. (2015). Incidence and factors associated with medication nonadherence in patients with mental illness: A cross-sectional study. *Journal of Postgraduate Medicine, 61*(4), 251–256. https://doi.org/10.4103/0022-3859.166514

Magura, S., Mateu, P. F., Rosenblum, A., Matusow, H., & Fong, C. (2014). Risk factors for medication non-adherence among psychiatric patients with substance misuse histories. *Mental Health and Substance Use, 7*(4), 381–390. https://doi.org/10.1080/17523281.2013.839574

Malik, M., Kumari, S., & Manalai, P. (2020, March). Treatment nonadherence: An epidemic hidden in plain sight. *Psychiatric Times, 37*(3), 25–26. https://www.psychiatrictimes.com/view/treatment-nonadherence-epidemic-hidden-plain-sight

Marcus, S. C., Chuang, C. C., Ng-Mak, D. S., & Olfson, M. (2017). Outpatient follow-up care and risk of hospital readmission in schizophrenia and bipolar disorder. *Psychiatric Services, 68*(12), 1239–1246. https://doi.org/10.1176/appi.ps.201600498

Marder, S. R., & Galderisi, S. (2017). The current conceptualization of negative symptoms in schizophrenia. *World Psychiatry, 16*(1), 14–24. https://doi.org/10.1002/wps.20385

Mert, D. G., Turgut, N. H., Kelleci, M., & Semiz, M. (2015). Perspectives on reasons of medication nonadherence in psychiatric patients. *Patient Preference and Adherence, 9*, 87–93. https://doi.org/10.2147/PPA.S75013

Mirhaj Mohammadabadi, M. S., Mohammadsadeghi, H., Eftekhar Adrebili, M., Partovi Kolour, Z., Kashaninasab, F., Rashedi, V., & Shalbafan, M. (2022). Factors associated with pharmacological and psychotherapy treatments adherence in patients with borderline personality disorder. *Frontiers in Psychiatry, 13*, 1056050. https://doi.org/10.3389/fpsyt.2022.1056050

Morisky, D. E., Green, L. W., & Levine, D. M. (1986). Concurrent and predictive validity of a self-reported measure of medication adherence. *Medical Care, 24*(1), 67–74. https://doi.org/10.1097/00005650-198601000-00007

Morrison, R. L., & Wixted, J. T. (1989). Social skills training. In A. S. Bellack (Ed.), *A clinical guide for the treatment of schizophrenia* (pp. 201–228). Plenum Press. https://doi.org/10.1007/978-1-4757-9730-8_9

National Alliance on Mental Illness (NAMI). (2024). *Adherence*. https://www.nami.org/wp-content/uploads/2024/09/adherence.pdf

National Institute of Mental Health (NIMH). (n.d.). *RDoC matrix*. U.S. Department of Health and Human Services, National Institutes of Health. Retrieved July 10, 2025, from https://www.nimh.nih.gov/research/research-funded-by-nimh/rdoc/constructs/rdoc-matrix

National Institute on Drug Abuse (NIDA). (2020). *Sex differences in substance use. Substance use in women research report*. U.S. Department of Health and Human Services. https://nida.nih.gov/publications/research-reports/substance-use-in-women/sex-differences-in-substance-use

National Institute on Drug Abuse (NIDA). (n.d.). *Tobacco, alcohol, prescription medication, and other substance use (TAPS) tool*. U.S. Department of Health and Human Services. https://nida.nih.gov/taps2/

Ojo, S., Okoye, T. O., Olaniyi, S. A., Ofochukwu, V. C., Obi, M. O., Nwokolo, A. S., Okeke-Moffatt, C., Iyun, O. B., Idemudia, E. A., Obodo, O. R., Mokwenye, V. C., & Okobi, O. E. (2024). Ensuring continuity of care: Effective strategies for the post-hospitalization transition of psychiatric patients in a family medicine outpatient clinic. *Cureus, 16*(1), e52263. https://doi.org/10.7759/cureus.52263

Pacheco, J., Garvey, M. A., Sarampote, C. S., Cohen, E. D., Murphy, E. R., & Friedman-Hill, S. R. (2022). Annual research review: The contributions of the RDoC research framework on understanding the neurodevelopmental origins, progression and treatment of mental illnesses. *Journal of Child Psychology and Psychiatry, 63*(4), 360–376. https://doi.org/10.1111/jcpp.13543

Ritsher, J. B., Otilingam, P. G., & Grajales, M. (2003). Internalized stigma of mental illness: Psychometric properties of a new measure. *Psychiatry Research, 121*(1), 31–49. https://doi.org/10.1016/j.psychres.2003.08.008

Rozalski, V., & McKeegan, G. M. (2019). Insight and symptom severity in an inpatient psychiatric sample. *Psychiatric Quarterly, 90*(2), 339–350. https://doi.org/10.1007/s11126-019-09631-6

Semahegn, A., Torpey, K., Manu, A., Assefa, N., Tesfaye, G., & Ankomah, A. (2020). Psychotropic medication non-adherence and its associated factors among patients with major psychiatric disorders: A systematic review and meta-analysis. *Systematic Reviews, 9*, 1–18. https://doi.org/10.1186/s13643-020-1274-3

Skou, S. T., Mair, F. S., Fortin, M., Guthrie, B., Nunes, B. P., Miranda, J. J., Boyd, C. M., Pati, S., Mtenga, S., & Smith, S. M. (2022). Multimorbidity. *Nature Reviews Disease Primers, 8*(1), 48. https://doi.org/10.1038/s41572-022-00376-4

Smith, D., Lovell, J., Weller, C., Kennedy, B., Winbolt, M., Young, C., & Ibrahim, J. (2017). A systematic review of medication non-adherence in persons with dementia or cognitive impairment. *PLOS ONE, 12*(2), e0170651. https://doi.org/10.1371/journal.pone.0170651

Tattan, T. M., & Creed, F. H. (2001). Negative symptoms of schizophrenia and compliance with medication. *Schizophrenia Bulletin, 27*(1), 149–155. https://doi.org/10.1093/oxfordjournals.schbul.a006853

Tehrani, E., Krussel, J., Borg, L., & Munk-Jorgensen, P. (1996). Dropping out of psychiatric treatment: A prospective study of a first-admission cohort. *Acta Psychiatrica Scandinavica, 94*(4), 266–271. https://doi.org/10.1111/j.1600-0447.1996.tb09859.x

U.S. Department of Health and Human Services (HHS), National Institutes of Health (NIH). (2023). *Borderline personality disorder* (NIH Publication No. 23-MH-8083). National Institute of Mental Health (NIMH). https://www.nimh.nih.gov/health/publications/borderline-personality-disorder

Vaughn, C., & Leff, J. (1976). The measurement of expressed emotion in the families of psychiatric patients. *British Journal of Social and Clinical Psychology, 15*(2), 157–165. https://doi.org/10.1111/j.2044-8260.1976.tb00021.x

Vázquez-Bourgon, J., Mayoral-van Son, J., Gómez-Revuelta, M., Juncal-Ruiz, M., Ortiz-García de la Foz, V., Tordesillas-Gutiérrez, D., Ayesa-Arriola, R., Bioque, M., & Crespo-Facorro, B. (2021). Treatment discontinuation impact on long-term (10-year) weight gain and lipid metabolism in first-episode psychosis: Results from the PAFIP-10 cohort. *International Journal of Neuropsychopharmacology, 24*(1), 1–7. https://doi.org/10.1093/ijnp/pyaa066

Vega, D., Acosta, F. J., & Saavedra, P. (2020). Testing the hypothesis of subtypes of nonadherence in schizophrenia and schizoaffective disorder: A prospective study. *World Journal of Psychiatry, 10*(11), 260. https://doi.org/10.5498/wjp.v10.i11.260

Velligan, D. I., Sajatovic, M., Hatch, A., Kramata, P., & Docherty, J. P. (2017). Why do psychiatric patients stop antipsychotic medication? A systematic review of reasons for nonadherence to medication in patients with serious mental illness. *Patient Preference and Adherence, 11*, 449–468. https://doi.org/10.2147/PPA.S124658

Velligan, D., Salinas, G. D., Belcher, E., Franzenburg, K. R., Suett, M., Thompson, S., & Hansen, R. T., III. (2025). Clinician differences in attitudes and perceptions on the use of long-acting injectable antipsychotic agents in treating patients with schizophrenia: Results from the US DECIDE survey. *BMC Psychiatry, 25*(1), 232. https://doi.org/10.1186/s12888-025-06565-1

Vieira, M., Silva, B. F., & Ribeiro, J. S. (2023). Internalized stigma–how we view our mental illness. *European Psychiatry, 66*(S1), S1032–S1032. https://doi.org/10.1192/j.eurpsy.2023.2190

Viswanath, B., & Chaturvedi, S. K. (2012). Cultural aspects of major mental disorders: A critical review from an Indian perspective. *Indian Journal of Psychological Medicine, 34*(4), 306–312. https://doi.org/10.4103/0253-7176.108193

Vrijens, B., De Geest, S., Hughes, D. A., Kardas, P., Demonceau, J., Ruppar, T., Dobbels, F., Fargher, E., Morrison, V., Lewek, P., Matyjaszczyk, M., Mshelia, C., Clyne, W., Aronson, J. K., & Urquhart, J. (2012). A new taxonomy for describing and defining adherence to medications. *British Journal of Clinical Pharmacology, 73*(5), 691–705. https://doi.org/10.1111/j.1365-2125.2012.04167.x

Wells, J. E., Browne, M. O., Aguilar-Gaxiola, S., Al-Hamzawi, A., Alonso, J., Angermeyer, M. C., Bouzan, C., Bruffaerts, R., Bunting, B., Caldas-de-Almeida, J. M., de Girolamo, G., de Graaf, R., Florescu, S., Fukao, A., Gureje, O., Hinkov, H. R., Hu, C., Hwang, I., Karam, E. G., et al. (2013). Drop out from out-patient mental healthcare in the World Health Organization's World Mental Health Survey initiative. *The British Journal of Psychiatry, 202*(1), 42–49. https://doi.org/10.1192/bjp.bp.112.113134

World Health Organization (WHO). (2001). *International classification of functioning, disability and health (ICF)*. World Health Organization. https://doi.org/10.1037/t76403-000

Zimet, G. D., Dahlem, N. W., Zimet, S. G., & Farley, G. K. (1988). The multidimensional scale of perceived social support. *Journal of Personality Assessment, 52*(1), 30–41. https://doi.org/10.1207/s15327752jpa5201_2

Chapter 17
Problems with Suicide and Self-Harming Behaviors by Individuals Living with Serious Mental Illness

Introduction

Suicide and self-harming behaviors represent some of the most urgent and complex challenges encountered in the study and treatment of serious mental illness (SMI). These phenomena are not only markers of profound psychological distress but also significant contributors to global morbidity and mortality. It is imperative that mental health disciplines understand the interplay between suicidal behaviors, non-suicidal self-injury (NSSI), and the broader context of SMI so as to develop the clinical insights and research literacy required to address these issues. This chapter situates suicide and self-harm within the continuum of self-directed violence, emphasizing their definitions, prevalence, and the multidimensional risk factors that shape their occurrence.

The scope of suicidal and self-harming behaviors is vast, encompassing ideation, planning, attempts, and completed suicide, as well as non-lethal acts of self-injury undertaken without intent to die. Epidemiological data reveal striking disparities across age, gender, and cultural groups, with youth, males, and marginalized populations disproportionately affected. These behaviors are further complicated by the presence of psychiatric conditions such as major depressive disorder, bipolar disorder, schizophrenia spectrum disorders, and borderline personality disorder, alongside environmental stressors including trauma, stigma, and socioeconomic disadvantage. By examining these dimensions, the chapter underscores the necessity of precise definitions and standardized nomenclature to facilitate accurate assessment and effective intervention.

Beyond prevalence and classification, the neurobiological and psychological substrates that underpin suicidal and self-harming behaviors are explored. Research

Supplementary Information The online version contains supplementary material available at https://doi.org/10.1007/978-3-032-18372-9_17.

G. F. McKeegan, *Behavior Change Interventions for Serious Mental Illness*, Evidence-Based Practices in Behavioral Health,
https://doi.org/10.1007/978-3-032-18372-9_17

highlights the role of impulsivity, aggression, and serotonergic dysregulation, as well as the impact of trauma and adverse childhood experiences on emotional regulation and vulnerability. These findings illustrate how dispositional traits interact with environmental influences to shape risk trajectories. Importantly, the functional aspects of self-harm, particularly its role in affect regulation, are addressed, and consider how repetitive engagement in such behaviors may increase susceptibility to future suicide attempts.

The importance of safety planning and behavioral support strategies is emphasized as critical components of prevention and intervention. Effective approaches must integrate biological, psychological, and social domains, while remaining sensitive to cultural and contextual factors. By synthesizing definitions, prevalence data, risk factors, neurological and environmental influences, and practical strategies, this chapter provides a comprehensive framework for understanding and addressing suicide and self-harm in individuals living with SMI, equipping the individual with the conceptual and clinical tools necessary to engage with one of the most pressing issues in contemporary mental health practice.

> My relative sometimes threatens to hurt herself. She will cut her arms or legs when she is upset or angry; she uses whatever she can get to hurt herself. She hits her head against the floor, wall or furniture, anything that is hard. She has taken an overdose of her medications. At this point, we do not trust her to be by herself.

The Case of Susan

Susan is a 32-year-old woman who was admitted to a psychiatric hospital after exhibiting a variety of severe problem behaviors. Among these were frequent threats of suicide and acts of self-injury. These included cutting her wrists and forearms with sharp objects. She was first hospitalized when she was 19 years old after making threats of suicide to her parents and the local rescue squad. Since then, she has been hospitalized 11 times. During these hospitalizations, she had received a variety of psychiatric diagnoses including schizophrenia, depression, and schizoaffective mental health problems, and several forms of personality mental health problems. She has had neurological examinations to determine if there is an underlying physical reason for her behavior.

While she had many different behavioral problems, the most serious was the threats of suicide and acts of self-harm. At times, she would begin talking about hurting herself or other people. Her threats of harm toward others were primarily directed at hospital staff whom she said did not care about her. The attempts by staff to calm her down often just made the situation worse. When they tried to calm her, she would begin yelling and making louder threats. After a while, she began scratching and cutting her wrists, twisting clothes around her neck until she blacked out, or other acts which could result in serious injury or death. Some of the staff remarked that they had dreams of finding her dead and that it was inevitable that she would eventually succeed.

Over the years, Susan had been prescribed many psychiatric medications to keep her from getting out of control and hurting herself. These included medications that are normally given for anxiety, depression, and more serious psychiatric illnesses such as schizophrenia spectrum problems. However, none of these were very effective in keeping the self-injurious threats and acts from happening. The problem was so severe that the hospital staff resorted to putting her in "mechanical restraints" to prevent her from being able to hurt herself in any way. This strategy concerned many of the staff, however, and her case was brought to the attention of a hospital committee that reviewed such difficult management cases. They mandated that a plan be formally developed to address Susan's problem behaviors.

Definitions and Characteristics of Problems with Suicide and Self-Harming Behaviors by Individuals Living with Serious Mental Illness

Suicide is a serious public health problem (World Health Organization [WHO], 2025). Suicidal and self-harming behaviors represent urgent and complex phenomena with profound implications for public health, clinical care, and mental health research. Suicidal behaviors encompass a broad continuum of self-directed actions driven by an active or passive intent to die involving covert self-critical negative self-statements relating to loneliness, burdensomeness, belongingness, and social disengagement. Intent refers to the desire to end one's life, including the individual's knowledge of the risk and the means to achieve the desired outcome (American Psychiatric 2013; Hausmann-Stabile et al., 2012).

Suicide is a major public health concern across the globe, representing a leading cause of preventable mortality and impacting individuals, families, and societies in profound and lasting ways. According to global estimates, approximately 800,000 to 1 million individuals die by suicide each year, equating to one death every 40 seconds worldwide (Bachmann, 2018; WHO, 2025). The global suicide rate is estimated to range between 10.7 and 11.4 per 100,000 individuals, with nearly 80% of these deaths occurring in low- and middle-income countries although suicide does occur at a substantial rate in high-income countries as well (Nock et al., 2008).

Across the globe, the prevalence of suicidal behaviors demonstrates notable differences depending on the economic status of a country; yet, certain trends remain strikingly consistent. In low- and middle-income nations, the proportion of individuals who experience suicidal ideation ranges from 3.1% to 12.4%. Within these same contexts, 0.9–4.1% of people report having formulated a suicide plan, while 0.7–4.7% have attempted suicide (Nock et al., 2008). High-income countries show a similar pattern, with rates of suicidal ideation spanning 3.0–15.9%. Planning suicide in these countries is reported by 0.7–5.6% of individuals, and suicide attempts by 0.5–5.0%. These results show that the likelihood of progressing from thinking about suicide to planning or attempting it remains relatively stable regardless of a country's wealth.

Suicide continues to be a significant concern in the United States. National Institute of Mental Health (NIMH) (2025b) reported over 49,400 suicide deaths in 2022 alone, reflecting a national age-adjusted suicide rate of 14.2 per 100,000 people. Suicide stands as the second leading cause of death for youth aged 10–14 and young adults aged 25–34, third among those aged 15–24, and fourth among individuals aged 35–44, emphasizing the critical importance of identifying and managing risk factors in adolescents and working-age adults.

Suicide is a phenomenon deeply intertwined with mental health conditions, access to care, socioeconomic status, and systemic disparities. Demographic disparities are notable. Males account for nearly 80% of all suicide deaths in the United States, with a rate of 23.0 per 100,000 compared to 5.9 for females. Among specific racial and ethnic groups, American and Alaska Native males exhibit the highest suicide rate nationally, at 39.5 per 100,000, followed by White non-Hispanic males at 28.0 per 100,000. Among females, the highest rates are observed in American and Alaska Native women (14.6 per 100,000). In terms of age-related vulnerability, suicide ranks as the second leading cause of death for individuals aged 15–29 years globally, and the third among those aged 15–44 years, underscoring the urgency of suicide prevention efforts targeting youth and early adulthood, when neurobiological, psychosocial, and environmental stressors may converge (Substance Abuse and Mental Health Services Administration [SAMHSA], 2020).

A comprehensive understanding of suicidal-related behaviors is critical for accurate classification and effective intervention. Consistent definitions of suicide and related behaviors (i.e., self-harming behaviors) are critical for suicide prevention and treatment. Variability in terminology complicates the comparison of international prevalence rates. The Center for Disease Control and Prevention (CDC) and the National Academy of Medicine (NAM) (formerly known as the Institute of Medicine (IOM)) emphasize the need for a common language in suicide research (Posner et al., 2014).

Suicidal behaviors are multidimensional and heterogeneous, categorized by intent, method, degree of planning, and outcome (American Psychiatric Association, 2022c). The method of suicidal behaviors and the intensity of violence associated with the method, the amount and detail of planning (versus impulsivity), and the desire to die are essential elements in determining suicidal behaviors (American Psychiatric Association, 2022c).

Suicidal behaviors are comprised of various behaviors that include death by self-inflicted means, nonfatal attempts, and passive or active suicidal ideations. Ideation may manifest as fleeting thoughts or evolve into detailed planning. Completed suicide is death resulting from intentional self-injurious behavior, where there is a clear or inferred intent to die (Bachmann, 2018; NIMH, 2025b). In contrast, a suicide attempt refers to nonfatal, self-directed, potentially injurious behavior that is undertaken with some intent to die by engaging in the behaviors (NIMH, 2025b). A suicide attempt might not result in death or injury. Distinctions are made for interrupted and self-interrupted (or aborted) attempts (Posner et al., 2014). An interrupted attempt occurs when an individual begins to engage in behaviors toward a suicide attempt but is stopped by external circumstances before any injury or potential injury can occur. Conversely, a self-interrupted or aborted attempt is characterized by the individual halting their own actions before any injury or potential injury takes place (Posner et al., 2014). Notably, injury does not have to occur, but there must be a potential for harm in terms of the lethality of the topography of the intended self-harming behaviors and the intent to die; an example would be a person who puts a loaded gun into his mouth and the gun misfires—the lethality of the behavior is severe and the person would have died if the gun had discharged. Lethality of the behavior is defined as degree of dangerousness or likelihood of death associated with a particular behavior (American Psychological Association, n.d.-c; Hausmann-Stabile et al., 2012; Kar et al., 2014).

Methods of suicide are significant factors in both epidemiologic trends and prevention strategies as accessibility to highly lethal methods of intentional self-harm contributes to the occurrence of completed suicide (Hausmann-Stabile et al., 2012). Firearms were involved in more than half of the completed suicides in the United States (Miller et al., 2013); in 2022, firearms accounted for approximately 54–55% of cases of completed suicides (CDC, 2024b). Other prevalent methods include hanging or suffocation, and poisoning—particularly through drug overdose or pesticide ingestion. The lethality and accessibility of these methods play a central role in outcome severity and the success of preventive interventions (Hausmann-Stabile et al., 2012; Kar et al., 2014).

Preparatory acts or behaviors also play a significant role in risk assessment. These involve actions or preparations taken toward making a suicide attempt, such as writing a suicide note, giving away possessions, or assembling the means for self-harm (Posner et al., 2014). The clear delineation of intent is essential for distinguishing between suicidal and non-suicidal self-injurious behavior. Such classifications underscore the necessity of nuanced assessment in clinical practice and contribute to the development of effective prevention and intervention strategies (Silverman et al., 2007). This distinction is critical within clinical and research contexts, where confusion between suicidal actions and non-suicidal acts can undermine accurate assessment and intervention.

Non-suicidal self-injurious behavior (NSSIB) refers to deliberate and self-directed bodily harm inflicted likely to induce bleeding, bruising, or pain without the intention to die (American Psychiatric Association, 2022e). Common forms of self-harm include cutting, burning, hitting, scratching, wound interference, and hair pulling (Fliege et al., 2009; Klonsky, 2007; Lorentzen et al., 2022; National Alliance on Mental Illness [NAMI], 2025). These behaviors typically arise in response to intense psychological distress, serving intrapersonal functions such as emotional regulation (i.e., avoidance or diminution of aversive respondents), relief from numbness, or self-punishment (Klonsky, 2007).

Unlike suicidal behavior, which is defined by intent to die (NIMH, 2025b), self-harming behaviors are not driven by the desire to end life. Instead, they are often linked to affective instability, trauma histories, low emotional expressivity, and mental health problems such as borderline personality (BPD) (American Psychiatric

Association, 2022e) and major depressive (MDD) mental health problems, and post-traumatic stress disorder (PTSD) (Fliege et al., 2009; Sadath et al., 2023). Klonsky (2007) reported that the function of deliberate self-harming behaviors has a predominant role in affect regulation as well as other underlying psychological mechanisms. Self-harming behaviors are found to serve multiple functions across both clinical and non-clinical populations, with affect regulation being the most reported. Before engaging in self-harm, individuals often experience intense negative emotional states such as anger toward others, feelings of hurt, or a sense of emptiness. The act of self-injury frequently results in the individual feeling relief, with acute negative respondents decreasing afterward, resulting in self-harming behavior being negatively reinforced as the person avoids or escapes the high-intensity adverse respondents.

Interpersonal conflict frequently appears as an antecedent to self-injurious behavior, further underscoring the complexity of factors that may precipitate such actions. Studies have shed additional light on the psychological and physiological effects associated with self-injury or its proxies. Research indicates that individuals who engage in self-harming behaviors display elevated physiological arousal and increased negative affect prior to the act, both of which decrease following the behavior. Experimental evidence supports these findings, as physiological measures during self-injury imagery revealed the anticipated patterns (Brain et al., 1998; Haines et al., 1995).

A synthesis of the research shows that the primary function of self-injury is affect regulation with the objective of reducing the intensity of adverse respondents. Typically, individuals experience acute negative emotions before self-injury and relief or decreased intensity of negative respondents afterward. The self-punishment function also received strong backing, while functions such as anti-dissociation (i.e., conflicting or threatening impulses and self-statements are occurring simultaneously), interpersonal influence, sensation seeking, anti-suicide, and establishing interpersonal boundaries were found to have limited support. Importantly, findings regarding the functions of self-injury have shown consistency across diverse sample types, including clinical, forensic, and community populations (Klonsky, 2007).

Despite the absence of suicidal intent, NSSIB is strongly associated with increased risk for future suicide attempts and thus warrants clinical attention (Miller et al., 2013). The relationship between self-harm and suicidal behaviors is both complex and dynamic. While most individuals who engage in NSSIB do not intend to die, longitudinal research reveals that repetitive self-harm may desensitize individuals to physical pain or foster maladaptive coping behaviors that evolve toward suicidal action (Edgcomb et al., 2021; Gvion & Apter, 2012; Joiner, 2005). Method switching—from low-lethality self-harm (e.g., cutting) to high-lethality suicidal acts (e.g., hanging or suffocation)—has been documented as a serious progression with fatal outcomes (Miller et al., 2013).

The distinction also carries implications for the presence of mental health problems. The DSM-5-TR (American Psychiatric Association, 2022a) does not currently include NSSIB or suicidal behavior disorder as standalone problems, despite evidence suggesting that they represent clinically significant phenomena (American

Psychiatric Association, 2022c; Xu et al., 2023). "Suicide behavior disorder" is defined as an individual engaging in a purposeful attempt to end their life within the last two years. The behavior must be intentional and driven by a genuine expectation of death and not impulsive self-harm, confused mental states, or ideological acts (American Psychiatric Association, 2022c).

Ongoing research underscores the importance of implementing standardized nomenclature and precise operational definitions to advance surveillance, inform treatment planning, and guide policy development (Goodfellow et al., 2019; Silverman & De Leo, 2016). Although self-harming behaviors are distinct from suicidal behaviors with respect to motivation and intent, their association is complex and significant. NSSIB should not be regarded as benign or disconnected from suicidality; rather, it serves as an indicator of emotional distress with the potential for escalation. Accurate differentiation, standardized classification, and targeted interventions are essential for mitigating morbidity and mortality among individuals impacted by one or both forms of self-directed violence.

Suicidal ideations are multidimensional private behaviors that are linked and are part of the phenomenon of suicidal behaviors. They refer to thinking about and/or planning suicide (Beck et al., 1976; Ghasemi et al., 2015; NIMH, 2025b; Posner et al., 2011; Steer et al., 1993). Suicidal ideations usually precede the occurrence of violent behaviors associated with suicide attempts and involve aversive self-statements related to belongingness and burdensomeness. These two concepts are viewed as dynamic cognitive-affective states that can change over time and context (Espinosa-Salido et al., 2021). Belongingness refers to a perception of social belonging, where individuals feel connected to others and experience reciprocally caring relationships (Chu et al., 2017; Espinosa-Salido et al., 2021; Joiner, 2005). It is influenced by interpersonal and intrapersonal factors, such as the current interpersonal environment, active beliefs or thoughts about one's social surroundings, and prevailing emotional states. Perceptions of disengagement, being disconnected from others, and lacking caring relationships result in "thwarted belongingness" and has been postulated as a motivating factor for the occurrence of suicidal behaviors and is closely related to social isolation (Chu et al., 2017; Cornwell & Waite, 2009; Espinosa-Salido et al., 2021; Joiner, 2005) which is a significant problem in individuals living with SMI (Song et al., 2020). Burdensomeness is defined as a cognitive, dimensional, and dynamic state. It refers to an individual's perception of being a burden on others, such as family, friends, or society (Espinosa-Salido et al., 2021; Joiner, 2005). This feeling can be triggered by negative circumstances like unemployment, family conflicts, or physical illness. It encompasses two dimensions of interpersonal functioning: (a) a feeling of not being suitably capable of taking responsibility for others; and (b) private events (cognitions) that are antecedent conditions for aversive affective respondents (Chu et al., 2017; Espinosa-Salido et al., 2021; Joiner, 2005), like dysphoria and depression.

Suicidal behavior encompasses a broad spectrum of ideation, planning, and action rooted in a complex interplay of psychological, social, biological, and clinical determinants. Risk factors for suicidal and self-harming behaviors span general and clinical populations. In the general population, mental health problems identified with SMI, including major depressive (MDD), bipolar (BD), borderline personality (BPD), and schizophrenia spectrum mental health problems, are consistently associated with elevated risk for the occurrence of suicidal behaviors (Brådvik, 2018; Masango et al., 2008; Fu et al., 2023). Substance use, involving alcohol and opioids, further exacerbates suicidal behaviors (Turecki & Brent, 2016). Demographic vulnerabilities include male gender, adolescence, older age, trauma exposure, and adverse childhood experiences (CDC, 2024b). Social factors, including isolation, unemployment, and discrimination, have been identified as contributing to risk (Silverman & De Leo, 2016). The link between suicide and mental health problems (in particular, depression and alcohol use problems) and previous suicide attempts are well established in high-income countries. However, many suicides happen impulsively in moments of crisis with a breakdown in the ability to deal with life stresses, such as financial problems, relationship disputes, or chronic pain and illness. Exposure to conflict, disaster, violence, abuse, loss, or social isolation is strongly correlated with suicidal behaviors. Additionally, suicide rates are elevated among vulnerable populations who face discrimination, including refugees and migrants, Indigenous peoples, lesbian, gay, bisexual, transgender, intersex (LGBTI) individuals, and incarcerated persons (WHO, 2025).

Research suggests an association between living with SMI and increased likelihood of suicide (Moitra et al., 2021). Living with mental health problems represents significant risk factors for the manifestation of suicidal behaviors across different age groups in the general populations. Approximately 46% of people who die by suicide had a known mental health condition, though other research suggests that this may be an undercount due to cases not recognized (Conner et al., 2013). Among these, MDD, BD, and schizophrenia spectrum mental health problems are associated with higher relative risks for suicidal behaviors. Individuals living with MDD, for example, have over seven times the risk compared to those without such problems, while BD and schizophrenia spectrum mental health problems have elevated risks. Dysthymia and anxiety disorders present lower relative risks but still contribute to overall suicide vulnerability (Moitra et al., 2021; Uebelacker et al., 2013).

Living with MDD raises suicide risk by approximately 17 times when compared to age- and sex-adjusted rates. According to Moitra et al. (2021), meta-regression analysis found that MDD ranked among the highest in pooled relative risks for suicide. In high-income countries, up to 80% of suicide deaths are associated with a mental or substance use disorder, while in low-income countries, the figure is about 70%. Findings from the National Comorbidity Survey Replication (NCS-R) (Kessler & Merikangas, 2006) indicate that individuals with six or more concurrent mental health conditions face a 29-fold increased risk of suicide attempts relative to those without any diagnosis. Nock et al. (2010) noted that depression was a strong predictor of suicidal ideation, and impulse-control or substance use problems were stronger predictors of suicide attempts, particularly in the presence of multiple mental health problems.

Individuals living with MDD frequently experience anhedonia, hopelessness, and social disconnectedness (Joiner 2005), which mediate the emergence and escalation of suicidal ideation and attempts (American Psychiatric Association, 2022b;

Brådvik, 2018). Living with a BD is similarly associated with elevated risk. Lifetime suicide deaths in people living with BD occur in approximately 5–6% cases, with the episode of mood polarity and substance use influencing lethality and recurrence (American Psychiatric Association, 2022c). Among those diagnosed with schizophrenia spectrum disorders, suicide risk persists chronically, particularly during early illness stages, hospital discharge periods, or in the presence of co-occurring depressive symptoms (Radomsky et al., 1999; American Psychiatric Association, 2022b). Personality mental health problems, especially BPD, demonstrate high rates of nonfatal suicidal behavior, often serving as a chronic marker of emotional dysregulation and interpersonal instability (Albert et al., 2019; American Psychiatric Association, 2022d).

Co-occurring conditions—both psychiatric and physical—exert a strong amplifying effect on suicide risk. Individuals with chronic pain, HIV, epilepsy, or cancer show substantially higher suicide intent and rates, especially when psychological distress coexists with somatic burden (Fu et al., 2023; Sadath et al., 2023). Substance use problems (SUD), notably alcohol and opioid use, further heighten this risk by impairing cognitive control and augmenting impulsivity (American Psychiatric Association, 2022c; Xu et al., 2023).

Research consistently demonstrates that a history of suicide attempts remains the most potent proximal predictor of future suicidal behavior. Following hospitalization for self-harm, nearly one in five adults living with SMI were readmitted for subsequent suicidal behavior, particularly those with prior attempts, impulsivity traits, or medical comorbidities (Edgcomb et al., 2021). Method choice during initial self-harm episodes has prognostic implications; individuals using low-lethality methods such as drug overdose or cutting may switch to more lethal strategies (e.g., hanging or firearm use) in fatal attempts (Miller et al., 2013).

Demographic variables compound clinical vulnerability. Males are nearly four times more likely to die by suicide than females, while females engage in more nonfatal suicidal behaviors (CDC, 2024b; NIMH, 2025b). Age-specific patterns reveal suicide as a leading cause of death among individuals aged 10–34, with high rates observed in older adults, particularly males aged 85 and older (WHO, 2025). Suicide health disparities are prominent in American Indian/Alaska Native populations and individuals residing in rural areas, and in sexual minorities experiencing discrimination and isolation (CDC, 2025). Social stressors such as unemployment, poverty, and limited healthcare access exacerbate risk across subgroups.

Psychological and behavioral constructs like impulsivity and aggression serve as dispositional vulnerabilities. These traits interact with environmental stressors and mental health conditions, contributing to the likelihood, timing, and severity of suicide attempts requiring medical intervention. Contrary to common assumptions, impulsive attempts can carry higher lethality scores than planned ones, as ideation and lethality are not always correlated. For example, someone may have high intent but choose a low-lethality method due to access or impulsivity. Research also suggests that lethality may be influenced by personality dimensions, such as impulsivity or aggression, rather than ideation alone (Harvard T.H. Chan School of Public Health, n.d.; Kar et al. 2014).

Mann et al. (1999) demonstrated that impulsivity and aggression profiles serve as predictors of suicide attempts, irrespective of the presence of mental health conditions. Subsequent neurobiological research supports these findings, highlighting the role of serotonergic dysregulation, prefrontal cortical dysfunction, and genetic polymorphisms associated with emotional regulation and decision making (Mann, 2003; Xu et al., 2023). These factors are fundamental components of executive functions, which have been observed to be compromised in individuals who live with SMI (Regev & Josman, 2020).

Trauma, adversity, and stigma remain pivotal contextual risk factors (Oexle et al., 2016). Individuals with adverse childhood experiences—such as sexual abuse, violence, or early loss—report higher rates of suicidal behavior, with these events functioning as both distal and proximal contributors to emotional dysregulation and mental pain (Brådvik, 2018; Sadath et al., 2023). Exposure to stigma, particularly among unemployed individuals living with SMI, was shown to mediate suicidal ideation through anticipated discrimination and social isolation (Oexle et al., 2018; Xu et al., 2023); social isolation has been found to be a behavioral antecedent to the occurrence of experiencing social disconnectedness that has been found to be a critical factor in suicidal behaviors (Cornwell & Waite, 2009; Espinosa-Salido et al., 2021; Joiner, 2005). The role of stigma-related stress further emphasizes the need for multifaceted prevention approaches targeting both public attitudes and individual resilience.

Access to means is a modifiable antecedent condition yet underappreciated factor in suicide prevention. Firearms remain the most prevalent method of suicide in the United States, accounting for over 50% of all deaths (Miller et al., 2013; NIMH, 2025b). Global patterns differ, with pesticide ingestion and hanging more common in low- and middle-income countries (WHO, 2025). The choice of methods is shaped by availability, cultural norms, and lethality. Instruments like the Scale for Assessment of Lethality of Suicide Attempt (SALSA) (Kar et al., 2014) enable service providers to evaluate risk based on method severity, intent, impulsivity and rescuer factors (Jang et al., 2025) that encompass: (a) the location of the attempt—whether it occurs in a remote setting like the outdoors or in familiar places such as the home or workplace; (b) the identity of the rescuer, who might range from anonymous passersby or professionals to those closest to the individual, such as family or close acquaintances; (c) the probability that the attempt will be discovered plays, varying from situations where discovery is almost certain to those where it is purely accidental; (d) the individual's behavior regarding help-seeking, which might include not asking for help at all, dropping subtle clues, or directly reaching out; and (e) the delay until discovery focusing on how much time elapses before the attempt is found that shapes the potential for rescue (e.g., whether more than four hours, less than four hours, or immediately within an hour) Together, these dimensions interweave to determine the rescue potential, highlighting how method, context, relationships, and timing critically influence outcomes in moments of a suicidal crisis (Jang et al., 2025; Kar et al., 2014).

Taken together, these findings highlight the importance of integrated risk models that account for the presence and severity of a mental health problem (Mann &

Arango, 1999), psychosocial context (including stigmatization), dispositional traits, and behavioral history. Ongoing suicide prevention efforts should emphasize routine screening for prior attempts and ideation, the development of culturally sensitive interventions, and targeted approaches for high-risk groups, including those with comorbid mental health problems, chronic illness, and limited social support.

Research suggests that mental health conditions are significant risk factors for the occurrence of suicidal behaviors across the lifespan (Masango et al., 2008). Between 60% and 98% of suicides have been associated with mental health conditions, with depression identified as a major contributor (NIMH, 2024; Bachmann, 2018; Brådvik, 2018). Over 90% of individuals who die by suicide have mental health challenges, yet over 98% of those with mental disorders do not die by suicide (Klonsky et al., 2016).

Mental health problems, including MDD, BPD, BD, and schizophrenia spectrum mental health problems, are consistently associated with elevated risk (Brådvik, 2018; Fu et al., 2023). Substance use, especially involving alcohol and opioids, further exacerbates suicidal behavior (Turecki & Brent, 2016). Individuals living with SMI face higher risk, shaped by complexity of the mental health problem and systemic factors. In schizophrenia spectrum mental health problems, suicide risk is especially high in the early years of the condition, exacerbated by depressive features and psychotic symptoms such as command hallucinations (American Psychiatric Association, 2022b; Radomsky et al., 1999). Comorbid mood or personality mental health problems and co-occurring substance use problems compound the suicide risk in SMI populations (Sadath et al., 2023). Recurrent hospitalizations and periods following discharge are considered high-risk intervals. Similarly, neurobiological factors, such as serotonergic dysregulation and pronounced stress-reactive diathesis, are also recognized as significant vulnerabilities (Mann et al., 1999; Mann, 2003). Traits such as impulsivity and aggression span diagnostic categories, increasing both attempt frequency and lethality.

Suicidal behaviors are observed at notably high rates among individuals living with SMI, influenced by a range of psychological, biological, social, and diagnostic factors that are specific to various mental health conditions associated with SMI (Bachmann, 2018). The presence of SMI, particularly schizophrenia spectrum and personality mental health problems, and co-occurring substance use (such as alcohol consumption), constitutes significant risk factors for the manifestation of suicidal behaviors (Masango et al., 2008; Song et al., 2020).

The likelihood of suicidal behavior increases in proportion to the severity of problem behaviors associated with SMI, the number of concurrent mental health conditions, medical comorbidities (Fu et al., 2023; Mann & Arango, 1999; Sadath et al., 2023), and co-occurring substance use problems (American Psychiatric Association, 2022b; Xu et al., 2023). Data from the NCS-R (Kessler & Merikangas, 2006) demonstrate that individuals with six or more co-occurring mental health conditions have a 29-fold greater risk of suicide attempts compared to those without any diagnoses. Individuals living with SMI frequently experience symptoms such as anhedonia, hopelessness, social disconnection, and isolation, which can mediate the onset and progression of suicidal thoughts and behaviors (American Psychiatric

Association, 2022a; Brådvik, 2018; Klonsky et al., 2016). People living with MDD have a suicide risk about 17 times higher than the general population. Those with BD face a lifetime suicide mortality rate of 5–6% (American Psychiatric Association, 2022b; Kamali et al., 2021). For individuals diagnosed with schizophrenia spectrum disorders, suicide risk remains elevated. Personality disorders, notably BPD, are characterized by high rates of nonfatal suicidal behavior, often reflecting persistent emotional dysregulation and interpersonal instability (Albert et al., 2019; American Psychiatric Association, 2022d). Co-occurring physical and substance use problems add to the psychological burden of the individual contributing to the increased risk of suicide.

The highest suicide risks occur among inpatients with psychotic or mood disorders, particularly when combined with substance abuse or personality mental health problems. Risk of suicide in an outpatient setting involves mood, substance, personality, anxiety-related mental health problems, and PTSD. Risk increases further with comorbid psychiatric or physical illnesses; chronic conditions like cancer or HIV can double suicide risk even without the presence of a mental health problem (Bachmann, 2018).

Distinct from suicidal behaviors, nonsuicidal self-injury behaviors (NSSIB) are defined as purposeful injuries to the body without intent to die. These behaviors, such as cutting, burning, or hitting, are often employed to regulate intolerable emotional states. Studies have shown that NSSIB typically reflects dysregulated coping strategies, particularly among youth and individuals with mood or personality mental health problems (Fliege et al., 2009; NAMI, 2025).

Central to understanding both suicide and NSSIB is the concept of lethality, which refers to the capacity of a chosen method to result in death. Highly lethal methods, such as firearms, hanging, or suffocation, tend to be selected in more planned or impulsive suicide attempts, particularly among individuals with certain mental health problems (Kar et al., 2014; Miller et al., 2013). Miller et al. (2013) reported that a clear pattern emerges in the use of methods among individuals with a history of self-harm: those who initially employed low-lethality means, such as drug overdose or cutting, often transition to more lethal methods in fatal episodes with 81% of overdose cases and 71% of cutting cases switched to higher lethality methods before their deaths. In contrast, individuals who began with high-lethality methods tended to persist with similar means. These observations underscore the critical importance of assessing the dimensions of method used in NSSIB for both the potential for method switching and the inherent danger in certain methods when designing prevention strategies (Miller et al., 2013). Furthermore, mental health comorbidities play a significant role in the repetition of NSSIB. Those with two or more mental health problems face a substantially heightened risk of repeating self-harm behaviors compared to individuals with one or no diagnoses. Specific psychiatric conditions, including personality, bipolar, drug-related, and alcohol-related mental health problems also confer greater risk for repeated self-harm compared to depressive disorders (Miller et al., 2013). These findings reflect the complex interplay between method choice, mental health comorbidities, and the recurrence of NSSIB, emphasizing the need for detailed and thorough assessment of the dimension of suicidal behaviors tailored to individual risk profiles, especially with individuals living with SMI.

Suicidal and self-harming behaviors present a multifaceted challenge across mental health problems and population groups. While these behaviors occur in the general domain, individuals living with SMI exhibit elevated prevalence, higher lethality, and greater complexity. The presence of mental health and medical comorbidities, biological vulnerability, trauma exposure, and sociodemographic stressors intersect to drive risk in people living with SMI. To mitigate the public health burden, mental health systems and service providers must emphasize clarity in terminology, depth in assessment, and precision in intervention that is tailored to the needs of the individual.

Dimensions of Suicidal and Self-Harming Behaviors

Current approaches to classifying mental health issues often utilize dimensional frameworks. Dimensional measures for mental health conditions typically include identifying observable and covert behaviors, as well as assessing frequency, duration, intensity or magnitude, relevant contexts (such as environmental antecedents and consequences), and the hypothesized function of behaviors associated with mental health behaviors. Using a dimensional framework for suicidal behaviors includes identifying, defining, and assessing areas such as the method and lethality of the injurious behaviors, the covert suicidal ideations, frequency and duration of planning, intent of the overt behaviors, and preventive actions (Beck et al., 1976; Diaz et al., 2003; Steer et al., 1993). Assessment instruments like the Columbia Suicide Severity Rating Scale (C-SSRS) systematically evaluate these behaviors, providing structured assessment of ideation severity, behavioral intent, and lethality, bringing essential data to inform clinical decision making (Posner et al., 2011).

Progress in suicide research is often constrained by inconsistent terminology. The absence of standardized definitions impedes data synthesis, clinical translation, and policy implementation (Goodfellow et al., 2019; Silverman et al., 2007). Suicidal ideation should be categorized as passive (e.g., wishing to be dead) or active (e.g., planning suicide), while behaviors must be defined with precision, distinguishing between attempts, aborted efforts, interrupted actions, and preparatory acts to obtain a comprehensive assessment of the targeted behaviors and develop individualized tailored interventions.

Suicidal and self-harm behaviors are complex, multidimensional, and multidirectional. "Multidimensionality" is defined as a concept not being explained by a single trait or attribute (American Psychological Association, n.d.-d). Multidirectionality refers to the capacity to change, progress, or function in various ways, not just along one linear path but in complex ways (Institute for Functional Medicine [IFM], 2023). Using this framework for suicidal behaviors, a change in one behavioral dimension would influence changes in one or more other covert and overt dimensions of suicidal behaviors in complex and heterogeneous ways. An example would be if an individual attempted intentional self-harm after being terminated at her place of employment. Her attempt was interrupted by friends who were concerned about her welfare. Attempting suicide increased her risk for suicidal behaviors in the future but the aborted attempt also resulted in a perception by the person that she has support in the community, resulting in a change and lessening of perceived isolation and burdensomeness, thereby mitigating the risk of future suicidal behaviors in the immediate future. Studies show that ideation, suicidal attempts, and lethality are not always correlated as more people think about suicide who attempt and complete suicide (Klonsky et al., 2016). For example, someone may have high intent but choose a low method of lethality due to factors related to the availability of method or impulsivity. Research indicates that lethality may be affected by personality characteristics, including impulsivity and aggression, in addition to ideation. Higher levels of physical aggression have been associated with an increased capacity for highly lethal suicide attempts (Brokke et al., 2022).

Dimensions of suicidal behaviors are both covert, overt, and observable response classes of behaviors. These dimensions require both self-reports and observational data. Dimensions of covert private events of suicidal behaviors are thoughts associated with a desire to die (e.g., intent), planning for suicide, and the intensity of distressing covert respondents such as depression. Self-reports include cognitive experiences and associations (self-talk) and perceptual experiences including hopelessness, social disconnectedness (e.g., marked by a lack of social relationships and low levels of participation in social activities), perceived isolation (i.e., feelings of loneliness and a perception of lack of social support), and perceived burdensomeness to others. Self-reports can include reports from collateral sources such as informants who are familiar with the individual. For example, an informant can corroborate reports by the person who describes a lack of engaging in social activities with others (Martinez-Rives et al., 2025). Observational data can be accessed from records, reports, and watching and recording actual events. Electronic sleep, activity, and mood logs can support self-reports from respondents with depressive symptoms.

Within each domain, dimensions can be categorized by frequency, duration, intensity/severity, and contextual variables. Based on psychometric analyses, covert dimensional frameworks indicate underlying elements in suicidal ideation, such as how often, how intensely, and for how long thoughts about dying occur (i.e., desire to die), as well as planning and intent (Diaz et al., 2003; Steer et al., 1993). For ideation, relevant dimensions include passive versus active thoughts, intent to die, and planning. For lethality, dimensions involve method selection, level of medical severity, and comparisons between perceived and actual danger.

Suicidal ideation and the lethality of method can be distinct domains within the broader construct of suicidal behavior. Ideation is a covert domain while lethality is an overt domain of suicidal response classes. Ideation reflects cognitive and emotional processes (e.g., frequency, intensity, and intent) that can be accessed by self-reports and categorized as passive or active. Assessed dimensions of suicidal ideations ought to include distressing cognition and perceptions like loneliness, social disengagement, burdensomeness, hopelessness, and helplessness.

Lethality is a measurable aspect that can be evaluated using different tools (Kar et al., 2014). It refers to the method used during suicidal behavior and the associated likelihood of death, as well as the medical severity, such as the degree of medical intervention required. Defining lethality in overt suicidal behaviors requires precise and detailed criteria, including distinctions among attempts, aborted efforts, interrupted actions, and preparatory acts. Differentiating between individuals with suicidal ideations and those who have made actual attempts involves validated assessment tools and comprehensive psychosocial evaluation. Evidence indicates that the history of NSSIB is associated with increased concern for subsequent suicidal behavior, as such patterns may develop into more severe attempts (Edgcomb et al., 2021).

Suicide risk assessment must be routine and multidimensional across all mental health settings (Xu et al., 2023). Dimensional models such as the ideation-to-action framework (Klonsky & May, 2014) further clarify the transition from self-harming ideation to observable suicidal behavior. Empirical studies suggest that specific behavioral components—such as access to lethal means, levels of impulsivity, and exposure to trauma—may interact with emotional dysregulation to escalate risk (Campos et al., 2021; Mann et al., 1999). Factor analytic work with the Suicide Intent Scale (Beck et al., 1976; Diaz et al., 2003) identifies planning and perceived lethality as critical constructs for distinguishing self-harm from suicide attempts.

Suicidal and self-harming behaviors in people living with SMI are multifaceted and are a complex interplay of psychological, behavioral, social, cultural, and environmental factors at individual and societal levels. The dimensions of suicidal and self-harming actions consist of overt and covert behavioral response classes that can be assessed on topography (that includes the description of the suicidal and self-harming behaviors, amount of effort in engaging in the suicidal behaviors, latency between the suicidal ideation and engaging in overt suicidal and self-harming behaviors), the frequency, duration, intensity/magnitude, and the context when engaging in the suicidal behaviors, including the function, reinforcing consequences, and motivating operations (MO) (e.g., antecedent conditions that change the value of the consequence of the behavior) (Cooper et al., 2020). Understanding these behaviors involves recognizing them as complex phenomena that are influenced by various dimensions rather than a single factor. Several of the dimensions contain both covert and overt response classes of behaviors, necessitating a multimodal, multimethod approach of comprehensive assessment. Research has identified several dimensions that play a role:

- Suicidal ideation: Thoughts of wanting to die. Passive ideation is wishing for death without intent or plan (Steer et al., 1993), while active ideation includes intent (Posner et al., 2011).
- Desire for death: An urgency and commitment to die often driven by hopelessness, "psychache" (Shneidman, 1993), and emotional pain (Steer et al., 1993; Turecki & Brent, 2016). Psychache is defined as a subjective experience of adverse respondents such as dread, despair, fear, grief, shame, guilt, frustrated love, loneliness, and loss (American Psychological Association, n.d.-e;

Shneidman, 1993). These aversive respondents may function as MOs for the covert behavior of self-criticism that is defined as distressing and negative statements about oneself.

- Negative and positive ideations: Risk-enhancing (e.g., thoughts of escape from distressing respondents) vs. protective factors (Ghasemi et al., 2015).
- Experiencing hallucinations and delusions: Hallucinations, especially auditory hallucinations such as hearing voices, are strongly associated with increased suicidal ideation and risk of suicide attempts. Persons living with SMI frequently report that derogatory, distressing, or commanding voices intensify psychological pain, contributing not just to passive death wishes, but to more active planning or attempts (Freeman et al., 2019). Auditory hallucination can be persecutory, derogatory, or commanding, often leading individuals to feel overwhelmed, worthless, or hopeless. Commanding or persecutory voices are often implicated in more impulsive suicide attempts or active planning, driven by acute distress or a desire to escape overwhelming auditory experiences. Visual and tactile hallucinations may amplify overall distress and isolation, indirectly increasing suicide risk (Harris et al., 2020). Delusions, especially of a persecutory or paranoid nature, are closely linked to heightened suicidal ideation and behaviors. Individuals who believe they are being plotted against or persecuted often experience profound defeat, entrapment, and psychological distress, feelings that are strongly associated with suicidal thinking (Freeman et al., 2019).
- Cognitive impairments and presence of negative symptoms: Cognitive impairments and negative symptoms such as slowed thinking and impaired executive functions are both linked to increased suicidal ideations as well as behavioral symptoms of apathy and impulsivity that further elevates risk (Kułak-Bejda et al., 2021).
- Suicide attempt: Nonfatal self-injurious behavior with intent to die.
- Completed suicide: Fatal self-directed act with intent to die.
- Preparatory behavior: Actions taken before a suicide attempt (e.g., acquiring means, writing a note, and giving away possessions) (Beck et al., 1976; Campos et al., 2021).
- Interrupted attempt: Suicide attempt stopped by external factors (e.g., someone intervenes).
- Self-aborted attempt: Individual halts the attempt before harm occurs (Barber et al., 1998).
- Non-suicidal self-injurious behaviors (NSSIB): Self-harm without intent to die (e.g., cutting, burning). NSSIB can only be classified when there is an absence of suicidal intent linked to the self-harming behaviors of an individual (Hooley et al., 2020). NSSIB and suicidal thoughts and behaviors frequently co-occur. In addition to strong associations, NSSIB longitudinally predicts suicidal thoughts and behaviors, and the strength of this relationship is as strong as (or even stronger than) that observed for suicidal thoughts and behaviors (Hooley et al., 2020). Many individuals participate in NSSIB during times of suicidal ideation, and in some cases, their actions are intended or hoped to result in death. However, the prevalence of suicidal thoughts and hopes for death is generally higher in sui-

cidal behaviors compared to NSSIB, indicating a difference in degree. Research indicates that individuals may engage in NSSIB as a strategy to avoid acting on suicidal thoughts. Multiple studies (Hooley et al., 2020) have shown that NSSIB can serve as a coping mechanism and a way to prevent acting on such thoughts.

- Suicide plans: Developing a detailed method or strategy for carrying out a suicide attempt.
- Lethality: Cognitions related to method of self-harming and magnitude of self-harm and injury.
- Access to lethal means: Availability of methods that could be used for suicide, such as firearms, medications, or dangerous objects.
- Rescuability: The situational and interpersonal likelihood of intervention. Factors such as attempt location, proximity to others, and the time until discovery heavily influence the probability of survival. Jang et al. (2025) operationalized these variables through the Risk-Rescue Rating Scale (RRRS), demonstrating how external variables moderate lethality irrespective of internal intent.
- Hopelessness: The belief that improvement in a situation is unlikely and that solutions are not available. Research has identified hopelessness as a significant predictor of suicide risk (Beck et al., 1985).
- Self-criticism: Distressing and aversive covert statement about oneself; this dimension is defined as the evaluation of one's own behavior and attributes, with recognition of one's weaknesses, errors, and shortcomings and maybe a risk factor for the presence of a depressive mental health problem (American Psychological Association, n.d.-f).
- Emotional dysregulation: Characterized by emotional instability, anxiety, and negative emotions; this dimension possibly increases intensity and frequency of suicidal ideation and impulsivity (Giner et al., 2016).
- Impulsivity: Tendency to act on sudden urges or thoughts without considering potential consequences (Brokke et al., 2022). Duration between the thought of emitting a behavior and manifesting the behavior is "latency" (Cooper et al., 2020). This dimension includes the frequency, duration, and organization of covert planning (e.g., premeditation) to engage in suicidal behaviors that range from impulsive to elaborate plans for suicidal behaviors (Gomez et al., 2023; Kar et al., 2014).
- Social isolation: The objective absence or paucity of contacts and interactions between a person and a social network. The experience of social isolation is the antecedent condition for loneliness, which is a subjective covert state of being alone, separated or apart from others, and has been conceptualized as an imbalance between desired social contacts and actual social contacts (Veazie et al., 2019).
- Relationship problems: Difficulties and conflicts within relationships, particularly intimate partner problems and family issues.
- Perceived burdensomeness: Self-statements of being a burden on others and believing that one's death would be a relief to them (Espinosa-Salido et al., 2021; Joiner, 2005).

- Thwarted belongingness: Feeling disconnected from others and lacking a sense of belonging or acceptance (Espinosa-Salido et al., 2021; Joiner, 2005).
- Family environment: Having and/or living with parents with mental health problems, family history of suicide, family conflict, loss of a parent due to death or divorce, poor parent–child relationship quality, and maltreatment.
- Communication: Communication of suicidal intents serves several vital purposes; it helps individuals seek support, reduces isolation, enables early intervention, challenges stigma, provides emotional relief, and strengthens social connections. Communication such as verbal disclosures, indirect threats, or suicide notes serves as both a warning signal and a behavioral dimension linked to premeditation or desire for intervention. Campos et al. (2021) note that these communicative acts can sometimes demarcate interrupted or self-aborted attempts from completed ones, adding further to risk assessment.
- Cultural norms, beliefs, and attitudes toward suicide and help seeking: Societal views on suicide, including whether it is stigmatized or considered acceptable under certain circumstances and stigma associated with seeking mental health support in certain cultures (Goldsmith et al., 2002).
- Cultural differences in expression of distress: The ways in which emotional pain is communicated differ among cultural groups (Goldsmith et al., 2002).
- Impact of discrimination: Experiences of discrimination based on race, ethnicity, sexual orientation, or other factors can significantly increase suicide risk (Goldsmith et al., 2002).
- Prolonged stress: Ongoing stressors like unemployment, financial strain, relationship problems, or bullying can be compounded by acute stressful life events like rejection, divorce, financial crisis, or loss of a loved one.
- Acculturation stress: Challenges faced by individuals adjusting to a new culture (Goldsmith et al., 2002).
- Historical trauma: Intergenerational trauma experienced by certain communities, such as those affected by colonization or human rights abuses (Goldsmith et al., 2002).
- Exposure to suicide: Exposure to another person's suicide, particularly through media or in one's community, can increase risk (Swanson & Colman, 2013) and can function as a MO for the individual engaging in suicidal ideation.
- Protective factors: Variables that mitigate against suicidal behaviors including coping behaviors, positive perceptions of oneself, being physically active and participating in social activities, and attachment to others (Bakken et al., 2024; CDC, 2024a; Hutchinson, 2023).

Dimensional models of suicidal behavior offer a comprehensive framework that transcends binary categorizations like ideation versus attempt. These models reveal multifaceted constructs encompassing psychological motivation, behavioral engagement, and contextual risk. The ideational spectrum is strongly shaped by covert class of respondents like hopelessness, "psychache," and perceived burdensomeness (Espinosa-Salido et al., 2021; Turecki & Brent, 2016).

Intent to die represents another crucial dimension, reflecting the degree of emotional commitment and decisiveness involved in the suicide process. Individuals may exhibit strong intent, yet select methods of low lethality due to impulsivity, cognitive impairments, or limited access to means (Hausmann-Stabile et al., 2012; Lara et al., 2015). This disjunction is noted in individuals who attempted suicide and whose understanding of medical consequences may be incomplete (for example, taking a bottle of aspirin or 25 tablets of acetaminophen).

Preparation behaviors—such as acquiring lethal means, leaving suicide notes, or rehearsing the act—form a distinct behavioral dimension that often co-occurs with elevated intent. Factor analyses of the Suicidal Intent Scale (SIS) highlighted this preparatory cluster, aligning with Beck's original classification of premeditative versus impulsive attempts (Beck et al., 1976; Campos et al., 2021; Diaz et al., 2003). Yet, impulsivity itself constitutes another vulnerability dimension, particularly in stress–diathesis models where trait aggression and poor inhibition amplify suicide risk across mental health problems (Mann et al., 1999).

Lethality—the medical seriousness of an attempt—is often treated as an independent dimension, despite common assumptions linking high intent with high lethality. Studies show that individuals with low intent may use highly lethal methods due to method availability or transient emotional crises (Hausmann-Stabile et al., 2012; Miller et al., 2013). Conversely, highly intentional attempts may involve less lethal means when restriction of methods or internal ambivalence is present.

Beyond cognitive and behavioral facets, mental pain or "psychache" emerges as an experiential dimension with predictive relevance (Shneidman, 1993). Individuals reporting unbearable psychological distress often display elevated scores on ideation and intent scales, regardless of the presence of a mental health problem (Gvion & Apter, 2012; Klonsky, 2007). This subjective torment frequently intersects with hopelessness, self-punishment drives, and emotional detachment, especially in populations with borderline traits or trauma histories.

Together, these dimensions—ideation, intent, preparation, lethality, "rescuability," communication, impulsivity, and psychological pain—form an integrative model that accommodates variability across individual cases. Such a framework is reflected in tools like the Columbia Suicide Severity Rating Scale (C-SSRS) and Beck's SIS, which analyze suicidal behaviors into measurable elements with clinical and research utility (Beck et al., 1976; Posner et al., 2011). Dimensional assessment allows for stratified suicide risk profiles and intervention matching, enabling clinicians to move beyond static categories and toward dynamic, person-centered evaluations.

Assessment of suicidal behavior is a major core aspect of mental health evaluation and crisis intervention. Accurate identification of ideation, intent, behavior, and lethality allows for appropriate classification of the relevant dimensions of suicidal behaviors for an individual and individualized treatment planning. A variety of validated scales and structured instruments have been developed to measure distinct dimensions of suicidality, ranging from passive ideation to medically serious attempts.

Table 17.1 Commonly used assessment tools for suicidal behaviors and dimensions assessed

Name of tool	Dimension(s) measured
Columbia–Suicide Severity Rating Scale (Posner et al., 2011)	Severity and intensity of ideation, behavioral subtypes (actual, aborted, preparatory), and lethality
Beck Scale for Suicide Ideation (BSI) (Beck et al., 1976)	Active suicidal desire, planning, intent, and motivation
Suicide Intent Scale (SIS) (Beck et al., 1974; Diaz et al., 2003)	Lethality, planning, precautions, communication, and medical seriousness
Modified Scale for Suicide Ideation (MSSI) (Ghasemi et al., 2015)	Severity and cognitive structure of ideation
Positive and Negative Suicide Ideation (PANSI) (Ghasemi et al., 2015)	Protective factors and negative ideation structure
Risk-Rescue Rating Scale (RRRS) (Jang et al., 2025; Kar et al., 2014)	Lethality of method, probability of discovery, access to rescuers, and time to discovery
Lethality of Suicide Attempt Rating Scale (LSARS/LSARS-II) (Hausmann-Stabile et al., 2012)	Medical consequences and likelihood of death

Conducting a comprehensive assessment on all the dimensions of suicidal behaviors would be cumbersome, time consuming, and aversive not only for the service provider doing the evaluation but the individual who has exhibited suicidal behaviors. There have been several assessment tools that are commonly used with individuals presenting with suicidal behaviors. An assessment tool is a structured approach to assess the critical dimensions that influence the occurrence of suicidal behaviors and may assist in identifying and evaluating the criticality of the dimensions of suicidal behaviors that need to be the point of intervention and prevention. The best assessment begins with a focused psychosocial interview assessment using a compassionate, empathic, and person-centered approach; using the obtained data, the service provider can expand the assessment using those tools that are salient for the individual and would clarify the clinical picture so as to get a more complete understanding of the person in need and possible interventions and preventive measures.

Table 17.1 presents a summary of key assessment instruments commonly used and applied in clinical and research contexts, along with the dimensions they assess. The tools presented in Table 17.1 vary in scope and granularity. For instance, the Columbia Suicide Severity Rating Scale (C-SSRS) offers a comprehensive framework for delineating ideation severity, behavioral typology (e.g., actual, aborted, or interrupted attempts), and lethality. The Beck Scale for Suicide Ideation (BSI) and Suicide Intent Scale (SIS) provide psychometrically robust measures of suicidal thoughts and intent in clinical populations. Meanwhile, the Risk-Rescue Rating Scale (RRRS) emphasizes medical lethality and contextual discovery potential, making it useful for evaluating attempt severity post-crisis.

Dimensions such as desire to die, cognitive planning, emotional ambivalence, and method selection are central constructs measured across these tools. Importantly, research supports the clinical utility of multidimensional models that delineate ideation from intent and preparation, strengthening the predictive capacity of these assessments (Campos et al., 2021; Diaz et al., 2003; Steer et al., 1993).

Origins of Suicidal and Self-Harming Behaviors

Suicide is a complex issue, often linked to mental health problems, with about one million suicides and ten million attempts globally each year. Suicide is the 11th leading cause of death in the United States in 2023 with over 49,000 people completing suicide (CDC, 2024b). There are 10–20 suicide attempts for every completed suicide, indicating a significant prevalence of suicidal behavior. Over 90% of people who completed suicide lived with severe mental health problems with mood-related problems accounting for 60% of suicides (Mann, 2003).

A complex interplay of genetic, environmental, and neurobiological factors influences suicidal behaviors across the lifespan. The concept of diathesis, or a predisposition to suicidal behavior (American Psychological Association, n.d.-a), is significant; while many individuals may possess multiple risk factors, not all attempt suicide. Diathesis refers to a genetic or biological predisposition, but the manifestation of suicidal behaviors typically requires the interaction of one or more environmental variables, reflecting the diathesis–stress model (American Psychological Association, n.d.-b).

Genetics appear to significantly contribute to suicidal thoughts and behaviors (STBs), including suicidal ideation, suicide attempts, and completed suicide. Research has reported that STBs are moderately heritable, with estimates ranging from 30% to 55% of variability (DiBlasi et al., 2021). Genetic factors play a primary role in the intergenerational transmission of STBs, independent of mental health comorbidities. Genetic studies indicate overlap between STBs and mental health problems associated with SMI like MDD and BD mental health problems, and schizophrenia spectrum mental health problems. However, STBs are not solely attributable to these genetic variables, suggesting unique genetic factors (DiBlasi et al., 2021) indicating that familial environmental variables like trauma and role modeling of STBs could be influential in the occurrence of both covert and overt suicidal behaviors. Mental health conditions can exacerbate environmental psychosocial stressors, complicating the relationship between mental health and suicide. Environmental factors such as rural living, poverty, unemployment, social isolation, substance use, and stigmatization/discrimination have a pronounced impact on suicide risk (Lengvenyte et al., 2019; Mann, 2003; Oexle et al., 2016). Postmortem studies indicate abnormalities in serotonergic, noradrenergic, and dopaminergic systems in individuals who completed suicide. Lower serotonin levels and altered receptor binding in the prefrontal cortex (PFC) are associated with increased suicide risk. Imaging studies show reduced prefrontal activity in individuals with suicidal behavior, highlighting the importance of this brain region (Mann, 2003). Genetic variations can influence serotonergic activity and predispose individuals to impulsive aggression and suicidal behavior. The relationship between serotonin function and impulsivity/aggression is significant, with low serotonergic activity linked to higher aggression (Mann, 2003).

Nevertheless, biology is not destiny. Research has demonstrated the effectiveness of various interventions in preventing and treating suicidal behaviors. Psychotherapeutic approaches such as Dialectical Behavioral Therapy (DBT) and Cognitive Behavioral Therapy (CBT) are among the most effective, with CBT capable of halving the risk of new suicide attempts (Sufrate-Sorzano et al., 2023). Pharmacological treatments, including lithium and intravenous ketamine, as well as internet-based interventions like online CBT and self-help platforms, also show positive outcomes, though the latter require careful monitoring. Brief contact interventions, such as follow-up calls or emails, and community strategies that improve healthcare access and restrict lethal means further contribute to risk reduction. Building a strong therapeutic alliance, teaching coping skills, and addressing depression are protective measures. Méndez-Bustos et al. (2019) further support these findings, noting that DBT, CBT, Acceptance and Commitment Therapy (ACT), group therapies, mindfulness training, and collaborative care models are effective in reducing suicidal ideation and attempts across diverse populations and settings.

Biological and Neurological Substrates

Suicidal and self-harming behaviors are investigated as outcomes of complex neurobiological mechanisms. Research into structural, functional, and molecular characteristics, utilizing neuroimaging, neurotransmitter studies, and genetic analysis, has contributed to understanding the biological substrates related to suicidality and self-injury.

These behaviors are associated with dysfunction in several brain regions involved in emotion regulation, decision making, impulse control, and cognitive flexibility. These regions include the following:

- Prefrontal cortex (PFC): Structural and functional neuroimaging studies have identified the PFC, particularly the ventromedial (vmPFC), dorsolateral (dlPFC), and orbitofrontal (OFC) regions, as being involved in the biological mechanisms associated with suicidality. Research indicates that structural differences, such as decreased gray matter volume, and functional alterations in these areas are correlated with changes in judgment, decision making, and emotional regulation. These regions mediate executive functioning, inhibition, and planning, and their dysfunction contributes to impaired judgment, emotional dysregulation, and impulsivity in individuals at risk for suicide (Balcioglu & Kose, 2018; Mann, 2003). Damage to the vmPFC affects decision making and social behavior, increasing suicide risk. Impaired emotional responses and poor decision making are linked to PFC dysfunction (Mann, 2003).

- Cingulate cortex (CC): Abnormalities in the cingulate area, which is involved in emotion formation and processing, have been observed in individuals with a history of suicidal behavior (Lengvenyte et al., 2021). The anterior cingulate cortex (ACC) has shown increased activity during emotional tasks in suicidal individuals, particularly those with mood disorders. Abnormalities in the amygdala (amygd) and insular cortex (IC) further indicate disruptions in affective processing and pain sensitivity, often observed in those with self-injurious tendencies (Lengvenyte et al., 2021).
- Insular cortex (IC): The IC is connected to pain sensitivity and emotional awareness. Alterations here are linked to disrupted emotional regulation, processing, and heightened psychological pain in those at risk for suicide (Lengvenyte et al., 2021).
- Striatal regions: Changes in the striatum, associated with reward and motivation, may underlie impulsivity and altered responses to stress, both of which are relevant to suicidality (Lengvenyte et al., 2021).
- Default mode network (DMN): The DMN connects several brain regions and is involved in self-referential thought and future planning. Functional connectivity changes, especially in the posterior cingulate cortex (PCC) and orbitomedial (ORBm) regions, have been associated with rumination and hopelessness, which elevate suicide risk (Balcioglu & Kose, 2018; Lengvenyte et al., 2021).

Neurotransmitter Systems The serotonergic system plays a pivotal role in the regulation of mood, aggression, and impulsivity. Reduced serotonin activity has been consistently associated with increased suicidal ideation and attempts. Postmortem studies have demonstrated decreased serotonin metabolite levels in cerebrospinal fluid and lower serotonin transporter densities in key brain regions among suicide victims (DiBlasi et al., 2021; Mann, 2003). Altered expression of serotonin receptor subtypes (5-HT1A) have been linked to suicide risk with fMRI studies showing that individuals with high-lethality attempts exhibit reduced binding of this receptor in prefrontal regions, suggesting deficits in serotonergic modulation of executive functions and emotional regulation (Lengvenyte et al., 2021).

Other neurotransmitter systems including dopaminergic, noradrenergic, and glutamatergic pathways have also been implicated. Dysfunctions in reward processing and stress response mechanisms contribute to suicidal behaviors, especially in adolescents and individuals with mood disorders (Mann et al., 1999).

Neuroendocrine and Inflammatory Correlates Dysregulation of the hypothalamic–pituitary–adrenal (HPA) axis is another biological marker associated with suicidality. Low basal salivary cortisol levels and altered secretion patterns have been identified in depressed patients with a history of suicide attempts, pointing to an impaired stress response system (Lengvenyte et al., 2021). Inflammatory markers are elevated in individuals displaying suicidal behavior, suggesting a role for immune dysregulation. Certain immunological pathways, influenced by inflammation, is thought to deplete serotonin and contribute to depressive and suicidal symptomatology (Lengvenyte et al., 2021).

Genetic Influences on Suicide and Self-Harm Genetic research has provided compelling evidence for heritability in suicidal thoughts and behaviors. Estimates suggest that suicide-related traits are 30–55% heritable, indicating a significant risk among first-degree relatives of suicide victims, supporting the intergenerational transmission of vulnerability (DiBlasi et al., 2021).

Genome-wide association studies (GWAS) have identified chromosomes and other regions related to suicide risk. Genetic variants have been found that affect serotonin transport and receptor function, as well as genes involved in DNA repair, cell cycle regulation, and neuroplasticity have been implicated (Balcioglu & Kose, 2018; DiBlasi et al., 2021).

Epigenetic mechanisms, such as DNA methylation patterns in certain genes and changes in the telomeres of genes due to stress (Lin & Epel, 2022), reflect gene–environment interactions that may mediate suicide risk, particularly following early-life adversity (Lengvenyte et al., 2021).

Biological and neurological substrates of suicidal and self-harming behaviors reveal a convergence of structural brain abnormalities, neurotransmitter deficits, endocrine dysregulation, inflammatory changes, and genetic vulnerability. These findings underscore the importance of multilevel, interdisciplinary approaches in understanding, assessing, and preventing suicide.

Behavioral and Psychological Substrates

The mental health literature indicates that biological factors, including heredity and neurological mechanisms, are important in influencing suicidal and self-harm behaviors among individuals living with SMI. The brain regions and neurotransmitters associated with these behaviors, such as the frontal lobes, limbic system, dopamine, and serotonin, are also related to other behavioral issues observed in SMI. While biological factors may contribute to both suicidal and self-harming behaviors, as well as other behavioral challenges in this population, a definitive causal pathway has not yet been identified.

Environmental and psychological aspects, supportive social networks, loss, depression, unemployment, poverty, lack of educational opportunities, discrimination and stigmatization, and trauma are critical factors as to whether suicidal and self-harm behaviors occur. Using familial data, researchers postulate that people living with SMI engage in suicidal behaviors due to genetic risk factors that result in a genotypic liability to self-harm and commit suicide. The heritability of STBs, including ideation, attempts, and death, is moderate, with genetics accounting for approximately 30% to 55% of the variance in risk across general populations (DiBlasi et al., 2021) which leaves 70% to 45% accounted for by other variables including environmental conditions.

Genetic influences on suicide risk are more complex in individuals who live with SMI. Current research indicates that suicidality may possess unique genetic factors that are not solely attributable to the genetics associated with specific mental health conditions and may exist independently of these disorders. There is no evidence that STBs that are used are a function of the determinants of specific mental health problems, like delusions, hallucinations, and neurocognitive impairments (DiBlasi et al., 2021). STBs may be viewed as a coping mechanism, where focusing on STBs could help individuals avoid or lessen the distress related to hallucinations and delusions. This may result in a reduction in certain aspects of these experiences, such as their frequency and intensity, with the decrease in distress serving as negative reinforcement for engaging in STBs (Borges et al., 2019).

People living with SMI encounter many of the known environmental and psychological risk factors for STB that increase the chances of them occurring in response to certain overt and covert antecedent conditions. Important contributing factors in the development of STB in people living with SMI is the role of social learning, respondent conditioning, and operant learning processes in the genesis and maintenance of STBs by an individual living with SMI.

Emotions including depression are basic tendencies to detect and respond to significant events (LeDoux, 2012). Emotional states and their related memories are considered private events that can be examined through behavioral analysis, and these subjective experiences may play roles similar to motivating operations (MOs), antecedent stimuli, and functional consequences within a behavioral framework (Friman et al., 1998; Skinner, 1945; Skinner, 1969; Tourinho, 2006). Depression and its associated dysphoric respondents and cognitions (e.g., despair, guilt, hopelessness, apathy, and STBs) serve as conditioned stimuli to motivate the individual to engage in certain behaviors. Depressive respondents and associated covert behaviors function as an MO, which acts as an establishing operation (EO) by increasing the effectiveness of certain contingencies and, consequently, the likelihood of specific behaviors such as suicidal or self-harming actions. Alternatively, it can serve as an abolishing operation (AO), diminishing the impact of these contingencies (Cooper et al., 2020).

Based on the analysis of experienced emotions, dysphoria is a conditioned stimulus and could be understood as tracking a consequential contingency where the individual faces aversive conditions or fails to meet certain behavioral or social requirements (Layng, 2017). Dysphoria may describe a situation where the contingencies involve punishment, a change in the frequency or lack of reinforcement, or unmet expectations, leading to feelings of discomfort or dissatisfaction (Skinner, 1953). Identifying and addressing the contingencies responsible for the dysphoric feelings could help the person understand and alter their responses effectively. An appropriate intensity of dysphoric respondents may serve as an MO, as it enhances performance in certain tasks like analytical reasoning, problem solving, and persistence—useful behaviors in complex tasks (Clarkson University, 2011). Experiencing dysphoric-related respondents may facilitate the person to effectively seek out and acquire other reinforcing stimuli. An example would be the proverbial "empty nest syndrome" in which a parent experiences a decrease in the schedule of reinforcement for a variety of childcare behaviors. The parent "feels lost" as the behaviors that have been emitted over a prolonged period are not reinforced at the same frequency. The dearth of reinforcing stimuli for behaviors habitually emitted results in self-statements of uselessness, rejection, and aimlessness unless the parent engages in behaviors that may be novel in the behavioral repertoire like joining a club, seeking out new acquaintances, going to school, or starting a business, thereby acquiring new opportunities to be reinforced.

Dysphoric behaviors exhibited by an individual can serve as a MO for an observer. Such behavioral expressions, which include both covert and overt actions, may involve withdrawal, apathy, crying, disruptions in sleep and eating patterns, and subjective discomfort. These behaviors may function to obtain or avoid certain responses from others. The observed behaviors within this group of conditioned responses can sometimes be directed toward others to seek additional reinforcement, such as assistance or support. There is a reciprocal relationship between depression and dysphoric behavior; however, experiencing neither guarantees nor excludes the possibility of STBs, as individuals with depressive conditions may or may not exhibit STBs (Lara et al., 2015).

Observing the display of behaviors that are the result of dysphoric respondents can result in behaviors on the part of the observer expressing empathy and caring, offering solutions, and social engagement. It could also result in the observer removing oneself from the situation, stopping the interaction, or emitting counter-control behaviors, such as ridiculing, shaming and other punitive responses; punitive responses to the display of dysphoric behaviors could act as an MO for more frequent and intense self-critical self-statements, including burdensomeness, increased social isolation, and STBs. These consequences may affect the frequency and intensity of dysphoric-related behaviors, contingent upon the individual's history of risk factors that include trauma, discrimination, loss, self-harming behaviors, and previous suicide attempts. Using the "empty nester" example, others familiar with the individual may offer contexts in which new reinforcing contingencies can be established; on the other hand, observers can engage in punitive behaviors, telling the person to "snap out of it," "find something to do," "stop feeling sorry for yourself," and other dismissive and critical statements that may result in a furtherance of negative statements and a lessening of available reinforcers.

Dysphoric and depressogenic behaviors are associated with a wide range of mental health problems and affect the occurrence of STBs in people living with SMI. Private events and processes such as self-critical thoughts, grief, rumination about losses or negative outcomes, blame, and guilt are factors that can influence the onset and continuation of dysphoric responses and associated conditioned internal responses. Sadness, disappointment, and frustration are normal emotional responses; however, these emotions may be considered dysregulated if they occur with increased frequency or intensity, or in situations where such reactions are not typically expected—for example, experiencing profound depression following a minor event such as receiving a parking ticket.

Dysphoria-related emotions are unlearned physiological and covert responses triggered by environmental stimuli. These behaviors, influenced by neurological structures like the frontal lobes and limbic system, occur when an individual experiences acute or chronic deprivation of reinforcing stimuli. Depression arises when individuals fail to secure positive reinforcement due to limited or a lack of stimuli functioning as reinforcers in the environment or an inability to perform behaviors that access reinforcement (Skinner, 1953). This leads to behavioral suppression and emotional responses like sadness and despair (Dygdon & Dienes, 2013). Depression has been associated with a tendency to give greater significance to perceived losses compared to equivalent gains (Sediyama et al., 2020). When individuals perceive more losses—whether real, imagined, or exaggerated—they may focus increased attention on environmental stimuli related to negative outcomes (Sediyama et al., 2020). Loss aversion refers to this heightened sensitivity to losses, which can affect risk and reward evaluation by leading individuals to avoid situations seen as potentially harmful or risky, even when potential benefits are equal to or greater than the risks. For instance, people with higher loss aversion might overestimate the likelihood or severity of negative outcomes, influencing their decision-making processes. This pattern is observed in clinical groups, including those diagnosed with MDD or anxiety-related mental health problems, where loss aversion is linked to changes in decision making and processing of negative information (Sediyama et al., 2020). Individuals experiencing dysphoric responses may be motivated to avoid situations they perceive as likely to result in failure or negative outcomes, thus reducing encounters with potential negative consequences.

Nevertheless, depressive emotions can be conditioned and modified through interactions with the environment in which the individual learns how to mediate and modulate the experiences of depressogenic variables and, in so doing, alters the dimensions of experiencing dysphoria and aversive respondents; that is, altering the frequency, intensity, and the conditions in which the dysphoria is experienced (Goldiamond, 2022). The modulation of the experience of dysphoric-related respondents by an individual develops through associative learning which is a process by which a person learns to associate two stimuli or a behavior and a stimulus (Lind, 2018). This type of learning involves forming connections between different elements of the environment, leading to changes in behavior based on these associations. Associative learning is fundamental in understanding how organisms adapt their behaviors based on experiences and environmental cues.

There are two main types of associative learning:

- Classical (Pavlovian or respondent) conditioning refers to the process by which a neutral stimulus becomes associated with a significant stimulus, leading to the neutral stimulus eliciting a similar response. For instance, a child engages in rough play with a younger sibling who then begins to cry; the parent responds by expressing distress, attributing feelings of anxiety and personal inadequacy to the child's actions, conveying statements such as "I cannot trust you." The result of this interaction may be that the child internalizes the guilt and shame by engaging in covert self-critical statements (e.g., "I am a bad girl"). Through repeated occurrences, the child becomes conditioned to associate certain stimuli such as disappointing authority with guilt, shame, and the occurrence of critical self-statements. Additionally, the child learns to respond to situations involving frustration, punishment, or induced guilt from adults with sadness. As an adult, this individual subsequently experiences feelings of sadness and guilt when encountering obstacles imposed by authority figures, such as not obtaining a desired employment position.

Prolonged dysphoric respondents increase the chances that sadness will be conditioned to other situations that are out of context and inappropriate to the situation. An example may be a person who was admonished by his supervisor at work. While driving after work, he continues to engage in subvocal speech about this encounter and engages in critical self-statements (Tourinho, 2006). The result is that he experiences sadness with situations related to perceived criticism and rejection from others. He becomes more depressed and sadder when his significant other blames him for the non-payment of a bill, or a friend cancels going to the movies. Depressogenic covert events transfer to other similar situations, resulting in a cascade of intensifying negative and adverse self-statements that result in increasing the intensity of respondents. The MOs associated with reducing the intensity of the experienced aversive stimuli change the probability of the certain behaviors occurring, including self-harm and suicidal behaviors.

- Instrumental (operant) conditioning: This involves learning to associate behavior with a consequence that is reinforcing or punishing that results in an increase or decrease in the frequency, intensity, or the contextual display of the behavior. The behaviors of self-harm and suicide are negatively reinforced by the temporary reduction of the aversiveness of the respondents; these behaviors also result in positive consequences for the individual by an increase in caring and empathic responses on the part of others in the community.

Individuals may acquire knowledge about suicidal and self-harming behaviors through social learning processes. By observing the actions of others in their environment, particularly individuals with perceived authority or influence, people notice the outcomes, whether the behaviors are reinforced or punished. For example, if a person witnesses a parent engaging in self-harm or suicidal behavior following a loss or disappointment (such as the end of a significant relationship), and subsequently observes positive reinforcement like reconciliation between the parent and the former partner, the observer may learn to replicate similar behaviors in comparable situations due to both the modeled individual's status and the observed consequences.

The dimensions of the experience of depression and STBs are subject to environmental influences. The regulation of these variables entails modulating the emotional dimensions to achieve instrumental benefits, such as positive reinforcement, or being negatively reinforced by diminishing the discomfort associated with negative experiences. Individuals may modify unpleasant emotions to alleviate distress or in anticipation of perceived long-term advantages, such as eliciting supportive responses from others.

The experience of depression and the display of dysphoric behaviors are intertwined in complex manners, involving biological innate responses, perception, covert responses, and learning, resulting in a complex behavioral chain with multiple determinants. Depression and related respondents significantly influence the display of suicidal and self-harming behaviors through various mechanisms. Biological factors may provide a foundation for the class of dysphoric respondents, while associative and social learning shape and regulate how suicidal and self-harm behaviors are manifested.

The STBs act as a form of negative reinforcement by providing temporary relief from distressing emotions or situations by the individual focusing on the STBs (Borges et al., 2019). Focusing on STBs reduces contact with the distressing respondents of shame, hopelessness, and increased physiological arousal an individual experienced before engaging in STBs. As these emotions are experienced as undesirable, STBs that provide escape from them are likely to occur at greater frequency and intensity in the future. The display of suicidal behaviors is impacted by the environmental consequences of the behavior. Overt suicidal behavior is maintained through negative reinforcement as the suicidal behaviors cause an individual to be removed in some way from aversive internal/external environments. This relief can increase the likelihood of these thoughts or behaviors occurring again in similar circumstances, both to escape internal pain and to avoid difficult external environments (Borges et al., 2019).

Using a structural behavioral approach, signs and symptoms of suicidal ideation and behaviors are identified and categorized, resulting in an analysis of the behaviors, hypothesized functions of the STBs, and the designated level of suicide risk. For example, an individual who is living with a bipolar type of mental health problem gets terminated from his job because of frequent absences, timeliness, and impulsive and rash behaviors at work toward co-workers. He initially reacts with anger and threatens his supervisor. Following a day of being rejected by places of employment, he sees a group of former co-workers at a "happy hour." He is acknowledged by his peers, but receives no invitations to participate. Upon returning to his apartment, he notices the prescribed medication for his mental health condition, which he has discontinued. He takes all the pills and drinks a bottle of vodka. He wakes up in the ED and is informed that his girlfriend called the police when he did not answer the phone.

A chain analysis could be conducted on this situation to determine the behaviors that resulted in the suicide attempt of overdosing on prescription medications. The person has risk factors that include living with a mental health problem, discontinuing treatment, and impulsivity. The prompting event is that he was fired from his job that is then followed by self-statements of self-criticisms, shame, and anxious thoughts about his future, resulting in conditioned respondents of anxiety and dysphoria related to losses and perceived failures in the past. The self-deprecating self-statements increase in intensity and frequency following repeated rejections of finding a job. Self-statements of being socially isolated, disconnected from others, and alone are emitted following his perceived rejection by friends and acquaintances. Seeing the bottles of psychiatric medications elicits more negative self-statements about self-stigmatization, burdensomeness, and hopelessness. He takes the pills after taking a few shots of vodka with the plan of not waking up and escaping from his experience of despair. His suicide attempt was interrupted by his girlfriend who contacted the police after no answer to her repeated calls. Although embarrassed by his STBs, he engages in self-statements about his girlfriend caring about him.

Given this scenario, analyses of the chain of behavior place his behavior as a moderate risk of suicide. His attempt at suicide by overdosing was impulsive when he took the overdose with alcohol because of availability of means; the lethality of overdosing by using alcohol and medications was moderate. He did not communicate or engage in any preparatory behaviors before the attempt. He reported that he had never attempted to harm or kill himself before. He does have friends and a close intimate relationship. The significant risk factors for the display of suicidal behaviors in the future is: (a) he is living with an SMI, and he is not adherent to treatment recommendations; (b) impulsivity is a problem behavior linked to the mental health condition of BD; and (c) his suicide attempt was reinforced by a caring response by his girlfriend. Further assessment would need to be conducted to ascertain the dimensions of the STBs and other possible risk factors, like family history, history of loss and trauma, and presence of coping behaviors as risk factors modulate the dimensions of STBs.

STBs may be reinforced when consequences lead to the avoidance or removal of unpleasant emotional states or environmental situations (such as incarceration), which can increase the likelihood of future occurrence. Additionally, STBs are reinforced if their outcomes result in obtaining a desired response or exerting control over internal and external stimuli (Pavulans et al., 2012).

Consequences also act to inhibit the display and intensity of STBs. STBs are regulated by inhibitory control mechanisms that are influenced by internal and external cues. These include physical constraints, expectations of punishment or retaliation, empathy, consideration of consequences, and prosocial values. When individuals consider the potential negative outcomes of STBs, they may be more likely to inhibit them and engage in alternative response class of self-management behaviors. However, inhibition of STBs can be impaired if the frequency and intensity of STBs overwhelm the covert cognitive and metacognitive processes, thinking about one's thinking (e.g., theory of mind), consideration of the other person (i.e., empathy), and prosocial values, making it difficult to consider other alternative behaviors that would mitigate and replace the distressing respondents.

Epidemiological Considerations

The prevalence of suicidal and self-harming behaviors is shaped by a complex interplay of biological, psychological, social, and systemic factors. Epidemiological trends underscore the urgency of developing culturally sensitive, psychologically informed, and socially attuned interventions for prevention and care. Statistical data reinforce the clinical urgency of these phenomena. In the general US population, suicide rates hover around 14.2 per 100,000 individuals, while NSSIB prevalence among adolescents and young adults ranges between 18% and 25% (Fliege et al.,

2009; NIMH, 2025b). Among people living with schizophrenia spectrum mental health problems, approximately 5–6% die by suicide, and up to 31% engage in lifetime self-injury (American Psychiatric Association, 2022b; Lorentzen et al., 2022). Suicide mortality in people living with BD mirrors that of individuals living with schizophrenia spectrum mental health problems, while attempts may affect half of all individuals living with BD (Xu et al., 2023). Individuals living with BPD present the highest self-harm and attempt rates, with nearly 79% reporting past suicidal behavior (American Psychiatric Association, 2022b). Across groups of people living with mental health problems, specific clinical and demographic subtypes—including males, indigenous populations, and individuals with comorbid depression—appear to carry disproportionate risk.

Suicidal and self-harming behaviors are recognized as significant public health issues that affect various populations globally, regardless of cultural or socioeconomic differences. According to WHO (2025), suicide results in approximately 800,000 deaths per year worldwide, equating to one death every 40 seconds, with an estimated global mortality rate of 10.7 per 100,000 people. The lifetime prevalence of suicide attempts is between 1% and over 7%, while 12-month rates have been reported to range from 0.2% to 2.6% (IOM, 2001).

In the United States, suicide was the eleventh leading cause of death in 2022, accounting for over 49,000 deaths (NIMH, 2025b). Suicide rates vary significantly by region in the United States, with the highest rates found in western and frontier states like Alaska and the lowest in mid-Atlantic states such as New Jersey (NIMH, 2025b).

Socioeconomic factors are associated with variations in suicide rates, with higher rates documented among groups experiencing economic challenges, unemployment, or lower levels of education (De Leo & Altin, 2025). Internationally, the occurrence of suicidal behaviors differs based on a country's economic classification, though some trends are consistent. In low- and middle-income countries, reported suicidal ideation ranges from 3.1% to 12.4%, while suicide planning ranges from 0.9% to 4.1%, and attempts range from 0.7% to 4.7% (Nock et al., 2008). In high-income nations, suicidal ideation is reported between 3.0% and 15.9%, suicide planning from 0.7% to 5.6%, and suicide attempts from 0.5% to 5.0%. Across different economic categories, the probability of progressing from ideation to planning or attempting suicide remains relatively consistent (Nock et al., 2008).

Cross-national research indicates considerable variation in suicide rates across different geographic regions. The highest rates are observed in Eastern Europe, South-East Asia, and sub-Saharan Africa; Hungary reports the highest national rate, while Mexico ranks among the lowest. These trends are strongly influenced by the presence and robustness of social networks, familial relationships, and religious norms that discourage suicide, factors which serve as protective elements in communities with comparatively lower rates. The lowest suicide rates are typically found in Middle Eastern and Caribbean countries (Bachmann, 2018; WHO, 2025).

The NIMH (2025b) reported over 49,400 suicide deaths in 2022 alone, reflecting a national age-adjusted suicide rate of 14.2 per 100,000 people. Suicide stands as the second leading cause of death for youth aged 10–14 and young adults aged

25–34, third among those aged 15–24, and fourth among individuals aged 35–44. Among males aged 15–24, countries such as New Zealand, Australia, and Canada report the highest suicide rates, whereas Hungary consistently exhibits the highest prevalence among older males aged 75 and above. For young females within the same age group, Finland and New Zealand report the highest rates, with Hungary again leading among older women (De Leo & Altin, 2025).

Latin countries, including Spain, Italy, and Portugal, report the lowest suicide rates among young males, while Greece and Ireland demonstrate notably low rates among older males and females. In younger populations, particularly males, suicide rates in Latin nations are four to five times lower than those observed in Anglo-Saxon countries. This disparity diminishes among middle-aged adults, with Latin countries displaying less than twice the difference compared to Anglo-Saxon regions. However, in older age groups, this pattern reverses, with suicide rates in Latin countries surpassing those in their Anglo-Saxon counterparts (De Leo & Altin, 2025).

Bachmann (2018) reports that suicide contributes to 1.4% of all premature deaths worldwide, with approximately 78% of suicides occurring in low- and middle-income countries. Within these nations, limited access to mental health services, stigma, and underreporting compound the public health burden. The global frequency of suicide attempts is estimated to be 5 to 30 times higher than completed suicides (WHO, 2025), and this disparity underlines the scale of nonfatal self-harming behavior.

Suicide presents with demographic patterns and methods in the United States. Males account for nearly 80% of all suicide deaths in the United States, with a rate of 23.0 per 100,000 compared to 5.9 for females. Among specific racial and ethnic groups, American Indian and Alaska Native males exhibit the highest suicide rate nationally, at 39.5 per 100,000, followed by White non-Hispanic males at 28.0 per 100,000. Among females, the highest rates are observed in American Indian and Alaska Native women (14.6 per 100,000).

Firearms remain the predominant means, especially among men, followed by hanging and self-poisoning. Firearms were involved in more than half of suicides in the United States in 2022, accounting for approximately 54–55% of cases (CDC, 2024b; Miller et al., 2013). Other prevalent methods include hanging or suffocation, and poisoning, particularly through drug overdose or pesticide ingestion. The lethality and accessibility of these methods play a central role in outcome severity and the success of preventive interventions.

While men are more likely to die by suicide, women tend to report more attempts over their lifetime, though recent attempt rates between genders are similar. Age and ethnicity further shape these patterns. Gender differences are pronounced with suicide rates being generally much higher among males than among females, regardless of age group. Yet, the highest rates for young females are found in Anglo-Saxon countries, while older females in Latin countries—especially Portugal and Spain—are at greater risk (De Leo & Altin, 2025).

Suicide rates peak among older Caucasian men, whereas younger age groups are more at risk in other racial and ethnic groups. African American men, Native

Americans and Native Alaskan males have the highest racial/ethnic suicide rate, with rate of suicidal behaviors 39.5 per 100,000 for Native Americans followed closely by White non-Hispanic males at 28.0 (IOM, 2001; NIMH, 2025b). Notably, African American women, particularly in midlife, have some of the lowest rates. Marital status also matters, as widowed individuals face higher rates compared to those who are married. These findings underscore the multifaceted nature of suicide risk, shaped by gender, age, ethnicity, and social circumstances (IOM, 2001).

Culture and gender play influential roles in suicidal behavior patterns. In some cultures, suicide is shaped by religious, ceremonial, or honor-based motives, for example, ritual suicide in East Asian contexts (Giner et al., 2016). In others, stigma surrounding suicide impedes disclosure and prevention efforts (Oexle et al., 2018). Cultural norms also mediate gender disparities. While men die by suicide nearly four times more often than women globally, women attempt suicide more frequently (Bachmann, 2018). This pattern holds across many societies but varies in places like Bangladesh and China, where female suicide rates exceed male rates due to culturally embedded gender expectations and limited rights. Among individuals identifying as LGBTQ+, rates of suicidal ideation and behavior are significantly elevated, attributed to stigma, discrimination, and minority stress (CDC, 2024a; WHO, 2025). Religious involvement and participation in cultural rituals are associated with lower suicide rates. For example, Protestants in Chicago had double the suicide rates of Catholics after controlling for race, sex, and age (De Leo & Altin, 2025).

Most suicides are associated with the presence of mental health conditions. Certain clinical and demographic groups, such as males, indigenous populations, and individuals with comorbid depression, have been identified as having a higher risk across various mental health conditions. Mental health conditions are implicated in approximately 60–98% of completed suicides (Brådvik, 2018; Nock et al., 2008; Turecki & Brent, 2016). Elevated risks are particularly noted in MDD, BD, schizophrenia spectrum mental health problems, BPD, and substance use mental health problems (Fu et al., 2023; Xu et al., 2023). For instance, people with major depressive mental health problems have up to a 17-fold increased risk of suicide compared to the general population (American Psychiatric Association, 2022b), while lifetime suicide attempt rates in BD mental health problems range from 25% to 50%. In individuals with schizophrenia spectrum mental health problems, suicide completion occurs in roughly 5–6% of cases, with up to 20% attempting suicide at least once (American Psychiatric Association, 2022b). Among those with BPD mental health problems, 79% report previous suicide attempts, and long-term mortality rates approach 6% (Albert et al., 2019). Co-occurring psychiatric and physical illnesses—including chronic pain, HIV, and cancer—further compound suicide risk (Brådvik, 2018; Sadath et al., 2023).

Self-harming behaviors, notably NSSIB, are prevalent among both clinical and non-clinical populations. Fliege et al. (2009) note that self-harm occurs in 14–57% of individuals with schizophrenia spectrum mental health problems, while Lorentzen et al. (2022) estimate lifetime self-harm prevalence at 31% in individuals living with schizophrenia spectrum mental health problems and 39.7% among individuals at clinical high risk for psychotic-related problems. Cutting is the most frequently reported method, followed by burning, scratching, and hair pulling. Importantly, the presence of self-harm substantially increases the likelihood of subsequent suicide attempts, particularly when co-occurring psychiatric conditions such as MDD and BPD mental health problems, or substance use mental health problems are present (Hausmann-Stabile et al., 2012; Miller et al., 2013).

Socioeconomic status and income levels contribute meaningfully to both suicidal and self-harming behaviors. Economic instability, unemployment, poverty, and lack of access to affordable housing and mental healthcare serve as critical stressors (CDC, 2025). Individuals experiencing high unemployment, financial hardship, or educational disadvantage are more vulnerable, particularly when such challenges interact with mental health conditions. A study by Lara et al. (2015) found elevated suicide attempt risk among individuals with elementary-level education, those unable to work, and those lacking religious affiliation. These disparities are compounded by racial and ethnic minority populations, rural communities, and veterans, who often experience elevated suicide rates due to structural inequality and limited support systems (CDC, 2025).

Temporal analyses have revealed a concerning rise in suicide rates. Between 2000 and 2018, suicide rates in the United States increased by approximately 35%. Although a slight decline was observed in 2019 and 2020, rates subsequently rebounded to their previous peak by 2022. Emergency department surveillance data further underscore the growing burden. Between 2017 and 2018, the United States saw a 25.5% increase in emergency department visits for suicidal ideation and self-directed violence, with the highest spike (62.3%) observed among males aged 10–19 years (Zwald et al., 2020).

Certain environmental context influences the prevalence of suicidal behaviors. Suicide rates increase temporarily following published stories of suicides, particularly among teenagers and when the suicide is glorified (IOM, 2001). Limited social contact, such as living alone or being divorced, increases suicide risk. Extended families, religious involvement, and other types of social support reduce risk. Suicide is the leading cause of death in jails and prisons in the United States, with most suicides occurring within the first 48 hours of confinement (IOM, 2001).

These figures not only highlight the pervasiveness of suicidal behavior across lifespans, cultures, and contexts but also call attention to the necessity of region-specific interventions, demographic sensitivity, and longitudinal data monitoring. Suicide is a phenomenon deeply intertwined with mental health conditions, access to care, socioeconomic status, and systemic disparities.

Classifications and Types of Suicidal and Self-Harming Behaviors

Developing a precise classification system for mental health problems is essential, as it significantly enhances the ability of service providers to reliably identify and address problem behaviors more effectively. Classification systems enhance consistency in clinical reporting and facilitate risk assessment across settings. The system also supports research by providing a systematic framework to study mental health problems, fosters clearer communication among professionals and policymakers, and informs public health strategies through accurate tracking of prevalence and impact. An accurate classification system reduces the likelihood of errors in determining the presence of mental health problems, thereby promoting more appropriate care and decreasing the stigma often associated with mental health conditions (Basso, 2021).

Developing accurate mental health classification systems presents significant challenges, including the lack of consistent terminology and operationalized definitions, the complexity of mental health problems, and the absence of universal organizing principles or external standards for validation. The variety of disciplinary perspectives, ranging from psychology to neuroscience, adds complexity by introducing differing criteria, terminology and focus. Additionally, the absence of universally accepted tools for assessing mental health issues—tools that are standard in other health-related fields—renders the determination of measurement accuracy challenging. Classifications must also remain flexible to accommodate new findings, negotiating the tension between conventional, symptom-based approaches, and frameworks based on etiology (Basso, 2021). The DSM-5-TR (American Psychiatric Association, 2022a) is the present classification system and is primarily descriptive in the determination of the presence and severity of a mental health problem.

Efforts to classify suicidal and self-harming behaviors have spanned decades, reflecting a persistent struggle with developing clear, operational definitions of suicidal and self-harming behaviors capable of guiding clinical, legal, and research practices. The lack of universally agreed-upon terminology has long impeded both cross-study comparisons and clinical precision (Goodfellow et al., 2019). Classification frameworks have varied widely in scope, intent, focus, and utility.

Before the advent of modern science, classical philosophers attempted to classify suicides (Mueller et al., 2021). Durkheim (1897) proposed a framework for analyzing suicide by investigating its causes in connection with imbalances within societal and cultural structures where individuals exist (Mueller et al., 2021). Durkheim argued that suicide is related to the level of social cohesion and moral regulation present in society. He identified four types of suicide, each associated with different levels of social integration and regulation:

- Egoistic suicide: Occurs when social integration is low; individuals may feel isolated or disconnected from their community (Mueller et al., 2021).

- Altruistic suicide: Develops when social integration is high; individuals may prioritize group interests over personal ones, potentially leading to self-sacrifice (Mueller et al., 2021).
- Anomic suicide: Associated with weak or unstable social norms; individuals can experience uncertainty in periods of significant societal change or loss of established norms, such as during divorce or job loss (Giner et al., 2016; Mueller et al., 2021).
- Fatalistic suicide: Linked to excessive regulation; individuals may perceive oppression or lack of autonomy due to strict rules and expectations (Giner et al., 2016; Mueller et al., 2021).

Other classifications that may be affected by societal and cultural factors, such as religion, are referred to as culturally sanctioned suicide and encompass the following:

- Ceremonial suicide: Referred to as "seppuku" or "hara-kiri" in Japan, is a ritualized act of self-killing, typically performed to uphold or regain honor in the face of disgrace, failure, or impending defeat (Pierre, 2015).
- Euthanasia: Suicide in the context of a terminal illness is increasingly accepted to preserve autonomy and dignity in the West (Pierre, 2015).
- Terrorist martyrdom: Suicide as an act of murder and terrorism is a practice currently popular with Islamic militants who regard it as martyrdom in the context of war (Pierre, 2015).
- Cultural suicide: Motivated by honor, duty, or tradition (e.g., ritual suicide) (Giner et al., 2016).
- Mass suicide: Group-based, often ideological or religious (e.g., cults) (Giner et al., 2016).
- Heroic suicide: Seen as noble sacrifice (e.g., wartime acts) (Giner et al., 2016).

Early comprehensive systems aimed to categorize the range of suicidal behavior and its precursors. Devries (1968) introduced a hierarchical scheme that includes normal behavior, emotional disturbance, suicidal ideation, threatened suicide, attempted suicide, and completed suicide, with the intention of classifying based on risk and observable behaviors. Cohen (1969) introduced a dual-process model dividing "suicidation" (the mental process) and "suicidaction" (the behavioral process), alongside "self-assault" representing physical harm. Ellis (1988) incorporated multiple dimensions—including method, lethality, communication, and motivational context—underscoring the complexity of suicide-related behaviors.

Beck et al. (1973) made a pivotal contribution by offering operational definitions: (a) completed suicide was defined as a fatal act of self-injury with intent to die; (b) suicide attempts were nonfatal acts with the same intent; and (c) suicidal ideation encompassed thoughts related to engaging in such behaviors. O'Carroll et al. (1996) expanded on this by introducing "instrumental suicide-related behaviors" such as suicide threats or accidental death under conditions of suicidal intent. These frameworks emphasize observable behaviors as a crucial correlation of intent, bridging conceptual gaps between ideation and action.

Restricted systems, while narrower in scope, offer valuable behavioral stratification. Litman (1968) proposed degrees of suicide based on intentionality, emphasizing the spectrum from impulsivity to sustained planning. Rosenberg et al. (1988) focused on standardizing forensic criteria for determining suicide causes, aiding medical examiners in classification tasks. Lester (1990) concentrated on differentiating self-harm behaviors, specifically in the absence of clear suicidal intent, a precursor to the present conceptualizations of NSSIB.

Several classifications have introduced novel behavior types that supplemented existing types. Barber et al. (1998) advanced the term "aborted suicide attempt" to describe individuals who halted their own suicidal action before harm occurred—a behavior later incorporated into the Columbia-Suicide Severity Rating Scale (C-SSRS) (Posner et al., 2011).

A comprehensive understanding of suicidal and self-harming behaviors necessitates an integrated framework encompassing cognitive, behavioral, and contextual factors (Beck et al., 1979, 1985; Giner et al., 2016; Goodfellow et al., 2019; Steer et al., 1993). Suicidal behaviors may be classified into interrelated domains, each offering awareness and understanding of the diverse presentations and risk profiles observed in both clinical and research contexts. Classification of suicidal and self-harming behaviors can also be informed by topographical descriptions, including distinctions between covert and overt dimensions of these behaviors.

At the cognitive and motivational level, individuals may encounter various private psychological and emotional states characterized by suicidal ideation. Such ideation can manifest passively or actively, with deliberate intention and preparation (Beck et al., 1979; Giner et al., 2016). Hopelessness often appears as a significant cognitive indicator, associated with elevated suicide risk and frequently preceding more explicit actions (Beck et al., 1985; Steer et al., 1993). The typologies proposed below are derived from hypothesized internal states and motivations (Giner et al., 2016), including the following:

- Depressive suicide: arising from profound sadness, feelings of guilt, or hopelessness
- Impulsive suicide: occurring amid acute emotional crises and lacking prior planning
- Psychotic suicide: precipitated by hallucinations or delusions associated with severe mental illness
- Escape suicide: an effort to end intolerable psychological or physical pain (e.g., "psychache")
- Existential suicide: resulting from a perceived absence of meaning or purpose in life

Suicide-related behaviors exist on a spectrum, encompassing varied degrees of intent, lethality, and covert motivational variables. Behavioral and preparatory acts represent observable manifestations of suicidal risk. These behaviors span from acquiring the means to attempt suicide or writing farewell notes, to rehearsing the act itself. In some instances, individuals may initiate an attempt but abort the process before harm occurs, or their attempts may be interrupted by external intervention (e.g., rescuers) (Goodfellow et al., 2019). Suicide attempts—nonfatal acts performed with the intention of dying—are distinguished from completed suicides, which result in death and for which a clear suicidal intent is confirmed (Beck et al., 1979; Giner et al., 2016; Goodfellow et al., 2019).

Operational and nomenclature-based classifications further organize these phenomena. Systematic reviews have identified categories including self-injurious behavior (which may occur with or without intent to die), non-suicidal self-injurious behavior (NSSIB, defined as intentional harm without suicidal intent), and suicide-related thoughts and behaviors (SRTBs), a broad category that includes ideation, planning, and attempts (Giner et al., 2016; Goodfellow et al., 2019). There is ongoing debate regarding the possible classification of suicide-related mental health concerns, such as suicidal ideation, as a distinct entity. The types of suicide classified using this classification system include the following:

- Interrupted and aborted attempts: Broadly defined as ambivalence in pursuing the behaviors that comprise suicidal attempts. Interrupted suicide attempts occur when an external condition—such as another person (i.e., "rescuer") or circumstance—halts the occurrence or completion of a suicidal act. Though physical harm is averted, psychological distress may intensify due to the uncompleted act and subsequent emotional repercussions. By contrast, aborted suicide attempts are self-interrupted (Barber et al., 1998); the individual willingly halts the process before harm occurs. This often reflects a dynamic balance between a desire to die and residual survival instincts or cognitive re-evaluation.
- Preparatory acts: Signals of imminent risk. Behavioral signals such as giving away possessions, drafting suicide notes, or securing lethal means represent preparatory acts toward suicide. While these acts do not result in immediate self-harm, they signal increased risk and typically accompany heightened ideation or planning. Identifying these behaviors allows clinicians to intervene preemptively, potentially averting future attempts.
- Actual attempts: Clear intent and consequences. An actual suicide attempt involves a deliberate act with intent to die. Suicide attempts can be categorized based on whether the act was interrupted by external factors or individuals, or if the method used was non-fatal in its lethality. Outcomes may range from survival without injury to severe medical consequences. The defining criterion is "non-zero intent"—a purposeful desire to die at the time of the act (Posner et al., 2014). Recognition and documentation of intent remain essential for risk stratification and tracking.
- Non-suicidal self-injury behavior (NSSIB): Refers to deliberate self-inflicted harm without suicidal intent, including self-mutilation (American Psychiatric Association, 2022b; Klonsky, 2007), and self-poisoning (Bachmann, 2018; Miller et al., 2013). Though not considered a suicide attempt, its presence is clinically relevant, as it often coexists with mood dysregulation and predicts future suicidal behavior. It is imperative to differentiate NSSIB from suicidal acts to avoid a co-mingling of NSSIB and actual attempts.

- Ambiguous and sub-intentional attempts: Some behaviors exhibit unclear or ambivalent intent. These sub-intentional acts may involve high-risk conduct without overt suicidal goals, driven by unconscious distress or passive death wishes. Their classification requires nuanced understanding and often depends on post-event interviews and analyses of the data obtained concerning the behaviors.

Tables 17.2 and 17.3 summarize the types of suicidal behaviors and self-harm behaviors that are presented in the literature.

Modern classification systems have prioritized standardization and practical utility. The Columbia Classification Algorithm of Suicide Assessment (C-CASA), developed by Posner et al. (2007) and widely utilized, provides standardized categories for suicidal behaviors: completed suicide, suicide attempt, preparatory acts, suicidal ideation, and non-suicidal self-injury (Posner et al., 2014). Similarly, Brenner et al. (2011) developed the Self-Directed Violence Classification System (SDVCS), which distinguishes suicidal self-directed violence, non-suicidal self-directed violence, and preparatory behaviors, improving surveillance in certain contexts. Psychometric research, notably by Beck et al. (1973, 1976) and Steer et al., (1993), highlights the dimensional nature of suicidal intent. Using instruments like the Scale for Suicide Ideation (SSI), researchers have identified constructs such as the desire for death, the degree of preparation for suicide, and the intensity of active suicidal desire. These constructs not only help distinguish between those who experience suicidal thoughts and those who act upon them but also guide clinicians in stratifying risk and tailoring intervention strategies (Beck et al., 1979; Steer et al., 1993). A summary of classification schemes is presented in Table 17.4

Table 17.2 Types and definitions of suicidal behaviors

Type of behavior	Definition	References
Suicidal ideation	Thoughts of ending one's life; may be passive (wish to die) or active (plan or intent)	C-SSRS (Posner et al., 2011), Campos et al. (2021), American Psychiatric Association (2022b)
Suicide attempt	Self-inflicted potentially injurious behavior with some intent to die. May or may not result in injury	Posner et al. (2011), Lara et al. (2015), American Psychiatric Association (2022b)
Completed suicide	Death caused by self-directed injurious behavior with intent to die	NIMH (2025b), Silverman et al. (2007), American Psychiatric Association (2022b)
Interrupted suicide attempt	Attempt interrupted by an external force before harm occurs	Posner et al. (2011), Goodfellow et al. (2019)
Self-aborted attempt	A person stops themselves before harm occurs	Forte et al. (2025), Posner et al. (2011)
Preparatory behavior	Actions taken toward suicide (e.g., collecting pills and writing notes) without actual attempt	C-SSRS; Beck et al. (1976), Silverman et al. (2007)
Instrumental behavior	Suicide-related behavior without direct intent to die (e.g., gestures)	O'Carroll et al. (1996), Goodfellow et al. (2019)

Table 17.3 Types and definitions of self-harm behaviors

Type of self-harm	Definition	References
Non-suicidal self-injury behavior (NSSIB)	Direct bodily harm without intent to die; used to regulate affect or express distress	Klonsky (2007), Fliege et al. (2009), Goodfellow et al. (2019)
Deliberate self-harm (DSH)	Broad term encompassing NSSIB and suicide attempts, sometimes without clear differentiation	Fliege et al. (2009), Silverman and De Leo (2016)
Self-mutilation (burning and cutting	Severe physical harm to the body often associated with psychiatric conditions by using sharp objects or applying heat to skin	Klonsky (2007), American Psychiatric Association (2022b)
Biting	Self-inflicted bites, often on hands or arms	Fliege et al. (2009)
Hitting/punching	Striking oneself or objects to cause pain or injury	Fliege et al. (2009), NAMI (2025)
Hair-pulling	Pulling out hair from scalp or body (can overlap with trichotillomania)	Lorentzen et al. (2022)
Ingesting substances (i.e., self-poisoning)	Consuming harmful items (e.g., bleach, detergent) with or without suicidal intent	Bachmann (2018), Miller et al. (2013)
Covert self-harm	Less visible behaviors like food restriction, over-exercising, or substance misuse	Brådvik (2018), Klonsky (2007), Oexle et al. (2018)

Table 17.4 Classification systems for type of suicidal behaviors

Classification system	Key categories	References
C-SSRS (Columbia scale)	Ideation severity, ideation intensity, behavior (actual/aborted/interrupted), and lethality	Posner et al. (2011)
SIS (suicidal intent scale)	Expected lethality, planning, precautions, final acts, and communication	Beck et al. (1976), Diaz et al. (2003)
RRRS (risk-rescue rating scale)	Combines lethality (method, outcome) and rescue potential (location, time to discovery, and help-seeking)	Jang et al. (2025)
Silverman's nomenclature	Ideation, plans, communication, preparatory behaviors, attempts, and completions	Silverman et al. (2007), Goodfellow et al. (2019)
SDVCS (self-directed violence classification system)	Suicidal behavior, non-suicidal self-injury, and preparatory acts	Brenner et al. (2011)
Diagnostic systems (DSM-5)	Suicide-related behaviors under mood, personality, and psychotic disorders	American Psychiatric Association (2022a)

Finally, contextual and risk modifiers play a crucial role in shaping the likelihood and expression of suicidal behavior. Hopelessness stands out as a robust predictor of eventual suicide, while presence of mental health problems such as depression, psychosis, and personality mental health conditions further elevate risk (Beck et al., 1985; Steer et al., 1993). The perception of burdensomeness and social disengagement are additional variables identified by Joiner (2005) (Espinosa-Salido et al., 2021). Social isolation, as described in classical sociological models, is associated with egoistic forms of suicide, and emotional dysregulation can amplify both ideation and impulsivity (Giner et al., 2016). By synthesizing these domains and appreciating their interdependence, mental health service providers can more accurately identify, assess, and intervene with individuals at risk for suicide, thus advancing both clinical care and research in this critical area.

What Are the Problematic Behaviors Associated with Self-Harm or Talk of Suicide?

Problems with self-harm or suicide may take a variety of forms. In some situations, a person may harm herself with a clear idea of ending her life. For example, shooting herself in a vital organ is very likely fatal. Some behaviors are dangerous but not lethal, such as taking 10–15 tablets for a fever. It is important to determine if the person had the intent to die or if it was an impulsive act. Sometimes it is hard to determine. Behaviors such as these are recognized as attempts at suicide which require the attention and oversight of a mental health service provider.

In other situations, the person may do harm to herself but there may be uncertainty about whether she wanted to end her life. For example, she may make shallow cuts on her wrists. This may draw a lot of blood but, in some cases, not be life threatening. Mental health professionals refer to some self-harmful acts as a "cry for help" rather than an attempt to commit suicide. For example, Susan harmed herself in several ways (such as making cuts on her wrists and forearms or twisting clothes tightly around her neck). Many hospital staff questioned whether she really was trying to commit suicide or, instead, wanted to make sure that other people would take care of her. People engaging in self-harming behaviors sometimes report that hurting themselves relieves the emotional distress they may be experiencing.

In many situations, mental health service professionals and caregivers may find it challenging to determine whether certain behaviors are indicative of self-harm, even when injury occurs. For instance, if an individual consumes excessive alcohol and engages in dangerous driving, it may be unclear whether this constitutes suicidal intent or mere recklessness. Similarly, when someone combines medications with alcohol, distinguishing between suicidal behavior and a misunderstanding of medical instructions can be difficult. This ambiguity can create significant confusion and stress for those involved in the individual's care.

In addition to acts of self-harm, problems with self-harm and suicide may also take the form of talking about it. Many people who attempt suicide will provide some form of warning or clue before doing something. This will often involve comments about it. Some comments may be very clear, such as "I'm going to kill myself." However, other statements such as "I wish I was dead," "I just wish the world would go away," "I hope I don't wake up tomorrow," may indicate that the person is thinking about self-harm or suicide but also may be ways of expressing frustration or anger. Some people who attempt suicide will not say anything before the attempt; if asked beforehand, the person may even deny it. While difficult to predict, mental health service professionals view all attempts and statements of suicide as serious; because of the seriousness of the suicidal and self-harm behaviors, mental health service professionals treat it accordingly.

The potential for self-harm or suicide can present significant stress for individuals providing support. It is often challenging to determine with certainty whether the person has a genuine intent to cause harm. Given the risks involved, it is not advisable to make assumptions. Furthermore, even if it appears unlikely that the individual intends to end their life, there remains a possibility of accidental fatality resulting from self-harming behavior. For example, the person may take an overdose of medication with the idea that another member of the family will soon get home and find her. If the relative doesn't get home on time, the situation can become much more dangerous. Therefore, any self-harmful act or talking about it represents potentially dangerous behavior which should not be ignored. Because of this, the advice of a mental health service professional should be sought.

Suicide is a significant concern among individuals who live with SMI. Research indicates that approximately 46% of individuals who die by suicide had a diagnosed mental health condition; however, this figure may underestimate true prevalence due to undiagnosed cases (Conner et al., 2013). Major depressive (MDD), bipolar (BD), and schizophrenia spectrum mental health problems are particularly associated with increased risks for suicidal behaviors. While dysthymia and anxiety-related problems exhibit comparatively lower relative risks, they nonetheless contribute to overall suicide risk. These findings underscore the association between SMI and heightened suicide vulnerability (Moitra et al., 2021).

Individuals diagnosed and living with BD are at risk of suicide. Even when "manic" and appearing energetic and enthusiastic, suicide may still be a concern. The moods of such people can suddenly change from enthusiasm to deep despair. The energy of a manic phase can persist as feelings of hopelessness and despair develop. This can enable a person to carry through on a plan for suicide which would be much less likely if the person was lethargic and depressed. This mental health problem is strongly associated with elevated suicide risk. Individuals with this condition face a 10–30 times greater risk of dying by suicide compared to the general population. Research suggests that up to 20% of people with this mental health problem may die by suicide, and 20–60% will attempt suicide at least once in their lifetime. This risk surpasses that of MDD, with an individual living with BD being twice as likely to die by suicide as those with a unipolar mental health problem (NIMH, 2025a).

Why Do Problems with Self-Harm and Talk of Suicide Happen?

Part of the Reason May Be Biological or Physical

- SMIs are thought to be strongly influenced by biochemical imbalances in the brain. In certain imbalances, there may be a deficit in the chemical (i.e., neurotransmitter); the result is that the person experiences very little pleasure or satisfaction. People who attempt suicide often report that they don't feel pleasure from situations that used to make them happy. They experience little or no little pleasure in doing daily tasks that give "purpose" to most people's lives. In other cases, there may be an excessive amount of the neurotransmitter (Mann et al., 1999; Mann, 2003). The effect of this imbalance in people may result in "command hallucinations" in which the person hears voices that tell them to do certain things. These may include commands to do something harmful to their welfare.
- Suicide attempts are often connected to alcohol abuse in a person who is periodically depressed. The effect of alcohol will often make feelings of depression worsen and inhibit the person's ability to think clearly and find more acceptable ways of resolving problems. Mixing alcohol with some medications can be hazardous, even if there is no intention of self-harm.
- Even if the person living with SMI doesn't have a history of depression, suicide may still be a concern. Suicide or self-harmful acts may be a danger in other forms of SMI, including in a person living with personality types of mental health problems. Occasionally, the medications that are required for treatment of the SMI may produce or worsen feelings of depression as a side effect. This can complicate the treatment of the person living with SMI.

Part of the Reason May Be Psychosocial

- Self-harm behavior may also occur in patients who are living with severe "characterological" conditions, or personality mental health problems in addition to other forms of SMIs. These conditions are referred to as "Borderline Personality Disorder" (BPD) in the DSM-5-TR (American Psychiatric Association, 2022d). Such individuals often desire to have other people show concern for them but feel that they cannot get it. In this way, self-harm can become a maladaptive way of ensuring that other people remain concerned about them. As stated previously, some people living with this type of mental health problem experience self-harming behaviors as resulting in some relief for the distressing emotions and private events that they are experiencing at the moment.
- Ironically, the possibility of suicide is sometimes more likely after a person living with SMI has begun to improve. In the example above, Susan would sud-

denly do something that was self-harming after several weeks of improvement. It was difficult for the staff to identify a situation that preceded the self-harming behaviors. As the person improves, there may be an increased awareness of difficult problems that lie ahead. Also, an increase in energy level, which may happen as the person improves with treatment, can intensify feelings of hopelessness. For instance, a young person living with a schizophrenia spectrum mental health problem and multiple hospitalizations may realize that goals like finishing school or getting a good job are now harder to achieve. Adjusting these goals can be discouraging, but this does not mean everyone with SMI cannot achieve them—though it is often more challenging.
- A person who is depressed and is complaining of helplessness or hopelessness may have faced many setbacks. Loss of a job, the breakup of a relationship, loneliness, not having enough money to pay the bills, and many other stressful situations will discourage almost anyone. People with SMI often face great stressors and challenges. For instance, Susan had never worked or lived independently before leaving the hospital; starting a new job and living alone made things harder for her to manage.

Recognizing the Warning Signs of Suicide

Clinicians have identified a variety of behaviors which may signal a possible suicide attempt. While these may not apply in all cases, they represent relatively important indicators that there is an increased chance of the person living with a SMI may attempt suicide.

- Depression often includes persistent talk about hopelessness, helplessness, or worthlessness. A person living with SMI can become overwhelmed and lose all ability to rationally assess her situation. She may begin to believe that what she does is never enough and that it simply makes no difference. She may believe that there is nothing that she can do to change the situation. Even though other people point out positive aspects about her, she feels that there is little gratification or pleasure from her efforts.
- A history of previous attempts or a family history of suicide. If the person living with SMI had had thoughts of suicide or tried in the past, this is more likely to happen again. A higher frequency of attempts is associated with an increased likelihood that a person living with an SMI will make another attempt. Service providers should consider the way that past attempts were made. For example, it is more difficult to overdose on medication or drugs than to commit suicide with a gun. If previous attempts have involved methods with high potential for harm, future attempts may present a significant risk. Additionally, non-lethal methods could potentially lead to the use of more dangerous means in subsequent incidents. It is also relevant to assess whether any other family members have a history of such attempts and the availability of lethal means.

- A sudden improvement in the mood of a person who recently has talked about suicide when depressed. Clinicians report that a person who has struggled with suicidal thoughts will sometimes appear more composed and energetic when he has decided to end his life. To other people, it will often appear that he has improved and is getting better. If the person has swings of mood between periods of depression and euphoria and high energy, the transition from depression to increased energy can be a critical time. In people living with schizophrenia spectrum mental health problems, the danger is greater for young people who are becoming aware of the problems of living with SMI. The person who is more aware of the problems associated with living with a SMI may be more likely to feel hopeless about the future yet still have the energy and motivation to take his own life.
- Visiting old friends and setting affairs in order. A person who has decided to end her life will sometimes make attempts to set her affairs in order by visiting friends that she hasn't seen in a while. Such a person may check her will or give away items that she believes other people would like to have. If the person has a pet, she may make arrangements for the care of the pet.
- Circumstances where the person living with an SMI has little or no support system. An adult person living with an SMI can be in a living arrangement with very little access to supportive people. For example, the lack of appropriate housing means that she may live in an adult home or rooming house that is in a different town from her family and friends. She may be unemployed and unmarried. She may not have developed a trusting relationship with people from the community mental health center. Family members may live far away and have little time to visit. When the person has a history of self-harm or suicide attempts and has little support, the situation is dangerous for a repeat of past attempts as social isolation and loneliness contribute to risk of suicide (Espinosa-Salido et al., 2021; Joiner, 2005).
- Abuse of alcohol or other drugs. The use of mood-altering drugs such as alcohol will usually make problems worse. Alcohol, for example, can make depression more serious. Individuals experiencing depression may sometimes engage in alcohol and antidepressant medication overdose. This combination poses health risks and is considered hazardous. In addition, someone who is using drugs will experience more difficulty in reasoning and thinking out the consequences of her actions. Such a person will be more likely to go ahead and do something that may cause self-harm when her judgment is impeded by the effects of the drugs that are used.

Although these indicators do not necessarily mean a suicide attempt will occur, they suggest that closer attention may be needed. In such cases, it is recommended to consult a mental health service professional promptly.

Behavioral Support Strategies for Individuals Living with Serious Mental Illness Who Express Self-Harm or Suicidal Thoughts

- Clearly articulate the observed behaviors that indicate concerns regarding self-harm or suicide. There are many different behaviors that may cause concern about the possibility of self-harm or suicide by the person living with SMI. Service providers may sometimes conflate the terms "self-harm" and "suicidal," which can add complexity to the accuracy of an assessment of the suicidal behaviors. It is important to accurately distinguish between these behaviors when assessing concerns regarding the individual living with SMI. Clearly identifying specific statements or actions—both current and historical—that raise concern enables the development of an effective intervention plan. When consulting with a mental health service professional, these behaviors need to be clearly specified prior to assisting in collaborative planning.
- Seek professional assistance. Talk of self-harm or suicide is serious and the situation should be evaluated by a mental health service professional. In some cases, it will be necessary to commit the person to a hospital against their will. If this seems to be even a remote possibility, consider consulting a mental health service professional who is authorized to make such a commitment in the legal jurisdiction. This will usually be a licensed clinical psychologist or a psychiatrist. In some jurisdictions, only a psychiatrist can perform such a commitment (see Chap. 19, Hospitalization, Involuntary Commitment, and Guardianships).
- It is important to carefully manage medications for individuals living with SMI, as these prescriptions often exert significant physiological effects. Although individuals are generally encouraged to manage their medication regimen independently, exceptions may be necessary if there is an increased risk of suicide. Certain medications can be life-threatening if overdosed or combined with alcohol. Consultation with the person's prescribing psychiatric service provider is advised to determine whether temporary assistance in administering medications is appropriate until the suicide risk has subsided.
- Directly inquire about suicidal thoughts and plans. Do not avoid the topic; if there is reason to think someone living with SMI may be considering suicide, it is important to ask clearly whether they are having such thoughts and whether they have considered specific means. If there is evidence of suicidal thoughts or planning, seek a professional evaluation promptly. It is recommended not to leave the person alone or allow them to go independently until further assessment of safety has been made.
- Convey to individuals living with SMI that their safety and well-being are valued. Individuals experiencing suicidal thoughts may believe that others would not be affected by their death. It should not be assumed that they are aware of the concern for their welfare. In the example of Susan above, this was especially difficult for the hospital staff to do. They were not only angry with her for her acts of self-harm, but they were also fearful that someday she might kill herself; the

staff avoided her as they were concerned about doing or saying something that would result in self-harm or a suicide attempt. Their fear and anger motivated them to avoid her whenever they could. Take the opportunity to communicate to the individual that she is important and valued. Provide specific examples highlighting how her contributions are appreciated and demonstrate her worth to others.

- Clarify what the person living with SMI is doing if he is losing control and make a "safety plan." If the person has talked of suicide or has attempted suicide, consider establishing a contract with him to not engage in any behavior that is intentionally harmful to self. This contract should specify what he should do (such as call the suicide hot line or call a friend) if he feels that he is losing control. The contract can incorporate a written "Safety Plan." The safety plan usually is completed by a mental health service professional and the individual living with SMI. The "Safety Plan" identifies any factors that precede thoughts of suicide and establish alternative behaviors that the individual can do to avoid or lessen the impact of the preceding factors. The "Safety Plan" outlines specific actions to take when suicidal thoughts become more severe. It provides step-by-step guidance on strategies the individual can use to manage these thoughts and reduce the risk of suicide attempts (see Appendix I for steps and a form in developing a Safety Plan (Stanley & Brown, 2012)). Assistance from a mental health service professional may be needed to develop the safety plan and the contract. The safety plan needs to be done with the engagement and cooperation of the person living with SMI. Complement the person living with SMI for following through and cooperating. Using the example of Susan above, the hospital staff made an agreement with her to come to them if she felt that she was about to lose control and hurt herself. When she did this, they were willing to either sit with her and help her calm herself or let her stay alone in an area where they could frequently check on her. They made sure to compliment her when she followed through on this agreement.
- If possible, discuss the feelings associated with talk of self-harm or suicide. When suicide is not considered an imminent risk, it may be helpful to inquire about the feelings that seem to be expressed when talking of self-harm. Discussing feelings, such as anger or discouragement, is more productive than asking why the person would want to harm himself. The ability to discuss these feelings may require considerable skill and may require the assistance of a mental health service professional to do it well.
- Watch for circumstances which provoke the problem. Try to be aware of the circumstances in which the person living with SMI makes such statements. Watch for any variation that may be due to the situation, mood, or any other factors which might be noticed. For example, the person may become more discouraged and be more likely to think about self-harm when other people talk about their careers or have access to family. This information might be very important in developing ways to manage the problem.
- Do not overlook other desired behaviors that the person living with SMI is doing already. Be careful not to focus attention and concern just on the comments of

possible self-harm. Watch for periods when the person is in a calm and stable mood or when the person living with SMI engages in activities that she performs well. Remember to show interest or provide compliments at such times. For Susan, the inclination of the hospital caregivers was to stay away from her if possible. As we noted earlier, hospital staff had to remind themselves to pay attention to what Susan did well and compliment her during those times.

- Minimize access to lethal objects. Think about the possible ways that the person living with SMI might hurt herself. Access to items that are potentially lethal (such as knives, guns, certain medications, and poisons) should be controlled. Many objects may pose greater risks than initially apparent. While it may not be possible to eliminate every potential hazard, it is imperative to address and remove any dangers that can be identified. It may be helpful to have an experienced mental health service provider assist with making the living environment as "self-harm proof" as possible. The mental health service professional can provide a review of items to avoid having in the person's living situation or if needed to make sure that access to these items is secured.
- It is essential to establish a comprehensive plan with an individual who may pose a risk of self-harm. If the person who lives with SMI has a history of self-injurious behavior or suicide attempts, it is critical to prepare strategies to address any potential recurrence. Engage with mental health service professionals to identify and clarify possible warning signs, and proactively determine appropriate actions, such as obtaining an order for commitment if necessary. Service providers and caregivers often face uncertainty regarding the correct steps to take in crisis situations; developing a thorough safety plan can provide guidance. Although there are no simple solutions, seeking expert advice can help mitigate uncertainty and enhance preparedness.

Conclusion for Behavioral Support Strategies for Individuals Living with Serious Mental Illness Who Express Self-Harm or Suicidal Thoughts

If the person living with SMI has deliberately hurt himself or talked about suicide in the past, consider the following points. While not all of these will apply in all cases, it is likely that several of these can be helpful.

1. Take any mention of suicide seriously and consult with a mental health service professional for guidance. This is a critical issue that should not be managed alone.
2. Limit access to potentially harmful items or substances within the residence, ensuring that weapons or dangerous objects are not readily available.
3. Prepare a plan of action in case a serious suicide attempt occurs. Keep emergency contact numbers accessible for quick communication with medical professionals or emergency services.

4. If the individual living with SMI expresses thoughts of suicide, address the topic directly. Encourage him to commit to his safety and seek professional support. Implement any existing "Safety Plan" as appropriate.
5. Monitor factors that may influence the individual's well-being, such as mood changes, time of year, time of day, or interactions with specific people. These elements may help inform effective responses to emerging issues.
6. Acknowledge periods of stability and positive behavior. Engage with the person during times when self-harm or suicidal behaviors are not present and provide positive reinforcement for improvements.

What About Susan?

At the hospital, a psychologist was requested to consult on Susan's situation and try to develop a plan that would improve the situation. The consultant recognized the fear and frustration that the hospital staff felt toward her. Because of her unpredictable behavior, and because she often attributed her self-injurious acts to the fact that the staff did not care about her; the staff tried to avoid interacting with her as much as possible for concern that the interaction might "trigger" self-harm behaviors or a suicide attempt. They felt that it was safer not only for Susan but also for them to keep away from her, place her in restraints when she did any self-harm and allow her little opportunity to hurt herself. Ironically, their detachment from her seemed to result in more complaints about them by Susan and in more efforts by Susan to severely hurt herself. It seemed that the staff were trying as hard as they could to ignore her and that she was trying as hard as she could not to allow them to ignore her.

The hospital staff became tired of trying to keep track of her to make sure that she wouldn't hurt herself. Some wanted to put her into mechanical restraints and keep her there "round the clock." She developed a reputation as being a "manipulator" who knew how to get staff to do what she wanted them to do.

The consultant worked with them to emphasize several points. First, he tried to help them recognize that Susan seemed to value having them show concern for her. Even when she was hurting herself and saying that she was trying to kill herself, she did it in a way that she made sure that the staff were very aware that she was doing self-harm behaviors. He also tried to help them recognize that, despite her serious behavioral problems, there were long periods of time that she was being in control and was doing well. However, because of her severe problematic behaviors and the fact that she often blamed the staff for her problems, they stayed away from her as much as they could. When the problems started, they would be forced to interact with her. This often began with attempts to reason with her and typically resulted in an argument, with Susan yelling and blaming the staff for a variety of problems. She would threaten to lose control and "kill myself." This would continue until she was placed in mechanical restraints.

The plan that the staff and Susan developed collaboratively had several important points. The psychologist educated the staff about the personality problems that

Susan was displaying. He pointed out that the behavior of "ignoring her" was the condition for the self-harm behaviors to occur as Susan would get attention of staff one way or the other; it was pointed out to give her attention when she was in control and not displaying the self-harm behaviors. Because there were long periods of time when Susan wasn't a problem and she seemed to care about how concerned the staff was about her, they agreed to try to spend time with Susan at those times. They would begin by just saying hello and making a comment of interest about what Susan was doing. If Susan responded well to the interaction, the staff would try to keep the interaction going if Susan seemed interested. If Susan didn't seem interested, they simply went on with their duties. When Susan began hurting herself, they would not reason or cajole her to stop; the staff applied the restraints quickly and with as little conversation as possible, even with each other. When Susan calmed down, she was quickly released. Therefore, there were several times when she was put in restraints for only 5 minutes. After she was released, the staff again watched for acceptable behavior and tried to spend more time with her then. As increasing amounts of time passed without a severe incident, they made plans with her to do activities which she identified as desirable, such as trips to a local shopping mall or going to a specific fast-food restaurant. She also received a variety of smaller items that she wanted for doing her daily self-care behaviors without problem. There were other plans directed toward other behaviors, but this was the plan which was primarily directed toward her self-injurious behavior and threats of suicide.

While this plan was difficult for the staff to carry out consistently; they succeeded over the next several months in helping Susan stop talking about suicide or hurting herself. Within a year, she was discharged to a supervised home placement.

In this example, the staff took several steps to reduce Susan's talk and acts of self-harm.

1. Using observational data and graphs, the consultant helped them to recognize that there were long periods of time when Susan wasn't a problem.
2. The consultant assisted them in understanding that their responses to Susan—such as avoiding her when no issues were present or engaging in arguments and then physically intervening during more serious incidents—impacted the situation. Furthermore, it became evident that Susan was attentive to whether they demonstrated genuine care and concern for her.
3. They made a conscious effort to spend time with her when she was doing well (or at least not talking about hurting herself or some other serious problem behavior). They tried to respond as she responded. If she seemed interested, they tried to spend more time with her. If she seemed uninterested, they politely moved on.
4. They decided to ignore much less serious problem behaviors. These included several problems that had aggravated them and which they had angrily responded to in the past.
5. The staff also started to respond to threats and acts of self-injury rapidly and with a minimum of arguing and other demands. They also sought to release her as soon as she displayed calm behaviors that were well defined.

6. As she had longer periods of time without threats or acts of self-injury, they planned with her to do things that she enjoyed.
7. The staff also used the consultant to examine how their frustration with Susan and their fear that she would eventually succeed in killing herself affected their own behavior.

When it came time for discharge, many of these staff were able to work with the foster family to help them predict problems that they might encounter and how to respond to those problems. In the way, the foster family continued to carry out many of the plans that were developed by the hospital caregivers.

Summary

Suicidal self-harming behaviors are complex phenomena with significant public health implications, requiring urgent attention and intervention. Suicide is a major public health issue, with approximately 800,000 to 1 million deaths annually. Global suicide rates range from 10.7 to 11.4 per 100,000 individuals. In the United States, over 49,400 suicide deaths were reported in 2022, with a rate of 14.2 per 100,000. Males account for nearly 80% of suicide deaths in the United States, with the highest rates among American Indian/Alaska Native males.

Numerous risk factors contribute to suicidal behaviors. Mental health conditions, including major depressive and borderline personality mental health problems, are significantly associated with an increased risk of suicide. Substance use, particularly involving alcohol and opioids, further elevates this risk. Demographic factors such as male gender, adolescence, exposure to trauma, and social isolation present heightened vulnerabilities. Additionally, discrimination toward marginalized populations is recognized as a factor that increases the risk of suicide.

Suicidal ideation refers to thoughts or plans concerning suicide and is frequently associated with perceptions of burdensomeness and experiences of social isolation. Suicidal ideation is categorized as passive (wishing to be dead) or active (planning suicide). Non-suicidal self-injurious behavior (NSSIB) describes deliberate self-harm without suicidal intent, typically utilized as a coping strategy for emotional distress. NSSIB has been identified as a predictor of increased future suicide risk, underscoring the importance of clinical intervention.

Establishing consistent definitions and classifications of suicidal behaviors is critical for developing effective prevention and treatment strategies. The availability of lethal means, particularly firearms, plays a substantial role in influencing suicide rates. Furthermore, a comprehensive understanding of the underlying functions of self-harm can guide the development of targeted interventions aimed at reducing morbidity and mortality associated with self-directed violence.

Mental health problems are closely associated with an elevated risk of suicide, and multiple factors contribute to suicidal behaviors across various populations. Approximately 46% of individuals who died by suicide had a diagnosed mental health condition. Major depressive mental health problems are linked to a 17-fold increase in suicide risk compared to rates adjusted for age and sex. The lifetime suicide mortality rate among individuals with bipolar mental health problems ranges from 5% to 6%. Schizophrenia spectrum mental health problems are also correlated with persistent suicide risk, particularly during the early stages of the illness and shortly after discharge following a psychiatric inpatient admission.

Co-occurring conditions are associated with an elevated risk of suicide. Individuals presenting with six or more concurrent mental health problems exhibit a 29-fold increase in the likelihood of suicide attempts. The presence of co-occurring physical conditions, such as chronic pain or cancer, also substantially increases suicide risk. Moreover, mental health problems involving substance use—especially those related to alcohol and opioids—further intensify the propensity for suicidal behaviors.

Demographic, contextual, environmental, and behavioral factors contribute to suicide risk. Males have a suicide mortality rate nearly four times higher than females. Suicide is the leading cause of death among those aged 10–34 years. Impulsivity and aggression are significant predictors of suicide attempts, independent of mental health status. Adverse childhood experiences and stigma of living with SMI are associated with elevated rates of suicidal behaviors. Access to lethal means, such as firearms, remains a critical consideration in prevention efforts. Social stressors, including unemployment and poverty, further increase suicide risk across diverse population subgroups.

Hopelessness is a robust predictor of suicide risk. Mental health issues, social disengagement, and burdensomeness elevate risk levels. Emotional dysregulation can amplify suicidal ideation and impulsivity.

Prevention and intervention strategies should incorporate integrated risk models that account for the severity of mental health conditions, psychosocial factors, and individual characteristics. Routine assessment for previous suicide attempts and suicidal ideation is critical to effective prevention efforts. Culturally competent interventions are also necessary for high-risk populations, particularly individuals with co-occurring conditions.

Non-suicidal self-injury behaviors (NSSIB) are characterized by intentional self-harm without suicidal intent, including actions such as cutting or burning. These behaviors are commonly associated with the regulation of acute emotional distress and are considered maladaptive coping mechanisms. NSSIB is particularly prevalent among youth with mood or personality-related mental health problems, and demonstrates a complex association with both mental health challenges and an elevated risk of suicidal behaviors.

Lethality denotes the likelihood that a particular method will result in death. Methods with high lethality, such as firearms or hanging, are frequently employed in both premeditated and impulsive suicide attempts. Notably, 81% of overdose incidents and 71% of cutting cases involved a transition to higher lethality methods prior to death.

Individuals experiencing multiple mental health problems are at a markedly elevated risk of recurrent non-suicidal self-injurious behavior (NSSIB). The presence of specific mental health problems such as personality, bipolar, and substance-related conditions further exacerbates the likelihood of self-harm. The relationship between method selection and mental health comorbidities is multifaceted and necessitates comprehensive clinical evaluation.

Suicidal behaviors present significant challenges across diverse population groups, particularly among individuals living with SMI. Contributing factors include co-occurring mental health and medical conditions, biological vulnerabilities, trauma, and sociodemographic stressors, all of which may elevate risk. It is imperative that mental health systems prioritize the use of precise terminology, conduct comprehensive assessments, and implement tailored interventions to effectively address individual needs.

Suicide and self-harming behaviors are intricate, multidimensional phenomena that underscore the necessity of dimensional frameworks for effective assessment and intervention within mental healthcare. Contemporary approaches to understanding suicidal behavior employ dimensional models to evaluate both overt and covert actions. Dimensional metrics include the frequency, duration, intensity, and context of suicidal behaviors. The Columbia Suicide Severity Rating Scale (C-SSRS) is a prominent assessment instrument that measures the severity of ideation, behavioral intent, and potential lethality. Inconsistent terminology in suicide research impedes data integration and clinical application. Suicidal ideation is classified as either passive (expressing a wish to be dead) or active (formulating plans for suicide). Precise definitions of behaviors are essential to distinguish between attempts, aborted efforts, and preparatory acts.

Suicidal and self-harming behaviors are complex, multidimensional, and influenced by various psychological and social factors. Multidimensionality indicates that behaviors cannot be explained by a single trait or attribute. Multidirectionality reflects the capacity for behaviors to change in complex ways. Studies show that ideation, attempts, and lethality are not always correlated, indicating variability in risk factors.

Suicidal and self-harming behaviors are complex, multifaceted phenomena shaped by various psychological and social determinants. Their multidimensional nature indicates that these behaviors cannot be ascribed to a single trait or factor. Moreover, their multidirectionality underscores the potential for diverse and intricate progressions; for example, an interrupted suicide attempt may lead to increased perceived community support, thereby reducing subsequent risk. Empirical studies demonstrate that suicidal ideation, attempts, and lethality do not always align, reflecting notable variability among risk factors.

These behaviors comprise both covert (internal cognitive and emotional processes) and overt (observable actions) dimensions, necessitating thorough assessment. Covert components include suicidal thoughts, planning, and emotional distress, while overt elements encompass actual attempts and preparatory behaviors. Comprehensive evaluation requires the integration of self-reports and observational data. Additionally, these dimensions can be further classified according to frequency, duration, intensity, and contextual variables.

Multiple factors contribute to the risk of suicidal behaviors, encompassing psychological, social, and environmental dimensions. Suicidal ideation encompasses both passive and active thoughts related to wishing for death. Emotional distress, termed "psychache," serves as a significant indicator of suicide risk. Additionally, cognitive impairments and negative symptoms are associated with heightened suicidal ideation. Conversely, coping strategies, social connectedness, and positive self-concept function as protective factors.

Numerous validated assessment instruments are available to evaluate specific aspects of suicidality. Tools such as the Columbia-Suicide Severity Rating Scale (C-SSRS) and the Beck Scale for Suicide Ideation (BSI) offer systematic approaches to assess suicidal ideation and intent. The Risk-Rescue Rating Scale (RRRS) focuses on evaluating medical lethality and contextual variables. A comprehensive evaluation should commence with a targeted psychosocial interview, supplemented by appropriate assessment measures. Employing multidimensional frameworks enhances predictive accuracy and supports the development of individualized treatment plans.

Suicide and self-harming behaviors arise from a complex interplay of neurobiological mechanisms, genetic predispositions, mental health conditions, and environmental factors. Suicide is a multifaceted issue, primarily associated with mental health problems, and demonstrates significant global prevalence with numerous contributing elements. Annually, approximately 1 million suicides and 10 million attempts are reported worldwide. In the United States, suicide ranks as the 11th leading cause of death, accounting for over 49,000 completed suicides in 2023. For every completed suicide, there are estimated 10–20 attempts, reflecting the high rate of suicidal behavior. More than 90% of individuals who die by suicide lived with SMI, with mood mental health problems responsible for about 60% of these cases. Suicidal behaviors are shaped by genetic, environmental, and neurobiological influences, consistent with the diathesis–stress model. Genetic factors account for 30–55% of the variability in suicidal thoughts and behaviors (STBs). Additionally, environmental stressors such as poverty, unemployment, and social isolation substantially elevate suicide risk.

Suicidal and self-harming behaviors are associated with distinct brain regions and neurotransmitter systems implicated in emotional regulation and decision-making processes. Key regions involved include the prefrontal cortex (PFC), cingulate cortex (CC), insular cortex (IC), striatal areas, and the default mode network (DMN). Dysfunction of the PFC has been correlated with compromised judgment and emotional dysregulation, thereby elevating suicide risk (Balcioglu & Kose, 2018). The CC often demonstrates abnormalities in emotion processing, especially among individuals experiencing mood-related mental health problems. The serotonergic system plays a pivotal role in mood regulation, as diminished serotonin activity is linked to increased suicidal ideation and attempts. Additionally, other neurotransmitter systems, such as dopaminergic and noradrenergic pathways, have also been shown to contribute to suicidal behavior.

Dysregulation of the hypothalamic–pituitary–adrenal (HPA) axis and inflammatory processes serve as key biological markers correlated with suicidality, reflecting the intricate interplay of physiological mechanisms. Research indicates that individuals with depression and a history of suicide attempts often exhibit reduced cortisol levels and irregular secretion patterns. Elevated inflammatory markers have also been noted among those displaying suicidal behaviors, underscoring the potential involvement of immune dysregulation in suicide risk. Additionally, genetic factors contribute to suicide risk, with heritability estimates ranging from 30% to 55% and certain genetic variants associated with serotonin transport and receptor function.

Environmental and psychological factors, in addition to biological influences, are critical determinants in the emergence of suicidal and self-harming behaviors among individuals with SMI. Elements such as the presence of supportive social networks, exposure to trauma, and experiences of discrimination substantially affect the risk of suicidal thoughts and behaviors (STBs). While genetic predispositions play a role in increasing vulnerability to self-harm and suicide, environmental variables are responsible for 45–70% of the observed variance in risk. Emotional states such as dysphoria and depression may act as conditioned stimuli, prompting individuals to engage in STBs as maladaptive coping strategies. Furthermore, social learning processes contribute to the development of STBs, as individuals may adopt behaviors modeled by others within their environment.

Dysphoric emotions and their regulation are closely linked to suicidal and self-harming behaviors, with these relationships being influenced by biological, environmental, and learning factors. Dysphoria may serve as a motivating operation that increases the probability of suicidal thoughts and behaviors (STBs), as individuals seek to alleviate emotional distress. Emotional reactions to perceived losses can result in increased sensitivity and avoidance behavior, thereby affecting decision-making processes. Mechanisms of associative learning, including both classical and operant conditioning, contribute to how individuals manage dysphoric states and influence the expression of STBs. The interaction among biological processes, individual perception, and learned responses form a complex behavioral sequence that impacts the emergence of suicidal and self-harming behaviors.

A systematic examination of the sequence of events preceding suicidal behavior facilitates the identification of risk factors and the development of targeted intervention strategies. Chain analysis enables the categorization of behaviors, the formulation of hypotheses regarding the functions of STBs, and the assessment of suicide risk based on individual circumstances. A comprehensive understanding of the dynamics underlying STBs supports the design of effective, individualized prevention and intervention measures.

Multiple complex factors contribute to suicidal behavior, underscoring the importance of targeted interventions. In the United States, suicide rates are reported at 14.2 per 100,000 individuals, with the prevalence of non-suicidal self-injurious behavior among adolescents ranging from 18% to 25%. Among individuals living with schizophrenia spectrum mental health problems, 5–6% die by suicide and 31% engage in self-injury. Regional variation is observed, with the highest suicide rates in western states such as Alaska and the lowest in New Jersey. Globally, approximately 800,000 individuals die by suicide each year, translating to a worldwide rate of 10.7 per 100,000.

Elevated suicide risk is associated with economically disadvantaged populations, with unemployment and lower educational attainment serving as significant risk factors. Economic instability and limited access to mental healthcare are significant contributors to suicide risk. Structural inequalities have resulted in disproportionately higher suicide rates among racial and ethnic minorities, veterans, and rural populations.

In low- and middle-income countries, the prevalence of suicidal ideation ranges from 3.1% to 12.4%, compared to 3–15.9% in high-income nations. Socioeconomic and cultural determinants significantly influence suicide rates internationally. Males comprise 80% of suicide deaths in the United States, with the highest rates observed among American and Alaskan Native males (39.5 per 100,000). Firearms are involved in 54–55% of suicides in the United States, with hanging and poisoning also being commonly employed methods. Higher rates are noted among young females in Anglo-Saxon countries, while older females exhibit greater risk in Latin regions. Cultural norms and stigmatization of living with SMI can impact both suicide rates and their reporting; religious participation has been linked to reduced suicide incidence. LGBTQ+ populations experience significantly higher rates of suicidal ideation, primarily due to discrimination and stigma.

Approximately 60–98% of completed suicides are associated with mental health conditions. Major depressive (MDD), bipolar (BD), and borderline personality (BPD) mental health problems are linked to particularly elevated risks. Individuals diagnosed with BPD report a 79% lifetime rate of suicide attempts, while those within the schizophrenia spectrum mental health problems experience completion rates of 5–6%. The prevalence of non-suicidal self-injurious behavior (NSSIB) among individuals living with schizophrenia spectrum mental health problems ranges from 14% to 57%, with cutting identified as the most common method. The presence of self-harming behaviors significantly increases the likelihood of future suicide attempts, especially in the context of co-occurring mental health problems.

Media reporting on suicides has been associated with subsequent increases in the occurrences of suicidal behaviors, while social isolation is also a recognized risk factor. Suicide remains the leading cause of death in jails in the United States, particularly during the initial 48 hours of incarceration. In the United States, suicide rates rose by 35% between 2000 and 2018, experienced a slight decrease in 2019–2020, and then increased again by 2022. Emergency department visits for suicidal ideation grew by 25.5% from 2017 to 2018, with a 62.3% increase observed among males aged 10–19 years.

Accurate classification systems play a critical role in the identification and management of mental health conditions. However, challenges persist, such as inconsistent terminology and the absence of universally accepted standards. The DSM-5-TR (American Psychiatric Association, 2022a) adopts a primarily descriptive approach, emphasizing the presence and severity of mental health problems.

Classical philosophers sought to systematically classify suicidal behaviors. Emile Durkheim, a nineteenth-century sociologist, analyzed and classified suicide within the context of societal structures, distinguishing four primary types: egoistic, altruistic, anomic, and fatalistic. Culturally sanctioned suicides may encompass ceremonial suicide, euthanasia, and terrorist martyrdom. Mass and heroic suicides often stem from ideological beliefs or considerations of honor. Initial classification systems ranged from normative suicidal thoughts to completed suicide. Beck et al. (1973, 1976) delineated completed suicide, attempted suicide, and suicidal ideation, focusing on observable indicators. The Columbia Classification Algorithm of Suicide Assessment (C-CASA) provides standardized categories for suicidal behavior, while the Self-Directed Violence Classification System (SDVCS) differentiates between suicidal and non-suicidal self-directed violence.

Self-harm and suicide risk, along with their underlying causes and warning signs, especially among individuals who live with SMI, necessitate timely mental health intervention. Self-harming behaviors can range from non-lethal acts to potentially fatal incidents, all of which require careful clinical oversight. The covert intent for the self-harm may not always be clear, as some actions serve as "cries for help" rather than direct expressions of suicidal ideation. For certain individuals, self-injury may function as a means of alleviating emotional distress. Distinguishing between reckless conduct and actual suicidal intent is often complex. Communication about suicidal thoughts frequently precedes attempts; thus, all expressions regarding suicide must be addressed with appropriate seriousness. Individuals living with SMI, particularly those with bipolar mental health problems, can experience an increased risk of suicide, especially during times of increased irritability, impulsiveness, agitation, and accelerated speed of thinking (e.g., mania)

Suicidal and self-harming behaviors arise from multiple contributing factors. Biological influences, such as neurotransmitter imbalances, can affect pleasure regulation and decision-making processes. Alcohol misuse may further aggravate depressive symptoms and impair judgment, thereby elevating the risk of suicide. Psychosocial elements include personality traits, underlying mental health conditions, and ineffective coping strategies. Notably, an improvement in mood can paradoxically heighten suicide risk as individuals may gain increased clarity regarding their challenges. Additionally, stressors such as unemployment or relationship difficulties can intensify feelings of hopelessness.

Behavior associated with suicidal ideation includes persistent feelings of hopelessness and worthlessness, which are commonly observed in individuals with depression. The history of previous suicide attempts is a strong predictor of future risk. Notably, a sudden improvement in mood among previously depressed individuals may indicate an increased risk for suicide. Individuals at risk may also demonstrate behaviors such as reconnecting with old acquaintances or organizing personal affairs. Social isolation and a lack of support systems further elevate suicide risk.

Effectively addressing self-harm and suicide concerns in individuals who live with SMI requires service providers to follow specific, evidence-based practices. It is essential to clearly define behaviors indicative of self-harm or suicidal ideation, and to differentiate between these behaviors for accurate assessment. Identifying statements or actions that may signal risk is critical for developing effective intervention strategies.

For indications of serious self-harm or suicidal intent, prompt evaluation by qualified mental health service professionals is recommended. In situations warranting it, involuntary hospitalization should be considered in consultation with authorized service providers. Medication management is crucial, as medication changes can significantly impact those with SMI; if suicide risk escalates, consultation with the prescribing service provider and temporary support with medication administration may be necessary.

Direct inquiry regarding suicidal thoughts and plans should not be avoided. If an individual confirms such thoughts, immediate professional evaluation is indicated. Emphasize the individual's safety and well-being, offering concrete examples of their value to others to help counteract feelings of isolation and burdensomeness.

Developing a safety plan or behavioral contract to prevent self-harming and suicidal behaviors is recommended. This plan should include alternative coping strategies and steps to take when suicidal ideation intensifies. When imminent risk is not present, inquire about the emotional context surrounding self-harm or suicidal thoughts—discussing feelings such as anger or discouragement may yield more insights than questioning motives. Remain aware of situational triggers and variations in mood that could influence self-harm risk. Recognize and reinforce positive behaviors and stable moods during non-crisis periods to encourage ongoing engagement.

To further reduce risk, restrict access to potentially lethal means and work with mental health service professionals to enhance environmental safety. A comprehensive care plan is essential for individuals with a history of self-harm or suicide attempts, including collaboration with mental health service professionals to proactively identify warning signs and outline appropriate interventions.

References

Albert, U., Pellegrini, L., Maina, G., & Aguglia, A. (2019). Suicide in obsessive-compulsive related disorders: Prevalence rates and psychopathological risk factors. *Journal of Psychopathology, 25*, 139–148. https://www.jpsychopathol.it/article/suicide-in-obsessive-compulsive-related-disorders-prevalence-rates-and-psychopathological-risk-factors/

American Psychiatric Association. (2013). *Diagnostic and statistical manual of mental disorders* (5th ed.).

American Psychiatric Association. (2022a). *Diagnostic and statistical manual of mental disorders* (5th ed., text rev.). https://doi.org/10.1176/appi.books.9780890425787

American Psychiatric Association. (2022b). Schizophrenia spectrum and other psychotic disorders. In *Diagnostic and statistical manual of mental disorders* (5th ed., text rev.). https://doi.org/10.1176/appi.books.9780890425787.x01

American Psychiatric Association. (2022c). Suicidal behavior and nonsuicidal self-injury. In *Diagnostic and statistical manual of mental disorders* (5th ed., text rev.). https://doi.org/10.1176/appi.books.9780890425787.x06

American Psychiatric Association. (2022d). Anxiety disorders. In *Diagnostic and statistical manual of mental disorders* (5th ed., text rev.). https://doi.org/10.1176/appi.books.9780890425787.x05

American Psychiatric Association. (2022e). Borderline personality disorder. In *Diagnostic and statistical manual of mental disorders* (5th ed., text rev.). https://doi.org/10.1176/appi.books.9780890425787.x06

American Psychological Association. (n.d.-a). Diathesis. In *APA Dictionary of Psychology*. https://dictionary.apa.org/diathesis

American Psychological Association. (n.d.-b). Diathesis-stress model. In *APA Dictionary of Psychology*. https://dictionary.apa.org/diathesis-stress-model

American Psychological Association. (n.d.-c). Lethality. In *APA Dictionary of Psychology*. https://dictionary.apa.org/lethality

American Psychological Association. (n.d.-d). Multidimensionality. In *APA Dictionary of Psychology*. https://dictionary.apa.org/multidimensionality.

American Psychological Association. (n.d.-e). Psychache. In *APA Dictionary of Psychology*. https://dictionary.apa.org/psychache

American Psychological Association. (n.d.-f). Self-criticism. In *APA Dictionary of Psychology*. https://dictionary.apa.org/self-criticism.

Bachmann, S. (2018). Epidemiology of suicide and the psychiatric perspective. *International Journal of Environmental Research and Public Health, 15*(7), 1425. https://doi.org/10.3390/ijerph15071425

Bakken, V., Lydersen, S., Skokauskas, N., Sund, A. M., & Kaasbøll, J. (2024). Protective factors for suicidal ideation: A prospective study from adolescence to adulthood. *European Child & Adolescent Psychiatry, 33*(9), 3079–3089. https://doi.org/10.1007/s00787-024-02379-w

Balcioglu, Y. H., & Kose, S. (2018). Neural substrates of suicide and suicidal behaviour: From a neuroimaging perspective. *Psychiatry and Clinical Psychopharmacology, 28*(3), 314–328. https://doi.org/10.1080/24750573.2017.1420378

Barber, M. E., Marzuk, P. M., Leon, A. C., & Portera, L. (1998). Aborted suicide attempts: A new classification of suicidal behavior. *American Journal of Psychiatry, 155*(3), 385–389. https://doi.org/10.1176/ajp.155.3.385

Basso, A. (2021). From measurement to classificatory practice: Improving psychiatric classification independently of the opposition between symptom-based and causal approaches. *European Journal for Philosophy of Science, 11*(4), 104. https://doi.org/10.1007/s13194-021-00424-y

Beck, A. T., Kovacs, M., & Weissman, A. (1973). Assessment of suicidal intention: The scale for suicide ideation. *Journal of Consulting and Clinical Psychology, 47*(2), 343–352. https://doi.org/10.1037/h0035567

Beck, A. T., Weissman, A., Lester, D., & Trexler, L. (1974). The measurement of pessimism: The Hopelessness Scale. *Journal of Consulting and Clinical Psychology, 42*(6), 861–865. https://doi.org/10.1037/h0037562

Beck, A. T., Weissman, A., Lester, D., & Trexler, L. (1976). Classification of suicidal behaviors: II. Dimensions of suicidal intent. *Archives of General Psychiatry, 33*(7), 835–837. https://doi.org/10.1001/archpsyc.1976.01770070065006

Beck, A. T., Kovacs, M., & Weissman, A. (1979). Assessment of suicidal intention: The Scale for Suicide Ideation. *Journal of Consulting and Clinical Psychology, 47*(2), 343–352. https://doi.org/10.1037/0022-006X.47.2.343

Beck, A. T., Steer, R. A., Kovacs, M., & Garrison, B. (1985). Hopelessness and eventual suicide: A 10-year prospective study of patients hospitalized with suicidal ideation. *American Journal of Psychiatry, 142*(5), 559–563. https://doi.org/10.1176/ajp.142.5.559

Borges, L. M., Nazem, S., Matarazzo, B. B., Barnes, S. M., & Wortzel, H. S. (2019). Therapeutic risk management: Chain analysis of suicidal ideation and behavior. *Journal of Psychiatric Practice, 25*(1), 46–53. https://doi.org/10.1097/PRA.0000000000000358

Brådvik, L. (2018). Suicide risk and mental disorders. *International Journal of Environmental Research and Public Health, 15*(9), 2028. https://doi.org/10.3390/ijerph15092028

Brain, K. L., Haines, J., & Williams, C. L. (1998). The psychophysiology of self-mutilation: Evidence of tension reduction. *Archives of Suicide Research, 4*, 227–242. https://doi.org/10.1023/A:1009630801238

Brenner, L. A., Breshears, R. E., & Betthauser, L. M. (2011). Implementation of a self-directed violence classification system for data collection and clinical care. *Suicide and Life-Threatening Behavior, 41*(3), 330–340. https://doi.org/10.1111/j.1943-278X.2011.00033.x

Brokke, S. S., Landrø, N. I., & Haaland, V. Ø. (2022). Impulsivity and aggression in suicide ideators and suicide attempters of high and low lethality. *BMC Psychiatry, 22*(1), 753. https://doi.org/10.1186/s12888-022-04398-w

Campos, R. C., Holden, R. R., Spínola, J., Marques, D., & Lambert, C. E. (2021). Dimensionality of suicide behaviors: Results within two samples from two different countries. *Omega - Journal of Death and Dying*. https://doi.org/10.1177/0030222819882849

Centers for Disease Control and Prevention (CDC). (2024a, April 25). *Risk and protective factors for suicide*. https://www.cdc.gov/suicide/risk-factors/index.html

Centers for Disease Control and Prevention (CDC). (2024b, December 20). *Suicide data and statistics*. U.S. Department of Health and Human Services. https://www.cdc.gov/suicide/facts/data.html

Centers for Disease Control and Prevention (CDC). (2025, January 30). *Health disparities in suicide*. https://www.cdc.gov/suicide/disparities/index.html

Chu, C., Buchman-Schmitt, J. M., Stanley, I. H., Hom, M. A., Tucker, R. P., Hagan, C. R., Rogers, M. L., Podlogar, M. C., Chiurliza, B., Ringer-Moberg, F. B., Michaels, M. S., Patros, C. H. G., & Joiner, T. E., Jr. (2017). The interpersonal theory of suicide: A systematic review and meta-analysis of a decade of cross-national research. *Psychological Bulletin, 143*(12), 1313–1345. https://doi.org/10.1037/bul0000123

Clarkson University. (2011, May 4). *Positive effects of depression*. ScienceDaily. https://www.sciencedaily.com/releases/2011/05/110504155113.htm

Cohen, M. (1969). *Suicide and attempted suicide: A study of causation and prevention*. Charles C. Thomas. https://doi.org/10.1037/10544-000

Conner, K. R., Bohnert, A. S., McCarthy, J. F., Valenstein, M., Bossarte, R., Ignacio, R., Lu, N., & Ilgen, M. A. (2013). Mental disorder comorbidity and suicide among 2.96 million men receiving care in the Veterans Health Administration health system. *Journal of Abnormal Psychology, 122*(1), 256–263. https://doi.org/10.1037/a0030163

Cooper, J. O., Heron, T. E., & Heward, W. L. (2020). *Applied behavior analysis* (3rd ed.). Pearson Education. https://psycnet.apa.org/record/2020-62773-000

Cornwell, E. Y., & Waite, L. J. (2009). Social disconnectedness, perceived isolation, and health among older adults. *Journal of Health and Social Behavior, 50*(1), 31–48. https://doi.org/10.1177/002214650905000103

De Leo, D., & Altin, M. (2025). Revisiting cultural issues in suicide rates: The case of western countries. *International Journal of Environmental Research and Public Health, 22*(4), 596. https://doi.org/10.3390/ijerph22040596

Devries, A. G. (1968). Prediction of suicide by means of psychological tests. In *Fourth international conference for suicide Prevention*. Delmar. https://doi.org/10.1037/e400352009-001

Diaz, F. J., Baca-Garcia, E., Diaz-Sastre, C., García Resa, E., Blasco, H., Braquehais Conesa, D., Pérez-Rodríguez, M. M., Saiz-Ruiz, J., & de Leon, J. (2003). Dimensions of suicidal behavior according to patient reports. *European Archives of Psychiatry and Clinical Neuroscience, 253*(4), 197–202. https://doi.org/10.1007/s00406-003-0436-0

DiBlasi, E., Kang, J., & Docherty, A. R. (2021). Genetic contributions to suicidal thoughts and behaviors. *Psychological Medicine, 51*(13), 2148–2155. https://doi.org/10.1017/S0033291721001720

Durkheim, É. (1897). *Le suicide: Étude de sociologie*. Félix Alcan. https://doi.org/10.1037/12275-000

Dygdon, J. A., & Dienes, K. A. (2013). Behavioral excesses in depression: A learning theory hypothesis. *Depression and Anxiety, 30*(6), 598–605. https://doi.org/10.1002/da.22111

Edgcomb, J. B., Shaddox, T., Hellemann, G., & Brooks, J. O., III. (2021). Predicting suicidal behavior and self-harm after general hospitalization of adults with serious mental illness. *Journal of Psychiatric Research, 136*, 515–521. https://doi.org/10.1016/j.jpsychires.2020.10.024

Ellis, T. E. (1988). Toward a multidimensional understanding of suicidal behavior. *Suicide and Life-Threatening Behavior, 18*(4), 396–406. https://doi.org/10.1111/j.1943-278X.1988.tb00169.x

Espinosa-Salido, P., Perez Nieto, M. A., Baca-García, E., & Provencio Ortega, M. (2021). Systematic review of the indirect relationships of thwarted belongingness and perceived burdensomeness in suicide. *Clínica y Salud, 32*(1), 29–36. https://doi.org/10.5093/clysa2020a27

Fliege, H., Lee, J. R., Grimm, A., & Klapp, B. F. (2009). Risk factors and correlates of deliberate self-harm behavior: A systematic review. *Journal of Psychosomatic Research, 66*(6), 477–493. https://doi.org/10.1016/j.jpsychores.2008.10.013

Forte, A., Orri, M., Golay, P., Armando, M., Costanza, A., Saillant, S., & Michaud, L. (2025). Comparison between aborted/interrupted and actual suicide attempt: An observational study on clinical and sociodemographic characteristics. *Journal of Affective Disorders, 378*, 373–380. https://doi.org/10.1016/j.jad.2024.12.080

Freeman, D., Bold, E., Chadwick, E., Taylor, K. M., Collett, N., Diamond, R., Černis, E., Bird, J. C., Isham, L., Forkert, A., Carr, L., Causier, C., & Waite, F. (2019). Suicidal ideation and behaviour in patients with persecutory delusions: Prevalence, symptom associations, and psychological correlates. *Comprehensive Psychiatry, 93*, 41–47. https://doi.org/10.1016/j.comppsych.2019.07.001

Friman, P. C., Hayes, S. C., & Wilson, K. G. (1998). Why behavior analysts should study emotion: The example of anxiety. *Journal of Applied Behavior Analysis, 31*(1), 137–156. https://doi.org/10.1901/jaba.1998.31-137

Fu, X. L., Qian, Y., Jin, X. H., Yu, H. R., Wu, H., Du, L., Chen, H. L., & Shi, Y. Q. (2023). Suicide rates among people with serious mental illness: A systematic review and meta-analysis. *Psychological Medicine, 53*(2), 351–361. https://doi.org/10.1017/S0033291721001549

Ghasemi, P., Shaghaghi, A., & Allahverdipour, H. (2015). Measurement scales of suicidal ideation and attitudes: A systematic review article. *Health Promotion Perspectives, 5*(3), 156–168. https://doi.org/10.15171/hpp.2015.019

Giner, L., Guija, J. A., Root, C. W., & Baca-Garcia, E. (2016). Nomenclature and definition of suicidal behavior. In P. Courtet (Ed.), *Understanding suicide: From diagnosis to personalized treatment* (pp. 3–17). Springer. https://doi.org/10.1007/978-3-319-26282-6_1

Goldiamond, I. (2022). *A programing contingency analysis of mental health.* Routledge. https://doi.org/10.4324/9781003260103

Goldsmith, S. K., Pellmar, T. C., Kleinman, A. M., & Bunney, W. E. (Eds.). (2002). *Reducing suicide: A national imperative.* National Academies Press. https://doi.org/10.17226/10398.

Gomez, S. H., Overholser, J., McGovern, C., Silva, C., & Stockmeier, C. A. (2023). The role of premeditation in suicide: Identifying factors associated with increased planning among suicide decedents. *Journal of Clinical Psychology, 79*(12), 2768–2780. https://doi.org/10.1002/jclp.23577

Goodfellow, B., Kolves, K., & De Leo, D. (2019). Contemporary nomenclatures of suicidal behaviors: A systematic literature review. *Suicide and Life-Threatening Behavior, 48*(3), 353–366. https://doi.org/10.1027/0227-5910/a000622

Gvion, Y., & Apter, A. (2012). Suicide and suicidal behavior. *Public Health Reviews, 34*(2), 9. https://doi.org/10.1007/BF03391688

Haines, J., Williams, C. L., Brain, K. L., & Wilson, G. V. (1995). The psychophysiology of self-mutilation. *Journal of Abnormal Psychology, 104*, 471–489. https://doi.org/10.1037/0021-843X.104.3.471

Harris, K., Gooding, P., Peters, S., & Haddock, G. (2020). Investigating the perceived impact of psychosis on suicidal thoughts and behaviors. *Schizophrenia Bulletin Open, 1*(1), sgaa038. https://doi.org/10.1093/schizbullopen/sgaa038

Harvard T.H. Chan School of Public Health. (n.d.). *Method choice and intent.* Means Matter. https://hsph.harvard.edu/research/means-matter/means-matter-basics/method-choice-and-intent/

Hausmann-Stabile, C., Kuhlberg, J. A., Zayas, L. H., Nolle, A. P., & Cintron, S. L. (2012). Means, intent, lethality, behaviors, and psychiatric diagnosis in Latina adolescent suicide attempters. *Professional Psychology: Research and Practice, 43*(3), 241–247. https://doi.org/10.1037/a0026258

Hooley, J. M., Fox, K. R., & Boccagno, C. (2020). Nonsuicidal self-injury: Diagnostic challenges and current perspectives. *Neuropsychiatric Disease and Treatment, 16*, 101–112. https://doi.org/10.2147/NDT.S198806

Hutchinson, G. (2023). Protective factors in suicidal behavior. In *Suicide risk assessment and prevention* (pp. 77–84). Springer. https://link.springer.com/referenceworkentry/10.1007/978-3-030-42003-1_10

Institute for Functional Medicine (IFM). (2023, September 22). *The multidirectional nature of mental illness, chronic disease, & sleep*. https://www.ifm.org/articles/the-multidirectional-nature-of-mental-illness-chronic-disease-sleep

Institute of Medicine (IOM). (2001). *Risk factors for suicide: Summary of a workshop*. National Academy Press. https://doi.org/10.17226/10215

Jang, S. Y., Choi, H. J., Kim, H., & Kim, H. J. (2025). Analyzing the impact of social distancing policies during covid-19 on the risk and rescue of suicide attempters presenting to the emergency department: applying the Risk-Rescue Rating Scale. *Psychiatry Investigation, 22*(2), 175–185. https://doi.org/10.30773/pi.2024.0095

Joiner, T. (2005). *Why people die by suicide*. Harvard University Press. https://doi.org/10.4159/9780674038825

Kamali, M., Pegg, S., Janos, J. A., Bobo, W. V., Brody, B., Gao, K., Tohen, M., McIntyre, R. S., Calabrese, J. R., Thase, M. E., Ketter, T. A., Goldberg, J. F., Sachs, G. S., & Nierenberg, A. A. (2021). Illness stage and predominant polarity in bipolar disorder: Correlation with burden of illness and moderation of treatment outcome. *Journal of Psychiatric Research, 140*, 205–213. https://doi.org/10.1016/j.jpsychires.2021.05.082

Kar, N., Arun, M., Mohanty, M. K., & Bastia, B. K. (2014). Scale for assessment of lethality of suicide attempt. *Indian Journal of Psychiatry, 56*(4), 337–343. https://doi.org/10.4103/0019-5545.146512

Kessler, R. C., & Merikangas, K. R. (2006). The national comorbidity survey replication (NCS-R): Background and aims. *International Journal of Methods in Psychiatric Research, 13*(2), 60–68. https://doi.org/10.1002/mpr.166

Klonsky, E. D. (2007). The functions of deliberate self-injury: A review of the evidence. *Clinical Psychology Review, 27*(2), 226–239. https://doi.org/10.1016/j.cpr.2006.08.002

Klonsky, E. D., & May, A. M. (2014). Differentiating suicide attempters from suicide ideators: A critical frontier for suicidology research. *Suicide and Life-Threatening Behavior, 44*(1), 1–5. https://doi.org/10.1111/sltb.12068

Klonsky, E. D., May, A. M., & Saffer, B. Y. (2016). Suicide, suicide attempts, and suicidal ideation. *Annual Review of Clinical Psychology, 12*(1), 307–330. https://doi.org/10.1146/annurev-clinpsy-021815-093204

Kułak-Bejda, A., Bejda, G., & Waszkiewicz, N. (2021). Mental disorders, cognitive impairment and the risk of suicide in older adults. *Frontiers in Psychiatry, 12*, 695286. https://doi.org/10.3389/fpsyt.2021.695286

Lara, D. R., Ottoni, G. L., de Araújo, R. M. F., & Mazzochi, L. (2015). Thinking about dying and trying and intending to die: Results on suicidal behavior from a large web-based sample. *The Journal of Clinical Psychiatry, 76*(3), e20944. https://doi.org/10.4088/JCP.14m09117

Layng, T. J. (2017). Private emotions as contingency descriptors: Emotions, emotional behavior, and their evolution. *European Journal of Behavior Analysis, 18*(2), 168–179. https://doi.org/10.1080/15021149.2017.1304875

LeDoux, J. (2012). Rethinking the emotional brain. *Neuron, 73*(4), 653–676. https://doi.org/10.1016/j.neuron.2012.02.004

Lengvenyte, A., Conejero, I., Courtet, P., & Olié, E. (2021). Biological bases of suicidal behaviours: A narrative review. *European Journal of Neuroscience, 53*(1), 330–351. https://doi.org/10.1111/ejn.14635

Lester, D. (1990). Classification of self-harm behaviors. *Perceptual and Motor Skills, 70*(2), 432–434. https://doi.org/10.2466/pms.1990.70.2.432

Lin, J., & Epel, E. (2022). Stress and telomere shortening: Insights from cellular mechanisms. *Ageing Research Reviews, 73*, 101507. https://doi.org/10.1016/j.arr.2021.101507

Lind, J. (2018). What can associative learning do for planning? *Royal Society Open Science, 5*(11), 180778. https://doi.org/10.1098/rsos.180778

Litman, R. E. (1968). The degree of suicide. *International Journal of Social Psychiatry, 14*(2), 105–116. https://doi.org/10.1177/002076406801400204

Lorentzen, E. A., Mors, O., & Kjær, J. N. (2022). The prevalence of self-injurious behavior in patients with schizophrenia spectrum disorders: A systematic review and meta-analysis. *Schizophrenia Bulletin Open, 3*(1), sgac069. https://doi.org/10.1093/schizbullopen/sgac069

Mann, J. J. (2003). Neurobiology of suicidal behaviour. *Nature Reviews Neuroscience, 4*(10), 819–828. https://doi.org/10.1038/nrn1220

Mann, J. J., & Arango, V. (1999). Neurobiology of suicidal behavior. In D. G. Jacobs (Ed.), *The Harvard Medical School guide to suicide assessment and intervention* (pp. 98–114). Jossey-Bass/Wiley. https://doi.org/10.1002/9781118269633.ch6

Mann, J. J., Waternaux, C., Haas, G. L., & Malone, K. M. (1999). Toward a clinical model of suicidal behavior in psychiatric patients. *American Journal of Psychiatry, 156*(2), 181–189. https://doi.org/10.1176/ajp.156.2.181

Martinez-Rives, N. L., Chaparro, M. P. M., Kotera, Y., Dhungel, B., & Gilmour, S. (2025). The role of communication and social support in suicidal behaviour in adults aged between 18–40 years: A systematic review. *The European Journal of Psychiatry, 39*(1), 100266. https://doi.org/10.1016/j.ejpsy.2024.100266

Masango, S. M., Rataemane, S. T., & Motojesi, A. A. (2008). Suicide and suicide risk factors: A literature review. *South African Family Practice, 50*(6), 25–29. https://doi.org/10.1080/20786204.2008.10873774

Méndez-Bustos, P., Calati, R., Rubio-Ramírez, F., Olié, E., Courtet, P., & Lopez-Castroman, J. (2019). Effectiveness of psychotherapy on suicidal risk: A systematic review of observational studies. *Frontiers in Psychology, 10*, 277. https://doi.org/10.3389/fpsyg.2019.00277

Miller, M., Hempstead, K., Nguyen, T., Barber, C., Rosenberg-Wohl, S., & Azrael, D. (2013). Method choice in nonfatal self-harm as a predictor of subsequent episodes of self-harm and suicide: Implications for clinical practice. *American Journal of Public Health, 103*(6), 61–68. https://doi.org/10.2105/AJPH.2013.301326

Moitra, M., Santomauro, D., Degenhardt, L., Collins, P. Y., Whiteford, H., Vos, T., & Ferrari, A. (2021). Estimating the risk of suicide associated with mental disorders: A systematic review and meta-regression analysis. *Journal of Psychiatric Research, 137*, 242–249. https://doi.org/10.1016/j.jpsychires.2021.02.053

Mueller, A. S., Abrutyn, S., Pescosolido, B., & Diefendorf, S. (2021). The social roots of suicide: Theorizing how the external social world matters to suicide and suicide prevention. *Frontiers in Psychology, 12*, 621569. https://doi.org/10.3389/fpsyg.2021.621569

National Alliance on Mental Illness (NAMI). (2025). *Self-harm*. https://www.nami.org/about-mental-illness/common-with-mental-illness/self-harm/

National Institute of Mental Health (NIMH). (2024, December). *Depression*. U.S. Department of Health and Human Services, National Institutes of Health. Retrieved July 30, 2025, from https://www.nimh.nih.gov/health/publications/depression

National Institute of Mental Health (NIMH). (2025a, March). *Bipolar disorder*. U.S. Department of Health and Human Services, National Institutes of Health. Retrieved August 3, 2025, from https://www.nimh.nih.gov/health/statistics/bipolar-disorder

National Institute of Mental Health (NIMH). (2025b, March). *Suicide statistics*. U.S. Department of Health and Human Services (HHS), National Institutes of Health (NIH). Retrieved July 20, 2025, from https://www.nimh.nih.gov/health/statistics/suicide

Nock, M., Borges, G., Bromet, E., Alonso, J., Angermeyer, M., Beautrais, A., & Williams, D. (2008). Cross-national prevalence and risk factors for suicidal ideation, plans and attempts. *British Journal of Psychiatry, 192*(2), 98–105. https://doi.org/10.1192/bjp.bp.107.040113

Nock, M. K., Hwang, I., Sampson, N. A., & Kessler, R. C. (2010). Mental disorders, comorbidity and suicidal behavior: Results from the National Comorbidity Survey Replication. *Molecular Psychiatry, 15*(8), 868–876. https://doi.org/10.1038/mp.2009.29

O'Carroll, P. W., Berman, A. L., Maris, R. W., Moscicki, E. K., Sherill, J. T., & Joiner, T. E. (1996). Beyond the tower of Babel: A nomenclature for suicidology. *Suicide and Life-Threatening Behavior, 26*(3), 237–252. https://doi.org/10.1111/j.1943-278X.1996.tb00431.x

Oexle, N., Rüsch, N., Viering, S., Wyss, C., Seifritz, E., Xu, Z., & Kawohl, W. (2016). Self-stigma and suicidality: A longitudinal study. *European Archives of Psychiatry and Clinical Neuroscience*. https://doi.org/10.1007/s00406-016-0698-1

Oexle, N., Waldmann, T., Staiger, T., Xu, Z., & Rüsch, N. (2018). Mental illness stigma and suicidality: The role of public and individual stigma. *Epidemiology and Psychiatric Sciences, 27*(2), 169–175. https://doi.org/10.1017/S2045796016000949

Pavulans, K., Bolmsjö, I., Edberg, A. K., & Öjehagen, A. (2012). Being in want of control: Experiences of being on the road to, and making, a suicide attempt. *International Journal of Qualitative Studies on Health and Well-Being, 7*(1), 16228. https://doi.org/10.3402/qhw.v7i0.16228

Pierre, J. M. (2015). Culturally sanctioned suicide: Euthanasia, seppuku, and terrorist martyrdom. *World Journal of Psychiatry, 5*(1), 4–11. https://doi.org/10.5498/wjp.v5.i1.4

Posner, K., Oquendo, M. A., Gould, M., Stanley, B., & Davies, M. (2007). Columbia Classification Algorithm of Suicide Assessment (C-CASA): Classification of suicidal events in the FDA's pediatric suicidal risk analysis of antidepressants. *American Journal of Psychiatry, 164*(7), 1035–1043. https://doi.org/10.1176/ajp.2007.164.7.1035

Posner, K., Brown, G. K., Stanley, B., Brent, D. A., Yershova, K. V., Oquendo, M. A., Currier, G. W., Melvin, G. A., Greenhill, L., Shen, S., & Mann, J. J. (2011). The Columbia–Suicide Severity Rating Scale: Initial validity and internal consistency findings from three multisite studies with adolescents and adults. *American Journal of Psychiatry, 168*(12), 1266–1277. https://doi.org/10.1176/appi.ajp.2011.10111704

Posner, K., Brodsky, B., Yershova, K., Buchanan, J., & Mann, J. J. (2014). The classification of suicidal behavior. In M. K. Nock (Ed.), *The Oxford handbook of suicide and self-injury* (pp. 7–22). Oxford University Press. https://doi.org/10.1093/oxfordhb/9780195388565.013.002

Radomsky, E. D., Haas, G. L., Mann, J. J., & Sweeney, J. A. (1999). Suicidal behavior in patients with schizophrenia and other psychotic disorders. *The American Journal of Psychiatry, 156*(10), 1590–1595. https://doi.org/10.1176/ajp.156.10.1590

Regev, S., & Josman, N. (2020). Evaluation of executive functions and everyday life for people with severe mental illness: A systematic review. *Schizophrenia Research: Cognition, 21*, 100178. https://doi.org/10.1016/j.scog.2020.100178

Rosenberg, M. L., Davidson, L. E., Smith, J. C., Berman, A. L., Buzbee, H., Gantner, G., Jobes, D. A., & McIntosh, J. L. (1988). Operational criteria for the determination of suicide. *Journal of Forensic Sciences, 33*(6), 1445–1456. https://doi.org/10.1520/JFS12426J

Sadath, A., Troya, M. I., Nicholson, S., Cully, G., Leahy, D., Ramos Costa, A. P., Benson, R., Corcoran, P., Griffin, E., Phillip, E., Cassidy, E., Jeffers, A., Shiely, F., Alberdi-Páramo, Í., Kavalidou, K., & Arensman, E. (2023). Physical and mental illness comorbidity among individuals with frequent self-harm episodes: A mixed-methods study. *Frontiers in Psychiatry, 14*, 1121313. https://doi.org/10.3389/fpsyt.2023.1121313

Sediyama, C. Y. N., de Castro Martins, C., & Teodoro, M. L. M. (2020). Association of loss aversion, personality traits, depressive, anxious, and suicidal symptoms: Systematic review. *Clinical Neuropsychiatry, 17*(5), 286–294. https://doi.org/10.36131/cnfioritieditore20200505

Shneidman, E. S. (1993). Commentary: Suicide as psychache. *Journal of Nervous and Mental Disease, 181*(3), 145–147. https://doi.org/10.1097/00005053-199303000-00001

Silverman, M. M., & De Leo, D. (2016). Why there is a need for an international nomenclature and classification system for suicide. *Crisis*. https://doi.org/10.1027/0227-5910/a000419

Silverman, M. M., Berman, A. L., Sanddal, T. L., O'Carroll, P. W., & Joiner, T. E. (2007). Rebuilding the tower of Babel: A revised nomenclature for the study of suicide and suicidal behaviors part 1: Background, rationale, and methodology. *Suicide and Life-Threatening Behavior, 37*(3), 248–263. https://doi.org/10.1521/suli.2007.37.3.248

Skinner, B. F. (1945). The operational analysis of psychological terms. *Psychological Review, 52*(4), 270–277. https://doi.org/10.1037/h0062535

Skinner, B. F. (1953). *Science and human behavior*. Macmillan. https://doi.org/10.1037/11149-000

Skinner, B. F. (1969). *Contingencies of reinforcement: A theoretical analysis*. Appleton-Century-Crofts. https://doi.org/10.1037/11496-000

Song, Y., Rhee, S. J., Lee, H., Kim, M. J., Shin, D., & Ahn, Y. M. (2020). Comparison of suicide risk by mental illness: A retrospective review of 14-year electronic medical records. *Journal of Korean Medical Science, 35*(47). https://doi.org/10.3346/jkms.2020.35.e402

Stanley, B., & Brown, G. K. (2012). Safety planning intervention: A brief intervention to mitigate suicide risk. *Cognitive and Behavioral Practice, 19*(2), 256–264. https://doi.org/10.1016/j.cbpra.2011.01.001

Steer, R. A., Rissmiller, D. J., Ranieri, W. F., & Beck, A. T. (1993). Dimensions of suicidal ideation in psychiatric inpatients. *Behaviour Research and Therapy, 31*(2), 229–236. https://doi.org/10.1016/0005-7967(93)90090-H

Substance Abuse and Mental Health Services Administration (SAMHSA). (2020). *Treatment for suicidal ideation, self-harm, and suicide attempts among youth* (SAMHSA Publication No. PEP20-06-01-002). National Mental Health and Substance Use Policy Laboratory. https://store.samhsa.gov/product/Treatment-for-Suicidal-Ideation-Self-Harm-and-Suicide-Attempts-Among-Youth/PEP20-06-01-002

Sufrate-Sorzano, T., Santolalla-Arnedo, I., Garrote-Cámara, M. E., Angulo-Nalda, B., Cotelo-Sáenz, R., Pastells-Peiró, R., Juárez-Vela, R., Bellon, F., Blanco-Blanco, J., & Molina-Luque, F. (2023). Interventions of choice for the prevention and treatment of suicidal behaviours: An umbrella review. *Nursing Open, 10*(8), 4959–4970. https://doi.org/10.1002/nop2.1820

Swanson, S. A., & Colman, I. (2013). Association between exposure to suicide and suicidality outcomes in youth. *Canadian Medical Association Journal, 185*(10), 870–877. https://doi.org/10.1503/cmaj.121377

Tourinho, E. Z. (2006). Private stimuli, covert responses, and private events: Conceptual remarks. *The Behavior Analyst, 29*(1), 13–31. https://doi.org/10.1007/BF03392115

Turecki, G., & Brent, D. A. (2016). Suicide and suicidal behaviour. *The Lancet, 387*(10024), 1227–1239. https://doi.org/10.1016/S0140-6736(15)00234-2

Uebelacker, L. A., Weisberg, R., Millman, M., Yen, S., & Keller, M. (2013). Prospective study of risk factors for suicidal behavior in individuals with anxiety disorders. *Psychological Medicine, 43*(7), 1465–1474. https://doi.org/10.1017/S0033291712002504

Veazie, S., Gilbert, J., Winchell, K., Paynter, R., & Guise, J.-M. (2019). *Addressing social isolation to improve the health of older adults: a rapid review* (AHRQ Publication No. 19-EHC009-EF). Agency for Healthcare Research and Quality. https://doi.org/10.23970/AHRQEPC-RAPIDISOLATION

World Health Organization (WHO). (2025, March 25). *Suicide* [Fact sheet]. https://www.who.int/news-room/fact-sheets/detail/suicide

Xu, Y. E., Barron, D. A., Sudol, K., Zisook, S., & Oquendo, M. A. (2023). Suicidal behavior across a broad range of psychiatric disorders. *Molecular Psychiatry, 28*(7), 2764–2810. https://doi.org/10.1038/s41380-022-01935-7

Zwald, M. L., Holland, K. M., Annor, F. B., Kite-Powell, A., Sumner, S. A., Bowen, D. A., Vivolo-Kantor, A. M., Stone, D. M., & Crosby, A. E. (2020). Syndromic surveillance of suicidal ideation and self-directed violence - United States, January 2017–December 2018. *Morbidity and Mortality Weekly Report, 69*(4), 103–108. https://stacks.cdc.gov/view/cdc/85140

Chapter 18
Problems with Expressions of Problematic Personality-Based Behaviors by Individuals Living with Serious Mental Illness

Introduction

Serious mental illness (SMI) encompasses a range of conditions that profoundly disrupt functioning, often extending across social, occupational, and personal domains. Within this broad category, personality-related problems occupy a particularly complex and challenging space. Personality represents the enduring configuration of traits and behavioral tendencies that shape how individuals perceive, respond to, and interact with their environments. When these traits become rigid, maladaptive, and distressing, they can contribute to significant impairment and exacerbate the difficulties already associated with SMI. Understanding personality in this context requires moving beyond categorical labels toward dimensional frameworks that capture the nuanced variability of human behavior.

The study of personality has long been informed by temperament and trait-based theories, with the lexical hypothesis and the Five-Factor Model (FFM) serving as foundational approaches. These models emphasize that personality traits exist along continua, ranging from adaptive to maladaptive expressions. Contemporary psychiatric classification systems, such as the DSM-5-TR Alternative Model for Personality Disorders (AMPD) and the ICD-11, have increasingly adopted dimensional perspectives. These frameworks assess both the severity of dysfunction and the presence of maladaptive traits, including negative affectivity, detachment, antagonism, disinhibition, psychoticism, and anankastia. Such approaches provide greater clinical utility by recognizing the heterogeneity of personality problems and their overlap with other mental health conditions.

Personality-related mental health problems are shaped by multiple influences, including neurological substrates, genetic predispositions, and environmental contexts. These factors interact dynamically across the lifespan, contributing to the emergence, persistence, or modification of personality traits. While maladaptive traits may appear early and remain stable, they are not immutable; interpersonal

G. F. McKeegan, *Behavior Change Interventions for Serious Mental Illness*, Evidence-Based Practices in Behavioral Health,
https://doi.org/10.1007/978-3-032-18372-9_18

relationships, educational and occupational experiences, and targeted interventions can foster adaptive change. The dimensional approach thus highlights both vulnerability and resilience, underscoring the importance of situating personality within broader biopsychosocial frameworks.

This chapter will examine the expression of problematic personality-based behaviors among individuals living with SMI, integrating perspectives from personality science and clinical psychiatry. It explores the conceptualization of personality and temperament, the dimensional assessment of traits, and the relevance of the lexical hypothesis in trait identification. The discussion will compare categorical and dimensional models, with particular attention to the DSM-5 AMPD and ICD-11 frameworks and will situate these within the broader FFM. Consideration will also be given to the severity of personality problems, their biological and environmental underpinnings, and the behavioral strategies that support adaptive functioning. By aligning personality research with clinical practice, the chapter aims to provide a comprehensive understanding of how personality-related difficulties intersect with serious mental illness and inform individualized approaches to care.

> My daughter overreacts to any conflictual problem with friends or relatives. She becomes very dramatic; if she has a problem at work or school, she says that she has nothing to live for and threatens to kill herself or others. There have been times she has cut herself after a bad day. She overreacts to any disappointment. It is like she has no coping skills and has "thin skin." She has problems dealing with stress and her negative emotions.

Definitions and Characteristics of Personality Traits

Personality refers to the collection of enduring traits, manifested as both overt and covert behaviors in a wide range of social and personal contexts, encompassing patterns of thinking, perceiving, feeling, and acting that are distinctive to everyone (American Psychiatric Association, 2022a). Personality is defined as follows:

"The enduring configuration of characteristics and behavior that comprises an individual's unique adjustment to life, including major traits, interests, drives, values, self-concept, abilities, and emotional patterns. Personality is generally viewed as a complex, dynamic integration or totality shaped by many forces, including hereditary and constitutional tendencies; physical maturation; early training; identification with significant individuals and groups; culturally conditioned values and roles; and critical experiences and relationships. Various theories explain the structure and development of personality in different ways, but all agree that personality helps determine behavior" (American Psychological Association, n.d.-a).

All individuals possess unique personality traits; for example, some may be sociable and approachable, while others may prefer solitude and introspection. Certain individuals exhibit a natural propensity for leadership in challenging situations, whereas others may seek direction from their peers. It is important to note that these traits are often habitual and static, being displayed in different contexts and making them challenging to change.

These behavioral traits that are linked to personality are manifested across various situations and environmental contexts. Personality traits can have varying impacts depending on the context. For instance, an individual who prefers to take charge may demonstrate effective leadership when they are knowledgeable about a situation. In contrast, if that person assumes a leadership role without sufficient understanding, challenges may arise. Similarly, someone who typically follows directions can be a reliable assistant in many scenarios. However, such individuals may be less likely to lead even when they possess relevant knowledge, which could limit the advantages others might gain from their expertise.

In many circumstances, individuals demonstrate an ability to adapt to the situations they encounter. Effective leaders recognize when it is appropriate for others to assume leadership roles in response to specific demands, while competent followers may take the initiative in situations where their expertise is most relevant. This reflects a capacity to adjust behavior according to situational requirements. Although personality traits are challenging to alter, targeted interventions focusing on the behavioral expression of the traits can support individuals in adopting more adaptive behaviors. Such approaches enable people to leverage their strengths to benefit both themselves and those around them. Problems arise when the behaviors that are displayed across situations by the person result in aversive consequences for the person and others in the environment. Personality traits that demonstrate rigid maladaptive patterns that diverge from culturally accepted standards, leading to functional impairment and significant distress for individuals are recognized as personality-related problems (American Psychiatric Association, 2022a).

Personality is a psychological construct that is multidimensional and heterogeneous. The dimensions of personality typically refer to the broad, overarching categories used to describe and analyze individual differences in behavior, thoughts, and feelings (Kapur, 2021). Research has found various factors of personality-based behaviors that are driven by the theory from which they are defined. The number of factors comprising different models of personality functioning range from three to 16 according to the most popular theories. The most common and well-researched model of personality is the five-factor model of personality (FFM) often called the "Big Five" which is predominant and has become a cornerstone in the understanding of human personality (Costa & McCrae, 1992; Feher & Vernon, 2021; Soto & Jackson, 2020; Widiger & Crego, 2019). This model describes personality along five broad domains as follows:

Factor I: Openness to experience (imaginative/curious/creative vs. conventional/cautious/unimaginative): This dimension is characterized by qualities such as inventiveness, curiosity, consistency, and caution. It encompasses a broad interest in culture aspects, emotions, adventure, unconventional ideas, and diverse experiences. Individuals demonstrating openness typically exhibit intellectual curiosity, creativity, and an inclination toward novelty and variety. The precise interpretation of this dimension is debatable and is occasionally referred to as "intellect," instead of openness to experience. Individuals scoring high in openness tend to be imaginative, intellectually curious, and receptive to novel ideas and experiences. They often enjoy artistic pursuits and abstract thinking. Conversely, those with low scores are typically more conventional, favor routine, and may resist change or unfamiliar concepts (Costa & McCrae, 2008; Lim, 2025; Widiger & Crego, 2019).

Factor II: Conscientiousness (efficient/organized vs. easy-going/careless). This dimension describes the tendency to demonstrate consistent self-discipline, fulfill responsibilities, and maintain a strong focus on goal attainment. It encompasses methodical, deliberate behaviors, as well as an inclination toward organization and dependability. High scorers on conscientiousness are organized, dependable, and goal oriented. They exhibit strong self-discipline and are often meticulous in planning and execution. Low scorers, in contrast, may be impulsive, disorganized, and prone to procrastination, often struggling with follow-through and reliability (Costa & McCrae, 2008; Lim, 2025; Widiger & Crego, 2019).

Factor III: Extraversion (vs. introversion): This dimension reflects the extent to which an individual exhibits outgoing and energetic behavior, in contrast to being solitary and reserved. It includes traits such as energy, positive disposition, assertiveness, sociability, a preference for stimulation within social environments, and communicative tendencies. Extraverted individuals are sociable, energetic, and assertive. They thrive in social settings and often seek stimulation through interaction. Those with low extraversion (i.e., introverts) tend to be reserved, introspective, and prefer solitary activities, often finding social engagement taxing (Costa & McCrae, 2008; Lim, 2025; Widiger & Crego, 2019).

Factor IV: Agreeableness (vs. antagonism): This dimension reflects an individual's propensity to be compassionate, cooperative, and considerate toward others, as opposed to being suspicious or antagonistic. It encompasses the spectrum from friendliness and empathy to coldness and unkindness. Individuals who have high scores on agreeableness are characterized as compassionate, cooperative, and trusting in others. These individuals are empathetic and value harmonious relationships. Low scorers may be more skeptical, competitive, and critical, often prioritizing personal goals over social cohesion (Costa & McCrae, 2008; Lim, 2025; Widiger & Crego, 2019).

Factor V: Neuroticism (sensitive/nervous/instability vs. secure/confident/stability): This trait reflects an individual's propensity to experience negative emotions, such as anger, anxiety, depression, or vulnerability. Neuroticism also pertains to the level of emotional stability and impulse control and may be described at its lower end as 'emotional stability.' Individuals scoring high on neuroticism are more emotionally reactive and prone to anxiety, mood swings, and stress. They may have trouble coping with adversity. Low scorers are typically calm, emotionally stable, and resilient, showing less susceptibility to psychological distress (Costa & McCrae, 2008; Lim, 2025; Widiger & Crego, 2019).

These factors are considered to account for much of the primary human variation in typical ways of thinking, feeling, and behaving. Each factor encompasses multiple lower level personality facets. Facets are viewed as conceptually situated between broad factors and specific behavioral patterns and are described as fundamental components of personality (Hong & Paunonen, 2015). The factors are defined along a continuum from "high" to "low." FFM views personality traits along spectrums and not the presence or absence of a factor or trait. Each of these domains includes more specific facets; for example, facets of gullible vs. cynical, meek vs. aggressive, soft-hearted vs. callous, and selfless vs. exploitative are within the domain of agreeableness vs. antagonism. FFM is rooted in the lexical paradigm, reflecting role of language in describing personality by other people in the person's environment (Widiger & Crego, 2019).

Each of these dimensions captures a spectrum of traits—such as sociability, emotional resilience, and cognitive flexibility—that together paint a comprehensive picture of individual differences. Personality traits tend to be stable over short time intervals but can change considerably over years or decades. Research indicates that personality development is influenced by life experiences, such as work and relationships (Soto & Jackson, 2020).

Definitions and Characteristics with the Expression of Problematic Personality Traits

Personality emerges from birth and is shaped by both genetic predispositions and environmental influences that evolve further through individual lifespan experiences. Disruptions in personality development, leading to pronounced and inflexible characteristics, can give rise to personality-related difficulties. Such challenges have a broad impact within clinical contexts, often affecting the presentation and management of both mental and physical health conditions. Nevertheless, the problems with personality traits and characteristics frequently remain under-recognized and inadequately addressed in standard clinical practice. Recent studies have advanced understanding by demonstrating that maladaptive personality traits—when severe and associated with significant distress or functional impairment—are prevalent, can be detected early in life, and may continue to change across the lifespan (Newton-Howes et al., 2015).

Personality mental health problems were once seen as categorically distinct and stable; however, current evidence supports a dimensional and dynamic model. Personality traits, both adaptive and maladaptive, are now viewed as existing on a continuum and subject to change due to interactions with the environment. For example, personality can change for better or worse due to significant interpersonal relationships, job and educational experiences, experiencing trauma, the result of targeted interventions (Newton-Howes et al., 2015; Swinson Evans et al., 2016).

Problems with personality mental health problems (PDs) are defined as pervasive patterns of thought, feeling, and behavior that deviate markedly from the expectations of an individual's culture (American Psychiatric Association, 2022a). These patterns are stable over time, have an onset in adolescence or early adulthood, and lead to significant distress or impairment in personal, social, or occupational functioning. PDs are characterized by extreme personality traits that interfere with everyday life, contribute to experiencing distress, and often result in difficulties in building and maintaining healthy interpersonal relationships (Ekselius, 2018).

SMI includes PDs if the degree of functional impairment is severe. SMI is defined as "a mental, behavioral, or emotional problem resulting in serious functional impairment, which substantially interferes with or limits one or more major life activities" (National Institute of Mental Health [NIMH], 2024) that often results in the experiences of lifelong disability (American Psychiatric Association, 2022a; NIMH, 2024; Swinson Evans et al., 2016).

The DSM-5-TR (American Psychiatric Association, 2022a) identifies 10 distinct personality mental health problems, grouped into three broad clusters based on shared characteristics. These mental health problems are enduring patterns of covert and overt experiences and behaviors that deviate markedly from cultural expectations and cause significant distress or impairment in functioning (American Psychiatric Association, 2022a).

The personality mental health problems are grouped into three clusters that share similarities in the description of individuals living with the specific personality mental health problem. Cluster A describes individuals who display odd, eccentric, and idiosyncratic covert and overt behaviors. Cluster B describes individuals who appear dramatic, impulsive, erratic, and emotional. Cluster C includes those people who manifest behaviors that would be labeled as anxious, uncertain, and fearful (American Psychiatric Association, 2022a).

According to the DSM-5-TR (American Psychiatric Association, 2022a), the personality mental health problems (PDs) in the three clusters are as follows:

Cluster A

- Paranoid personality disorder: Characterized by pervasive distrust and suspiciousness of others, interpreting their motives as malevolent.
- Schizoid personality disorder: Marked by detachment from social relationships and a restricted range of emotional expression.
- Schizotypal personality disorder: Involves acute discomfort in close relationships, cognitive or perceptual distortions, and eccentric behavior.

Cluster B

- Antisocial personality disorder: A pattern of disregard for and violation of the rights of others, often involving deceit and impulsivity.
- Borderline personality disorder: Characterized by instability in interpersonal relationships, self-image, and affect, with marked impulsivity.
- Histrionic personality disorder: Involves excessive emotionality and attention-seeking behavior.
- Narcissistic personality disorder: Defined by grandiosity, need for admiration, and lack of empathy.

Cluster C

- Avoidant personality disorder: Marked by social inhibition, feelings of inadequacy, and hypersensitivity to negative evaluation.
- Dependent personality disorder: Characterized by a pervasive need to be taken care of, leading to submissive and clinging behavior.

- Obsessive-compulsive personality disorder: Involves preoccupation with orderliness, perfectionism, and control at the expense of flexibility and efficiency.

The presence of an individual living with PD is based on specific criteria sets outlined in the DSM-5-TR. The type of PD that is present shares overlapping features with and co-occur with other PDs. Both the DSM and ICD historically classified PDs categorically, assigning individuals to one of several distinct PDs based on descriptive symptoms and behavioral checklists. This approach has long been criticized for its high comorbidity rates, poor inter-rater reliability, and limited clinical utility (American Psychological Association, 2024; American Psychiatric Association, 2022b; Widiger & Hines, 2022; World Health Organization [WHO], 2022). These limitations prompted the development of alternative models that conceptualize PDs as patterns of maladaptive traits and functional impairments distributed along spectrums of dimensions as in personality theories, like the FFM (American Psychological Association, 2024; Widiger & Hines, 2022).

As the PD categories are not supported by evidence, the mental health field has shifted toward empirically derived, dimensional models of personality mental health problems. The most prominent models are the DSM-5 section III Alternative Model for Personality Disorder (AMPD) and the ICD-11 (Chanen, 2024). New measures have been developed to assess personality pathology according to the dimension in the AMPD and ICD-11. Various assessment tools include the Level of Personality Functioning Scale (LPFS) (Hopwood et al., 2015a; Hopwood et al., 2015b; Hopwood et al., 2018; Natoli & Rodriguez, 2024) and the Personality Inventory for DSM-5 (PID-5) (Krueger et al., 2012a, 2012b). The LPFS assesses severity through a structured scale, while the PID-5 evaluates maladaptive traits across five domains (Zimmermann et al., 2019).

The DSM-5-TR includes the Alternative Model for Personality Disorders (AMPD) in Sect. III (American Psychiatric Association, 2022b), which conceptualizes personality problems dimensionally through impairments in personality functioning and maladaptive trait domains. The AMPD identifies a PD based on assessed evidence of personality dysfunction, which includes challenges related to self and interpersonal interactions, as well as the presence of dysfunctional personality traits such as negative affectivity, detachment, antagonism, disinhibition, or psychoticism. These difficulties are required to be long-standing, persistent, pervasive, and must cause significant distress or impairment. This AMPD allows for both traditional categorical diagnoses and more dimensional approaches via the PD–trait-specified method. The AMPD describes problematic personality using dimensions rather than categories, representing variation from typical to atypical presentations and explaining covariation through dimensional analysis. In doing so, the AMPD addresses validity concerns found in the PD categories as outlined in the DSM-5-TR (American Psychiatric Association, 2022a).

The AMPD comprises two core components, the level of personality functioning and problematic (pathological) traits of an individual's personality. The level of personality functioning incorporates the assessment of the following dimensions:

- Self-functioning covers personal identity and self-direction. Personal identity refers to knowing oneself as unique, maintaining self-esteem, evaluating oneself accurately, and handling emotions. Self-direction is about pursuing meaningful goals, upholding positive standards, and engaging in productive reflection (American Psychiatric Association, 2022b).
- Interpersonal functioning includes empathy and intimacy in relationships. Empathy is defined as the ability to comprehend others' experiences, motivations, perspectives, and the consequences of one's actions. Intimacy refers to the capacity for sustained connections and reciprocal regard within close relationships (American Psychiatric Association, 2022b).

The component of problematic (pathological) personality traits and the polar opposites of the trait are grouped into five main categories:

- Negative affectivity (vs. emotional stability): Characterized by frequent, intense negative emotions such as anxiety, depression, guilt, and anger, as well as related behaviors like self-harm or dependency (American Psychiatric Association, 2022b).
- Detachment (vs. extraversion): Marked by avoiding social experiences and limited expression of emotion, including withdrawal from interactions and reduced ability to experience pleasure (American Psychiatric Association, 2022b).
- Antagonism (vs. agreeableness): Involves acting against others, inflated self-importance, expectation of special treatment, and disregard for others' needs and feelings.
- Disinhibition (vs. conscientiousness): Driven by impulsivity and immediate gratification, with little consideration for past learning or future outcomes (American Psychiatric Association, 2022b).
- Psychoticism (vs. lucidity): The display of culturally unusual, eccentric behaviors and beliefs affecting cognition and perception (American Psychiatric Association, 2022b).

As with the FFM, each of the five domains encompasses 25 lower level personality facets. Facets are viewed as conceptually situated between broad factors and specific behavioral patterns and expressions of personality characteristics. The factors are defined along a continuum from "high" to "low." These facets were developed through reviews of trait models and research with mental health service users, informed by meta-analyses and data on their links to DSM-IV personality disorders (American Psychiatric Association, 2022b). The problematic traits and facets of personality in the AMPD are operationalized and assessed through tools like the Personality Inventory for DSM-5 (PID-5), which has demonstrated robust psychometric properties and clinical validity (Krueger et al., 2012a, 2012b). At least one trait must be clinically significant to determine the presence of a personality mental health problem. The AMPD also allows six specific PD types (e.g., borderline and narcissistic) that can be determined as present in an individual or assigning a "personality disorder trait specified" (PDTS) mental health problem for non-prototypical patterns (Zimmermann et al., 2019).

The ICD-11 (WHO, 2022) adopts a fully dimensional model for personality-linked mental health classifications. It eliminates specific categories and instead evaluates personality mental health problems according to dimensions of severity and behavioral expressions of problematic traits across five domains that include: (a) negative affectivity; (b) detachment; (c) dissociality; (d) disinhibition; and (e) anankastia. The dimensions of severity are rated as mild, moderate, or severe, with an optional specifier for borderline pattern, acknowledging clinical continuity with prior ICD constructs of borderline personality mental health problem (BPD). The borderline pattern specifier attempts to define features consistent with the BPD construct consisting of emotional instability, fear of abandonment, and self-harming behaviors (Bach & First, 2018).

Rather than viewing personality disorders as fixed types, the ICD-11 emphasizes a spectrum of severity, recognizing that difficulties can range from mild disruptions to pervasive dysfunction across all aspects of life (WHO, 2022) as follows:

- Mild personality mental health disorders are defined by the presence of personality disturbances resulting in limited functional impairment. While individuals may encounter some distress or interpersonal challenges, they generally sustain effective daily functioning. The effects of these disorders are observable but do not significantly compromise an individual's capacity to meet social, occupational, or personal obligations, with minimal disruption to everyday activities (Bach & First, 2018; WHO, 2022).
- Moderate personality mental health problems are characterized by noticeable impairments in specific domains, such as relationships or the accomplishment of personal goals. These challenges are more evident, although not all aspects of an individual's life are affected. The person may retain certain adaptive capacities, but difficulties with emotional regulation, identity, and interpersonal interactions can result in significant obstacles in particular situations (Bach & First, 2018; WHO, 2022). For instance, an individual may struggle to maintain close and intimate relationships, yet still have acquaintances or friends at work.
- Severe personality mental health disorder is characterized by pervasive dysfunction that impacts nearly all aspects of an individual's life. Emotional stability may be compromised; interpersonal relationships are frequently turbulent or difficult to sustain and achieving life goals can become highly challenging. This degree of severity is reflected in significant disturbances in self-concept, persistent difficulties in social interactions, and notable behavioral dysregulation, including instances of self-harming behaviors (Bach & First, 2018; WHO, 2022).

To determine severity, clinicians consider several core factors that incorporate (a) self-functioning (i.e., identity, self-worth, sense of purpose, and self-directedness); (b) interpersonal functioning (i.e., capacity for intimacy, empathy, and conflict resolution); and (c) behavioral, emotional, and cognitive regulation. This severity-based approach helps clinicians customize treatment to match individual needs and levels of impairment, offering a flexible and evidence-based way to support those with personality-related mental health problems (WHO, 2022).

ICD-11 identifies five trait domain qualifiers that may be used to characterize the nature of personality problems. These domains are conceptually independent and may co-occur to varying degrees. Each domain reflects maladaptive variants of normal-range personality traits and contributes to the clinical presentation and functional impairment of the individual (Bagby & Widiger, 2020; Swales, 2022). The five domains are listed below:

- Negative affectivity indicates strong emotional reactions and stress sensitivity, similar to neuroticism and DSM-5 traits like mood swings and anxiety (Bagby & Widiger, 2020; Swales, 2022; WHO, 2022).
- Detachment describes social and emotional withdrawal, resembling introversion and DSM-5 features such as intimacy avoidance (Bagby & Widiger, 2020; Swales, 2022; WHO, 2022).
- Dissociality involves hostility and lack of empathy, mirroring low agreeableness and callousness on the FFM (Bagby & Widiger, 2020; Swales, 2022; WHO, 2022).
- Disinhibition signifies poor impulse control and irresponsibility, relating to low conscientiousness and impulsivity on the FFM (Bagby & Widiger, 2020; Swales, 2022; WHO, 2022).
- Anankastia is characterized by strict control and perfectionism, as identified in ICD-11, and is associated with obsessive-compulsive traits as well as high conscientiousness on the FFM (Bagby & Widiger, 2020; Swales, 2022; WHO, 2022).

The ICD-11 model is supported by the Personality Inventory for ICD-11 (PiCD) (Oltmanns & Widiger, 2021) and the Standardized Assessment of Severity of Personality Disorder (SASPD), both of which have shown strong reliability and cross-cultural applicability (Bach & First, 2018; Oltmanns & Widiger, 2018).

The ICD-11 and DSM-5-TR have overlapping domains—particularly negative affectivity, detachment, and disinhibition—but diverge in key areas. The DSM-5-TR (American Psychiatric Association, 2022b) includes psychoticism, reflecting more extreme perceptual and cognitive distortions, whereas the ICD-11 includes anankastia, capturing rigid perfectionism and overcontrol. Additionally, dissociality in ICD-11 parallels antagonism in DSM-5-TR, but emphasizes interpersonal disregard and callousness (Bagby & Widiger, 2020; Swales, 2022).

Recent approaches to the classification of mental health problems now favor dimensional frameworks; personality-related conditions are described in terms of spectrums of maladaptive traits and aspects of functioning that can result in impaired outcomes for individuals. The Five-Factor Model (FFM), the DSM-5 AMPD, and the ICD-11 all utilize this dimensional concept, though each defines traits in different ways (Hualparuca-Olivera et al., 2023). There is trait-based alignment across the FFM, DSM-5 AMPD, and ICD-11 models of PDs.

The FFM is the normative framework for the AMPD and ICD-11 models of PDs. The FFM organizes personality across five domains—neuroticism, extraversion, agreeableness, conscientiousness, and openness to experience—each comprising specific facets. Widely used for normal personality research, it has increasingly served as a comparative referent for maladaptive and problematic traits (Samuel & Widiger, 2008; Widiger & Simonsen, 2005).

DSM-5 AMPD is a hybrid trait-and-function model. The AMPD defines personality disorder through two components, Criteria A and B (American Psychiatric Association, 2022b). Criterion A is based on the degree of impairment in self/interpersonal functioning that is measured by the Level of Personality Functioning Scale-Self Report (LPFS-SR). The LPFS-SR is self-report inventory in which the respondents rate 80 statements on a 4-point scale from "totally false" to "very true." Each item is weighed differently, affecting the total score. The assessment evaluates four core functions of personality: identity, self-direction, empathy, and intimacy (Hopwood et al., 2015a, 2015b). Criterion B consists of five maladaptive trait domains—negative affectivity, detachment, antagonism, disinhibition, and psychoticism. Psychoticism is particularly notable for its alignment with maladaptive openness, capturing eccentricity and perceptual dysregulation (Krueger et al., 2012a, 2012b; Hopwood et al., 2015a, 2015b). The domains are assessed by the Personality Inventory for DSM-5 (PID-5). The PID-5 assesses 25 personality trait facets, each consisting of 4–14 items. These facets are grouped into broader domains that are the five maladaptive trait domains of personality functioning.

The model used by the ICD-11 is completely dimensional. The ICD-11 eliminates categories of PDs in favor of severity-based classifications (mild, moderate, and severe), supplemented by optional trait domain specifiers: negative affectivity, detachment, dissociality, disinhibition, and anankastia, with an optional borderline pattern specifier (McCabe & Widiger, 2020). Unlike DSM-5, ICD-11 excludes psychoticism and includes anankastia, a domain reflecting overcontrolled and perfectionistic traits, aligning with high conscientiousness.

Research consistently demonstrates substantial convergence and concordance with the FFM between DSM and ICD trait domains and FFM dimensions. Meta-analytic findings confirm the FFM's utility in describing DSM-IV personality disorder profiles with strong facet-level correspondence, especially for borderline, antisocial, and avoidant PDs (Samuel & Widiger, 2008). Openness, however, showed limited relevance in earlier DSM conceptualizations. The convergence between the DSM, ICD and FFM trait domains and dimensions are presented in Table 18.1.

Table 18.1 Concordance with the FFM between DSM and ICD trait domains and FFM dimensions

DSM-5 / ICD-11 Trait domain	FFM Counterpart	Description
Negative affectivity	Neuroticism	Emotional instability
Detachment	Low extraversion	Social withdrawal
Antagonism/Dissociality	Low agreeableness	Hostility and callousness
Disinhibition	Low conscientiousness	Impulsivity
Psychoticism (DSM only)	High openness (maladaptive)	Odd beliefs and cognitive-perceptual issues
Anankastia (ICD only)	High conscientiousness (rigid)	Overcontrol and perfectionism

(Bach & Simonsen, 2021; Hong & Paunonen, 2015; Soto & Jackson, 2020)

Empirical studies comparing instruments such as the PID-5 (DSM-5) (Krueger et al., 2012a, 2012b) and PiCD (ICD-11) (Hopwood et al., 2015a, 2015b) show high convergent validity with FFM measures like the NEO PI (Neuroticism, Extraversion, Openness Personality Inventory) (Costa Jr & McCrae, 1978) and the NEO PI-R (or Revised NEO PI) (Costa & McCrae, 2008). The ICD-11's SASPD (WHO, 2022) and DSM-5's LPFS-SR (American Psychiatric Association, 2022b) demonstrate consistent functional assessment across systems (McCabe & Widiger, 2020). ICD-11 showed stronger discriminant validity between trait domains, suggesting clearer structural separation.

Despite structural nuances, both DSM-5 AMPD and ICD-11 draw heavily from the FFM. While DSM-5 offers greater detail via trait facets and functioning levels, ICD-11 prioritizes diagnostic parsimony. The alignment of both systems with the FFM underscores the dimensional continuity between normal and pathological personality, supporting trait-based diagnostic clarity.

Both dimensional models for PDs have garnered empirical support. The PID-5 and PiCD demonstrate strong internal consistency, convergent validity with established trait models (e.g., Five-Factor Model), and predictive utility for clinical outcomes (Hong & Paunonen, 2015; Soto & Jackson, 2020). Moreover, dimensional assessments allow clinicians to tailor interventions based on trait severity and configuration rather than rigid diagnostic thresholds, enhancing treatment planning and prognosis (Bach & Simonsen, 2021).

The shift from categorical to dimensional models in the DSM-5-TR and ICD-11 marks an advancement in the conceptualization of personality mental health problems. By conceptualizing personality traits as existing along continuums and considering functional impairments, these models provide enhanced accuracy, increased clinical adaptability, and consistency with modern approaches to personality theory. As research continues to validate these frameworks, their integration into practice promises to improve both assessment and intervention for individuals living with personality mental health problems.

PDs are enduring patterns of covert and overt behaviors and experiences of an individual that deviate markedly from cultural and societal expectations and impair functioning across various domains, especially interpersonal relationships. Research has found that there is a high rate of comorbidity between PDs and other mental health conditions, which complicates the recognition, treatment, and outcome of personality mental health problems (Newton-Howes et al., 2015; Zimmerman et al., 2005).

There is a high prevalence of co-occurring mental health problems who have been identified as living with a PD. Up to 50% of individuals with an recognized mental health problem meet the criteria for a PD, and many of these individuals also present with mood, anxiety, psychotic, or substance use mental health problems (Chanen, 2024; Ekselius, 2018; Newton-Howes et al., 2015). Symptoms of PDs often resemble or exacerbate the mental health problems linked to SMI (e.g., depression and schizophrenia spectrum), leading to confusion and ambiguity unless PDs are identified as premorbid or trait-based (Fok et al., 2014). Individuals with co-occurring PDs and SMI show increased rates of inpatient hospitalization and involuntary admission (Fok et al., 2014; Lay et al., 2006), supporting the supposition that living with PD exacerbates the problems of living with SMI.

PDs often present with complex clinical pictures due to their frequent comorbidity with other mental health problems and at times an ambiguous clinical presentation. Understanding these overlapping mental health problems is essential for effective assessment and treatment planning (Leichsenring et al., 2024). Recent research has shown that there are common occurring comorbidities, distinguishing features, and clinical implications for specified PDs according to the DSM-5-TR nomenclature.

BPD has been extensively studied and is notable for its high rates of co-occurring mental health-related problems. Common comorbidities include major depression, bipolar, anxiety (particularly post-traumatic stress disorder [PTSD]), substance use, and eating mental health problems. Psychotic-like experiences such as paranoia and dissociation are not uncommon and may overlap with features seen in schizophrenia spectrum mental health problems (Balaratnasingam & Janca, 2015; Leichsenring et al., 2024). The complexity inherent in BPD's comorbidity profile necessitates integrated, multimodal assessments and interventions. Of particular concern is the elevated risk of suicide and self-harm behaviors in people living with BPD.

Avoidant personality mental health condition (AvPD) frequently coexists with social anxiety, generalized anxiety, and depressive conditions. There is growing evidence supporting a spectrum model where AvPD and social anxiety represent varying levels of severity within a shared underlying clinical condition (Fok et al., 2014). Clinically, avoidant traits can blur the presentation of anxiety, increasing challenges of recognizing the problematic condition and complicating treatment.

Obsessive-compulsive personality mental health problem (OCPD) is commonly comorbid with major depressive, anxiety, and other somatic symptomatic syndromes (American Psychiatric Association, 2022c). OCPD's defining features of rigidity and perfectionism distinguish it from obsessive-compulsive disorder, which is characterized by intrusive thoughts and compulsions.

Antisocial personality mental health condition (ASPD) is associated with significant externalizing behaviors, including impulsivity, aggression, and criminality. ASPD frequently presents with the co-occurring problems of substance use, attention-deficit/hyperactivity (ADHD), and mood mental health conditions (Fariba et al., 2024). The behavioral patterns associated with co-occurring mental health problems may obscure underlying affective symptoms and limit treatment engagement by the person living with ASPD; however, approaches such as behavioral strategies and motivational interviewing have shown some efficacy.

Schizotypal personality disorder (STPD) shares core features with schizophrenia and schizoaffective spectrum and bipolar conditions with psychotic features. As part of the broader schizophrenia spectrum, STPD conveys an increased risk for transition to displaying overt psychotic behaviors like hallucinations and delusions (Balaratnasingam & Janca, 2015). Early recognition and continuous monitoring are therefore critical for prevention and timely intervention.

Dependent personality mental health problems (DPD) frequently co-occur with depressive and anxiety conditions, and PTSD. Clinical considerations include increased interpersonal sensitivity, particularly regarding perceived rejection, a marked fear of abandonment, and challenges in maintaining therapeutic boundaries. These factors may contribute to an increased risk of exploitation.

Narcissistic personality conditions (NPD) are linked to mood disorders (particularly dysthymia), substance use and intermittent explosive mental health problems. Grandiosity or denial associated with NPD can mask coexisting mental health conditions, requiring the need for thorough clinical assessment.

The high prevalence of comorbid conditions among individuals living with personality mental health conditions underscores the importance of comprehensive evaluation using psychometrically sound assessments as structured interviews yield higher PD prevalence rates than unstructured evaluations (Zimmerman et al., 2005). The assessment results can be used to develop and formulate the integration of effective treatment strategies. Awareness of comorbidity profiles improves accuracy in the detection of problems of personality and informs more effective management approaches across clinical settings.

Dimensions of Problematic Personality-Based Behaviors

Individuals vary in temperament, attitudes, and personality traits, which are shaped by factors including cultural and family environment, spiritual beliefs, age, gender, and socioeconomic background. Identifying and acknowledging personality traits can contribute to the development of communication skills and interactive abilities relevant to personal and professional contexts. Approaching problems and challenges with adaptable strategies may reduce potential negative impacts on personality and support general well-being. Assistance from family, community members, and professionals can be important in addressing obstacles to personality development.

The five key dimensions of functional personality are openness, conscientiousness, extraversion, agreeableness, and neuroticism (OCEAN). Openness involves honesty and directness, conscientiousness is diligence and attention to detail, and extraversion is fulfilment from social interaction. Agreeableness means sociability and kindness, and neuroticism refers to anxiety and self-doubt, which can be managed with effective coping strategies and at times is useful and adaptive in certain contexts. A comprehensive understanding of the five dimensions of personality and the application of improvement measures enable individuals to achieve personal and professional success and improve their overall quality of life.

In mental health, "dimensional" refers to the concept of assessing mental health conditions on a continuum rather than categorizing them into distinct groups. A dimension is a homogeneous variable that is continuous and can be measured according to frequency, duration, and intensity/severity (Hopwood et al., 2023). It implies that symptoms or traits are measured in terms of measurable construct, like severity or degree, allowing for a more detailed understanding of individual differences. Dimensional approaches focus on quantitative gradations, capturing variations in symptoms across a spectrum rather than making binary distinctions like "having" or "not having" a mental health problem. This perspective is increasingly favored for its ability to reflect the complexity of mental health conditions and improve the precision of identification and treatment (Hopwood et al., 2023).

Dimensions of mental health are evaluated and measured through a range of standardized instruments and scales that quantify the severity, duration, and extent of impairments related to behavioral issues and symptoms. Assessments typically encompass behavioral, emotional, and neurobiological evaluations, including psychological testing, neuroimaging techniques, and neurochemical analyses (Phillips, 2016). These models view problematic behaviors as existing on a continuum, where individuals vary in the degree or severity of symptoms and behaviors (Hopwood et al., 2023). For example, in a categorical model, a person with six out of nine problem behaviors related to depressive mental health condition might be identified as living with this problem, while someone with three behaviors would not. In a dimensional model, both individuals would be assessed based on the severity and number of problematic behaviors, providing a more detailed picture of their mental health (Hopwood et al., 2023).

Dimensional measures help monitor and track problem behaviors, changes, and treatment outcomes, offering a detailed view of progress. Though appealing for their reflection of the spectrum of mental health-related problems, these measures are often inconsistent and highly intercorrelated, limiting their reliability for predicting outcomes or guiding specific treatments. Identifying mental health problems based on dimensional scores could result in a plethora of complex categories, making routine use difficult (Phillips, 2016).

PDs are described as extreme versions of normal personality dimensions (Costa & Widiger, 1994; Widiger & Costa Jr., 1994) that are expressed at maladaptive levels persisting for a long time and are associated with difficulties in functioning and individual distress (Saulsman & Page, 2004). PDs are typically defined as patterns of perceiving, relating to, and thinking about the environment and oneself that affect long-term functioning and can be habitually expressed. These patterns persist over time and are apparent across different situations and contexts, rather than occurring only during specific episodes (American Psychological Association, n.d.-c). The classification and identification of PDs have undergone a paradigm shift from rigid categorical typologies to empirically grounded dimensional models using widely accepted theories of personality functioning and traits, like the FFM. The DSM-5-TR AMPD and the ICD-11 framework represent this evolution, emphasizing impairments in personality functioning and the overt expression of maladaptive traits. These models offer complementary perspectives on the structure and dynamics of personality problems, enabling more detailed clinical assessment and individualized intervention.

Both AMPD and ICD-11 conceptualize personality disorder as a unified construct characterized by impairments in self and interpersonal functioning and the presence of maladaptive trait expression. These impairments manifest across domains such as identity, self-direction, empathy, and intimacy, and are considered central to the severity of personality dysfunction (Swales, 2022; Zimmermann et al., 2019).

The dimension of severity is a foundational in both models. It enables the mental health service provider to assess the depth and breadth of personality dysfunction in a systematic, dimensional fashion. The AMPD employs the Level of Personality Functioning Scale (LPFS) to evaluate functioning across four dimensions within two domains: self-functioning, which includes identity and self-direction; and interpersonal functioning, comprised of empathy and intimacy (Krueger & Hobbs, 2020). The scale provides an operational framework for assessing impairments in self and interpersonal functioning, which are the core features distinguishing personality disorders from normative personality variation. Self-functioning encompasses self-identity, characterized by coherence, stability, and emotional regulation, and self-direction, which involves goal setting, reflective thinking, and adherence to behavioral standards. Impairments in identity may manifest as a fragmented sense of self, unstable self-image, or altered self-appraisal, while difficulties in self-direction can present as lack of clear goals, unrealistic aspirations, or limited introspection. Interpersonal functioning comprises empathy and intimacy; empathy reflects the capacity to understand others' experiences, and deficits may include misinterpreting intentions or diminished awareness of others' needs. Intimacy refers to the depth and quality of relationships, with dysfunction evident in superficial or opportunistic interactions and difficulty establishing enduring connections.

The severity of personality impairment can be conceptualized across five distinct levels, ranging from no impairment to extreme impairment. At level 0, individuals display adaptive functioning throughout all domains, exhibiting resilience and flexibility in self-concept as well as relationships. Mild impairment (level 1) may be characterized by occasional struggles with identity formation or maintaining relationships, though these difficulties are generally transient and do not significantly disrupt daily life. As impairment becomes moderate (level 2), dysfunction in self-concept or reciprocity within interpersonal relationships becomes more noticeable. Individuals at this level may experience persistent challenges with self-direction or empathy, leading to ongoing interpersonal difficulties. Severe impairment (level 3) is marked by significant instability in self-identity, poor ability to set or pursue goals, and relationships that are often exploitative or emotionally detached. At the most extreme end, level 4, individuals experience profound confusion about their own identity, a striking absence of empathy, and are largely unable to maintain meaningful relationships. Functioning is deeply compromised across all areas, with little capacity to adapt or recover from interpersonal or internal challenges.

ICD-11 classifies severity as mild, moderate, or severe based on the pervasiveness and impact of dysfunction in self and interpersonal domains (Bach & First, 2018; Lee, 2025; WHO, 2022). The ICD-11 uses a dimensional approach for classifying PDs, assessing the level of impairment rather than fitting individuals into strict categories. This method recognizes a spectrum from mild-to-severe difficulty as follows:

- Mild PD involves limited impairment where individuals may have relationship issues but can generally manage daily tasks and responsibilities.

- Moderate PD indicates significant problems in specific areas, such as relationships or personal goals, though some adaptive abilities remain intact.
- Severe PD is marked by broad dysfunction affecting most aspects of life, with major challenges in emotional stability, self-concept, and relationships.

Clinicians determine severity based on self-functioning, interpersonal skills, and behavioral regulation. This framework enables more targeted treatment aligned with each individual's level of impairment, replacing rigid categories with a flexible, evidence-based model. The level of severity guides treatment intensity and prognostic expectations, with severe PD often overlapping with BPD pathology (Chanen, 2024).

AMPD assesses five core domains of personality impairments: negative affectivity (emotional instability and distress), detachment (social withdrawal and anhedonia), antagonism (hostility and manipulativeness), disinhibition (impulsivity and lack of control), and psychoticism (eccentricity and unusual beliefs). Psychoticism is unique to AMPD.

ICD-11 also uses five domains: Negative affectivity (negative emotions), detachment (interpersonal distance), dissociality (callousness and manipulativeness aligning with AMPD's antagonism), disinhibition (recklessness), and anankastia (perfectionism and rigidity that is unique to ICD-11).

AMPD requires at least one significant trait for identification and includes psychoticism; ICD-11 treats traits as optional and omits psychoticism. These differences highlight the evolving nature of dimensional personality models.

Research shows moderate overlap among the dimensions of maladaptive personality in the AMPD model and the ICD-11. Negative affectivity and detachment are strongly aligned across systems; antagonism (AMPD) matches dissociality (ICD-11); anankastia is unique to ICD-11 but somewhat similar to the PID-5 facets of "rigid perfectionism" and "perseveration" (Strus et al., 2021); psychoticism in AMPD has no ICD-11 counterpart.

Assessing the expression of a problematic personality traits begins with a clinical interview usually employing a scale that is tailored to determine the presence of problematic behaviors that an individual displays. The Structured Clinical Interview for DSM-5 (SCID5) is a semi-structured interview used by professional mental health service providers and researchers to detect mental health problems based on the DSM-5 (American Psychiatric Association, 2013; Boberg et al., 2020; Krueger & Eaton, 2015). To obtain a more detailed assessment of the presence of a personality mental health problem, a self-report inventory can be used. The Personality Inventory for DSM-5 (PID5) is a self-report measure assessing maladaptive personality traits within AMPD in the DSM-5 (American Psychiatric Association, 2013; Krueger et al., 2012a, 2012b). It consists of 220 items that evaluate 25 facets across the five higher order domains of personality mental health problems that are listed above. It provides a more comprehensive assessment of a person's personality assisting in gaining a more objective insight into specific personality traits and how they might be contributing to the individual's distress and mental health problems (Krueger et al., 2012a, 2012b). A shorter, 100-item version is also available.

Research indicates that maladaptive traits correlate with general personality traits, with significant overlap observed. The PID-5 organizes personality traits into five broader trait domains, each composed of specific contributing facets. Studies have demonstrated the incremental validity of maladaptive traits in predicting treatment planning and psychosocial impairment (Krueger & Eaton, 2015). Table 18.2 presents the facet assessed by PID5, description of facet, and AMPD domain associated with the facet.

The Level of Personality Functioning Scale-Self Report (LPFS-SR) for is an 80-item self-report scale that assesses personality functioning in adults using the AMPD framework of the DSM5. Respondents rate 80 statements on a 4-point scale from "totally false" to "very true." The assessment evaluates four core functions: identity, self-direction, empathy, and intimacy (Hopwood et al., 2015a; Hopwood et al., 2015b). Each item is weighed differently, affecting the total score. Subcomponent scores are summed to yield a total score indicating the severity of maladaptive personality functioning. Norms are based on a sample of 306

Table 18.2 Facet assessed by PID5, description of facet, and AMPD domain associated with facet

PID5 Facet	Description	AMPD Domain
Anhedonia	Lack of enjoyment in life	Detachment
Anxiousness	Excessive worry and fear	Negative affect
Attention seeking	Desire for admiration and recognition	
Callousness	Lack of empathy or concern for others	
Deceitfulness	Tendency to lie or manipulate	Antagonism
Depressivity	Persistent feelings of sadness and hopelessness	
Distractibility	Difficulty maintaining focus	Disinhibition
Eccentricity	Odd or unusual behavior and thoughts	Psychoticism
Emotional lability	Unpredictable and intense emotional changes	Negative affect
Grandiosity	Inflated sense of self-importance	Antagonism
Hostility	Aggressiveness and irritability	
Impulsivity	Acting without thinking about consequences	Disinhibition
Intimacy avoidance	Reluctance to form close relationships	Detachment
Irresponsibility	Neglect of obligations and duties	Disinhibition
Manipulativeness	Using others for personal gain	Antagonism
Perceptual dysregulation	Distorted perceptions or experiences	Psychoticism
Perseveration	Difficulty stopping repetitive behaviors	
Restricted affectivity	Limited emotional expression	
Rigid perfectionism	Obsession with order and perfection	
Risk taking	Preference for dangerous or risky activities	
Separation insecurity	Fear of being abandoned	Negative affect
Submissiveness	Excessive compliance with others	
Suspiciousness	Distrust of others' intentions	
Unusual beliefs & experiences	Belief in extraordinary or implausible phenomena	Psychoticism
Withdrawal	Avoidance of social interactions	Detachment

non-clinical respondents, with average scores provided for comparison (Hopwood et al., 2015a, 2015b). LPFS-SR demonstrated strong validity with the PID-5, with many correlations on the PID scales exceeding 0.50. The LPFS-SR demonstrated notable associations with specific maladaptive traits measured by the PID-5. For instance, the identity component showed strong relationships with traits such as depressivity and emotional lability. Likewise, self-direction was connected to irresponsibility and distractibility, while empathy exhibited links to callousness and manipulativeness. Intimacy, on the other hand, was associated with withdrawal and avoidance of close relationships. Across its domains, the LPFS-SR reliably captured the severity of personality-based problems as reflected in the various maladaptive traits assessed by the PID-5 (Hopwood et al., 2015a; Hopwood et al., 2015b).

The Personality Inventory for ICD-11 (PiCD) centers on five major domains of maladaptive personality traits, as defined within the ICD-11 framework. The PiCD employs 60 items, 12 for each of the five domains, providing a comprehensive assessment of the personality traits in the ICD-11. Negative affective traits reflect a tendency toward distressing emotions, such as anxiety, irritability, and vulnerability, often triggered by minor stressors. Detachment is characterized by emotional distance, social withdrawal, and a lack of interpersonal engagement. The dissociality domain encompasses traits like callousness, aggression, manipulativeness, and a disregard for others, highlighting a significant impairment in being empathic. Disinhibition is linked to impulsivity and a lack of behavioral control, marked by irresponsibility and distractibility. In contrast, anankastic traits are defined by a preoccupation with order, perfectionism, and strict adherence to rules, focusing on self-regulation and control. The PiCD underscores a bipolar relationship between anankastic and disinhibition, viewing them as opposite ends of a behavioral spectrum.

The dimensions of personality mental health problems in AMPD (DSM-5) and ICD-11 frameworks share similarities while also presenting unique traits. Both models assess PDs based on impairments in self-functioning (identity, self-direction) and interpersonal functioning (empathy, intimacy), emphasizing severity levels ranging from mild to extreme impairment. Both the AMPD and ICD-11 use dimensional models to assess PDs, focusing on domains like negative affectivity (emotional instability and distress); detachment (social withdrawal and lack of experienced pleasure); antagonism/dissociality (hostility, manipulativeness, and callousness); and disinhibition (impulsivity, lack of control, and reckless behaviors). Other unique dimensions are psychoticism (eccentricity and unusual beliefs) in the AMPD and while ICD-11 features anankastia (perfectionism and rigidity). The dimensions of the severity, facets and traits of personality mental health problems can be assessed and measured by various structured, semi-structured, and self-report inventories that have been shown to have adequate psychometric properties.

Personality assessment is most frequently conducted through self-report inventories, wherein individuals are asked to indicate, rank, or acknowledge specific traits, attitudes, beliefs, or behaviors they perceive that they possess. There are hundreds of personality assessment instruments that are commercially available in the United States (Weiner & Greene, 2017). These instruments typically present respondents with targeted stimulus materials in the form of questions, statements, or descriptor lists. Self-report inventories have evolved to encompass not only descriptive items but also inquiries regarding beliefs, attitudes, and behaviors, covering broad assessments such as the Minnesota Multiphasic Personality Inventory (MMPI), 16 Personality Factors Questionnaire (16PF), and California Personality Inventory (CPI), as well as more focused assessments like the Beck Depression Inventory (BDI), State-Trait Anxiety Inventory (STAI), and State-Trait Anger Expression Inventory (STAXI). When selecting a self-report personality measure, it is essential to consider the characteristics of the standardization sample used for norming the instrument and its applicability to relevant populations. It should be noted that self-report inventories may not be suitable for certain groups, such as older adults, or individuals with impaired neurocognitive functioning as well as individuals living with SMI. In such cases, alternative assessment strategies including interviews, behavioral observations, or informant-based inventories completed by informants, caretakers and service providers may be warranted (Gregory, 2008).

Origins of Problems with Expressions of Problematic Personality-Based Behaviors

Personality develops from birth through adulthood. Individual differences in personality traits are recognized at birth and these differences are understood to arise from genetic endowment and neurobiological variables, changing with maturation and environmental factors until adulthood (Newton-Howes et al., 2015).

The expression of behaviors associated with personality is the result of complex interactions with genotypes, phenotypes, neurobiological variables, and environmental experiences. Continuous change and development occur with experiences across the entire life course in both the healthy and problematic ranges, as genotypes and phenotypical characteristics interact with environmental factors. PDs are influenced by genetic, biological, and environmental factors, including temperament, trauma, and socioeconomic conditions (Fariba et al., 2024). The pervasive effect of PDs when personality traits are extreme, and personality development is arrested, delayed, or derailed is many times overlooked in clinical practice. However, recognition of PDs has the potential to deepen understanding of individuals living with SMI and to enhance the ability to support them in managing their lives. PD is clinically significant throughout life, with potential effects on all mental and physical health problems.

Neurological Substrates

Understanding the neurobiological underpinnings of personality, especially maladaptive traits and features of personality problems, require examining how specific brain regions contribute to emotional, cognitive, and behavioral disturbances associated with PDs. Numerous studies (Allen et al., 2020; Gawda et al., 2016) have highlighted the nature of these neural mechanisms, revealing that personality is not localized to a single brain area, but instead emerges from intricate networks distributed throughout the brain.

The regions of the brain and how maladaptive personality facets and traits are impacted are as follows:

- Prefrontal cortex (PFC): Areas in the PFC influence maladaptive traits like impulsivity, emotional instability, and loss of executive control. Neurobiological impairments in prefrontal and limbic connectivity may underlie emotional dysregulation in response to perceived rejection or abandonment, resulting in separation insecurity that is linked to impairments in interpreting social norms and managing interpersonal relationships. The dorsolateral and dorsomedial prefrontal cortex (DLPFC/DMPFC) are central to executive functions (EFs) and cognitive control of emotions and covert events like evaluating perceptions, and the planning and execution of behaviors. Abnormalities in these regions are frequently observed in mental health problems, such as borderline personality (BPD) and antisocial personality mental health problems (ASPD). For instance, individuals with BPD may exhibit reduced volume in the anterior cingulate cortex (ACC) and orbitofrontal cortex (OFC), contributing to emotional instability, impulse control difficulties, and disorganized identity (Gawda et al., 2016). Similarly, ASPD is associated with diminished gray matter in the ventromedial prefrontal cortex (vmPFC) and ACC, which has been linked to deficits in moral reasoning, empathy, and impulse regulation. Other findings have shown increased influence on behaviors in regions such as the thalamus (thal), caudate nucleus (CN), and ACC (Allen et al., 2020; Gawda et al., 2016).
- Amygdala (amyg) and limbic structures: The amyg plays a critical role in emotional processing and threat detection. In maladaptive personality presentations, such as BPD, structural reductions and hyperactivity in this region are noted. The heightened amygdaloid responsivity is associated with emotional dysregulation, hypersensitivity to social threats, and intense emotional reactions. In combination with impaired prefrontal modulation, this can manifest as impulsivity and unstable relationships (Gawda et al., 2016).
- Medial temporal regions: Functional impairments in these regions—including the middle and inferior temporal gyri (MTG/ITG) and the amyg—have been linked to traits related to depressive covert behaviors. They are also part of the negative affectivity domain. These areas are critical for emotion regulation and impulse control, highlighting differences in depressive features between BPD and major depressive mental health problems (D'Adda et al., 2025). As with other areas associated with emotional regulation, findings have shown reduced control of behaviors in these areas (Allen et al., 2020; Gawda et al., 2016).
- Mesolimbic dopamine system: Impairments in this area are correlated with impulsive reward-seeking, risk-taking, and extremes of extraversion and sensation-seeking behaviors that can become maladaptive. These traits are linked to the dopaminergic system, particularly the ventral tegmental area (VTA),

nucleus accumbens (NAc), and OFC. Overactivity in these circuits may underlie impulsive reward-seeking and diminished capacity for delayed gratification, often observed in antisocial and substance use-prone personalities (Allen et al., 2020).

- Serotonergic system: The global serotonergic tone is believed to underpin trait stability, with individual differences in serotonin functioning influencing susceptibility to maladaptive traits. Low serotonergic activity may contribute to impulsivity, aggression, and emotional instability, as seen in BPD and ASPD (Allen et al., 2020).
- White matter integrity and neural connectivity: Research highlights reduced white matter integrity in the frontal lobes of individuals with traits that are high in openness (e.g., imaginative, curious, and creative) or psychoticism (e.g., odd thinking and eccentric) as defined in the FFM and AMPD, respectively, and have been linked to individuals living with schizotypal personality mental health problem (SPD). Such disruptions may lead to impaired communication between brain regions, manifesting as perceptual anomalies, disorganized thinking, and problems with reality testing (Allen et al., 2020; Gawda et al., 2016).
- Default and frontoparietal networks: The default mode network (DMN) and frontoparietal control network are implicated in self-referential processing and cognitive flexibility. Altered functional connectivity in these networks can contribute to maladaptive personality features, such as rigid thinking or excessive preoccupation with internal experiences, often seen in SPD and individuals with high openness.

Cumulatively, these findings underscore the importance of distributed brain circuits in shaping maladaptive personality expressions and highlight key targets for psychological and biological interventions (Allen et al., 2020; Gawda et al., 2016).

The inheritance of personality traits is influenced by genetic variance, which is typically measured through heritability estimates that represent the proportion of variance in liability to PDs that can be attributed to genetic factors. Twin studies suggest that personality traits have moderate heritability, with estimates ranging from 30% to 60% depending on the trait and study design. For example, identical twins show higher concordance in personality traits compared to non-identical twins, with heritability estimates around 40% predicted from parental trait values. Studies involving family membership and adoption have found lower heritability estimates (about 30%) (Sanchez-Roige et al., 2018).

Genome-wide association studies (GWAS) and polygenic analyses have demonstrated that personality traits are highly polygenic, meaning they are influenced by many genetic variants, each with small effects. SNP heritability, which measures the proportion of phenotypic variance explained by common genetic variants, ranges from 5% to 18% for personality traits. Environmental factors also play a role, interacting with genetic influences shaping personality traits. Gene–environmental interactions and non-shared environmental factors contribute to the variability in personality traits across individuals (Sanchez-Roige et al., 2018).

Research focusing on genetic heritability of PDs varies depending on the specific mental health problem and methodology. Generally, heritability estimates range from approximately 21% to 77% for different PDs. For personality mental health problems in Cluster A, estimates range from 21% to 72%, reflecting considerable variability depending on the specific disorder. Cluster B PDs show heritability estimates between 24% and 77%, while Cluster C PDs range from 27% to 77%. These findings underscore the significant role that genetics and environmental factors play in susceptibility to various PDs, though the extent of genetic influence can differ substantially (Reichborn-Kjennerud, 2010).

Behavioral and Environmental Substrates

The development of personality traits and mental health problems are a dynamic interplay between biological predispositions, environmental contexts, and learning histories. Contemporary dimensional models, such as the DSM-5 AMPD and the ICD-11 framework, emphasize impairments in self and interpersonal functioning alongside maladaptive trait expressions. Personality traits and their behavioral expression are influenced by genetic, evolutionary, and social variables. Genetic and environmental factors significantly influence traits, with about 40% of individual differences attributed to genes (Soto & Jackson, 2020). Shared family environment plays a substantial role in developing similar traits and the behavioral expression of the traits among individuals raised together, indicating importance of the role of role modeling and learning. Traits are also shaped by cultural influences and historical changes, with gender differences observed across various cultures (Araiba, 2020; Behaviorism, 1993).

Empirical research indicates that personality development is influenced by life experiences, encompassing professional roles and interpersonal relationships (Soto & Jackson, 2020). While personality traits tend to remain stable over short periods, extended timeframes may result in notable changes due to such experiences. Traits including neuroticism and conscientiousness are particularly susceptible to environmental factors, which can impact both mental health and behavioral patterns. Studies have shown that mean levels of traits such as agreeableness and conscientiousness typically rise with age, whereas neuroticism frequently decreases (Hopwood & Bleidorn, 2018; Soto & Jackson, 2020). Moreover, there is evidence suggesting that personality traits generally demonstrate greater stability than personality-related difficulties, with maladaptive traits often identified at an early stage and displaying more plasticity than previously assumed (Newton-Howes et al., 2015). Early interventions addressing trait vulnerabilities (for instance, elevated neuroticism or reduced conscientiousness) may mitigate progression toward recognizable personality mental health problems in individuals (Santesteban-Echarri et al., 2021). Acute stress, major life transitions, and therapeutic interventions are among the factors that can facilitate meaningful change. Developmental phases play a significant role; young adulthood is typically associated with increased instability, while middle adulthood is marked by improved emotional resilience and responsibility. These observations suggest that environmental exposures and educational opportunities across the lifespan contribute to the integration and evolution of both adaptive and maladaptive individual personality traits (Hopwood & Bleidorn, 2018).

Chess and Thomas (1977) identified that interactions between organisms and their environment shape new behavioral patterns in each succeeding age period as individuals develop even though certain factors appear to be determined at birth, such as temperament. Temperament is the foundation of personality traits and facets that are assumed to be biologically determined and present early in life; it includes such characteristics as energy level, emotional responsiveness, demeanor, mood, response tempo, behavioral inhibition, and willingness to explore (American Psychological Association, n.d.-b). Depending on environmental changes, some temperament factors remain influential, and others become dominant or lose significance. Chess and Thomas (1977) recognized that child–parent relationships are bi-directional, introducing the "goodness of fit" model, which states that optimal development occurs when environmental demands align with individual traits; poor fit—including cultural, economic, and familial contexts—can lead to maladaptation (McClowry et al., 2008). "Goodness of fit results when the properties of the environment and its expectations and demands are in accord with the organism's own capacities, characteristics, and style of behaving" (Chess & Thomas, 2013, pp. 3). If there is a match between an individual's temperament and the environment, optimal development can be achieved.

The environment is a significant factor in the development of personality and its expression, depending on the topography and the dimensions of the environmental events. Alterations in behavioral expression of personality traits can be sudden and intense if the salient environmental event is extreme. In 1848, Phineas Gage, a 25-year-old railroad worker, experienced a serious brain injury that affected his frontal lobes. Following his recovery, notable changes were observed in his personality. Before the accident, he was regarded as moderate and even-tempered; however, after the injury, the physician who treated him, noted, "He is fitful, irreverent, indulging at times in the grossest profanity, which was not previously his custom." His accident and subsequent recovery revealed the crucial role certain areas of the brain has in personality and social behavior, providing early evidence for brain localization, demonstrating the brain's capacity for healing, and highlighting the importance of secondary brain damage (Hamilton, 2017).

While not as severe as traumatic brain injury (TBI), the causes of PDs are diverse, involving factors such as adverse childhood experiences, relational trauma, and sociocultural influences (Chanen, 2024; Ekselius, 2018). Neuroimaging research shows that environmental stressors may alter neural circuits involved in emotion regulation and social cognition, which can contribute to trait expression linked to personality trait impairments (Ekselius, 2018). These environmental factors interact with genetic predispositions and help shape consistent patterns of thought, emotion, and behavior. Multiple traumatic events over a lifetime may play a role in the development of personality traits and expressions. Early challenges and trauma show a strong association with increased risk for PDs, particularly BPD, characterized by emotional dysregulation, unstable interpersonal relationships, and identity disturbance.

Although genetic contributions to severe PDs are notable, environmental factors are also important in their manifestation and progression. Early intervention and supportive environments have potential to reduce risk and foster adaptive functioning, highlighting the capacity for change in personality traits (Chanen, 2024; Ekselius, 2018).

Trauma does not create traits "ex nihilo," but it can amplify, distort, or entrench existing predispositions. The FFM provides a useful scaffold for examining these effects. High neuroticism, for instance, is associated with emotional instability and vulnerability to stress—traits that may be exacerbated by trauma, leading to chronic anxiety, depression, or dissociative tendencies (Soto & Jackson, 2020). Conversely, traits like agreeableness and conscientiousness may be suppressed in individuals exposed to betrayal or neglect, resulting in interpersonal mistrust or impulsivity.

Both the AMPD and ICD-11 frameworks conceptualize PDs as impairments in functioning coupled with maladaptive traits, many of which are shaped or intensified by trauma. Criterion A of the AMPD assesses severity through domains like identity and intimacy, which are often compromised in trauma survivors. Criterion B includes traits such as negative affectivity, disinhibition, and detachment, which may reflect learned responses to chronic stress or relational harm (Krueger & Hobbs, 2020).

The ICD-11 similarly identifies trait domains that resonate with trauma-linked adaptations. For instance, negative affectivity may stem from chronic emotional invalidation or fear-based conditioning while detachment may reflect learned avoidance of intimacy following relational trauma. Dissociality may emerge in contexts of exploitation or neglect, fostering callousness or mistrust; disinhibition may be reinforced by chaotic environments lacking structure or safety, and anankastia may develop as a compensatory strategy for control in unpredictable settings (Bach & First, 2018). These traits represent enduring adaptations to adverse environments, often with significant clinical implications. PDs are generally less stable than normative traits, particularly in adolescence and young adulthood, a period marked by heightened vulnerability to trauma. This developmental window is critical; traumatic experiences during these developmental phases can derail normative personality maturation, entrenching maladaptive traits and impairments in functioning (Hopwood & Bleidorn, 2018).

Research suggests that personality is modifiable. Maladaptive personality traits may change over the lifespan and could be more flexible than previously assumed. Environmental factors such as therapeutic interventions, supportive relationships, and corrective experiences have been observed to influence trait expression, including individuals with significant problematic expression of personality traits (Chanen, 2024).

The development of personality traits and facets that are represented in the domains and dimensions of personality assessment tools are based on the psycholexical approach to personality. This approach is called the "lexical hypothesis," which posits that the significant individual differences in personality are encoded in natural language and involve constructing comprehensive lists of person-descriptive terms. There is a close connection between important personality traits and behavior-descriptive adjectives that people use to represent their intentions, beliefs, characteristics, and thoughts. (Morin, 2011; Piedmont & Aycock, 2007; tailcalled, 2023; Volungevičienė et al., 2022). The FFM, most common personality theory, was developed using this approach.

Skinner (1965) postulated that personality or an individual's statements about oneself is based on unified systems of covert and overt responses that are shaped by environmental contingencies. Personality may be defined as set of responses based on topographical subdivisions of behavior within the single individual. For instance, the person may be described as a "social butterfly" as he manifests behaviors such as meeting other people, enjoying social situations, and participates in activities with others, but his main interest is in pursuing fishing by himself in a boat in the middle of a lake. Although topographically dissimilar, these descriptors are about the same person.

Personality can be associated with specific situations in which a system of responses is organized around a particular discriminative stimulus (S^D). Behaviors that are effective for obtaining reinforcement in one context are grouped together and differentiated from a response class of behaviors that are effective in response to other stimuli. For instance, an individual may be perceived as a highly driven CEO who is exacting and unyielding with colleagues, yet exhibit distinctly different behaviors and expressions of personality within a family environment.

A set of responses which lead to a common reinforcement regardless of the situation may also comprise a functional system as well. A person who is described as "always thinking about her own needs" is an individual where the motivating operation of deprivation is the organizing stimuli for displayed behaviors. However, the manifested behaviors may be different when the person is able to attain satiation of the deprived stimulus (e.g., food, social attention, and money) and is said to be "easygoing, relaxed and tolerant."

Covert respondents or emotional variables also can establish the expression of personality traits in certain contexts and S^Ds. The person who is seen as a "peace maker" may engage in violent behavior to protect his loved ones when they are threatened. The effects of environmental stimuli like drugs or trauma can also impact the expression of personality traits. The use of certain drugs like methamphetamine can result in behaviors that have a low probability of occurrence and reinforcement in many contexts. An example would be a lawyer who is under the physiological condition of a stimulant who attempts to leave a restaurant while not paying the bill. These organized sets of responses or repertoires in language, cognitive, emotional-motivational, and sensory-motor behaviors are acquired through cumulative-hierarchical learning, where simpler behaviors scaffold the development of more complex ones. Personality is both a dependent variable (shaped by learning conditions) and an independent variable (influencing future behavior and learning) (Staats, 1993).

Environmental contingencies and reinforcement histories determine which repertoires are strengthened or inhibited. For example, emotional responses learned through repeated exposure to specific stimuli become motivational drivers, influencing preferences and aversions. Similarly, language-cognitive repertoires enable individuals to interpret and respond to private events, shaping internal narratives and self-concept (Staats, 1993).

Expressions of personality traits and PDs can be understood as learned behavioral repertoires shaped by environmental contingencies (Skinner, 1965; Staats, 1993). For example, avoidant behavior may be maintained by negative reinforcement (e.g., escape from social anxiety), while attention-seeking behavior may be positively reinforced by social validation (e.g., in histrionic PD); perfectionism in OCPD (e.g., anankastia in ICD-11) reflects rigid rule-governed behavior that is shaped by reinforcement history.

The integration of multiple responses can lead to the personification of behaviors that are influenced by environmental factors. While a relatively consistent response system may give rise to expectations of behavioral uniformity and functional integrity, such consistency may not always be present. Alternatively, it is preferable to address observed covariations in response strength or frequency across varying antecedent conditions and reinforcing outcomes within a given context instead of inferring consistency in trait expression.

The absence of self-knowledge can influence the concept of personality. Self-knowledge functions because of self-awareness, which may be limited when reinforcing stimuli are not connected to behaviors associated with self-awareness. An individual may not recognize their actions, past behavior, intentions, or be aware of the factors and outcomes linked to their actions (Skinner, 1965). Self-awareness is described as the ability to focus on the stimuli that influences the occurrence of covert and overt behaviors of oneself. In this state, a person identifies, processes, and retains information about himself, including experiences, emotions, thoughts, traits, preferences, goals, and other aspects. It also encompasses a sense of continuity over time and the perception of being disparate from one's surroundings (Morin, 2011).

Self-knowledge involves understanding one's own self-concept, which includes covert self-talk about traits, abilities, emotions, and behaviors. This understanding covers personal characteristics, behaviors, and mental states. Individuals with self-awareness typically provide more accurate self-reports and display better insights into their physical and psychological traits.

Self-awareness can be acquired and developed through life. It appears during infancy and is sustained by mechanisms such as social reinforcement, exposure to self-focused stimuli (for example, mirrors and media), imitation, internal processes like inner speech and imagery, and activation of particular brain regions (Morin, 2011). Practices such as self-evaluation, self-regulation, perspective-taking, and environments promoting self-reflection can contribute to improving self-awareness.

The social effects of personality are the psychological (emotional, cognitive, and motivational) reactions evoked in other people by the observed expression of personality traits in behavior and emotion (Volungevičienė et al., 2022). From the transactional view on personality, the psycholexical structures of social effects can help to discover unique vs. common thought and behavior patterns, affects, and motivations, which are primarily related to personality dispositions (Soto & Jackson, 2020). Psychological structure of social effects are the covert and overt verbal adjectives and descriptors that occur in reference to another's behaviors. Social effects are temporary psychological reactions to the expression of dispositions, which means social effects are states by their nature. When recurrent relationships and consistent patterns of social effects are observed, persoanlity dispositions are manifested by repeated behavioral patterns. These interact with common emotional, motivational, and cognitive reponses associated with the expressed traits by others. (Volungevičienė et al., 2022).

Self-awareness is defined as the capacity to become the object of one's own attention (Morin, 2011). Self-awareness entails an individual intentionally identifies, "thinks about," and remembers information about himself. While one may consciously experience sensory input, self-awareness arises when a person recognizes and considers his own experience (for example, acknowledging that "I see a blue object" or "I am eating food, and it tastes good").

Self-awareness is a complex, multidimensional phenomenon that encompasses numerous aspects of the self. It includes the ability to think about one's past as well as to anticipate the future. Furthermore, individuals can direct their focus toward a wide range of self-focused domains such as their emotions, thoughts, beliefs, personality traits, preferences, goals, attitudes, perceptions, sensations, and intentions (Morin, 2011).

A distinction can be made between private and public dimensions of self-awareness. Private self-aspects, such as emotions and traits, are internal and not directly observable, while public self-dimensions include visible characteristics such as physical appearance, mannerisms, and behaviors. This multifaceted understanding of self-awareness highlights the complexity of how individuals come to know, reflect on, and self-report about themselves—that is, describing their personality.

The expression of behaviors by an individual is subject to individual face-to-face interactions as well as the wider social audience from which the person receives feedback. Verbal and non-verbal feedback during the social interaction becomes an aspect of the individual "thinking about" her behavior that can result in the feedback becoming part of the person's awareness about herself. If she thinks that the feedback is valid or reinforcing, then it may be incorporated into the verbal repertoire of describing the type of person she is. She may find the feedback onerous and distressing and escape from the aversive respondents associated with the feedback by making self-statements that she "is not like that." Negative feedback then will not be used in self-descriptors.

Observed patterns of topographically and functionally related behaviors by the social audience can be correlated with a person's self-reports of traits. This positive or negative correlation results in the social audience labeling the person as deficit in self-awareness, using descriptors as "being in denial," "lack of insight," "not willing to accept," and "lying."

It should be noted that personality assessment tools have been criticized for being prone to influence by response styles such as social desirability and acquiescence, thereby compromising the measurement of the trait-related contents of the scales (Bäckström & Björklund, 2013) including the FFM and other instruments.

The expression of behaviors (e.g., traits) is the function of antecedent and consequential environmental stimuli. How an individual describes herself or another person is environmentally determined through learning. Everyone receives and reads or hears feedback about their behaviors that are displayed. This feedback then "labels" the behaviors, making inferences about causality, antecedent, and discriminative stimuli, and generalization of the behavior across contexts, resulting in personality traits that are presumed to occur across multiple situations.

Verbal statements provided by the social audience of a person's behaviors serve as tools through which individuals verbally articulate their behaviors in specific contexts; these "labels" or descriptors form a component of self-statements that emerge when one is prompted or reflects on their actions, thus shaping self-concept through language. In certain cases, individuals may encounter linguistic environments characterized by limited vocabulary (lexical limitation) and constrained grammatical structures (syntactic limitation). Such restrictions can impede self-knowledge by reducing the availability of descriptive terms for expressing behaviors under particular circumstances (Rezaii et al., 2022). The findings may explain the challenges of some of the descriptors used in dimensions of personality traits as pre-industrial non-western cultures have limited contexts that are connected to the descriptors in established theories of personality (Piedmont & Aycock, 2007). These limitations can also arise in socially deprived settings, within some cultural backgrounds and when the person has neurocognitive impairments.

The social effects of behavior represent the psychological (emotional, cognitive, and motivational) reactions evoked in other people by the expression of traits in behavior and emotion. From the view on personality, studying the psycholexical structures of social effects can help to discover unique vs. common thought and behavior patterns, affects, and motivations, which are primarily related to personality dispositions (Soto & Jackson, 2020).

As stated previously, personality is a complex multidimensional construct that involves interactions with others in one's environment. For example, a person becomes frequently emotionally distressed and displays this distress by crying and stating to the social audience that she is "upset and cannot control myself." The social audience responds by making compassionate and empathetic statements to her with the intent of calming her down and helping her regain control. The social audience engages in verbal statements that she "overreacts and makes a big deal out of everything" and that "she is just doing it for attention." This person may tell others that she is "high strung and emotional" and relates that her mother was the same way. If a comprehensive functional behavioral assessment was conducted, it may be discovered that her father was an alcoholic who was unemotional and unavailable to other family members; he would abuse the mother, stopping only when this person would cry and behave "hysterically" when the father's response class of abusive behaviors were displayed. The person's "hysterical" behaviors were negatively reinforced by the father terminating his abusive behaviors towards the mother. She has had difficulty maintaining close relationships because of her emotionally reactive behavior. She has described herself as "emotional and sensitive," while the social audience has labeled her as "histrionic, easily overwhelmed, and emotionally unstable." Using the traits and facets of personality of the FFM, the AMPD, and the ICD-11, she would be described as high in neuroticism, as she has a propensity to experience negative emotions, such as anger, anxiety, depression, exhibiting emotional instability, and lack of impulse control. Individuals high in neuroticism are more emotionally reactive and prone to anxiety, mood swings, and stress, having trouble coping with adversity.

Based on the traits of personality disorders as described in the AMPD and ICD-11, this individual presents with elevated negative affectivity, which involves recurring and intense experiences of negative emotions such as anxiety, depression, guilt, and anger, along with dependency (American Psychiatric Association, 2022b). The person also exhibits a moderate level of disinhibition, indicated by impulsivity and a tendency toward immediate gratification (American Psychiatric Association, 2022b). According to ICD-11 severity criteria (WHO, 2022), the level of impairment is considered moderate, affecting specific domains such as relationships or achieving personal goals, while not impacting all areas of life. If the individual were to seek support from a mental health provider, they may be identified with histrionic personality disorder per the DSM-5-TR (American Psychiatric Association, 2022a), which encompasses patterns of pronounced emotional expression and attention-seeking behavior.

Epidemiology and Cultural Considerations

Personality mental health problems (PDs) are enduring patterns of overt and covert behaviors and private events (i.e., self-talk, perceptions, and emotional respondents) that deviate from cultural norms and impair functioning. Despite their clinical significance, PDs remain under-recognized in global mental health frameworks.

Personality disorders (PDs) are defined by persistent maladaptive patterns of cognition, affectivity, interpersonal functioning, and impulse control (American Psychological Association, n.d.-c; American Psychological Association, 2024; American Psychiatric Association, 2022b, 2024). These disorders often emerge in adolescence or early adulthood and are associated with significant distress, functional impairment, and increased healthcare utilization. Despite their chronicity and impact, PDs have historically been marginalized in mental health classification and global health policy (Chanen, 2024; Ekselius, 2018).

Recent shifts toward dimensional models, such as the DSM-5 Alternative Model for Personality Disorders (AMPD) and ICD-11, have reframed PDs as impairments in functioning modulated by maladaptive traits (Swales, 2022; Zimmermann et al., 2019).

A systematic review and meta-analysis by Winsper et al. (2020) estimated the global pooled prevalence of any PD at 7.8% with a confidence interval of 6.1–9.5%.

Volkert et al. (2018) reported a higher prevalence of 12.16% in Western adult populations. Cluster-specific rates include 2.8% for Cluster B (dramatic/emotional), 5.0% for Cluster C (anxious/fearful), and 3.8% for Cluster A (odd/eccentric) (American Psychiatric Association, 2024). Notably, prevalence estimates vary based on diagnostic methodology, with structured interviews yielding higher rates than unstructured assessments (Zimmerman et al., 2005).

Prevalence rates differ markedly across regions and income levels. High-income countries report a prevalence of 9.6%, compared to 4.3% in low- and middle-income countries (Winsper et al., 2020). For example:

- United States: Estimated prevalence of 9.1%, with obsessive-compulsive PD (OCPD) and borderline PD (BPD) among the most common (Fariba et al., 2024)
- Western Europe: England (10.7%), Norway (13.4%) (Gawda, 2018)
- Asia: China (4.1%), Lebanon (6.2%)
- Africa: Nigeria (2.7%), South Africa (6.5%)

These disparities may reflect differences in mental health services' accessibility, cultural stigma, and mental health prioritization. Cultural norms influence the expression and recognition of PDs, with collectivist societies less likely to pathologize traits such as dependency or submissiveness (Gawda, 2018; Loranger et al., 1997).

Socioeconomic status (SES) is a significant determinant of PD risk. Individuals from lower SES backgrounds are more likely to experience early adversity, chronic stress, and limited access to care, factors that contribute to maladaptive personality development (Newton-Howes et al., 2015). Cultural context also shapes the perception and recognition of PDs. For instance, traits like emotional expressiveness may be pathologized in Western settings but normalized in Latin American cultures (Caballo et al., 2024).

Cross-cultural studies reveal that PDs are both universal and culturally modulated. While the underlying neurobiological mechanisms may be consistent, their behavioral manifestations and clinical interpretations vary (Gawda, 2018; Piedmont & Aycock, 2007).

PDs frequently co-occur with SMIs such as schizophrenia spectrum, bipolar (BD), and major depression (MDD) mental health problems (Table 18.3). Zimmerman et al. (2005) found that 45.5% of psychiatric outpatients met criteria for a PD according to the criteria in the DSM-IV, with avoidant, borderline, and OCPD being most prevalent. It has been reported that 45% of individuals living with both PDs and BPD had increased psychological symptoms and reduced treatment efficacy (Barbato & Hafner, 1998). It is noted that up to half of individuals living with a major mental health problem can be identified as living with a PD, making it one of the most common mental health problems (Newton-Howes et al., 2015). Fok et al. (2014) reported that people living with co-occurring PD and SMI were 2.3 times more likely to be high inpatient service users and 1.56 times more likely to experience involuntarily hospitalization. Comorbid PDs are associated with higher psychiatric service use, poorer treatment outcomes, and greater functional impairment (Tyrer & Simmonds, 2003). Routine assessment of personality

Table 18.3 Summary of comorbidity patterns of PD and SMI mental health problems

SMI Mental health problem	Common comorbid PDs	Clinical implications
Schizophrenia	Schizotypal, paranoid	Diagnostic overlap complicates treatment
Bipolar disorder	Borderline, narcissistic	Increased suicidality, poor medication response (Barbato & Hafner, 1998)
Major depression	Avoidant, dependent	Chronicity and treatment resistance (Khan et al., 2005)

functioning in people living with SMI is recommended to improve intervention, planning, and reduce relapse (Chanen, 2024).

Early intervention is critical, particularly in youth and marginalized populations. Despite evidence supporting the validity of the detection of PD in adolescents, stigma and reluctance persist in the recognition of PDs in younger individuals (Newton-Howes et al., 2015). Culturally informed assessment and treatment approaches are essential to reduce misidentification and improve access to care; they are essential for accurate, effective treatment, and equitable care. Future research should prioritize longitudinal studies, cross-cultural validation, and integration of personality assessment routinely into mental health services.

Types of Personality Mental Health Problems

Personality mental health problems (PDs) have typically been described using categorical models, which may result in overlapping identification of maladaptive personality traits, limited clinical relevance, and challenges with cross-cultural applicability. Recent frameworks such as ICD-11, DSM-5 Alternative Model for Personality Disorders (AMPD), and the Five-Factor Model (FFM) employ dimensional approaches, conceptualizing PDs as impairments in personality functioning shaped by maladaptive characteristics (McCabe & Widiger, 2020; Oltmanns & Widiger, 2018). While these models broadly agree on structural features and classifications of PDs, notable differences exist concerning their implementation within mental health systems. Each framework provides unique, yet intersecting, perspectives on PD typologies, outlining methods for distinguishing personality impairments and offering possibilities for translating categorically defined PD types across different models.

The ICD-11 model eliminated most of the identification of categorical-based PDs in favor of the detection of "Personality Disorder," specified by the following dimensions:

- Severity levels: Ranging as mild, moderate, and severe. Severity is determined by impairments in self-functioning (e.g., identity and self-worth) and interpersonal functioning (e.g., intimacy and conflict resolution), with traits serving as descriptors rather than diagnostic thresholds (Bach & First, 2018).

- Trait domains: These include the dimensional traits of negative affectivity; detachment; dissociality; disinhibition; and anankastia. A borderline pattern qualifier is included, which is an addition to preserving the recognition of borderline features displayed by an individual.

The detection and identification of PD using the ICD-11 criteria are done by first identifying persistent, pervasive disturbances in self-functioning (e.g., identity and self-worth) and/or interpersonal functioning (e.g., relationships and empathy). If these impairments are significant and meet the criteria, a general personality mental health problem is determined and then specified by a severity level (mild, moderate, or severe) (Mulder, 2021; Swales, 2022). Additionally, the identification is further described by one or more five maladaptive trait domains such as negative affectivity, detachment, dissociality, disinhibition, anankastia, and possibly a borderline pattern. For example, a PD using the ICD-11 could be a "moderate personality disorder with negative affectivity and dissociality" (Swales, 2022). The borderline pattern modifier consists of the nine features to identify the presence of borderline PD that is outlined in the DSM-5-TR (American Psychiatric Association, 2022a). Bach and First (2018) outlined the use of the borderline pattern qualifier. This descriptive qualifier "may be applied to individuals whose pattern of maladaptive personality behavioral expression is characterized by a pervasive pattern of instability of interpersonal relationships, self-image, and affects, and marked impulsivity" (Bach & First, 2018, p. 6), as indicated by five (or more) of the following:

- Frantic efforts to avoid real or imagined abandonment.
- A pattern of unstable and intense interpersonal relationships, typically characterized by alternating between extremes of idealization and devaluation.
- Identity disturbance, manifested in markedly and persistently unstable self-image or sense of self.
- Impulsivity manifested in potentially self-damaging behaviors (e.g., risky sexual behavior, reckless driving, excessive alcohol or substance use, and binge eating).
- Recurrent episodes of self-harm (e.g., suicide attempts or gestures, and self-mutilation).
- Emotional instability due to marked reactivity of mood. Fluctuations of mood may be triggered either internally (e.g., by one's own thoughts) or by external events. As a consequence, the individual experiences intense dysphoric mood states, which typically last a few hours but may last up to several days.
- Chronic feelings of emptiness.
- Inappropriate intense anger or difficulty controlling anger manifested in frequent displays of temper (e.g., yelling or screaming, throwing or breaking things, and getting into physical fights).
- Transient dissociative symptoms or psychotic-like features (e.g., brief hallucinations and paranoia) in situations of high affective arousal.

Other manifestations of borderline patterns, not all of which may be present in a given individual at a given time, include the following:

- A view of the self as inadequate, bad, guilty, disgusting, and contemptible

- An experience of the self as profoundly different and isolated from other people
- A painful sense of alienation and pervasive loneliness
- Proneness to rejection hypersensitivity
- Problems in establishing and maintaining consistent and appropriate levels of trust in interpersonal relationships
- Frequent misinterpretation of social signals

The DSM-5-TR (American Psychiatric Association, 2022a, 2024) differentiates nine types of maladaptive personality mental health problems which include the following:

- Antisocial personality disorder (ASPD): Marked by a persistent disregard for others' rights, requiring evidence of conduct disorder before age 15 and at least three ongoing traits such as lawbreaking, deceit, impulsivity, aggression, irresponsibility, or lack of remorse; identification is limited to adults, especially males. It is often missed due to co-occurring conditions and reluctance to seek help. Symptoms may lessen over time, but functional issues remain. Behavior-analytic methods targeting maladaptive behaviors through assessment and reinforcement strategies have some beneficial effect.
- Avoidant: Defined by extreme shyness and sensitivity to criticism, leading to difficulty forming relationships and avoiding social or career opportunities.
- Borderline personality disorder (BPD): Involves unstable emotions, intense relationships, fear of abandonment, impulsivity, and self-destructive behaviors. Identity and mood are frequently unstable.
- Dependent: Characterized by reliance on others for decisions and support, fear of being alone, and urgent pursuit of new relationships when one ends.
- Histrionic: Marked by dramatic, attention-seeking behavior, emotional exaggeration, discomfort without central attention, and superficial relationships.
- Narcissistic: Features an inflated sense of self-importance, entitlement, lack of empathy, need for admiration, and exploitation of others.
- Obsessive-compulsive personality disorder (OCPD): Displays a pattern of perfectionism, orderliness, inflexibility, workaholism, and difficulty discarding useless items (distinct from obsessive compulsive mental health problem).
- Paranoid: Displays distrust and suspicion towards others, interpreting benign actions as threats, holding grudges, and fearing disloyalty.
- Schizoid: Exhibits emotional detachment, prefers solitude, indifferent to both criticism and praise, and has little interest in social or sexual interactions.
- Schizotypal: Characterized by eccentric behavior, odd beliefs, paranoia, social anxiety, few close relationships, and distorted perceptions of reality.

The DSM-5 AMPD (American Psychiatric Association, 2022b, 2024) is a hybrid framework that is comprised of both categorical and dimensional frameworks, using severity rating of impairments, categorical classification of PD types, and dimensions of maladaptive personality traits along the lines of the FFM and the ICD-11 (American Psychiatric Association, 2024). AMPD uses a two-part process to provide a more nuanced diagnosis than the standard categorical system. A mental health service provider evaluates (1) if the individual is living with impairments in the level of personality functioning (LPF) (i.e., Criterion A) and the degree of severity rated on a continuum and (2) determines the pathological personality traits (i.e., Criterion B) that are being expressed (American Psychiatric Association, 2024).

The LPF (Criterion A) assesses the severity of a person's difficulties in two core areas, rated on a continuum from little to no impairment (=0) to extreme impairment (=4). The identification of a PD requires at least a moderate (=2) or greater impairment in at least two of the following four subdomains as follows:

- Self-functioning: This includes (a) identity which is a person's stable sense of self, including their self-esteem, self-appraisal, and emotional regulation; and (b) self-direction, that is, the ability to set and achieve goals, reflect on one's behavior, and use constructive internal standards.
- Interpersonal functioning: This is comprised of (a) empathy which is the capacity to understand and appreciate others' experiences and perspectives; and (b) intimacy which is the ability to form and maintain deep, mutual, and satisfying relationships.

If the determination is made that the person is living with impairment in two or more of the subdomains (i.e., meeting impairment criteria for Criterion A), then the mental health service provider assesses the person for the presence on five broad problematic trait domains, which are maladaptive versions of the traits in the FFM (Criterion B). Each domain is composed of several specific trait "facets."

- Negative affectivity: Experiencing frequent and intense negative emotions (e.g., anxiety, anger, and shame)
- Detachment: Withdrawal from social interactions and emotional expression (e.g., social withdrawal and anhedonia)
- Antagonism: Behaviors that put a person at odds with others (e.g., manipulativeness, deceitfulness, and grandiosity)
- Disinhibition: Impulsive behaviors aimed at immediate gratification rather than long-term planning (e.g., irresponsibility and risk-taking)
- Psychoticism: Unusual or eccentric beliefs, perceptions, and behaviors (e.g., eccentricity and odd thoughts).

Trait profiles are assessed using instruments like the PID-5, which operationalize 25 facets of maladaptive traits (Krueger et al., 2012a, 2012b).

Based on the severity of impairment (Criterion A) and the constellation of problematic expression of traits (Criterion B), a mental health service provider can arrive at one of two following conclusions regarding the identification of a mental health problem:

- A specified PD: The AMPD defines six specific personality disorder categories (antisocial, avoidant, borderline, narcissistic, obsessive-compulsive, and schizotypal) based on specific combinations of functional impairment and characteristic trait profiles. For example, a diagnosis of narcissistic personality disor-

der requires moderate impairment in at least two areas of functioning (Criterion A) combined with specific traits of grandiosity and attention-seeking (Criterion B).
- Personality disorder–trait specified (PD-TS): This identification of a mental health problem is used when a person meets the general criteria for a PD, but their specific pattern of traits does not align with one of the six named types. In this case, the mental health service provider lists the specific trait domains and facets that are clinically significant.

The FFM conceptualizes maladaptive personality types across a continuum of five domains. FFM enables cross-cultural and lifespan assessment but lacks formal diagnostic thresholds. The following are the FFM domains and the behavioral expression of the maladaptive FFM variant that impairs an individual's functioning and adjustment:

- Neuroticism: Emotional lability, anxiousness, and hostility
- Extraversion: Withdrawal and attention seeking
- Openness: Perceptual dysregulation and eccentricity
- Agreeableness: Callousness and manipulativeness
- Conscientiousness: Rigid perfectionism and irresponsibility

Meta-analytic studies (Bagby & Widiger, 2020; Samuel & Widiger, 2008) confirm that the DSM PDs can be understood as maladaptive extremes of FFM traits. For example, borderline PD aligns with high neuroticism and low agreeableness, while obsessive-compulsive PD reflects high conscientiousness and low openness. Table 18.4 illustrates how categorical PDs listed in the DSM-5-TR translate across ICD-11, AMPD, and FFM domains.

Table 18.4 demonstrates the substantial convergence across the PD identification systems, particularly in the domains of negative affectivity and detachment. However, differences in trait definitions (e.g., anankastia vs. conscientiousness) and trait dimensionality and polarity complicate direct translations across the models and frameworks.

Integrating these models can improve precision of identifying PDs, reduce comorbidity artifacts, and support personalized treatment. For example, the borderline pattern specifier in ICD-11 captures core features of BPD, but PID-5 facets add dimensional specificity in assessing impulsivity and emotional lability (McCabe & Widiger, 2020).

The dimensional reconceptualization of personality disorders within the ICD-11, DSM-5 AMPD, and FFM frameworks represents a notable development in the identification and classification of PDs and typologies. Although each model offers distinct advantages, their alignment concerning trait domains and severity highlights a collective emphasis on empirical validity and clinical applicability. Ongoing research should prioritize the harmonization of trait definitions, the validation of dimensional convergence, and the advancement of cultural sensitivity in personality assessment.

Table 18.4 Categorical PDs in the DSM-5-TR translated across ICD-11, AMPD, and FFM domains

DSM-5-TR PD type	ICD-11 traits	AMPD traits	FFM profile
Antisocial	Dissociality, disinhibition	Antagonism, disinhibition	Low agreeableness, low conscientiousness
Avoidant	Detachment, negative affectivity	Detachment, negative affectivity	High neuroticism, low extraversion
Borderline	Negative affectivity, disinhibition	Negative affectivity, disinhibition	High neuroticism, low agreeableness
Narcissistic	Dissociality	Antagonism	High extraversion, low agreeableness
OCPD	Anankastia	Rigid perfectionism, perseveration	High conscientiousness, low openness
Schizotypal	Detachment, psychoticism	Detachment, psychoticism	High openness, low extraversion
Paranoid	Dissociality, negative affectivity	Suspiciousness, hostility	Low agreeableness, high neuroticism
Dependent	Negative affectivity	Submissiveness	High agreeableness, high neuroticism
Histrionic	Disinhibition, attention seeking	Attention seeking, emotional lability	High extraversion, high neuroticism
Schizoid	Detachment	Withdrawal, restricted affectivity	Low extraversion, low openness

Why Are Problems with Expressions of Personality Traits Important in Understanding and Treating Individuals Living with SMI?

Individuals who exhibit extreme personality traits often encounter greater challenges when adapting to difficult circumstances. For example, Daniel, discussed below, demonstrated strong qualities as a dependable person who adhered to the hospital routine; he consistently fulfilled expectations within the hospital setting due to structured routines and reminders from staff, such as assistance with getting out of bed or attending group sessions. Hospital mental health service professionals and staff frequently described him as an exemplary patient. However, Daniel struggled in situations that demanded personal initiative. Outside the hospital environment, he did not adhere to treatment recommendations, primarily because there was no one available to guide or prompt him regarding necessary behaviors. It is not uncommon for individuals to face difficulties resulting from an inability to adjust specific behavioral manifestations of their personality traits to varying contexts.

Personality characteristics can become pronounced and maladaptive due to the impact of significant life stressors. Individuals encountering substantial challenges, such as unemployment, inadequate housing, financial constraints, limited social support, isolation, or substance use, may find it more difficult to respond in an adaptive manner. Those living with SMI may experience cognitive difficulties, memory issues, and various other complications associated with their condition. When multiple stressors accumulate, individuals who are typically agreeable and cooperative might withdraw from social interactions, resulting in an inability to make independent decisions without external guidance, and permitting others to exploit them repeatedly. Others may develop feelings of anger or suspicion, perceiving a lack of trust from those around them. Consequently, certain personality traits become less adaptive, and their behavioral manifestations may exacerbate existing challenges.

The most significant challenge faced by mental health service providers and staff is that certain personality traits can hinder the effectiveness of support efforts. Since these traits typically develop during childhood and adolescence, modifying them often requires considerable time. This issue is especially pertinent to professionals in mental health settings, who frequently encourage individuals living with SMI to engage in behaviors they may not currently perform at typical frequency, duration, or magnitude, or may be exhibiting in inappropriate contexts. Personality characteristics can influence how an individual responds to expectations such as taking medication, attending club activities, participating in recovery planning and treatment, or adhering to reminders to maintain daily routines. For instance, someone with an identity of being independent may become argumentative or resistant when encouraged to undertake actions they do not wish to pursue. Conversely, individuals like Dan may demonstrate high levels of cooperation within supportive, structured environments, but are less likely to adhere to treatment recommendations outside of such settings.

Problems with the expression of personality traits likewise relate to the behaviors of mental health service providers and staff as well. Giving support to a person living with SMI is a stressor. This will challenge the person's ability to be adaptive when faced with the many challenges of interacting with a person living with SMI. Individual personality traits may influence one's approach, potentially resulting in either excessive persistence or premature withdrawal; some individuals may react strongly and discontinue their efforts. The conduct of mental health service providers and staff plays a significant role in shaping adaptive behaviors, ongoing recovery, and reducing the risk of re-hospitalization for those living with SMI. Seeking guidance from support groups or qualified mental health service professionals and obtaining ongoing supervision and training will help in overcoming personal challenges when interacting with individuals living with SMI.

Common Personality Problems Seen in People Living with Serious Mental Illness

The types of challenges faced by mental health service providers and staff when supporting individuals with SMI are influenced by these characteristics. Furthermore, individuals with varying personality traits may respond differently to interactions with others. Understanding a person's personality can assist mental health professionals in determining the most effective approach for working with individuals living with SMI, which may help minimize complications and promote positive adaptive behaviors.

Personality mental health problems represent pronounced manifestations of typical personality traits. Individuals with SMI may also experience co-occurring PD. When personality traits become so extreme that adaptation to everyday situations is impaired, those with PD may engage in behaviors that are significant and potentially harmful. Mental health professionals may find that working with individuals with PD presents unique challenges compared to those with SMI, such as schizophrenia spectrum or bipolar mental health problems.

Personality traits have long been recognized as central components in the understanding and classification of SMI. Dimensional approaches emphasize the significance of specific trait domains in both risk and expression of problem behaviors in people living with SMI. Among these, high neuroticism is notable for its association with emotional instability, anxiety, and heightened vulnerability. Individuals exhibiting this trait often experience frequent mood fluctuations and are more susceptible to stress-related symptoms. Low extraversion, manifesting as social withdrawal, reduced engagement, and introversion, is similarly prominent, especially within clinical presentations marked by detachment (Simonsen & Newton-Howes, 2018).

Avoidant characteristics, such as social anxiety and reduced engagement in interpersonal interactions, are significant factors in the overall assessment. Additionally, features indicative of BPD, including emotional instability and heightened sensitivity to others' perspectives, provide additional specificity in evaluations. Recognizing these traits is crucial for comprehending the intricate relationship between personality and the progression of mental health problems (Simonsen & Newton-Howes, 2018). These traits interact with problematic behaviors exhibited by people living with SMI over time, potentially worsening its course and increasing the risk of relapse (Donat et al., 1992; Simonsen & Newton-Howes, 2018). .

Research has shown that there are commonalities of personality traits that have been identified as problematic for individuals living with SMI. Below are three types of combinations of maladaptive personality traits that are problematic for a person living with SMI (Donat et al., 1992).

Type One: Cooperative and Controlled

Individuals exhibiting these behavioral traits are classified as high in agreeableness and neuroticism according to the FFM (Costa & McCrae, 2008; Lim, 2025; Widiger & Crego, 2019), and as high in negative affectivity and submissiveness based on the AMPD traits (American Psychiatric Association, 2022b). Individuals with these characteristics are generally emotionally sensitive, frequently experiencing anxiety, worry, or tension, and anticipating negative outcomes. They may have difficulty coping with stress, sometimes defer to others even if it conflicts with their own needs, and tend to be empathetic, cooperative, and considerate. Additionally, they prioritize harmonious relationships but may face increased susceptibility to psychological distress and fluctuations in mood (American Psychiatric Association, 2022b; Costa & McCrae, 2008; Lim, 2025; Widiger & Crego, 2019).

Individuals who possess these characteristics tend to demonstrate better adjustment compared to those with differing personality traits. They are attentive to the way others interact with them and strive to present themselves in a socially acceptable way, often aligning their behavior with perceived social expectations. Consequently, they are more inclined to adhere to common norms, such as maintaining punctuality, practicing basic self-care, and interacting courteously with others.

This inclination toward "normal behavior" is motivated by a desire to conform to perceived social standards. However, individuals may possess a limited understanding of the experiences of others and frequently do not recognize that those around them also encounter challenges and concerns. Often, they interpret any indication of difficulty as something to minimize or avoid discussing. There is a prevailing perception that acknowledgment of serious issues will result in others perceiving them as less normal and living with SMI.

Because they minimize their problems, it is particularly challenging when mental health service providers try to help with the challenges of living with SMI. People with these personality characteristics will tend to perceive living with SMI as something to be minimized rather than actively managed. They will, therefore, be inclined to downplay and deny problems caused by living with SMI and show a lack of concern about the importance of such basic treatments as taking medication and maintaining contact with treatment providers.

Individuals with these characteristics may experience challenges in chaotic environments and can be sensitive to changes in routine. For example, Daniel was cooperative and agreeable when the hospital ward was quiet and stable. If the environment became noisy or if he was asked to do more than he felt capable of, he became upset and tended to withdraw from others. People with these personality traits often attempt to act as though nothing is wrong and work to avoid displaying distressing behaviors. This approach typically does not address the underlying issues, and frustration may gradually develop until it results in an expression of anger. This response may be unexpected by others due to the individual's usual success in managing frustrations. After such episodes, the person is generally embarrassed and regains composure quickly.

Behavioral Support Strategies to Approach and Interact with Individuals Living with SMI Who Exhibit Type One Personality Traits

- Approach individuals living with SMI with sensitivity, recognizing the challenges they face and acknowledging their difficulties. Individuals exhibiting these personality traits often demonstrate greater stability and cooperation compared to others who live with SMI. As a result, mental health professionals may perceive these individuals as more open to discussions regarding SMI or related concerns. However, this perception is often inaccurate, as these individuals typically prefer not to be identified as "persons with a problem." Therefore, it is generally advisable to refrain from making assertive attempts to engage them in conversations about perceived problems.

- Even if an individual who lives with SMI is reluctant to acknowledge her challenges, it remains important to recognize and commend her strengths and skills. Avoid letting the difficulty in admitting problems overshadow an appreciation for her capabilities. Individuals with these personality traits benefit from feeling valued by others, and acknowledging genuine strengths can create an environment where they are more comfortable addressing concerns. This consideration does not suggest that mental health professionals should refrain from working to enhance the individual's awareness of the problems living with SMI; however, interventions are generally more effective when individuals feel respected for their competencies and abilities and are an equal partner in their recovery.
- Engage openly in discussions, even regarding topics that may appear trivial. Individuals exhibiting these personality traits often seek acknowledgment from others, yet prefer to avoid conflict and may fear that deeper interactions will reveal insecurities they wish to conceal. As a result, their conversations are frequently brief and focused on neutral subjects such as the weather, rather than personal matters. They tend to refrain from disclosing their own concerns or inquiring into those of others, which can make them seem reserved or "difficult to get to know." Nevertheless, fostering familiarity with such individuals is essential for increasing influence with them. Engaging with individuals during moments when they are receptive to conversation, regardless of the perceived significance of the topics, can foster openness and support the development of more substantive dialogue over time.
- Observe instances when individuals living with SMI demonstrate a willingness to discuss challenges or emotional concerns. Although people exhibiting these traits often avoid conversations about difficulties and distress, there are occasions when they become upset and may be more open to communication. Mental health service providers and staff, having had limited opportunities for such discussions in the past, might not always initiate these conversations. It is important to recognize and utilize moments when the individual appears more receptive, and to engage with them at these times. This approach can facilitate gradual rapport-building; as trust develops and the person feels comfortable sharing, discussing similar topics in the future may become easier. Nonetheless, it remains crucial to proceed sensitively, as pressing the individual too much may halt progress if they perceive the conversation as intrusive. With patience, advancement is achievable. Additionally, guidance from a mental health service professional can assist in determining appropriate boundaries for these interactions.
- For professional appointments, establish a consistent schedule to maintain engagement. Individuals exhibiting these personality traits may demonstrate reduced commitment to addressing their concerns and participating in treatment.

If attendance is left solely to their discretion, they may be unlikely to comply. Adherence improves when appointments are scheduled at regular, frequent intervals. Mental health professionals and staff are encouraged to acknowledge and reinforce the individual's effort to attend appointments, even if the individual does not perceive the value in doing so.
- Highlighting the importance of adhering to treatment can contribute significantly to maintaining stability in an individual's life. For people exhibiting these personality traits, it is beneficial to be recognized by others as demonstrating sound judgment and composure. When individuals living with SMI consistently take prescribed medication and follow recommended treatments, it is important to periodically acknowledge how these actions support ongoing recovery and help prevent hospital readmission. Conveying this message is essential for their well-being and recovery.

Example of Cooperative and Controlled Personality: Daniel is a hospitalized individual. Upon admission, he tried hard to act in a friendly and cooperative way. This was a problem because it helped him to effectively "cover up" many of his problems. He gave the impression that he was doing fine but didn't really take his problems seriously. For example, Daniel told his family that he was going to attend college to get a degree. For 2 years, he went to college and sat in the library while telling his wife that he was attending classes.

After being hospitalized, Daniel was discharged very quickly after admission because he apparently "responded well" to treatment and did not pose any serious problem. It took several admissions to the same hospital before the staff understood that his desire to "look good" was really a problem. Subsequently, the hospital staff tailored their interventions according to their assessment of his personality traits. This approach enabled Daniel to minimize attention on issues related to his alcohol use, marital challenges, depression, and other difficulties. They thoughtfully considered strategies that would support Daniel's ability to remain out of the hospital. Recognizing the need for balance, they committed to providing patient, compassionate, and sustained support aimed at facilitating his progress. The team encouraged ongoing participation in Alcoholics Anonymous and supported his transition to a community placement, ensuring continued engagement with treatment providers.

Type Two: Energetic and Self-Centered

Individuals exhibiting these behavioral characteristics are typically classified as low in agreeableness and conscientiousness according to the FFM (Costa & McCrae, 2008; Lim, 2025; Widiger & Crego, 2019), and as high in antagonism and disinhibition based on the AMPD trait model (American Psychiatric Association, 2022b).

According to the ICD-11 typology (WHO, 2022), such individuals are characterized by elevated levels of dissociality and disinhibition. These individuals may be identified as living with ASPD.

People living with SMI who are described as energetic and self-centered would be classified as individuals high in antagonism and disinhibition, behavioral expressions of traits that result in interpersonal conflict due to self-importance, expectation of special treatment, and disregard for others' feelings. Low disinhibition is associated with impulsive actions aimed at immediate gratification, with little thought for past or future consequences. People low in agreeableness are typically skeptical, competitive, and prioritize personal goals over group harmony (Costa & McCrae, 2008; Lim, 2025; Widiger & Crego, 2019). Those with low conscientiousness may struggle with impulsivity, disorganization, and follow-through, affecting their reliability (Costa & McCrae, 2008; Lim, 2025; Widiger & Crego, 2019).

Individuals exhibiting these personality traits may present as communicative and energetic, often described as "glib and gregarious" in interpersonal interactions However, such individuals may place limited emphasis on the preferences or perceptions of others, prioritizing personal needs over those of mental health service providers and staff. They tend to demonstrate initiative in pursuing their own interests. They may frequently seek to have their needs met, which can manifest as demanding behavior and complaints regarding sources of dissatisfaction. These dynamics may occasionally contribute to conflict, including arguments or even physical confrontations with service providers and staff.

Individuals exhibiting these personality traits generally prefer self-reliance and may view dependence on others as undesirable. They often prioritize personal autonomy, sometimes perceiving those who seek assistance as lacking strength. Consequently, they are less likely to pursue support from others and may not recognize the necessity of medication and following treatment recommendations. These individuals may express concerns regarding side effects or discomfort related to prescribed medications. It is not uncommon for them to discharge themselves from treatment facilities without medical approval or discontinued medication contrary to the guidance of mental health professionals. Additionally, they may voice dissatisfaction with mental health service providers, feeling that their needs are unmet or that the providers are overly involved in personal matters.

Individuals exhibiting these traits may appear approachable and enthusiastic, particularly when their needs are met. However, they often assert themselves promptly when seeking something new or expressing dissatisfaction. Mental health service providers and staff may learn to acquiesce to such demands for the sake of maintaining a pleasant environment. Over time, this pattern can result in providers conceding more frequently. As requests escalate, frustration among mental health professionals may increase, sometimes leading to establishing stricter boundaries, additional limit setting, and punitive consequences as necessary to encourage greater consideration for others. Nevertheless, this approach is typically ineffective, as individuals with these characteristics often tend to engage in prolonged arguments or confrontations.

Behavioral Support Strategies to Approach and Interact with Individuals Living with SMI Who Exhibit Type Two Personality Traits

- Avoid arguments. Individuals exhibiting these personality traits may have expectations of mental health service providers and staff that exceed reasonable bounds. As a result, they may make demands that are difficult to satisfy and initiate confrontations. Staff may reactively want to enforce strict boundaries to encourage respectful interactions. However, those with such maladaptive traits can be resistant to reconsidering their viewpoints, and persistent efforts to persuade them often escalate disputes and potentially increase risk of aggressive behaviors. It is essential for mental health professionals to master the skill of appropriately disengaging from conversations when necessary. This approach can be challenging and may require support from trained mental health practitioners. For example, Charles frequently expressed concerns that others were seeking to take advantage of him. When staff attempted to reassure him otherwise, he became argumentative and increasingly loud and demanding. The team learned to respond calmly, stating, "I am not yelling at you. When you are calm, we can continue our discussion." This was delivered in a neutral, non-judgmental manner. Afterward, the staff would disengage and, whenever feasible, refrain from interacting further until Charles had regained composure.
- Practice effective limit setting. Developing the ability to set appropriate limits is a vital skill for mental health service providers, especially when engaging individuals with the personality characteristics described above. Recognizing unrealistic requests or expectations and implementing suitable boundaries are crucial. Failing to assert oneself can result in an individual perceiving acquiescence, making it increasingly challenging to redirect behavior. On occasion, Charles expressed feelings of being insulted and, without clear limits, his agitation would intensify, sometimes resulting in aggressive behavior directed at property or staff. Staff were trained to address such incidents by stating, "I'm not going to listen to you when you yell about this. You need to go to the mood room and calm yourself down. When you are calm, I will speak with you. Please go now; I'll check on you in a few minutes." Upon Charles successfully calming himself, staff provided positive reinforcement regarding his self-control. Although complaints persisted, proper boundary-setting helped minimize escalation. As with de-escalating arguments, developing proficiency in setting limits may necessitate guidance from experienced mental health professionals.
- Demonstrate respect for the strengths and positive behaviors exhibited by individuals living with SMI and maladaptive personality traits. Individuals with these characteristics may present themselves as domineering or entitled to mental health service providers and staff. As a result, some professionals may feel discouraged or inclined to avoid interacting with them entirely; however, avoidance is not beneficial and can exacerbate challenges. Effecting change in the behavior of someone living with SMI typically requires establishing rapport and

influence, which is best achieved by acknowledging genuine accomplishments and appropriately setting boundaries when necessary. Avoidance diminishes the opportunity to build rapport.

- It is important to recognize instances when the individual who lives with SMI demonstrates effective management of frustration or anger. Managing anger can be challenging for many individuals exhibiting these personality characteristics, and there may be numerous situations where improvement is possible. Nonetheless, it is equally essential to acknowledge occasions where anger is managed appropriately. Providing positive feedback for these achievements may encourage continued progress in future situations.
- Recognize instances in which individuals living with SMI demonstrate consideration for others or display a willingness to compromise. While such individuals may often prioritize their own needs over those of others, it is important to acknowledge occasions when they express concern for others or adapt to different perspectives. Providing positive feedback in these situations can encourage similar behaviors in the future.
- When offering compliments, it is advisable to focus on the individual's capacity for self-control. The way praise is delivered can significantly impact its effectiveness, as certain phrasings are more influential than others. Individuals exhibiting these personality traits tend to value autonomy and agency and prefer not to feel dependent on others. They are more likely to recall statements such as, "I was impressed with the way you maintained control," rather than, "I think you're doing better with your anger." Additionally, adherence to treatment recommendations may be enhanced by highlighting how these actions support their personal goals (e.g., "Taking your medication helps you remain out of the hospital").
- Implementing regular behavioral contracts can facilitate the promotion of desired behaviors. Individuals who respond well to structured environments often benefit from clearly defined formal or informal agreements that outline expectations. These contracts delineate the responsibilities of both the individual and mental health service providers or staff, as well as outcomes that are meaningful for individuals with SMI and maladaptive personality traits and within the influence of the mental health recovery team. Utilizing such agreements allows providers to effectively motivate engagement in recommended actions while supporting individuals in maintaining a sense of agency through access to preferred outcomes contingent upon their cooperation.

Example of Energetic and Self-Centered Personality: Charles would occasionally become "pushy" with other people. When other people tried to help him calm down, he would continue to complain about the situation and sometimes the situation would worsen, by Charles threatening and, sometimes, attacking them. Charles often could get something he wanted by getting loud and intimidating. Other people were both angry and scared about his "tough guy" behavior. Most of them simply tried to stay away from him as much as they could.

The staff eventually became more familiar with how to work with him. When he was in control, they complimented him for "carrying himself well and looking good." They also began to point out to him how his self-control capabilities were keeping other people "out of his hair." They became familiar with things that he enjoyed, such as playing cards. They were willing to do this with him if he exhibited self-control. As he became friendly to them, he became reluctant to act in a threatening or intimidating way. Much of what the staff did with Charles was based on his tendency to show "angry, aggressive" behaviors. However, what they did with him was also based on their understanding of his personality features.

Type Three: Negative and Moody

Individuals exhibiting these behavioral characteristics would be identified as high in neuroticism and low in agreeableness according to the FFM (Costa & McCrae, 2008; Lim, 2025; Widiger & Crego, 2019), and as high in negative affectivity and disinhibition based on the AMPD trait dimensions (American Psychiatric Association, 2022b). Consistent with the ICD-11 typology (WHO, 2022), such individuals display traits aligning with those described in the AMPD. These individuals may be identified as living with BPD.

Individuals with low scores in agreeableness may demonstrate greater skepticism, competitiveness, and critical thinking, often placing personal objectives above group harmony (Costa & McCrae, 2008; Lim, 2025; Widiger & Crego, 2019). Neuroticism, characterized by sensitivity, nervousness, and emotional instability versus security, confidence, and stability, reflects one's susceptibility to negative emotions such as anger, anxiety, depression, or vulnerability. This trait encompasses emotional stability and impulse control, with those exhibiting high neuroticism being typically more emotionally reactive and may experience frequent anxiety, mood fluctuations, and stress, potentially facing challenges in coping with adversity (Costa & McCrae, 2008; Lim, 2025; Widiger & Crego, 2019).

Individuals with elevated disinhibition tend to seek immediate gratification, resulting in impulsive behaviors influenced by transient thoughts, emotions, and external stimuli, while minimally considering previous experiences or future outcomes. Additionally, those with high levels of negative affectivity frequently encounter anxiety, nervousness, tension, or panic across various situations. Such individuals may become preoccupied with concerns about past adverse events (e.g., trauma) and the prospect of future difficulties, resulting in persistent apprehension towards uncertainty and a heightened tendency to anticipate unfavorable outcomes (American Psychiatric Association, 2022b).

Individuals exhibiting these personality characteristics may alternate between cooperative behavior and periods of negativity or criticism. They often conform to perceived expectations over extended durations but eventually experience frustration, perceiving an imbalance in effort within the relationship. Such behavioral inconsistency can present challenges for mental health service professionals and staff, who may find it perplexing and, at times, respond with criticism and being judgmental. This dynamic may contribute to the emergence of interpersonal conflicts.

Individuals exhibiting these personality characteristics may initially resemble those who are "energetic but self-centered" (i.e., type two). While individuals with type two traits are generally unconcerned with others' opinions, those with type three traits are highly sensitive to how others perceive and treat them. They often strive to appear cooperative and be regarded as pleasant by others; yet, they may experience significant anxiety during social interactions, which can hinder their communication effectiveness. This often results in frustration, and instead of attributing difficulties to themselves, they may blame others for being indifferent or unfair.

Such personality traits can evoke strong emotional responses from mental health professionals and staff. Providers may initially feel empathy and dedicate substantial time and effort to supporting the individual. When efforts to demonstrate concern are met with increased expectations from the individual, providers may begin to feel overwhelmed or frustrated. If this frustration is expressed, the therapeutic relationship may deteriorate with the individual living with SMI and maladaptive personality traits perceiving a lack of genuine care and becoming more negative, while providers may respond critically, withdrawing from engagement and acting punitively.

Despite having clear strengths and abilities, these individuals may not recognize or utilize their skills effectively. As a result, service providers may become discouraged when progress appears limited, often concluding that the individual lacks motivation for improvement or "is not ready for change."

Behavioral Support Strategies to Approach and Interact with Individuals Living with SMI Who Exhibit Type Three Personality Traits

- Remain calm and patient. People with these personality features can be very frustrating because of their periods of inconsistent moody and "negative" behaviors. Many mental health service providers and staff will be motivated to either "tell them to grow up" or just avoid them as much as possible. Mental health service providers and staff must remember that they are sensitive to how others react and want others to appreciate them. Critical reactions by mental health service providers and staff and attempts to avoid them usually make them anxious; they are likely to complain that other people don't care. It is important to stay calm despite an inclination to criticize them and their behaviors. A mental health professional can help with managing harsh and punitive behaviors born out of frustration.
- Refrain from engaging in complaints. Individuals displaying these personality traits may frequently express dissatisfaction, believing that others are not treating them fairly or demonstrating sufficient concern. Compared to other individu-

als living with SMI, they may be more likely to voice criticism regarding their mental health service providers and staff. This situation may prompt staff to feel the need to defend themselves or attempt to encourage the individual to consider circumstances from a more positive perspective; however, such efforts often result in further complaints and additional objections to proposed solutions. As a result, mental health professionals may perceive that the person is not genuinely interested in recovery. It is typically more effective to avoid participating in extended discussions of grievances. Mental health service providers should strive to disregard persistent complaints while maintaining an attitude of interest and support. For example, Juan occasionally expressed fatigue, claiming he was unable to participate in group activities at the clubhouse or complete chores at the group home. Staff permitted him to remain in the room with his head down on the table. After 2 weeks, Juan began to engage in activities again. On other occasions, when greeted by others, Juan would respond loudly with "Don't talk to me." While it is understandable that others might take offense and wish to address his behavior, staff were encouraged to move forward and attempt interaction again later.
- Direct comments toward the strengths demonstrated by individuals living with co-occurring SMI and maladaptive personality traits. Individuals exhibiting these personality characteristics may display tendencies to complain or act negatively, which can result in mental health service providers and staff choosing to limit interactions. Nevertheless, consistently providing brief, specific recognition for their current positive behaviors can contribute to their development. Many individuals with these traits may not readily acknowledge their own abilities; therefore, it is beneficial for others to affirm their competencies. Such feedback encourages more accurate self-assessment and fosters greater self-appreciation like complimenting a person's communication skills during periods of emotional and behavioral stability.
- Demonstrate an interest in the preferences of the individual who is living with SMI and personality problems. A common challenge faced by individuals with these personality features is difficulty recognizing and acknowledging their own sources of enjoyment or strengths. Mental health providers and staff should remain attentive to activities in which they engage, bring enjoyment to the person, and strive to participate in or support these pursuits. Such moments also provide opportunities to offer positive and specific feedback regarding their capabilities. When individuals are engaged in intrinsically enjoyable activities, they are less likely to experience intrusive thoughts regarding others' motives for expressing interest in them.
- Avoid excessive compliments or undue attention. While it is important to recognize current strengths and interests, the manner of delivering praise can significantly influence its impact. Individuals with certain personality traits may express that others are indifferent toward them, yet they might also experience discomfort when their achievements are acknowledged. Self-critical responses, such as, "I don't think it was so good," are not uncommon. Increasing the enthusiasm of praise to reassure them may inadvertently heighten their discomfort. In these

situations, offering a sincere but succinct compliment is typically most effective. For instance, Juan reported enjoying positive feedback with his artwork; however, when accolades were overly emphasized, he began to question his ability to maintain high performance, leading to anxiety and discouragement. This perceived pressure sometimes resulted in complaints about heightened expectations from others and his perception that he could not meet the expectations.
- Establish a plan in case the individual exhibits aggressive behavior. Certain personality traits may increase the likelihood of argumentative or physically dangerous actions. While many of the strategies previously discussed can help prevent such situations, there may be occasions when the person becomes uncontrollable and poses a risk. Typically, these episodes are brief, and the individual may express remorse afterwards; however, recurrence cannot be ruled out. Prior to any incident, ensure that you have a clear course of action, such as seeking assistance from others or contacting emergency services (e.g., 911).
- Develop a plan to address situations where the individual may pose a risk to themselves. Certain personality characteristics can increase the likelihood of self-harm, which may be manifested through excessive alcohol consumption, misuse of medication, self-injurious behaviors such as cutting or head-banging, or expressions of suicidal ideation. It is important to establish a clear and actionable strategy for responding if the person exhibits behaviors that indicate they may be a danger to self.

Example of Moody and Negative Personality: Juan developed a reputation of being unpredictable in how he interacted with other people. Sometimes he would act friendly and cooperative. At other times, he would pace the floor and complain that they were holding him against his will. He accused them of refusing to do anything for him. Then he would stay off by himself and refuse to participate in ward activities. Many staff wanted to tell him to "grow up." After understanding his personality features, however, they remained calm and patient with him. They ignored many complaints that he made but made sure to attend to his necessary daily needs. They discussed ways to avoid getting into an argument with him. When he was friendly, they spent time with him. With this approach Juan gradually became more stable and had fewer negative and moody episodes.

Summary

Personality traits are enduring characteristics that influence individual behavior, thoughts, and emotions across various contexts. Personality is a collection of traits that shape behavior and is influenced by genetic and environmental factors. The Five-Factor Model (FFM), also known as the "Big Five," is a widely recognized framework for understanding personality, comprising five dimensions: openness, conscientiousness, extraversion, agreeableness, and neuroticism. Each dimension of the FFM includes specific facets that provide a more detailed understanding of personality traits. Personality traits are generally stable but can change over time due to life experiences and targeted interventions.

The Five-Factor Model categorizes personality traits into five broad domains that describe individual differences.

- Factor I: Openness to experience reflects creativity and curiosity versus conventionality.
- Factor II: Conscientiousness indicates organization and dependability versus carelessness.
- Factor III: Extraversion measures sociability and energy versus introversion.
- Factor IV: Agreeableness encompasses compassion and cooperation versus antagonism.
- Factor V: Neuroticism relates to emotional stability and sensitivity versus resilience.

Personality mental health problems (PDs) are pervasive patterns of behavior that deviate from cultural norms and cause significant distress or impairment. The DSM-5-TR identifies 10 distinct personality mental health problems grouped into three clusters: A (odd/eccentric), B (dramatic/emotional), and C (anxious/fearful). Cluster A includes paranoid, schizoid, and schizotypal personality mental health problems. Cluster B includes antisocial, borderline, histrionic and narcissistic personality mental health problems. Cluster C includes avoidant, dependent, and obsessive-compulsive personality mental health problems.

Recent approaches favor dimensional models for understanding personality mental health problems, moving away from categorical classifications. The DSM-5 Alternative Model for Personality Disorders (AMPD) and International Classification of Diseases 11th Revision (ICD-11) emphasize a dimensional approach based on severity and trait domains. The AMPD assesses personality dysfunction through self and interpersonal functioning and identifies maladaptive traits. The ICD-11 evaluates personality mental health problems based on severity (mild, moderate, severe) and includes trait domain qualifiers. Both models align with the FFM, highlighting the continuum between normal and pathological personality traits.

There is a high prevalence of comorbidity between personality mental health problems and other mental health conditions. Up to 50% of individuals with a recognized mental health problem also meet the criteria for personality mental health problems. Co-occurring personality mental health problems can exacerbate symptoms of other mental health issues, complicating treatment and outcomes. Individuals with personality mental health problems and SMI often experience increased rates of hospitalization and involuntary admission.

Understanding the complex interplay of personality mental health problems and their frequent comorbidities is essential for effective assessment and treatment planning. PDs often present with overlapping mental health issues. Comorbidities complicate clinical presentations and necessitate integrated assessments. High rates of co-occurring mental health problems are common in various PDs, especially in persons living with borderline personality mental health problems (BPD).

BPD is characterized by a high prevalence of co-occurring mental health issues, necessitating comprehensive treatment approaches. Common comorbidities include major depression, bipolar, anxiety (especially PTSD), substance use, and eating mental health problems. Psychotic-like experiences such as paranoia and dissociation may occur. There is an elevated risk of suicide and self-harm behaviors in individuals with BPD.

Avoidant personality mental health problem (AvPD) frequently co-occurs with anxiety and depressive mental health problems, which can complicate both diagnosis and treatment. It is often associated with social anxiety disorder and generalized anxiety disorder. Current evidence supports a spectrum model connecting AvPD and social anxiety, and avoidant traits may mask presentations of anxiety, further challenging accurate identification and appropriate intervention.

Obsessive-compulsive personality mental health problem (OCPD) is characterized by rigidity and perfectionism and may occur alongside other mental health conditions. It is commonly comorbid with major depressive and anxiety mental health problems. OCPD differs from obsessive-compulsive disorder, which involves intrusive thoughts and compulsive behaviors.

Features of antisocial personality disorder (ASPD) are associated with externalizing behaviors and a range of co-occurring mental health conditions. ASPD is related to impulsivity, aggression, and involvement with criminal activity. It commonly appears alongside substance use mental health problems, ADHD, and mood mental health problems. Behavioral patterns can sometimes mask affective symptoms, which may complicate engagement in treatment.

Schizotypal personality disorder (STPD) exhibits characteristics similar to those found in schizophrenia spectrum mental health problems and is associated with an elevated risk for progression to overt psychotic symptoms. There is an increased likelihood of transitioning to hallucinations and delusions. Early identification and ongoing monitoring are essential for effective prevention and intervention.

Dependent personality mental health problem (DPD) often co-occurs with depressive and anxiety conditions, impacting interpersonal relationships with increased sensitivity to perceived rejection and fear of abandonment. Challenges in maintaining therapeutic boundaries may lead to risk of being exploited.

Narcissistic personality mental health problem (NPD) is linked to various mood mental health problems and can mask coexisting mental health conditions. It is commonly associated with mood mental health problems, particularly dysthymia, and substance use. Grandiosity or denial may obscure the presence of other mental health issues.

A thorough evaluation is crucial for accurate diagnosis and effective treatment planning in personality mental health problems. High prevalence of comorbid conditions necessitates comprehensive assessments. Structured interviews yield higher PD prevalence rates compared to unstructured evaluations. Awareness of comorbidity profiles enhances detection and management strategies across clinical settings.

Dimensions of problematic personality-based behaviors is essential to understanding and assessing mental health conditions and personality functioning. Individuals' personality traits are influenced by various factors and can be assessed to improve communication and well-being. Personality traits are shaped by cultural, familial, spiritual, and socioeconomic factors. The five key dimensions of functional personality are openness, conscientiousness, extraversion, agreeableness, and neuroticism (OCEAN). Understanding these dimensions can enhance personal and professional success and overall quality of life. Assistance from family, community, and professionals is crucial for addressing personality development obstacles.

The dimensional approach evaluates mental health conditions along a continuum rather than within fixed categories, facilitating a more nuanced understanding of individual differences. "Dimensional" denotes the assessment of mental health symptoms based on severity, duration, and intensity. This methodology effectively captures symptom variability, acknowledging the inherent complexity of mental health conditions. Standardized instruments are employed in dimensional assessments to quantify symptom severity and monitor treatment outcomes. In contrast, categorical models may oversimplify mental health concerns, whereas dimensional models offer a comprehensive perspective on individual functioning.

Personality mental health problems (PDs) are extreme versions of normal personality traits that lead to significant functional impairments and distress. PDs are characterized by persistent patterns of perception, relating, and thinking that affect long-term functioning. The classification of PDs has shifted from categorical to dimensional models, emphasizing impairments in personality functioning. The DSM-5-TR, AMPD, and ICD-11 frameworks focus on self and interpersonal functioning impairments. Severity levels range from no impairment to extreme impairment, guiding treatment and intervention strategies.

Severity of impairment in personality functioning is evaluated through structured dimensional frameworks, which facilitate the development of targeted interventions. The AMPD employs the Level of Personality Functioning Scale (LPFS) to systematically assess both self and interpersonal domains. Severity is classified across five gradations: no impairment, mild, moderate, severe, and extreme. In contrast, ICD-11 delineates severity as mild, moderate, or severe, according to the extent of dysfunction present. Clinical evaluation of severity informs both the intensity of therapeutic approaches and anticipated prognostic outcomes.

Both AMPD and ICD-11 frameworks assess personality mental health problems based on core domains of impairments. AMPD identifies five core domains: negative affectivity, detachment, antagonism, disinhibition, and psychoticism. ICD-11 includes five domains: negative affectivity, detachment, dissociality, disinhibition, and anankastia. Both models emphasize the importance of self-functioning and interpersonal functioning in assessing personality mental health problems. Unique traits such as psychoticism (AMPD) and anankastia (ICD-11) highlight differences between the two frameworks.

Personality assessments utilize various structured and self-report inventories to evaluate maladaptive traits and functioning (Furnham & Crump, 2005). The Structured Clinical Interview for DSM-5 (SCID-5) is used for detecting mental health problems. The Personality Inventory for DSM-5 (PID-5) assesses maladaptive personality traits with 220 items across five domains. The Level of Personality Functioning Scale-Self Report (LPFS-SR) evaluates personality functioning with

80 items. The Personality Inventory for ICD-11 (PiCD) assesses five major domains with 60 items, focusing on maladaptive traits.

Self-report inventories are commonly used for personality assessment, but their applicability varies across populations. Hundreds of personality assessment instruments are available, including broad and focused assessments. Self-report measures may not be suitable for certain groups, such as older adults or those with cognitive impairments. Alternative assessment strategies, like interviews and informant-based inventories, may be necessary for specific populations.

The ontogenesis of problematic personality-based behaviors and their expression is a dynamic interplay of neurobiological and genetic underpinnings with phenotypic expression significantly influenced by environmental conditions and stimuli. Personality develops from birth through adulthood. Extreme personality traits can lead to PDs, affecting mental and physical health. Recognition of PDs can enhance support for individuals living with SMI.

Maladaptive personality traits are linked to specific brain regions, including the prefrontal cortex, amygdala, and medial temporal regions. Impairments in the prefrontal cortex are associated with impulsivity and emotional instability. The amygdala plays a critical role in emotional processing and threat detection, with hyperactivity linked to emotional dysregulation.

Heritability estimates for personality traits range from 30% to 60%, with identical twins showing higher concordance. Genome-wide association studies indicate that personality traits are polygenic, influenced by many genetic variants. Heritability estimates for personality mental health problems vary from 21% to 77%, with Cluster B PDs showing 24% to 77% heritability.

The emergence of personality traits and mental health conditions results from an interplay of biological predispositions, environmental factors, and individual learning experiences. Genetic, evolutionary, and social influences contribute to personality development, with research indicating that roughly 40% of variation among individuals is attributable to genetic factors. Shared family environments also play a substantial role in fostering similarities in traits among those raised together. Furthermore, cultural contexts and historical developments impact personality characteristics, and notable gender differences persist across diverse societies.

Personality traits generally remain stable over short periods but can change significantly over extended timeframes due to life experiences. Traits like neuroticism and conscientiousness are particularly susceptible to environmental influences. Mean levels of agreeableness and conscientiousness tend to increase with age, while neuroticism often decreases. Maladaptive traits may exhibit more plasticity than previously thought, with early interventions potentially mitigating the progression toward personality mental health problems.

Temperament, which is biologically determined and present early in life, serves as the foundation for personality traits. The "goodness of fit" model suggests that optimal development occurs when environmental demands align with individual traits. Poor environmental fit can lead to maladaptive behaviors and impaired personality development. Environmental events, like trauma, can lead to sudden and intense changes in behavioral expression of personality traits.

Trauma and adverse childhood experiences significantly influence the development of PDs. Neuroimaging research indicates that environmental stressors can alter neural circuits related to emotion regulation and social cognition. Early challenges and trauma are strongly associated with an increased risk for PDs, particularly BPD. Environmental factors interact with genetic predispositions to shape consistent patterns of thought, emotion, and behavior.

PDs are characterized by impairments in functioning and maladaptive traits shaped by trauma. The AMPD and ICD-11 frameworks assess personality mental health problems through domains like identity and intimacy, often compromised in trauma survivors. Traits such as negative affectivity, disinhibition, and detachment may reflect learned responses to chronic stress or relational harm. PDs are generally less stable than normative traits, particularly during adolescence and young adulthood.

Research suggests that personality traits are modifiable and can change over a person's lifespan. Environmental factors, including therapeutic interventions and supportive relationships, can influence trait expression. Maladaptive personality traits may be more flexible than previously assumed, allowing for potential change and adaptation.

The psycholexical approach to personality assessment posits that meaningful individual differences in personality are reflected within natural language. The FFM was developed based on this methodology, correlating personality traits with behavior-descriptive adjectives. It should be noted that personality assessment instruments may be affected by response tendencies such as social desirability, which have the potential to impact on the accuracy of trait measurement.

Self-awareness is crucial for understanding one's personality and involves recognizing and processing personal experiences. It encompasses private self-aspects (emotions, traits) and public self-dimensions (observable characteristics). Self-awareness can be developed through life experiences and is influenced by social reinforcement and exposure to self-focused stimuli.

The expression of personality traits evokes psychological reactions in others, influencing social interactions. Social effects are temporary psychological reactions to observed behaviors and can reveal common thought and behavior patterns. Feedback from the social audience can shape an individual's self-concept and influence their self-reports of traits.

PDs are enduring patterns of behavior and cognition that deviate from cultural norms. They often emerge in adolescence or early adulthood and are associated with significant distress and functional impairment. PDs have been historically marginalized in mental health classification and global health policy.

Global pooled prevalence of any PD is estimated at 7.8% (CI: 6.1–9.5%). Higher prevalence in Western adult populations at 12.16%. Specific cluster rates: 2.8% for Cluster B, 5.0% for Cluster C, and 3.8% for Cluster A. Prevalence varies by region: 9.1% in the United States, 10.7% in England, and 4.1% in China.

Cultural norms influence the expression and recognition of PDs, with collectivist societies less likely to pathologize certain traits. Socioeconomic status is a significant determinant of PD risk, with lower SES linked to early adversity and chronic stress. Emotional expressiveness may be viewed differently across cultures, affecting diagnosis and treatment.

PDs frequently co-occur with SMIs such as schizophrenia spectrum and major depressive conditions. Over 45% of psychiatric outpatients met criteria for PD, with avoidant and borderline PDs being most prevalent. Individuals with co-occurring PDs and SMIs are 2.3 times more likely to be high inpatient service users.

Early intervention is critical, especially in youth and marginalized populations. Stigma and reluctance persist in recognizing PDs in younger individuals. Culturally informed assessment and treatment approaches are essential for effective care and reducing misidentification.

Several frameworks exist for conceptualizing personality mental health problems, with emphasis on dimensional models and their relevance to clinical practice. PDs are traditionally categorized but recent models favor dimensional approaches for better clinical relevance. ICD-11 emphasizes severity levels (mild, moderate, and severe) and identifies traits like negative affectivity and detachment. DSM-5-TR outlines nine specific PD types, including antisocial, avoidant, and borderline, each with distinct characteristics. AMPD combines categorical and dimensional frameworks, assessing personality functioning and maladaptive traits for nuanced identification. FFM conceptualizes maladaptive traits across five domains, aiding cross-cultural assessments but lacking formal diagnostic thresholds.

ICD-11 model focuses on identifying disturbances in self and interpersonal functioning to determine general personality mental health problems. Severity is rated based on impairments, with traits serving as descriptors rather than diagnostic thresholds. Borderline pattern includes nine features, such as fear of abandonment and emotional instability, for identifying borderline PD.

DSM-5-TR structure differentiates nine types of maladaptive personality mental health problems, each with specific criteria and symptoms. ASPD requires evidence of impairment and dysfunction in conduct before age 15 and ongoing traits like impulsivity and aggression. BPD is characterized by unstable emotions, intense relationships, and self-destructive behaviors.

The AMPD framework employs a two-step approach to assess personality functioning and identify problematic traits. The identification of personality mental health problems requires moderate impairment in at least two functional domains. The framework delineates six specific categories of personality mental health problems and provides for a PD–trait-specified (PD-TS) problematic condition when an individual's traits do not correspond with established types.

FFM conceptualizes maladaptive personality types within five domains: neuroticism, extraversion, openness, agreeableness, and conscientiousness. It underscores how DSM personality mental health problems may be interpreted as maladaptive extremes of these FFM traits. While the model offers a comprehensive framework for cross-cultural and lifespan assessment, it does not establish formal diagnostic thresholds for determination and identification of impairment and dysfunction in expressions of personality.

Integrating various models for recognizing and identifying personality traits, as well as expressions of maladaptive traits, underscores the importance of harmonizing trait definitions and enhancing precision in the identification of PDs. This integration can improve clinical utility and promote tailored treatment strategies. Continued research should prioritize validating dimensional convergence and advancing cultural sensitivity within personality assessment practices.

Problems with the expressions of personality traits are important for understanding and treating SMI. Extreme personality traits can hinder adaptation to difficult circumstances. Individuals who excel in structured environments can struggle outside them. Significant life stressors can exacerbate maladaptive personality traits. Cognitive difficulties in SMI may lead to withdrawal or anger in response to stress. Mental health professionals face challenges in encouraging adaptive behaviors due to entrenched personality traits.

Personality traits can manifest as pronounced mental health problems. Co-occurring personality mental health problems complicate treatment for individuals living with SMI. High neuroticism is linked to emotional instability and stress vulnerability. Low extraversion often results in social withdrawal and detachment. Avoidant characteristics and features of BPD are significant in assessments. Understanding these traits is crucial for effective treatment and minimizing relapse risks.

Research has shown that there are commonalities of personality traits that have been identified as problematic for individuals living with SMI. Below are three types of combinations of maladaptive personality traits that are problematic for a person living with SMI:

- Type one features: Individuals living with SMI exhibiting type one personality features are characterized by cooperative and controlled behaviors. They often score high on measures of agreeableness and neuroticism, frequently experiencing anxiety and tension. While they prioritize harmonious relationships, they may also experience notable psychological distress. These individuals tend to minimize their difficulties and may avoid discussing significant concerns.

- It is recommended to approach these clients with sensitivity, acknowledging their challenges without pressuring them to disclose personal issues. Recognizing and affirming their strengths help foster a supportive therapeutic environment. Establishing rapport through open discussion, even about non-essential topics, can facilitate trust over time. Consistency in scheduling appointments is beneficial for treatment adherence. Emphasizing the importance of following prescribed treatment regimens is crucial for maintaining stability and preventing hospital readmissions. Acknowledging attendance and engagement reinforces positive behaviors that support recovery.
- Type two features: Individuals living with SMI and exhibiting type two personality features are characterized by energetic and self-focused behaviors that may present unique challenges in interpersonal interactions. These individuals typically demonstrate low agreeableness and conscientiousness, while displaying elevated antagonism and disinhibition. As a result, their traits can contribute to interpersonal conflict due to heightened self-importance and limited consider-

ation for others' feelings. Impulsivity and the prioritization of personal goals over group cohesion are common.

- Effective interaction strategies should include minimizing confrontation and withdrawing from potentially escalating situations when appropriate. Employing clear limit-setting techniques is advised to address unrealistic demands and expectations. Building rapport involves recognizing and reinforcing strengths and positive behaviors, such as effective management of frustration and anger. Acknowledging demonstrations of consideration for others can encourage the repetition of such behaviors. Additionally, providing praise for instances of self-control may support adherence to treatment plans.
- Implementing regular behavioral contracts that specify expectations and responsibilities can foster engagement in recommended activities while supporting individual autonomy. Structured environments, featuring transparent agreements and predictable outcomes, are generally beneficial for these individuals.
- Type three features: Individuals living with serious mental illness SMI who display type three personality characteristics are typically characterized by negative and moody traits. They tend to score high on neuroticism and low on agreeableness, frequently exhibiting negative affectivity and disinhibition. These attributes are consistent with borderline personality disorder (BPD), including emotional instability, impulsivity, and skepticism. Such individuals may alternate between cooperative and critical behaviors, which can contribute to interpersonal difficulties.

Effective interaction strategies include maintaining a calm and patient approach to help minimize anxiety and frustration. It is advisable to avoid engaging in complaints to reduce negativity, and to focus comments on individual strengths to promote self-recognition and appreciation of abilities. Demonstrating genuine interest in personal preferences can support greater engagement in meaningful activities. When managing feedback, it is recommended to avoid excessive praise that may cause discomfort and to instead provide sincere, concise commendations. A clear plan should be established to address risks related to aggressive behavior and self-harm, prioritizing safety at all times. It is important to recognize that while individuals may express regret following aggressive incidents, the potential for recurrence remains.

References

Allen, T. A., Schreiber, A. M., Hall, N. T., & Hallquist, M. N. (2020). From description to explanation: Integrating across multiple levels of analysis to inform neuroscientific accounts of dimensional personality pathology. *Journal of Personality Disorders, 34*(5), 650–676. https://doi.org/10.1521/pedi.2020.34.5.650

American Psychiatric Association. (2013). *The personality inventory for DSM-5 (PID-5)—Adult*. https://www.psychiatry.org/File%20Library/Psychiatrists/Practice/DSM/APA_DSM5_The-Personality-Inventory-For-DSM-5-Full-Version-Adult.pdf

American Psychiatric Association. (2022a). Personality disorders. In *Diagnostic and statistical manual of mental disorders* (5th ed., text rev.; DSM-5-TR). https://doi.org/10.1176/appi.books.9780890425787.x06_Personality_Disorders

American Psychiatric Association. (2022b). Alternative model for personality disorders. In *Diagnostic and statistical manual of mental disorders* (5th ed., text rev.; DSM-5-TR). https://doi.org/10.1176/appi.books.9780890425787.x06_Alternative_Model_for_Personality_Disorders

American Psychiatric Association. (2022c). *Somatic symptom and related disorders*. In *Diagnostic and statistical manual of mental disorders* (5th ed.). https://doi.org/10.1176/appi.books.9780890425787.x10

American Psychiatric Association. (2024, November). *What are personality disorders?* Psychiatry.org. Retrieved August 10, 2025, from https://www.psychiatry.org/patients-families/personality-disorders/what-are-personality-disorders

American Psychological Association. (n.d.-a). *Personality*. In *APA dictionary of psychology*. Retrieved August 10, 2025, from https://dictionary.apa.org/personality

American Psychological Association. (n.d.-b). *Temperament*. In *APA Dictionary of Psychology*. https://dictionary.apa.org/temperament

American Psychological Association. (n.d.-c). *Personality disorder*. In *APA Dictionary of Psychology*. https://dictionary.apa.org/personality-disorder

American Psychological Association (2024, April). *Spotlight on personality disorders: Issue 244*. APA Highlights. Retrieved August 14, 2025, from https://www.apa.org/pubs/highlights/spotlight/issue-244

Araiba, S. (2020). Current diversification of behaviorism. *Perspectives on Behavior Science, 43*(1), 157–175. https://doi.org/10.1007/s40614-019-00207-0

Bach, B., & First, M. B. (2018). Application of the ICD-11 classification of personality disorders. *BMC Psychiatry, 18*, 351. https://doi.org/10.1186/s12888-018-1908-3

Bach, B., & Simonsen, E. (2021). Personality disorder severity and traits predict clinical severity and functioning across diagnostic systems. *Journal of Personality Disorders, 35*(2), 175–197. https://doi.org/10.1521/pedi_2020_35_427

Bäckström, M., & Björklund, F. (2013). Social desirability in personality inventories: Symptoms, diagnosis and prescribed cure. *Scandinavian Journal of Psychology, 54*(2), 152–159. https://doi.org/10.1111/sjop.12015

Bagby, R. M., & Widiger, T. A. (2020). Assessment of the ICD-11dimensional trait model: An introduction to the special section. *Psychological Assessment, 32*(1), 1. https://doi.org/10.1037/pas0000785

Balaratnasingam, S., & Janca, A. (2015). Normal personality, personality disorder and psychosis: Current views and future perspectives. *Current Opinion in Psychiatry, 28*(1), 30–34. https://doi.org/10.1097/YCO.0000000000000124

Barbato, N., & Hafner, R. J. (1998). Comorbidity of bipolar and personality disorder. *Australian and New Zealand Journal of Psychiatry, 32*(2), 276–280. https://doi.org/10.3109/00048679809062739

Behaviorism, A. P. (1993). Personality theory, abnormal psychology, and psychological measurement. *Behavior Modification, 17*(1), 8–42. https://doi.org/10.1177/01454455930171002

Boberg, M., Felding, S., Jansson, L. B., & Nordgaard, J. (2020). Challenges assessing personality disorders with the SCID-5-PD in psychiatric patients [preprint]. *Research Square*. https://doi.org/10.21203/rs.3.rs-22789/v1

Caballo, V. E., Fernández, A. L., & Salazar, I. C. (2024). Personality disorders, fact or fiction? The dark future of their diagnosis. *Behavioral Psychology/Psicologia Conductual, 32*(1). https://doi.org/10.51668/bp.8324101n

Chanen, A. M. (2024). National Mental Health Research Strategy background paper: Personality disorders (session 3A). *National Mental Health Commission.*. https://www.mentalhealthcommission.gov.au/sites/default/files/2024-03/background-paper-personality-disorders-session-3a.pdf

Chess, S., & Thomas, A. (1977). Temperamental individuality from childhood to adolescence. *Journal of the American Academy of Child Psychiatry, 16*(2), 218–226. https://doi.org/10.1016/S0002-7138(09)60038-8

Chess, S., & Thomas, A. (2013). *Goodness of fit: Clinical applications, from infancy through adult life*. Routledge. https://doi.org/10.4324/9780203727607

Costa, P. T., Jr., & McCrae, R. R. (1992). The five-factor model of personality and its relevance to personality disorders. *Journal of Personality Disorders, 6*(4), 343–359. https://doi.org/10.1521/pedi.1992.6.4.343

Costa, P. T., Jr., & McCrae, R. R. (1978). Objective personality assessment. In I. M. Lubin (Ed.), *The clinical psychology of aging* (pp. 119–143). Springer. https://doi.org/10.1007/978-1-4684-3342-5_5

Costa, P. T., Jr., & McCrae, R. R. (2008). The revised NEO personality inventory (NEO-PI-R). In G. J. Boyle, G. Matthews, & D. H. Saklofske (Eds.), The SAGE handbook of personality theory and assessment, Vol. 2. Personality measurement and testing (pp. 179–198). Sage Publications, doi:https://doi.org/10.4135/9781849200479.n9

Costa, P. T., Jr., & Widiger, T. A. (Eds.). (1994). Personality disorders and the five-factor model of personality. American Psychological Association. doi:https://doi.org/10.1037/10140-000

D'Adda, F., Sighinolfi, G., Mitolo, M., Scala, M., Guidi, L., Motta, L., Cirignotta, I., Manners, D. M., Tonon, C., Lodi, R., & Menchetti, M. (2025). Neurobiological correlates of personality dimensions in borderline personality disorder using graph analysis of functional connectivity. *Scientific Reports, 15*(1), 12623. https://doi.org/10.1038/s41598-025-85989-x

Donat, D. C., Geczy, B., Jr., Helmrich, J., & LeMay, M. (1992). Empirically derived personality subtypes of public psychiatric patients: Effect on self-reported symptoms, coping inclinations, and evaluation of expressed emotion in caregivers. *Journal of Personality Assessment, 58*(1), 36–50. https://doi.org/10.1207/s15327752jpa5801_4

Ekselius, L. (2018). Personality disorder: A disease in disguise. *Upsala Journal of Medical Sciences, 123*(4), 194–204. https://doi.org/10.1080/03009734.2018.1526235

Fariba, K. A., Gupta, V., Torrico, T. J., & Kass, E. (2024, July 17). Personality disorder. In *StatPearls*. StatPearls Publishing. Retrieved August 10, 2025, from https://www.ncbi.nlm.nih.gov/books/NBK556058

Feher, A., & Vernon, P. A. (2021). Looking beyond the big five: A selective review of alternatives to the big five model of personality. *Personality and Individual Differences, 169*, 110002. https://doi.org/10.1016/j.paid.2020.110002

Fok, M. L. Y., Stewart, R., Hayes, R. D., & Moran, P. (2014). The impact of co-morbid personality disorder on use of psychiatric services and involuntary hospitalization in people with severe mental illness. *Social Psychiatry and Psychiatric Epidemiology, 49*(10), 1631–1640. https://doi.org/10.1007/s00127-014-0874-4

Furnham, A., & Crump, J. (2005). Personality traits, types, and disorders: An examination of the relationship between three self-report measures. *European Journal of Personality, 19*(3), 167–184. https://doi.org/10.1002/per.543

Gawda, B. (2018). Cross-cultural studies on the prevalence of personality disorders. *Current Issues in Personality Psychology, 6*(4), 318–329. https://doi.org/10.5114/cipp.2018.80200

Gawda, B., Bernacka, R., & Gawda, A. (2016). The neural mechanisms underlying personality disorders. *NeuroQuantology, 14*(2), 348–356. https://doi.org/10.14704/nq.2016.14.2.948

Gregory, R. J. (2008). Personality tests. In N. J. Salkind (Ed.), *Encyclopedia of educational psychology* (Vol. 2, pp. 740–743). SAGE Publications. https://sk.sagepub.com/ency/edvol/statistics/chpt/personality-tests

Hamilton, J. (2017, May 21). *Why brain scientists are still obsessed with the curious case of Phineas gage*. NPR. https://www.npr.org/sections/health-shots/2017/05/21/528966102/why-brain-scientists-are-still-obsessed-with-the-curious-case-of-phineas-gage

Hong, R. Y., & Paunonen, S. V. (2015). Five factor model of personality, facets of. In *International encyclopedia of the social & behavioral sciences* (2nd ed.). Elsevier. https://doi.org/10.1016/B978-0-08-097086-8.25063-0

Hopwood, C. J., & Bleidorn, W. (2018). Stability and change in personality and personality disorders. *Current Opinion in Psychology, 21*, 6–10. https://doi.org/10.1016/j.copsyc.2017.08.034

Hopwood, C. J., Good, E. W., & Morey, L. C. (2018). Validity of the DSM–5 levels of personality functioning scale–self report. *Journal of Personality Assessment, 100*(6), 650–659. https://doi.org/10.1080/00223891.2017.1420660

Hopwood, C. J., Morey, L. C., & Markon, K. E. (2023). What is a psychopathology dimension? *Clinical Psychology Review, 106*, 102356. https://doi.org/10.1016/j.cpr.2023.102356

Hopwood, C. J., Zimmermann, J., Pincus, A. L., & Krueger, R. F. (2015a). Connecting personality structure and dynamics: Insights from the personality inventory for DSM-5 (PID-5). *Journal of Personality Assessment, 97*(5), 478–490. https://doi.org/10.1080/00223891.2015.1045067

Hopwood, C. J., Zimmermann, J., Pincus, A. L., & Krueger, R. F. (2015b). *Level questions for PID-5 facets* [Supplemental material]. https://supp.apa.org/psycarticles/supplemental/pas0000450/LevelQuesFor

Hualparuca-Olivera, L., Caycho-Rodríguez, T., Torales, J., & Ramos-Campos, D. (2023). Convergence between the dimensional PD models of ICD-11 and DSM-5: A meta-analytic approach. *Frontiers in Psychiatry, 14*, 1325583. https://doi.org/10.3389/fpsyt.2023.1325583

Kapur, R. (2021). *Understanding the dimensions of personality*. ResearchGate. Retrieved August 10, 2025, from https://www.researchgate.net/publication/353331440_Understanding_the_Dimensions_of_Personality

Khan, A. A., Jacobson, K. C., Gardner, C. O., Prescott, C. A., & Kendler, K. S. (2005). Personality and comorbidity of common psychiatric disorders. *The British Journal of Psychiatry, 186*(3), 190–196. https://doi.org/10.1192/bjp.186.3.190

Krueger, R. F., & Eaton, N. R. (2015). Transdiagnostic factors of mental disorders. *World Psychiatry, 14*(1), 27–29. https://doi.org/10.1002/wps.20175

Krueger, R. F., & Hobbs, K. A. (2020). An overview of the DSM-5 alternative model of personality disorders. *Psychopathology, 53*(3–4), 126–132. https://doi.org/10.1159/000508538

Krueger, R. F., Derringer, J., Markon, K. E., Watson, D., & Skodol, A. E. (2012a). Initial construction of a maladaptive personality trait model and inventory for DSM-5. *Psychological Medicine, 42*(9), 1879–1890. https://doi.org/10.1017/S0033291711002674

Krueger, R. F., Derringer, J., Markon, K. E., Watson, D., & Skodol, A. E. (2012b). *Personality inventory for DSM-5 (PID-5)* [database record]. APA PsycTests. https://doi.org/10.1037/t30042-000

Lee, S. (2025, June 15). *ICD-11 essentials for personality disorder diagnosis*. Number Analytics. https://www.numberanalytics.com/blog/icd-11-essentials-personality-disorder-diagnosis

Leichsenring, F., Fonagy, P., Heim, N., Kernberg, O. F., Leweke, F., Luyten, P., Salzer, S., Spitzer, C., & Steinert, C. (2024). Borderline personality disorder: A comprehensive review of diagnosis and clinical presentation, etiology, treatment, and current. *World Psychiatry, 23*(1), 4–25. https://doi.org/10.1002/wps.2115

Lim, A. G. Y. (2025, March 20). *Big five personality traits: The 5-factor model of personality*. Simply Psychology. https://www.simplypsychology.org/big-five-personality.html

Loranger, A. W., Janca, A., & Sartorius, N. (Eds.). (1997). Assessment and diagnosis of personality disorders: The ICD-10 international personality disorder examination (IPDE). Cambridge University Press.

McCabe, G. A., & Widiger, T. A. (2020). A comprehensive comparison of the ICD-11 and DSM–5 section III personality disorder models. *Psychological Assessment, 32*(1), 72–84. https://doi.org/10.1037/pas0000772

McClowry, S. G., Rodriguez, E. T., & Koslowitz, R. (2008). Temperament-based intervention: Re-examining goodness of fit. *European Journal of Developmental Science, 2*(1–2), 120–135. https://doi.org/10.3238/ejds.2008.0120

Morin, A. (2011). Self-awareness part 1: Definition, measures, effects, functions, and antecedents. *Social and Personality Psychology Compass, 5*(10), 807–823. https://doi.org/10.1111/j.1751-9004.2011.00387.x

Mulder, R. T. (2021). ICD-11 personality disorders: Utility and implications of the new model. *Frontiers in Psychiatry, 12*, 655548. https://doi.org/10.3389/fpsyt.2021.655548

National Institute of Mental Health (NIMH). (2024, May). *Mental illness*. U.S. Department of Health and Human Services (HHS), National Institutes of Health (NIH). Retrieved August 13, 2025, from https://www.nimh.nih.gov/health/statistics/mental-illness

Natoli, A. P., & Rodriguez, C. M. (2024). A new performance-based measure of personality functioning impairment: Development and preliminary evaluation of reliability and validity. *Discover Mental Health, 4*, 6. https://doi.org/10.1007/s44192-024-00059-4

Newton-Howes, G., Clark, L. A., & Chanen, A. (2015). Personality disorder across the life course. *The Lancet, 385*(9969), 727–734. https://doi.org/10.1016/S0140-6736(14)61283-6

Oltmanns, J. R., & Widiger, T. A. (2018). A self-report measure for the ICD-11 dimensional trait model proposal: The personality inventory for ICD-11. *Psychological Assessment, 30*(2), 154–169. https://doi.org/10.1037/pas0000459

Oltmanns, J. R., & Widiger, T. A. (2021). The self- and informant-personality inventories for ICD-11: Agreement, structure, and relations with health, social, and satisfaction variables in older adults. *Psychological Assessment, 33*(4), 300. https://doi.org/10.1037/pas0000982

Phillips, M. R. (2016). Would the use of dimensional measures improve the utility of psychiatric diagnoses? *World Psychiatry, 15*(1), 38. https://doi.org/10.1002/wps.20289

Piedmont, R. L., & Aycock, W. (2007). An historical analysis of the lexical emergence of the big five personality adjective descriptors. *Personality and Individual Differences, 42*(6), 1059–1068. https://doi.org/10.1016/j.paid.2006.09.015

Reichborn-Kjennerud, T. (2010). The genetic epidemiology of personality disorders. *Dialogues in Clinical Neuroscience, 12*(1), 103–114. https://doi.org/10.31887/DCNS.2010.12.1/trkjennerud

Rezaii, N., Mahowald, K., Ryskin, R., Dickerson, B., & Gibson, E. (2022). A syntax–lexicon trade-off in language production. *Proceedings of the National Academy of Sciences, 119*(25), e2120203119. https://doi.org/10.1073/pnas.2120203119

Samuel, D. B., & Widiger, T. A. (2008). A meta-analytic review of the relationships between the five-factor model and DSM-IV-TR personality disorders: A facet level analysis. *Clinical Psychology Review, 28*(8), 1326–1342. https://doi.org/10.1016/j.cpr.2008.07.002

Sanchez-Roige, S., Gray, J. C., MacKillop, J., Chen, C. H., & Palmer, A. A. (2018). The genetics of human personality. *Genes, Brain, and Behavior, 17*(3), e12439. https://doi.org/10.1111/gbb.12439

Santesteban-Echarri, O., MacQueen, G., Goldstein, B. I., Wang, J., Kennedy, S. H., Bray, S., Lebel, C., & Addington, J. (2021). Personality and risk for serious mental illness. *Early Intervention in Psychiatry, 15*(1), 133–139. https://doi.org/10.1111/eip.12921

Saulsman, L. M., & Page, A. C. (2004). The five-factor model and personality disorder empirical literature: A meta-analytic review. *Clinical Psychology Review, 23*(8), 1055–1085. https://doi.org/10.1016/j.cpr.2005.01.001

Simonsen, E., & Newton-Howes, G. (2018). Personality pathology and schizophrenia. *Schizophrenia Bulletin, 44*(6), 1180–1184. https://doi.org/10.1093/schbul/sby053

Skinner, B. F. (1965). *Science and human behavior*. Free Press. https://archive.org/details/scienceandhumanbehavior

Soto, C. J., & Jackson, J. J. (2020). Five-factor model of personality. In D. S. Dunn (Ed.), *Oxford bibliographies in psychology*. Oxford University Press. https://doi.org/10.1093/obo/9780199828340-0120

Staats, A. W. (1993). Personality theory, abnormal psychology, and psychological measurement: A psychological behaviorism. *Behavior Modification, 17*(1), 8–42. https://doi.org/10.1177/01454455930171002

Strus, W., Łakuta, P., & Cieciuch, J. (2021). Anankastia or psychoticism? Which one is better suited for the fifth trait in the pathological big five: Insight from the circumplex of personality metatraits perspective. *Frontiers in Psychiatry, 12*, 648386. https://doi.org/10.3389/fpsyt.2021.648386

Swales, M. A. (2022). Personality disorder diagnoses in ICD-11: Transforming conceptualisations and practice. *Clinical Psychology in Europe, 4*(Spec Issue), e9635. https://doi.org/10.32872/cpe.9635

Swinson Evans, T., Berkman, N., Brown, C., Gaynes, B., & Palmieri Weber, R. (2016). *Disparities within serious mental illness* (Technical Brief No. 25). Agency for Healthcare Research and Quality. https://effectivehealthcare.ahrq.gov/products/mental-illness-disparities/technical-brief

tailcalled. (2023, March 22). *Which personality traits are real?* Stress-testing the lexical hypothesis. Substack. https://tailcalled.substack.com/p/which-personality-traits-are-real

Tyrer, P., & Simmonds, S. (2003). Treatment models for those with severe mental illness and comorbid personality disorder. *The British Journal of Psychiatry, 182*(Suppl. 44), s15–s18. https://doi.org/10.1192/bjp.182.44.s15

Volkert, J., Gablonski, T.-C., & Rabung, S. (2018). Prevalence of personality disorders in the general adult population in Western countries: Systematic review and meta-analysis. *The British Journal of Psychiatry, 213*(6), 709–715. https://doi.org/10.1192/bjp.2018.202

Volungevičienė, A., Mlacić, B., & Gorbaniuk, O. (2022). The impact of our personality on others: The Lithuanian comprehensive lexical taxonomy of social effects. *Frontiers in Psychology, 13*, 869920. https://doi.org/10.3389/fpsyg.2022.869920

Weiner, I. B., & Greene, R. L. (2017). *Handbook of personality assessment*. John Wiley & Sons. https://doi.org/10.1002/9781119505101

Widiger, T. A., & Costa, P. T., Jr. (1994). Personality and personality disorders. *Journal of Abnormal Psychology, 103*(1), 78–91. https://doi.org/10.1037/0021-843X.103.1.78

Widiger, T. A., & Crego, C. (2019). The five factor model of personality structure: An update. *World Psychiatry, 18*(3), 271. https://doi.org/10.1002/wps.20658

Widiger, T. A., & Hines, A. (2022). The diagnostic and statistical manual of mental disorders, fifth edition alternative model of personality disorder. *Personality Disorders: Theory, Research, and Treatment, 13*(4), 347–355. https://doi.org/10.1037/per0000524

Widiger, T. A., & Simonsen, E. (2005). Alternative dimensional models of personality disorder: Finding a common ground. *Journal of Personality Disorders, 19*(2), 110–130. https://doi.org/10.1521/pedi.19.2.110.62627

Winsper, C., Bilgin, A., Thompson, A., Marwaha, S., Chanen, A. M., Singh, S. P., Wang, A., & Furtado, V. (2020). The prevalence of personality disorders in the community: A global systematic review and meta-analysis. *The British Journal of Psychiatry, 216*(2), 69–78. https://doi.org/10.1192/bjp.2019.166

World Health Organization (WHO). (2022). *International classification of diseases for mortality and morbidity statistics (11th Revision)*. https://icd.who.int

Zimmerman, M., Rothschild, L., & Chelminski, I. (2005). The prevalence of DSM-IV personality disorders in psychiatric outpatients. *The American Journal of Psychiatry, 162*(10), 1911–1918. https://doi.org/10.1176/appi.ajp.162.10.1911

Zimmermann, J., Kerber, A., Rek, K., Hopwood, C. J., & Krueger, R. F. (2019). A brief but comprehensive review of research on the alternative DSM-5 model for personality disorders. *Current Psychiatry Reports, 21*, 92. https://doi.org/10.1007/s11920-019-1079-z

Chapter 19
Mental Health Crises, Capacity, and Confinement: Legal and Clinical Pathways for Individuals Living with SMI

Introduction

Serious mental illness (SMI) presents profound challenges not only for affected individuals but also for the systems of care and governance tasked with ensuring safety, autonomy, and recovery. Beyond the clinical manifestations of psychiatric disorders, the lived experience of SMI often intersects with legal structures, ethical dilemmas, and social policies that shape the trajectory of treatment and support. Mental health crises, relapses, and the potential need for involuntary interventions highlight the delicate balance between protecting individuals and respecting their rights. This chapter situates these issues within a broader framework that integrates clinical insights with legal safeguards, underscoring the complexity of decision making in contexts where autonomy and protection may appear in tension.

A central focus of this discussion is the management of mental health crises that are acute episodes of psychological distress that demand immediate intervention. Crises are frequently precipitated by stress, trauma, or psychiatric instability, and they carry significant risks for both the individual and the community. Relapses, defined as the recurrence of symptoms after a period of improvement, further complicate the course of illness, often necessitating renewed treatment strategies and sometimes legal involvement. The chapter examines how these phenomena are addressed through clinical planning, behavioral interventions, and, when necessary, commitment procedures that invoke the authority of the state to ensure safety.

Equally critical are the mechanisms designed to preserve autonomy and informed participation in care. Psychiatric advance directives (PADs) provide individuals with the opportunity to articulate treatment preferences prior to crisis, while assessments of decision-making capacity distinguish between informed consent and assent in clinical practice. The roles of representative payees and guardianship are explored as forms of substituted decision making, raising important questions about the boundaries of autonomy and the responsibilities of caregivers and institutions.

G. F. McKeegan, *Behavior Change Interventions for Serious Mental Illness*, Evidence-Based Practices in Behavioral Health,
https://doi.org/10.1007/978-3-032-18372-9_19

These processes highlight the ethical dilemmas inherent in balancing individual rights with protective oversight.

Involuntary commitment and guardianship are legal avenues that, although at times essential, have profound effects on individual dignity, justice, and human rights. This analysis reviews the trajectory from crisis intervention to confinement, highlighting the importance of collaborative, person-centered strategies that incorporate both clinical judgment and robust legal protections. Building on the preceding overview of symptoms and challenges associated with SMI, this chapter moves from the clinical presentation to the systemic responses that shape treatment, autonomy, and protection in practice and presents a comprehensive understanding of how mental health systems navigate the intersection of care, law, and ethics in supporting individuals living with SMI.

Definition and Characteristics of Mental Health Crises

The convergence of mental health crises, involuntary treatment, decision-making capacity, guardianship determinations, and the incarceration of individuals living with SMI reflects systemic gaps at the interface of healthcare, law, and social policy. Responses to mental health crises that involve coercive treatment, substituted decision making, and custodial detention raise profound ethical and human rights questions about autonomy, dignity, and justice for people with SMI. Mental health crises, involuntary interventions, capacity and guardianship processes, and incarceration represent interconnected points along a continuum where clinical care, legal authority, and societal protection intersect and have profound consequences for the individual living with SMI, their families and caretakers, and mental health service providers,

There may be situations when a behavior needs to either stop or decrease in intensity, frequency, or duration. An action plan has not been developed to deal with a particular problematic behavior as the behavior may be unexpected or occur at a low frequency and intensity. The behavior may be dangerous to the person or to others or may become dangerous if it continues and worsens.

A mental health crisis can manifest in various ways for individuals living with SMI. It is generally defined as a situation in which a person who lives with SMI is unable to manage safely on their own and requires intervention from trained mental health service professionals. Individuals experiencing a crisis may present with intense fear, overwhelming negative emotions and thoughts, or a loss of behavioral control (National Alliance on Mental Illness [NAMI] Wisconsin, n.d.). A mental health crisis can be precipitated by factors such as heightened stress, bereavement, the loss of a relationship, disappointment, traumatic events, significant life changes, and less visible situations like severe depression, hopelessness, anxiety, anger, and panic (NAMI Wisconsin, n.d.). Indicators that an individual living with SMI may be experiencing a mental health crisis include attempts or plans to inflict self-harm or suicide, threats to harm oneself or others, verbal or physical aggression, marked social withdrawal, prolonged periods without sleep or food, and evidence of increased frequency or intensity of psychological distress, which may be associated with hallucinations or delusional beliefs (NAMI Wisconsin, n.d.). When the behaviors accompanying the crisis becomes dangerous to the person or others, mental health service professionals need to be contacted so they can assess the crisis and determine the extent of the intervention to ensure safety for the person and the public.

There are essential steps to follow during a mental health crisis. Initially, it is important to remain composed and avoid reacting emotionally, criticizing, or using negatively charged language (i.e., criticism). Service providers working with individuals living with SMI should strive to de-escalate the situation by maintaining a calm tone, moderate pace, and appropriate volume when speaking. It is crucial not to dismiss or minimize the individual's subjective experience during a crisis, including delusions or hallucinations, as this may undermine trust. Instead, focus on understanding what would increase their sense of safety and control.

Service providers should engage individuals using person-centered and reflective communication techniques, such as asking respectful, open-ended questions regarding their experience, and offering choices whenever possible to support autonomy, particularly by inquiring about what measures might help them feel safe and what has helped in similar situations (i.e., problem solving). Maintaining a non-judgmental, reality-oriented stance and refraining from making promises outside the provider's control can assist in reducing intensity of the crisis. Presenting realistic options empowers the individual to make informed decisions regarding their care.

If the person is willing to seek care, a plan of increased support can be developed and implemented. The person experiencing a crisis needs to be engaged and asked if there is someone on the recovery team who can help during the crisis by seeking advice. An individual experiencing the crisis may have a support plan for a mental health crisis or have ideas about what works for them.

The written plans for people living with mental health problems are called "psychiatric advance directives (PADs)." They are legal instruments that enable individuals living with SMI to articulate their treatment preferences prior to the onset of a mental health crisis. PADs support the autonomy of those with mental health conditions, facilitating appropriate care when it is most needed. Individuals who complete PADs are more likely to engage collaboratively with the recovery team and service providers, experience fewer involuntary interventions during crises, and report greater satisfaction with their mental health services (NAMI, 2020). PADs have been found to decrease the frequency of involuntary admissions for mental health treatment (Tinland et al., 2019). When properly implemented, PADs allow medical professionals, hospitals, law enforcement agencies, and caregivers to deliver care that reflects the individual's stated preferences.

If an individual is in immediate danger and unwilling to seek care, mental health service providers must prioritize the safety of both the individual and those around them. It is advisable to relocate the person to a calm and secure environment to minimize sensory overload or emotional triggers. Remove potentially harmful objects from the vicinity and ensure that someone remains present with the individual. Providers should implement self-control strategies aimed at de-escalating extreme emotional responses and alleviating feelings of being overwhelmed.

Recognizing when a mental health crisis exceeds one's capacity to manage is critical; seeking support from additional professionals may be necessary. Should the individual continue to pose a risk to themselves or others and lack a PAD, it may become necessary to contact a mental health service provider professional to consider involuntary admission to a psychiatric facility.

To reduce the likelihood of relapses or mental health crises, mental health service providers and recovery team members working with individuals who live with SMI should engage the person in developing comprehensive support plans addressing problematic behaviors that, if escalated, may pose risks to the individual or others. This consideration is particularly important when such behaviors have the potential to result in interactions with law enforcement.

Behaviors that are an aspect of living with SMI that have shown improvement or decreased in intensity or frequency for a period may reappear; this is defined as "relapse" (Shahrokh & Hales, 2003). Occasionally, a behavior may persist despite comprehensive intervention efforts. This phenomenon is frequently observed, especially when maladaptive behavior has persisted over time and has functioned efficiently and effectively for the individual. For people who live with SMI, maladaptive problematic behaviors are often reinforced by consistently leading to preferred outcomes or by permitting avoidance of undesirable covert or overt situations or demands.

An individual may increase the likelihood of receiving reinforcement if their actions convey an implicit message such as "Do this, or else." The "or else" component often represents problematic, potentially harmful behaviors, which can be distressing to mental health service professionals and staff. Consequently, over time, the mere threat of such challenging behaviors can lead service providers to comply with the individual's requests to prevent escalation, including instances of self-harm or aggression.

For example, Susan likes to smoke frequently; she smokes one cigarette, throwing away an unfinished cigarette followed shortly by smoking another. Her caregivers have developed a plan to cut down on the frequency of her smoking and limit the number of cigarettes and the places and times that she can smoke. This plan has been working, but Susan has recently been leaving the house and going to neighbors, banging on doors and requesting cigarettes. This has resulted in complaints to the police. Restricting cigarettes or ignoring her requests for "another smoke" has resulted in her screaming and then leaving the house to knock on doors or ask strangers for a cigarette.

At this point, one must consider what the goal of the intervention is. A comprehensive analysis of the problematic behavior is a good starting point. As stated before, first define the behavior that is the problem. By "define," describe the topography of the behavior—defining a behavior based on its physical form or shape, describing what the behavior looks, sounds, or feels like, rather than its function or purpose (Cooper et al., 2020). The definition needs to be understood so that everyone observing the behavior agrees when the behavior occurs and when it does not.

The definition should be concise and clear to all mental health service providers and stakeholders. A behavior that is targeted for change must be clearly described through an operational definition that makes it objective, so it can be observed, and measurable, allowing for consistent data collection and analysis of treatment effectiveness (Cooper et al., 2020).

After clearly defining the problematic behavior, each occurrence ought to be systematically documented by noting the time, location, and individuals present, as well as instances when the behavior does not occur. This approach facilitates a comprehensive understanding of the conditions under which the behavior is exhibited. For example, does Susan's "demands" for another cigarette only happen around certain staff? Do the demands occur at certain times or in certain situations (such as after meals, when there is less to do, in the morning)? Does it happen when she sees someone else smoking, even on a TV program? A change in the schedule of the "cigarette breaks" may be beneficial. If this behavior arises exclusively in the presence of a specific individual, it is important to determine whether that person has become a potential antecedent condition prompting Susan to request another cigarette. Has that person "given in to her" or promised her a cigarette as a "pay-off" for something else? Does that person smoke and the smell is retained in their clothes? This may be a condition for Susan to have "cravings." Could it be that Susan asking for another cigarette sets up a "chain of behaviors" that results in her yelling and leaving the house and engaging in the problematic behaviors stated above? Given that smoking is an addictive behavior, implementing an alternative activity for Susan—such as using nicotine gum or lozenges—between smoking sessions may help maintain consistent nicotine levels. This approach also provides a constructive option during periods when she might otherwise seek cigarettes.

At times, mental health service providers and staff must think about stopping the problematic behavior once it gets started to protect the person from harming himself or others or preventing legal problems and incarceration. To stop the behavior displayed by Susan, her mental health service providers and staff can give her a cigarette; even then, certain conditions can be developed for Susan, such as obtaining a cigarette after she engages in another alternative behavior that she may like to do, such as helping to cook, do laundry, or riding a stationary bike. A plan also can be considered that reinforces a time delay between Susan making a request for another cigarette and when she gets the cigarette. The service provider staff may say, "Susan, I will get you the cigarette but only after you ride the bike for 10 min. I will set a timer and when it rings, I can give you the cigarette. When you are smoking, you need to smoke it outside on the patio and sit down at the table." The mental health service providers also must reinforce Susan doing what she is asked to with verbal praise as well and specify the behavior for which she is receiving verbal praise.

Despite the best efforts in implementing plans, there will be times that the behavior will re-occur. During these times, mental health service providers and staff may become frustrated and "throw the baby out with the bathwater." They may give in, allowing Susan to "do what she wants" or just give her cigarettes (despite the safety concerns). At this stage, it is advisable to convene all members of Susan's recovery team to review the assessment and evaluation of the problem behavior and identify any potential oversights. Such a meeting would provide an opportunity to address outstanding questions and ensure that staff are thoroughly trained in the implementation of the developed plan.

While the aim of the intervention is to avoid the use of negative consequences, such as taking something away, there are situations for which it may be necessary. Behaviors such as smoking present significant treatment challenges due to the addictive properties of nicotine and the wide variety of circumstances in which individuals engage in smoking—both external and internal. When asked about their smoking habits, most smokers report using cigarettes numerous times during the day: upon waking, in the bathroom, after meals, while drinking coffee, socializing with friends over drinks, or before and after entering a store, among other situations. Additionally, individuals may smoke in response to a range of emotional states, including happiness, sadness, boredom, fatigue, anger, or excitement. Consequently, the ubiquity of these triggers makes cessation particularly challenging for many smokers. Giving a cigarette as a reinforcer may appear contradictory and may be seen as "giving in" or "bribing" because an item that is the focus of being limited and controlled for the safety of the person is being used to reinforce a behavior. Smoking may also be so "automatically reinforcing," as it does not respond to many social contingencies or other types of reinforcers such as verbal praise, food, and activities.

It is at this point that mental health service providers and staff must "think out of the box." While eliminating smoking would be extremely difficult, the mental health service providers and staff may want to consider delivering and withholding reinforcement for another response for the problem behavior. Using the example of Susan, her mental health service providers and staff would give her a cigarette after she engaged in another more adaptive behavior first, such as folding laundry, or riding on the stationary bike for 10 min. The goal would be that by using these interventions, there will be an increase in the frequency of requested appropriate responding, while keeping the occurrence of the problematic targeted behavior at a relatively low frequency.

For example, Susan has problems taking her medications. It is a challenge many times for her to take her medications. She will do other behaviors such as saying she has to go to the bathroom or "wait a minute" when it is time for the medication to be taken to avoid taking them; sometimes, this becomes a crisis, in that she will be loud and threatening to the staff. A plan can be developed that uses Susan's "smoking times" to be right after she takes her medications. A timer can be set that allows her to see how much time she has before the "cigarette break" is no longer available. If the individual does not take her prescribed medications and subsequently misses her scheduled smoke break, the next opportunity for a smoke break will be provided 30 min later when she takes her medications. This approach may be characterized as implementing a brief period during which reinforcement—in this case, the cigarette—is withheld following noncompliance, while compliance with medication administration is positively reinforced by rescheduling the smoke break to coincide with medication adherence after the designated interval.

The preceding plan presupposes comprehensive knowledge of both the conditions and reinforcers associated with the problematic behavior. It is possible that the individual living with SMI experiences certain situations resulting from the occurrence of challenging behavior as either reinforcing or aversive. Therefore, a thorough assessment is essential to accurately identify relevant stimuli and antecedent conditions. The most effective approach involves systematically testing each condition, closely monitoring behavioral outcomes, and meticulously documenting results. Repetition of these trials is critical, as initial changes or novel conditions may produce only temporary effects. Over time, the reinforcing value of a stimulus tends to diminish as novelty subsides; for example, individuals often experience decreased desire for a new food or beverage after repeated consumption. The primary objective of such assessments is to generate a greater number of competing positive scenarios or reinforcers, thereby expanding the range of effective treatment options for reducing problematic behaviors.

The initial phase involves identifying a diverse range of potential reinforcers for inclusion in the assessment. This process generally starts by soliciting input from individuals most familiar with the person engaging in the challenging behavior, as well as from mental health professionals and support staff. The recovery team—those who are stakeholders in helping the person recover—may have to implement a systematic procedure for identifying conditions (reinforcers) that effectively competes with the problem behavior. Sometimes, many reinforcers must be identified that can effectively compete with the reinforcer that is maintaining the problematic behavior. During this assessment, team members are encouraged to employ creativity and occasionally introduce novel stimuli that may serve as effective reinforcers for the individual. One strategy to identify preferences is to pose a "fantasy question"—asking what activities or items the individual has considered but has not realistically pursued. However, it is important to maintain practical expectations; any suggested stimulus or activity should be realistically attainable. For example, while a world cruise might be highly desirable, it is generally not feasible for individuals with limited financial resources or other obligations. Furthermore, the reward should be readily available and deliverable in a timely manner.

For optimal effectiveness, reinforcers should be easily provided by the caretaker after the individual demonstrates the desired adaptive behavior. The reinforcer then can be presented to the person systematically and observe if it can effectively compete as a reinforcer for an alternative behavior or be as effective as a reinforcer that is problematic, such as smoking or drinking too much coffee.

Once the reinforcers or conditions have been identified, the next step is to develop a plan in which the person living with SMI can gain access to what they find reinforcing. It is very important to clearly identify what behavior needs to happen to access the reinforcer. Clearly identifying the behavior will help everyone involved in supporting the person living with SMI to understand and implement the plan successfully. For instance, while the phrase "a change in attitude" is ambiguous, specifying behaviors such as "rising within 15 min after being called and adhering to prescribed medication instructions" provides greater clarity.

The key to any plan is consistency in implementation. Using football as an example, if the players decide "to do their own thing" during a game, it is doubtful if the team will score. More than likely, those players will not be with the team for very long. The only way the team scores in football is when the players implement the "game plan"—run, block, and throw—as it was written up by the coaching staff and rehearsed in practice. If the plan does not work, then it is up to the team and coaches to "go back to the drawing board" and try something different with the talent on the team that they have. A treatment plan to deal with problem behaviors requires all stakeholders to be on the same page and understand what is in the "game plan." If it is unclear, then it will not be implemented consistently; the person living with SMI will continue with the problem behavior and may get worse if the staff inadvertently reinforce the problem behavior.

Step-by-Step Summary for Developing a Behavioral Support Plan for Challenging Behaviors

1. If a new challenging behavior occurs or another behavior changes suddenly, make sure that there are no medical reasons for the change. People living with SMI may be more susceptible to physical problems, especially with the side effects of the psychiatric medications that are prescribed. The best practice is to have the person evaluated by a primary care physician as well as the prescribing psychiatric service provider.
2. Define the behavior that is of concern. Describe the behavior in concrete terms—basically what is seen, heard, and sensed. Do not use labels or assume intentions about the behavior; avoid the use of labels. For instance, instead of saying, "Carlos gets mean as a snake," define what is seen/and heard: "Carlos hits others in the face with his closed fist."
3. Describe concretely what happens before the behavior occurs. Provide a detailed description of the antecedent conditions leading to the targeted behavior. Clearly document the observable actions and environmental context that immediately precede the behavior that is targeted to be modified. Specificity is essential—describing the situation and the individual's actions with precision. For example, rather than stating, "When Carlos gets mad and frustrated," offer a concrete account such as: "When Carlos is informed that he cannot have a cigarette or that he must wait, he responds by loudly stating, 'Why? I have my rights!' He then begins pacing quickly, striking his fist into the palm of his other hand while audibly mumbling. If another individual approaches him during this time, Carlos fixes his gaze on them and asserts in a raised voice, 'You better stay out of my way,' while shaking his fist and issuing verbal threats of physical aggression."
4. Identify and document potential antecedent conditions that may serve as precursors to the targeted behaviors. Record observable patterns or situational

factors that appear to consistently precede the behavior in question. These may include specific interactions, environmental triggers, or unmet expectations. For example, Carlos exhibits specified problematic behaviors when he requests a cigarette outside of his scheduled smoking times. Additionally, these behaviors have been observed in response to denial of his requests—particularly by newly assigned or female staff members at the group home—such as when he is not permitted to visit fast food establishments for coffee.

5. Monitor and document each occurrence of the behavior. Be sure to note relevant details such as the context, time of day, and individuals present during the incident, as these conditions are essential for accurate data collection.
6. Behavior does not occur all the time. It may be important to also observe and record when the behavior does not occur in the situations. Carlos is told "No" or is delayed in getting the cigarette and does not display the behaviors described above—what is different about those situations? Again, record when, where, and with whom the behavior does not occur.
7. Members of the recovery team may know what Carlos likes. It is important to engage with Carlos and ask him. If there are not many items that Carlos prefers that can be easily accessible and obtained, then develop a list based on experience. At times, novel items and activities must be tried—just like new food items—to see if they can be a preferred item.
8. Identify and promote adaptive replacement behaviors. It is essential not only to reduce or eliminate the targeted behavior but also to encourage the development of appropriate, adaptive alternatives. Staff should identify specific behaviors that can serve as constructive replacements. For example, rather than engaging in aggressive behavior when frustrated, Carlos should be supported in developing adaptive strategies to manage his emotions when he is required to wait for a cigarette or is denied a request. This may include offering him choices, reminding him of scheduled times for smoking or outings, and reinforcing his ability to tolerate delays or refusals.
9. Develop a collaborative and comprehensive behavior support plan. A unified behavior support plan should be created with input and agreement from all relevant parties, including the person living with SMI, staff, and mental health service professionals. The plan must contain and outline the following:

   - Strategies for reinforcing desirable behaviors such as attending structured activities (e.g., clubhouse participation), adhering to medication regimens, and following established routines.
   - Specific skill-building interventions aimed at enhancing emotional regulation and adaptive abilities. These may include relaxation techniques, mindfulness exercises, or other therapeutic modalities.
   - Procedures for responding to occurrences of the targeted behavior, including the implementation of appropriate consequences such as temporary loss of privileges or restricted access to preferred items.

10. Monitor implementation and collect behavioral data. Ongoing observation and documentation are critical to evaluating the effectiveness of the plan. Staff should record the following:

    - The time, location, and individuals present during both the occurrence and the non-occurrence of the targeted behavior and the demonstration of adaptive skills.
    - Instances where the individual successfully utilizes adaptive alternative behaviors and strategies, such as practicing deep breathing when denied a request even if the alternative behaviors is prompted by mental health service providers.
    - Scheduled opportunities for the individual to rehearse appropriate responses to triggering situations. Role-playing practice sessions as to when and how to engage in adaptive alternative behaviors should be a part of the support plan. For example, staff may prompt Carlos to take deep breaths in a private space when he is informed that he must wait or cannot access a desired item.

11. Ensure staff engagement and modify interaction strategies. The behavior support plan must also address the responsibilities of mental health service providers and staff. Their role includes the following:

    - Adjusting their communication and interaction styles to prevent escalation of the targeted behavior.
    - Supporting the individual in practicing adaptive skills, such as guiding Carlos through deep breathing exercises and encouraging him to consult his personalized schedule for smoking times or outings.
    - Avoiding language that may be provoking a negative response. For instance, staff should refrain from using the word "No," and instead say, "Carlos, I'm not sure if that's possible right now. Let me check and I'll get back to you." When feasible, staff should provide a specific time when the request can be fulfilled.
    - Implementing proactive interventions when early signs of agitation and distress appear, such as instructing Carlos to go to his room to calm down and regain control.
    - Responding appropriately in emergency situations, including contacting support personnel, ensuring the safety of others, directing Carlos to a safe space, and administering PRN medication as prescribed.

Hospitalization, Involuntary Treatment, and Guardianship

Despite best efforts, there are times when mental health service providers and staff may have to get other care teams involved, such as inpatient psychiatric facilities. Relapse in people living with SMI is defined as the recurrence of a mental health-related condition after a period of improvement or apparent cure (American

Psychological Association, n.d.-c). Relapse is of critical concern because of its associations with poor psychosocial outcomes, increased healthcare utilization, diminished quality of life (QoL), interruption of the recovery process in the community, higher rates of future relapses, increases in stigmatization, higher frequency and intensity of problematic behaviors, lower levels of employment, and elevated economic burden (American Psychiatric Association, 2022; Emsley 2013; Lin et al., 2021; Pinto et al., 2020; Rivelli et al., 2024).

Despite advances in pharmacological and psychosocial treatments, there is a persistent risk of relapse among people living with SMI emphasizing the need for sustained interventions and systemic support to reduce recurrence and improve long-term outcomes. Relapse rates remain high across types of mental health problems. Research has shown that about a third of individuals who are living with SMI will relapse within a year even if treatment has continued and adherence to treatment is not an issue (Emsley et al., 2013).

Nonadherence—not complying with treatment recommendations—is a factor that impacts the frequency of relapse and the duration between relapses. Experts have considered that relapses are an aspect of the course of living with an SMI. Relapses often occur early during the occurrence of the mental health problem, with approximately 81.9% of individuals experiencing a relapse within 5 years of their first episode of schizophrenia spectrum mental health problem. Relapses frequently occur following the cessation of treatment, and extended treatment durations before discontinuation have not been shown to decrease the likelihood of relapse. The shift from remission to relapse may be sudden and typically presents with minimal early warning signs. Upon relapse, symptom severity often returns to levels observed during the initial psychotic episode (Emsley et al., 2013; Gignac, A., et al., 2015; Lin et al., 2021; Pinto et al., 2020; Rivelli et al., 2024.)

Psychiatric readmission is influenced by multiple factors, including the type of mental health problem, demographics, and treatment adherence. Short inpatient stays, younger age, unemployment, socioeconomic deprivation, prior admissions, and certain mental health problems like schizophrenia spectrum, bipolar and depressive mental health problems, and alcohol-related psychotic mental health problems are linked to higher readmission rates (Osborn et al., 2021). Nonadherence to medication and limited psychosocial support further elevate risk . Suicidal ideation and co-occurring PTSD are notable predictors. Effective interventions, such as comprehensive care, residential treatment, and coordinated discharge planning and management by service providers can reduce readmissions for high-risk individuals (Owusu et al., 2022).

A recent retrospective cohort study involving over 8000 individuals identified as living with schizophrenia spectrum mental health problems found that approximately 31% experienced relapses during an average follow-up period of slightly more than 2 years. These individuals were also more likely to have frequent emergency room visits and hospitalizations (Rivelli et al., 2024). In those with bipolar-type mental health problems, recovery following the first episode of mania remains challenging; only 62% attained symptomatic recovery within the initial year. Relapse rates are notable, with 41% experiencing recurrence after 1 year and nearly 60% within 4 years (Gignac et al., 2015; Pinto et al., 2020). For individuals aged

15–24 years who undergo a first episode of psychosis, relapse rates remain high despite early intervention strategies. Approximately 38% experience at least one relapse during care, and long-term relapse rates may reach up to 80% within 5 years (Brown et al., 2020).

Relapses in people living with SMI is multifactorial, shaped by an interplay of demographic, socioeconomic, clinical, and neurobiological influences. Demographic variables and socioeconomic status shape the risk of relapses in SMI. Insurance coverage emerges as a powerful predictor: individuals insured by Medicaid and Medicare experience relapse at rates 33% and 22% higher, respectively, compared to those with private insurance. Age also plays an important understated role, with each additional year conferring a modest 1% decrease in relapse risk. Racial and ethnic background further influences vulnerability, as relapse rates are disproportionately higher among Black Non-Hispanic, Hispanic, and Other Pacific Islander populations compared to White Non-Hispanic individuals (Rivelli et al., 2024). These disparities may be rooted in differential access to care, social determinants of health, and cultural contexts around mental health (Rivelli et al., 2024).

Clinical history and co-occurring disorders play a significant role in relapse risk. Substance use mental health problems stand out as a major factor for relapse (Brown et al., 2020; Owusu et al., 2022). The presence of extrapyramidal symptoms (EPS), a side effect of antipsychotic medications (APS), also increases relapse prevalence by 78%. A history of prior relapse shapes future risk with a single past episode raising the probability of subsequent recurrence by 5%. Medication nonadherence is the most frequent context in which relapses occur, accounting for more than a quarter of relapses in first-episode psychosis, often intertwined with substance use (Rivelli et al., 2024).

Securing a psychiatric inpatient admission for an individual in a mental health crisis may require court involvement. Individuals living with SMI frequently exhibit impaired awareness regarding behaviors that could compromise their own safety or the safety of others; the result is a reluctance and refusal to pursue hospitalization when it is necessary. This is comparable to what is sometimes observed in those experiencing physical health issues: some may delay seeking medical attention due to concerns about receiving unfavorable health information, hoping that symptoms or discomfort will diminish over time. Others may avoid hospitalization because it represents a loss of autonomy, including restrictions on personal routines such as time to get out of bed, eating, and other activities. Hospitals, as institutions, operate according to established protocols, and individuals admitted are required to adhere to these policies, which can be challenging for those who value independence.

The outcome is that the person living with SMI will not admit herself voluntarily into a hospital for care that is needed. There are times when going to the hospital for treatment is involuntary—the mental health recovery and support teams may have to decide to have the person living with SMI to be admitted to a hospital for treatment against her wishes. Involuntary treatment or commitment is typically justified under conditions of severe mental health conditions, with variations in definitions across countries. The World Health Organization (WHO) outlines that involuntary treatment in a psychiatric facility should only be used for the well-being or safety of the person experiencing a mental health crisis, or to protect others (World Health Organization & Office of the United Nations High Commissioner for Human Rights, 2023). Nevertheless, a meta-analysis indicated that 23% of people living with SMI experience involuntary hospitalization.

However, getting a person involuntarily admitted or committed to a hospital for evaluation and treatment is a legal matter, as it is temporarily depriving the person of her constitutional rights to make decisions of her own. The consideration of involuntary commitment of a service user by the recovery team results in ethical and clinical quandaries for the mental health service providers. Mental health care is characterized by a collaborative relationship between professional providers and consumers. Healthcare professionals contribute specialized knowledge in human behavior while consumers offer perspectives based on their individual experiences, preferences, and objectives. This partnership is anchored in ethical standards—most notably, beneficence and respect for autonomy—and frequently utilizes a shared decision-making approach. The process begins when the mental health user communicates their concern, prompting the mental healthcare service professional to assess the issue. Together, they engage in a discussion about the problem and potential treatments. Ultimately, the consumer decides whether to proceed with an action or decline intervention; treatment is only carried out if the mental health service user gives consent (Stallman & Gupta, 2025), which is the voluntary assent or approval given by an individual after being fully informed about risk and benefits of the proposed treatment (American Psychological Association, n.d-a).

The ethical principles that are the focus of concerns in involuntary mental health treatment include the four core principles related to the care of individuals by service providers including the following:

- Beneficence: The obligation to act in the individual's best interest, promoting his well-being and recovery. Ethical dilemmas occur when coercive measures are justified as beneficial but may harm the therapeutic alliance or the person's dignity (Laureano et al., 2024; Varkey, 2021).
- Autonomy: The principle of respecting an individual's ability to make decisions about his treatment. Ethical concerns arise when involuntary treatment restricts autonomy, especially for people deemed capable of making informed decisions (Laureano et al., 2024; Varkey, 2021).
- Non-maleficence: The principle of avoiding harm. Ethical concerns include whether coercive measures, such as involuntary hospitalization or administration of medication, cause more harm than good (Laureano et al., 2024; Varkey, 2021).
- Justice: Ensuring fairness and equity in treatment. Ethical concerns include potential discrimination against vulnerable and marginalized populations, such as ethnic and gender minorities or socioeconomically disadvantaged individuals in the application of involuntary measures (Laureano et al., 2024; Varkey, 2021).

In addition, other ethical principles that are related to and support the core ethical principles need to be considered in the implementation of involuntary treatment for a person living with SMI are as follows:

- Human dignity: protecting the inherent dignity of the individual, which can be compromised by coercive practices (Laureano et al., 2024).
- Relational ethics: Emphasizing the importance of maintaining ethical relationships between the service user and mental health service providers, including communication respect, and shared decision making (Laureano et al., 2024).
- Informed consent: This is directly rooted in the principle of autonomy. Autonomy emphasizes that all individuals have intrinsic worth and the right to make rational decisions about their own bodies and healthcare (Varkey, 2021).
- Truth-telling: This supports autonomy and informed consent by providing service users with the information they need to make informed decisions about their healthcare (Varkey, 2021).
- Professional competence: The service professional considering commitment for involuntary treatment requires specialist knowledge, training, skill, and experience, and should not provide service if the requisite skills and knowledge are lacking (American Psychological Association, 2017).

Involuntary treatment encompasses a range of ethical, legal, and clinical factors. Service providers may encounter ethical dilemmas when involuntary commitment conflicts with adherence to established ethical principles, particularly in cases where an individual's clinical circumstances create tension between two or more moral imperatives (American Psychological Association, n.d.-b).

Balancing an individual's autonomy with care and safety remains central to the ethics of involuntary mental health treatment. Core principles like autonomy, beneficence, non-maleficence, and justice guide decisions about when involuntary measures are justified, emphasizing that coercion should only occur when there is a serious risk of harm and always prioritize the well-being of the person. Establishing clear criteria for involuntary treatment is essential to protect individual rights; however, ongoing discussions persist regarding the definitions of "danger," "imminent," "grave danger," and what constitutes treatable conditions (Laureano et al., 2024).

The personal values of mental health service providers frequently influence decision-making processes. Individuals living with SMI and their families may experience exclusion from these processes, which can result in diminished dignity as well as increased disenfranchisement, marginalization, and stigmatization. Additionally, limited resources may contribute to higher rates of involuntary hospitalization, particularly among marginalized populations (Laureano et al., 2024).

Assertive community treatment (ACT), individualized planning, crisis intervention, and PADs can reduce reliance on involuntary care and improve the engagement of the person living with SMI (Tinland et al., 2019). Evidence-based practices highlight transparent oversight, shared decision making, and PADs are ways to foster trust and respect autonomy. Ethical reflection and collaboration among professionals are vital for humane and effective approaches.

Involuntary treatment typically entails mandatory mental health assessments and/or interventions for individuals deemed incapable of providing informed consent due to impaired decision-making capacity (Stallman & Gupta, 2025). Such treatments may be administered in hospital settings or within the community and are governed by legislation that varies across jurisdictions (Mental Illness Policy. Org., 2024; Organization for Economic Cooperation and Development [OECD], 2021). The person living with SMI and experiencing a crisis may decline treatment, refuse medications and other treatments that are recommended to her to assist in stabilization and recovery. A person who is administered medication involuntarily must meet the same criteria that result in getting committed to a psychiatric facility. This again is a legal matter and may involve the courts if a person is administered medication against her wishes.

At other times, the person living with SMI is discharged after a few days. Sometimes, the person who gets committed agrees to become a voluntary admission, meaning that the individual gives consent to being admitted to a psychiatric treatment facility. Being "voluntary" gives the person more control over their treatment and discharge; the person living with SMI who is hospitalized voluntarily can give "notice" to the hospital and treatment team that he wants to be discharged. The treatment team may agree that he can be discharged; if the team disagrees with the person's request, then the team must petition the court for a commitment and go through the process stated above.

Insurance administrators also have a say in the person's discharge; the insurance administrators may have determined that the person no longer benefits from being in the hospital and needs to get treatment in the community. This sometimes results in the "revolving door" of a person living with SMI being committed and released repeatedly with little to no improvement. Studies have found that short periods of inpatient hospitalizations are a risk factor for future relapses and readmissions (Owusu et al., 2022).

The mental health service providers and the recovery teams may have to resort to the courts for someone living with SMI. The following are some legal issues that may involve a person living with SMI and the care team:

1. Involuntary admission to a hospital for evaluation and treatment.
2. Treatment over objection.
3. Capacity to independently make decisions (i.e., financial, health, and living arrangements).

There is no one set of rules to the above. Each state has regulations that govern the above-stated legal issues. The regulations in some states are complex; some are restrictive. There are websites available that summarize—and evaluate—each state's regulations on mental health issues (Center for Public Health Law Research, n.d.; Mental Illness Policy.Org., 2024). The commonalities of the regulations will be summarized in the following section. It is advised that the service providers and recovery teams become familiar with the mental health regulations of the state in which the individual living with SMI resides.

Involuntary Admission to a Psychiatric Facility

When someone is living with SMI and is at imminent risk of harming themselves or others, involuntary treatment may be required, especially when no less restrictive options are available. In these cases, mental health service professionals must act within strict legal frameworks, evaluating the immediate risks and aiming to stabilize the individual's condition. The nature of this intervention is inherently coercive, as it proceeds without the person's consent and is governed by laws designed to protect both the individual and the community. The goal follows the core ethical principle of beneficence—that is, to promote the person's well-being and safety, even if treatment must take place against their wishes (Stallman & Gupta, 2025).

Criteria for involuntary admission to a psychiatric facility for evaluation and treatment are known as an involuntary commitment. It is a civil commitment, and the procedures and regulations are established by laws, which vary between states and jurisdictions, although there are some commonalities; there is, however, a range of what the commonalities mean among the states. In all states, commitment is a legal civil procedure rather than a criminal one. This process involves a court-appointed, qualified mental health professional evaluating an individual living with SMI who exhibits behaviors of a serious mental health condition. If deemed necessary, the individual may be involuntarily admitted to a psychiatric or general inpatient hospital for mental health assessment and treatment.

The nature of involuntary treatment is inherently coercive, proceeding without the individual's consent and often involving mandatory hospitalization or community-based treatment orders. These interventions may entail restrictive practices, such as seclusion, physical, mechanical, chemical restraints and the involuntary administration of medications (i.e., "medications over objection"), which are employed as a last resort and accompanied by safeguards to prevent misuse and minimize harm (Stallman & Gupta, 2025).

Evaluation and treatment may be part of the commitment, or it may just entail a "temporary detention order (TDO)" in a mental health treatment facility to assess the individual for her safety. Detention is limited in duration, typically measured in hours, with the exact period of emergency detainment differing by jurisdiction. Such orders are generally short term, ranging from 48 to 72 hours, and are subsequently followed by a judicial hearing to evaluate the individual's mental health status.

In many jurisdictions, people presenting with SMI also can have compulsory treatment while in the community; this is sometimes referred to as involuntary commitment to outpatient treatment commonly known as assisted outpatient treatment (AOT). AOT shares legal processes with commitment to an inpatient facility, but the person is committed by the courts to participate in outpatient treatment. The problem with AOT is that there is no consequence if a person drops out of treatment. A review of studies found that the effectiveness of compulsory community treatment did not significantly improve service use, social functioning, mental state, or quality of life compared to standard voluntary care (Segal & Badran, 2024).

The legal standards for civil commitment vary across states. However, all states fundamentally include the criterion of "future dangerousness," meaning there is a risk that an individual with a mental health condition may exhibit behaviors (or the absence of behaviors) that could pose a danger to themselves or others if they do not receive appropriate treatment. Some states have now extended the criterion to include that the person poses a physical threat to himself through an inability to care for her basic needs, such as eating, hygiene, and taking medically indcated medications. This standard is referred to as the "grave disability" standard, which indicates that an individual who lives with SMI is unable to provide for their own essential needs required for survival. This does not include being homeless as a person does not pose a threat to her basic well-being and safety even if the person is "unhoused" and living on the streets; she can make decisions to take care of basic needs (i.e., going to shelters, having some kind of protection from the weather, and seeking out social services). However, if she is unable to appreciate, understand, and avoid the risks of taking care of chronic physical problems—winter freezes or storms, and starvation—then she may be dangerous to herself although not having thoughts of intentionally harming herself or committing suicide.

Certain states employ a more stringent criterion referred to as "the need for treatment." This commitment standard emphasizes harm prevention, acknowledging that individuals who live with SMI may, at times, lack the capacity to recognize or comprehend their need for intervention. Consequently, untreated symptoms associated with SMI can lead to significant impairment in functioning and pose unacceptable risks to the individual's psychiatric and physical well-being.

Commitment proceedings often follow a period of involuntary emergency hospitalization (TDOs) during which an individual with acute behaviors linked to living with SMI is confined for a short duration in a treatment facility for evaluation and stabilization by mental health professionals who may then determine whether further civil commitment for a longer period is appropriate or necessary. All states have a process for this under the law. In most states, the maximum period of a TDO is 72 hours or less.

Civil commitment procedures may occur either within a courtroom setting or through proceedings held at a hospital. In situations where commitment is carried out without a court hearing, an appeals process typically exists that involves judicial oversight, often using a specialty court. Within such courts, a magistrate with limited judicial authority presides over specific matters. During these hearings, the individual subject to commitment retains the right to present witnesses and to be represented by legal counsel. The decision regarding involuntary commitment to a psychiatric facility is rendered by a judge, as juries are not utilized in this process.

Behaviors that Are Considered for Commitment

The basic behavioral criteria for consideration of involuntary commitment for treatment are if a person is a danger to self or others or does not have the ability to take care of basic needs that in all probability would result in harm to the person due to the problem behaviors of their mental health condition, this "disability" places the person's physical well-being in jeopardy. The nuances of the commitment law for each state may differ but dangerousness to self or others—in any way—is the nexus of the commitment laws. Basically, the question is whether the behavior of the person living with a SMI is a threat to their own life or is jeopardizing the physical safety of others by their behavior. The problem lies in the interpretation or the opinion of the person in authority who judges that the person's life is in danger or that the person living with SMI is putting the lives of others at risk. The petitioner who is asking for the person living with SMI to be involuntarily committed must state and give examples of how that person's mental health condition and problematic behaviors are putting their physical well-being in danger. Just because the behavior or lack of behavior—such as taking care of one's physical well-being—may result in the person living with SMI developing a life-threatening illness is not sufficient to deprive that person of their liberties and freely make decisions. The question is if the person's behavior imminently places their life in danger, such as walking into traffic on a highway or jumping in front of a train. The person who is using street drugs that impairs their judgment and is jumping into traffic is not considered a danger to herself or others; the assumption is that once the effect of the drug "wears off," the life-threatening behaviors would abate. The person using drugs can be taken to an emergency room and be evaluated; if the life-threatening behavior is the result of "intoxication" from any substance, then that person would not be considered for involuntary commitment to a mental health treatment facility.

There is an inherent tension between protecting the rights of the individual living with SMI and protecting their well-being and that of others. Judges and the courts take infringement of constitutional rights very seriously; there must be very good reasons for taking away a person's liberty and autonomy even for a short period, especially if that person has not broken the law.

Although the mental health service providers and staff might be concerned about the person living with SMI talking to themselves incessantly in public, this is not a criterion for commitment. Having a belief that one owns the World Bank also is not a reason for commitment unless the beliefs result in potential harm to self in some way or to others. Unfortunately, the above behaviors may result in problematic interactions with law enforcement.

Length of Time that the Behaviors Need to Be Witnessed

In some states, a petitioner who is asking for the person living with SMI to be committed to a treatment facility against their will must give eyewitness testimony and examples of the behavior; the eyewitness testimony and examples have to be about that the person living with SMI and related to how the manifested behaviors are dangerous to self or others or unable to care for self; the testimony and examples have to meet the criteria for commitment. The testimony, eyewitness accounts, and examples must be within a certain time frame, usually within the past few days to a month. Examples of unsafe and dangerous behaviors that occurred in the past are not taken into consideration. For example, it may not be admissible as evidence of dangerousness if the person attacked a family member or threatened to kill himself 2 months ago. The phrase "imminent danger" is a term often used when it comes to deciding if a person living with a mental health problem needs commitment to a treatment facility.

Who Can Initiate the Commitment Process?

In all states, anyone can petition the courts for commitment. Hospital staff, family members, and police are often the ones who begin the commitment proceedings. It also is important that whoever does initiate the proceedings has witnessed the behaviors that the person is doing that cause concerns about the safety of the person and others. It is essential to describe explicitly the observable actions of individuals living with SMI, rather than speculating about their intentions. The determination of whether these actions meet the criteria for commitment is solely within the jurisdiction of the courts.

Length of Time that a Person Can Be Committed

Commitment can last a few weeks (2–3 weeks) to a few months (3–6 months). Commitment is different from an emergency detention; during TDO, the time of being involuntarily confined is 2–3 days. The person living with SMI is evaluated to see if further treatment is necessary. At the end of the temporary confinement, the treatment team can decide if the person is well enough to be discharged or additional time is needed for further treatment. Again, the criterion for discharge is determined by state regulations—if the person living with SMI does not meet criteria to be held involuntarily at a treatment facility, then they must be discharged. The mental health service providers and other stakeholders may disagree with the mental health facility and the treating professionals' decision to discharge the person living with SMI. The mental health service providers and staff want the person to improve and may have expectations that are beyond what can be done in a mental health facility. The treatment teams are under the limitation of the legal regulations.

Appeal of the Involuntary Commitment Decision

If a person living with SMI is committed to a psychiatric facility, that person has a right to challenge and appeal the commitment. The appeal usually is held in a courtroom, and the person who is being considered for commitment can hire an attorney and call witnesses to support the appeal. Testimony and cross examination of witnesses can be done. The judge (or hearing officer) hears the evidence and decides about the involuntary commitment.

Less Restrictive Interventions (e.g., AOT)

Involuntary commitment to treatment is a serious matter—both for mental health service providers and staff and for the legal system. There is inherent tension in the commitment process. The mental health service providers and staff want what is best for the person living with SMI; the legal system hesitates to take away or suspend a person's liberties and rights to make their decision. This sometimes results in a frustrating process, and the outcome may not be what the mental health service providers and staff expect. The person living with SMI may not be committed as the judge is of the opinion that the person does not meet the criterion for commitment.

At times, it may be best to consider a less restrictive alternative such as Assertive Outpatient Treatment (AOT). AOT provides community-based services to people living with SMI. The person eligible for AOT has a history of hospital admissions—voluntary or involuntary—and/or has exhibited dangerous behaviors towards themselves or others. The goal of AOT is to reduce the manifestation of dangerous behaviors for any offense and to get the person into a treatment setting to reduce the possibility of being a danger to self or others before resorting to involuntary commitment or possible incarceration. A person living with SMI can be committed to AOT the same way as to a hospital. It is seldom used; the person committed can refuse to attend the treatment being offered without any legal consequence.

This may not be acceptable to mental health service providers and staff as the person living with SMI and the mental health service providers and staff are in the same position as before. The refusal to accept treatment voluntarily is an aspect of living with SMI. This problematic behavior is called "anosognosia" or lack of insight. It is the lack of awareness that one has a mental health problem and is prominent symptom of an SMI; it is not a denial but a lack of awareness by the person that he is manifesting behaviors that are inappropriate for the context and that his behaviors are dangerous to himself or others. This behavioral phenomenon is the primary reason individuals living with SMI may decline medication or refrain from seeking treatment. In certain circumstances, involuntary admission to a mental health facility may be considered as the sole viable option.

Treatment over Objection

All people living in the United States have constitutional right to decide they take into their bodies, including medications. A person living with a SMI has that right. If that person refuses medications, it may take a court order to force the person to take medication—usually using intramuscular injections (IMs). In the hospital, a person who is delusional or paranoid about being harmed by medications may refuse medications. Hospitals must follow the legal statutes of the state to administer medication over objection. The procedure may be for another mental health service provider to make an opinion that the person has met the standard of being a danger to self or others (or whatever the standard is in the state). In some states, it may take a court order signed by a judge to make that decision. Certain jurisdictions stipulate that, prior to the consideration of involuntary medication administration, the individual must have previously experienced positive outcomes from the prescribed treatment and, based on reasonable assessment, is likely to benefit from its use again.

Websites Pertaining to State Commitment Laws

There are useful websites that provide helpful information about commitment laws for each state; more importantly, these sites provide step-by-step instructions as to what to do and the requirements for any involuntary commitment to proceed. The information is available through the Policy Surveillance Program at the Center for Public Health Law Research, Beasley School of Law, Temple University (2024), as well as in the Standards for Involuntary Commitment (Assisted Treatment) State-by-State, provided by the Treatment Advocacy Center and Mental Illness Policy Org. (2024).

Guardianships: Capacity to Independently Make Decisions (i.e., Financial, Health, and Living Arrangements)

Many problems and possible solutions that face the person living with SMI have been identified in the previous chapters. However, it is not just the person living with SMI facing these problems but also the mental health service providers and staff. The mental health service providers and staff are concerned about the safety and welfare of the person living with SMI for whom they support.

There may come a time when the members of the support and recovery team for the individual living with SMI realize that the problematic behaviors being manifested by the person will not improve to the point that the person can live and make life choices independently. The choices involve making decisions about health care, recognizing physical and mental health problems, getting treatment for the problems, knowing the risks and benefits of treatment and abiding by the demands of treatment. Financial decisions also can be problematic; the person living with SMI can be taken advantage of by others, spend money recklessly and impulsively purchase items that either they cannot afford or is not needed; for instance, buying a car and the person cannot drive, the loan rates are exorbitant, or the car needs major repairs. As pointed out previously, many problems associated with living with SMI include problems with memory, language, social skills, wanting to be left alone, understanding what is being said, and dependent on others for completing daily independent living skills (e.g., making sure medication sure taken correctly, eating healthy food). Many people living with SMI may live in neighbors that have crime rates; at times the person living with SMI may be a target for financial and sexual exploitation by others who reside in the vicinity of the person living with SMI.

Definitions of Capacity, Legal Competence, and Consent

Capacity is when a person has the demonstrated ability to receive information about a specific matter, understand the information, reason and deliberate, maintain appropriate values and objectives, appreciate one's situation, comprehend provided information, and make and communicate independent decisions. An informed independent choice is a dynamic attribute that may fluctuate in degree over time (American Bar Association [ABA], 2018; Buchanan, 2004). Being incapacitated is that the person has not demonstrated the ability to comprehend information given to him and use it to decide himself about himself. Legal competence, by contrast, is both task-specific and dichotomous; it determines whether an individual is legally empowered to have their healthcare choices honored. This status relies on possessing adequate mental capacity for the specific decision at issue. While mental capacity can vary in extent, legal competence represents a definitive judgment. Consent to treatment denotes an individual's authorization to proceed with a medical procedure or therapy after receiving sufficient information regarding associated risks, benefits, and alternatives (American Psychological Association, n.d.-a). Valid consent presupposes that the person possesses both the requisite mental capacity and legal competence to reach an informed choice (Buchanan, 2004).

The issue with capacity–incapacity is not the decision the person makes but the process of making that decision. Determining the capacity of an individual who is living with SMI to make decisions is crucial. This capacity hinges on four key elements. First, the person must truly understand the information about their condition, the proposed treatments, and the potential risks and benefits. Next, they need to appreciate how this information applies to their own circumstances, recognizing the personal impact of each choice. Reasoning is equally vital: the patient should be able to thoughtfully compare options and weigh possible consequences, focusing on their decision-making process rather than on the outcome. Finally, the individual must be able to clearly communicate their decision, whether directly or through a proxy. If any of these components are lacking, the ability to make informed mental healthcare choices is compromised. Only when all four are present can an individual be considered capable of making decisions about their treatment (Palmer & Harmell, 2016).

A lack of capacity occurs when an individual living with SMI is unable to make informed decisions due to impairments. Capacity may be affected by difficulties in hearing, comprehending, and retaining relevant information about a given situation, as well as challenges in recognizing and evaluating available alternatives based on that information. Additionally, it involves understanding the potential consequences and making choices independently, free from undue influence. Typically, concerns regarding capacity arise when an individual's decisions place them at risk of danger or harm.

For example, a person crosses a busy street using information that she is receiving and has received in that situation. She understands that crossing the street with cars approaching will put her in danger and possible harm. She waits until that traffic light is in her favor, and no cars are approaching; she then steps into the street. She hurries across if the light begins to change. Most people cross the street independently without being influenced by others, understanding the risks of going into traffic and the possible outcomes if the person darts into oncoming traffic. If a person has a mental or emotional impairment (which could be temporary such as being intoxicated) and does not consider the information being received from the environment, does not remember past instructions about crossing the street, and walks into a busy intersection putting himself into immediate danger, then that person may be incapacitated. The person may not perceive the danger of crossing a busy street against the light and may have no understanding of the danger of doing so. The person may be incapacitated because of a delusion (i.e., a false belief) that she is "a spirit" and cannot be hurt; perhaps the person lives with hallucinations that tell him to walk into the street. The person may be experiencing suicidal thoughts and the having the intention of being killed by walking into traffic. A person living with SMI may be considered incapacitated as the symptoms and problematic behaviors of living with a SMI prevent her from making adequate life decisions and putting herself at risk for harm.

Warning Signs for Diminished Capacity

Here is a list of "red flags" that service providers of a person living with SMI should be aware:

1. The person is disabled and the symptoms and problematic behaviors linked to living with SMI are chronic and resistive to medications and treatments.
2. The person living with SMI depends on others for help or care in daily life.
3. The person living with SMI has problems with hearing, vision, or speaking. If the person can speak, do others understand him when he speaks?
4. Problems with memory. Can the person recall what he has been told recently?
5. Problems communicating and understanding. Can the person communicate by speaking, using gestures, sign language, writing, or a communication device? Does she make sense to others when she does communicate? Can she communicate and understand what she has been told and informed of?
6. Problems in understanding the consequences of decisions. Does she understand the pros and cons of her decisions either by the manifestation of behavior or speaking about her decision?
7. Developmental disability. Does the person living with SMI have problems with learning new information?
8. Dependent or passive behavior. Does the person not make decisions, allows others to make decisions for her, or avoids making decisions?
9. Emotional distress (e.g., grief, anxiety, fear, and depression). Does severe emotional distress contribute to understanding, communicating, remembering, and being able to reach a decision based on what information has been given? Is the person able to communicate the pros and cons of her decision?
10. Language/literacy barriers. Can the person read, write, and comprehend what they hear or read?
11. Isolated from others. Does the person socialize and to what extent? Do they have anyone on whom they can rely for help if needed?
12. Lives in a chaotic or dysfunctional setting where victimization is possible. Does the person with SMI live in a community where exploitation can occur?

People living with SMI may have the problems and impairments noted above. If that is the case, the mental health service providers and staff consider guardianship to assist the person living with SMI to function as best and as independently as possible without putting the person at risk for harm. Guardianship is a legal process in which one individual (the guardian) is appointed to make decisions on behalf of another individual (the ward) who has been determined to lack decision-making capacity (Zietlow et al., 2022).

Capacity Determination

Capacity requires a comprehensive evaluation by a healthcare professional. It requires an extended evaluation by a licensed psychologist or a psychiatrist to make the determination. It is important to understand that there is a presumption of capacity of the person in question (Buchanan, 2004; Palmer & Harmell, 2016). The evaluation requires (a) a comprehensive history of the person being evaluated; (b) the health-related condition that the person is living with; and (c) health-related documents supporting the identification of the health condition. An interview with mental health service providers and staff is needed to get examples of the "red flags' 'that they have observed with the person who is being evaluated. An assessment of the person's level of functioning may be asked of the mental health service providers and staff. The healthcare professional will meet face to face with the individual whose capacity is being evaluated by interviewing the individual to ascertain if any problems with cognitive functioning are evident. Sometimes, a neuropsychological performance evaluation is done to find out the specific areas in which the person may have diminished or impaired capacities.

Capacity and Need for Guardianship

All states have regulations concerning diminished capacity and guardianship. The regulations in each state vary but all require the following:

1. An individual experiences significant difficulty in comprehending and retaining information provided, conveying their understanding effectively, and applying the given information to analyze the advantages and disadvantages of decisions made.
2. The problems described above are because the person has a documented physical or mental health condition.

Diminished capacity is a legal concept determined by a judge or magistrate. It constitutes a significant legal issue, as an individual's fundamental rights to make personal decisions may be restricted and transferred to another party. In accordance with standard legal procedures, both parties present evidence which the judge evaluates to determine its validity and whether the individual satisfies the statutory criteria. Typically, assessment of capacity arises in the context of petitions seeking to appoint a guardian for individuals living with diminished capacity (Zietlow et al., 2022). A guardian is defined as a person whom the court appoints to protect the rights and manage the affairs of an incapacitated person or a minor; the appointed person must agree to be the guardian for that person. The courts attempt to appoint a guardian who has a familial relationship with the incapacitated person. In some cases, families are not available or do not want this responsibility. The guardian can then be a public guardian who agrees to the appointment and is paid by the state to manage the affairs of the incapacitated person.

All guardians are responsible for managing the affairs of the person with the interest and welfare of the incapacitated person always in consideration. Until the guardianship is terminated, the guardian must file and send to the court a report every year that describes what has happened to the incapacitated person and their income and assets.

There are guardians with different powers and responsibilities that are again decided by the courts as to the limits of the incapacitation of the person. Guardians are encouraged to use "substituted judgment," making decisions based on the known preferences and values of the "ward" (who is the person for whom guardianship is established person) rather than paternalistic "best interest" decision making (Zietlow et al., 2022).

There are different types of guardianships. Each type of guardianship varies in scope and duration, and the process is regulated at the state level (Zietlow et al., 2022):

- Full guardianship: The person if fully incapacitated; a guardian is appointed to have total decision-making responsibilities for medical, housing, services, legal, and financial areas for the incapacitated person.
- Conservatorship: The term is often used synonymously with guardianship but typically refers to guardianship limited to financial matters.
- Partial or limited guardianship: This type of guardianship is based upon a court's finding that the person alleged to be incapacitated lacks the capacity to do some, but not all, of the tasks necessary to care for themselves. It is a less restrictive and more individualized type of guardianship in which a guardian is appointed with authority in identified areas of impairment. The areas that are selected for guardianship can be decision making around health, finance, and housing, but not all areas are included. The "ward" has more independence to make her own decisions. Many states now strive for limited guardianship when the individual retains some ability to manage affairs.
- Temporary guardianship: This type is established by the court on an interim basis in emergency situations, granting authority to a guardian for a defined period or specific decision-making areas. For instance, the court may issue an emergency appointment to address an urgent, life-threatening medical matter, or designate a guardian for a limited duration, such as 6 months, to assist with decisions.
- Emergency guardianship refers to a temporary arrangement established swiftly to address urgent medical or safety concerns regarding the ward's condition.

The Social Security Administration (SSA) has a website listing the specific criteria for diminished capacity and guardianship for each state. It is listed under Guardianship Laws on the SSA website.

Difference Between a Guardian and a Payee

Many people living with SMI receives monetary benefits from the Social Security Administration (SSA) in the form of Social Security Disability Benefits (SSDI) or Supplemental Security Income (SSI); what type of benefits the person gets depends on prior work history and contributing and paying social security taxes. Some people living with SMI may obtain money through trust funds and/or inheritances. Due to challenges associated with managing finances, family members, caregivers, and other stakeholders may express concerns regarding an individual living with SMI independently handling their financial affairs. Consequently, it is often necessary to designate a representative to oversee the financial matters of the individual living with SMI.

As stated previously, a full or limited guardian of finances would have complete control over making financial decisions for the person living with SMI. A representative payee is an individual (or organization, such as a group home, mental health center) that receives Social Security and/or SSI payments for someone else who cannot competently manage their money. Payees use the funds for the needs of the person and save any remaining funds for the person's future use (SSA, 2023).

Both the payee and the guardian must report annually on the monies that are received and allocated to the person for whom they have been appointed to oversee his finances. Most living expenses are paid by the payee and the guardian. The person living with SMI usually receives a small allowance for other personal needs.

Jails as Treatment Facilities

Psychiatric hospital beds have declined since the middle 1950s. The decline coincides with the advent of psychiatric medications that have been effective in managing the most serious symptoms and problematic behaviors related to living with SMI. In addition, the legislation known as the Community Mental Health Act of 1963 (also known as the Mental Retardation and Community Mental Health Centers Construction Act of 1963) provided federal funding for community mental health centers and research facilities devoted to the causes and treatment of developmental disabilities and mental health problems (Rochefort, 1984). Large state facilities were seen as "warehousing" people without providing any effective treatment. Several landmark legal decisions established the right to "least restrictive environment" in which there must be a consideration if a person living with SMI or other serious neurodevelopmental conditions can be treated in the community.

State psychiatric and developmental centers were gradually closed, leading to the emergence of private psychiatric hospitals and general hospitals that offered short-term treatment. These services primarily focused on stabilization through medication management, basic psychoeducational groups, and subsequent referral of individuals living with SMI to community providers. This sounds like a good plan; the only problem is that insurance companies do not pay at the same rate as physical and medical conditions. Insurance policies for mental health problems have many exceptions. Sometimes, there are large co-payments for care and medications, and pre-authorization paperwork must be completed before treatment is provided. Given the less than welcoming economic picture and bureaucratic hurdles to receive care, providers of mental health services "opt out" and provide limited services; these services often provide the bare minimum in treatment with staff that are not experienced or have competencies in working with individuals living with SMI, face physical injury from combative individuals, and are poorly compensated. Although there has been a recent decrease in turnover among mental health treatment staff, the rate is still stubbornly high; research has shown that the turnover is over 30% (OPEN MINDS, 2023). Due to challenging working conditions, high staff turnover and low wages, employees often hold multiple jobs and are required to work overtime, which can contribute to staff burnout. Additionally, many staff members experience compassion fatigue, characterized by diminished empathy and sensitivity, feelings of helplessness when addressing the needs of the person living with SMI, emotional detachment, increased anxiety and depression, difficulty concentrating and making decisions, and various physical symptoms (Substance Abuse and Mental Health Services Administration [SAMSHA], 2022). Consequently, numerous inpatient and residential care providers have discontinued their services and ceased operations.

With the changing sociopolitical climate and the use of medications, hospital beds for serious mental health conditions have declined. Both state and private psychiatric facilities as well as general hospitals have closed psychiatric beds. However, as the beds available to treat problems linked to SMI have decreased, the rate of people living with SMI being incarcerated has increased dramatically since 1975.

Jail and prisons have become the largest providers of mental healthcare (Cherson, 2025). About two in five people who are incarcerated have a history of living with SMI with estimates of 37% in state and federal prisons and 44% held in local jails (NAMI, n.d.; NAMI, 2024). This is twice the prevalence of mental health problems within the overall adult population. Given these rates, jails and prisons in the United States have become de facto mental health providers, at great cost to the well-being of people with mental health conditions.

There are headlines in the news that the county jails in large cities have become the largest de facto mental health facilities. Housing many people living with SMI does not mean that jails and prisons provide comprehensive mental health treatment. Only the most rudimentary care is given, usually in the form of medications. Staff are not trained adequately to identify and treat a person in a mental health crisis. Mental health staff who work in correctional settings are overwhelmed with the sheer number of people that require intervention (NAMI, n.d.). In addition, the philosophy of the correctional setting is "correctional"; it is not a treatment facility, providing therapeutic interventions. Mental health staff in correctional facilities often face challenges, as their efforts may lack support or be undermined by correctional staff, whose primary role is to enforce rules, maintain order, and prevent escapes. In the news, there are reports of jails and prisons being understaffed to the extent that it is not a safe place to work or be an inmate; recent reports of inmates escaping or being killed are blamed on understaffing. The same economic and work conditions that plague centers that provide mental healthcare are common in jails and prisons—lack of staff, dangerous conditions, and lack of work–life balance. Burnout and compassion fatigue are a common occurrence in these settings.

Jails have effectively become the provider of last resort for mental health services, with staff often struggling to secure appropriate care for individuals living with SMI. National news sources have reported cases where families are compelled to have their relatives arrested to prevent potential harm to themselves or others (Herman, 2023). This situation arises when courts determine that an individual does not meet the criteria for involuntary commitment, or when individuals with SMI decline voluntary treatment. As noted previously, refusal to seek voluntary treatment is frequently a symptom of the illness, as people living with SMI may lack awareness of their condition referred to as lack of insight or anosognosia.

Summary

The intersection of mental health crises, legal authority, and social policy raises ethical and clinical concerns regarding the treatment of individuals living with SMI. Mental health crises can manifest in various ways and require immediate professional intervention. Crises may be triggered by stress, trauma, or significant life changes. Indicators include self-harm, aggression, social withdrawal, and severe psychological distress. The continuum of care during a mental health crisis includes crisis intervention, guardianship, and potential incarceration, which negatively impact the individual living with SMI, families, and stakeholders. Coercive treatment and involuntary interventions pose ethical questions about autonomy and dignity.

Mental health crises often require intervention from trained professionals when individuals cannot manage safely on their own. Professionals must assess the situation to ensure safety for the individual and the public. Effective crisis intervention involves maintaining composure and employing de-escalation techniques. Service providers should use calm communication and avoid dismissing the individual's experiences. Engaging individuals with open-ended questions and offering choices supports their autonomy during crises. If the individual is unwilling to seek care, relocating them to a calm environment is advisable.

Psychiatric Advance Directives (PADs) are legal documents that permit individuals living with SMI to specify their preferences regarding future mental healthcare and treatment. PADs also provide the option to designate a healthcare proxy authorized to make decisions on the individual's behalf during times when they are incapacitated. Through the establishment of PADs, individuals with SMI can communicate their treatment preferences prior to a crisis, fostering greater collaboration with recovery teams, minimizing involuntary interventions, and enhancing overall satisfaction with mental health services.

Effectively addressing challenging behaviors among individuals living with SMI and experiencing a mental health crisis necessitates a systematic approach. Behaviors should be precisely defined and thoroughly documented to promote clarity and guide appropriate interventions. Identifying antecedent conditions is important for recognizing triggers associated with challenging behaviors. Comprehensive support plans must be developed in collaboration with all relevant stakeholders.

The successful implementation of behavioral intervention strategies during a crisis is essential for supporting those living with SMI. Prioritizing the reinforcement of adaptive behaviors over punitive measures is recommended. The introduction of alternative activities and structured routines can assist in managing and minimizing problematic behaviors. Consistent application of behavior support plans is vital for achieving positive outcomes.

Ongoing evaluation and adjustment of support plans are necessary for effective intervention. Staff should document occurrences of both targeted behaviors and adaptive responses when they occur. Regular team meetings can help address challenges and ensure that all members are aligned with the intervention strategies. Engaging individuals in the process and soliciting their preferences can enhance the effectiveness of the support plan.

When an individual living with SMI is at imminent risk of harming themselves or others, involuntary treatment may become necessary, particularly if less restrictive alternatives are unavailable. Involuntary commitment, also known as civil commitment, is a legal procedure applied to individuals with SMI who present immediate risks to themselves or others, decline alternative treatments, and are unable to provide informed consent due to impairment. This process includes evaluation by a qualified mental health professional and may involve hospitalization for further assessment and intervention. Commitment can be ordered as a temporary detention (TDO) for a period of 48–72 hours. During this time, a mental health evaluation is conducted to assess the individual's need for treatment, which may lead to a judicial hearing to determine subsequent actions. Commitment proceedings may occur in courtrooms or hospital settings, with individuals retaining rights to legal representation and witness presentation. Decisions are made by a judge, without jury involvement, ensuring judicial oversight in the commitment process.

Mental health professionals are obligated to evaluate the risk of harm associated with untreated mental health conditions. State regulations mandate the presence of a "dangerousness" criterion, which refers to the potential for imminent or foreseeable harm should the individual remain untreated. In addition, some states consider "grave disability," defined as the inability to provide for one's basic needs, while others highlight "the need for treatment" as a preventative measure against potential harm.

An alternative to compulsory inpatient treatment for individuals living with mental health conditions deemed potentially dangerous is Assisted Outpatient Treatment (AOT). AOT permits mandated community-based care without imposing legal consequences for non-compliance. It is designed to support individuals with a history of hospitalizations or high-risk behaviors, aiming to prevent escalation to involuntary commitment or incarceration. However, the absence of enforceable sanctions may present challenges, particularly in cases involving anosognosia, where individuals lack awareness of their condition and problematic and dangerous behaviors. Research, however, indicates that AOT does not demonstrate significant improvements in outcomes when compared to voluntary care.

Involuntary commitment is considered when a person poses a danger to themselves or others or cannot care for their basic needs, risking harm due to their mental health condition. Behaviors by the individual being considered for commitment must clearly indicate immediate risk, including acts of self-harm or threats, rather than referencing prior incidents. Individuals affected by substance intoxication may not meet commitment criteria if their dangerous behaviors are anticipated to resolve upon regaining sobriety. Any individual, including family, hospital staff, or police, can petition for commitment, provided they have witnessed the challenging and concerning behaviors. Eyewitness testimony must be recent and directly related to the individual's dangerous actions. Commitment can last from a few weeks to several months, differing from emergency detentions, which are shorter. Individuals have the right to appeal their commitment in court, where they can present evidence and challenge the decision.

Involuntary commitment poses significant legal and ethical issues, balancing the rights and dignity of the person living with SMI with the need for treatment. Mental health service providers are guided by ethical principles that include beneficence, autonomy, non-maleficence, and justice. Mental health providers aim to assist and support individuals with SMI with the intention of doing no harm to the individual while the legal system is cautious about restricting personal liberties. A judge may determine that a person does not meet the criteria for commitment, leading to frustration among providers and family.

Individuals have the constitutional right to refuse medication, even if they are living with an SMI. In some cases, court orders may be necessary to administer medication against a person's will, particularly if they pose a danger to themselves or others. Legal statutes vary by state regarding the administration of involuntary medication, often requiring prior positive treatment outcomes from the medication.

People living with SMI may have difficulty understanding, processing, or making decisions after receiving important information. These challenges can affect their ability to make and communicate independent decisions. Incapacity means not being able to understand and use information for personal choices, while legal competence is a specific, binary judgment about a person's authority to make healthcare decisions based on sufficient mental capacity. Mental capacity varies, but legal competence is clear-cut. Consent to treatment requires both mental capacity and legal competence, ensuring that the person understands risks, benefits, and options before agreeing.

Decision making requires the capacity to understand information, appreciate its relevance, reason through available options, and effectively communicate decisions. Diminished capacity may arise from impairments affecting comprehension, memory, and decision making, often leading to risks of harm. The concern regarding capacity and incapacity lies not in the specific decision a person makes, but rather in the process by which that decision is reached. Decision-making impairments may be affected by problematic behaviors linked with living with an SMI that are resistant to treatment, reliance on others for daily care and decision making, communication challenges such as difficulties with memory and understanding consequences, emotional distress influencing decision-making abilities, and isolation or chaotic living conditions that heighten vulnerability to exploitation.

Capacity assessment require comprehensive evaluations by licensed professionals, including interviews and possibly neuropsychological performance testing. Legal determination of diminished capacity is made by a judge, based on evidence presented by both parties. Guardianship is a legal process where a guardian is appointed to manage the affairs of an incapacitated individual, prioritizing their welfare.

Guardianships differ according to the extent of decision making granted to a proxy. Full guardianship provides complete authority over decisions. Conservatorship generally pertains to financial affairs. Partial guardianship enables decision making in designated areas while allowing some independence. Temporary and emergency guardianships are used for urgent circumstances over restricted time periods.

There is a significant difference between a guardian and an authorized payee. A guardian has comprehensive authority over an individual's affairs, while a payee manages specific financial benefits, ensuring that funds are used for the individual's needs. Both must report annually on financial management, ensuring accountability and transparency.

Since the 1950s, psychiatric hospital beds have decreased due to effective medications and the Community Mental Health Act of 1963, which promoted community-based care. Legal decisions established the right to treatment in the least restrictive environment, leading to the closure of state psychiatric facilities and the rise of private and general hospitals focused on short-term stabilization. Insurance limitations and economic challenges have led to inadequate mental health services, high staff turnover, and burnout among providers.

As psychiatric beds have diminished, incarceration rates for individuals living with SMI have surged, with jails becoming the largest providers of mental healthcare in the United States. Approximately 37% of state and federal prison inmates and 44% of local jail inmates have a history of SMI, significantly higher than the general population. Jails offer minimal mental health treatment, primarily medication, and staff often lack adequate training to manage mental health crises, leading to further challenges in care delivery. Correctional facilities are understaffed and prioritize order over therapeutic interventions, contributing to burnout and compassion fatigue among mental health staff. Families sometimes resort to having relatives arrested to secure care when voluntary treatment is declined, often due to a lack of insight and awareness associated with living with SMI.

References

American Bar Association (ABA). (2018, December). *Assessment of older adults with diminished capacity: A handbook for psychologists*. American Bar Association commission on law and aging–American Psychological Association.

American Psychiatric Association. (2022). *Diagnostic and statistical manual of mental disorders* (5th ed., text rev.). https://doi.org/10.1176/appi.books.9780890425787

American Psychological Association. (n.d.-a). *Relapse*. In *APA Dictionary of Psychology*. https://dictionary.apa.org/relapse

American Psychological Association. (n.d.-b). *Consent*. In *APA dictionary of psychology*. https://dictionary.apa.org/consent

American Psychological Association. (n.d.-c). *Ethical dilemma*. In *APA dictionary of psychology*. https://dictionary.apa.org/ethical-dilemma

American Psychological Association. (2017). *Ethical principles of psychologists and code of conduct* (2002, amended effective June 1, 2010, and January 1, 2017). https://www.apa.org/ethics/code

Brown, E., Bedi, G., McGorry, P., & O'Donoghue, B. (2020). Rates and predictors of relapse in first-episode psychosis: An Australian cohort study. *Schizophrenia Bulletin Open, 1*(1), sgaa017. https://doi.org/10.1093/schizbullopen/sgaa017

Buchanan, A. (2004). Mental capacity, legal competence and consent to treatment. *Journal of the Royal Society of Medicine, 97*(9), 415–420. https://doi.org/10.1177/014107680409700902

Center for Public Health Law Research, Beasley School of Law, Temple University. (n.d.). *The policy surveillance program*. Temple University. https://phlr.org/topics

Cherson, J. (2025, May 14). *America's three largest mental health facilities are jails*. The Bail Project. https://bailproject.org/learn/americas-three-largest-mental-health-facilities-are-jails/#:~:text=Jail%20is%20not%20a%20place,receive%20the%20help%20they%20need

Cooper, J. O., Heron, T. E., & Heward, W. L. (2020). *Applied behavior analysis* (3rd ed.). Pearson Education. https://www.pearson.com/en-us/subject-catalog/p/applied-behavior-analysis/P200000003382/9780134752556

Emsley, R., Chiliza, B., Asmal, L., & Harvey, B. H. (2013). The nature of relapse in schizophrenia. *BMC Psychiatry, 13*, 50. https://doi.org/10.1186/1471-244X-13-50

Gignac, A., McGirr, A., Lam, R. W., & Yatham, L. N. (2015). Recovery and recurrence following a first episode of mania: A systematic review and meta-analysis of prospectively characterized cohorts. *Journal of Clinical Psychiatry, 76*(9), 1241–1248. https://doi.org/10.4088/JCP.14r09267

Herman, C. (2023). *Families take drastic steps to help children in mental health crises*. Center for Public Integrity. https://publicintegrity.org/health/health-parity/families-help-children-mental-health-crises/#:~:text=If%20you%20or%20someone%20you%20know%20may,Text%20Line%20by%20texting%20HOME%20to%20741741

Laureano, C. D., Laranjeira, C., Querido, A., Dixe, M. A., & Rego, F. (2024). Ethical issues in clinical decision-making about involuntary psychiatric treatment: A scoping review. *Healthcare, 12*(4), 445. https://doi.org/10.3390/healthcare12040445

Lin, D., Joshi, K., Keenan, A., Shepherd, J., Bailey, H., Berry, M., Wright, J., Meakin, S., Benson, C., & Kim, E. (2021). Associations between relapses and psychosocial outcomes in patients with schizophrenia in real-world settings in the United States. *Frontiers in Psychiatry, 12*, 695672. https://doi.org/10.3389/fpsyt.2021.695672

Mental Illness Policy.Org. (2024). *Standards for involuntary commitment (assisted treatment) state-by-state (source treatment advocacy center)*. Retrieved from https://mentalillnesspolicy.org/national-studies/state-standards-involuntary-treatment.html

NAMI Wisconsin. (n.d.). *Mental health crisis overview*. NAMI Wisconsin. https://namiwisconsin.org/resources/mental-health-crisis-overview/

National Alliance on Mental Illness (NAMI). (n.d.). *Mental health treatment while incarcerated*. NAMI. https://www.nami.org/advocacy/policy-priorities/improving-health/mental-health-treatment-while-incarcerated/#:~:text=Too%20often%2C%20jails%20and%20prisons,successful%20reentry%20to%20the%20community

National Alliance on Mental Illness (NAMI). (2020, December 3). *Psychiatric advance directives*. NAMI. https://www.nami.org/advocacy/policy-priorities/responding-to-crises/psychiatric-advance-directives/.

National Alliance on Mental Illness (NAMI) (2024). *National Alliance on Mental Illness (NAMI)*. Retrieved from https://www.nami.org/Home

OPEN MINDS. (2023, June 29). 2023 turnover at behavioral health facilities decreases to 27.5%. *OPEN MINDS weekly news* Wired https://openminds.com/market-intelligence/news/2023-turnover-at-behavioral-health-facilities-decreases-to-27-5/#:~:text=2023%20Turnover%20At%20Behavioral%20Health%20Facilities%20Decreases%20To%2027.5%25%20%2D%20OPEN%20MINDS

Organization for Economic Cooperation and Development (OECD). (2021). *A new benchmark for mental health systems*. OECD Publishing. https://doi.org/10.1787/4edc92d4-en

Osborn, D. P. J., Favarato, G., Lamb, D., Harper, T., Johnson, S., Lloyd-Evans, B., Marston, L., Mathieson, F., Forsyth, R., Hunter, R., Davidson, M., Piotrowicz, A., Smith, J., McNicholas, S., Harrison, V., Lavelle, M., & Weich, S. (2021). Readmission after discharge from acute mental healthcare among 231,988 people in England: Cohort study exploring predictors of readmission including availability of acute day units in local areas. *BJPsych Open, 7*(4), e136. https://doi.org/10.1192/bjo.2021.961

Owusu, E., Oluwasina, F., Nkire, N., Lawal, M. A., & Agyapong, V. I. (2022). Readmission of patients to acute psychiatric hospitals: Influential factors and interventions to reduce psychiatric readmission rates. In *Healthcare*. (Vol. 10, 9, p. 1808). MDPI. https://doi.org/10.3390/healthcare10091808

Palmer, B. W., & Harmell, A. L. (2016). Assessment of healthcare decision-making capacity. *Archives of Clinical Neuropsychology, 31*(6), 530–540. https://doi.org/10.1093/arclin/acw051

Pinto, J. V., Saraf, G., Kozicky, J., Beaulieu, S., Sharma, V., Parikh, S. V., Cervantes, P., Daigneault, A., Walji, N., Kauer-Sant'Anna, M., & Yatham, L. N. (2020). Remission and recurrence in bipolar disorder: The data from health outcomes and patient evaluations in bipolar disorder (HOPE-BD) study. *Journal of Affective Disorders, 268*, 150–157. https://doi.org/10.1016/j.jad.2020.03.018

Rivelli, A., Fitzpatrick, V., Nelson, M., Laubmeier, K., Zeni, C., & Mylavarapu, S. (2024). Real-world predictors of relapse in patients with schizophrenia and schizoaffective disorder in a large health system. *Schizophrenia, 10*(1), 28. https://doi.org/10.1038/s41537-024-00448-2

Rochefort, D. A. (1984). Origins of the "third psychiatric revolution": The community mental health centers act of 1963. *Journal of Health Politics, Policy and Law, 9*(1), 1–30. https://doi.org/10.1215/03616878-9-1-1

Segal, S. P., & Badran, L. (2024). Cochrane meta-analysis fuels invalid skepticism about compulsory community treatment effectiveness. *Psychiatry Research, 342*, 116218. https://doi.org/10.1016/j.psychres.2024.116218

Shahrokh, N. C., & Hales, R. E. (2003). *American psychiatric glossary* (8th ed.). American Psychiatric Publishing. https://doi.org/10.1176/appi.books.9781585621809

Social Security Administration (SSA). (2023). *Digest of state guardianship laws*. (Program Operations Manual Systems, Publication No. GN 00502.300). Retrieved from http://policy.ssa.gov/poms.nsf/lnx/0200502300

Stallman, H. M., & Gupta, V. (2025, January 20). Involuntary commitment. In *StatPearls* [internet]. StatPearls Publishing. https://www.ncbi.nlm.nih.gov/books/NBK557377/

Substance Abuse and Mental Health Services Administration (SAMHSA). (2022). *Addressing burnout in the behavioral health workforce through organizational strategies* (SAMHSA Publication No. PEP22–06–02-005). National Mental Health and Substance Use Policy Laboratory. https://www.samhsa.gov/resource-search/pep-22-06-02-005

Tinland, A., Leclerc, L., Loubière, S., Mougeot, F., Greacen, T., Pontier, M., Girard, V., Boucekine, M., Pelletier, J.-F., Rowe, M., & Auquier, P. (2019). Psychiatric advance directives for people living with schizophrenia, bipolar I disorders, or schizoaffective disorders: Study protocol for a randomized controlled trial—DAiP study. *BMC Psychiatry, 19*, 422. https://doi.org/10.1186/s12888-019-2416-9

Varkey, B. (2021). Principles of clinical ethics and their application to practice. *Medical Principles and Practice, 30*(1), 17–28. https://doi.org/10.1159/000509119

World Health Organization, & Office of the United Nations High Commissioner for Human Rights. (2023). *Mental health, human rights and legislation: Guidance and practice*. World Health Organization. https://iris.who.int/bitstream/handle/10665/373126/9789240080737-eng.pdf

Zietlow, K., Dubin, L., Battles, A., & Vitale, C. (2022). Guardianship: A medicolegal review for clinicians. *Journal of the American Geriatrics Society, 70*(11), 3070–3079. https://doi.org/10.1111/jgs.17797

Appendix A: Functional Assessment Interview—Mental Health Version (FAI-MH)

Name of Individual:	Age:
Gender:	Location
DOB:	Date of Interview:
Interviewer(s):	Respondents:

A. DESCRIBE THE TARGET BEHAVIORS:
   1. ADAPTIVE STRENGTHS

For each of the behavioral strengths (i.e. communication skills, positive coping skills, or any other socially appropriate skills the client performs), define the topography (how it is performed), occurrence (in what situations or contexts), duration (how long it lasts when it occurs), and goal (what is this person trying to achieve or get).

a. Behavior:
   Topography:
   Occurrence:
   Duration:
   Goal:
b. Behavior:
   Topography:
   Occurrence:
   Duration:
   Goal:

B. CHALLENGES TO RECOVERY

A. For each of the behaviors of concern, define the topography (how it is performed), frequency (how often it occurs per day, week, or month), duration

G. F. McKeegan, *Behavior Change Interventions for Serious Mental Illness*, Evidence-Based Practices in Behavioral Health,
https://doi.org/10.1007/978-3-032-18372-9

(how long it lasts when it occurs), and severity (how damaging or destructive are the behaviors are when they occur).

a. Behavior:
   Topography:
   Frequency:
   Duration:
   Severity:
b. Behavior:
   Topography:
   Frequency:
   Duration:
   Severity:

Which of the behaviors described above are likely to occur together in some way? Do they occur at about the same time? In some kind of predictable sequence or "chain" of behaviors? In response to the same type of situation?

B. Define the environmental events (setting events) that may predict or set the scene for the problem behavior to occur.

   1. If this person is on medication (psychotropic and others), do you think they may affect their problem behavior?
   2. What mental illness (e.g., hallucinations, delusions) does this person experience that may affect their problem behavior?
   3. If this person has medical or physical conditions (e.g., asthma, allergies, rashes, sinus infections, and seizures), do you think they may affect their problem behavior?
   4. Describe the sleep patterns of the individual and the extent to which these patterns may affect their problem behavior?
   5. Describe the eating routines and diet of the person and the extent to which these may affect their problem behavior?
   6. Briefly list below the person's typical daily schedule of activities. (Check the boxes by those activities the person enjoys and those activities most associated with problem behaviors).

Enjoys	Problems	Time	Activity

7. To what extent are the activities on the day schedule predictable for the person, about what will be happening, when it will occur, with whom, and for how long?
8. To what extent does the person have the opportunity during the day to make choices about their activities and reinforcing events? (e.g., food, clothing, social companions, leisure activities).
9. How many other people are typically around the individual during the day? Does the person typically seem bothered in situations that are more crowded and noisier?
10. What is the pattern of support that the person receives where they live and other settings? Do you believe that the support people, the training, or their social interactions with the person affect the problem behaviors?

C. Define specific immediate antecedent events that predict when the behaviors are likely and not likely to occur.
   1. Times of day: When are the behaviors most and least likely to happen?
      Most likely:
      Least likely:
   2. Settings: Where are the behaviors most and least likely to happen?
      Most likely:
      Least likely:

3. People: With whom are the behaviors most and least likely to happen?
   Most likely:
   Least likely:
4. Activity: What activities are most and least likely to produce the behaviors?
   Most likely:
   Least likely:
5. Briefly describe how the person's behavior would be affected if ...
   A. You asked them to perform a difficult task.
   B. You interrupted a desired activity, such as eating ice cream or watching TV.
   C. You unexpectedly changed their typical routine or schedule of activities.
   D. They wanted something but wasn't able to get it (e.g., a food item up on a shelf).
   E. You didn't pay attention to the person or left them alone for a while (e.g., 15 minutes).
   F. What behaviors should you avoid or not do when interacting with the person?
      1. What things can you do to improve the likelihood that ward, training, or other activities will go well with this person?
      2. What things should you avoid that might interfere with or disrupt ward, training, or other activities with this person?
   G. What is reinforcing to the person? What does the person prefer?
      1. Food items:
      2. Tangibles:
      3. Activities available:
      4. Activities/outings in the community:
      5. Others (specify):

Appendix B: Open-Ended Functional Assessment Interview

Date of Interview: ____________________

Client: ______________________________

Respondent:___________________________

Respondent's relation to client: ___________________

Interviewer: __________________________

Relevant background information

1. Their date of birth and current age: ____-_____-_________ _____yrs ____mos Male/Female
2. Describe their language abilities.
3. Describe their preferred activities (what does the person do most of the time) or leisure activities (what does the person prefer doing).
4. What else do they prefer?

   Questions to inform the design of a functional analysis

   To develop objective definitions of observable problem behaviors:
5. What are the problem behaviors? What do they look like?

   To determine which problem behavior(s) will be targeted in the functional analysis:
6. What is the single-most concerning problem behavior?
7. What are the top 3 most concerning problem behaviors? Are there other behaviors of concern?

   To determine the precautions required when conducting the functional analysis:
8. Describe the range of intensities of the problem behaviors and the extent to which they or others may be hurt or injured from the problem behavior.

G. F. McKeegan, *Behavior Change Interventions for Serious Mental Illness*, Evidence-Based Practices in Behavioral Health,
https://doi.org/10.1007/978-3-032-18372-9

To assist in identifying precursors to dangerous problem behaviors that may be targeted in the functional analysis instead of more dangerous problem behaviors:

9. Do the different types of problem behavior tend to occur in bursts or clusters and/or does any type of problem behavior typically precede another type of problem behavior (e.g., yelling preceding hitting)?

To determine the antecedent conditions that may be incorporated into the functional analysis test conditions:

10. Under what conditions or situations are the problem behaviors most likely to occur?
11. Do the problem behaviors reliably occur during any particular activities?
12. What seems to trigger the problem behavior?
13. Does problem behavior occur when you break routines or interrupt activities? If so, describe.
14. Does the problem behavior occur when it appears that they won't get their way? If so, describe the things that the person often attempts to control.

To determine the test condition(s) that should be conducted and the specific type(s) of consequences that may be incorporated into the test condition(s):

15. How do you and others react or respond to the problem behavior?
16. What do you and others do to calm them down or mitigate the behavior once they engaged in the problem behavior?
17. What do you and others do to distract them from engaging in the problem behavior?

In addition to the above information, to assist in developing a hunch as to why problem behavior is occurring and to assist in determining the test condition(s) to be conducted:

18. What do you think they are trying to communicate with their problem behavior, if anything?
19. Does this behavior occur when the person is experiencing hallucinations, is maniac or depressed? Does the behavior occur because the person is responding to voices, smells, sights that are not there? Does the behavior occur because the person is acting on a false belief/delusions? If so, what gives you that impression?
20. Why do you think they are engaging in the problem behavior?

Appendix C: Scatterplot

Time	Behavior:							Behavior:						
	Definition:							Definition:						
	Mon	**Tues**	**Wed**	**Thurs**	**Fri**	**Sat**	**Sun**	**Mon**	**Tues**	**Wed**	**Thurs**	**Fri**	**Sat**	**Sun**
6 am														
7 am														
8 am														
9 am														
10 am														
11 am														
12 noon														
1 pm														
2 pm														
3 pm														
4 pm														
5 pm														
6 pm														
7 pm														
8 pm														
9 pm														
10 pm														
11 pm														
12 midnight														
1 am														
2 am														
3 am														
4 am														
5 am														

G. F. McKeegan, *Behavior Change Interventions for Serious Mental Illness*, Evidence-Based Practices in Behavioral Health,
https://doi.org/10.1007/978-3-032-18372-9

Appendix D: Instructions for Using a Scatterplot

Below is a completed scatterplot for aggression and verbal aggression. The two behaviors are behaviors that sometimes happen in the same time-period—but not always—so both are defined as to what the observer is to look for.

Instructions For Using Scatterplot:

1. During a one-hour period, place a "hash mark" or slash in the box when the behavior occurs. /
2. If person is sleep, put an "S" in box

SCATTERPLOT DATA COLLECTION SHEET

G. F. McKeegan, *Behavior Change Interventions for Serious Mental Illness*, Evidence-Based Practices in Behavioral Health,
https://doi.org/10.1007/978-3-032-18372-9

Time	Behavior: Verbal Aggression							Behavior: Physical Aggression						
	Definition: Yelling, cursing, threats to harm others							Definition: Physical aggression toward staff, peers, or property (objects). Hitting, kicking others or any other type of physical aggression toward staff, peers, or himself.						
	Mon	**Tues**	**Wed**	**Thur**	**Fri**	**Sat**	**Sun**	**Mon**	**Tues**	**Wed**	**Thur**	**Fri**	**Sat**	**Sun**
6 am	/					/								
7 am														
8 am		//				/			/		/			
9 am														
10 am			/											
11 am							/							/
12 noon														
1 pm	/											//		
2 pm					/									
3 pm														
4 pm														
5 pm			///								/			/
6 pm														
7 pm	S	S	S	S	S	S	S	S	S	S	S	S	S	S
8 pm	S	S	S	S	S	S	S	S	S	S	S	S	S	S
9 pm	S	S	S	S	S	S	S	S	S	S	S	S	S	S
10 pm	S	S	S	S	S	S	S	S	S	S	S	S	S	S
11 pm	S	S	S	S	S	S	S	S	S	S	S	S	S	S
12 midnight	S	S	S	S	S	S	S	S	S	S	S	S	S	S
1 am	S	S	S	S	S	S	S	S	S	S	S	S	S	S
2 am	S	S	S	S	S	S	S	S	S	S	S	S	S	S
3 am	S	S	S	S	S	S	S	S	S	S	S	S	S	S
4 am	S	S	S	S	S	S	S	S	S	S	S	S	S	S
5 am	S	S	S	S	S	S	S	S	S	S	S	S	S	S

Appendix E: ABC Log

Client name: ____________________

Targeted behavior:____________________

No.	Date	Time	Setting	Person Recording	Antecedent	Behavior	Consequence
1							
2							
3							
4							
5							
6							
7							
8							
9							
10							

G. F. McKeegan, *Behavior Change Interventions for Serious Mental Illness*, Evidence-Based Practices in Behavioral Health,
https://doi.org/10.1007/978-3-032-18372-9

Appendix F: Maladaptive Behavior Record

Name:	Date:	Time:
For each occurrence, mark all items that apply in each column		
What happened before	Behavior	What happened after
☐ ☐Loud/disruptive environment ☐ No scheduled activities ☐ Waiting ☐ Changing activities/location ☐ Shift Change ☐ Mealtime ☐ Interaction with staff ☐ Staff makes request ☐ Asked to return item taken ☐ Did not get desired item ☐ Interaction w/peer ☐ Other Observer________________	☐ Hitting/kicking ☐ Screaming/yelling ☐ Threats ☐ Cursing ☐ Refuses request of staff ☐ Teasing/provoking others ☐ Stealing ☐ Other______ Location:________________	☐ Ignore ☐ Complies with request ☐ Victim yelled/reacted ☐ Staff stopped request ☐ Given break ☐ Told to stop ☐ Redirected to activity ☐ Restore environment/ apologize ☐ Blocked ☐ Separated within environment ☐ Directed to quiet area ☐ Holding Restraint ☐ PRN ☐ Other______

G. F. McKeegan, *Behavior Change Interventions for Serious Mental Illness*, Evidence-Based Practices in Behavioral Health,
https://doi.org/10.1007/978-3-032-18372-9

Appendix G: Example of Maladaptive Behavior Record Scale

Name: Peter	Date: 7/8	Time: 3:20PM
For each occurrence, mark all items that apply in each column		
What happened before	Behavior	What happened after
☐ Loud/disruptive environment ☐ No scheduled activities ☐ Waiting ☐ Changing activities/location ☐ Shift Change ☐ Mealtime ☐ Interaction with staff ☐ Staff makes request ☐ Asked to return item taken ☐ Did not get desired item ☐ Interaction w/peer ■ Other: walked past Peter Observer: Sue	☐ Hitting/kicking ☐ Screaming/yelling ☐ Threats ☐ Cursing ☐ Refuses request of staff ☐ Teasing/provoking others ☐ Stealing ■ Slapping ☐ Other______ Location: Work area	■ Ignored ☐ Complies with request ☐ Victim yelled/reacted ☐ Staff stopped request ☐ Given break ☐ Told to stop ☐ Redirected to activity ☐ Restore environment/ apologize ☐ Blocked ■ Client separated himself ☐ Separated within environment ☐ Directed to quiet area ☐ Holding Restraint ☐ PRN ☐ Other_______

G. F. McKeegan, *Behavior Change Interventions for Serious Mental Illness*, Evidence-Based Practices in Behavioral Health,
https://doi.org/10.1007/978-3-032-18372-9

Appendix H: Questions About Behavioral Function—Mental Illness Version (QABF-MI)

Name: ____________________ Responder: ____________________

Date: ____________________

Behavior: ____

Rate how often the indexed person demonstrates the behavior in situations where they might occur. Be sure to rate how often each behavior occurs, not what you think a good answer would be.

X = Doesn't apply, 0 = Never, 1 = Rarely, 2 = Some, 3 = Often

Score	Number	Behavior
	1	Engages in the behavior to get attention.
	2	Engages in the behavior to get out of group, medical appointments, leisure activities, or learning situations.
	3	Engages in the behavior because it makes them feel good emotionally or physically (e.g., aggression, sexual behaviors).
	4	Engages in the behavior because they are in pain (e.g., headache, toothache).
	5	Engages in the behavior to get things and activities that they like (e.g., cigarettes, beverages, snacks).
	6	Engages in the behavior to get into trouble so they can get attention.
	7	Engages in the behavior when asked to do something (get dressed, engage in activities of daily living, work).
	8	Engages in the behavior even if they think no one is watching them.
	9	Engages in the behavior more frequently when they are physically ill.
	10	Engages in the behavior when you take something away from them.

G. F. McKeegan, *Behavior Change Interventions for Serious Mental Illness*, Evidence-Based Practices in Behavioral Health,
https://doi.org/10.1007/978-3-032-18372-9

	11	Engages in the behavior to draw attention to themselves.
	12	Engages in the behavior when they do not want to do something.
	13	Engages in the behavior because they are bored.
	14	Engages in the behavior when there is something physically wrong with them.
	15	Engages in the behavior when you have something that they want.
	16	Engages in the behavior to try to get a reaction from you.
	17	Engages in the behavior to try to get people to leave them alone.
	18	Engages in the behavior in a highly repetitive manner, ignoring their surroundings.
	19	Engages in the behavior because they are physically uncomfortable.
	20	Engages in the behavior when another person has something that they want.
	21	Do they seem to be saying, "come see me" or "look at me" when engaging in the behavior?
	22	Do they seem to be saying, "leave me alone" or "stop asking me to do this" when engaging in the behavior?
	23	Do they seem to enjoy engaging in the behavior over and over regardless of what is going on around him?
	24	Does the behavior seem to indicate to you that they are not feeling well?
	25	Do they seem to be saying, "give me that item" when engaging in the behavior?

Scoring

Attention	Escape	Non-social	Physical	Tangible
1.Attention	2. Escape	3. Self-stim	4. In pain	5. Access to items
6. Reprimand	7. Do something	8. Thinks alone	9. When ill	10. Takes away
11. Draws	12. Not do	13. Boredom	14. Physical problem.	15. You have
16. Reaction	17. Alone	18. Repetitive	19. Uncomfortable	20. Peer has
21."Come see"	22. "Leave alone"	23. Enjoy by self	24 Not feeling well	25. "Give me that"
Total	Total	Total	Total	Total

Appendix I: Step-By-Step Guidance on Developing a Safety Plan for Individuals to Manage Suicidal Ideations and Reduce the Risk of Suicide Attempts.

What Is a Safety Plan?

A Safety Plan is a written list of coping strategies and sources of support that individuals can use who have been assessed to be at high risk for suicide. By using the form below, individuals and support staff can use these strategies before or during a suicidal crisis. The plan is brief and is in the individual's own words. It needs to be completed with the engagement of the individuals who is at risk of self-harm.

Who Should Have a Safety Plan?

Any individual who has a suicidal crisis should have a comprehensive suicide risk assessment. Service providers should then collaborate with the individual on developing a safety plan.

How Should a Safety Plan Be Drawn Up?

Safety Planning is a clinical process. Listening to, empathizing with, and engaging the individual in the process can promote the development of the Safety Plan and the likelihood of its use.

What are the steps after the Safety Plan is developed?

1. Assess the likelihood that the overall safety plan will be used and problem solve with the individual to identify barriers or obstacles to using the plan.
2. Discuss where the individual will keep the safety plan and how it will be located during a crisis.
3. Evaluate if the format is appropriate for individual's understanding and living circumstances.

Implementing the Safety Plan

There are six steps involved in the development of a Safety Plan.

Step 1: Warning Signs

G. F. McKeegan, *Behavior Change Interventions for Serious Mental Illness*, Evidence-Based Practices in Behavioral Health,
https://doi.org/10.1007/978-3-032-18372-9

- Ask: "How will you know when the safety plan should be used?"
- Ask: "What do you experience when you start to think about suicide or feel extremely depressed?"
- List warning signs (thoughts, images, thinking processes, mood, and/or behaviors) using the individual's own words.
- Discuss situations that may trigger suicidal ideation using empathetic listening skills. Ask for examples of warning signs and use the examples in the development of the safety plan.

Step 2: Internal Coping Strategies

- Ask: "What can you do, on your own, if you become suicidal again, to help yourself not to act on your thoughts or urges?"
- Ask for examples if the individual engaged in alternative coping behaviors that were successful during past suicidal crises.

Step 3: Social Contacts Who May Distract from the Crisis

- Ask: "Who or what social settings help you take your mind off your problems at least for a little while?" "Who helps you feel better when you socialize with them?"
- Ask for safe places they can go to be around people (i.e. coffee shop, clubhouse).
- Ask individual to list several people and social settings in case the first option is unavailable.

Step 4: Family Members or Friends Who May Offer Help

- Review safety plan with family members or friends that will hold the individual accountable for following the plan. If alone, request that the individual informs a relative or friend about the plan.
- Ask: "Among your family or friends, who do you think you could contact for help during a crisis?" or "Who is supportive of you and who do you feel that you can talk with when you're under stress?"

Step 5: Professionals and Agencies to Contact for Help

- Ask: "Who are the mental health service professionals that we should identify to be on your safety plan?" and "Are there other health care providers?"
- List names, numbers, and/or locations of service providers, local urgent care services.

Step 6: Making the Environment Safe

- Ask individuals which means they would consider using during a suicidal crisis. For methods with low lethality, clinicians may ask individuals to remove or limit their access to these methods themselves. Restricting the individual's access to a highly lethal method, such as a firearm, should be done by a designated, responsible person—usually a family member or close friend, or the police.
- Ask: "Do you own a firearm, such as a gun or rifle??" and "What other means do you have access to and may use to attempt to kill yourself?"

- Collaboratively identify ways to secure or limit access to lethal means by asking "How can we go about developing a plan to limit your access to these means?"

Stanley-Brown Safety Plan

Step 1: Warning signs
1.
2.
3.
Step 2: Internal coping strategies—things I can do to take my mind off my problems without contacting another person
1.
2.
3.
Step 3: People and social settings that provide distraction
1. Name: ____________________ Contact:
2. Name: ____________________ Contact:
3. Place: ______________ Address:
4. Place: ______________ Address:
Step 4: People whom I can ask for help during a crisis
1. Name: ____________________ Contact:
2. Name: ____________________ Contact:
3. Name: ____________________ Contact:
Step 5: Professionals or professional services I can contact during a crisis
1. Professional/services name ______________ Contact: Emergency contact:
2. Professional/services name ______________ Contact: Emergency contact:
3. Emergency department: Emergency department address: Emergency department phone:
Crisis line phone (e.g. 988)
Step 6: Making the environment safer (plan for lethal means safety):
1.
2.

Index

G. F. McKeegan, *Behavior Change Interventions for Serious Mental Illness*, Evidence-Based Practices in Behavioral Health,
https://doi.org/10.1007/978-3-032-18372-9

B

C

D

J

K

L

M

The manufacturer's authorised representative in the EU is Springer Nature Customer Service Centre GmbH, Europaplatz 3, 69115 Heidelberg, Germany. If you have any concerns regarding our products, please contact ProductSafety@springernature.com

Printed and bound by CPI Group (UK) Ltd, Croydon, CR0 4YY
05/10/2026
02228030-0003